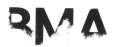

D1324562

ESSENTIALS OF
INTERNAL MEDICINE

Fourth Edition

WITHDRAWN FROM

BRITISH MEDICAL ASSOCIATION

1007729

ESSENTIALS OF
INTERNAL MEDICINE

Fourth Edition

Nicholas J. Talley
AC, MD, PhD, FRACP, FAFPHM, FRCP (Lond.), FRCP (Edin.), FACP, FAHMS
Laureate Professor, University of Newcastle and Senior Staff Specialist, John Hunter
Hospital, NSW, Australia; Adjunct Professor, Mayo Clinic, Rochester, MN, USA; Adjunct
Professor, University of North Carolina, Chapel Hill, NC, USA;
Foreign Guest Professor, Karolinska Institutet, Stockholm, Sweden

Brad Frankum
OAM, B. Med (Hons), FRACP, FAMA
Senior Staff Specialist and Consultant in Immunology and Allergy, Campbelltown
and Camden Hospitals, NSW, Australia; Conjoint Professor, School of Medicine,
Western Sydney University, NSW, Australia

Simon O'Connor
FRACP, DDU, FCSANZ
Cardiologist, Canberra Hospital; Clinical Senior Lecturer,
Australian National University Medical School, Canberra, ACT, Australia

ELSEVIER

Elsevier Australia. ACN 001 002 357
(a division of Reed International Books Australia Pty Ltd)
Tower 1, 475 Victoria Avenue, Chatswood, NSW 2067

This edition © 2021 Elsevier Australia.
First edition © 1990; Second edition © 2000; Third edition © 2015

All rights reserved. No part of this publication may be reproduced or transmitted in any form or by any means, electronic or mechanical, including photocopying, recording, or any information storage and retrieval system, without permission in writing from the publisher. Details on how to seek permission, further information about the Publisher's permissions policies and our arrangements with organizations such as the Copyright Clearance Center and the Copyright Licensing Agency, can be found at our website: www.elsevier.com/permissions.

This book and the individual contributions contained in it are protected under copyright by the Publisher (other than as may be noted herein).

ISBN: 978-0-7295-4312-5

Notice

Practitioners and researchers must always rely on their own experience and knowledge in evaluating and using any information, methods, compounds or experiments described herein. Because of rapid advances in the medical sciences, in particular, independent verification of diagnoses and drug dosages should be made. To the fullest extent of the law, no responsibility is assumed by Elsevier, authors, editors or contributors for any injury and/or damage to persons or property as a matter of products liability, negligence or otherwise, or from any use or operation of any methods, products, instructions, or ideas contained in the material herein.

National Library of Australia Cataloguing-in-Publication Data

A catalogue record for this book is available from the National Library of Australia

Head of Content: Larissa Norrie
Content Project Manager: Shubham Dixit
Edited by Annabel Adair
Proofread by Tim Learner
Internal design by Tania Gomes
Cover design by Alice Weston
Index by Innodata Indexing
Typeset by New Best-set Typesetters Ltd
Printed in Singapore by KHL Printing Co Pte Ltd

Last digit is the print number: 9 8 7 6 5 4 3 2 1

CONTENTS

Chapter 4
GENETICS

Chapter 5
MEDICAL IMAGING FOR INTERNISTS

Chapter 10
ENDOCRINOLOGY 261

David Simmons, Rohit Rajagopal, Milan K Piya,
Sue Lynn Lau and Mark McLean

Chapter 15
PALLIATIVE MEDICINE 493
Meera Agar, Katherine Clark and David Currow

Chapter 16
IMMUNOLOGY 507
Brad Frankum, Monique Wei Meng Lee and Jessie A Lee

Chapter 17
MUSCULOSKELETAL MEDICINE 563
Carlos El Haddad and Kevin Pile

Chapter 18
NEUROLOGY 599
Christopher Levi and Thomas Wellings

Chapter 19
PSYCHIATRY FOR THE INTERNIST 657
Brian Kelly and Lisa Lampe

Chapter 20
CLINICAL INFECTIOUS DISEASES 667
Iain Gosbell and D Ashley R Watson

GETTING BACK TO THE 'WHY'

Medicine is in a time of disruption and transformation. Artificial intelligence and other technologies are turning care models upside down. We are in the midst of the greatest disease crisis since the onset of HIV/AIDS, now with COVID. Unfortunately, despite this challenge, physician burn-out is at record high levels. To address these challenges, it is opportune that we take a step back and remember why we went into medicine. Medicine was, is, and always has been 'a calling'. It's about changing the world one patient at a time through relationships and giving all of ourselves to help others. Our greatest medical role models have always been individuals who pursued this selfless path.

This takes us to our topic at hand, *Essentials of Internal Medicine* 4th Edition by Nick Talley and his team. A quick read through this book reinvigorates our purpose as doctors. Whether it is to prepare for a clerkship or a test, to enhance knowledge, or, most importantly, just to be a better doctor, this book reminds us of our greatest role models in medicine, those with comprehensive knowledge which could be applied to individual patients at hand and used as a vehicle to disseminate knowledge to others. With so many decades of expertise in their pockets, Nick Talley and his team are the ideal ones to pursue this clarion call—and they fully deliver, exceeding all expectations.

Vijay Shah, M.D
Chair, Department of Medicine, and
Professor of Medicine and
Physiology, Mayo Clinic, Rochester, MN, USA

'A good physician treats the disease, the great physician treats the patient who has the disease.' Anonymous

'The definition of a specialist is one who "knows more and more about less and less".' Dr. Charlie Mayo

The American Board of Internal Medicine describes an internist as 'a personal physician who provides long-term, comprehensive care in the office and in the hospital, managing both common and complex illnesses of adolescents, adults and the elderly'. We have never needed excellent physicians more than today. At the time we are writing this Preface, the world is engaged in a desperate fight against a pandemic viral infection SARS-CoV-2 that has claimed the lives of doctors and their patients around the world; general physicians with their subspecialty colleagues have played a vital role in the response, and their work has saved many lives and alleviated much suffering.

In order to practice safely and competently, specialist physicians must master a set of clinical core competencies and acquire a deep knowledge of diseases in all the body systems as well as an understanding of prevention. This short textbook has been written to guide mastery of the required key knowledge and highlights the essential clinical facts you must learn.

We have included difficult to master topics from medical genetics to poisoning and acid–base balance, biostatistics, and interpreting cross-sectional imaging. Each chapter is written by experts in the field and multiple-choice questions are included to enhance learning.

While journal articles and more detailed textbooks will complement this volume, we have striven to highlight what must be known, and avoid waffle or less relevant material. In our experience, the concepts presented in the book are frequently tested in knowledge-based internal medicine examinations.

We are delighted *Essentials of Internal Medicine* has proven popular with physician trainees around the world. Medical students have also found the book valuable although it is aimed at those sitting barrier examinations such as The Royal Australasian College of Physicians Basic Physician Training and the American Board in Internal Medicine.

We wish you every success in your learning and practice.

Nicholas J. Talley, AC
Brad Frankum, OAM
Simon O'Connor

The authors and publishers wish to thank the following for their assistance with the preparation of *Essentials of Internal Medicine* 4th edition:

Dr Mudar Irani MD, Advanced Trainee in General Medicine, John Hunter Hospital, Newcastle; Conjoint Fellow, School of Medicine and Public Health, University of Newcastle, NSW, Australia;

Jasmine Wark BBiomedSci, Administrative and Research Assistant, School of Medicine and Public Health, University of Newcastle, NSW, Australia.

Meera R Agar MBBS, MPC, FRACP, FAChPM, PhD
Professor of Palliative Medicine; IMPACCT – Improving Palliative, Aged and Chronic Care through Clinical Research and Translation; Faculty of Health, University of Technology Sydney, Australia

Vimalan Ambikaipaker FRACP
Consultant Gastroenterologist and General Physician, NSW, Australia

David Arnold BMed, FRACP, FCCP
Respiratory Physician, John Hunter Hospital, University of Newcastle, NSW, Australia

John Attia MD, PhD, FRCPC, FRACP
School of Medicine and Public Health, Faculty of Health and Medicine, University of Newcastle, NSW, Australia

Ramdeep Bajwa MBChB, BMedSc, MRCP (UK)
The Prince Charles Hospital, Internal Medicine Services, QLD, Australia

Victoria Bray MBBS, FRACP, PhD
Liverpool Hospital, NSW, Australia

Will Browne FRACP
Eastern Health, VIC, Australia

Wei Chua BAppSci, MBBS, FRACP, PhD
Professor of Oncology and Cancer Care, Western Sydney University, NSW, Australia; Staff Specialist in Medical Oncology, Liverpool Hospital, NSW, Australia

Katherine Clark MBBS, MMed, FRACP, FAChPM
Director of Palliative Care, Calvary Mater Newcastle, NSW, Australia; Adjunct Professor, Faculty of Health and Medicine, University of Newcastle; Adjunct Professor, University of Wollongong, Australia

Elisa Cornish BMedSc (Hons), MBBS, GradDipMed (OphthalSc), PhD, FRANZCO
Senior Clinical Lecturer, The University of Sydney, Discipline of Clinical Ophthalmology and Eye Health, NSW, Australia

David Currow BMed, MPH, PhD, FRACP
Professor of Palliative Medicine, University of Technology Sydney, NSW, Australia

Matthew Doogue MBChB, FRACP
Associate Professor, Department of Medicine, University of Otago, Christchurch; Clinical Director, Department of Clinical Pharmacology, Canterbury District Health Board, New Zealand

Tracy Dudding-Byth BMed, PhD, FRACP
Senior Staff Specialist in Clinical Genetics, Hunter New England Health Service, NSW, Australia; Associate Professor, School of Medicine and Public Health, University of Newcastle, NSW, Australia

Georgia C Edwards BSc (Biochem), MBBS (Hons), FRACP
John Hunter Hospital, Newcastle and Conjoint Fellow, University of Newcastle, NSW, Australia

Carlos El Haddad FRACP
Rheumatologist, Liverpool Hospital & Senior Lecturer, School of Medicine, Western Sydney University, NSW, Australia

Randall Faull MBBS, FRACP, FRCP, PhD
Senior Consultant Nephrologist, Royal Adelaide Hospital, SA, Australia; Clinical Professor of Medicine, University of Adelaide, SA, Australia

Stephen James Fuller MBBS, PhD, FRACP, FRCPA
Associate Professor and Head of Clinical School, The University of Sydney, Faculty of Medicine and Health, Sydney Medical School, Nepean Clinical School, NSW, Australia

Robert Gibson BMed, FRACP
Hunter New England Health – Local Health District, NSW, Australia; University of Newcastle, NSW, Australia

Iain Bruce Gosbell MBBS, MD (Research, UNSW), FRACP, FRCPA, FASM
School of Medicine, Western Sydney University, Penrith, NSW, Australia; Clinical Services and Research, Australian Red Cross Lifeblood, Sydney, Australia

Magnus Halland BMed, BMedSci (Hons), MPH
Conjoint Lecturer, School of Medicine and Public Health, Faculty of Health and Medicine, University of Newcastle, NSW, Australia

Annemarie Hennessy MBBS, PhD, FRACP, MBA
Foundation Professor of Medicine, School of Medicine Western Sydney University, NSW, Australia; Clinical Academic Professor, Campbelltown Hospital, Sydney; Dean, School of Medicine, Western Sydney University; Honorary Professor, University of Sydney; Honorary Professor, University of New South Wales, NSW, Australia

Michael Hennessy BMedSc, MBBS, MBioMedE, FRANZCO
Prince of Wales Hospital, Sydney, NSW, Australia; Specialist in General and Surgical Ophthalmology, private practice, Sydney, NSW, Australia

Michael J Hensley MBBS, PhD
Head, Department of Respiratory and Sleep Medicine, John Hunter Hospital, NSW, Australia; Emeritus Professor of Medicine, University of Newcastle, NSW, Australia; Adjunct Professor of Medicine, University of New England, NSW, Australia

Alison L Jones MD, FRCPE, FRCP, CBiolFSB, FRACP, FACMT, FAACT, GAICD
Deputy Vice-Chancellor (Health and Communities) & Executive Dean, Faculty of Science, Medicine and Health, University of Wollongong, NSW, Australia

Christos S Karapetis MBBS, FRACP, MMedSc
Associate Professor, Flinders University, Adelaide, SA, Australia; Regional Clinical Director, Cancer Services, Southern Adelaide Local Health Network; Head, Department of Medical Oncology, Flinders Medical Centre, Adelaide; Director of Cancer Clinical Research, Flinders Centre for Innovation in Cancer, SA, Australia

Paven Preet Kaur MBChB, MRCP (UK)
The Prince Charles Hospital, Internal Medicine Services, QLD, Australia

Brian J Kelly BMed, PhD, FRANZCP, FAChPM
Professor of Psychiatry and Head, School of Medicine and Public Health, University of Newcastle, NSW, Australia

Andrew Korda AM MA, MHL, MBBS, FRCOG, FRANZCOG, CU
Professor of Obstetrics and Gynaecology, School of Medicine, Western Sydney University, NSW, Australia; Consultant Emeritus, Royal Prince Alfred Hospital, Sydney, NSW, Australia

Lisa Lampe MBBS, PhD, FRANZCP
Associate Professor and Discipline Lead, Psychiatry, School of Medicine and Public Health, University of Newcastle, NSW, Australia; Program Convenor, Joint Medical Program, Universities of Newcastle and New England, NSW, Australia; Staff Specialist (Academic), Hunter New England Local Health District, NSW, Australia

Sue-Lynn Lau MBBS, FRACP, PhD
Staff Specialist Endocrinology, Westmead Hospital, Sydney, NSW, Australia; Senior Lecturer Endocrinology, University of Sydney; Senior Lecturer Endocrinology, Western Sydney University, NSW, Australia

Monique Wei Meng Lee MBBS, BSc (Med) Hons, FRACP
Staff Specialist Immunologist, Campbelltown Hospital, NSW, Australia

Jessie A Lee BSc (Med), MBBS, FRACP, FRCPA
Department of Immunology, Concord Repatriation General Hospital, Sydney, NSW, Australia; Lecturer, Central Clinical School, Faculty of Medicine and Health, The University of Sydney, NSW, Australia

Christopher R Levi BMedSci, MBBS, FRACP
The Sydney Partnership for Health, Education, Research & Enterprise (SPHERE), NSW, Australia; Conjoint Professor, School of Medicine and Public Health, University of Newcastle, NSW, Australia

Angela Makris MBBS, FRACP, PhD, MMed
Nephrologist and Obstetric Physician, Liverpool Hospital, NSW, Australia; School of Medicine, Western Sydney University, NSW, Australia

Jennifer H Martin MBChB, MA (Oxon.), FRACP, PhD, GAICD
Physician and Director, Centre for Drug Repurposing and Medicines Research, School of Medicine and Public Health, University of Newcastle, NSW, Australia; Visiting Adjunct Professor, University of Queensland, QLD, Australia and Visiting Adjunct Professor, Monash University, VIC, Australia

Peter McCluskey AO, MBBS, MD, FRANZCO, FRACS
Professor & Chair of Ophthalmology, Director Save Sight Institute, The University of Sydney, Discipline of Clinical Ophthalmology and Eye Health, NSW, Australia

Mark McLean MBBS, FRACP, PhD
Head of Department of Medicine and Staff Specialist Endocrinology, Blacktown & Mount Druitt Hospital, NSW, Australia; Conjoint Professor of Medicine, Blacktown Clinical School, Western Sydney University, NSW, Australia

Melissa Moore BA, BSc, MBBS (Hons), FRACP, PhD
St Vincent's Hospital Melbourne & Department of Medicine University of Melbourne, VIC, Australia

Lucy Catriona Morgan BMed, PhD, FRACP
Concord Clinical School and Nepean Clinical School, The University of Sydney, NSW, Australia; Macquarie University Hospitals, NSW, Australia

Balakrishnan Kichu R Nair AM MBBS, MD (Newc), FRACP, FRCPE, FRCPG, FRCPI, FANZSGM, GradDip Epid
Professor of Medicine and Associate Dean, School of Medicine and Public Health, NSW, Australia; Director, Educational Research, Health Education and Training Institute, NSW, Australia; Director, Centre for Medical Professional Development, Hunter New England Health, NSW, Australia; Director, Academy of Clinical Educators, John Hunter Hospital Campus, NSW, Australia

Robert W Pickles BMed, FRACP
Department of Infectious Diseases, John Hunter Hospital, New Lambton Heights, NSW, Australia; Conjoint Associate Professor, School of Medicine and Public Health, University of Newcastle, NSW, Australia

Kevin Pile MBChB, MD, FRACP
Conjoint Professor of Medicine, Western Sydney University, Sydney, NSW, Australia

Milan K Piya MBBS, MRCP, PhD, FRACP
Senior Lecturer in Diabetes, School of Medicine, Western Sydney University; Camden and Campbelltown Hospitals, NSW, Australia

Michael Potter MBBS (Hons)
Department of Gastroenterology, John Hunter Hospital, University of Newcastle, NSW, Australia

Rohit Rajagopal BSc (Med), MBBS, FRACP
Senior Staff Specialist in endocrinology, Campbelltown and Camden Hospitals; Conjoint Senior Lecturer, Western Sydney University, NSW, Australia

Steve Robson MD, PhD, FRANZCOG, FRCOG
Professor, Australian National University Medical School, ACT, Australia

Lindsay Rowe (Deceased) MAppSci, BMed, FRANZCR
Associate Professor, School of Medicine and Public Health, University of Newcastle, NSW, Australia; Visiting Adjunct Professor, Murdoch University, Perth, WA, Australia; Visiting Adjunct Professor, North Western Health Sciences University, Minneapolis, MN, USA; Senior Staff Specialist Radiologist, John Hunter Hospital, Newcastle, NSW, Australia

Jeffrey Rowland MBBS, MPH, Grad Cert Hlth Sci (Health Innovation), FRACP, FANZSGM
Associate Professor of Medicine, University of Queensland, QLD, Australia; Executive Director of Medicine Stream, Medical Director of Acute Medicine & Sub-Specialties (Internal Medicine), The Prince Charles Hospital, QLD, Australia

David Simmons MA (Cantab), MBBS, FRACP, FRCP, MD (Cantab)
Professor of Medicine, School of Medicine, Western Sydney University and Campbelltown Hospital; Head of Department, Endocrinology, Campbelltown Hospital; Director, Diabetes Obesity and Metabolism Translational Research Unit, School of Medicine and South Western Sydney Local Health District; Co-Lead, Healthy and Connected, NSW Public Policy Institute, Sydney, NSW, Australia; Professorial Fellow, University of Melbourne, VIC, Australia; Visiting Professor, University of Örebro, Sweden; Guest Professor, First Affiliated Hospital, Zhengzhou University, China

Saxon D Smith MBChB, MHL, PhD, GAICD, FAMA, FACD
The Dermatology and Skin Cancer Centre, St Leonards, New South Wales, Australia

Peter L Thompson MD, FRACP, FACP, FACC, FCSANZ, MBA
Cardiologist and Director of Department of Research, and Director of Heart Research Institute, Sir Charles Gairdner Hospital, Nedlands, WA, Australia; Clinical Professor of Medicine and Population Health, University of Western Australia; Deputy Director, Harry Perkins Institute for Medical Research, WA, Australia

Peter AB Wark BMed, PhD, FRACP
Conjoint Professor, University of Newcastle, NSW, Australia; Senior Staff Specialist Department of Respiratory and Sleep Medicine John Hunter Hospital, NSW, Australia

D Ashley R Watson MBBS, Grad Cert Ed, MPH, FRACP
Senior Staff Specialist, Infectious Diseases, Canberra Health Services; Associate Professor, ANU Medical School, ACT, Australia

Thomas P Wellings BSc (Med) MBBS (Hons) FRACP PhD
Neurologist, John Hunter Hospital, Newcastle, NSW, Australia; Conjoint Lecturer, University of Newcastle, NSW, Australia

Elizabeth Whiting BA, MB BCh BAO, FRACP, FANZSGM
Staff Specialist Geriatric Medicine and General Medicine, The Prince Charles Hospital, QLD, Australia; Senior Lecturer, School of Medicine, University of Queensland, QLD, Australia; Executive Director Clinical Services, Metro North Hospital and Health Service, QLD, Australia

Jane Young MBBS, MPH, PhD, FAFPHM
Professor in Cancer Epidemiology, Sydney School of Public Health, Faculty of Medicine and Health, The University of Sydney and Sydney Local Health District, NSW, Australia

As this edition of *Essentials of Internal Medicine* goes to print, the world is experiencing an unprecedented pandemic due to the coronavirus disease 2019 (COVID-19). The first cases of this viral infection appeared in Hubei Province in China in December 2019, and were reported to the World Health Organization at the end of that month. Since then, the virus has spread across the globe and new case numbers (and deaths) rapidly increased in many parts of the world.

The virus responsible for the pandemic is a single-stranded RNA virus and is termed SARS-CoV-2 (severe acute respiratory syndrome coronavirus 2). It is transmitted through respiratory droplets, and is highly contagious. It can be transmitted from asymptomatic individuals. The incubation period may be up to 2 weeks, with a median of around 5 days.

COVID-19 infection occurs via the respiratory route. The virus enters pneumocytes through its viral structural spike protein, via the angiotensin-converting enzyme 2 receptor.

CLINICAL FEATURES

- Infection may be asymptomatic.
- Disease is mild in the majority of cases.
- Around 15% will develop severe disease, and 5% of cases will develop critical illness.
- Death rates may be between 1–4%.
- Symptoms include fever, cough, dyspnea, fatigue, myalgia and malaise, loss of sense of taste and smell, sore throat, headache, nasal congestion, conjunctivitis, skin rash, nausea, vomiting, and diarrhea.
- Dyspnea that begins several days after initial symptoms is suggestive of the diagnosis.
- Fever may be absent at the time of hospital admission.
- Pneumonia and Acute Respiratory Distress Syndrome (ARDS) are most lethal complications of the disease.
- The median onset of ARDS from the time of first symptoms is reported to be around 8 days.

RISK FACTORS FOR SEVERE DISEASE AND MORTALITY

- Advancing age
- Lung disease (e.g. chronic obstructive pulmonary disease, interstitial lung disease)
- Cardiovascular disease
- Diabetes mellitus
- Chronic kidney disease
- Obesity
- Cancer
- Immunocompromised patients
- Hypertension
- Cerebrovascular disease
- Dementia
- Cigarette smoking

LABORATORY FACTORS ASSOCIATED WITH POOR OUTCOMES

- Lymphopenia
- Elevated D-dimer
- Elevated lactate dehydrogenase
- Elevated CRP and ferritin
- Increased prothrombin time
- Increased creatine kinase and troponin
- Increased prothrombin time
- Abnormal liver enzymes
- Acute kidney injury

RADIOLOGICAL LUNG FINDINGS

- Ground glass opacities, especially in the lung peripheries
- Consolidation
- ARDS

DISEASE COMPLICATIONS

- Pneumonia, ARDS, and respiratory failure
- Hypercoagulability with venous and arterial thrombosis
- Stroke
- Myocardial injury and arrhythmias

- Acute kidney injury
- Concurrent viral and bacterial infection is relatively common in hospitalized patients

DIAGNOSIS

Diagnosis can be confirmed by polymerase chain reaction performed on respiratory secretions:

- Nasal swab
- Tracheal aspirate
- Bronchoalveolar lavage

Sensitivity of the test may depend on the viral load in the sample. Seroconversion may not occur until later in the disease course, making antibody testing unreliable for early diagnosis.

TREATMENT

Only two pharmacological treatments have achieved consensus as effective for the treatment of severe SARS-CoV-2 infection at the time of publication:

- Dexamethasone at 6 mg daily for hypoxemic patients, resulting in modestly lower mortality rates
- Remdesivir, resulting in reduced time to hospital discharge

The mainstay of treatment for severely affected individuals is respiratory support with supplemental oxygen and mechanical ventilation if required. Multi-organ failure will require typical intensive care management. Many questions remain regarding a variety of other pharmacological agents that are undergoing clinical trials, both in terms of efficacy, and in timing of their use. Statins and angiotensin-converting enzyme inhibitors are continued if there is no contraindication.

Prevention of SARS-CoV-2 infection remains paramount in attempts to limit the spread of infection. Isolation of infected individuals, social distancing, diligent hand-washing, mask wearing in public spaces, and appropriate use of personal protective equipment by those in contact with infected individuals are key strategies.

Peter Wark and Brad Frankum

Table: Clinical manifestations of COVID-19

	SYMPTOMS	LABORATORY FINDINGS	RADIOLOGICAL FINDINGS	SUPPORT AND TREATMENT
Mild	Commonly: fever can be intermittent, dry cough, fatigue, myalgia, loss of taste and smell. Less commonly: rash, headache and abdominal pain and diarrhea.		Chest radiograph and CT scans are usually normal.	Symptomatic treatment in the community.
Moderate to severe (hospitalized)	Persistent fever >37.5°C, severe dry cough, more likely to experience confusion, severe muscle pains, and shortness of breath.	Increased white cell count, neutrophilia, lymphopenia, rising CRP and LDH.	Chest radiographs/CT chest bilateral ground glass opacities.	May require support with oxygen, at flow rates 4 l/min sufficient to maintain SaO2>93%.
Severe disease	As above but more severe dyspnea.	Increasing white cell count, neutrophilia and platelets, fall in haemoglobin. Rising D-dimer, rising CRP, fall in albumin. Rise in troponin and creatine kinase. Deranged liver function.	Worsening chest radiograph/CT findings of ground glass opacification, and more confluent areas of consolidation.	Increasing requirements for respiratory support, with high flow nasal oxygen or non-invasive ventilation.
Critical illness	Severe dyspnea, signs of shock. Increased complications such as severe weakness, disseminated intravascular coagulation, acute renal failure, myocarditis, and encephalopathy.	Rising white cell count and neutrophilia. Proportion develop a rise in procalcitonin. Acute renal failure, rising troponin, creatine kinase, myoglobinuria.	Extensive pulmonary infiltrates that are widespread and increasingly confluent. Increased prevalence of severe pulmonary thromboembolic disease.	Support required in intensive care. Intubation and mechanical ventilation, with protective ventilatory strategies. Need for extracorporeal membrane oxygenation (ECMO). Requirement for hemodynamic support, renal replacement therapy.

CHAPTER 1

INTERNAL MEDICINE IN THE 21st CENTURY—BEST PRACTICE, BEST OUTCOMES

Brad Frankum, Simon O'Connor and Nicholas J Talley

The 21st century is a time of rapid change because of many challenges that impact on health from pandemics to over-population, environmental decline, pollution, climate change, food and water insecurity, dangerous technologies, and anti-science (e.g. anti-vaccine) movements. On the other hand the technological tools available to the modern internist allow us to understand and investigate disease in our patients in great depth. In the 21st century, targeted therapy now offers enormous capacity to alleviate suffering, but challenges us to be absolutely precise with diagnosis, and with the use of evidence in decision-making. Deciding when and how to employ resources that are limited and expensive raises questions of ethics, equity, and where the balance lies between the science of human biology and the art of caring for sick people.

Computer technology (including sophisticated approaches to dredging big data to rapidly identify the likely diagnosis), ready access to information (for physicians, their patients and families), and increasing use of molecular and genetic diagnostic techniques are rapidly changing the practice of modern internal medicine. Physicians need to be able to use these tools, and we need to be flexible in the way we learn. Perhaps surprisingly in this internet-driven world the textbook, with its synthesis of information and perspective on what is clinically important, retains its relevance as a cornerstone of medical education. We must also, however, recognize that the experience and expertise of our colleagues remains absolutely crucial to guide our ongoing learning and development.

GENERAL VERSUS SUB-SPECIALTY MEDICINE

There is a dichotomy in the practice of internal medicine. On the one hand is the lure of specialization, of becoming expert and authoritative in very narrow fields. On the other hand is the need to retain the ability to treat patients in a holistic manner.

Many patients present with undifferentiated illness, often accompanied by multiple comorbidities. These people require a physician with the skills to sort out multiple problems in the context of their overall health, both physical and psychological, while taking into account their social and cultural background. Too often the sub-specialist has lost the will or confidence to manage a patient's problems when they fall outside a particular organ system. Patients with multiple medical problems can become the victims of an unseemly conflict between medical teams as to who should take responsibility for their overall care, while each specialty is absolute about how their body system should be treated. For best outcomes, care must be highly coordinated; fragmented care puts patients at risk. Physicians as medical experts must take a leadership role here; it is not the responsibility of someone else.

As life expectancy increases in populations globally, as a result of both improved living conditions and longer survival due to the course of much chronic disease being ameliorated, physicians need to maintain the skills to manage the elderly. There is no doubt that the elderly experience unique physiological and pathological changes, but too often physicians fail to factor this into their decision-making. As an example, there is good evidence that polypharmacy is detrimental to the prognosis of elderly patients regardless of which drug combinations are being prescribed, yet most physicians are more comfortable adding medications to a patient's treatment than removing them. Similarly, the care provided must be appropriate for each individual, and toward the end of life withholding potential treatment may be a much better choice than attempting heroic but clinically futile measures.

Arguments are made that there should be a renaissance of generalism, particularly in the hospital setting, to allow for more holistic and rational treatment of patients. Perhaps a better alternative would be for all of us in the field of internal medicine to strive to practice as internist first and sub-specialist second. We also help patients more effectively when we work as part of a healthcare team, recognizing and employing the unique skills of colleagues as well as nursing and allied health staff.

Most importantly, the care of patients should be conducted in a partnership with the patient, and often also with their family. No amount of technical knowledge and procedural expertise on the part of the physician can treat patients effectively in the absence of trust and empathy. Communication skills need to be increasingly sophisticated as people's health literacy increases. Poor outcomes for patients occur much more frequently through failures of communication than due to a lack of scientific knowledge on the part of physicians.

THE IMPORTANCE OF DIAGNOSIS

Rational treatment of patients can only occur after rational diagnosis. When diagnosis proves elusive, a sensible differential diagnosis can allow for the formulation of an appropriate plan of investigation and management. 'Non-cardiac chest pain', 'dyspnea', or 'abdominal pain for investigation' are not diagnoses—they are symptoms. The internist needs to do better than allocating broad symptomatic labels to patients. Internal medicine is the branch of medicine for the expert diagnostician, and the discipline of committing to a refined provisional and differential diagnosis identifies the path forward for both clinician and patient.

Too often in modern medicine, physicians make cursory attempts to form a diagnosis based on limited history and physical examination, and then rely on investigations to refine the diagnosis. A defensive approach often results in excessive numbers of tests and more mistakes; this trap should be avoided. An investigation is only helpful diagnostically if there is a reasonable pre-test probability that it will be positive.

As an example, an 'autoimmune screen' is often performed for a patient with fatigue as a presenting problem but no other features of a systemic autoimmune disease. What, then, to do when the antinuclear antibody (ANA) comes back detectable in a titer of 1:160? Is this within the range of normal? How many asymptomatic patients will have a detectable ANA in low titer? How many extra tests should

now be performed to ensure that the ANA is not of significance? How do we deal with the inevitable anxiety of our patient who consults the internet to find that ANA is found in systemic lupus erythematosus, as indeed is the symptom of fatigue? How will we look in the eyes of the patient when we say to them that the 'positive' test was really negative and unimportant? If so, why was it ordered in the first place?

Furthermore, the larger the number of investigations performed, the higher the likelihood that a result will fall outside the reference range as a matter of chance. This is the statistical nature of a normal distribution curve. An abnormal result may be of no clinical significance, but still needs to be explained to a patient. As diagnostic techniques become more sensitive, especially imaging modalities, increasing numbers of incidental findings result. The physician needs to be able to discern between when this needs further investigation and when it can be dismissed. Most investigations are not innocuous and run the risk of potential harm. Physicians have a societal responsibility to be cost-conscious and all investigations should be ordered judiciously.

THE PHYSICIAN'S ROLE IN PUBLIC HEALTH

In the era of personalized medicine, there remains a critical role for the physician as an advocate for, and guardian of, public health. The SARS-COV2 pandemic is an excellent illustration of why this is important.

The greatest impact on health that we can make as physicians remains in the area of global preventative medicine. The world population's health will only continue to improve with concentrated, ongoing efforts to implement vital measures such as large-scale vaccination against infection; tobacco, alcohol, and recreational drug control; screening for pre-cancerous lesions, and earlier-stage cancers that can be cured; obesity and diabetes mellitus prevention; protection from war, violence, and road trauma; reduction in the spread of HIV, malaria, and tuberculosis; and minimalization of climate change. Even at a local level, it is essential for physicians to argue the case for these measures, especially in the face of ever-pressured health budgets, anti-scientific misinformation from vested interests, and governments intent on spending vastly more money on military defenses than on preventative health.

As physicians we generally treat patients on a one-on-one basis. Most feel, quite appropriately, duty-bound to facilitate the best possible care for each individual patient. There is, however, an opportunity cost for every dollar spent on healthcare. It is an obligation for each of us to spend this money appropriately and not waste valuable resources. Appropriate care is not necessarily the same as the most expensive care. Sometimes, simplifying investigations and treatments serves patients' interests far better.

THE PHYSICIAN AS SCHOLAR

Scholarly activity continues to define the essence of internal medicine. Scientific analysis of material, education of others, and ongoing research into basic and clinical mechanisms of health and disease are the cornerstones of practice for the internist.

The sources of information available to the physician continue to expand. The temptation to be influenced by vested interests is ever-present, whether that be from pharmaceutical companies trying to market drugs, researchers trying to maintain grant funding, colleagues trying to boost referrals, or even textbook authors trying to sell their books! Critical analysis of information through understanding the many factors influencing and biasing the production and presentation of data is the only way to guard against poor decision-making. All physicians need to exercise the intellectual discipline of critical appraisal in these settings.

Most medical graduates understand the importance of teaching and role-modeling provided by their senior colleagues. There is no more powerful lesson than seeing an expert in action in a clinical setting, or having a complex concept explained in an insightful and succinct fashion. As learning becomes increasingly blended between the classroom, the internet, and the clinical setting, the physician remains the central reference point for students and junior doctors to comprehend what is really important to understand and master. Physicians must take this responsibility as educators seriously. They must strive for excellence as teachers just as they do as clinicians.

To research is to improve. If we do not strive for new knowledge and understanding, our patients will not be able to look forward to better healthcare in the future. Research may involve an audit of an individual's current practice, or may involve participation in a multinational trial of a new therapy. Whatever form it takes, it underpins the practice of internal medicine. Our participation in research such as a clinical trial is likely to improve our practice, no matter what the outcome of the clinical trial.

As physicians, we must remain curious, vigilant, and sceptical. If we remain inspired by the scholarship of medicine, we can no doubt be an inspiration to our patients and colleagues.

CHAPTER 2

EVIDENCE-BASED MEDICINE AND CRITICAL APPRAISAL OF THE LITERATURE

Jane Young and John Attia

CHAPTER OUTLINE

INTRODUCTION

In order for patients to benefit from gains in knowledge achieved by medical science, the findings of research must be integrated into routine clinical practice. Evidence-based medicine is an approach to clinical practice in which there is an explicit undertaking to incorporate the best available scientific evidence into the process of clinical decision-making. Achievement of this requires skills in the identification, critical appraisal and interpretation of relevant research studies in order to assess the strengths, limitations and relevance of the evidence for the care of an individual patient.

ASSESSING THE EVIDENCE

When assessing the findings of scientific research, one of the first considerations is whether the results of a study are **accurate**. The accuracy of a study is also referred to as its 'internal validity'. To assess internal validity, potential sources of error or bias in the study must be considered.

Sources of error

There are two major sources of error that affect research studies. **Random error** arises due to chance variations in study samples and can be thought of as adding 'noise' to the data. It reduces the precision of the findings but can be minimized by increasing the sample size of the study.

In contrast, **systematic error** is due to the way in which the study was designed or conducted and will always deviate a research finding away from the truth in a particular direction, resulting in an under- or over-estimate of the true value. Systematic error may arise from the way in which study participants were selected into the study ('selection bias'), the accuracy of study measures ('information bias' or 'measurement bias') or the concomitant effect of other factors on the outcome in question ('confounding') (Box 2-1, overleaf). It should be recognized that different sources of systematic

---

Box 2-1
Types of systematic error

Selection bias

Error in the study's findings which arises from the methods used to select and recruit study participants.

- If the relationship between the study factor and the outcome is different for participants and non-participants (those excluded, omitted or who declined to participate), the study's results will be inaccurate. This affects the 'generalizability' of the study, otherwise known as the 'external validity'.
- Recruitment of random, population-based samples with high consent rates minimizes potential selection bias in a study.
- Be alert to potential selection bias in studies which:
  » recruit volunteers
  » recruit other non-representative groups
  » have low participation or consent rates
  » have high losses to follow-up.

Information bias

Errors in the study's findings due to inaccurate collection of information.

- Accuracy is how well the measure represents the true value.
- Reliability is the ability of a measure to provide consistent results when repeated.
- Measures that rely on the judgment of an individual can be influenced subconsciously by knowledge of the research question.
- In clinical trials, blinding of outcome assessors, clinicians and patients to treatment allocation reduces

the potential for awareness of group allocation to influence study measures.

- In case-control studies, cases may have heightened awareness of possible causes of their disease and so have different recall of exposure to factors of interest than controls ('recall bias').

Confounding

Error in the study's findings owing to mixing up of effects due to the study factor with those due to other factors.

- Occurs when there is an uneven distribution of prognostic factors between the groups being compared.
- In clinical trials, randomization aims to produce groups which are equally balanced for both known and unknown prognostic factors.
- Randomization will usually control for confounding if the sample size of the trial is large enough for the comparison groups to have similar distributions of prognostic factors.
- Potential confounding is a major issue in non-randomized studies that can be minimized by:
  » restricting study participation to exclude potential confounding factors
  » matching participants in different study groups for prognostic factors
  » stratifying participants by the prognostic factor and analyzing each stratum separately
  » statistical modeling to adjust for the effect of confounding.

---

error within the same study may work in the same or opposing directions. However, as the true value of interest is generally not known, the size of any error cannot be measured directly. Whereas random error is an issue of precision and can be handled by the use of statistics, systematic error is an issue of validity and can only be addressed by good study design. Increasing the sample size only increases precision not validity. Assessment of the potential for systematic error requires consideration of the potential for selection bias, information bias and confounding within each study.

Assessing potential biases in different study designs

A number of different types of study are used in clinical research and each is susceptible to varying sources of systematic bias. An understanding of the key features of each study design, and the most important sources of bias, provides the basis for critical appraisal of the scientific literature. Furthermore, once the design of the study has been identified, there are design-specific critical appraisal checklists, such as those developed by the Critical Appraisal Skills Programme

(CASP) in the United Kingdom, or the Users' Guides published by JAMA, that are readily available online to provide a step-by-step guide to the assessment of the methodological quality of research studies.

Randomized controlled trials

In randomized trials, participants are randomly allocated to treatment groups, for example to new treatment or placebo. The randomization process should achieve treatment groups in which patients are similar for both known and unknown prognostic factors (confounders) so that any differences in outcome can be attributed to differences in treatment.

Well-designed randomized trials use a method to allocate patients to treatment groups that is truly random and that ensures that the sequence cannot be known or guessed in advance by patients or those recruiting them ('allocation concealment'). Random number tables or computer-generated sequences are the best methods to obtain a truly random sequence. Inappropriate methods of 'randomization' are those in which the group allocation is not truly random, such as alternating patients between treatment groups or selecting the treatment group based on a patient characteristic (such as date of birth) or day of clinic attendance. In addition to generating a truly random sequence, the trial methods need to ensure allocation concealment so that a clinician's decision to recruit a particular patient to a trial and the patients' decisions whether or not to participate cannot be influenced by knowledge of the treatment group to which they will be allocated. Trial methods must ensure that the randomization schedule is not freely available to those involved in the actual recruitment of patients. This can be achieved by use of a central randomization service in which clinicians contact the service by phone, fax or email to register a patient who has already consented to be in the study, and to find out which treatment the patient has been randomly allocated to receive.

Intention-to-treat (ITT) analysis is a method used to preserve the randomization of participants at the analysis stage of a clinical trial. In ITT analysis, patients are analyzed in the groups to which they were originally allocated, regardless of what may have happened in practice. So any patients who decline the treatment to which they were randomized, those who cross over to another group for any reason, and those who drop out are analyzed as part of their original allocated group. As all patients who were randomized must be accounted for at final follow-up, the trial methods should attempt to minimize any drop-outs or losses to follow-up. Furthermore, the statistical methods should describe how any losses to follow-up were dealt with in the statistical analysis.

The use of **blinding** is a method to guard against information bias in randomized trials that also can be used in non-randomized studies. 'Blinding' or concealment of a study participant's treatment group ensures that preconceived attitudes or expectations of the relative effectiveness of the treatments being compared cannot influence the study data. Blinding of patients can guard against a placebo effect, in which patients report better outcomes due to the psychological effect of receiving a treatment that they perceive as being more effective than a control treatment. Blinding of clinicians reduces the potential for overt or subconscious differences in patient management that could arise from knowledge of the treatment that has been received. Blinding of other study staff such as outcome assessors, data collectors and biostatisticians can minimize the risk that measurement or analysis decisions are influenced by awareness of treatment group. As blinding addresses any information bias that results from participants' attitudes and expectations of the likely benefits of the treatment being tested, blinding is particularly important for study outcome measures that are subjective, such as pain, quality of life or satisfaction. Blinding is less important for objective measures such as mortality.

Key points to consider in the assessment of a randomized trial are summarized in Box 2-2.

Pseudo-randomized or quasi-experimental trials

In these trials, the method of developing the treatment allocation sequence is not truly random. For example, alternate patients could be allocated to different treatment groups, or treatments could be offered according to days of the week or last digit of a medical record number. A major concern is

---

> ## Box 2-2
> ## Key points for appraisal of a randomized controlled trial
>
> - How was the randomization schedule developed?
> - Was this a truly random process?
> - Could patients, or those recruiting them, have been able to know or deduce the next treatment allocation?
> - Were patients concealed to their treatment allocations?
> - Were clinicians concealed to the patients' treatment allocations?
> - Were those responsible for measurement of study outcomes blinded to the patients' treatment allocations, or were objective measures used?
> - Were all patients who were randomized accounted for in the final analysis in the groups to which they were allocated (regardless of whether they actually received this treatment)?
> - Were there any other factors that could have influenced the results of the study (e.g. poor compliance with allocated treatment, large numbers of patients crossing over to a non-allocated treatment group, contamination between treatment groups, co-interventions or changes in healthcare delivery during the trial that may have influenced outcomes)?
>
> Adapted with permission from Macmillan Publishers Ltd. Young JM and Solomon MJ. How to critically appraise an article. Nature Clinical Practice Gastroenterology 2009;6(2):82–91.

whether there is any relationship between the method of allocation and specific types of patient. For example, it may be that older or sicker patients attend a clinic on a particular day for reasons relating to clinical, administrative, access or transport issues. In addition to careful consideration of potential pitfalls of the group allocation method, other points to consider in the assessment of a pseudo-randomized study are the same as for randomized trials.

Cohort studies

Cohort studies involve the longitudinal follow-up of groups of individuals to identify those who develop the outcome of interest.

- In a prospective cohort study, the individuals are identified at the start of the study and data are collected about the study factors or exposures of interest as well as all potential confounding factors. The cohort is then followed, usually for several years, with regular assessment of study outcomes over this period.

- In a retrospective cohort study, individuals are usually identified at some point in the past from existing databases or records, and information about study factors, potential confounders and outcomes through to the present day is also obtained from existing data sources.

Retrospective cohort studies are usually much quicker to complete than prospective studies, but a major disadvantage

Box 2-3

Key points for appraisal of a cohort study

- Is the study prospective or retrospective?
- Is the cohort well-defined in terms of person, time and place?
- Is the cohort population-based?
- Were data collected on all important confounding factors?
- Were study outcomes and potential confounders measured in the same way for all members of the cohort?
- Was the length of follow-up sufficient to identify the outcomes of interest?
- Were there large losses to follow-up?
- Were those lost to follow-up likely to have different outcomes to those who continued in the study?

Adapted with permission from Macmillan Publishers Ltd. Young JM and Solomon MJ. How to critically appraise an article. Nature Clinical Practice Gastroenterology 2009;6(2):82–91.

Box 2-4

Ten questions to ask about a research article

1 Is the study question relevant?
2 Does the study add anything new?
3 What type of research question is being asked?
4 Was the study design appropriate for the research question?
5 Did the study methods address the most important potential sources of bias?
6 Was the study performed according to the original protocol?
7 Does the study test a stated hypothesis?
8 Were the statistical analyses performed correctly?
9 Are the conclusions justified from the data?
10 Are there any conflicts of interest?

Adapted with permission from Macmillan Publishers Ltd. Young JM and Solomon MJ. How to critically appraise an article. Nature Clinical Practice Gastroenterology 2009;6(2):82–91.

is that information about potential confounders may not have been collected at the time the original data were obtained. Box 2-3 summarizes key points to consider in the assessment of a cohort study.

Case-control studies

In case-control studies, cases are selected because they have already developed the outcome of interest, for example a disease, and their history of exposure, risk factors or treatment are compared with similar people who have not developed the outcome of interest ('controls'). Case-control studies are particularly useful to investigate risk factors when the clinical condition of interest is rare, as it would take too long to recruit and follow up a prospective cohort of patients. Selection of appropriate controls and the possibility of recall bias are major concerns with case-control studies.

Cross-sectional studies

In cross-sectional studies, information about the study factors and outcomes of interest are collected at one point in time. The purpose of this type of study is to investigate associations between these factors, but it is not possible to draw conclusions about causation as a sequence of events cannot be established. A survey is an example of a cross-sectional study.

CRITICAL APPRAISAL OF THE LITERATURE

While a focus of the critical appraisal of a research study is an assessment of the potential for bias in the design and conduct of the research, there are a number of other important factors that should be considered (Box 2-4).

Two important considerations are whether the specific research question addressed in the study is relevant to the clinical question of interest, and whether the appropriate study design was used to answer this question. While it is widely recognized that well-designed randomized controlled trials provide the best quality evidence about the effectiveness of medical therapies, other study designs are optimal for different types of research question. For example, an evaluation of the accuracy of a new diagnostic test would be best investigated using a cross-sectional study design in which a consecutive sample of patients received both the new test and an existing 'gold standard' test simultaneously. The accuracy of the new test could then be established by comparing the results with the 'gold standard' test. Questions about prognosis are best answered using prospective cohort studies.

Many studies are conducted that are not the optimal design for the research question being addressed. This can be because the optimal design is not acceptable or is not feasible with the time and resources available. For example, it can be very difficult to conduct randomized trials to test new surgical procedures, particularly when there is a large difference in the extent of surgery between the experimental and standard approaches. Patients are likely to refuse to have a non-reversible treatment option decided essentially on the basis of the toss of a coin. Another circumstance where randomized trials are difficult is when the condition of interest is very rare so that it would be impossible to achieve the required sample size within a reasonable timeframe. Many organizations, such as those involved in the development of evidence-based clinical practice guidelines, have developed hierarchies of evidence that rank study designs from strongest to weakest for questions relating to therapeutic effectiveness, prognosis or diagnostic test accuracy. For therapeutic effectiveness, for example, one hierarchy from strongest to weakest would be: randomized trial; a comparative study with concurrent controls (pseudo-randomized trial, prospective cohort study, case-control study, controlled time series); comparative study with historical controls; uncontrolled (single-arm) studies such as uncontrolled time series or uncontrolled case series.

Systematic review is an explicit process whereby evidence on a particular question is identified and assessed in terms of suitability for pooling. This assessment is usually based on the algorithm PICOD, i.e. population, intervention, comparator, outcome and design, that is to say an assessment is made whether these factors are similar enough that it makes sense to pool data together or different enough that pooling would not make sense (clinical heterogeneity).

Meta-analysis is a statistical technique in which the findings of several studies can be pooled together to provide a summary measure of effect. Meta-analysis should always follow a comprehensive systematic review of the literature to identify all relevant primary studies and to assess the quality and comparability of these studies. When conducted according to strict protocols, such as those developed by the Cochrane Collaboration to minimize bias, systematic review and meta-analysis can provide the strongest evidence on a topic as it incorporates all the relevant scientific evidence from individual studies. Hence, most evidence hierarchies have meta-analysis as the highest-ranked study design. In the case of questions of therapeutic effectiveness, meta-analysis of individual randomized controlled trials would be considered the strongest evidence on the topic. After pooling, one can check the assumption of similarity by doing a test of heterogeneity (statistical heterogeneity). Key points to consider when assessing a systematic review or meta-analysis are summarized in Box 2-5.

INTERPRETING A STUDY'S FINDINGS

Clinical studies use a variety of measures to summarize their findings.

- A '**point estimate**' is the single value or result that is obtained from the study sample. It is the best estimate of the underlying true value that has been obtained from the study data. Different studies that address the same clinical question may yield slightly different point estimates due to small differences between the study methods and samples and the play of chance.

- **Incidence** and **prevalence** are measures commonly used to describe the burden of disease in the community.

- A **rate** is the number of events occurring in a defined population over a specific time period, such as one year.

Incidence and prevalence are often mixed up, but shouldn't be! An **incidence rate** is the number of *new* cases per population in a given time period, and is a measure of the risk of developing the condition of interest. For example, cancer incidence rates are usually reported as the number of new cases per 100,000 people per year. In contrast, **prevalence** is

---

> **Box 2-5**
>
> **Key points for appraisal of a systematic review or meta-analysis**
>
> - Was the literature review sufficiently comprehensive to identify all the relevant literature?
> - Were specific inclusion and exclusion criteria used to select articles to be included in the review?
> - Were important types of article excluded (e.g. those in foreign languages, unpublished articles)?
> - Was the quality of the included articles assessed using explicit criteria by two independent reviewers?
> - Were numerical results and key findings extracted from the included articles by two independent reviewers?
> - Was sufficient detail about the included studies provided to enable comparisons of patient characteristics, treatments and outcomes between studies?
> - If a meta-analysis was conducted, was an assessment of heterogeneity and the appropriateness of calculating a summary measure assessed?
>
> Adapted with permission from Macmillan Publishers Ltd. Young JM and Solomon MJ. How to critically appraise an article. Nature Clinical Practice Gastroenterology 2009;6(2):82–91.

---

the number of people in the population with the condition of interest during a specified time period or at a specific time point and is a good measure of the effect of the disease in the community. Prevalence includes cases that were diagnosed prior to but continue to exist during the time period, as well as the new cases that occur for the first time during the time period. **Point prevalence** is the number of people in the population with the disease at a single point in time.

Rates can be **standardized** to allow valid comparisons to be made between two or more different populations. For example, the risk of most cancers increases with advancing age. A comparison of cancer incidence rates between two regions with different age structures would be misleading if age were not taken into account, as a higher cancer incidence rate would be expected in the region with the older population. The incidence rates for the different regions can be age-standardized by calculating what the rates would be if each region had the age structure of a standard population (direct standardization). In this way, the effect of age is removed as much as possible from the comparison of the cancer incidence rates.

Many clinical studies investigate the relationship between a study factor (e.g. risk factor or type of treatment) and an outcome. The results can be presented in a 2×2 contingency table, from which various measures of association or effect can be calculated (Figure 2-1, overleaf). These measures can be reported in *absolute* or *relative* terms.

- The **absolute** effect is simply the difference in means, medians, proportions or rates between groups. Imagine that in a hypothetical trial, 200 patients are randomly allocated to either a new treatment for cancer

Consider a hypothetical trial comparing a new treatment for cancer (intervention group) with the standard treatment (control group), with 200 patients in each group. The primary outcome is the proportion of patients who are disease-free at 12 months. Twenty patients are disease-free at 12 months in the intervention group compared with 10 in the control group. The results can be presented in a 2 × 2 table:

	Disease-free	Not disease-free	Total
Treatment	20(a)	180(b)	200
Control	10(c)	190(d)	200
Total	30	370	400

Event rate (proportion disease-free) in treatment group
= a/(a+b) = 20/200 = 10%
Event rate (proportion disease-free) in control group
= c/(c+d) = 10/200 = 5%
Absolute risk reduction (ARR) = difference in event rates
= (a/(a+b)) − (c/(c+d) = 10 − 5 = 5%
Number needed to treat (NNT) = 20 (1/ARR)
Relative risk = (a/(a+b))/(c/(c+d)) = 10/5 = 2
Odds ratio = (ad)/(bc) = (20 × 190)/(180 × 10) = 2.11

Figure 2-1 Example of a 2 × 2 table for calculating measures of association

Adapted from Young JM. Understanding statistical analysis in the surgical literature: some key concepts. Australian and New Zealand Journal of Surgery 2009;79:398–403.

(intervention group) or standard treatment (control group) and the proportion who are disease-free at 12 months is the primary outcome measure (Figure 2-1). If 20 (10%) patients in the intervention group and 10 (5%) patients in the control group are disease-free at 12 months, the **absolute risk reduction** is 10 − 5 = 5%. The number needed to treat (NNT) is the number of people who need to be treated based on the trial to prevent 1 additional event over a specified period of time. The NNT is calculated by taking the inverse of the absolute risk reduction. In this example, the NNT is 1/(5/100) = 20, showing that 20 people would need to be treated to prevent 1 additional recurrence at 12 months. Remember that the NNT always needs to be qualified by the time period on which it is based.

- These results can also be presented in terms of the outcome of the intervention group **relative** to the control group. The **relative risk** (sometimes called the risk ratio) compares the probability, or risk, of the event (being disease-free at 12 months) in the two groups. In this example, the event rate in the intervention group is 10% compared with 5% in the control group, giving a relative risk of 10/5 = 2. This means that patients in the intervention group are twice as likely to be disease-free at 12 months compared with those in the control group.

The **odds** of an outcome are the ratio of it occurring (numerator) to it not occurring (denominator). In contrast to a proportion, individuals who are counted in the numerator are not also counted in the denominator. For example, if 5 out of 20 patients develop a complication, the odds of the complication are 5:15 or 0.33 whereas the corresponding proportion is 5:20 or 0.25 (or 25%). An **odds ratio** (OR) is the ratio of the odds of the outcome occurring in one group compared with the odds of it occurring in a second group. The odds ratio will be very close to the relative risk when the outcome of interest is rare. However, for common outcomes, the odds ratio will depart from the relative risk. See Figure 2-1 for how to calculate a relative risk and an odds ratio from a 2 × 2 table.

For both odds ratios and relative risks, the **null value**, or value at which there is no difference between groups, is 1.

- If the likelihood of the outcome is greater in the intervention or exposure group compared with the control group, the odds ratio or relative risk will be greater than 1. The larger the value of the odds ratio or relative risk, the stronger the association is between the study factor (treatment or exposure) and the outcome. An OR of 5.0, for example, indicates that patients in the treatment or exposed group were 5 times more likely to develop the outcome than patients in the control group, and an OR of 1.3 means that they were 30% more likely to do so.

- Conversely, if the outcome is less likely in the treatment or exposed group than the control group, the odds ratio or relative risk will be less than 1 (but cannot be below 0). A value of 0.8 means that patients in the study group were 20% less likely to develop the outcome of interest compared with controls, and a value of 0.5 means that they were half as likely to do so.

INTERPRETING STATISTICAL ANALYSIS

Part of the critical appraisal of a research study is assessment of the logic and appropriateness of the statistical methods used. In clinical research, the focus of much statistical analysis is **hypothesis testing**. Therefore, it is imperative that the study's hypotheses are clearly stated. The purpose of hypothesis testing is to make a judgment as to whether the study's findings are likely to have occurred by chance alone. The choice of appropriate statistical tests to achieve this is unrelated to the design of the study but is determined by the specific type of data that have been collected to measure the study outcomes ('endpoints').

- Where individuals can be grouped into separate categories for a factor (e.g. vital status can only be 'dead' or 'alive'), the data are *categorical*. There are different types of categorical data. *Binary* data occur when there are only two possible categories. Where there are more than two possible categories, the data are *nominal* when there is no particular order to the categories (e.g. blue, green or brown eye color), and *ordinal* when a natural order is present (e.g. stage of cancer).

- *Continuous* data occur when a measure can take any value within a range (e.g. age). Within a group of individuals, the values of continuous data can follow a

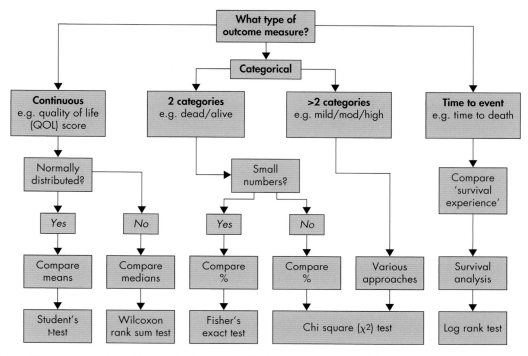

Figure 2-2 Algorithm to select statistical tests for analyzing a surgical trial (two independent groups)

Reprinted by permission from John Wiley and Sons. Young JM. Understanding statistical analysis in the surgical literature: some key concepts. Australian and New Zealand Journal of Surgery 2009;79:398–403.

bell-shaped curve that is symmetrical around the mean value (a normal distribution), or follow an asymmetrical distribution with a larger proportion of people having high or low values (a skewed distribution).

In addition to the type of outcome data, the number of patient groups being compared dictates the most appropriate statistical test. A third consideration is whether the comparison groups are made up of different individuals and are therefore independent of each other (e.g. treatment and control groups in a two-arm randomized trial), or are the same individuals assessed at different time points (e.g. in a randomized cross-over study). In the latter case, study data relate to pairs of measurements on the same individual.

Slightly different statistical tests are used depending on whether the data are independent or paired, and a biostatistician can advise about the best approaches. An example of an algorithm to choose the most appropriate statistical test for two independent groups is given in Figure 2-2.

Correlation is used to assess the strength of association between two continuous variables. The Pearson correlation coefficient (r) ranges from −1 to +1. A value of +1 means that there is a perfect positive linear relationship between the two variables, so as one increases, the other increases. In contrast, a value of −1 means that there is a perfect negative linear relationship, with one variable decreasing as the other increases. A value of 0 means that there is no linear relationship between the two variables.

Statistical tests of hypotheses generate a **probability** or **p value** that indicates the likelihood of obtaining the result seen in the study if the truth is that there is no effect or no difference between groups. A conventional cut-off for p of 0.05 or less to indicate statistical significance means that there is a 5% (or 1 in 20) chance or less of obtaining the observed finding or one more extreme in the study if there is truly no difference between groups.

Due to natural variability, the results from different samples will vary and each study provides an estimate of the true value. **Confidence intervals** provide a range of values around the study finding where the true value is likely to lie. A 95% confidence interval indicates that the true value will lie within this range in 95% of samples.

INTERPRETING TEST RESULTS

An everyday task for clinicians is to order and interpret tests in light of a patient's history and clinical examination. Whenever a test is undertaken there are four possible results:

1 the patient has the disease and the test is positive—true positive

2 the patient has the disease but the test is negative—false negative

3 the patient doesn't have the disease but the test is positive—false positive

4 the patient doesn't have the disease and the test is negative—true negative.

This can be illustrated using a 2 × 2 table (Figure 2-3, overleaf).

Sensitivity and specificity are used to describe the **accuracy** of the test.

		DISEASE	
		Truly present	**Truly not present**
TEST	**Positive**	TRUE POSITIVE *a*	FALSE POSITIVE *b*
	Negative	FALSE NEGATIVE *c*	TRUE NEGATIVE *d*

Sensitivity $= a/(a + c)$
Specificity $= d/(b + d)$
Positive predictive value (PPV) $= a/(a + b)$
Negative predictive value (NPV) $= d/(c + d)$
Likelihood ratio—positive test result (LR+) $=$ sensitivity $/ (1 -$ specificity$)$
$= (a/(a + c)) / (1 - d/(b + d))$
$= a/(a + c) / (b/(b + d))$

Likelihood ratio—negative test result (LR−) $= (1 -$ sensitivity$) /$ specificity
$= 1 - a /(a + c) / d/(b + d)$
$= (c/(a + c)) / d/(b + d)$

Post-test odds = pre-test odds × LR
Post-test probability = post-test odds / (post-test odds +1)

Positive LR (rule in disease)	Increased probability of disease (approximate)
2	15%
5	30%
10	45%

Figure 2-3 Interpretation of test results using a 2 × 2 table

- **Sensitivity** is the percentage of affected persons with a positive test (true positive proportion). Sensitivity therefore means positive in disease (PID).
- **Specificity** is the percentage of unaffected persons with a negative test (true negative proportion). Specificity therefore means negative in health (NIH) (Figure 2-3).

Test sensitivity and specificity are *not* related to how common the disease is in the community (prevalence). The prevalence of disease in a population, or pre-test probability of the disease, will alter how useful the test is for an individual patient. The **positive predictive value** (PPV) of a test is the probability of disease in a patient with a positive test, whereas the **negative predictive value** (NPV) is the probability of no disease in a patient with a negative test result. Figure 2-3 demonstrates how to calculate these values from a 2 × 2 table and shows that both PPV and NPV are dependent on the underlying prevalence of the disease. This means that a patient who has a positive test result and who is from a group with a low prevalence of the disease has a lower probability of having the disease than a patient with a positive test result who is from a group with a high prevalence of the disease in question.

The **likelihood ratio** (LR) is another measure of the usefulness of a diagnostic test. It provides a way of combining the sensitivity and specificity of a test into a single measure (see Figure 2-3). As sensitivity and specificity are characteristics of the test itself and are not influenced by prevalence, the LR is not influenced by the prevalence of disease in the population.

- Imagine that a diagnostic test has a sensitivity of 0.95 and a specificity of 0.85. The likelihood ratio for a positive test (LR+) is calculated by dividing the sensitivity by $(1 -$ specificity$)$. In this example, the LR+ is $0.95/(1 - 0.85) = 6.3$. The best test to **rule in** a disease is the one with a LR+ near to or exceeding a value of 10. The hypothetical test in this example does not meet this criterion and so is only of limited value in ruling in the disease for a patient with a positive test result.
- The likelihood ratio for a negative test (LR−) is calculated by dividing $(1 -$ sensitivity$)$ by the specificity, which is $(1 - 0.95)/0.85 = 0.058$ in this example. The best test to **rule out** a disease is the one with a small LR− (<0.1). The hypothetical test meets this criterion, suggesting that the disease can be ruled out in a patient with a negative test result.
- Likelihood ratios around 1.0 indicate that the test results provide no useful information to rule in or rule out the disease.

Likelihood ratios can be used to calculate the probability that a patient has the disease taking into account the test result (**post-test probability**).

- In the above example, imagine that the prevalence of the disease (**pre-test probability**) in the community is 10% or 0.1. The pre-test odds of the disease are calculated by dividing the prevalence by (1 − prevalence), which in this case is $0.1/(1 − 0.1) = 0.1/0.9 = 0.11$ or 11%.
- The post-test odds are then calculated by multiplying the pre-test odds by LR+. In our example, this is $0.11 \times 6.3 = 0.693$.
- To convert this to a post-test probability, the post-test odds are divided by (post-test odds + 1). In our example, this is $0.693/1.639 = 0.409$ or 40.9%.

So for a patient with a positive test result, the probability of disease has risen from 10% to 41% on the basis of the test result.

SCREENING

A test's sensitivity and specificity are particularly important when evaluating a screening test. Screening is used to detect disease in affected individuals before it becomes symptomatic. For example, Papanicolaou (Pap) smears and mammograms are used to detect cervical and breast cancer, respectively, to facilitate early treatment and reduce morbidity and mortality from these cancers. Before screening is introduced, it must fulfill the following criteria:

- there must be a presymptomatic phase detectable by the screening test

- intervention at this time will change the natural history of the disease to reduce morbidity or mortality
- the screening test must be inexpensive, easy to administer and acceptable to patients
- the screening test will ideally be highly sensitive and specific (although this is not usually possible)
- the screening program is feasible and effective.

CONCLUSION

Critical appraisal is a systematic process to identify the strengths and limitations of research evidence that can assist clinicians to base their clinical practice on the most relevant, high-quality studies. Critical appraisal skills underpin the practice of evidence-based medicine.

ACKNOWLEDGMENTS

This chapter is based on the papers Young JM and Solomon MJ. How to critically appraise an article. Nature Clinical Practice Gastroenterology 2009;6(2):82–91, and Young JM. Understanding statistical analysis in the surgical literature: some key concepts. Australian and New Zealand Journal of Surgery 2009;79:398–403. We acknowledge and thank Dr. David Currow who was a contributing author to this chapter in the third edition.

SELF-ASSESSMENT QUESTIONS

1 A randomized controlled trial demonstrates that a new drug for cystic fibrosis reduces age-adjusted 10-year mortality by 50% but does not cure the disease. The new drug has few side-effects and is rapidly adopted into the clinical care of patients with cystic fibrosis in the community. Which of the following statements is correct?

A   The incidence of cystic fibrosis will increase but prevalence will be unaffected.
B   Both incidence and prevalence of cystic fibrosis will increase.
C   Prevalence will increase but incidence will be unaffected.
D   Neither incidence nor prevalence will change.

2 A randomized controlled trial was conducted to investigate the effectiveness of a new chemotherapy drug to improve 1-year survival for people diagnosed with advanced lung cancer. Overall, 300 people were randomized, 150 to the new drug and 150 to standard treatment. However, 10 people who were allocated to receive the new drug decided not to take it as they were worried about potential side-effects. These 10 people were all alive at 1 year. At 1 year, 80 people in the new treatment group had died, compared with 92 in the standard treatment group. How many patients need to be treated with the new drug to prevent 1 additional death at 12 months?

A   280
B   12.5
C   12.23
D   0.125

3 Alzheimer disease is a common condition in the community, affecting 13% of North Americans aged over 65 years. A new test for Alzheimer disease has a sensitivity of 65% and a specificity of 80%. What is the probability that a 70-year-old with a positive test result has Alzheimer disease?

A   0.084
B   0.104
C   0.206
D   0.326

4 Which of the following statements about randomized controlled trials (RCTs) is/are correct?

i   RCTs are always the optimal study design in clinical research.
ii   Randomization ensures that equal numbers of patients receive the intervention and control treatments.
iii Randomization reduces information bias.
iv   Randomization reduces random error.

A   (i) only
B   (ii) only
C   (ii) and (iii)
D   None

5 In the methods section of a trial, the sample size calculation states that they had 80% power to detect a 10% difference in the incidence of heart attacks over the 3-year follow-up period at a type I error rate of 5%. What is the chance of type II error, i.e. concluding that there is no effect even if the real effect is a 10% difference or more?

A   5%
B   10%
C   15%
D   20%
E   25%

6 In the above example, what is the chance of concluding that there is an effect of 10% or more when the reality is that there is no effect?

A   5%
B   10%
C   15%
D   20%
E   25%

7 The best way to increase internal validity is through:

A   better study design
B   increased sample size
C   increased power
D   adjustment for more variables
E   better selection of participants

8 Blinded allocation refers to blinding during the process of:

A selection
B randomization
C measurement
D adjudication of outcomes
E analysis

9 A study is comparing median hospital length of stay between older patients randomized at admission to a physical activity maintenance program and those receiving usual care. Comparing the 2 medians should be done with what statistical test?

A t-test
B Wilcoxon rank sum test
C Fisher's exact test
D chi-squared test
E McNemar's test

ANSWERS

1 **C.**

People who take the new drug are less likely to die, so the number of existing cases will increase, thereby increasing prevalence (new plus existing cases in the community). However, the number of new cases is not affected, so the incidence will remain unchanged.

2 **B.**

The results of the study are summarized in the following 2 × 2 contingency table.

VITAL STATUS AT 1 YEAR	NEW TREATMENT	STANDARD TREATMENT
Dead	80	92
Alive	70	58
Total	150	150

Intention-to-treat (ITT) analysis should be used to preserve randomization. Using ITT analysis, it is irrelevant whether people who were randomized to receive the new treatment actually took the drug, as all study participants are analyzed in their original group. The proportion who died in the new treatment group is 80/150 = 0.533 = 53.3%. The proportion who died in the standard treatment group is 92/150 = 0.613 = 61.3%. Therefore, the absolute risk reduction (ARR) is 0.613 − 0.533 = 0.08 = 8%. The number needed to treat is 1/ARR = 1/0.08 = 12.5.

3 **D.**

This calculation requires four steps. First, calculate the likelihood ratio of a positive test (LR+) which is given by sensitivity/(1 − specificity). For this test, LR+ =0.65/(1 − 0.80) = 0.65/0.20 = 3.25.

Next, calculate the pre-test odds of this patient having the disease, which is given by prevalence/(1 − prevalence). In this situation, this is 0.13/0.87 = 0.149.

Next, calculate the post-test odds by multiplying the pre-test odds by LR+. In this case, this is 3.25 × 0.149 = 0.484.

Last, convert this to a post-test probability which is post-test odds/(post-test odds + 1). Here, this is 0.484/1.484 = 0.326.

Therefore, this patient with a positive test has a 32.6% probability of having Alzheimer disease.

4 **D.**

None are correct. The optimal study design depends on the research question. RCTs are the optimal study design to test the effectiveness of new treatments, but other study designs are optimal for questions of prognosis or diagnostic test accuracy. While trials in which equal numbers of participants are randomized to each treatment group are common, different proportions of patients can be randomized to each arm of an RCT (e.g. 1:2 or 1:3). The purpose of randomization is to achieve treatment groups that are equivalent, so as to reduce the potential for selection bias and confounding. Information bias (e.g. recall bias or measurement error) would not be affected by the randomization process. Random error is chance variation or noise, and this can only be addressed by increasing the size of the study.

5 D.

Power is the likelihood of detecting an effect as big or bigger than hypothesized at the *p*-value threshold stated. This is 80%, hence the complement is that there is a 20% likelihood of missing this effect size.

6 A.

This is the type I error rate, otherwise known as the *p*-value. A *p*-value of 0.05 means that we would see an effect size of 10% or greater purely by chance 5 times out of a 100 (imagining that we repeated our trial 100 times) assuming there was no effect; this is low enough (or rare enough) that we say we are happy to reject chance as an explanation and say there is a true effect.

7 A.

Validity is maximized through good design. Both sample size and power reflect the same concept and increase precision. Adjustment for more variables cannot ensure lack of confounding; only randomization can do this. Selection of participants will influence mainly external validity or generalizability, not internal validity.

8 B.

Allocation refers to blinding during the process of randomization, i.e. the physician cannot tell which arm the participant is getting randomized to, otherwise there might be the temptation to withhold randomization if the participant is getting the placebo (and the physician wants treatment) or the treatment arm (and the physician doesn't believe in the new intervention).

9 B.

Comparing medians means the data is not normally distributed and hence a non-parametric test is required, i.e. Wilcoxon rank sum test. t-test and Fisher's exact are for continuous, normally distributed data and chi-square is for dichotomous data. McNemar's test is for matched pairs.

CHAPTER 3

CLINICAL PHARMACOLOGY AND TOXICOLOGY

Matt Doogue, Jennifer Martin and Alison Jones

CHAPTER OUTLINE

- Acetaminophen (paracetamol)
- Non-steroidal anti-inflammatory drugs (NSAIDs)
- Tricyclic antidepressants
- Newer antidepressants
- Newest antidepressants
- Newer antipsychotics
- Benzodiazepines
- Insulin and oral hypoglycemics

- **DRUGS OF ABUSE OR MISUSE**
  - Amphetamines
  - Cocaine and crack cocaine
  - Gammahydroxybutyrate (GHB)
  - Opioids, e.g. heroin or morphine
  - Prescription drug abuse
  - Synthetic cathinones, e.g. 'vanilla sky', 'ivory wave'

- Synthetic cannabinoids, e.g. 'spice', 'K2'
- Drink spiking

- **CHEMICALS**
  - Acids and alkalis
  - Chlorine
  - Pesticides
  - Lead poisoning

- **SPIDER BITES**

- **SNAKE BITES**

- **MARINE ENVENOMATION**

- **TERRORISM, AND USE OF MEDICAL COUNTERMEASURES**
  - Chemical agents
  - Biological agents

Clinical pharmacology is the clinical and scientific discipline that involves all aspects of the relationship between drugs and humans. In considering this relationship, it is useful to consider drugs both in individual patients (pharmacotherapy) and in populations (pharmacoepidemiology). This chapter on clinical pharmacology has three sections.

1. Principles of clinical pharmacology—the steps from drug ingestion to drug effects; 'what the body does to the drug' (pharmacokinetics) and 'what the drug does to the body' (pharmacodynamics).
2. Quality use of medicines (QUM)—the tools of safe, effective and rational use of drugs in individuals and in populations.
3. Clinical toxicology—understanding and managing supratherapeutic (toxic) doses of drugs and other substances.

1. PRINCIPLES OF CLINICAL PHARMACOLOGY

INTRODUCTION

Pharmacotherapy has two components, patient and drug(s); and two processes, pharmacokinetics and pharmacodynamics. Pharmacokinetics (PK)—*what the body does to the drug*—is about the factors affecting drug exposure. Pharmacodynamics (PD)—*what the drug does to the body*—is about the factors affecting drug effects.

Drug effects differ between individuals. Understanding and managing therapeutic variability requires consideration of both drug and patient.

- In clinical practice, patients are treated with therapeutic intent using drugs at doses
  - » to maximize potential benefit, and
  - » to minimize potential harm.

- In clinical studies, groups of patients are studied:
  - » to define therapeutic doses for a population
  - » to consider whether there are sub-populations of response (for future pharmacokinetic and dynamic research)
  - » to describe drug disposition, and
  - » to describe and quantify drug effects.

Applying the information derived from clinical studies to clinical practice is based on a thorough understanding of pharmacokinetic and pharmacodynamic variability and therefore the relevance of trial data to an individual patient—these usually vary greatly from the average of the population studied.

Treatment of a patient with a drug can be described by the interaction between drug and patient through multiple steps (Figure 3-1).

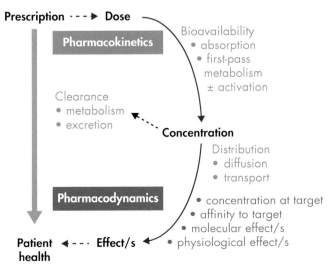

Figure 3-1 Pharmacotherapy, from prescription to health

PHARMACOKINETICS

Pharmacokinetics, what the body does to the drug, is mainly about the relationship between drug dose and drug concentration *at steady state* (C_{ss}). This can be understood by considering the active drug from administration to excretion and all points in between. Inactive drug metabolites are not biologically important and can usually be ignored.

To understand and apply pharmacokinetics, some math is necessary. For example, doubling a drug dose usually results in doubling the drug concentration.

CLINICAL PEARLS

The ABCD of pharmacokinetics:
A Administration—drug dose and route
B Bioavailability—percentage of the drug dose reaching the systemic circulation
C Clearance—removal of drug from the systemic circulation
D Distribution—transport of drug to the site(s) of action and distribution within the body

---

Administration

Administration of a drug involves dose and route.

- **Dose** is amount per time and is usually given by drug mass (e.g. mg) and frequency (e.g. daily). Duration of dose is important, as it takes time (4–5 lives) to reach steady-state concentration, and can take longer to achieve therapeutic effects.

- **Route** of administration is important to drug disposition. The most common route is oral, but every conceivable route is used to administer drugs, depending on the physico-chemical characteristics of the drug. The route of administration affects both the rate and the extent of the drug reaching the systemic circulation.

Bioavailability (*F*)

Bioavailability is the proportion of the drug dose that reaches the systemic circulation. For orally administered drugs, bioavailability is made up of absorption and first-pass hepatic extraction. For orally administered drugs, there are three steps in reaching the systemic circulation:

1 Ingested drug must remain intact in the gastrointestinal (GI) tract to reach the apical membrane of the enterocytes.

2 The drug must cross the gut wall into the portal circulation—drug absorption. The proportion absorbed is determined by drug transport (discussed later) across both the apical and the basolateral membranes of the enterocyte and by any drug metabolism within the enterocyte.

3 The drug must pass from the portal circulation through the liver to the systemic circulation. First-pass hepatic extraction is the proportion removed by the liver.

Bioavailability is expressed as a percentage. For a drug with high bioavailability (>70%), variability between individuals is not usually important. However, for a drug with low bioavailability, variability causes some patients to be exposed to more drug and others to less drug. For example, for a drug with 10% bioavailability, 90% of the drug is removed before reaching the systemic circulation. If this is halved (i.e. only 45% is removed), then 55%, or about five times as much, of the drug will reach the circulation. Conversely, if the proportion of drug removed is only marginally increased from 90%, all the drug may be removed and hence no drug will reach the target. Food–drug interactions (e.g. grapefruit juice and simvastatin, or food and oral bisphosphonates) can affect absorption, and drug–drug interactions can affect absorption and/or first-pass metabolism. These are particularly an issue for drugs with low bioavailability. A particular case in hospitalized patients is enteral feeding with the potential for interactions affecting drug absorption.

Clearance (CL)

At steady state, the rate the drug enters the circulation (bioavailability × dose amount × dose frequency) equals the rate the drug leaves the circulation (elimination). Elimination is dependent on both drug concentration and the capacity of the body to remove the drug, which can vary greatly. The capacity of the body to remove the drug from the circulation is drug clearance, or more accurately **apparent drug clearance**.

Clearance (L/h) is defined experimentally as dose amount (mg) divided by area under the concentration–time curve (AUC) (h.mg/L). Clinically this corresponds to dose (mg/h) divided by average concentration (mg/L). If a patient has reduced clearance of a drug, the maintenance dose should usually be reduced proportionally, e.g. half the normal clearance = half the usual dose. Likewise, if a patient has high clearance of a drug, the maintenance dose should usually be increased proportionally, e.g. twice the normal clearance = twice the usual dose.

$$\text{clearance} = \frac{\text{dose} \times \text{bioavailability}}{\text{average steady-state concentration}}$$

$$\text{volume/time} = \frac{\text{amount/time} \times \text{percent}}{\text{amount/volume}} \qquad \textit{Equation 1}$$

Equation 1 illustrates that clearance and bioavailability determine steady-state drug concentration for any given dose. Hence changes in clearance and bioavailability need to be considered when choosing a maintenance drug dose.

Drugs are cleared from the body in two ways:

1 by metabolism to inactive metabolites

2 by excretion of active drug.

The most important method of clearing active drug is by metabolism, and most drug metabolism occurs in the liver. Excretion of active drug is most commonly in urine but may also be in feces, in breath or in other body fluids.

Drug metabolism

Drug metabolism usually involves converting a biologically active molecule to one or more biologically inactive molecule(s). Some drugs have an active metabolite, and occasionally drugs have several active metabolites. All active drug moieties are eventually cleared by metabolism or excretion. In most cases there is one drug moiety responsible for most of the activity and others can largely be disregarded.

Drug metabolism is mediated by enzymes that evolved in the biological 'arms race' between animals and plants. These enzymes serve as the defense against toxic xenobiotics ingested when animals eat plants, and their importance to drug treatment is that they inactivate drugs ingested by patients.

The cytochrome P450 enzymes (CYPs) catalyze oxidation and reduction reactions (Figure 3-2). Other enzymes catalyze conjugation reactions such as glucuronidation by the uridine diphosphate (UDP)-glucuronosyltransferases (UGTs). Oxidation/reduction and conjugation are the two major methods of drug metabolism. Proteases are responsible for protein catabolism, and most 'biologicals' (e.g. monoclonal antibodies) are eliminated by a combination of protein catabolism and target binding, which is followed by catabolism of the complex.

Pro-drugs

Some drugs are administered as inactive pro-drugs and are metabolized to the active form, for example aspirin, the angiotensin-converting enzyme (ACE) inhibitors, and azathioprine. It is the pharmacokinetics of the active drug moiety, whether this be the parent drug or a metabolite, that is clinically important.

Drug excretion

Some active drug moieties are excreted from the body unchanged, not metabolized. Renal excretion is the most important route and is a combination of two processes:

1 glomerular filtration
2 renal tubular transport.

The liver also excretes drugs in the bile via bile transporters. After biliary excretion, some of these drugs are resorbed from the gut (enterohepatic recirculation), although eventually they are either excreted in the feces or metabolized.

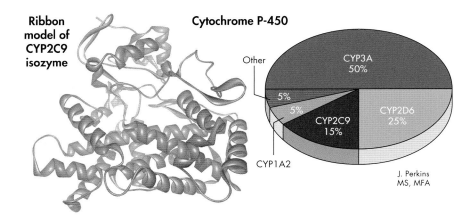

CYP	Substrate
1A2	Acetaminophen, antipyrine, caffeine, clomipramine, olanzapine, ondansetron, phenacetin, rilozole, ropinirole, tamoxifen, theophyline, warfarin
2A6	Coumarin
2B6	Artemisinin, buprorion, cyclophosphamide, S-mephobarbital, S-mephenytoin, (**N**-demethylation to nirvanol), propofol, selegiline, sertraline
2C8	Pioglitazone
2C9	Carvedilol, celecoxib, fluvastatin, glimepiride, hexobarbital, ibuprofen, losartan, mefenamic, meloxicam, montelukast, nateglinide, phenytoin, tolbutamide, trimethadone, sulfaphenazole, warfarin, ticrynafen, zafirlukast
2C19	Citalopram, diazepam, escitalopram, esomeprazole (**S**-isomer of omeprazole), irbesartan, S-mephenytoin, naproxen, nirvanol, omeprazole, pantoprazole, proguanil, propranolol
2D6	Almotriptan, bufuralol, bupranolol, carvedilol, clomipramine, clozapine, codeine, debrisoquin, dextromethorphan, dolasetron, fluoxetine (**S**-norfluoxetine), formoterol, galantamine, guanoxan, haloperidol, hydrocodone, 4-methoxy-amphetamine, metoprolol, mexiletine, olanzapine, oxycodone, paroxetine, phenformin, phenothiazines, propoxyphene, risperidone, selegiline, (deprenyl), sparteine, thioridazine, timolol, tolterodine, tramadol, tricyclic antidepressants, type 1C antirhythmics (e.g. encainide, flecainide, propafenone), venlafaxine
2E1	Acetaminophen, chlorzoxazone, enflurane, halothane, ethanol (minor pathway)
3A4	Acetaminophen, alfentanil, almotriptan, amiodarone, astemizole, beclomethasone, bexarotene, budesonide, **S**-bupivacaine, carbamazepine, citalopram, cocaine, cortisol, cyclosporine, dapsone, delavirdine, diazepam, dihydroergotamine, dihydropyridines, dilitiazem, escitalopram, ethinyl estradiol, fentanyl, finasteride, fluticasone, galantamine, gestodene, imatinib, indinavir, itraconazole, letrozole, lidocaine, loratidine, losartan, lovastatin, macrolides, methadone, miconazole, midazolam, mifepristone (RU-486), montelukast, oxybutynin, paclitaxel, pimecrolimus, pimozide, pioglitazone, progesterone, quinidine, rabeprazole, rapamycin, repaglinide, ritonavir, saquinavir, spironolactone, sulfamethoxazole, sufentanil, tracrolimus, tamoxifen, terfenadine, testosterone, tetrahydrocannibinol, tiagabine, triazolam, troleandomycin, verapamil, vinca alkaloids, ziprasidone, zonisamide
27	Doxercalciferol (activated)
No/ minimal involvement	Abacavir, acyclovir, alendronate, amiloride, benazepril, cabergoline, digoxin, disoproxil, hydrochlorothiazide, linezolid, lisinopril, olmesartan, oxaliplatin, metformin, moxifloxacin, raloxifene, ribavirin, risedronate, telmisartan, tenofovir, tiludronic acid, valacyclovir, valsartan, zoledronic acid

Figure 3-2 Cytochrome P450 drug-metabolizing enzymes. The proportion of drugs metabolized by each CYP isozyme is shown. Known polymorphisms in these enzymes require a drug dosage adjustment. If two drugs are metabolized by the same CYP enzyme, the normal routes or rates of metabolism can be affected and plasma drug concentrations may be altered

From Raffa RB, Rawls SM and Beyzarov EP. Netter's Illustrated pharmacology, updated ed. Philadelphia: Elsevier, 2014.

There are also other routes of excretion, for example volatile anesthetics excreted via the lungs.

Variation in drug clearance

Drug clearance varies considerably between patients. Most clinicians are aware that renal drug clearance is proportional to glomerular filtration rate (GFR) and that drug metabolism can be increased or decreased by other drugs (see section on drug interactions below). However, there is also large variability in the clearance of metabolized drugs and hence their concentrations. This becomes apparent when drug concentration or drug effect is monitored. One example is tacrolimus in renal transplant patients, where inter-individual variability in metabolism by CYP3A means that about a 10-fold range in dose is required to achieve the same drug concentration in different patients. Another example is warfarin and the wide range of doses used to achieve a target INR (international normalized ratio). While variability between individuals is obvious in these cases, variability in clearance is present for all drugs and is clinically most important for the outliers, those patients with very low or very high clearance.

Distribution

When drugs reach the systemic circulation, they are not evenly distributed about the body. Hydrophilic drugs are usually found predominantly in extracellular fluid, and lipophilic drugs predominantly in cells. Most drugs are present at different concentrations at different sites within the body. The apparent volume of distribution (V_d) of a drug is the volume the drug would occupy given the amount of drug in the body (A_B) and the steady-state concentration. For example, a drug with a V_d of 0.2 L/kg is likely to be contained within the extracellular fluid, whereas a drug with a V_d of 10 L/kg is likely to be at higher concentrations in cells than in plasma.

Importantly, volume of distribution allows estimation of a **loading dose**—the amount of drug needed to quickly reach a target concentration.

volume of distribution
= drug amount in the body × concentration   *Equation 2*

volume = amount × amount/volume

CLINICAL PEARLS

- A loading dose is useful when rapid onset of drug effect is desirable, e.g. acute pain, some infections.
- In treating a chronic illness, start with a low dose and titrate to effect—*start low, go slow.*

Distribution is about drug concentration at the site of action. However, this can be hard to measure, and the relationship between plasma drug concentration and concentration at the site of action is not captured by a single metric.

For example, metformin has a short half-life in the circulation and is thus sometimes dosed three times daily. However, the concentration in the hepatocyte mitochondria changes slowly, allowing dosing twice daily or even daily. Another, more extreme, example is the bisphosphonates

that have half-lives of a few hours but remain in bone for months or even years.

Half-life ($t_{1/2}$)

The half-life is the time taken for the drug concentration to fall by a half. Experimentally it is calculated from the slope (k) of the elimination phase of the log (ln) concentration–time curve. Drug half-life is important to dose interval. The ideal dose interval is once daily, but drugs with short half-lives usually need to be dosed more frequently, for example most antibiotics.

$$\text{half-life} = \frac{\ln 2 \times \text{volume of distribution}}{\text{clearance}} \quad \textit{Equation 3}$$

The relationships between the major pharmacokinetic parameters are shown in Begg's pharmacokinetic triangle (Figure 3-3).

CLINICAL PEARL

At steady state, amount in = amount out, i.e. drug dose = drug elimination.

The above discussion applies to first-order pharmacokinetics, which applies to most drugs most of the time. For drugs with first-order pharmacokinetics, doubling the dose doubles the concentration.

Pharmacokinetics are illustrated graphically by concentration–time curves (Figure 3–4, overleaf).

Zero-order pharmacokinetics occurs when there is constant elimination (rather than constant clearance). Ethanol is an example, familiar to many, of a drug that exceeds (saturates) the body's capacity for elimination at 'therapeutic doses'; phenytoin is another example. In drug overdose, elimination capacity is often exceeded and first-order principles, such as half-life, do not apply.

Drug transport

Drug transporters move drugs across cell membranes. Understanding drug transport helps explain drug distribution

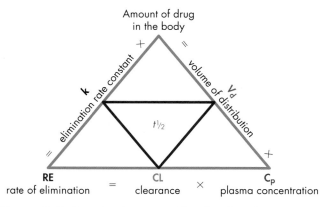

Figure 3-3 Begg's pharmacokinetic triangle. The sides of the triangle show how the major pharmacokinetic variables are related

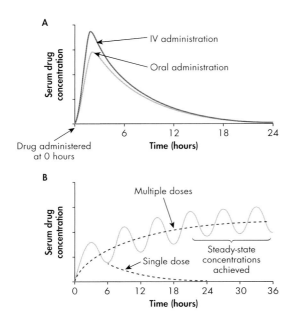

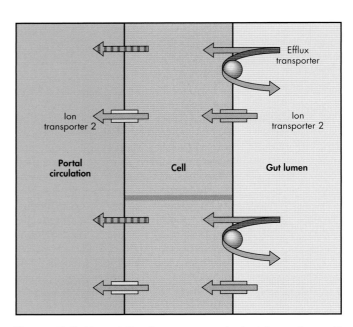

Figure 3-4 Drug concentration–time curves for (**A**) administration of the same drug by oral and IV routes; and (**B**) multiple doses of an oral drug administered every 6 hours and with first-order elimination. As the drug accumulates in the body, excretion eventually balances absorption and this results in steady-state concentrations being achieved

Figure 3-5 Lipophilic drugs are excluded from the cell by efflux transporters; some are metabolized in the cell. These systems protect us from environmental xenobiotics (mostly plant toxins). Polar drugs require transporters to enter and leave cells. These systems provide us with access to micronutrients (e.g. essential amino acids) and the ability to move endogenous molecules in and out of cells.

and hence drug concentration at the site of action. Drug transport is also important to absorption and excretion.

Functionally, there are three main groups of drug transporters:

1. Efflux transporters take drugs that have diffused across cell membranes into cells out of cells.
2. Anion and cation transporters move polar drugs across cell membranes bi-directionally.
3. Vesicular transporters move large drug molecules across cell membranes by endocytosis and exocytosis.

Transporters that allow drugs to cross cell membranes (groups 2 and 3) can be grouped as facilitative transporters. Like drug-metabolizing enzymes, drug transporters are not only there to transport drugs but have endogenous substrates. Figure 3-5 illustrates the role of drug transporters in the gastrointestinal epithelium.

CLINICAL PEARL

At steady-state conditions, the net effect of drug transport is to maintain a concentration gradient across one or more cell membrane(s). For example, efflux transporters result in low cerebrospinal fluid concentrations of many drugs. Transporters are particularly important to drugs that act on intracellular targets.

There are many drug transporters, each expressed to different extents in different tissues. Similarly, drugs are often substrates of multiple transporters. Hence, for any particular drug different transporters are important in different tissues. Our current understanding of the role of transporters in pharmacokinetics is not as well developed as our understanding of drug-metabolizing enzymes. The clinical questions related to drug transport are: What is the likely drug concentration at the site of action? What is the bioavailability and clearance? Both of these can be affected by drug transport.

Other pharmacokinetics

Protein binding is only important in the interpretation of drug concentrations. At steady state, the free drug concentration in the circulation is in equilibrium with concentrations in tissues; but free concentration is seldom measured directly. The measured plasma concentration of a drug is usually the total plasma concentration, i.e. free drug concentration + concentration of drug bound to plasma proteins. Hence, changes in protein binding or the concentration of plasma proteins can affect interpretation of the drug concentration.

The physico-chemical properties and structural characteristics of drugs are important to drug disposition and metabolism. One example is acidity/basicity, usually described by the pK_a of the drug. One clinical application of this is alkalinization of urine to increase the renal excretion of weak acids in some drug overdoses.

Altered pharmacokinetics

Drug pharmacokinetics vary substantially between individuals and are further altered in disease.

In clinical practice the dosing of most drugs is crude, e.g. going from 1 tablet a day to 2. To make most treatment decisions, relatively crude estimates of drug pharmacokinetics in the patient are sufficient. However, for a small number of drugs, relatively minor changes in clearance can be important (drugs with a narrow therapeutic index); these drugs should be monitored.

CLINICAL PEARL

Drugs with a narrow therapeutic index should be monitored using biomarkers of drug effect or drug concentrations.

Renal impairment

In dosing renally cleared drugs, there are good methods for estimating GFR and hence renal drug clearance. The relationship between GFR and drug dose is shown in Figure 3-6. Renal drug clearance is traditionally estimated using the Cockcroft and Gault equation, and most drug prescribing information is based on this equation. However, estimated GFR (eGFR) determined using other equations (e.g. CKD-epi) is routinely provided by most laboratories and may suffice as a guide, particularly if the patient is of average body size and composition.

Caution: laboratory estimates of GFR are standardized to a particular patient size (1.73 m²) and hence need to be corrected for patient size. An uncorrected eGFR will underestimate renal drug clearance in a larger patient and overestimate renal clearance in a smaller patient. For drugs with a narrow therapeutic index, estimates of GFR are not sufficient to guide dosing. Clinical monitoring, validated biomarkers of drug effect or drug concentrations should always pre-empt estimates of clearance.

CLINICAL PEARL

To adjust the dose of a drug in renal impairment, you need the glomerular filtration rate (GFR) of the patient and the fraction of the drug excreted unchanged (fe); see Table 3-1.

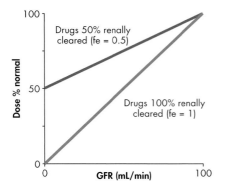

Figure 3-6 For a drug that is 100% renally cleared (fe = 1), clearance is proportional to GFR and the dose should be reduced proportionally to GFR. For a drug that is 50% renally cleared (fe = 0.5), clearance of the renally cleared component only is affected by GFR and the dose reduction is therefore smaller

Drug information often presents dosing in renal impairment in categories according to GFR. These arbitrary decision points can lead to arbitrary decisions. For example, when a decrease in drug dose is recommended at GFRs of 60 and 30 mL/min, is 31 mL/min different to 29 mL/min or the same as 57 mL/min? Some patients above the threshold may need a change in dose or a drug stopped, while other patients can still be treated rationally even after the threshold is crossed. A clinical decision should be based on clinical observations of effects (benefits and harms), available disease biomarkers and drug concentrations. These vary between diseases and drugs.

For a drug 100% renally cleared and a patient with a GFR half that of normal, a reasonable dose is half a normal dose. For a drug 50% renally cleared and patient with a GFR half that of normal, a reasonable dose is 75% of normal. Other factors such as patient health, drug response and tablet strengths are important to dose selection.

Some drugs are partially metabolized by proteases in the kidney, most notably insulin; metabolism by the kidney is not directly proportional to GFR.

Liver impairment

In dosing drugs that rely predominantly on metabolism for clearance, there is no equivalent to GFR to estimate changes in clearance. Hypoalbuminemia and international normalized ratio (INR) are late and imprecise markers of impaired metabolic capacity. Close attention to symptoms or signs of altered drug effect is needed when organ dysfunction is suspected.

Cardiac impairment

Cardiac impairment affects blood flow to the clearing organs and may further impair hepatic metabolism by 'liver congestion'. Right heart failure often causes clinically relevant reductions in absorption of drugs across the gut wall.

Metabolic impairment

Any change in physiology may affect the pharmacokinetics of a drug. For example, hypothyroidism decreases drug clearance and thyrotoxicosis increases drug clearance by altering cardiac output and cell metabolism. Acidosis or alkalosis can alter the bioavailability and clearance of acidic and basic drugs and, if severe, may impair hepatic function and thus decrease drug metabolism.

Patient size

Patient size is important, but in adults size is a minor contributor to variability in drug response, unless very big or very small. Both clearance and volume of distribution are proportional to body size. In most circumstances, lean body weight is the most valid descriptor of size.

In children, size differences also reflect physiological differences. In young children (neonates and infants), both maturation (age post-conception) and size need to be considered in selecting drug doses.

Obesity is a particular type of increased size and is increasingly common. With increasing obesity, fat mass increases a lot and lean mass a little. The main pharmacological

Table 3-1 Examples of renally cleared drugs grouped by therapeutic index

DRUG	fe
Narrow	
Aminoglycosides	1
Digoxin	0.7
Lithium	1
Dabigatran	0.9
Low-molecular-weight heparins	0.7
Intermediate	
Acyclovir and related antivirals	0.8
Allopurinol (active metabolite oxypurinol)	1
Atenolol	0.9
Clonidine	0.6
Gabapentin and pregabalin	0.9
Glycopeptides (e.g. vancomycin)	0.9
Levetiracetam	0.6
Memantine	0.7
Morphine-6-glucuronide	1
Paliperidone	0.6
Pramipexole	0.9
Topiramate	0.7
Wide	
ACEIs†	*
Baclofen	0.7
Carbapenems	1
Cephalosporins	*
Metformin	1
Penicillins	1
Sitagliptin	1
Varenicline	0.9

* Within-class variability—most are predominantly renally cleared.

† Most ACEIs are pro-drugs of a renally cleared active moiety (...prilat).

ACEIs, angiotensin-converting enzyme inhibitors; fe, fraction of dose excreted unchanged.

difference is increased volume of distribution of fat-soluble drugs. An important clinical difference is overdosing errors due to weight-based prescribing. Clearance is determined by lean body weight.

Drug clearance, along with most physiological parameters, can be compared across species ranging from ants to whales by weight to the power of 0.75 ($kg^{0.75}$).

PHARMACODYNAMICS

Pharmacodynamics, what the drug does to the body, is about the relationship between drug concentration and drug response. Broadly, pharmacodynamics can be considered at three levels.

1 **Health effects** for the patient are the ultimate measures of drug response. It is important to consider all drug effects, unwanted as well as wanted. These include global effects such as mortality or quality of life; disease-specific effects such as exercise tolerance or range of movement; and symptoms such as pain.

2 **Physiological effects** are often used clinically to monitor drug response and guide dosing, such as measuring blood pressure after antihypertensives have been commenced. Physiological effects can often be monitored by history and clinical examination or measured simply in the clinic. A change in physiological effect can be a useful marker of change in organ function in response to treatment.

3 **Molecular effects** are frequently studied in scientific experiments, as they are often specific to a particular drug and can be studied experimentally outside the body e.g. *in vitro*, in cell models or in gene expression arrays. Some molecular effects are also useful as biomarkers of drug response.

A drug response is caused by a drug molecule acting on a molecule or a group of molecules in the body. Any molecule in the body may be a drug **target**. A drug may either increase or decrease the molecular activity of the target(s).

Concentration–response relationships

A drug response may be anywhere from 0 to the maximum possible response (E_{max}). The E_{max} defines maximum efficacy. The greater the potential response, the greater the potential efficacy. The concentration of drug that has 50% of the maximum response is the EC_{50}. The EC_{50} defines drug potency—the lower the concentration required to achieve the response, the greater the potency. Note that the terms *potency* and *efficacy* are different concepts. A drug may have high potency (low EC_{50}) but low efficacy (E_{max}). Pharmacodynamics are illustrated graphically by concentration-response curves; see Figure 3-7.

CLINICAL PEARLS

- **Potency** is the drug concentration required to achieve a response.
- **Efficacy** is how much response there is to a drug.

All drugs have multiple effects, and hence multiple concentration–response curves can be plotted. This is particularly useful for comparing beneficial and harmful drug effects. This is shown in Figure 3-7B.

Therapeutic index

The therapeutic index of a drug is the ratio between the concentrations causing toxicity and efficacy. For a drug with

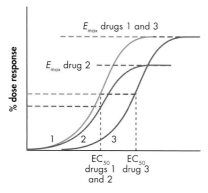

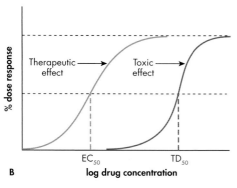

Figure 3-7 Sigmoidal concentration–response curves typical of many drugs. (**A**) Drugs 1 and 3 have the same maximum efficacy (E_{max}) but drug 1 has a higher potency (lower EC_{50}). Drug 2 has a similarly high potency (low EC_{50}) to drug 1 but a lower efficacy (E_{max}). (**B**) The therapeutic index is TD_{50}/EC_{50}, i.e. the ratio between the concentrations causing toxicity and efficacy. Note that toxic effect curves often have different slopes to therapeutic effect curves

Box 3-1

Examples of drug classes with a narrow therapeutic index

Antiarrhythmics

Anticoagulants

Anticonvulsants

Cytotoxics

Immunosuppressants

Some hormones, e.g. insulin

activity of intracellular signaling pathways, e.g. G-protein coupled receptors. In contrast, nuclear receptors increase or decrease gene expression.

An **agonist** acts on a receptor to increase the signal, whereas an **antagonist** decreases the signal. Strictly speaking, agonists and antagonists are drugs acting on a receptor, rather than on other drug targets. For example, beta-agonists and beta-blockers act on the beta-adrenergic receptors. Receptor signaling may also be modified by drugs changing the shape of the molecule rather than occupying the active site. This is called allosteric modulation.

CLINICAL PEARL

Drugs acting on nuclear receptors are more likely to have multiple effects than drugs acting on cell membrane receptors.

Enzymes catalyze reactions and are usually found inside cells. They are common drug targets and may be *induced* or *inhibited* (the latter is more common). Enzymes may catalyze reactions involved in signaling pathways directly or may produce or metabolize molecules important to cell function. For example, dihydrofolate reductase is inhibited by methotrexate in the treatment of some autoimmune diseases and some cancers.

Channels and transporters transport molecules across cell membranes. Blocking or increasing their function alters the concentration gradient of a molecule(s) across the cell membrane. For example, the gastric proton pump inhibited by proton pump inhibitors, or the potassium ATPase channel inhibited by sulfonylureas.

Signaling molecules may be directly targeted by drugs. For example, tumor necrosis factor alpha (TNF-alpha) is a cytokine targeted by several large molecule 'biological' drugs in the treatment of inflammatory diseases.

Other drug targets include structural molecules.

Some drug targets are difficult to classify, for example some inhaled anesthetics alter cell membrane function nonspecifically, with differing effects on a range of receptors, channels and transporters.

a wide therapeutic index, doses can be found that are likely to have the desired effect but are unlikely to have unwanted effects. Drugs with a narrow therapeutic index are loosely defined as drugs for which a halving or a doubling of the dose (or concentration) is likely to cause a significant change in effects. However, this definition is only a starting point and there are differences between patients as well as between drugs. For example, sulfonylureas have a wide therapeutic index in most circumstances, but in a frail elderly person a sulfonylurea may have a narrow therapeutic index due to the greater risk of hypoglycemia because of decreased counter-regulatory responses and decreased awareness of symptoms.

Drugs of narrow therapeutic index are hard to define but easy to recognize (usually). Examples of drug classes with narrow therapeutic indices are shown in Box 3-1.

Drug targets

Receptors of endogenous signaling molecules, such as neurotransmitters and hormones, are common drug targets. A receptor may be activated by an *agonist* or blocked by an *antagonist*. Cell membrane receptors increase or decrease the

Drug specificity

Specificity is how much more likely one response is than other responses. Specificity is often defined by relative affinity for different molecular targets. A highly specific drug will preferentially interact with one target molecule. However, no drug is completely specific and as concentration increases, other molecules will be affected.

Specificity differs from therapeutic index in that specificity generally refers to molecular response rather than the effect on the patient. Affecting multiple molecules is not necessarily bad, as the total effect may be beneficial. Conversely, an increase in one response may move from benefit to harm, for example anticoagulation.

Distribution and drug targets

To act on cytoplasmic enzymes or nuclear receptors, drugs have to get inside cells and their effect is therefore determined by *intracellular* concentration. In contrast, *extracellular* concentration is usually relevant for drugs acting on cell membrane receptors, channels and transporters, and signaling molecules. Cell membrane drug transport is thus particularly relevant to drugs targeting enzymes or nuclear receptors (see drug transport, below).

CLINICAL PEARLS

- Drug concentrations at intracellular targets are dependent on both circulating drug concentration and cell membrane transport.
- For drugs acting on extracellular targets, free plasma concentrations determine the concentration at the target.

Physiological effects

While the terms *agonist* and *antagonist* apply to drugs acting on receptors, the concept of stimulation or suppression is important and can be applied to physiological effects. Physiological effects are often primary or secondary outcomes of drug trials and are particularly useful in predicting the likely effects for individual patients. The physiological effects of the drug that are observed in the trials can be considered against the physiological state of the patient. For example, in treating diabetes, stimulating insulin production with a sulfonylurea is effective for type 2 diabetes but not for type 1 diabetes.

More about the patient

When choosing a drug therapy, the potential benefits and potential harms for a patient can be predicted to some extent from trial data. The probabilities of benefits and harms can be adjusted by considering the characteristics of this patient relative to the 'average patient'. Are they older or younger, male or female, fit or unfit? What are the states of their organs: heart, lungs, liver, kidneys, blood, bones, endothelium, gut, and (particularly) their brain?

THE INNOCENT BYSTANDER

While primarily treating one patient, the potential harm to others needs to be considered. The greatest risk of bystander drug exposure is to a fetus, with drug transfer to the fetus from the mother via the placenta. Other examples include drugs in breast milk, transfer via skin-to-skin contact, or radiation from a radiopharmaceutical. More indirect examples include a drug being administered to the wrong patient or the development of antibiotic-resistant organisms. Managing these risks is part of the quality use of medicines (part 2).

In evaluating the benefits and harms in a decision to treat a pregnant or breastfeeding mother, we need to consider: (1) the likely drug exposure of the fetus or infant and the potential consequent drug effects; (2) the effect of the mother's disease on the fetus or infant as well, especially if untreated (e.g. with epilepsy); and (3) any effect on the mother's ability to care for an infant.

In **pregnancy**, the rule of thumb is that fetal blood concentration equals maternal blood concentration. The second factor to consider is stage of fetal development, as the risks of drug exposure vary by trimester:

- 1st trimester—organogenesis
- 2nd trimester—maturation (especially neurological)
- 3rd trimester—maturation and the circulatory and respiratory changes that occur peripartum.

The third factor to consider is the risk of untreated disease to both fetus and mother. Consequently, pharmacotherapy in pregnancy is a specialized area with pregnancy risk classifications providing a useful starting point.

In **breastfeeding**, the rule of thumb is that infant drug exposure is usually much less than maternal drug exposure. To estimate likely infant drug exposure, there are three pharmacokinetic variables to consider.

1 The weight-adjusted maternal dose (WAMD), which provides a useful estimate of the infant's drug dose relative to that of the mother.

2 Oral bioavailability, given that many parenterally administered drugs have very low oral bioavailability with consequent negligible systemic exposure for the infant.

3 Drug clearance by the infant, which increases with maturation (post-conceptual age).

Consequently, if drug treatment is needed while breastfeeding, an option that poses minimal risk to the infant can often be found.

2. QUALITY USE OF MEDICINES

Quality use of medicines (QUM) is about using medicines safely, effectively and economically. There are multiple QUM tools deployed by communities in caring for groups of patients, and others deployed by healthcare professionals in the care of individual patients. Communities in healthcare can be grouped in several ways: by geography from the nation down to the local community; by disease types; and by sectors of healthcare.

QUM tools used by communities to support care across groups of patients include drug regulations, drug formularies, treatment guidelines and cost–effectiveness analyses. Those used by healthcare professionals for individual patients include drug profiles, prescriptions, drug interaction assessment tools, adverse reaction alerts and working in teams.

GETTING IT RIGHT

Prefacing any element of therapeutics with *right* can help to define QUM objectives and select QUM tools: right diagnosis, right drug, right route, right dose, right time, right patient. Figure 3-8 shows the **circle of care**: making the diagnosis; identifying treatment options; selecting treatment with the patient; and assessing the treatment response. Figure 3-9 shows the elements of the patient profile and the drug profile. Matching the patient profile with drug profiles is a QUM tool for individual patient care that can be used in any setting.

The circle of care

1 **The diagnosis.** Accurate characterization of patient problems for diagnosis of one or more disease(s) in a patient is necessary for scientific therapeutics. This allows application of the research literature to the individual case. Being based on diagnosis and pathophysiology is a strength of 'orthodox' medicine.

2 **Disease management**—identifying treatment options. In assessing the evidence for treatment(s), there are many decision-support tools to identify treatment options, such as evidence-based treatment guidelines. All good decision-support tools are traceable to the primary research information including relevant clinical trials.

3 **Patient management**—selecting the treatment with the patient. Sometimes this is more of an art than a science. It usually includes negotiation with the patient to match the treatment to the patient. Applying the principles outlined above supports rational treatment selection. Prescribing a drug or drugs is typically the final step in this process.

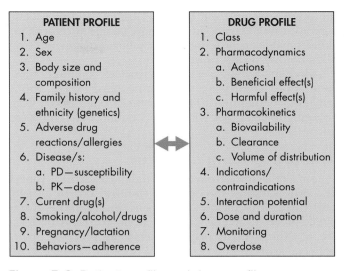

Figure 3-9 Patient profile and drug profile

4 **Assessing the treatment response.** Has the treatment addressed the presenting problems, and is the response consistent with the diagnosis? The response of each patient to treatment should be assessed in a planned manner. For most diseases and drug treatments, there are useful biomarkers to assess response to treatment. These range from changes in symptoms or signs to changes in biochemical or radiological test results. Many treatment guidelines include recommendations for monitoring and follow-up.

Drugs are the subject of this chapter, while diseases are the subjects of other chapters. QUM is about drugs and people (patients and prescribers), and about reducing errors.

Patient profile and drug profile(s)

The elements of the patient profile and the drug profile are shown in Figure 3-9. Matching the patient profile with for benefit and reduce the potential for harm. Simply selecting the 'best drug' on the basis of diagnosis is not sufficient.

Aligning the characteristics of the patient and the drug using headings allows assessment of the potential for benefit and harm to the individual. For example:

* Does the patient have any contraindications?
* Is the route appropriate?
* Are there potential drug–drug interactions?
* What is the likely adherence to the treatment plan?

PRESCRIBING

Prescribing is the communication of a written plan for drug treatment. Prescribing registered drugs is regulated in most countries. There are regulations governing who can prescribe, what can be prescribed, and who can dispense a registered drug. Prescribing, dispensing and administration of drugs are usually done by different people. Prescribers are mostly doctors, dispensers mostly pharmacists, and drugs

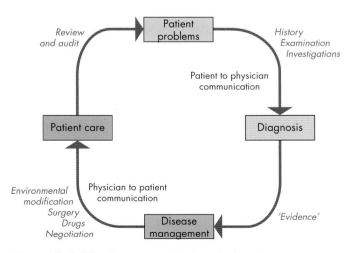

Figure 3-8 The four steps in the circle of care. Obtaining information from a patient, the history, is critical to diagnosis. Imparting information to a patient is critical to management, particularly in chronic care

are mostly administered by nurses (acute care) or patients (chronic care). Having three or more people, each bringing different skills to drug treatment, reduces treatment errors and improves quality of care.

Most prescribing errors are errors of communication, resulting in wrong drug, wrong dose, wrong route, wrong patient or wrong time. There are many other factors contributing to error, but with clear communication most can be avoided.

The prescribing checklist

Pharmacotherapy is complicated, and there are many patient and drug variables to consider before prescribing (or not prescribing) a medicine for a patient. In healthcare, therapeutic processes are complex and prone to error. Checklists are increasingly used to support therapeutic processes in surgery and there is good behavioral research to suggest that they can support good processes in other aspects of healthcare. Box 3-2 provides one example of a checklist to support the prescribing process.

DEPRESCRIBING

When to start drug treatments is covered in detail in almost every major guideline. However, when to *stop* drugs is not and, partly because of this, polypharmacy accumulates with multi-morbidity. Stopping drugs is hard and it is easy to justify the *status quo*, but a decision to continue is just as much a decision as a decision to stop.

We recommend that every drug treatment be formally reviewed at least annually. For every drug, ask yourself:

1 What are the potential benefits and potential harms for this person?
2 Are the potential benefits greater than the potential harms? If the answer is no, or uncertain, consider stopping the drug. One approach is the traffic light system for review shown in Figure 3-10.

Deprescribing requires all the same steps as prescribing. Sudden cessation can be dangerous and the results of deprescribing should be monitored and reviewed in the same way as the results of prescribing.

ADVERSE DRUG REACTIONS

An adverse drug reaction (ADR) is a harmful effect of a drug, or more precisely 'any response to a drug which is noxious, unintended, and which occurs at doses used in man for prophylaxis, diagnosis and therapy'. An adverse drug event (ADE) has a broader definition, including potential harm as well as actual harm. Drug safety has similarities to road safety: by reducing errors, we can reduce harm. For example, while wrong dose errors don't usually cause measurable harm, reducing dosing errors is likely to increase benefit and reduce harm across the community.

All drugs can cause adverse reactions, and some patients are at greater risk of these than others. A patient's ADR history and other characteristics, such as gender, age, ethnicity and physiological state, help to quantify the likely risk of a

---

Box 3-2

The prescribing checklist

Before prescribing, consider:

1 Goal/s of treatment and definitions of success and failure:
    a Symptom relief
    b Disease modification
2 Drug selection:
    a Drug for the problem?
    b Drug for this patient:
        » past adverse drug reactions?
        » prognosis?
        » frailty and vulnerabilities?
3 Potential effects: is net benefit likely for this patient?
    a Potential benefits for this patient?
    b Potential harms to this patient?
4 Dose regimen:
    a Loading dose or 'start low, go slow'?
    b Maintenance dose for this patient?
5 Potential drug interactions:
    a Pharmacodynamic?
    b Pharmacokinetic?

After prescribing, agree with the patient:

6 Monitoring for efficacy and toxicity—what, when, how and who?
    a By patient
    b By clinician
7 Risk management:
    a Potential harms
    b Treatment failures
    c Action if treatment failure or harm occurs
8 Patient and carer/s understanding:
    a Diagnosis/problem
    b Management
9 Review—when, where and who?

Finally, consider:

10 Problems not treated:
    a Are there untreated problems?
    b Should additional/alternative treatments be offered?

I used the prescribing checklist in prescribing for this patient ☐

---

given adverse reaction. Considering the potential for ADRs is part of prescribing assessment, and making plans with the patient (and any carers) to identify and manage potential ADRs is standard practice; for example, warning someone of the potential gastrointestinal effects of a drug and what to do if they occur.

CLINICAL PEARL

Anything that can do good can also do harm, and all drugs have harmful effects. Monitor treatment by monitoring patients for both benefits and harms to evaluate the net clinical effect.

ADRs have driven much of the current regulatory environment. The USA's 1938 Food, Drug and Cosmetic

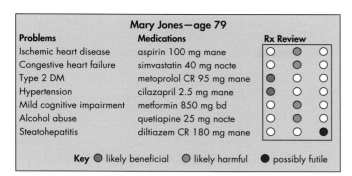

Mary Jones—age 79		
Problems	**Medications**	**Rx Review**
Ischemic heart disease	aspirin 100 mg mane	○ ◐ ○
Congestive heart failure	simvastatin 40 mg nocte	○ ◐ ○
Type 2 DM	metoprolol CR 95 mg mane	◐ ○ ○
Hypertension	cilazapril 2.5 mg mane	◐ ○ ○
Mild cognitive impairment	metformin 850 mg bd	○ ◐ ○
Alcohol abuse	quetiapine 25 mg nocte	○ ◐ ○
Steatohepatitis	diltiazem CR 180 mg mane	○ ○ ●

Key ◐ likely beneficial ◐ likely harmful ● possibly futile

Figure 3-10 Mary Jones is a hypothetical patient. Her current problems and current medications are shown side by side in one view. For each medication you, the prescriber, evaluate the likely net benefit for Mary. The selections in this case are not the point, and we have insufficient information to critique these. Each drug that is assessed as 'likely harmful' should be deprescribed, and deprescribing those assessed as 'possibly futile' should be discussed. We suggest that aiming to deprescribe half of the 'possibly futile' drugs is a good starting point

Act was a response to the deaths of many children from ingesting ethylene glycol used as the solvent for the elixir form of the antibiotic sulfanilamide. The 1962 Kefauver Harris amendment was a response to birth defects from thalidomide.

- A **type A (augmented) reaction** is one that is predictable from the pharmacological effect of the drug and may respond to dose adjustment.

- A **type B (bizarre) reaction** is usually due to a host reaction to a drug, e.g. anaphylaxis.

This simple classification is long-established, and is useful when prescribing drugs but is not sufficient to diagnose and manage ADRs.

Assessing an event in a patient as a potential ADR involves two steps. First, describing the event in relation to the drug and the patient. An ADR can be described using the DoTS and EIDOS method of Aronson and Ferner (Box 3-3). Second, as with any diagnosis, causality should be assessed. The Naranjo score (Box 3-4, overleaf) is one method of assessing causality. While assessment of ADRs is often neglected, clinical assessment using these tools is cheap and easy compared with radiological imaging and biochemical testing. All potential ADRs should be clearly documented in the patient's clinical record and reported to the relevant pharmacovigilance body.

Drug safety is not reliably assessed using the randomized controlled trials required for drug registration. To investigate drug safety, observational studies (e.g. case-control studies) usually provide more robust data. Pharmacovigilance is the science relating to the detection, assessment, understanding and prevention of adverse drug effects, and most countries have formal pharmacovigilance programs. *Spontaneous reporting of ADRs by prescribers is an essential component of pharmacovigilance.*

Box 3-3

Describing ADRs using DoTS[1] and EIDOS[2]

DoTS

Do Dose-relatedness—usual, very high or very low?

T Time-relatedness—immediately, or after hours, days, weeks or longer?

All drug effects are dose- and time-related. At what dose and after what duration did the reaction occur?

S Susceptibility—describe the patient. For example, disease states or family history of autoimmunity

EIDOS

E Extrinsic chemical species—what is the drug or related molecule responsible for the effect?

I Intrinsic chemical species—what is/are the molecule(s) that the drug affects?

D Distribution—where are those molecules in the body?

O Outcome—what is the pathophysiological effect?

S Sequelae—what are the consequences for the patient? The adverse effect

1. Aronson JK and Ferner RE. Joining the DoTS: new approach to classifying adverse drug reactions. BMJ 2003;327(7425):1222–5.

2. Ferner RE and Aronson JK. EIDOS: a mechanistic classification of adverse drug effects. Drug Saf 2010;33(1):15–23.

DRUG INTERACTIONS

A drug interaction occurs when a patient's response to a drug is modified by something else. The interaction may be due to other drugs, food or other substances, environmental factors, or disease. Drug–drug interactions (DDIs) are interactions between drugs. DDIs can either increase drug effect, potentially causing toxicity; or decrease drug effect, potentially leading to therapeutic failure. Elderly patients are especially vulnerable, with a strong relationship between increasing age, the number of drugs prescribed, and the frequency of potential DDIs.

Types of drug interaction

1 Behavioral: altered compliance
2 Pharmaceutical: outside the body
3 Pharmacokinetic: altered concentration:
　a bioavailability: absorption or first-pass metabolism
　b clearance: metabolism or excretion of active drug
　c distribution: cell membrane transport to the site of action
4 Pharmacodynamic; additive or opposing effect:
　a mechanism: molecular signal (e.g. receptor)
　b mode: physiological effect

One of the most common causes of significant DDIs is induction or inhibition of drug metabolism. In these interactions, there is a *perpetrator* (the drug causing the change in

---

Box 3-4

The Naranjo score for assessing causality of adverse drug reactions (ADRs)

1 Are there previous conclusive reports on this reaction?
Yes (+1); No (0); Do not know or not done (0)

2 Did the adverse event appear after the suspected drug was given?
Yes (+2); No (−1); Do not know or not done (0)

3 Did the adverse reaction improve when the drug was discontinued or a specific antagonist was given?
Yes (+1); No (0); Do not know or not done (0)

4 Did the adverse reaction appear when the drug was re-administered?
Yes (+2); No (−2); Do not know or not done (0)

5 Are there alternative causes that could have caused the reaction?
Yes (−1); No (+2); Do not know or not done (0)

6 Did the reaction reappear when a placebo was given?
Yes (−1); No (+1); Do not know or not done (0)

7 Was the drug detected in any body fluid in toxic concentrations?
Yes (+1); No (0); Do not know or not done (0)

8 Was the reaction more severe when the dose was increased, or less severe when the dose was decreased?
Yes (+1); No (0); Do not know or not done (0)

9 Did the patient have a similar reaction to the same or similar drugs in any previous exposure?
Yes (+1); No (0); Do not know or not done (0)

10 Was the adverse event confirmed by any objective evidence?
Yes (+1); No (0); Do not know or not done (0)

Score
- >9 = definite ADR
- 5−8 = probable ADR
- 1−4 = possible ADR
- 0 = doubtful ADR

Naranjo CA, Busto U, Sellers EM, et al. A method for estimating the probability of adverse drug reactions. Clinical Pharmacology and Therapeutics 1981;30(2):239–45.

---

metabolism) and an *object* (the drug whose concentration is changed). There are a relatively small number of perpetrator drugs that can cause large changes in the concentrations of other drugs. Of the object drugs, those with a narrow therapeutic index are particularly vulnerable; as are pro-drugs, given that pro-drugs are dependent on a single metabolic pathway for activation.

Patient harm from drug interactions can be reduced by:

- using a personal formulary—using few drugs and knowing them well
- recognizing drugs that are major perpetrators of interactions
- recognizing drugs with a narrow therapeutic index as vulnerable to interactions
- applying clinical pharmacology principles.

THERAPEUTIC DRUG MONITORING (TDM)

Therapeutic drug monitoring is the use of measured drug concentrations to inform drug treatment. TDM can be used in diagnosis:

1 In therapeutic failure there are three main differential diagnoses: low adherence, under-dosing and insufficient effect. TDM is a good discriminator of these three possible diagnoses.

2 In suspected drug toxicity or drug overdose, TDM can support or refute that symptoms are due to a drug or that a drug overdose has been taken.

3 When a patient is well, a drug may continue to be prescribed but not taken. TDM can identify that continued prescribing is unnecessary.

The other use of TDM is as a therapeutic tool to adjust a drug dose prospectively. Targeting a drug concentration can reduce potential harm and increase potential benefit by reducing pharmacokinetic variability.

CLINICAL PEARL

A target concentration is more precise than a target dose.

TDM is less useful if there is an accurate measure of drug effect(s), such as blood glucose and HbA_{1c} in the treatment of diabetes. However, there are relatively few drugs for which we have accurate measures of drug effect, and TDM is therefore a very cheap and an under-utilized tool.

Measuring drug concentrations is generally cheap and technically straightforward. To interpret a TDM result, other information is needed in addition to the drug concentration. This includes:

- drug dose (amount and frequency)
- duration of the current dose (to assess steady state)
- time after the last dose (concentration changes with time).

Knowing whether your patient has a drug concentration similar to, higher than, or lower than other patients treated with the same drug is valuable.

The greatest use of TDM is in transplant medicine, and to a lesser extent in neurology (epilepsy), infectious diseases, and psychiatry. Given the difficulties of adherence and inter-patient pharmacokinetic variability, TDM is one of the most under-used tools in 21st century medicine.

DRUG REGULATION

Drug regulation is a fundamental component of health systems aiming toward the societal goals of achieving safe, effective and economic use of drugs. Drug regulation has three main components in evaluating and regulating:

1 safety and efficacy—considered by drug registration bodies
2 cost-effective use of drugs—considered by funding, purchasing or advisory bodies
3 drug research—considered by registration bodies, ethics committees and public research funding bodies.

Drug registration bodies such as the Food and Drug Administration (FDA; USA), European Medicines Evaluation Agency (EMEA; Europe), Pharmaceutical and Medical Devices Agency (PMDA; Japan) and the Therapeutic Goods Administration (TGA; Australia) manage safety and efficacy in multiple ways. For example:

- regulating manufacture and distribution—is the right substance in the right place at the right time?
- evaluating new drugs by comprehensive review of their safety and efficacy for the treatment of particular diseases in particular patients
- evaluating the bioequivalence or biosimilarity of drugs
- co-ordinating pharmacovigilance.

Bodies that fund, or advise on funding, drugs operate at several levels. Some operate nationally, such as the United Kingdom's National Institute for Health and Care Excellence (NICE) or Australia's Pharmaceutical Benefits Advisory Committee (PBAC). Others consider spending for particular parts of the community, such as insurers for their policy-holders, or hospitals for their patients.

Pharmacoeconomics is the science of assessing costs and benefits to inform decisions about resource use and expenditure on drugs. To prioritize health spending, it is necessary to compare the costs, potential benefits and potential harms of treatment options. Benefits and harms may be compared subjectively; but for comparison across drugs, diseases and patients, objective or quasi-objective measures are needed.

One of the most widely used is the quality-adjusted life-year (QALY). While particular QALYs might be contentious, a strength is their transparency. This allows evaluation of uncertainty, open discussion and helps with the alignment of spending with societal values.

In making funding decisions about new drug treatments, a commonly used metric is the incremental cost–effectiveness ratio (ICER). The ICER is the difference in cost divided by the difference in net effectiveness (benefits minus harms) between the new drug treatment and existing care. While most clinicians do not undertake such analyses formally, these are implicit in every treatment decision. Cost minimization is more easily understood; when treatments do not significantly differ, costs can be compared. For example, a new generic drug that has demonstrated bioequivalence would be evaluated primarily on its relative costs.

Pharmacoepidemiology is the study of the use and effects of drugs on groups of people. The language of pharmacoepidemiology is statistics and to translate the information from clinical trials and other research, it is necessary to understand statistics!

DRUG RESEARCH

Medicine is research-based. A few words that mean a lot! Science requires the challenge and testing of ideas, whereas belief requires acceptance of ideas. The scientific consensus on the treatment of disease usually (although not always) reflects the existing evidence, and for a new treatment to be accepted it should be tested against the existing treatment. For an experiment to be valid, it should be *relevant* (what is measured matters) and *reliable* (the method is reproducible). Many research methods are used to gather the information needed to determine whether a drug is safe, effective and cost-effective.

In assessing drug efficacy, the final step is usually the randomized controlled trial (RCT). In a RCT the new treatment is compared with the existing treatment in a representative group of patients under conditions that minimize potential bias (e.g. randomization and blinding). Large RCTs are based on data from smaller clinical studies that establish estimates of dose–effect relationships (see the sections on pharmacokinetics and pharmacodynamics, above).

Before drugs are studied in people, multiple types of pre-clinical experiments are carried out. These include animal experiments (*in vivo*), laboratory experiments (*in vitro*) and computational experiments (*in silico*). Many different experiments are needed to describe a drug. For example, to predict the metabolism in humans of a new drug, multiple *in vitro* studies are conducted to develop data for use in *in silico* models before testing in selected *in vivo* models. Simultaneously, multiple other experiments are conducted to describe other variables, such as the potential effects of the drug on different tissues or its potential carcinogenicity.

Knowing which research methods can answer a particular question and understanding their limitations helps clinicians to interpret research. For example, RCTs are the 'gold standard' method for comparing the efficacy of two treatments. However, RCTs are poor at assessing drug safety, as they are usually not powered to quantify events occurring less commonly and vulnerable patients are often excluded.

Assessing drug safety has two components. First, toxicity can be studied in pre-clinical studies and in early human dose-finding studies. Second, adverse events—which may be rare or occur a long time after commencing treatment—should be systematically evaluated. Some observational study designs, such as case-control studies, are well suited to identifying and quantifying adverse events.

Cost–efficacy studies use efficacy and safety data from RCTs and observational studies, together with costs relevant to the study question(s), to inform policy-makers and clinicians. To assess cost–efficacy, it may be necessary to consider a number of efficacy and safety outcomes. Some outcomes can be quantified, e.g. time off work, resources required for independent living, but many are inherently subjective. To assign values (utilities) to different health states, it is necessary to ask people and there are a number of standardized methodologies used to assign utilities.

Drug research is conducted by people and organizations which, in addition to answering research questions, have other objectives such as career advancement or increasing shareholder value. Robust scientific research methods are required to be *transparent* (published) and *reproducible* so that others can repeat the experiment. In the long term, this provides protection from falsehood.

3. TOXICOLOGY

EPIDEMIOLOGY OF POISONING

Poisoned patients represent:
- 5–10% of an emergency department's workload
- 5–10% of medical admissions.

CLINICAL PEARLS
- In more developed countries, approximately 1% of people with poisoning are at serious risk and require intensive support.
- Distinguishing this 1% among all presentations with poisoning is difficult.

Mortality rates from poisoning remain relatively static in many countries. Severe poisoning in more developed countries occurs with a relatively small group of drugs which includes tricyclic antidepressants, anticonvulsants, opioids, amphetamines and cocaine.

Many patients co-ingest their drugs in overdose with alcohol, and the effects of both alcohol and the drug(s) in question are seen. Co-ingestions of multiple drugs may occur, and present a particular challenge. The frequently encountered substances in more developed countries are covered below.

SOURCES OF POISONS INFORMATION AND ADVICE

Toxicology information and advice is available from many sources, including poisoning information centers and websites for management (e.g. www.TOXINZ.com; WikiTox; www.atsdr.cdc.gov). Clinical reasoning and judgment can be augmented with expert advice, particularly for management in the more complex cases.

Most data are based on case series, given the extreme difficulty in conducting prospective trials. Even a single case report can be of value in managing unusual poisonings, as long as the limitations of lack of more data are understood.

CLINICAL ASSESSMENT OF POISONED PATIENTS

- Taking a history from a poisoned patient is critically important in determining:
  - » what substance?
  - » how much?
  - » the exact timing?
  - » by what route the person has been exposed, e.g. ingestion, inhalation?
- Corroborative evidence (empty packets of drugs, containers of chemicals, family/observer history) is

important. Finding out the source of the drug or toxin used in this instance of poisoning may help to prevent subsequent self-poisoning.

- Ask why the overdose was taken. A sympathetic non-judgmental approach works best with the majority of patients.
- Simple assessments of mental health are also required, with expert guidance from psychiatry. Serious suicidal intent is more likely with younger males, the elderly, where preplanning has taken place, where a note has been left and where the patient has taken trouble not to be discovered.
- The past medical history, especially asthma, jaundice, drug misuse (including alcohol), head injury, cardiovascular or renal problems, and past psychiatric illness and harm, are helpful to guide future clinical management. Ask about allergies.
- On clinical examination, first check airway, breathing, circulation (ABC) and institute necessary life-support measures.
- Complete a full physical examination, paying particular attention to the items listed in Table 3-2.

Investigations
- Check urea and electrolytes (UECs), arterial blood gases (ABGs) (where clinically indicated), and perform baseline electrocardiography (EKG) (where indicated). In the EKG, the heart rate, rhythm and any QTc or QRS prolongation should be particularly noted.
- Most patients have a metabolic acidosis, but if respiratory alkalosis is seen then salicylate (aspirin) poisoning should be suspected.
- Blood glucose and acetaminophen (paracetamol) concentrations must be checked in any patient who is unconscious. Rarely (e.g. in acetaminophen poisoning), drug blood concentrations are required to guide clinical management.

CLINICAL PEARLS
- If respiratory alkalosis is seen, then salicylate (aspirin) poisoning should be suspected.
- A blood sugar level estimation and acetaminophen (paracetamol) level must be carried out in any patient who is unconscious.

- Interpreting blood drug concentrations is complex—seek advice early. As a general rule of thumb, it takes 5 half-lives to fully eliminate a drug, and 4 half-lives to return to the therapeutic efficacy level. However, when toxic quantities of drugs have been ingested, the half-life of that drug may be extended due to saturation of enzymes involved in its metabolism, e.g. with carbamazepine.
- Currently, individual patient pharmacogenomic data are not routinely used in the management of overdose, but this may change in future. For example, mutations

Table 3-2 Physical examination of a suspected poisoned patient

BODY PART/SYSTEM	EXAMINE
Central nervous system	Check Glasgow Coma Scale (GCS), tone, power, reflexes and coordination (look for ataxic gait which can occur in toxic alcohol/anticonvulsant poisoning)
Eyes	Check pupil size (e.g. small with opioids or organophosphorus insecticide poisoning; large in tricyclic antidepressant overdose) Check presence (e.g. anticonvulsants) or absence of horizontal nystagmus
Cardiovascular system	Heart rate—elevated (e.g. tricyclic antidepressants, theophylline) or reduced (e.g. digoxin, beta-blockers) Blood pressure (e.g. reduced in tricyclic antidepressants, elevated after cocaine)
Respiratory system	Respiratory rate may be increased (salicylate poisoning) or decreased (e.g. opioid or benzodiazepine poisoning)
Skin	Look for needle marks, bruises, razor marks Check state of hydration Cyanosis (e.g. CNS-depressant drugs)
Gastrointestinal system	Check for bowel sounds before giving activated charcoal Feel for palpable liver to indicate possible liver disease and altered metabolism of drugs Right upper quadrant tenderness may indicate liver toxicity from acetaminophen (paracetamol) Epigastric tenderness may indicate gastrointestinal toxicity to NSAIDs
Weight	Helps determine whether toxicity is likely, given the dose ingested
Body temperature	Increased (e.g. ecstasy, SSRIs) or reduced (e.g. CNS depressants)

CNS, central nervous system; NSAIDs, non-steroidal anti-inflammatory drugs; SSRIs, selective serotonin reuptake inhibitors.

in CYP2CP and VKORC1 predict increased sensitivity to warfarin.

- Drugs of abuse are frequently detected in urine using detection strips that can identify opioids, cannabis, amphetamines and benzodiazepines, but may miss some of the newer drugs of abuse (see below). Rhabdomyolysis may be present with myoglobinuria in amphetamine or caffeine intoxication.
- A cranial computed tomography (CT) examination will be required to investigate coincident head injury or intracerebral events, if a patient presents unconscious or with focal neurological signs.

Risk assessment

All of the above clinical and investigation information (including the use of information and advice sources) is then integrated to formulate a 'risk assessment', i.e. a prediction of the most likely clinical course for the patient and any potential complications, and this informs the tailor-made management plan for that patient. This is the critical clinical judgment process in clinical toxicology.

PRINCIPLES OF MANAGEMENT OF POISONED PATIENTS

- Meticulous supportive care is critical to good outcome in poisoned patients. Doing simple things well, such as

administering intravenous fluids and giving oral activated charcoal (if the patient presents within an hour of the overdose), are sufficient to support most patients while they eliminate the drug(s). Only patients who have taken significant overdoses need further measures to prevent absorption or increase elimination of the drug.

- The American Academy of Clinical Toxicology recommends:
  - » oral activated charcoal 50 g (orally or by nasogastric tube) if ingestion of a substantial amount of drug has taken place within the past 1 hour
  - » multiple doses of activated charcoal to be given to adsorb the drug and enhance its elimination if drugs such as dapsone, theophylline, or carbamazepine have been ingested.
- Oral activated charcoal is *not* of value if:
  - » more than 1 hour has elapsed
  - » treating ingestion of acids, alkalis, alcohols or metals.

CLINICAL PEARL

Give oral activated charcoal 50 g (orally or by nasogastric tube) if ingestion of a substantial amount of drug has taken place within the past 1 hour.

- A nasogastric tube will be used very rarely to aspirate stomach contents if there has been recent ingestion of a toxic liquid. Gastric lavage with a large-bore tube to remove tablets is no longer recommended.

- Whole-bowel irrigation with polyethylene glycol can achieve bowel clearance of tablets if iron or slow-release preparations such as theophylline have been ingested in a potentially toxic dose. The dose is 500 mL/h in preschool children and 1 L/h if the person is above preschool age; its administration would usually be on the advice of a clinical toxicologist.
- Hemodialysis is occasionally used for serious poisoning with aspirin, lithium, methanol, valproate, carbamazepine, ethylene glycol or theophylline, again only on toxicology specialist advice.

CLINICAL PEARL

Hemodialysis is occasionally used for serious poisoning with aspirin, carbamazepine, ethylene glycol or theophylline.

- Intralipid 20% given as a bolus of 1.5 mL/kg followed by 0.25 mL/kg/min for 30–60 minutes has been used in the management of serious poisoning with lipophilic drugs such as bupivacaine. Its use is still considered experimental but is potentially life-saving.
- In young patients poisoned with cardiotoxic agents, maintain effective cardiopulmonary resuscitation (CPR) throughout because good neurological outcomes can be achieved even with an hour of CPR. In serious poisoning, management of seizures, coma and cardiovascular complications and intubation, where required, are also critical to good outcome.

- In contrast to the commonly held views, antidotes for poisoning are rare, with the exception of those listed in Table 3-3.
- Patients are usually discharged from medical care once the toxic effects of their overdose have worn off. This is a clinical judgment based on response to questions, lack of tachycardia or bradycardia, a demonstrated ability to walk safely, and no visual problems.
  - » Patients with sedative drug overdoses have residual cognitive deficits, even when the above parameters are normal, and should avoid driving for 3 days.

COMMON POISONS AND THEIR MANAGEMENT

Acetaminophen (paracetamol)

Acetaminophen (paracetamol) remains one of the most common drugs taken in overdose. Ingestion of more than 200 mg acetaminophen/kg bodyweight or 10 g (whichever is the less) in any one 24-hour period is associated with the risk of developing hepatotoxicity (and more rarely renal toxicity), unless the antidote **N-acetylcysteine** is given within 8–10 hours of the overdose being taken.

- If a patient presents more than 4 hours after an overdose, a plasma acetaminophen level should be requested regardless of the stated dose. If the plasma acetaminophen concentration is close to or above the treatment line on the acetaminophen nomogram currently in use (see Figure 3-11 for an example), then

Table 3-3 Poison antidotes

POISON	ANTIDOTE
Beta-blockers	IV glucagon, high-dose insulin euglycemic therapy
Calcium-channel blockers	10% calcium gluconate, 10% calcium chloride, glucagon, high-dose insulin euglycemic therapy
Cyanide	Oxygen, high-dose hydroxycobalamin
Digoxin	Digoxin-specific antibodies
Ethylene glycol/methanol	Ethanol, 4-methylpyrazole
Lead	DMSA, DMPS, disodium calcium edetate
Iron salts	Desferrioxamine/deferrioxamine
Opioids	Naloxone, naltrexone
Organophosphorus insecticides, nerve agents	Atropine, for nerve agents oximes (pralidoxime, obidoxime, H1-6): note that oximes are no longer recommended for routine use in organophosphorus insecticide poisoning
Acetaminophen (paracetamol)	N-acetylcysteine (preferred) or methionine
Thallium	Prussian blue

DMPS, 2,3-dimercapto-1-propanesulfonic acid; DMSA, dimercaptosuccinic acid; IV, intravenous.
Adapted from Jones AL, in JA Innes (ed), Davidson's Essentials of medicine. Edinburgh: Elsevier, 2009.

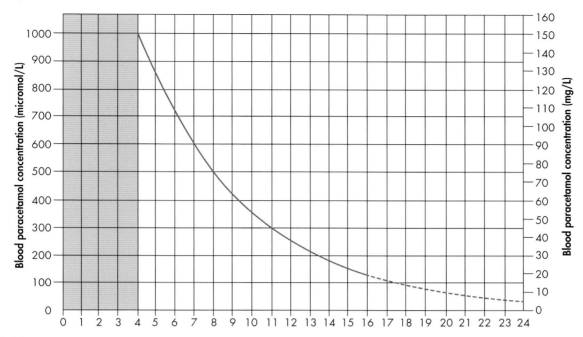

Figure 3-11 The Australian paracetamol (acetaminophen) treatment nomogram. Note that in some units the protocol for intravenous *N*-acetylcysteine has been altered, in particular to try to reduce the incidence of early anaphylactoid reactions—the approved protocol should be checked or a clinical toxicologist consulted if there is *any* doubt

Reproduced with permission from the Medical Journal of Australia. www.mja.com.au/journal/2008/188/5/guidelines-management-paracetamol-poisoning-australia-and-new-zealand-explanation

N-acetylcysteine should be administered intravenously (IV) over approximately 20 hours. If the concentration is below the line, this level is often rechecked at 4 hours to see if it subsequently crosses the line, indicating the need for *N*-acetylcysteine. The acetaminophen nomogram cannot be applied for repeat or staggered overdoses, or if the timing of ingestion cannot be determined with confidence. Alterations to this protocol may be required in cases with very high doses (> 30 g acetaminophen) or in cases involving ingestion of modified release acetaminophen.

- If the patient presents less than 4 hours after an overdose, then an acetaminophen level should be taken at 4 hours—if taken earlier than this, it cannot be interpreted.
- If the presentation is within 1 hour, give activated charcoal.
- If the timing of ingestion is unknown or the history is not clear, it is wise to err on the side of caution and treat with *N*-acetylcysteine according to the standard protocol (Table 3-4, overleaf).
- In approximately 1–2% of cases of administration of *N*-acetylcysteine an **anaphylactoid reaction** occurs within the first 2 hours of the infusion, characterized by skin flushing, rash, wheeze and, extremely rarely, by cardiac arrest. Management is supportive: administration of antihistamines and epinephrine (adrenaline) if needed, and stopping the infusion for at least 30 minutes; then the infusion can be restarted at the rate of 50 mg/kg/h, with monitoring.

- Recent evidence suggests that the shorter regimen (SNAP IV NAC 100 mg/kg over 2 hours followed by 200 mg/kg over 10 hours) has similar efficacy in regard to preventing liver injury with fewer ADRs compared to the 21-hour regimen. This is not yet under full recommendation despite successful trials in the UK and Australia.
- Tracking of repeat acetaminophen levels to ensure they don't cross the nomogram line and to ensure complete metabolism of acetaminophen has been recommended and has been adopted in some centers.

The most important risk factor for **liver damage** after acetaminophen ingestion is the extent of delay, beyond 8 hours, until treatment with *N*-acetylcysteine commences.

- Clinical or biochemical evidence of hepatic injury may not be apparent for up to 24 hours after an acute acetaminophen overdose. Developing an alanine aminotransferase (ALT) level >1000 IU/L within 12 hours of starting *N*-acetylcysteine is correlated with highest prothrombin time ratios (international normalized ratios) and poor prognosis.
- Hepatic failure, encephalopathy and death remain uncommon outcomes, although acetaminophen remains the most important single cause of acute liver failure in Western countries.
- Bernal's modification of the King's College London O'Grady criteria (pH <7.25 more than 24 hours after the overdose, prothrombin time in seconds, degree of acidosis and renal dysfunction) is used to determine the

Table 3-4 Standard protocol for administration of *N*-acetylcysteine in acetaminophen (paracetamol) overdose, according to the patient's weight

PATIENT'S LEAN BODYWEIGHT (KG)	INITIAL INFUSION BAG; mL VOLUME OF *N*-ACETYLCYSTEINE TO BE ADDED TO 200 mL OF 5% GLUCOSE: INFUSED OVER 15–60 MINUTES	SECOND INFUSION BAG; mL VOLUME OF *N*-ACETYLCYSTEINE TO BE ADDED TO 500 mL OF 5% GLUCOSE: INFUSED OVER 4 HOURS	THIRD INFUSION BAG; mL VOLUME OF *N*-ACETYLCYSTEINE TO BE ADDED TO 1000 ML OF 5% GLUCOSE: INFUSED OVER 16 HOURS
50	37.5	12.5	25
60	45.0	15.0	30
70	52.5	17.5	35
80	60.0	20.0	40
90	67.5	22.5	45
x	0.75*x*	0.25*x*	0.5*x*

Adapted from product information (Mayne Pharma Ltd, Melbourne,Vic) and Daly FFS et al. Guidelines for the management of paracetamol poisoning in Australia and New Zealand—explanation and elaboration. Med J Aus 2008;188(5)296–302.

need for transplantation, and additionally uses a lactate level of >3.0 mmol/L after resuscitation as an indicator. Persistent elevation of serum lactate is a bad sign. Markers of liver regeneration such as microRNA offer future promise as prognostic markers.

Non-steroidal anti-inflammatory drugs (NSAIDs)

Overdose with NSAIDs such as ibuprofen and naproxen are common. Mild abdominal pain, vomiting and occasional diarrhea are the common manifestations. Both are frequently self-limiting.

Urea, electrolytes and creatinine, and full blood count should be checked on every patient presenting with NSAID overdose. Ensure adequate hydration. Consider H_2 blockade (e.g. ranitidine) for symptomatic relief of gastric pain.

Tricyclic antidepressants

Tricyclic antidepressants such as amitriptyline remain commonly prescribed.

- Symptoms after overdose include dry mouth, blurred vision and impaired cognition (including anticholinergic delirium).
- Signs include reduced Glasgow Coma Scale (GCS) scores, tachycardia and seizures.
- An EKG should be taken, and monitoring continued. Look for tachycardia and QRS prolongation >120 ms, which predicts risk of seizures and arrhythmias; more so if the QRS >160 ms. If the QRS >160 ms or arrhythmias occur, administer 1 mmol/kg of IV sodium bicarbonate.

- Oral activated charcoal should be given only if the patient is seen within 1 hour of ingestion and has a secure airway due to risk of aspiration.
- Seizures should be treated with sodium bicarbonate (to reduce the central nervous system [CNS] penetration of the drug) and a benzodiazepine such as diazepam 10 mg IV or lorazepam.

Newer antidepressants

Selective serotonin reuptake inhibitors (SSRIs)

SSRIs such as fluoxetine, sertraline and citalopram are less toxic than tricyclic antidepressants in overdose. However, arrhythmias and seizures can occur. Rarely, but especially if a combination of serotonergic agents has been taken, then serotonin toxicity may occur (Figure 3-12).

Serotonin toxicity is a spectrum disorder, not a discrete syndrome as such. It is potentially life-threatening and can be caused by a mixture of serotonergic drugs (acting on 5-hydroxytryptamine [5-HT] receptors) in normal or overdose quantities.

It is managed by stopping any further doses of 5-HT drugs, meticulous supportive care and, where significant features occur, cyproheptadine (which blocks 5-HT$_2$ receptors in the CNS) is administered orally 12 mg stat then 4–8 mg every 4–6 hours.

Other antidepressants

- **SNRIs** (serotonin norepinephrine reuptake inhibitors) such as venlafaxine have drowsiness as the most common clinical feature in overdose. Other effects include

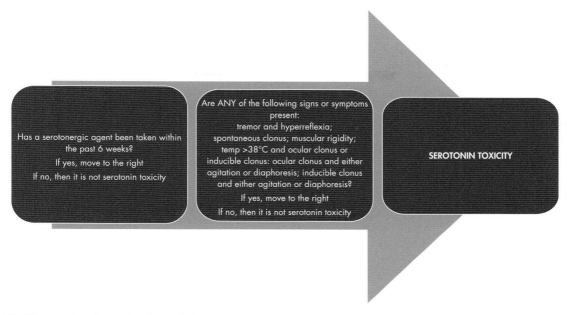

Figure 3-12 Diagnosis of serotonin toxicity

Adapted from Dunkley EJ et al. The Hunter Serotonin Toxicity Criteria: simple and accurate diagnostic decision rules for serotonin toxicity. QJM 2003;96(9):635-42.

seizures, tachycardia, hypotension or hypertension, and rarely arrhythmias. Venlafaxine overdoses are not associated with prolonged QTc or QRS. EKG monitoring and supportive care is all that is required in most cases.

- **NaSSAs** (noradrenergic and specific serotonergic antidepressants) such as mirtazapine are remarkably safe in overdose. EKG monitoring and supportive care is all that is required in most cases.
- **NRIs** (norepinephrine reuptake inhibitors) such as roboxetine also seem safer in overdose. No serious sequelae have been reported in two cases of taking up to 52 mg of roboxetine. EKG monitoring and supportive care is all that is required in most cases.

Second generation antipsychotics

These include drugs such as clozapine, risperidone, quetiapine and olanzapine. All antipsychotic drugs block dopamine receptors (D_2) and serotonin (5-HT blocking). Some, such as clozapine, olanzapine and quetiapine, also block H_1 histamine and alpha-adrenergic receptors. Clozapine is more toxic than other antipsychotics.

In overdose they can cause hypotension, seizure, tachycardia and drowsiness. Potentially life-threatening consequences include QT prolongation and respiratory depression. Death has been reported after an estimated overdose of 10,800 mg of quetiapine.

Benzodiazepines

Benzodiazepines taken alone in overdose are rarely fatal and present with drowsiness, cerebellar signs and confusion.

However, the patient's GCS score may be reduced for 24 hours. Some clinicians administer the antidote flumazenil, but it is seldom needed in clinical practice and is contraindicated in multiple drug overdose.

Meticulous supportive care, including maintenance of the airway, is required in those with an impaired GCS score.

Insulin and oral hypoglycemics

Overdose with these agents by diabetic patients is common. The key principles are to work out what dose of what has been taken, with what anticipated length of action, and to provide additional IV blood glucose support until the effects of the drug(s) or insulin have worn off. 50 mL IV of 50% dextrose is frequently followed by an infusion of 10–20% dextrose titrated to the patient's blood glucose level. Insulin is non-toxic if ingested.

Octreotide has been used as an antidote in severe sulfonylurea (gliclazide, glibenclamide) toxicity.

CLINICAL PEARLS

- In approximately 1–2% cases of administration of *N*-acetylcysteine, an anaphylactoid reaction occurs within the first 2 hours of the infusion.
- Up to 20% of patients who overdose on NSAIDs may experience seizures or renal dysfunction.
- In patients with a history of convulsions or toxin-induced cardiotoxicity, or those who have ingested tricyclic antidepressants, flumazenil may precipitate seizures or ventricular arrhythmias.

DRUGS OF ABUSE OR MISUSE

Amphetamines

Amphetamine-related presentations account for >1% of hospital admissions and often represent high-acuity patients with aggressive behavior. Inadequate or inappropriate sedation is a major clinical issue. All symptomatic patients should have EKG, blood pressure and temperature monitoring for >6 hours. Methamphetamine, or 'ice', may be injected intravenously, swallowed or smoked.

Ecstasy (MDMA; 3,4-methylenedioxy-*N*-methylamphetamine) produces feelings of euphoria and intimacy. Patients presenting to hospital are commonly intravascularly deplete and hot. The heat occurs due to local muscular production of heat and a central CNS (5-HT) source. The amount of time the patient's core spends at above 39°C is critical to poor clinical outcome. Management consists of sedation with benzodiazepines if required, cool IV fluids (often patients need 3–5 L) and management of complications (see Table 3-5).

Cocaine and crack cocaine

Cocaine is usually sniffed or snorted into the nose, or injected. Crack cocaine is heated and sniffed.

- Mild to moderate intoxication causes euphoria, agitation, cerebellar signs, dilated pupils, headache, tachycardia and hallucinations.
- Features of severe intoxication include convulsions, coma, severe hypertension and stroke.

Complications include the entire list above with amphetamines (Table 3-5). In addition, central chest pain due to coronary artery vasospasm and myocardial infarction (MI) can occur. All patients should be observed with EKG monitoring for >2 hours. It is important to consider the cocaine as a precipitant, as the investigation and management differs significantly from that of ischemic heart disease.

- Diagnosis of cocaine-related MI is difficult, as 84% of patients with cocaine-related chest pain have abnormal EKGs even in the absence of MI, and half of all cocaine users have elevated creatine kinase concentrations in the absence of MI; serum troponin is the most useful test to date.

The cornerstones of therapy for chest pain are generous doses of benzodiazepines to decrease central adrenergic stimulation (to manage hypertension or tachycardia), high-flow oxygen, nitrates (sublingual and intravenously) and aspirin. Patients with ongoing ischemia can be treated with low doses of calcium-channel blockers (verapamil) or alpha-blockers (phentolamine). Avoid beta-blockers because of the risk of enhancing coronary vasoconstriction.

Patients with continuing chest pain and/or EKG findings despite these measures should proceed to coronary angiography.

Gammahydroxybutyrate (GHB)

GHB is 'liquid Ecstasy' and has a mild seaweed flavor. It is taken in small amounts to achieve a high, but dosing is difficult and newer users in particular may experience sedation problems. Patients present with a diminished GCS score with small or midpoint pupils. They often recover spontaneously within a few hours, with airway and sometimes respiratory support.

Table 3-5 Complications of amphetamine intoxication (including Ecstasy)

COMPLICATION	HOW COMMON?	MANAGEMENT
Hyponatremia due to syndrome of inappropriate ADH secretion (SIADH)	Very rare	Water restriction
Intracerebral hemorrhage	Uncommon	CT/MRI required if any focal neurological signs are present or GCS score is reduced
Serotonin toxicity	Uncommon	Supportive care and cyproheptadine for serious cases (as above under SSRIs)
Hypertension	Uncommon	GTN infusion, benzodiazepines, labetalol (mixed alpha- and beta-antagonist) Avoid beta-blockers
Hyperthermia	Common	Cooling measures, diazepam, specific 5-HT agonists such as cyproheptadine
Rhabdomyolysis	Uncommon	IV fluids, cooling measures
Supraventricular and ventricular tachycardia	Uncommon	Short-acting antiarrhythmic drugs, e.g. esmolol for SVT
Seizures	Uncommon	IV diazepam

5-HT, 5-hydroxytryptamine; ADH, antidiuretic hormone; CT, computed tomography; GCS, Glasgow Coma Scale; GTN, glyceryl trinitrate; IV, intravenous; MRI, magnetic resonance imaging; SSRIs, selective serotonin reuptake inhibitors; SVT, supraventricular tachycardia.

CLINICAL PEARL

Patients with gammahydroxybutyrate toxicity present with a diminished GCS score with small or midpoint pupils. The differential diagnosis is opioid poisoning.

Opioids, such as heroin, morphine or fentanyl

Patients poisoned with opioids present with reduced GCS score, reduced respiratory rate and volume, and small pupils. Provision of an adequate airway and ventilation is critical to good outcome in most cases.

Reversal of the poisoning is achieved by administration of 0.8–2 mg IV naloxone (IV is better than IM—titrate against GCS score, respiratory rate and oxygen saturations). There is evidence that fentanyl and related highly potent synthetic opioids may require a more rapid administration of naloxone, higher doses of naloxone with more rapid escalation of additional doses and a longer period of observation following reversal. The half-life of the naloxone is much shorter than the opioid and to prevent return to toxic signs, further boluses or an infusion of naloxone are required. A common pitfall is giving inadequate doses as an infusion after the initial bolus. As a rule of thumb, this should be ⅔ of the dose required to initially rouse the patient, per hour. Intranasal naloxone is available for use in an outpatient setting e.g. drug injecting rooms.

CLINICAL PEARLS

- Reverse opioid poisoning by administering 0.8–2 mg IV naloxone boluses (IV is better than IM—titrate against GCS score, respiratory rate and oxygen saturations).
- In cases of intoxication with fentanyl or derivatives begin with 0.4 mg naloxone IV, followed by rapid escalation to higher doses (2 mg) if no response is observed within 2–3 minutes.
- A common pitfall is giving inadequate doses as an infusion after the initial bolus. As a rule of thumb, this should be ⅔ of the dose required to initially rouse the patient, per hour.

Prescription drug abuse

Prescription drug abuse in some countries is now overtaking illicit drugs as a cause of poisoning. There is high abuse and poisoning potential for oxycodone, methadone and other opioids, and for benzodiazepines such as alprazolam and oxazepam. In terms of risk of death per 100,000 single-substance exposures, methadone and morphine rank among the highest in the world.

Synthetic cathinones, e.g. 'vanilla sky', 'ivory wave'

Synthetic cathinones are a class of new psychoactive substances (NPS) often labeled as 'bath salts', 'plant food' or 'research chemicals'. Common examples include mephedrone (4-MMC; 4-methyl methcathinone), methylone (MDMC; 3,4-methylenedioxy-N-methylcathinone) and alphaPVP (alpha-pyrollidinovalerophenone).

Cathinones act to inhibit monoamine transporters for the reuptake of dopamine (DAT), serotonin (SERT) and norepinephrine (NET) blocking the reuptake of these neurotransmitters; however, their activity is complex due to varying selectivity for different transporters.

Clinical signs of synthetic cathinone intoxication include: tachycardia, hyperthermia, hypertension, agitation, with some patients experiencing elevated *serum creatine phosphokinase levels and acid–base imbalance*. Case reports indicate increased rates of paranoia, hallucinations, psychosis and suicidal ideation. Case reports demonstrate dependency and deaths, nose bleeds, high suicidality, CNS stimulation, and cardiac toxicity with possible QTc prolongation. Treatment should be symptomatic. Synthetic cathinones include mephedrone, 3,4-methylenedioxypyrovalerone and 3,4-methylenedioxy-N- methylcathinone (MDMC; also known as methylone). They are beta-ketone analogues of amphetamines. Sold as 'bath salts' or 'gas stations' on the internet, the packs usually say 'not for human consumption'. They are abused for stimulant effect and smoked or ingested orally. They may not cross-react with urine assays for amphetamines and need to be detected from blood samples using LC-MS/MS.

Synthetic cannabinoids, e.g. 'spice', 'K2'

Synthetic cannabinoids are cyclohexylphenolaminoalkylindoles and include many different products with a high affinity for CB_1 and CB_2 receptors with active metabolites. They are more potent than tetrahydrocannabinol (THC) from cannabis. They are sold as 'herbal incense' products on the internet or in shops. These are abused by smoking and there are case reports of tolerance, dependence and withdrawal, with attendant driving issues. Recently a case was reported in New York with seizures, sinus tachycardia and a creatine kinase level of 2700 IU/L.

Drink spiking

Most poisoning from drink spiking is due to alcohol. On rare occasions, drinks are spiked with additional drugs such as GHB or short-acting benzodiazepines. If samples of urine and blood are obtained from patients, they should be taken as soon as possible for toxicology screening, using legal precautions such as chain of custody.

CHEMICALS

Many toxic chemicals exist in household environments, such as bleaches, acids, alkalis, toxic alcohols and pesticides.

Acids and alkalis

These are corrosive, with oral cavity and pyloric injury more likely with acids and esophageal injury with alkalis. Endoscopy may be required to assess the degree of injury, and surgery may be necessary in a minority of cases. Do not empty the stomach, as this carries the risk of lung aspiration. Water should be given.

Table 3-6 Phases in organophosphorus poisoning

PHASE	TIME AFTER EXPOSURE	LASTS	CLINICAL FEATURES	MANAGEMENT
Acute cholinergic syndrome	Within 1 hour	48–72 hours	Miosis, muscle fasciculation, followed by limb, respiratory and sometimes extraocular muscle paralysis	Plasma cholinesterase confirms exposure Remove contaminated clothes, give oral activated charcoal, IV atropine reverses bronchorrhea, bradycardia and hypotension Role of oximes is contentious
Intermediate syndrome (IMS)	More than 48 hours		Progressive muscle weakness due to neuromuscular junction failure	Complete recovery is possible with ventilatory care
Organophosphate-induced delayed polyneuropathy (OPIDN)	1–3 weeks or with chronic exposure		Degeneration of long myelinated nerve fibers lead to paresthesiae and progressive limb weakness	Supportive care Recovery often incomplete

Modified from Karalliedes L, Chapter 3, in JA Innes (ed), Davidson's Essentials of medicine. Edinburgh: Elsevier, 2009.

Chlorine

This is commonly available for swimming pools, and may also be released when acid cleaners are combined with bleaches. Respiratory irritation, coughing and bronchospasm may occur, which are managed with nebulized bronchodilators such as salbutamol. Rarely, a delayed pulmonary edema may occur.

Pesticides

These are taken in overdose, especially in rural settings. They include organophosphorus (OP) insecticides, glyphosate and permethrins. Occasionally paraquat is taken, which is of particular concern because of the lack of effective treatment options.

Most pesticide poisoning is treated with meticulous supportive care, including ventilatory support as required. Atropine is the most commonly used antidote in organophosphorus insecticide poisoning. Oximes were once used to reactivate phosphorylated acetylcholinesterase at nerve endings. How effective oximes are is very much in question, resulting in their diminishing use globally.

The fatality rate following deliberate ingestion of OPs in developing countries may be as high as 70%. Three sequential phases are seen after ingestion; see Table 3-6.

Lead poisoning

Exposure to lead is common from mining and smelting sources. High lead levels are associated with neurological

(e.g. motor neuropathy), hematological (e.g. anemia, basophilic stippling) and gastrointestinal effects (e.g. abdominal pain). The World Health Organization's current blood lead action intervention level is 10 microg/dL. Evidence is building of neurocognitive deficits with chronic low lead levels (<10 microg/dL).

The primary management for lead intoxication is to reduce or prevent exposure, although in cases where lead concentration in the blood exceeds 45 microg/dL, chelation therapy with dimercaptosuccinic acid (DMSA) or 2,4-dimercapto-1-propanesulfonic acid (DMPS) is indicated. Specialist advice is needed for this.

SPIDER BITES

The majority of spider bites cause only minor effects (local swelling, pain, redness and itch). Most bites require no specific measures beyond analgesia, but a few species can cause severe and systemic features, in which case the appropriate antivenom is used.

SNAKE BITES

Snake bite is a common life-threatening condition in many countries; farmers, soldiers, rice-pickers and hunters are at particular risk, as are leisure travelers whose alcohol-fueled curiosity leads to unwanted encounters with snakes. Not all bites lead to envenomation, i.e. 'dry bites'.

First aid for snake bite is immobilization and appropriate pressure immobilization bandaging, although guidelines specific to country and species vary on this. Identification of the type of snake is made from direct visual identification of the snake, which is unreliable, and where available using venom detection kits from the wound's bite site (best) or urine (less good). This aids the choice of antivenom to be administered intravenously. In general, it is better practice to give specific snake antivenom than polyvalent antivenom, because of the higher risk of adverse reactions with the polyvalent antivenom. Additional tests such as coagulation and platelet counts are required in some cases, e.g. brown snake envenomation, and guidance on the management of snake bite from an experienced toxinologist is recommended.

Cardiovascular, respiratory and renal support may be needed, as may treatment for coagulopathies. Most patients who receive medical attention in developed countries survive their envenomation.

MARINE ENVENOMATION

- Bluebottle (*Physalia* spp.) stings are common and can be treated with warm water.

- Toxic jellyfish such as the box jellyfish (*Chironex fleckerii*) can cause death from acute respiratory failure or acute cardiac arrest. Acetic acid (vinegar) is used on the tentacles of adherent box jellyfish to inactivate nematocysts, but if not available then tentacles should be removed without delay, taking precautions to protect your skin as you do so. An antivenom is available for the box jellyfish.

- *Carukia barnesi* and other jellyfish can cause Irukandji syndrome—headache, hypertension, severe muscular and abdominal pain, elevated troponin I levels, cardiac dysfunction (with MI in about a third of patients). Systemic magnesium, in slow boluses of 10–20 mmol, may attenuate pain and hypotension in Irukandji syndrome.

- The blue-ringed octopus (*Hapalochlaena maculosa*) yields a potent neurotoxin which may first manifest itself with paresthesiae, tightness in the chest, cranial nerve palsies, e.g. bulbar palsy, followed by respiratory arrest. The best management is intubation if required and supportive care.

TERRORISM, AND USE OF MEDICAL COUNTERMEASURES

Chemical agents

As a hopefully never-in-a-lifetime event, physicians may be required to manage patients who have been exposed to terrorist activity. Mass sickness or fatalities occurring over a short period, all exhibiting the same types of symptoms and signs, or patients reporting unusual smells or tastes might alert clinicians to the possibility of an attack having occurred. Management of such situations requires resolve, calmness and specific knowledge, much of which is readily available and frequently updated on government preparatory and emergency websites, e.g. those of the Centers for Disease Control and Prevention (CDC), Agency for Toxic Substances and Disease Registry (ATSDR) and health departments. Diagnostic features and broad principles of care are discussed here.

If people have been exposed to toxic chemicals it is vital that thorough decontamination takes place before medical care can continue beyond the principles of airway, breathing and circulation support, and perhaps even antidote administration where early administration is critical to outcome (i.e. ABCD). Decontamination after a chemical terrorism event usually occurs near the incident site and is undertaken by the fire services (e.g. Hazmat teams) in most countries. In addition, minor decontamination facilities are available in key emergency departments for patients presenting directly to such facilities. After decontamination, it is important to look for signs of toxidromes (Table 3-7), while protecting staff with personal protective equipment (PPE) of the appropriate level (see local emergency department policy on PPE).

Biological agents

Unlike chemical attacks, where the features often develop within minutes, incubation times of biological agents often allow victims to spread far away and then present to their local healthcare providers. Diagnostic skills, attention to hygiene to avoid spread by respiratory or direct skin contact, and antimicrobials appropriate to the underlying diagnosis together with excellence in communication underpin effective clinical care (Table 3-8, overleaf).

Table 3-7 Possible toxidromes after chemical attack

SIGNS AND SYMPTOMS	LIKELY EXPOSURE	RELEVANT MANAGEMENT
Difficulty in seeing and breathing, miosis, bronchorrhea, reduced consciousness, weakness and fasciculation, i.e. acute cholinergic syndrome	Nerve agent*	Airway, breathing, circulation Atropine and antidote, e.g. DuoDote (contains atropine and oxime) to be given quickly after exposure. Note that not all nerve agents, e.g. sarin, respond to oximes Diazepam improves survival Intubation and ventilation as required Decreased plasma or red blood cell cholinesterase suggests a diagnosis of poisoning
Skin burns (mustards sometimes smell like garlic, onions or mustard)	Acids, alkalis, mustard agents	Decontaminate appropriately and treat as for burns
Bronchospasm, coughing, painful eyes, i.e. irritant syndrome	Chlorine	Skin decontamination, bronchodilators Beware the potential for late-onset pulmonary edema
Respiratory distress, fever, cough, nausea, chest tightness, pulmonary edema (if inhalational exposure), vomiting and diarrhea (if ingestion), low blood pressure, respiratory failure. Death within 72 hours	Ricin* (derived from castor beans)	Supportive medical care, e.g. intravenous fluids, ventilatory support No known antidote Activated charcoal if suspected recent ingestion
Very rapid symptoms after exposure, that include lightheadedness, rapid breathing, emesis, respiratory depression, opisthotonus, seizures and cardiac arrest	Hydrogen cyanide*	Supportive care, e.g. cardiopulmonary resuscitation—care is needed to avoid direct oral to oral contact The antidote of choice is hydroxycobalamin, and must be given as quickly as possible after exposure

* Management information sourced from the Emergency Preparedness and Response section of the website of the Centers for Disease Control and Prevention https://emergency.cdc.gov/.

Table 3-8 Clinical features and management of biological agents

CLINICAL SIGNS AND SYMPTOMS	LIKELY AGENT	MANAGEMENT
Bacillus anthracis infection occurs in three forms: 1. *Cutaneous*—itchy lump which develops into a vesicle, then a painless ulcer 1–3 cm in diameter with a typical black (necrotic) area in the center 2. *Inhalation*—common cold symptoms (EXCEPT rhinorrhea), followed by severe breathing difficulty and cardiovascular system shock. Usually fatal 3. *Gastrointestinal*—nausea, vomiting, fever followed by abdominal pain, hematemesis and severe diarrhea. Death occurs in 25–60% of cases	Anthrax (*B. anthracis*)	Meticulous supportive care, ciprofloxacin 500 mg twice daily or doxycycline pending sensitivity results*

CLINICAL SIGNS AND SYMPTOMS	LIKELY AGENT	MANAGEMENT
Acute generalized vesicular or pustular rash, deep-seated, hard and well-defined lesions in the same stage of development, with the greatest concentrations on the face and distal extremities, oral mucosa and soles Patient looks 'toxic' Note that a smallpox diagnostic risk calculator is available at www.bt.cdc.gov/agent/smallpox	Smallpox (*Variola major*)	Isolate all cases and face-to-face or household contacts after the onset of fever, and give supportive care No currently effective antibiotic or immune therapy Vaccination for contacts, including up to the first few days after exposure*
Bubonic plague is the most common manifestation with a painful 'bubo' occurring in the groin, axillae or cervical lymph nodes If untreated, septicemia and a pneumonic process results. Pneumonic plague is characterized by high fever, chills and breathing difficulty	Plague (*Yersinia pestis*)	Take laboratory samples (lymph node aspirate, blood cultures, sputum). Gram-negative organisms with a 'safety pin' appearance provide a rapid presumptive diagnosis Begin antibiotic immediately—streptomycin 1 g twice daily or gentamicin 5 mg/kg/day
With foodborne botulism, symptoms begin within 6 hours to 10 days after eating the toxin-containing food Symptoms include blurred vision, double vision, drooping eyelids, slurred speech, difficulty swallowing, and muscle weakness that moves down the body—first shoulders, then arms, then breathing Note that there is no person-to-person spread	Botulism (*Clostridium botulinum* toxin)	Meticulous supportive care, including ventilator support where necessary Antitoxin is available*
Severe hemorrhagic fever	Filoviruses (Ebola, Marburg)	Isolation to disrupt further transmission No known effective treatment#
Severe hemorrhagic fever	Arenaviruses (Lassa fever, Junin—Argentine haemorrhagic fever)	Supportive care

* Information sourced from the Emergency Preparedness and Response section of the website of the Centers for Disease Control and Prevention (CDC) https://emergency.cdc.gov/.

Information sourced from the CDC website: http://www.cdc.gov/ncidod/dvrd/spb/mnpages/dispages/vhf.htm (filovirus and arenavirus fact sheets).

SELF-ASSESSMENT QUESTIONS

For the following questions, one or more responses may be correct.

1 The bioavailability of an oral preparation of a new drug is assessed in a cross-over study. The summary results of the cross-over study are shown below.

Route	IV	Oral
Dose	20 mg	50 mg
C_{max}	2 mg/L	0.5 mg/L
AUC	60 mg.h/L	30 mg.h/L
AUC, area under the curve; C_{max}, maximum concentration; IV, intravenous.		

What is the oral bioavailability of this drug?
A 80%
B 60%
C 40%
D 20%
E 10%

2 A drug is 70% renally eliminated and 30% metabolized by cytochrome P450 3A4. The usual dose is 100 mg twice a day. Your patient has a stable creatinine clearance of 30 mL/min (normal is approximately 100 mL/min). What dose would achieve 'usual' drug concentrations? This drug is available in 30 mg and 100 mg scored tablets.
A 100 mg twice a day
B 100 mg daily
C 60 mg daily
D 30 mg twice a day
E 30 mg daily

3 A patient treated for hypertension comes for review. 24-hour blood pressure monitoring shows she is under-treated. You double the dose of her medication but there is minimal change in her blood pressure. What is the most likely explanation for the minimal response to the doubling of the drug dose?
A The patient is not taking the drug.
B The patient has secondary hypertension.
C The patient has very high drug clearance.
D There is a drug–drug interaction.
E The patient is already at the top of the dose–response curve.

4 Drug toxicity due to unintended drug–drug interactions is most commonly caused by what mechanism?
A Displacement from protein binding.
B Inhibition of p-glycoprotein efflux transporters.
C Inhibition of drug-metabolizing enzymes.
D Inhibition of renal drug transporters.
E Induction of drug absorption.

5 A 40-year-old tells you he had a rash when given penicillin as a child. He has not had penicillin since. What should you advise him?
A He is at high risk of anaphylaxis if exposed to penicillin antibiotics and should wear a Medic Alert bracelet.
B He should undergo desensitization to penicillin.
C He should undergo further assessment for penicillin allergy.
D He could be treated with penicillin if necessary but should also receive a corticosteroid and an antihistamine.
E He is at low risk of future adverse reactions and can have penicillin antibiotics if needed in the future.

6 Cost–efficacy analyses are frequently undertaken to assess whether a new drug should be funded by the government or an insurer. In a cost–efficacy analysis, what is the best description of efficacy?
A Improvement in primary outcome for patients treated with the new drug compared with placebo.
B Benefit–harm of the new drug compared with placebo.
C Benefit–harm of the new drug compared with usual care.
D Change in mortality of the new drug compared with placebo.
E Change in mortality of the new drug compared with usual care.

7 Which of the following is the best antidote for hydrogen cyanide poisoning?

  A Oxygen
  B Hydroxycobalamin
  C Sodium thiosulfate
  D Dicobalt edetate
  E Amyl nitrite

8 Which of the following is *not* a feature of late acetaminophen (paracetamol) poisoning in humans?

  A Right upper quadrant abdominal pain
  B Renal-angle tenderness on palpation
  C Prolonged prothrombin time
  D Methemoglobinemia
  E Nausea

9 Poisoning with which of the following does *not* cause mydriasis (dilated pupils)?

  A Benzodiazepines
  B Organophosphorus insecticides
  C Tricyclic antidepressants
  D Antihistamines
  E Ice (methamphetamine)

10 Which of the following is *not* true of snake bites?

  A The populations most at risk are rural farming ones.
  B Antivenins are almost always needed to treat victims.
  C Bite-site testing for venom detection is the preferred diagnostic tool.
  D Compression bandaging is recommended as a first aid measure.
  E Administration of antivenin may be associated with an anaphylactic reaction.

11 Which of the following is *not* true of ricin?

  A It is an extract from the castor bean.
  B It can cause pulmonary edema.
  C It has an antidote.
  D It can cause systemic hypotension.
  E It can cause vomiting and diarrhea.

ANSWERS

1 D

Bioavailability is the proportion of the dose reaching the systemic circulation. As all of an IV dose enters the systemic circulation, oral bioavailability can be calculated by comparing the drug exposure (AUC) of the oral dose vs the IV dose. The oral AUC is half the IV AUC, but only 40% of the oral dose was given IV. Half of 40% is 20%. Thus, 80% of the oral dose is either not absorbed or is metabolized before it reaches the circulation (first-pass metabolism).

2 B.

Metabolism is likely to be unchanged, and it is only the renally cleared portion that will be affected by the renal impairment. With 30% metabolic clearance and about 20% renal clearance (i.e. one-third of 70%), this patient will have about half normal clearance and the half-life will be doubled. Either the dose could be halved or the dose interval could be doubled. A single tablet once a day is simple, as well as being about the right dose. This will give this patient a starting dose that gives a similar drug exposure to other patients. The dose of every patient still needs to be adjusted based on patient response.

3 A or E.

Poor adherence to drug treatment is the most common cause of treatment failure in chronic care, particularly for asymptomatic conditions. Secondary hypertension occurs in a significant minority of patients with hypertension and should always be considered, but is not a good explanation for lack of dose response. Many drugs of *wide therapeutic index* are given in doses at the top of their dose–response curves, and therefore increasing the dose often has only a small effect on response. Variability in drug clearance and drug interactions always need to be considered, but are less likely explanations of the lack of response on increasing the dose.

4 C.

Drug interactions cause drug toxicity either by an additive effect or by increasing a drug concentration, as in this case. Inhibition of drug-metabolizing enzymes is the most common cause of drug toxicity due to a pharmacokinetic interaction. Displacement from protein binding only causes a minor transient increase in drug concentration. Increased drug absorption by inhibition of efflux transporters or decreased renal excretion can both cause clinically important drug toxicity.

5 C.

Anaphylaxis to penicillin is potentially fatal and is one of the most common drug causes of anaphylaxis. However, rashes at the time of febrile illnesses are common, especially in children. Many people are incorrectly labeled as being allergic to penicillin, and not having access to a major group of antibiotics can compromise the treatment of some conditions. It is not usually possible to make a diagnosis one way or the other on the basis of a distant history of rash. Investigation of drug allergy is a specialized area and suspected cases should be referred to an immunologist.

6 C.

In considering whether to fund a new drug, a comparison with current practice should always be made. If the drug were better than placebo but not as good as current care, it would not offer a clinical advantage. The correct comparator is thus usual care. In assessing the clinical value of the drug, we are interested in net efficacy, the sum of the benefits minus the sum of the harms. If the drug is more effective than current treatments, we may be prepared to pay more for it.

7 B.

While oxygen, sodium thiosulfate, dicobalt edetate and amyl nitrite have all been used in cyanide poisoning, hydroxycobalamin has the best benefit with the fewest side-effects and is the current antidote of choice.

8 D.

Methemoglobinemia occurs in cats but not humans after acetaminophen overdose. Right upper quadrant tenderness and nausea often reflect hepatic injury and the need to check liver function tests including clotting (prothrombin time or international normalized ratio). Renal-angle tenderness, while rarer, can indicate kidney injury and prompts the need to check renal function tests.

9 B.

Opioids, organophophorus insecticide exposures and nerve agents can cause miosis (pinpoint pupils).

10 B.

Bites from snakes may be 'dry' and antivenin is not usually administered unless signs of envenomation occur. Antivenin is potentially antigenic and reactions do occur. Where venom detection kits are available, e.g. in Australia, bite-site testing of venom for venom detection is preferred, together with positive identification of the snake if possible.

11 C.

There is no known antidote to ricin poisoning.

CHAPTER 4

GENETICS

John Attia and Tracy Dudding-Byth

CHAPTER OUTLINE

OVERVIEW

- There are 23 pairs of chromosomes in the human genome: 22 pairs of autosomes and 1 pair of sex chromosomes (Figure 4-1). One copy of each pair is inherited at fertilization, one from the father through the sperm and one from the mother through the egg.

- **Chromosomes** are made of deoxyribonucleic acid (DNA) complexed with various proteins (histones and non-histones); see Figure 4-2. Each chromosome has a *centromere*, where the DNA is tightly packed, and *telomeres*, which is the name given to the ends of the chromosome. The centromere is not quite in the center of the chromosome, creating a short arm (called p for 'petit', meaning 'small' in French) and a long arm (called q for 'queue', meaning 'tail' in French).

- **DNA** is a double-stranded helix (Figure 4-3) composed of nucleotides; each nucleotide is made up of a sugar and a phosphate group linked to one of four different bases: adenine or guanine (called purines), or cytosine or thymine (called pyrimidines).
  - » Adenine (A) on one DNA strand of the helix pairs with thymine (T), and guanine (G) pairs with cytosine (C).
  - » **RNA** (ribonucleic acid) has a different base, uracil (U), instead of thymine.

- The total **genome** (the DNA across all chromosomes) is 3.1 billion base pairs (bp).

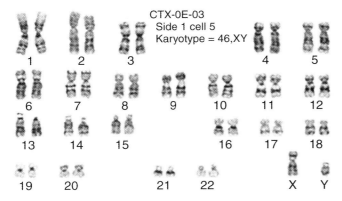

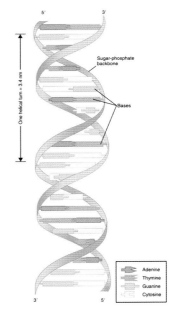

Figure 4-1 Human karyotype (male)

Courtesy of John Sinden, PhD, ReNeuron Group.

THE FLOW OF GENETIC INFORMATION

- The general flow of information was thought to be from one gene on the DNA to one on the RNA to one protein, although recent discoveries have substantially expanded this paradigm, described in the sections on transcription and translation, below.

- Only 1.1% of the genome (total DNA) consists of protein-coding genes; this represents around 20,000 genes in total. Another, smaller, portion of the genome consists of RNA-coding genes, of which around 6000 exist (see section on regulation, below). The function of the remaining vast majority of DNA is unclear.

Transcription

- A protein-coding gene is converted to messenger RNA (mRNA) by RNA polymerase II in a process called **transcription**. During this process, the DNA helix is unwound and a copy of the 'sense' strand is created. The process of transcription is upregulated by a number of proteins that bind to specific sequences at the start of each gene.

- These specific sequences at the start of each gene are called **promoters** and come in different forms (Figure 4-4):

Figure 4-3 DNA helix. A, adenine; C, cytosine; G, guanine; T, thymine

From Jorde LB, Carey JC and Bamshad MJ. Medical Genetics, 6th ed. Elsevier Inc., 2020.

  - » the 'TATA' box, found about 25 bp from the start of the gene (shown in orange)
  - » the 'GC'-rich box, found in place of TATA in some genes (shown in blue)
  - » the 'CAAT' box, found 80 bp from the start of the gene (shown in purple).

- **Enhancers** perform the same function as promoters but are typically found much further away from the gene and help to express genes in the right tissues. The DNA loops out to bring the promoter and the enhancer together to stimulate the transcription of a particular gene.

- Once the DNA has been transcribed into messenger RNA (mRNA), the mRNA moves to the cytoplasm to act as the blueprint for one or more protein(s).

- The coding sequences of genes can overlap so that a stretch of DNA can code for many different mRNAs; it is the promoters and enhancers that are responsible for deciding which gene is transcribed.

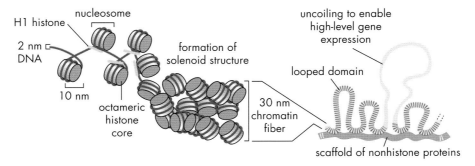

Figure 4-2 Packaging of deoxyribonucleic acid (DNA)

From Strachan T and Read A. Human molecular genetics, 4th ed. New York: Garland Science, 2011.

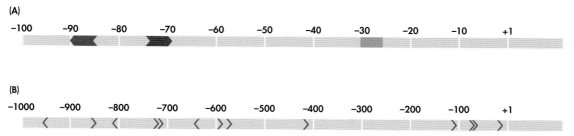

Figure 4-4 Location of promotors (**A**) and enhancers (**B**) relative to the start of a coding region (labeled +1)

From Strachan T and Read A. Human molecular genetics, 4th ed. New York: Garland Science, 2011.

Translation

- Not all of the mRNA molecule codes for protein. The mRNA sequence consists of coding sections (called **exons**) and 'intervening sections' (called **introns**). In a process of 'splicing', the introns are removed and the coding exons are brought together (Figure 4-5). This splicing is variable, such that different exons can be brought together to code for different forms of the same protein (called *isozymes* or *isoforms*) or to form completely different proteins. For example, the pro-opiomelanocortin gene codes for one mRNA that can be the blueprint for three different proteins and four related proteins.
  » Splicing is carried out by a complex of proteins and RNA (called small nuclear ribonucleoproteins (snRNPs), the 'spliceosome' (Figure 4-6).
  » Introns are usually recognized because they start with GT and end with AG (the GT-AG rule), although this is obviously not the only cue.
- The mRNA transcript also undergoes other changes, where the start of the transcript is 'capped' by a special

guanine and a long tail of adenines is added to the end of the transcript (a 'poly-A tail'). These modifications influence the location, function and degradation of the transcript.

- The sequence of the mRNA is translated into a chain of amino acids (a protein) via the **ribosome**, which is a complex of proteins and various ribosomal RNAs (rRNA, specified by RNA-coding genes); Figure 4-7.
  » The ribosome is composed of a large and a small subunit. Starting at the beginning of the mRNA, the ribosome looks for the start signal, the nucleotide

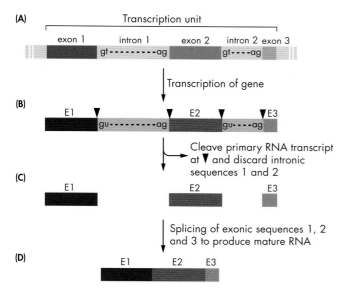

Figure 4-5 Splicing of a mRNA transcript, with (**B**) transcription, (**C**) cleaving and (**D**) splicing together of a transcript

From Strachan T and Read A. Human molecular genetics, 4th ed. New York: Garland Science, 2011.

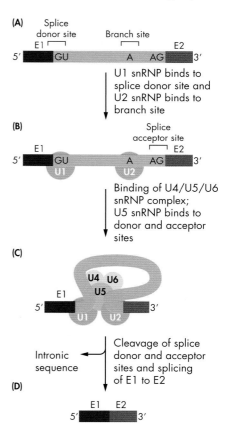

Figure 4-6 Mechanism for splicing a transcript, with (**B**) recognition of splice sites, (**C**) snRNP complex formation and (**D**) removal of intron

From Strachan T and Read A. Human molecular genetics, 4th ed. New York: Garland Science, 2011.

sequence AUG. This is the 'start codon' and codes for methionine; every protein therefore begins with this amino acid which is later cleaved off.

» The ribosome then reads each group of three nucleotides (codon) on the mRNA and brings in the corresponding amino acid. This amino acid is bound to a transfer RNA (tRNA), another in the family of RNAs specified by RNA-coding genes. The ribosome catalyzes the bonding of each amino acid to the previous one as it moves along the mRNA.

» When the ribosome hits a 'stop codon', it stops adding amino acids and releases the protein; there are three codons that signal a stop.

• Multiple ribosomes can bind a single mRNA, meaning that multiple protein molecules can be made from the one mRNA template.

Regulation

The greatest change in genetic dogma in the past 30 years has been the discovery of the role of RNA in gene expression.

We have mentioned that RNA-coding genes are the blueprint for RNA that will be part of the ribosome (rRNA) or form transfer RNA (tRNA) or be part of the spliceosome (snRNA). Another class of non-coding RNA is microRNA (miRNA) or small interfering RNA (siRNA). Both are short RNA molecules, about 20 nucleotides long, that interfere with mRNA translation. miRNA binds a complementary sequence on an mRNA molecule and causes its degradation, while siRNA binds and blocks the sequence, leading to repression of translation. Because of imperfect binding, one miRNA or siRNA can downregulate many different mRNAs (Figure 4-8).

Another mechanism of regulation is through epigenetic changes. 'Epigenetics' refers to heritable changes that are mediated through mechanisms other than a change in DNA sequence. The two main epigenetic mechanisms are:

• **Histone modification**—the most common modification is acetylation of the histone protein (addition of an acetyl group), but other mechanisms include methylation (addition of a methyl group), ubiquitylation (addition of ubiquitin, a 76 amino acid protein that tags proteins for destruction), phosphorylation (addition of a phosphoryl group) and sumoylation (addition of a SUMO protein, a class of small proteins that direct proteins in cellular traffic). These histone modifications are thought to affect the packing of the DNA and hence the ability to transcribe and translate DNA.

• **Methylation**—this consists of the addition of a methyl group to the DNA (not to protein, as in histone modification). The methyl group is attached to a cytosine that is next to a guanine, i.e. a CG sequence. Stretches of CG sequences are called CpG islands (where the p represents the phosphate group in the DNA backbone).

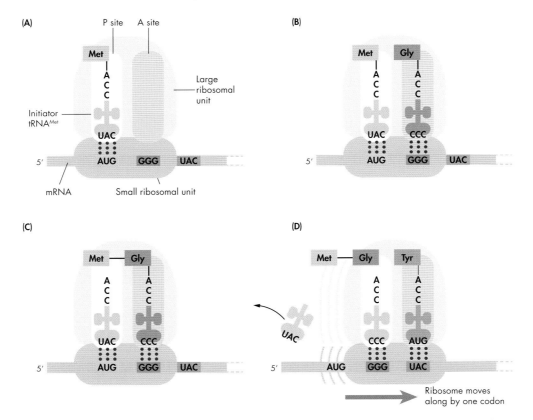

Figure 4-7 Process of translation with (**B**) binding of an amino acid, (**C**) covalent addition to the nascent protein and (**D**) progress along the mRNA transcript

From Strachan T and Read A. Human molecular genetics, 4th ed. New York: Garland Science, 2011.

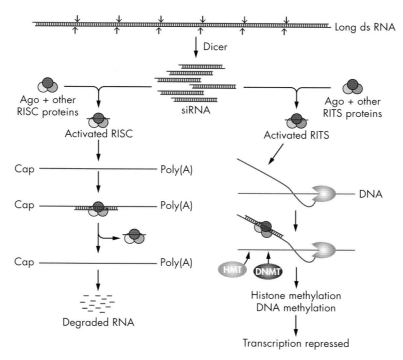

Figure 4-8 Mechanisms of regulation by small RNAs. DNMT, DNA methyltransferase, HMT, histone methyltransferase; RISC, RNA-induced silencing complex; RITS, RNA-induced transcriptional silencing

From Strachan T and Read A. Human molecular genetics, 4th ed. New York: Garland Science, 2011.

This methylation tends to 'silence' the gene and prevent transcription.

GENETIC VARIATION

The human genome contains over 3 billion bp, consisting of both protein-coding DNA (1%) and noncoding DNA (99%). There are an estimated 20,000 human protein-coding genes. The human 'reference genome' sequence is a template sequence derived from the DNA of a number of donors.

The Human Genome Project has revealed that humans are, on average, >99% identical in their DNA sequences, meaning that all the variation we see in appearance, color, height, build, etc. is due to the 1% difference (plus environmental differences). Although this sounds small, 1% of 3 billion bp is still 30 million bp.

In the era of genomic testing, the term 'DNA variant' refers to a difference in DNA sequence compared to the 'reference genome'. These DNA variants make each person's genome unique.

These differences, called **polymorphisms**, may take a number of different forms (Figure 4-9, overleaf):

- the presence or absence of an entire stretch of DNA (duplication or deletion), called *copy number variation* (CNV).

- repeating patterns of DNA that vary in the number of repeats; each repeating 'unit' may vary from 2–3 to hundreds of base pairs long and may repeat a few times to hundreds of times.

- a change in a single base pair, called a *single-nucleotide polymorphism* (SNP; pronounced 'snip'); this is by far the most common kind of variant.

What constitutes the difference between a benign variant and a pathogenic or disease-causing variant? Ultimately, it is the functional impact of the variant on the protein that provides the answer. However, frequency of the variant is often a surrogate, presumably because of selection against a poorly functioning or absent protein. A variant that is found at a frequency of 1% or more in the population is often judged to be a benign variant (polymorphism), whereas a variant found in less than 1% is more likely to be a pathogenic variant.

Some variants are present in parts of the gene that are translated, i.e. that code for proteins. Because the genetic code that governs the matching of codons to amino acids is redundant, a change in the DNA may mean that the same amino acid is coded for; this is called a **synonymous change**. However, a number of other possibilities arise:

- A **missense variant** means that a single nucleotide variant has changed a codon to specify a different amino acid, i.e. a non-synonymous change. The effect of this change will be smaller if the new amino acid is in the same class as the old one, or larger if the new amino acid is in a different class. This may lead to alteration, loss, or a completely new function of the protein.

- A **nonsense variant** means that the single nucleotide variant has created a premature stop codon, leading to loss of function of that protein.

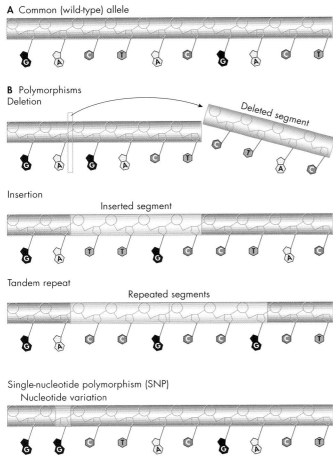

A Common (wild-type) allele

B Polymorphisms
Deletion

Deleted segment

Insertion

Inserted segment

Tandem repeat

Repeated segments

Single-nucleotide polymorphism (SNP)
Nucleotide variation

Figure 4-9 Common (wild-type) allele (**A**) and the four types of genetic polymorphism (**B**)

- A **frameshift variant** means that an insertion or a deletion has shifted the coding frame and how codons are read, usually creating a premature stop codon.
- A variant may change the **splice sites**, either blocking proper splicing or creating a new splice site.

A note about terminology and notation: the point along the DNA at which a genetic variant is found is called a locus. The 'normal' or wild-type sequence at that locus is denoted by a capital letter, and the variant sequence is denoted by a small letter: for example, someone who has the 'wild-type' base at a SNP locus on the maternal chromosome and the 'variant' base on the paternal chromosome is denoted Aa (heterozygote); someone with a wild-type sequence at both chromosomes is denoted AA (homozygote normal); and someone with a variant at both chromosomes is denoted aa (homozygote variant).

Complex traits such as height and intelligence are due to an interaction between variants at a number of different loci.

HUMAN DISEASE GENES

Mendelian conditions are typically rare, have predictable inheritance patterns and usually result from a pathogenic

variant in a single gene. Conversely, 'complex diseases' such as heart disease, asthma, type 2 diabetes, obesity and inflammatory bowel disease are common in the general population and result from a complex interaction between multiple rare and common susceptibility loci in combination with environmental factors.

MENDELIAN DISEASES

Some characteristics or functions depend on only a single gene; consequently, pathogenic variants in that gene are highly likely to cause disease. These are the traditional genetic diseases, e.g. cystic fibrosis or Huntington disease.

It is important to understand the patterns of inheritance for monogenic diseases and recognize these patterns on a pedigree. The symbols used for a genetic pedigree are shown in Figure 4-10.

1 **Autosomal dominant:** is where a pathogenic variant on only one gene allele is necessary for the person to be affected. The dominant allele is denoted by a capital letter (e.g. people with AA or Aa have the disease). Affected people are often seen in different generations. The parent may or may not express the condition (i.e. be affected by it), depending on the disease penetrance (see below). The condition may also be due to a de novo (new or spontaneous) dominant variant that occurred during or shortly after conception. A child with one 'affected' and one unaffected parent has a 50% chance of having the disease.

2 **Autosomal recessive:** a pathogenic variant on both copies of an allele are required for a person to be affected (aa). Those with Aa do not show the disease but are carriers for it. An affected person usually has unaffected parents, but they are very likely to be carriers of a pathogenic variant. A child born of two carriers has a 25% chance of having the disease.

3 **X-linked recessive:** refers to conditions where the pathogenic variant is carried on the X chromosome. X-linked recessive conditions are more common in males than females because males only have one X chromosome, but females can be affected if they are born of an affected father and a carrier mother. Females can also be affected, often more mildly, depending on the rate of expression of the X chromosome copy on which the pathogenic variant is located. This is because in females one copy of the X chromosome is randomly 'switched off' (inactivated; see below). Usually this inactivation is random, but if it is skewed toward inactivation of the X chromosome carrying the normal gene copy, the female can express the condition. An affected male is usually born of a carrier mother. In other cases, the variant is *de novo*. The pedigree shows no male-to-male transmission. X-inactivation: Although female embryos have two copies of the X chromosome, very early in development (at the blastula stage) one copy, either the maternal or the paternal copy of the X, is randomly inactivated, and this inactivation will be the same in all daughter cells. This means that a different X may be inactivated across different tissues, making

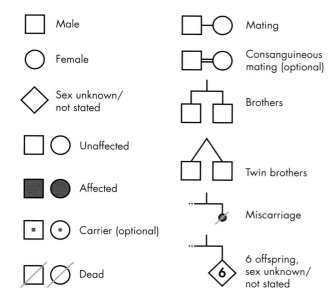

Figure 4-10 Symbols used in pedigree diagrams

From Strachan T and Read A. Human molecular genetics, 4th ed. New York: Garland Science, 2011.

the interpretation of an X-linked pedigree difficult. Males, having only one X chromosome, do not have this process.

4 **X-linked dominant:** an affected person usually has at least one affected parent. The children of an affected female have a 50% chance of having the disease, whereas only the daughters of an affected male have the disease (since the male only passes on his Y chromosome to a son and not his X chromosome). This is a rare form of inheritance.

5 **Y-linked inheritance:** only males are affected and they usually have an affected father. There are only a small number of genes on the Y chromosome.

There are a couple of issues that complicate the interpretation of pedigrees:

* The pathogenic variants may have reduced or incomplete penetrance, i.e. it may not manifest itself all the time. For example, in a pedigree, all those who are Aa for a dominant pathogenic variants would be expected to show disease but this may not be the case, partly because in some the disease may manifest later in life or not at all.

* Germline mosaicism or incomplete penetrance can account for an unaffected parent having a child with a dominantly inherited condition.

BREAST CANCER PREDISPOSITION GENES

Up to 10% of cancers occur through an inherited pathogenic variant within a cancer predisposition gene. Whereas sporadic cancers are due to somatic DNA changes, these inherited germline variants are within every cell of the body. Characteristics include a strong family history, moderate to high risk of cancer at a young age and the presence of multiple cancers in the same individuals. Penetrance is variable within and between families.

BREAST AND OVARIAN CANCER PREDISPOSITION GENES

* Both BRCA 1 and 2 are tumor-suppressor genes; this means they produce proteins involved in high-fidelity DNA repair.

* Pathogenic variants tend to be autosomal dominant because once one copy of the gene (and protein) malfunctions, the person is at high risk of getting a second pathogenic variants that knocks out the remaining wild-type copy.

* BRCA 1 and 2 are responsible for up to 10% of all breast cancers, i.e. the majority of sporadic breast cancer is not genetic.

* BRCA 1 and 2 are responsible for up to 50% of all hereditary breast and ovarian syndromes. Guidelines for recognizing familial risk and testing for BRCA 1 and 2 are shown in table below.

* Lifetime risk of having breast cancer (by age 80) is ~70% for both BRCA 1 and 2.

* Lifetime risk of ovarian cancer is ~40% for BRCA1 and ~20% for BRCA2.

* Pathogenic variants can be inherited from a father.

* Allele frequency is highest in the Ashkenazi Jewish population, where 3 specific pathogenic variants make up 90% of all cancer cases (Table 4-1).

CALCULATING THE RISKS OF DISEASE

It is important to be able to calculate the risk of disease in relatives or children, once a family member has been identified with a pathogenic variants. An important tool in doing these calculations is the Hardy-Weinberg distribution.

The **Hardy-Weinberg distribution** states that if the normal sequence 'A' has a frequency in the population of p and the variant sequence 'a' has a frequency of q, then the proportion of people in the population who are AA is $p \times p$ or p^2, and the proportion in the population who are aa is $q \times q$ or q^2. The proportion who are Aa is pq and the proportion who are aA is qp, and hence the proportion who are heterozygous is $pq + qp$ or $2pq$. The entire population is represented by these people, so $p^2 + 2pq + q^2 = 1$.

Some examples

Example 1
A male with an autosomal recessive disease marries a woman who is a carrier for the same disease. What is the risk of disease in their children?

The answer can be calculated using a Punnett square (a 2 × 2 table named after an early 20th-century

Table 4-1 Criteria for genetic risk evaluation and possible testing for breast and/or ovarian cancer

---

A. An individual with breast cancer (including invasive and ductal carcinoma) with any of the following:
- Breast cancer diagnosed ≤50 years
- Triple-negative breast cancer diagnosed ≤60 years
- Two breast cancers* (in a single patient)
- Male breast cancer
- Breast cancer diagnosed at any age, in addition to one of the following:
  - » ≥1 close blood relative¶ with breast cancer diagnosed ≤50 years, or
  - » ≥1 close blood relative¶ with ovarian, fallopian tube, or primary peritoneal cancer diagnosed at any age, or
  - » ≥1 close blood relatives¶ with male breast cancer, pancreatic, and/or prostate cancer (Gleason score ≥7), or advanced prostate cancer, diagnosed at any age
  - » ≥2 close blood relatives with breast cancer at any age¶

B. An individual of any age with a known or likely pathogenic variant in a cancer susceptibility gene within the family or found on tumor testing

---

C. Personal and/or family history of three or more of the following on the same side of the family:ᐃ
- Breast cancer, sarcoma, adrenocortical carcinoma, brain tumor or leukemia◊
- Colon, endometrial, thyroid, or kidney cancer, dermatologic manifestations of Cowden syndrome, macrocephaly, or hamartomatous polyps of the gastrointestinal tract§
- Lobular breast cancer, diffuse gastric cancer¥
- Breast cancer, gastrointestinal cancer or hamartomatous polyps, ovarian sex cord tumors, pancreatic cancer, testicular Sertoli cell tumors, or childhood skin pigmentation‡

D. Personal history of ovarian, pancreatic, metastatic prostate,† or male breast cancer

---

E. Ashkenazi Jewish ancestry and breast cancer or high-grade (Gleason score ≥7) prostate cancer

---

F. An individual with no personal history of cancer but with:**
- First- or second-degree relative with any of the following: breast cancer diagnosed ≤45 years, ovarian cancer, male breast cancer, pancreatic cancer, metastatic prostate cancer,† or ≥2 breast cancer primaries in a single individual or on the same side of the family with at least one diagnosed ≤50 years

---

* Two breast cancers indicates either bilateral disease or at least two separate ipsilateral primary tumor (that may have occurred at the same time or at different times).

¶ Close blood relatives are first-, second-, and third-degree relatives on the same side of the family. Maternal and paternal sides should be considered independently.

ᐃ Particularly if diagnosed ≤50 years. Can include multiple primary cancers in the same individual.

¥ For lobular breast cancer with a family history of diffuse gastric cancer, *CDH1* gene testing may be informative.

‡ For hamartomatous colon polyps in conjunction with breast cancer and hyperpigmented macules of the lips and oral mucosa, *STK11* testing may be informative.

† Including distant or nodal disease, but not biochemical recurrence.

** Whenever possible, testing of the affected family member should be performed first.

National Comprehensive Cancer Network, v2.2019 (www.nccn.org).

---

geneticist). The mother is Aa and the father is aa; assuming that the fertilization of a sperm and egg are random, and each parent contributes one copy of each chromosome/gene to their child, the risk to the children can be drawn as shown below:

	A	a
a	Aa	aa
a	Aa	aa

i.e. 50% of the children will be carriers Aa (²⁄₄) and 50% will have disease aa (²⁄₄).

Example 2
An autosomal recessive condition affects 1 person in 10,000. What is the expected frequency of carriers in the population?

Given that for a recessive disease a person must be 'aa' to show disease, then $\frac{1}{10,000}$ must be equal to q^2, or $q = \frac{1}{100}$. Because everyone is either p or q, the frequency of p must be $\frac{99}{100}$. Given

that carriers are the heterozygotes, their frequency is $2pq$, or $2 \times \frac{1}{100} \times \frac{99}{100} = $ about 1 in 50.

Example 3
A man who knows he is a carrier for cystic fibrosis (CF) is thinking of marrying a woman whose CF status is unknown. Given that the carrier frequency is 1 in 25, what is the risk to their children without any further testing?

If the woman is a carrier and we know the man is a carrier, then the risk to their children is ¼ (using a Punnett square like the one above). However, the risk that a woman is a carrier is ¹⁄₂₅; therefore, the risk that the woman is a carrier and that they pass CF on to their children is ¼ × ¹⁄₂₅ = 1 in 100.

Example 4
Red–green color blindness is an X-linked recessive disease. The frequency of the recessive variant is ¹⁄₁₂. What proportion of the population might be expected to be carriers?

The variant frequency, q, is $\frac{1}{12}$. There are no male carriers; since males only have one X chromosome, they either have the disease or not. Only females can be carriers and the Hardy-Weinberg distribution tells us that this group, $2pq$, is $2 \times \frac{1}{12} \times \frac{11}{12} = \frac{22}{144}$, or 15% of women are carriers. Women with the disease are $q^2 = \frac{1}{12} \times \frac{1}{12} = \frac{1}{144}$ or 0.7%.

GENETIC TESTING IN MEDICINE

It is important to be familiar with the different types of genetic tests and the answers they can provide, as well as their limitations.

Cytogenic karyotype

Given that the 23 pairs of chromosomes are tightly condensed in the nucleus of a cell, the best time to visualize them is when they have been 'untangled' during cell division. White blood cells are allowed to grow and divide in culture in the presence of an agent (colcemid) that blocks cells during mitosis, so that chromosomes have replicated and are maximally unfolded. The chromosomes are then stained with a dye that binds DNA (Giemsa) and differential staining leads to bands of DNA where dye has been bound (dark) and where it has not (light). Under the microscope, each chromosome has a distinct pattern of dark and light bands, called G-banding (Fig 4-11).

Analysis of chromosomes in this way can reveal different abnormalities:

- Deletion or duplication of an entire chromosome, e.g. Turner syndrome is a single copy (monosomy) of the X chromosome, while Down syndrome is three copies (trisomy) of chromosome 21.

- Formation of an abnormal chromosome, e.g. a ring chromosome (Figure 4-12).

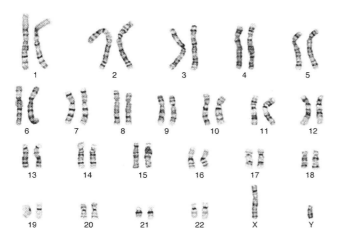

Figure 4-11 Karyotyping, Normal human male karyotype, showing 22 pairs of autosomes, one X chromosome, and one Y chromosome

From Chiang VW and Zaoutis LB. Comprehensive Pediatric Hospital Medicine. Elsevier Inc., 2007.

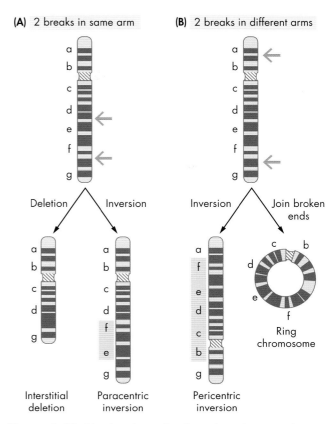

(A) 2 breaks in same arm   **(B)** 2 breaks in different arms

Figure 4-12 Mechanisms for forming abnormal chromosomes

From Strachan T and Read A. Human molecular genetics, 4th ed. New York: Garland Science, 2011.

- Re-arrangement of a section of a chromosome. A section of the chromosome can be removed, flipped and re-inserted back on the same chromosome, called an *inversion*; or can be re-inserted on a completely different chromosome, called a *translocation*. If a section on this second chromosome is also removed and 'exchanged' with the first chromosome, it is called a *reciprocal translocation* (Figure 4-13).

Fluorescence in situ hybridization (FISH)

This technique uses a DNA probe(s) labeled with a fluorescent marker, allowing a certain sequence or a certain section of a chromosome to be visualized when the probe binds to its target. All of the abnormalities described above can be detected at higher resolutions with FISH. An example of the use of FISH is to detect the *BCR-ABL1* translocation that is responsible for chronic myeloid leukemia (CML). A reciprocal translocation between the *BCR* oncogene on chromosome 22 and the *ABL1* oncogene on chromosome 9 leads to a fusion *ABL1–BCR* protein and a fusion *BCR–ABL1* protein (Figure 4-14); the latter is a protein kinase that is unregulated. The translocation leaves a longer than usual chromosome 9 and a shorter than usual chromosome 22, which has been labeled the Philadelphia chromosome.

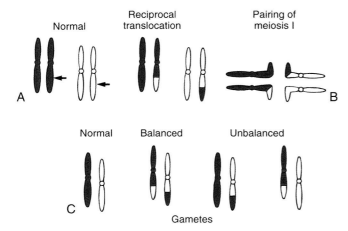

Figure 4-13 Mechanism for a reciprocal translocation. A, Normal chromosomes and reciprocal translocation. B, Pairing at meiosis. C, Consequences of translocation in gametes

From Jorde LB. Understanding Pathophysiology, 7th ed. Elsevier Inc., 2020.

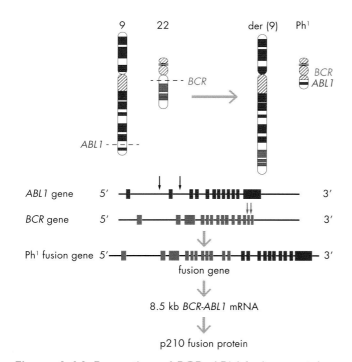

Figure 4-14 Formation of *BCR–ABL1* fusion protein

From Strachan T and Read A. Human molecular genetics, 4th ed. New York: Garland Science, 2011.

Chromosomal microarray (molecular karyotype)

A DNA microarray is a collection of microscopic DNA spots attached to a solid surface. Using a DNA hybridization process to compare the patient and control DNA, this advanced technique detects copy number variants (micro-deletions or micro-duplications) at a much higher resolution than conventional cytogenetic chromosomal karyotype. A molecular

karyotype is now used routinely for chromosome analysis; however, a cytogenetic karyotype is required to detect a balanced chromosomal translocation.

Genome-wide association studies

Single nucleotide polymorphisms (SNPs) contributing to complex diseases are identified through genome-wide association studies (GWAS).

These studies are made possible through microarrays, which are platforms the size of a microscope slide with millions of DNA templates dotted onto them; a person's DNA sample is then allowed to hybridise to these templates and then read automatically, generating information on up to 1 million SNPs on one person in one go. GWASs compare the genomic profile obtained by microarray in cases with a particular disease vs controls without that disease; any SNP that is overrepresented in cases vs controls is labeled as contributing to disease. Typically the individual contribution of each SNP is small in magnitude, i.e. relative risk or odds ratio of 1.02 to 1.3, and it is believed that the modest increase in disease risk across all of these thousands or millions of SNPs form part of an individual's overall risk of disease.

Indeed, polygenic risk scores (PRS) incorporating anywhere from 5 SNPs to millions of SNPs have been developed to predict disease risk. The performance of these PRSs is measured by the Area under the Receiver Operator Characteristic (AUROC) curve; scores that perform no better than chance have an AUROC of 0.5 while scores with perfect accuracy have an AUROC of 1.0. As a typical example, a clinical decision rule for type 2 diabetes using age, sex, and BMI has an AUROC of 0.79; adding 10 SNPs increases the AUROC to 0.80. This modest increase is typical of PRSs regardless of the number of SNPs used. PRS have not achieved sufficient predictive power to be clinically useful yet.

Polymerase chain reaction (PCR)

PCR is a method by which a small amount of DNA can be amplified by repeatedly separating the strands of the DNA helix and replicating the sequence *in vitro*. Using specific primers to guide the replication allows the presence of a specific point variant/SNP to be checked for. For example, testing for factor V Leiden, a pro-coagulant variant that predisposes to deep vein thrombosis and pulmonary embolism, is done using this method since the SNP that codes for this is unique and similar across the world (although the frequency of this SNP varies by ethnicity).

Sequencing

DNA sequencing is used to determine the sequence of nucleotides in a section of DNA. Regions of DNA up to about 900 bp in length are sequenced using a method called Sanger sequencing. Sanger sequencing provides a high-quality sequence for relatively long stretches of DNA, but is expensive and inefficient for larger scale projects, such as genome sequencing. For these tasks, new large-scale massively parallel (next generation) sequencing technology is faster and less expensive.

These methods can sequence the regions of the genome coding for proteins (exome sequencing) or the entire genome (whole genome sequencing). The rationale behind sequencing the coding regions only is that pathogenic variants affecting a phenotype are more likely to change the protein sequence and hence be found in the coding region of a gene, and testing is also cheaper. The reality, however, is that 85% of all 'hits' identified through GWASs lie in non-coding regions, indicating that what was previously thought to be 'junk' DNA are highly important regulatory regions. Current clinical practice is that people with phenotypes that appear to be highly heritable or consistent with Mendelian syndromes are those where whole genome/exome sequencing is performed. Another approach is to use a multi-gene panel containing a select set of genes known to be associated with a specific phenotype (e.g. cardiac gene panels).

The genomic sequences generated by these methods need extensive curation to classify DNA variants as benign, pathologic, or most commonly 'variant of unknown significance' (VUS). The current dilemma is how to interpret a VUS. Focusing on Mendelian disease allows family segregation studies.

Unlike microarrays, which are highly accurate, whole genome/exome sequencing is not as reliable and one needs to accumulate typically between 30 and 60 'reads' of any one stretch of DNA to be reasonably confident of the sequence; this is called the read 'depth'.

Mitochondrial DNA

Every cell within the body contains thousands of copies of mtDNA. Mitochondria containing a pathogenic mtDNA variant are frequently mixed with mitochondria containing normal mtDNA within a cell, a state known as heteroplasmy. The percentage heteroplasmy can shift during mitotic and meiotic cell division. The bioenergetics defect becomes more severe as the percentage of mutant mtDNA increases within a cell e.g. mitochondrial encephalopathy, lactic acidosis, and stroke-like episodes (MELAS) syndromes.

Imprinting

Most genes have biallelic expression. Genomic imprinting is an epigenetic mechanism whereby a gene or genomic domain is differentially expressed in a parent-of-origin manner. Most imprinted genes are found in clusters in the genome, and a given cluster often contains both paternal and maternally imprinted genes. The parent-of-origin epigenetic modifications including DNA methylation are erased and re-established during gametogenesis. For example, the SDHD tumor suppressor gene displays paternal parent-of-origin expression, and SDHD pathogenic variants inherited from a father cause highly penetrant hereditary paraganglioma-pheochromocytoma syndrome; whereas, maternal transmission, rarely, if ever leads to tumor development.

COMMON CHROMOSOMAL GENETIC CONDITIONS

Down syndrome

This is the most common chromosomal condition in liveborn infants and most often is the result of aneuploidy where there is a trisomy (three copies) of chromosome 21. Rarely, the additional copy of chromosome 21 is present as an unbalanced translocation. Babies with Down syndrome are born more frequently to women over the age of 35 years. The characteristic facial features are prominent epicanthal folds, flattened nose, small mouth and protruding tongue. Associated features include:

- congenital heart defects in about 45% of cases, including atrial septal defect (ASD) and ventricular septal defect (VSD)
- gastrointestinal abnormalities in approximately 5%, including duodenal atresia or stenosis
- obesity in approximately 50%
- hearing loss in 40–80%
- endocrine abnormalities, particularly hypothyroidism, and to a lesser degree hyperthyroidism and type 1 diabetes
- hematological disorders, especially polycythemia and leukemia
- obstructive sleep apnea
- early risk of Alzheimer disease.

Turner syndrome

This syndrome presents in women who are short and stocky; the karyotype is XO, i.e. one X chromosome. Associated features include:

- gonadal dysgenesis, presenting as reduced fertility, hypogonadism, and premature ovarian failure
- renal anomalies occurring in 30–50% of patients, particularly horseshoe kidney
- cardiovascular disease, especially coarctation and aortic valvular disease, along with hypertension
- endocrine disease, with elevated risks of premature osteoporosis, thyroid disease and diabetes.

Klinefelter syndrome

This syndrome occurs in males who have at least one extra X chromosome, typically XXY but potentially XXXY. The associated conditions include:

- hypogonadism and infertility
- neuropsychiatric problems, including lack of insight, poor judgment and mild cognitive impairment
- pulmonary disease: chronic bronchitis and bronchiectasis
- endocrine problems: higher risk of breast cancer and diabetes.

ACKNOWLEDGMENTS

Figures 4-1, 4-2, 4-3, 4-4, 4-5, 4-6, 4-7, 4-8, 4-10, 4-11, 4-12, 4-13, 4-14 and the figures appearing in the Self-assessment questions are © 2011 Garland Science from *Human Molecular Genetics*, 4th edition, by T Strachan and A Read. They are reproduced by permission of Garland Science/Taylor & Francis LLC.

SELF-ASSESSMENT QUESTIONS

1 The most common gene defect for cystic fibrosis (CF) is the delta-F508 variant in which three DNA bases coding for amino acid 508 of the CFTR protein are missing. This is an example of what kind of variant?
   A   Missense
   B   Nonsense
   C   Frameshift
   D   Deletion
   E   Splice site

2 In testing a patient for suspected cystic fibrosis (CF), you get back a report saying that they are negative for the delta-F508 variant. The correct interpretation is that:
   A   They probably do not have CF.
   B   They probably do have CF but the test is unreliable.
   C   They may have CF but have a different pathogenic variant in the CFTR gene.
   D   They need to have their parents and siblings tested in order to make a diagnosis.

3 How many genes are there in the human genome?
   A   5,000
   B   20,000
   C   100,000
   D   250,000
   E   500,000

4 RNA-coding genes code for all of the following except:
   A   mRNA
   B   rRNA
   C   tRNA
   D   snRNA
   E   miRNA

5 The function of siRNA is to:
   A   degrade mRNA
   B   block transcription
   C   block translation
   D   inhibit tRNA
   E   inhibit rRNA

6 The most common kind of genetic variant in the human genome is:
   A   insertion polymorphism
   B   deletion polymorphism
   C   microsatellite
   D   copy number variant
   E   single-nucleotide polymorphism

7 What mode of inheritance is evident in these pedigrees? (All images from Strachan T and Read A, Human molecular genetics, 4th ed. New York: Garland Science, 2011.)
   A   Autosomal recessive
   B   X-linked recessive
   C   Autosomal dominant
   D   X-linked dominant

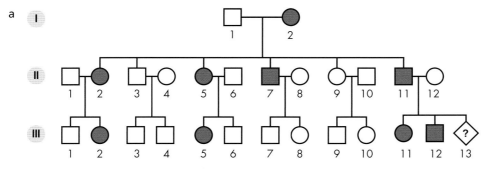

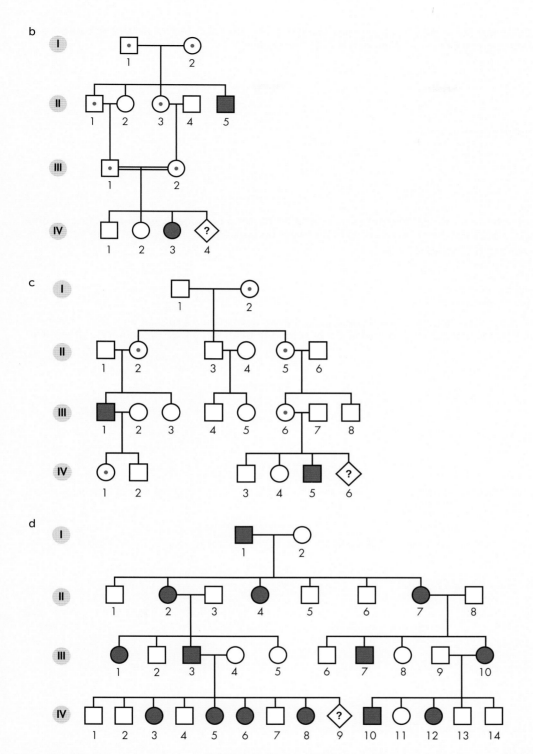

8 A patient has a typical appearance of Down syndrome but the karyotype shows only two copies of chromosome 21, i.e. no trisomy. In this case the explanation is likely:

A   A translocation between chromosome 21 and another chromosome in one of the parents
B   A deletion on chromosome 21 inherited from one of the parents
C   An inversion on chromosome 21 inherited from one of the parents
D   A ring chromosome 21
E   Monosomy in one of the parents

9 A genetics lab tests for the 10 most common CF pathogenic variant that together account for 80% of all pathogenic variant. What is the risk of still being a CF carrier if the genetic test is negative?

A 20%
B 10%
C 4%
D 1%
E <0.1%

10 The effect of methylation of DNA is to:

A Reduce transcription
B Reduce translation
C Increase transcription
D Increase translation
E Increase DNA turnover

11 For an autosomal dominant condition with paternal imprinting, a father passes a pathogenic variant on chromosome number 11 on to his daughter. What are the consequences of his daughter passing this gene variant on to her children?

A The chance of a daughter being affected is 100%.
B None of her sons will be affected.
C All of her children will be affected.
D None of her children will be affected.
E The chance of a child being affected is 50%.

12 The allele frequency of BRCA 1 or 2 pathogenic variants among Ashkenazi Jewish men and women is 2.5%. What is the likelihood that a person of Ashkenazi descent (with no disease or testing to date) will have 1 or 2 copies of the BRCA pathogenic variant?

A 2.5%
B 5%
C 7.5%
D 10%
E 12.5%

ANSWERS

1 D.

The deletion of three base pairs means that the encoded protein loses one amino acid but the rest of the reading frame is not affected, i.e. it is not shifted so missense and nonsense variants are not introduced.

2 C.

Delta-F508 is just the most common of hundreds of different pathogenic variants that have been described in CF.

3 B.

Most estimates are between 20,000 and 30,000.

4 A.

RNA-coding genes code for RNA molecules that are catalytically or enzymatically active. mRNA is translated to protein.

5 C.

Most regulatory RNAs work at the post-transcriptional level to affect mRNA stability and function.

6 E.

7 a   C.

An affected person usually has at least one affected parent, i.e. the disease does not skip generations. A child with one affected and one unaffected parent has a 50% chance of having the disease, i.e. 50% of each generation has the disease.

b   A.

An affected person usually has unaffected parents, but they are likely to be carriers, i.e. the disease skips generations. A child born of two carriers has a 25% chance of having disease, i.e. 25% of that generation is affected.

c   B.

Affected persons are mainly males, since they only have one X chromosome. An affected male is usually born of a carrier mother.

d **D.**

An affected person usually has at least one affected parent such as with an autosomal dominant disease, but all the daughters of an affected male have disease (since the male only passes on his Y chromosome to a son and not his X chromosome).

8 A.

Down syndrome is also a trisomy of some part of chromosome 21, if not the whole chromosome then some part of it; since parts of chromosomes are not able to survive on their own (except for ring chromosomes), they must exist by being attached to other chromosomes, e.g. translocation.

9 D.

Risk of being a CF carrier is $\frac{1}{20}$ and risk of being a false negative on the test is $\frac{1}{5}$, therefore risk of still being a carrier is $\frac{1}{20} \times \frac{1}{5} = \frac{1}{100}$ (1%).

10 A.

Methylation is involved in gene regulation, usually in reducing expression.

11 E.

The daughter is unaffected because the pathogenic variant inherited from her father is imprinted and not expressed. The DNA methylation patterns are erased and re-established during gametogenesis. When the daughter makes her gametes, 50% will contain the chromosome 11 she inherited from her father and 50% will contain the chromosome 11 she inherited from her mother. The region containing the pathogenic variant is now expressed. The chance of a child being affected is 50%.

12 B.

Using the HWE law, the frequency of people heterozygous for BRCA 1 or 2 will be $2pq$ or 2 (0.025)(0.985)= 4.9% and the frequency of those homozygous for BRCA 1 or 2 will be q^2 or $(0.025)^2$=0.06%; total of 4.96% or 5%.

CHAPTER 5

MEDICAL IMAGING FOR INTERNISTS

Lindsay Rowe

CHAPTER OUTLINE

- Technical review
- Initial image review
- Key image review
- Systematic review
- Review areas
- Summary

6. HEAD MAGNETIC RESONANCE

- **MRI PROTOCOLS**
  - T1
  - T2
  - Inversion recovery (IR)
  - Diffusion-weighted imaging (DWI)
  - Gradient echo (GRE)
  - Gadolinium-enhanced (GAD)
  - Magnetic resonance angiography/venography (MRA, MRV)

- MR spectroscopy (MRS)
- Magnetic resonance gated intracranial cerebrospinal dynamics (MR-GILD, CSF flow study)

- **PRINCIPLES OF INTERPRETATION IN BRAIN MR**
  - Patient demographics
  - Technical review
  - Initial image review
  - Key image review
  - Systematic review
  - Review areas
  - Summary

7. POSITRON EMISSION TOMOGRAPHY (PET)

1. CHEST RADIOGRAPHY

Plain-film chest radiography is the single most common imaging test obtained in clinical medicine, and has advantages and disadvantages (Box 5-1).

PRINCIPLES OF INTERPRETATION IN CHEST X-RAYS

The technique for systematic review of chest X-rays is akin to a clinical 'short case' examination. Initially steps are followed and practiced with a routine developed (Box 5-2).

Patient demographics

Patient details, including name, age and sex, as well as the date and time of exposure, are initially sought from the image.

Technical assessment

Four parameters of image technical adequacy need to be routinely assessed prior to interpretation to avoid artifacts being misconstrued as evidence of disease:

- patient position—anteroposterior (AP) or posteroanterior (PA)?
- exposure—under- or over-exposed?
- inspiratory effort—adequate or inadequate?
- rotation—neutral or rotated?

Patient position

Studies performed anterior-to-posterior (AP) or posterior-to-anterior (PA) appear very different, and diagnostic errors will be made if they are not recognized (Table 5-1, overleaf). Obvious clues to an AP study are identifying labels saying 'supine', 'sitting' or 'AP' and the presence of appliances such as endotracheal tubes and EKG leads. Reliable features for an AP include noting the chin low over the upper chest, the clavicles being steep and curved low in the

---

Box 5-1

Clinical utility of plain-film radiography of the chest

Advantages	**Disadvantages**
• Available	• False sense of security
• Cost-effective	• Premature termination of imaging investigations
• Small radiation dose	• Over-utilization
• Interpreter-friendly	• Low sensitivity for common disorders:
• Intermediate/high sensitivity for common conditions: » effusion, pneumothorax, pneumonia, mass >1 cm	» pulmonary embolism, nodule <1 cm, interstitial disease
	• Intermediate specificity for many findings
• Baseline study for monitoring of disease and treatment	• Radiographic lag time with clinical disease
• Rapid clinical triage for acute disease	• Image findings discordant with clinical findings

---

Box 5-2

Systematic interpretation of chest X-ray

Patient demographics
- Name and other details

Technical assessment
- Patient position (anteroposterior [AP], posteroanterior [PA])
- Exposure
- Inspiratory effort
- Rotation

Lines, tubes and implants
- Name
- Function
- Assess correct position
- Assess structural integrity
- Recognize complications

Anatomical review

Overview
- Gross perception

Systematic review
- Lungs
- Aeration
- Vascularity
- Hilum
- Lobar anatomy
- Pleura
- Peripheral
- Phrenic angles
- Fissures
- Heart
  - » Size (cardiothoracic ratio)
  - » Cardiac margin clarity
  - » Specific heart chambers

- Mediastinum
  - » Divisions
- Trachea
  - » Position
  - » Carina
  - » Main stem bronchi
- Diaphragm
  - » Position
  - » Shape
- Sub-diaphragmatic
  - » Stomach, bowel loops, liver/spleen enlargement
- Skeletal
  - » Spine
  - » Ribs, sternum
  - » Shoulder girdles
- Chest wall
  - » Breast contour
  - » Skin and muscle

Review areas
'The hard-to-see areas'
- Below the diaphragm
- Through the heart
- Chest wall
- Shoulder girdles
- Lung apices
- Trachea

Summary
- Comparison with previous study
- Correlation of findings and probable diagnosis
- Need for additional imaging

---

chest, arms straight by the sides and the scapulae clearly over the lung fields. Additional clues could include widening of the mediastinum, cardiomegaly with a raised cardiac apex, very concave elevated diaphragms and uniform upper-to-lower-lobe vascular prominence.

Exposure

A broad rule for adequate radiographic exposure is that the thoracic vertebrae should be discernible through the density of the heart. Overexposure renders the vertebrae very easily identified, while underexposure obliterates all detail. This rule is important to assess, as an overexposed chest X-ray mimics emphysema with dark lung fields and apparent decreased vascularity. An underexposed chest X-ray lightens the lung fields and enhances lung markings, simulating conditions such as pneumonia, interstitial lung disease and cardiac failure (Table 5-2, overleaf).

Inspiratory effort

A guideline for adequate inspiration is having at least 10 posterior and 7 anterior ribs visible above the diaphragm. The hallmarks of an expiratory study are elevation and exaggerated upward convexity of the diaphragms, cardiomegaly ('pancaking'), mediastinal widening and opacity of the lung bases commonly mimicking the appearance of congestive cardiac failure.

Rotation

Patient rotation induces apparent mediastinal shift, including the cardiac silhouette and the trachea. Rotation is assessed by comparing the distance of the medial ends of both clavicles relative to the thoracic spinous processes, usually around T4 (clavicle–spinous interval, CSI).

- In the presence of scoliosis, application of this method is invalid.
- When no rotation is present, the CSIs are equidistant; when there is rotation they will be unequal.

Lines, tubes and implants

These often provide clues on the underlying disease state and should be assessed by:

1. identifying the line or tube
2. knowing its function
3. confirming the normal position
4. assessing structural integrity
5. observing for complications.

Anatomical review

The sequence of anatomical review will vary with each case, but all components should be assessed (Box 5-2).

Overview

Review from a distance provides a wider perspective and aids perception of obvious findings such as disparity in lung size and opacity, mass lesions, mediastinal shift, mastectomy and shoulder girdle conditions such as fracture and malignancy.

Systematic review

A systems approach is used to simplify the search pattern—lungs, heart and mediastinum, skeletal and review areas.

Lungs

The lung contents are assessed globally, then specific details are sought. A simple 'ABCDEF' mnemonic may assist:

- **A** Aeration
- **B** Blood vessels
- **C** Costophrenic and cardiophrenic angles
- **D** Diaphragm
- **E** Endotracheal and endobronchial structures
- **F** Fissures.

Table 5-1 Features useful to differentiate AP from PA chest X-ray

FEATURE	AP (ANTERO-POSTERIOR)	PA (POSTERO-ANTERIOR)
Labels	AP, supine, sitting, mobile	Erect
Endotracheal tube	Present	Absent
EKG leads	Present	Absent
Arm position	Beside the thorax	Oblique to the thorax
Humeral length	Long, with shaft	Short, only the head
Scapula	Over lung fields	Off lung fields
Clavicle	Curved, steep, low	Straight, oblique
Chin	Visible	Absent
Gastric air	Gas in gastric body	Air–fluid level fundus
Mediastinum	Widened	Normal
Heart	Enlarged, elevated apex	Normal
Diaphragm	Elevated, more convex	Lower, gentle curve
Vascularity	Uniformly prominent. No vascular gradient	Narrow upper lobes. Dilated lower lobes ('vascular gradient')

Table 5-2 Chest exposure assessment guidelines

	NORMAL	UNDEREXPOSURE	OVEREXPOSURE
Spine	Perceptible	Not visible	Clear detail
Lung fields	Black	Whiter	Very black
Vascularity	Clear	Prominent	Absent
Mediastinum	Clear detail	Widened	Absent
Trachea	Clear	Very clear	Almost absent
Mimics	Vascular markings	Pneumonia. Interstitial disease. Pulmonary edema	Emphysema. Asthma. Pulmonary hypertension

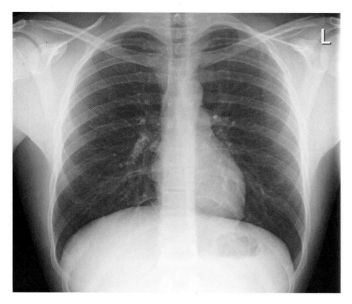

Figure 5-1 Normal chest X-ray

'Cover-up' method

A useful practical method to assist in the detection of subtle right-to-left changes in aeration, as well as subtle parenchymal disease, can be to cover the lung fields with a piece of paper. The paper is then slowly lowered as the viewer's eyes focus on the structures revealed at the edge of the descending paper, comparing the left-to-right structures.

Heart and mediastinum

The combined structures of the heart, great vessels and mediastinal contents are depicted as a composite radio-opaque structure referred to as the 'cardiac silhouette'. This is assessed by its size, definition of the heart borders and specific chamber analysis.

Size

The transverse dimension of the heart is expressed as a ratio to the transverse dimension of the thoracic cage ('cardio-thoracic ratio'), which should be less than 50%.

Heart border definition

The heart borders should be sharp and well defined at the heart–lung interfaces.

- If they are not, this may be a sign of opacifying disease such as pneumonia and atelectasis in the lung segments abutting the affected chamber ('silhouette sign').
- Loss of the left ventricular border is seen in lingula disease and of the right atrium in middle lobe disease.
- A common variant fat pad located at the cardiac apex often blurs its definition and is not to be confused with disease.

Heart chambers

The left heart border has five divisions:
- *left ventricle*—diaphragm to below the hilum
- *left atrium*—short, 2 cm segment above the left ventricle

- *pulmonary trunk*—marked by the left hilum pulmonary artery
- *aorto-pulmonary window*—above the left pulmonary artery and below the aortic arch
- *transverse aortic arch*—marked by the semicircular contour at the superior extent of the cardiac silhouette.

The right heart border has three divisions:
- *right atrium*—convex shadow from the diaphragm to the junction with the superior vena cava marked by the transition from the convex right atrium to the vertically straight superior vena cava
- *superior vena cava*—vertical, straight-edged opaque density beginning at the atrial–caval constriction and extending vertically over the right hilum and then curving laterally toward the lung apex
- *right paratracheal stripe*—a distinct opaque margin on the right side of the trachea which is a combination shadow of the right tracheal wall and azygous vein.

Skeleton

The thoracic spine, posterior and anterior ribs, as well as the shoulder girdles including clavicle, scapula and humerus, are reviewed to identify abnormalities that could be related to a chest abnormality. A destructive lesion in a rib, for example, may be relevant to a lung mass due to metastasis, symmetrical glenohumeral erosion as a sign of rheumatoid arthritis, and resorption of the distal clavicles in hyperparathyroidism.

Review areas ('hard to see areas')

Abnormalities away from the lung fields are readily overlooked but are often important.
- Below the diaphragm pneumoperitoneum, bowel obstruction, and a medially displaced gastric air bubble as a sign of splenomegaly may be identified.
- Through the cardiac silhouette, the air density of a hiatus hernia or a spinal mass may be seen.
- Evaluation of the chest wall for mastectomy, skin lesions and subcutaneous emphysema provide occasional but important clues to a chest disease process.
- The shoulders may show signs of lung-related disease such as rheumatoid arthritis or malignancy.
- Scrutiny of the often-obscured lung apex may elucidate a Pancoast tumor, tuberculosis or a pneumothorax.
- Finally, tracheal shift may be a feature of goiter, lymphoma or upper lobe volume loss.

Summary

Following the systematic review, relevant positive and negative findings can be correlated and final statements made (Table 5-3, overleaf). Named imaging signs of the chest should only be used when they are clearly present, as they often have specific meaning for a disease process or anatomical localization and, while useful, may be misleading when incorrectly applied (Table 5-4, see below). Comparison with a previous study, if not already viewed, should be made for assessing disease activity.

Table 5-3 Thumbnails of chest disease

FEATURES	PA	PA SPOT	OTHER	CT
PNEUMONIA Opacity Initially hazy or 'fluffy' with acinar nodules Rapidly confluent Lobar Air bronchogram (arrow) Silhouette sign				

ATELECTASIS
Opacity (arrow)
Lobar or segmental
Bronchovascular crowding
Air bronchogram
Shift
  —Fissures
  —Mediastinum
  —Diaphragm
  —Trachea				

EMPHYSEMA Increased lucency Low vascularity (arrow) Large hilar vessels Lower lobe compression Flat, low diaphragm Wide intercostal spaces Bullae Barrel chest Small tear-drop heart				

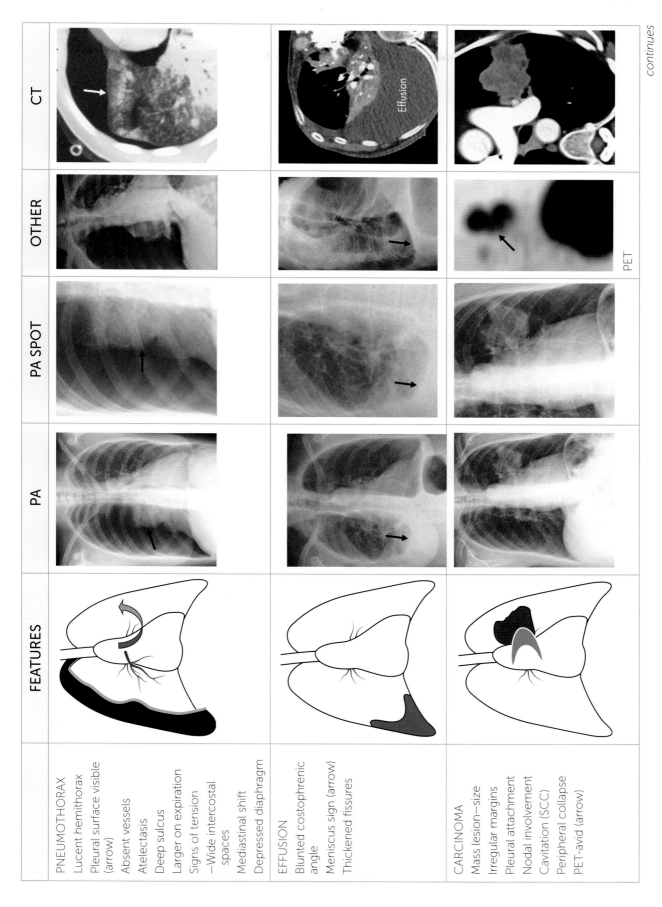

continues

	FEATURES	PA	PA SPOT	OTHER	CT
PNEUMOTHORAX Lucent hemithorax Pleural surface visible (arrow) Absent vessels Atelectasis Deep sulcus Larger on expiration Signs of tension —Wide intercostal spaces Mediastinal shift Depressed diaphragm					
EFFUSION Blunted costophrenic angle Meniscus sign (arrow) Thickened fissures					Effusion
CARCINOMA Mass lesion—size Irregular margins Pleural attachment Nodal involvement Cavitation (SCC) Peripheral collapse PET-avid (arrow)				PET	

Table 5-3 Thumbnails of chest disease *continued*

FEATURES	PA	PA SPOT	OTHER	CT
METASTASES Multiple nodules (arrow) Round Variable size Sharp margins Lower lobe dominance May cavitate				
INTERSTITIAL—NODULAR 1–5 mm nodules Well defined (arrow) May calcify				
ACUTE INTERSTITIAL—GROUND-GLASS OPACITY Mid–lower zones Hazy density (arrow) Poorly defined Vessels obscured Septal thickening Kerley lines				
CHRONIC INTERSTITIAL—RETICULAR Thin lines Honeycomb (arrow) Pleural contact Distortion Traction bronchiectasis Low lung volume				

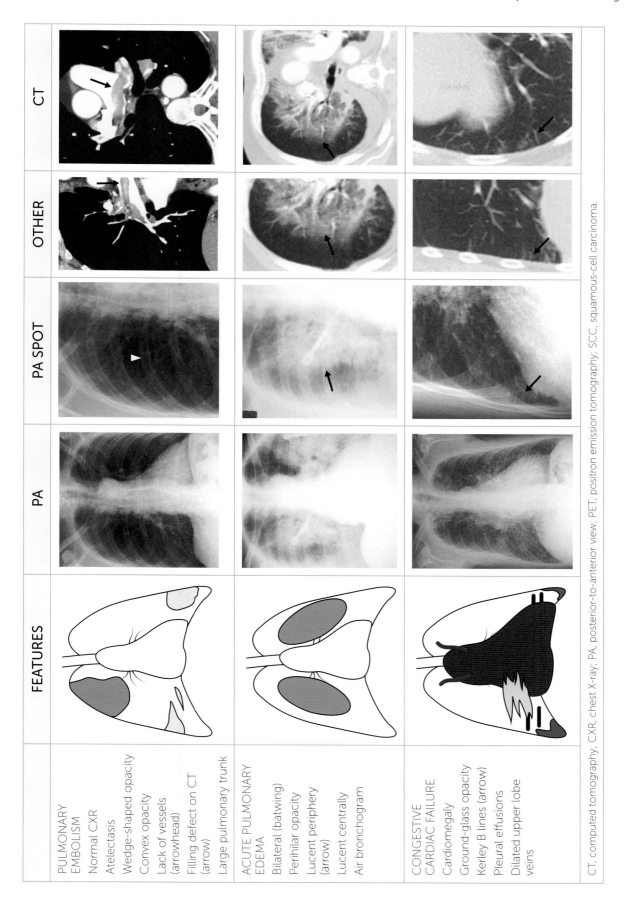

FEATURES	PA	PA SPOT	OTHER	CT

PULMONARY EMBOLISM
Normal CXR
Atelectasis
Wedge-shaped opacity
Convex opacity
Lack of vessels (arrowhead)
Filling defect on CT (arrow)
Large pulmonary trunk

ACUTE PULMONARY EDEMA
Bilateral (batwing)
Perihilar opacity
Lucent periphery (arrow)
Lucent centrally
Air bronchogram

CONGESTIVE CARDIAC FAILURE
Cardiomegaly
Ground-glass opacity
Kerley B lines (arrow)
Pleural effusions
Dilated upper lobe veins

CT, computed tomography; CXR, chest X-ray; PA, posterior-to-anterior view; PET, positron emission tomography; SCC, squamous-cell carcinoma.

Table 5-4 Common named imaging signs of chest disease

SIGN	DEFINITION	SIGNIFICANCE
Air bronchogram	Air-filled bronchi surrounded by fluid-filled alveoli	Pus: pneumonia Fluid: pulmonary edema Blood: hemorrhage Cells: bronchioalveolar carcinoma Protein: proteinosis
Cardiothoracic ratio	The ratio of the transverse diameter of the heart and the thorax	When greater than 50%, is due to cardiomegaly
Ground-glass opacity	Hazy lung density that does not obliterate vascular markings	Interstitial edema Alveolitis
Meniscus sign	Smooth, concave sweeping contour of the costophrenic sulcus	Pleural effusion
Silhouette sign	Cardiac border loses clear definition due to contact with opacified lung segment	Disease is in the lung segment abutting the heart (pneumonia, tumor, collapse)

2. THORACIC COMPUTED TOMOGRAPHY

Computed tomography (CT) of the chest is an integral component of chest evaluation and has broad applications. These include investigation of an abnormality found on chest X-ray, investigation of clinical signs and symptoms, tumor management from diagnosis to staging, biopsy planning and response to therapy. CT has unique application in the assessment of thoracic trauma. While there are many advantages, significant drawbacks—especially higher radiation dose—do exist (Box 5-3).

TECHNIQUES OF EXAMINATION

Different CT techniques are employed in specific clinical situations (Table 5-5). Knowledge of these techniques is pivotal in deriving the maximal information in different clinical scenarios.

PRINCIPLES OF INTERPRETATION IN CHEST CT

CT scans of the chest produce a large number of images to review in different planes. A systematic routine is necessary to avoid diagnostic error and maximize the derivation of information (Box 5-4).

Box 5-3

Clinical utility of CT scans of the chest

Advantages

- Available
- Fast
- Excellent anatomical detail
- Rapid reconstructions—multi-planar, 3D, vascular
- Wide areas of coverage
- Choice of vascular phase
- High sensitivity and specificity for most diseases
- Detection of small lesions
- Compatible with implanted devices

Disadvantages

- Higher radiation dose
- Higher cost
- Intravenous contrast reactions
- Extended breath-holding required
- Supine position occasionally not tolerated
- Over-utilization
- Large number of images
- Requires adequate computer systems for image display
- Competent technical staff for image acquisition
- False-positive diagnoses, especially benign nodules
- Rarely used in pregnancy
- Nursing mothers withhold breast feeds for 24 hours after IVI contrast study

CT, computed tomography; IVI, intravenous injection.

Table 5-5 Common techniques in CT scans of the chest

EXAMINATION	ACRONYM	TECHNIQUE	INDICATION
Non-contrast CT	NCCT	No IV contrast Helical mode Supine Suspended inspiration Neck to renal hilum	Contrast contraindication Poor venous access Identify calcification: —coronary artery calcium score —tuberculous granuloma —calcified lymph nodes —hamartoma Pneumothorax, pneumomediastinum Pleural calcification Bone disease Foreign body detection
High-resolution CT	HRCT	No IV contrast Non-helical, thin section Supine inspiration and expiration Supplemental prone inspiration Apices to below diaphragm	Interstitial lung disease Parenchymal scars Emphysema Bronchiectasis Foreign body localization
Routine contrast CT		Post IVI 20- to 30-second delay Helical mode Contrast in aorta and pulmonary arteries Neck to renal arteries	All chest disease
CT angiogram	CTA	Helical mode Post IVI 20- to 30-second delay Maximum contrast in aorta Neck to aortic bifurcation	Aortic disease: —aneurysm, dissection, coarctation Neck vessel disease: —occlusion, dissection Coronary artery disease Arteriovenous malformation Pulmonary sequestration SVC obstruction
CT pulmonary angiogram	CTPA	Post IVI 20-second delay Helical mode Maximum contrast in pulmonary trunk	Pulmonary artery disease Pulmonary embolism
CT perfusion		Post IVI at time intervals Helical mode Neck to aortic bifurcation	Arteriovenous malformations Nodule characterization
Cardiac CT	CCT	Post IVI 30-second delay Helical mode Maximum contrast in aorta Neck to cardiac apex	Coronary artery disease

CT, computed tomography; IV, intravenous; IVI, intravenous injection; SVC, superior vena cava.

Box 5-4

Systematic interpretation of chest CT

Patient demographics
- Name and other details

Technical review
- Non-contrast CT (NCCT)
- Contrast-enhanced CT (CECT)
- Clarify phase of contrast when scan performed:
  - » CT angiogram, CT pulmonary angiogram, routine

Initial image review
- Review the topogram (scanogram)
- Identify and review mediastinal and lung windows:
  - » axial followed by coronal
- Identify the first and last scans
- Conduct fast survey of all images (mediastinal and lung windows)

Key image review
- Review key images:
  - » thyroid
  - » aortic arch
  - » pulmonary arteries and carina
  - » hila
  - » four chambers of heart
  - » diaphragm

Systematic review
- Sequential assessment of all images:
  - » lung apices to sub-diaphragm abdomen
  - » trachea, mainstem and lobar bronchi
  - » pulmonary trunk, right and left pulmonary arteries
  - » aorta and branches
  - » superior vena cava
- Lung parenchyma
- Pleural surfaces, lung fissures
- Esophagus
- Heart, pericardium
- Diaphragm, retrocrural contents
- Skeletal, including spine, ribs, sternum, scapula

Review areas
- Thyroid gland
- Supraclavicular fossae and axillae
- Apices
- Mediastinal lymph nodes
- Sub-diaphragmatic organs and spaces

Summary
- Comparison with previous studies
- Correlation of findings and probable diagnosis
- Need for additional imaging

CT, computed tomography.

Patient demographics

Name, date of study and some scanning parameters can give diagnostic clues and the clinical relevance of the study.

Technical review

Identification of the vascular phase in which the images have been acquired should be done early in the diagnostic process by identifying the location and density of contrast within the superior vena cava, heart chambers, pulmonary arteries and aorta.

- Maximum density in the right ventricle and pulmonary arteries is expected in a CTPA, in the left ventricle and aorta in a CTA, and in all cardiac chambers, aorta and pulmonary vessels in a routine CT scan of the chest.
- Absence of contrast in any structure may be due to a NCCT, extravasation, or superior vena caval or thoracic outlet obstruction.

Initial image review

An overview can quickly identify major abnormalities and help focus the interpretation. This can be achieved with an initial four-step analysis.

1. Review the topogram (scanogram)

The image depicts the chest as a frontal chest X-ray, with at least 10% of diagnoses such as pleural effusion, mass and consolidation being visible.

2. Identify and review mediastinal and lung windows

Images depicting the lung parenchyma ('lung window') and mediastinal contents ('mediastinal window') are recognized in axial and coronal planes.

- Lung windows are photographically lighter and clearly demonstrate the branching vessels, bronchi, fissures and lung tissue.
- Mediastinal windows have black, featureless lung fields with clear definition of the mediastinal contents including the thyroid, trachea, superior vena cava, aorta and its branches, lymph nodes, esophagus, heart and pericardium.

3. Identify the first and last scans

Defining the upper and lower limits of the scan gives an overview of the anatomy to be reviewed and what has been excluded.

4. Conduct fast survey of all images (mediastinal and lung windows)

Rapid sequential review of all images provides the opportunity to appreciate gross abnormalities and normal anatomy.

Key image review

Isolating key levels in the chest can initially simplify interpretation (Table 5-6).

Table 5-6 Key landmarks in CT chest imaging

ANATOMY	MEDIASTINAL WINDOW	LUNG WINDOW
THYROID GLAND 1. Thyroid gland 2. Internal jugular vein 3. Common carotid artery 4. Trachea 5. Thoracic vertebra, T2		
AORTIC ARCH 1. Aortic arch 2. Superior vena cava 3. Trachea 4. Esophagus 5. Thymus 6. Sternum 7. Scapula 8. Pulmonary vessels 9. Oblique fissure 10. Anterior junction line 11. Upper lobe		
PULMONARY ARTERIES 1. Pulmonary trunk 2. Right pulmonary artery 3. Left pulmonary artery 4. Carina 5. Right main bronchus 6. Left main bronchus 7. Ascending aorta 8. Superior vena cava 9. Descending aorta 10. Esophagus 11. Oblique fissure 12. Lower lobe		
HEART 1. Right atrium 2. Right ventricle 3. Interventricular septum 4. Left ventricle 5. Left atrium 6. Pulmonary vein 7. Lower lobe bronchus 8. Descending aorta 9. Esophagus 10. Oblique fissure 11. Right middle lobe 12. Lower lobe		

continues

Table 5-6 Key landmarks in CT chest imaging *continued*

ANATOMY	MEDIASTINAL WINDOW	LUNG WINDOW
DIAPHRAGM 1. Right atrium 2. Right ventricle 3. Interventricular septum 4. Left ventricle 5. Descending aorta 6. Esophagus 7. Oblique fissure 8. Lower lobe 9. Lingula 10. Right middle lobe		
SUB-DIAPHRAGM 1. Liver, right lobe 2. Liver, left lobe 3. Stomach 4. Spleen 5. Inferior vena cava 6. Descending aorta 7. Lower lobes of lungs		

Thyroid gland

Beginning in the neck, the thyroid is marked by its high density due to its iodine content surrounding the trachea. A common routine is to then observe the trachea and its adjacent structures on sequential scans through to the carina and into the main stem bronchi.

Aortic arch

The transverse aorta dominates the image as an oblique right-to-left tubular structure. Branches to the neck and arms can be identified. A high concentration of contrast in the superior vena cava is visible to the right of the arch.

Pulmonary arteries and carina

The distinct Y-shaped structure of the pulmonary trunk originating out of the right ventricle and branching into the left and right pulmonary arteries lies immediately inferior to the aortic arch, separated by the aorto-pulmonary window. The trachea dominates this level where it bifurcates at the carina and the main stem bronchi diverge to the hilum.

Four chambers of the heart

The oblique long axis of the interventricular septum and cardiac apex are identified. Situated posteriorly behind the ventricles, the left atrium receives the pulmonary veins while the right atrium receives the superior and inferior vena cava. The normal pericardium is defined as a line 1 mm or less separated from the myocardium by a layer of fat.

Diaphragm

The dome of the diaphragm initially appears in the anterior to central hemithorax and then merges toward the lateral chest margin. At the posterior inferior extent of the diaphragm attachment, the crura become apparent near T12–L1 and the retrocrural space becomes identifiable where lymph nodes, cisterna chyli and azygous veins are located.

Systematic review

All images and their contents are systematically reviewed in both lung and mediastinal windows, initially on axial images and then on coronal images.

Review areas

At the end of interpretation, a last review of some key but often overlooked areas is undertaken.

- The thyroid gland is frequently abnormal, such as goiter, and effects on the superior mediastinal contents and trachea are common.
- Review of the neck, supraclavicular, axillary and mediastinal regions for lymphadenopathy requires careful scrutiny.
- The lung apices need to be re-inspected for pleural thickening, tuberculosis, lung bullae and Pancoast tumor.
- Sub-diaphragmatic organs such as the liver, spleen, pancreas, adrenal glands and kidneys are important to assess.
- Finally, select a bone window setting and review the skeleton for abnormalities such as fractures and neoplastic lesions.

Summary

Following the systematic review, relevant positive and negative findings can be correlated and final statements made. If contrast has not been administered appropriately for the clinical question being investigated and is deemed suboptimal this should be noted. Correlation of any findings with previous and additional imaging is also performed.

3. ABDOMINAL COMPUTED TOMOGRAPHY

A CT scan of the abdomen has similar advantages and disadvantages to chest CT. The use of oral contrast is considered integral to most examinations other than in acute emergencies, identification of renal system calculi and some selected organ evaluations such as that of the adrenal gland.

TECHNIQUES OF EXAMINATION

Different CT techniques are employed in specific clinical situations (Table 5-7).

Table 5-7 Common techniques in CT scans of the abdomen

EXAMINATION	ACRONYM	TECHNIQUE	INDICATION
Non-contrast CT	NCCT	No IV contrast Helical mode Supine Suspended inspiration Lung base to symphysis pubis	Contrast contraindication Poor venous access Identify calcification: —calculi —tuberculous granuloma —calcified lymph nodes —tumor calcification Gas: —pneumoperitoneum —pneumatosis intestinalis —emphysematous cholecystitis —intrahepatic gas —pneumothorax Fat—lipoma, myelolipoma Bone disease Foreign body detection
Non-contrast CT KUB	CT KUB	No IV contrast Non-helical, thin section Supine inspiration Supplemental prone scan if stone at VUJ Lung base to symphysis pubis	Renal calculi Same as for NCCT above
CT angiogram	CTA	Helical mode Post IVI 20-second delay Maximum contrast in aorta No oral contrast Lung base to symphysis pubis	Aortic disease: —aneurysm, dissection, coarctation Vessel disease: —occlusion, dissection Arteriovenous malformation IVC obstruction/fistula
Portal venous CT	CTPV	Helical mode Post IVI 50- to 70-second delay Maximum contrast in portal vein No oral contrast Lung base to symphysis pubis	Routine abdominal study Solid organ disease Obstruction of ducts Portal vein disease
Triple-phase abdominal CT	CTTP	Helical mode Three sequential studies obtained: —non-contrast —arterial —portal venous May add additional delayed study	Lesion characterization—liver, adrenal, renal Organ necrosis—pancreas Gastrointestinal hemorrhage
Delayed phase CT	CTD	Helical mode Delayed study 2–5 minutes or longer	Renal collecting system obstruction Active bleeding sites Liver lesions

CT, computed tomography; IV, intravenous; IVC, inferior vena cava; IVI, intravenous injection; KUB, kidneys–ureters–bladder; VUJ, vesico-ureteric junction.

Non-contrast CT abdomen

The study is performed from above the diaphragm to the inferior aspect of the symphysis pubis. No contrast is found in the aorta, inferior vena cava, portal vein or the kidneys, rendering them isodense with the adjacent organs.

Non-contrast CT KUB

A variation of a non-contrast abdominal CT is performed for the assessment of renal colic, focusing on the *kidneys, ureters* and *bladder* (KUB). Image acquisition is performed from the upper poles of the kidneys to the symphysis pubis, rather than going as high as the lung bases. Intravenous and oral contrast are not given as these can obscure opaque calculi.

Arterial phase CT abdomen (CT angiogram, CTA)

Image acquisition is performed 20–30 seconds post-injection, capturing contrast in the arterial system. Aneurysms, stenoses, occlusions and bleeding sites can be depicted.

Portal venous CT abdomen

Contrast perfuses the abdominal viscera and drains back to the portal vein and liver. This produces prominent enhancement of the liver parenchyma.

Triple-phase CT abdomen

Three successive scans are performed—non-contrast, arterial and portal venous—usually of the upper abdomen for the pancreas and liver. These are most commonly employed in the evaluation of liver, pancreatic and intestinal masses.

Delayed CT abdomen

A delayed study of 2–5 minutes allows contrast to accumulate in the collecting system of the kidneys, ureters and bladder, to assess lesions such as tumors and lacerations. Pooling in the intestine may be identified as a sign of hemorrhage.

PRINCIPLES OF INTERPRETATION IN ABDOMINAL CT

CT scans of the abdomen produce a large number of images to review in different planes. A systematic routine is necessary to avoid diagnostic error and maximize the derivation of information (Box 5-5).

Patient demographics

Name, date of study and some scanning parameters can give diagnostic clues and the clinical relevance of the study.

Technical review

The phase of vascular contrast can be identified by the location and density of contrast within the aorta, portal vein and

---

Box 5-5

Systematic interpretation of abdominal CT

Patient demographics
- Name and other details

Technical review
- Non-contrast CT (NCCT)
- Contrast-enhanced CT (CECT)
- Clarify phase of contrast when scan performed:
  » NCCT, CT KUB, CTA, PVCT, DCT, TPCT

Initial image review
- Review the topogram (scanogram)
- Identify axial and then coronal images
- Identify the first (lung bases) and last (lower pelvis) images
- Conduct fast survey of all images

Key image review
- Lung bases
- Liver, porta hepatis
- Renal hilum
- Iliac crest
- Mid-pelvis
- Symphysis pubis

Systematic review
- Cephalo-caudad progression
- Organ-by-organ assessment
- Slice-by-slice assessment

Review areas
- Para-aortic and pelvic lymph nodes
- Inguinal canals
- Abdominal wall and iliopsoas
- Lung bases
- Pneumoperitoneum search
- Skeletal (spine, ribs, sternum, scapula, pelvis)

Summary
- Comparison with previous studies
- Correlation of findings and probable diagnosis
- Need for additional imaging

CT, computed tomography; CTA, CT angiogram; KUB, kidneys–ureters–bladder; PVCT, portal venous CT; TPCT, triple-phase CT.

---

kidneys (Table 5-8). Knowledge of the various techniques is pivotal in deriving the maximal information in different clinical scenarios. Maximum density in the aorta and its branches signifies an arterial phase acquisition (CTA), in the portal vein the portal venous phase (PVCT), and contrast in the renal pelvis a delayed study (DCT).

Table 5-8 General criteria for identifying contrast phase in CT scan of the abdomen

	NON-CONTRAST	ARTERIAL (20-SECOND DELAY)	PORTAL VENOUS (50- TO 70-SECOND DELAY)	DELAYED (2–5 MINUTES DELAY)
Aorta	Neutral	Very dense	Slightly dense	Neutral
Vena cava	Neutral	Neutral	Slightly dense	Neutral
Portal vein	Neutral	Neutral	Dense	Neutral
Kidneys	Neutral	Cortex dense	Cortex and medulla dense	Dense pelvis, ureters

Initial image review

An overview can quickly identify major abnormalities and help focus the interpretation. This can be achieved with an initial four-step analysis.

1. Review the topogram (scanogram)

The image depicts the abdomen as a frontal abdominal X-ray with at least 10% of diagnoses such as obstruction and calculus being visible. Given its wide range of coverage, usually beyond that of the axial image acquisitions, incidental abnormalities of the lung bases, such as pleural effusion and masses, as well as those in the thighs can be seen.

2. Identify axial and coronal images

Axial images are recognizable by the depiction of organs in cross-section. There are fewer images in the coronal plane and these demonstrate the abdominal contents as an abdominal X-ray; for an overview it is often useful to review these first.

3. Identify the first and last scans

The upper limit of the scan is recognizable by the low-attenuating lung fields and their gradual reduction as the diaphragm comes into the image plane. The lowest extent of the scan, through to the pelvis, should be at least to the symphysis pubis to include the bladder and ano-rectal junction.

4. Conduct fast survey of all images

Rapid sequential review of all images, initially in the coronal plane, provides the opportunity to appreciate normal anatomy and gross abnormalities such as bowel obstruction, masses, aortic aneurysm and free fluid.

Key image review

It can be useful, especially for the inexperienced reader, to be able to identify a few key images and be familiar with their contents (Table 5-9, overleaf).

Lung bases

- With mediastinal window settings, the basal lung fields are black with very little vascular structure visible. The heart is typically evident, with the right and left ventricles separated by the interventricular septum. The aorta and esophagus are visible.
- On lung windows, the branching pulmonary vessels and bronchi are displayed.

Liver, porta hepatis

- The hallmark of the porta hepatis is contrast within the portal vein arcing over the inferior vena cava.
- The right and left lobes of the liver are usually identifiable, but the separating falciform ligament may not be evident at this level.
- The upper poles of both kidneys, the spleen, stomach and body of the pancreas are typically present at this level.

Renal hilum

- Both kidneys at their hilum in the portal venous phase show contrast in the draining renal veins entering into the inferior vena cava.
- The aorta is evident to the left side of the L3 vertebra.
- The inferior aspect of the right lobe of the liver dominates the right side.

Table 5-9 CT of the abdomen—key images

KEY IMAGE LEVEL	NORMAL	ABNORMAL
LUNG BASE—LUNG WINDOW 1. Right ventricle 2. Left ventricle 3. Right atrium 4. Descending aorta 5. Esophagus 6. Lower lobes of lungs		 Lung metastases (arrows)
LUNG BASE—ABDOMINAL WINDOW 1. Right ventricle 2. Left ventricle 3. Right atrium 4. Descending aorta 5. Lower lobes of lungs		 Pleural effusion (arrow) and pericardial effusion (arrowhead)
PORTA HEPATIS 1. Portal vein 2. Liver, right lobe 3. Liver, left lobe 4. Liver, caudate lobe 5. Stomach 6. Pancreas, tail 7. Pancreas, body 8. Spleen 9. Kidney 10. Aorta		 Liver cirrhosis (A), ascites (B) and splenomegaly (C)
RENAL HILUM 1. Renal hilum 2. Renal vein 3. Kidney 4. Inferior vena cava 5. Aorta 6. Superior mesenteric vein 7. Pancreas, head 8. Liver, right lobe 9. Stomach 10. Descending colon 11. Jejunum		 Transitional cell carcinoma, renal pelvis (arrow)

KEY IMAGE LEVEL	NORMAL	ABNORMAL
ILIAC CREST 1. Iliac crest 2. Right kidney 3. Psoas muscle 4. Aorta 5. Inferior vena cava 6. Cecum 7. Liver, right lobe 8 Colon, hepatic flexure 9. Jejunum 10. Descending colon		 Aortic aneurysm (arrow) with rupture (arrowhead)
MID-PELVIS 1. Bladder 2. Uterus 3. Rectum 4. Acetabulum 5. Coccyx 6. Gluteus maximus 7. Common femoral vein 8. Common femoral artery		 Carcinoma of the bladder (arrow)
SYMPHYSIS PUBIS 1. Rectum, anus 2. Cervix 3. Retropubic space 4. Symphysis pubis 5. Ischio-rectal fossa 6. Obturator internus 7. Gluteal crease 8. Gluteus maximus 9. Ischium 10. Femur 11. Femoral vein 12. Femoral artery		 Plasmacytoma, right pubis (arrows)

- The upper origins of the psoas muscle abut the posterior margin of both kidneys with an interposed layer of perinephric fat.

Iliac crest

- The ascending and descending colon and variable loops of the small bowel fill the majority of the anterior and lateral aspects of the abdomen.
- The inferior vena cava and the aorta lie anterior to the spine, and on occasions the aortic bifurcation becomes evident as two common iliac artery branches.
- The psoas muscle is readily identified, flanking the L4 vertebral body.
- Variably visible in many normal individuals, dependent on body habitus and degree of inspiration, will be the lower aspect of the right lobe of the liver and lower pole of the right kidney.

Mid-pelvis

- At the level of the hip joints, the thin-walled bladder lies in the midline anteriorly.
- In females the uterus is a solid structure sited anterior to the rectum.
- The external iliac artery and vein bilaterally lie lateral to the bladder, as does the muscle of the obturator internus.

Symphysis pubis

- The joint cavity of the symphysis pubis is a reliable indicator of an image low in the pelvis, with fat identifiable in the retropubic space. The anus and rectum are readily identifiable, and in males the prostate gland.
- The distinctive fat-filled ischio-rectal fossa flanked by the obturator internus, puborectalis and gluteus maximus is apparent.

Box 5-6

Clinical utility of ultrasound

Advantages

- Allows point examination in region of interest
- Performed in real time
- Non-ionizing radiation
- No contrast agents are employed
- Little to no patient preparation

Disadvantages

- Poor detail of air/gas structures (lung, bowel)
- Limited bone and intra-articular detail
- Not suitable for all patients
- Interpretation unfriendly
- Incomplete display of all anatomy/pathology
- Operator-dependent
- Can be time-consuming

Systematic review

Begin at the lung bases and progressively move caudally. Initially, an organ-by-organ assessment is done. Follow this with a slice-by-slice analysis with all depicted structures in the slice reviewed.

- With vascular structures such as the aorta and inferior vena cava, with their branches, selecting them for specific review by observing them over sequential slices is the best method.
- The colon is analyzed by beginning either at the cecum or the rectum and following the colon over sequential images. Due to its multiplicity of convolutions, the small bowel is similarly assessed from the duodenum or cecum.

Review areas

At the end of the interpretation, a last review of some key and often overlooked areas is undertaken.

- Lymph node evaluation is often neglected; specific locations need to be sought for, including para-aortic, aorto-caval, retrocrural, pelvic and inguinal regions.
- Inspecting the lower pelvic scans to exclude inguinal hernias can then be done.
- Scrutinize the abdominal wall and iliopsoas muscles for collections and abscess.
- As a last procedure, changing the image display to 'lung windows' demonstrates the lung parenchyma to view such abnormalities as pleural effusion, pneumothorax, masses and collapse. By reviewing the entire abdomen with this 'lung window', pneumoperitoneum can be confirmed. Select a 'bone window' setting to identify abnormalities such as fractures and neoplastic lesions.

Summary

Following the systematic review, relevant positive and negative findings can be correlated and final statements made. If contrast has not been administered appropriately for the clinical question being investigated and is deemed suboptimal, this should be noted. Correlation of any findings with previous and additional imaging is also performed.

Box 5-7

Contraindications for ultrasound

Obesity

Muscular body habitus

Excessive abdominal gas

Uncooperative patient

Inability to follow breathing instructions

Inability to suspend respiration

Large open wounds

Topical surgical dressings and drains

Unskilled operator and diagnostician

4. ABDOMINAL ULTRASOUND

Diagnostic ultrasound is a safe and rapid imaging technique. It is non-invasive, usually painless, and requires no contrast medium and limited or no patient preparation (Box 5-6). Not all patients are able to undergo ultrasound (Box 5-7).

BACKGROUND—ULTRASOUND PRINCIPLES

Ultrasound waves from a transducer pass through the underlying body tissues and are reflected back as returning 'echoes'. The time it takes for a generated wave to enter and then return is converted to a depth below the probe, while the number of returning echoes is converted to a displayed density ('echogenicity') which may be black, white or one of many shades of gray.

- Tissues which allow for through-transmission with little echo are displayed black ('hypo-echoic, anechoic').
- High numbers of returning echoes are displayed white ('hyper-echoic, echogenic').

Each organ is examined in the longitudinal and transverse planes (see Box 5-8 for an overview of the assessment procedure).

Box 5-8
Systematic interpretation of abdominal ultrasound

Patient demographics
- Name and other patient details

Technical assessment
- Longitudinal and transverse images
- Doppler examinations
- Patient position (erect, decubitus)

Anatomical review
- Overview
  » Gross perception
- Systematic organ review
  » Pancreas, liver, biliary ducts, gallbladder
  » Right and left kidneys, bladder
  » Spleen
  » Flanks, lung bases, pelvic contents

Summary
- Correlate organ findings
- Compare with previous study/other imaging

PRINCIPLES OF ULTRASOUND INTERPRETATION

Interpretation of ultrasound images initially appears confusing and daunting to the uninitiated. Applying basic principles will simplify interpretation, and with practice provides a framework for better understanding (Table 5–10).

Table 5-10 Ultrasound anatomy and pathological correlations

ANATOMY	NORMAL	ABNORMAL
LIVER METASTASES	Homogeneous liver parenchyma Smooth surface Normal branching portal vein (arrow)	Multiple hypo-echoic round masses (arrows) Mass effect on portal vessels
LIVER HEMANGIOMA	Homogeneous liver parenchyma Smooth surface Normal branching portal vein	Solitary round hyper-echoic mass (arrow) Peripheral vascularity

continues

Table 5-10 Ultrasound anatomy and pathological correlations *continued*

ANATOMY	NORMAL	ABNORMAL
LIVER DILATED BILIARY DUCTS	 Bile ducts not visible Normal portal vein branches visible	 Dilated ducts (arrows) Converge at the porta
LIVER CIRRHOSIS WITH ASCITES	 Smooth liver edge Sharp echogenic perihepatic fat interface	 Hypo-echoic perihepatic fluid (F) Nodular cirrhotic nodules (arrow)
PORTAL VEIN THROMBOSIS	 Doppler examination Flow direction toward the liver (arrow) Good wave above neutral flow line (arrowhead)	 Echogenic clot in portal vein (arrow) Very little flow detected (arrowhead)
GALLBLADDER CALCULI	 Thin-walled, hypo-echoic gallbladder (GB) Posterior acoustic enhancement	 Cholelithiasis with echogenic surfaces (arrows) Posterior acoustic shadowing (arrowheads) Thick-walled gallbladder (W) Pericholecystic fluid

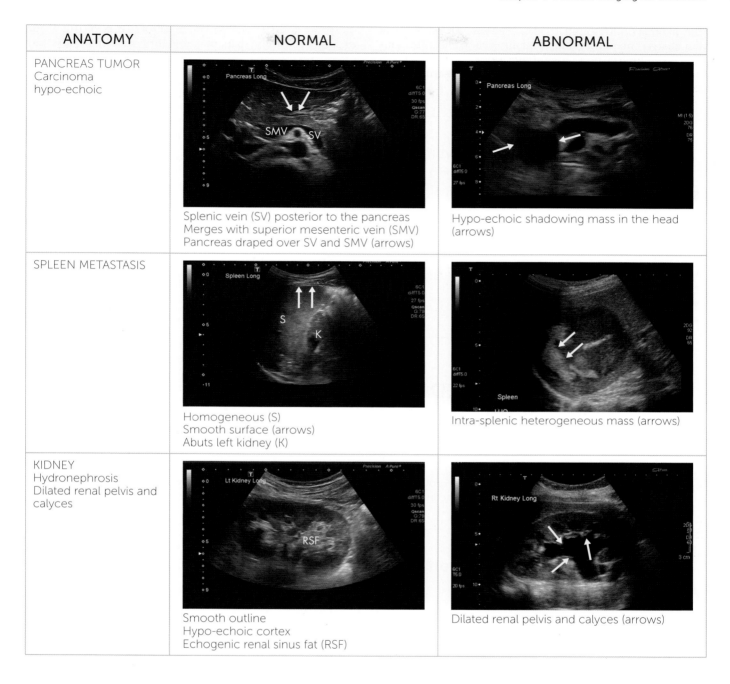

ANATOMY	NORMAL	ABNORMAL
PANCREAS TUMOR Carcinoma hypo-echoic	Splenic vein (SV) posterior to the pancreas Merges with superior mesenteric vein (SMV) Pancreas draped over SV and SMV (arrows)	Hypo-echoic shadowing mass in the head (arrows)
SPLEEN METASTASIS	Homogeneous (S) Smooth surface (arrows) Abuts left kidney (K)	Intra-splenic heterogeneous mass (arrows)
KIDNEY Hydronephrosis Dilated renal pelvis and calyces	Smooth outline Hypo-echoic cortex Echogenic renal sinus fat (RSF)	Dilated renal pelvis and calyces (arrows)

LOWER LIMB DUPLEX ULTRASOUND

Ultrasound is the 'gold standard' for identifying deep vein thrombosis (DVT), with sensitivity and specificity of greater than 95%. Patients with large calves, edematous calves, small vessels, marked skin sensitivity and pain limit the sensitivity of the study below the knee.

Duplex ultrasound is called 'duplex' because the veins are examined in two ways—structurally and flow ('Doppler').

- Each vein is imaged systematically in transverse and longitudinal planes, with and without compression.
- Doppler examination is then performed in quiet respiration and with calf compression ('augmentation') to confirm lack of blood movement when thrombosis occludes the vessel lumen. Both deep veins (external iliac, common and superficial femoral, popliteal, soleal and posterior tibial veins) and superficial veins (lesser and greater saphenous) are imaged.

The hallmark ultrasound triad of venous thrombosis is a vein that is incompressible, contains echogenic thrombus and lacks Doppler flow. Identifying DVT mimics, such as cellulitis, inguinal hernia, Baker's cyst and gastrocnemius tear, is important (Box 5-9).

Box 5-9

Ultrasound criteria for deep vein thrombosis (DVT)

Structural
- Incompressible vein
- Intraluminal thrombus
- Intraluminal echoes

Doppler
- No flow at rest
- No respiratory phasic flow fluctuation
- No augmented flow with calf compression

---

5. HEAD COMPUTED TOMOGRAPHY

CT scans of the brain are performed in a wide variety of clinical scenarios and are frequently pivotal in determining management. Selection of patients to undergo CT studies of the brain needs to be based on clear clinical grounds and an awareness of its deficiencies in diagnostic accuracy and radiation dose, as well as other factors (Box 5-10). Prior to any CT study, patient suitability should be assessed (Table 5-11).

CT BRAIN PROTOCOLS

Non-contrast (NCCT)
A CT brain study without contrast is the most common protocol to be used.
- It has high sensitivity for acute blood, whether this be extradural, subdural, subarachnoid, intracerebral or intraventricular, depicted as increased density. The increased density of acute blood is primarily due to clot retraction.
- Hydrocephalus, tumors, midline shift and features of cerebral edema can quickly and accurately be determined.

Contrast-enhanced (CECT)
Intravenous injection (IVI) of iodinated contrast increases the sensitivity for demonstration of brain pathology from 10% to 50%. Any lesion which induces increased vascular permeability and disrupts the blood–brain barrier will show enhancement ('MAGIC DR'; see Box 5-11).

CT angiography (CTA)
Image acquisition when contrast is maximal in the aorta opacifies the neck and intracranial arteries for the purpose of identifying stenoses, aneurysm, occlusions and other vascular disorders.

Box 5-10

Clinical utility of CT scans of the brain

Advantages
- Fast
  - » Rapid diagnosis
  - » Fewer motion artifacts
- Broad patient compatibility
- Body habitus, claustrophobia, metal implants
- Readily available
- Reader-friendly
- High sensitivity in acute intra-cerebral conditions
  - » Trauma, hemorrhage, midline shift, seizure
- CTA studies without complications of digital subtraction angiography (DSA) catheter
  - » Iatrogenic vascular and embolic disease
- Accurate base study for comparison
  - » Disease progression/complication/regression
  - » Multiplanar reconstructions

Disadvantages
- Radiation dose
  - » Acute injury, accumulated dose, pregnancy, cancer
- Complications of iodine contrast
  - » Anaphylaxis, allergy, renal failure, vasovagal
- False sense of security
- Premature termination of search
- Insensitive for infarction in first 4–24 hours
- Inconspicuous lesions not identified
  - » Small size, <1 cm—neuroma, aneurysm
  - » Isodense lesions to brain—subacute subdural/subarachnoid hemorrhage
  - » Leptomeningeal disease—meningitis, metastatic disease
  - » Diffuse disease—white matter: leukoencephalopathy, demyelination
  - » Hidden locations—vertex: high convexity; floor of middle cranial fossa; posterior fossa; foramen magnum

CTA, CT angiogram.

Table 5-11 Patient preparation checklist prior to CT

ITEM	RATIONALE
Definite CT scan indications	Correct modality selection, ensure coverage of correct area, correct scan technique
Assess need for contrast	Tumor, infection, CTA (aneurysm, arteriovenous malformation, occlusion)
Claustrophobia screening	Motion artifact, inability to complete the scan
Pregnancy screening	To avoid unnecessary radiation to the developing fetus
Renal function	May prevent administration of intravenous (IV) contrast to avoid renal failure
Contrast allergy	May prevent administration of IV contrast to avoid allergic reactions
Patient compliance	Any motion during scanning creates motion artifact image degradation
Patient safety	Vital sign assessment and in-scanner monitoring supervised when needed
Review of previous imaging	Assess cumulative radiation doses; identify abnormalities to guide present scan

---

Box 5-11

Differential diagnosis for contrast-enhanced brain lesions

'MAGIC DR'

M Metastasis, meningioma

A Abscess

G Glioma

I Infarct

C Contusion

D Demyelination

R Radiation

Perfusion CT

Rapid sequential brain scanning following IV contrast injection allows cerebral perfusion maps to be generated; these depict cerebral blood flow (CBF), cerebral blood volume (CBV) and mean transit time (MTT). From these maps, cerebral ischemia and infarction can be quantified.

PRINCIPLES OF INTERPRETATION IN BRAIN CT

Accurate interpretation of CT scans of the brain is based on knowledge of brain anatomy, key landmarks and development of a systematic approach (Box 5-12).

Box 5-12

Systematic interpretation of brain CT

Patient demographics
- Name and other details

Technical review
- Non-contrast CT (NCCT)
- Contrast-enhanced CT (CECT)

Initial image review
- Review the topogram (scanogram)
- Identify the first and last scans
- Conduct fast assessment of *all* images
- Identify normal calcifications
  » Pineal, choroid plexus, falx

Key image review
- Foramen magnum
- Posterior fossa
- Pituitary fossa
- Suprasellar
- Internal capsule—basal ganglia
- Lateral ventricles
- Vertex

Systematic review
- Sequential assessment of *all* images
  » Base to vertex

Review areas
- Brainstem
- Craniocervical junction
- Foramen magnum
- Mastoid sinuses
- Middle ear complex
- Orbits and contents
- Nasopharynx
- Bone—calvarium, skull base

Summary
- Comparison with previous studies
- Correlation of findings and probable diagnosis
- Need for additional imaging

Patient demographics

Name, date of study and some scanning parameters can give diagnostic clues and the clinical relevance of the study.

Technical review

Identifying whether contrast has been given and what vascular phase is being demonstrated allows specific details to be observed. Contrast in the circle of Willis may identify an aneurysm or arteriovenous malformation. A delayed contrast scan can depict a ring-enhancing lesion.

Initial image review

Early in the interpretive process it is crucial to gain an overview and quickly identify major abnormalities. This can be achieved with an initial four-step analysis.

1. Review the topogram (scanogram)

- The lateral view of the skull, at a minimum, is available for review, and skull fractures, calcifications and bony lesions can be identified.

- Intubation tubes confirm the acute status of the patient.
- Identify the atlanto-axial relationships to exclude unexpected dislocation or fracture.

2. Identify the first and last scans

This confirms the cephalad and caudad anatomy that has been included in the study, to ensure adequate coverage.

3. Conduct fast assessment of all images

Especially with digital viewing, a sequential, rapid display of each image is possible and will allow an appreciation of gradual changes in anatomy and the perception of gross pathology such as masses, bleeds, hydrocephalus and midline shift.

4. Identify normal calcifications

Physiological calcifications in the brain are common, especially of the pineal gland, choroid plexus and falx cerebri, and should be identified early so as to not be misconstrued as abnormalities (Table 5-12).

Table 5-12 Normal variant intracranial calcifications

LOCATION	AGE (Y)	INCIDENCE	DESCRIPTION	CT	DIFFERENTIAL DIAGNOSIS
PINEAL GLAND	10–90	<40 y: 60% >40 y: 100%	Dense Midline <1 cm Roof of aqueduct		Curvilinear–circular —aneurysm, cyst Dense, >1 cm —germinoma
CHOROID PLEXUS	10–90	>50 y: 100%	Bilateral Dense Arc-like Midline divergence Lateral ventricle Trigone		Focal dense calcification —papilloma —carcinoma

LOCATION	AGE (Y)	INCIDENCE	DESCRIPTION	CT	DIFFERENTIAL DIAGNOSIS
FALX CEREBRI	10–90	>50 y: 100%	Midline Thin Peripherally denser Often discontinuous		Focal thickening —meningioma Generalized thickening —subdural hematoma —venous thrombosis
TENTORIUM CEREBELLI	>40	>40 y: 50%	Thin Often discontinuous Petrous apex to posterior clinoid ('petro-clinoid ligament')		Focal thickening —meningioma Generalized thickening —subdural hematoma
BASAL GANGLIA	>60	>60 y: 10%	Fine, granular sand-like calcifications Basal ganglia lentiform nucleus		<60 y: metabolic disease Calcium: hyperpara-thyroidism Iron: Farr's disease Manganese: Hallervorden-Spatz disease
DENTATE NUCLEUS	>60	>60 y: 10%	Fine, granular sand-like calcifications Dentate nucleus of the cerebellum, usually bilaterally		<60 y: metabolic disease Hyperpara-thyroidism

continues

Table 5-12 Normal variant intracranial calcifications *continued*

LOCATION	AGE (Y)	INCIDENCE	DESCRIPTION	CT	DIFFERENTIAL DIAGNOSIS
HYPER-OSTOSIS FRONTALIS	>40	>60 y: 100%	Dense ossification Frontal bone Inner table Thickness 5–15 mm External cortex 'Tide-line' on inner table		Paget's disease —patchy sclerosis in dipole —broad lucent zone —cortical thickening

Key image review

To simplify the many structures and landmarks depicted on CT images, isolation of the following key image planes can simplify interpretation (Table 5–13).

Table 5-13 CT brain anatomy and pathological correlations

CT LANDMARKS	NORMAL	ABNORMAL	COMMON ABNORMALITIES
TOPOGRAM 1. Frontal bone 2. Parietal bone 3. Occipital bone 4. Sella turcica 5. Sphenoid sinus			Bone: —fracture —metastasis —myeloma —hemangioma —Paget's disease Brain: —calcifying tumor —meningioma (arrow) —oligodendroglioma —craniopharyngioma —pituitary mass —aneurysm
FORAMEN MAGNUM 1. Foramen magnum 2. Clivus 3. Medulla 4. Vertebral artery 5. Subarachnoid space 6. Ethmoid sinus 7. Nasal bones 8. Globe			Tumor: —glioma —meningioma Subarachnoid space: —coning (arrows) —hemorrhage Skull base tumor: —chordoma —glomus tumor

Table 5-13 CT brain anatomy and pathological correlations *continued*

CT LANDMARKS	NORMAL	ABNORMAL	COMMON ABNORMALITIES
POSTERIOR FOSSA 1. Cerebellum 2. Pons 3. Fourth ventricle 4. Petrous temporal bone 5. Temporal lobe 6. Cavernous sinus 7. Sphenoid sinus 8. Cribriform plate 9. Greater wing of sphenoid 10. Optic nerve			Bone: —metastasis —chondrosarcoma Cerebellum: —infarction —hemorrhage —glioma Pons: —basilar artery aneurysm —glioma —hemorrhage (arrow) Cerebello-pontine angle: —acoustic neuroma —subarachnoid hemorrhage Fourth ventricle: —intraventricular hemorrhage —ependymoma
PITUITARY FOSSA 1. Internal occipital protuberance 2. Cerebellum 3. Pons 4. Fourth ventricle 5. Cerebello-pontine cistern 6. Sigmoid venous sinus 7. Basilar artery 8. Posterior clinoid process 9. Sella turcica (pituitary fossa) 10. Temporal lobe 11. Gyrus rectus, frontal lobe 12. Orbital plate 13. Frontal sinus			Pituitary: —tumor —hemorrhage (arrow) Bone: —metastasis —chondrosarcoma Cerebellum: —infarction —hemorrhage —glioma Pons: —basilar artery aneurysm —glioma —hemorrhage Cerebello-pontine angle: —acoustic neuroma —subarachnoid hemorrhage Fourth ventricle —intraventricular hemorrhage —ependymoma
SUPRASELLAR 1. Venous confluence 2. Cerebellum, hemisphere 3. Cerebellum, vermis 4. Transverse venous sinus 5. Midbrain 6. Interpeduncular cistern 7. Basilar artery 8. Temporal lobe 9. Sylvian fissure 10. Frontal lobe			Cerebellum: —infarction —hemorrhage —glioma Midbrain: —tip of basilar aneurysm —glioma —subarachnoid hemorrhage (arrows) Frontal lobe: —glioma —infarction —hemorrhage Temporal lobe: —glioma —infarction —hemorrhage

continues

Table 5-13 CT brain anatomy and pathological correlations *continued*

CT LANDMARKS	NORMAL	ABNORMAL	COMMON ABNORMALITIES
BASAL GANGLIA 1. Occipital lobe 2. Posterior falx 3. Pineal gland 4. Third ventricle 5. Frontal horn, lateral ventricle 6. Septum pellucidum 7. Corpus callosum 8. Anterior falx 9. Caudate nucleus, head 10. Lentiform nucleus 11. Internal capsule, anterior limb 12. Internal capsule, genu 13. Internal capsule, posterior limb 14. External capsule 15. Insula 16. Sylvian fissure 17. Frontal lobe 18. Temporal lobe			Ventricles —hemorrhage —hydrocephalus —midline shift Cerebral hemisphere: —infarction (arrows) —hemorrhage —tumor —edema
LATERAL VENTRICLES 1. Body of lateral ventricle 2. Choroid plexus 3. White matter, corona radiata 4. Corpus callosum, genu 5. Corpus callosum, splenium 6. Posterior falx 7. Anterior falx 8. Frontal lobe 9. Parietal lobe			Ventricles: —hemorrhage (arrows) —hydrocephalus Cerebral hemisphere: —infarction —hemorrhage (arrowheads) —tumor —edema
VERTEX 1. Falx cerebri 2. Pre-central gyrus 3. Central sulcus 4. Post-central gyrus 5. Frontal lobe 6. Parietal lobe			Cerebral hemisphere: —infarction —hemorrhage (arrows) —tumor —edema (arrowhead) Falx —hemorrhage —meningioma —shift

Foramen magnum

- At the skull base, the large foramen magnum is readily identifiable.
- The medulla is centrally placed, flanked by the two vertebral arteries and surrounded by the low-attenuating cerebrospinal fluid (CSF).
- Loss of the subarachnoid space can be a sign of brainstem coning (see Table 5-13).

Posterior fossa

- The cerebellar hemispheres with the surface folia, superior cerebellar peduncle and fourth ventricle dominate the images.
- The transition from the smaller medulla to the larger pons is apparent, and the inferior aspect of the fourth ventricle comes into view.
- The cerebello-pontine angle is identifiable as a concave transition between the two structures and lies adjacent to the internal auditory meatus.

Pituitary fossa

The simultaneous depiction of the anterior, middle and posterior fossae produces a distinctive 'X' appearance, with the intersection at or adjacent to the pituitary fossa. The normal gland can be difficult to identify, although low-density CSF surrounds the pituitary stalk.

Suprasellar

Within a few images above the sella, the CSF density of the suprasellar cistern comes into view in which, even without contrast, the circle of Willis and its major branches can be defined. Subarachnoid hemorrhage often lies in this location as a high density.

Internal capsule—basal ganglia

- At this level, the distinctive periventricular bent band of low attenuation marking the internal capsule is surrounded by the higher-attenuating thalamus, lentiform and caudate nuclei.
- The Sylvian fissure delineates the temporal lobe.
- The lateral and third ventricles, cerebral aqueduct and corpus callosum dominate the midline structures.

Lateral ventricles

- The body of the lateral ventricle dominates this level.
- Additionally, the deep white matter of the corona radiata and sulci of the hemispheres are clearly visible.
- Both anterior and posterior edges of the falx, superior sagittal sinus and corpus callosum lie in the midline.

Vertex

- The distinctive thin, linear high density of the falx cerebri separates the two hemispheres.
- The dominant features of the hemispheres are the sulci and gyri as well as the gray and white matter. Each gyrus is surrounded by lower-attenuating sulci containing CSF.
- Gyral edema can erase the sulci, subarachnoid blood increases sulcal density, and sulcal widening is a sign of gyral atrophy.
- Subdural hemorrhage often is visible at this level.

Systematic review

Sequential assessment of all images from base to vertex can then follow, with attention to the same and other details.

Review areas

- Anatomical regions of the brain on CT require closer scrutiny, especially the brainstem.
- The transition from medulla to pons is marked by its increasing size and the appearance of the fourth ventricle.
- The midbrain is recognizable by its hallmark 'Mickey Mouse' appearance, with the 'ears' representing the cerebral peduncles, the 'nose' the cerebral aqueduct and the indented 'chin' the colliculi.
- Other regions requiring specific review include the craniocervical junction, foramen magnum, mastoid sinuses, middle ear complex, orbits and contents, nasopharynx and, importantly, 'bone windows' to evaluate the calvarium and skull base.

Summary

Following the systematic review, relevant positive and negative findings can be correlated and final statements made. If contrast has not been administered, its relevance for an additional study would be considered; as would an MRI study.

6. HEAD MAGNETIC RESONANCE

Magnetic resonance imaging (MRI, MR) is widely applied to many body systems and abnormalities including the brain, spine, joints, muscles, liver and biliary tree. MRI is the 'gold standard' for brain imaging and has a number of advantages over CT, especially regarding disease sensitivity and specificity (Box 5-13, overleaf). Safety issues for MRI are a major factor in many patients not able to undergo the study (Box 5-14, overleaf).

Box 5-13

Clinical utility of brain MRI

Advantages

- No ionizing radiation
- No demonstrable short-term or long-term complications
- Image in any plane ('multiplanar')
- High-resolution images for detail
- IV contrast often not required
- Vascular imaging without contrast (MRA, MRV)
- High sensitivity to neuronal disease and inflammation (DWI, IR)
- Characterizes chemical composition and metabolic activity (MRS)
- High sensitivity to hemosiderin as a marker of previous hemorrhage
- Differentiates acute from chronic disease (DWI)

Disadvantages

- Time-consuming
- Availability
- Higher cost
- Sequence selection specific
- Claustrophobia
- Many incompatible medical and bio-stimulation implants
- Prosthetic/hardware artifacts
- Limitations—bone, air, time, expertise

DWI, diffusion-weighted image; IR, inversion recovery; IV, intravenous; MRA, magnetic resonance angiography; MRS, magnetic resonance spectroscopy; MRV, magnetic resonance venography.

Box 5-14

Safety considerations for MRI

Magnetic fields

- Medical and bio-stimulation implants
  - » Pacemakers
  - » Neurostimulators
  - » Cardiac defibrillators
  - » Insulin pumps
  - » Cochlear implants
  - » Capsule endoscopy
  - » Some stents and clips
- Foreign bodies
  - » Explosive shell fragments
  - » Jewelry
  - » Some tattoos
  - » Acupuncture needles
  - » Orbit metal fragments
  - » Phones, watches
  - » Credit-card demagnetization
- Physiological issues
  - » Elevated body temperature
  - » Vertigo
  - » Peripheral nerve stimulation
  - » Pregnancy

Cryogenic liquids

- Emergency 'quench' causing room hypoxia

Noise

- Acoustic noise levels (<120 dB)

Claustrophobia

- Motion artifact

MRI PROTOCOLS

The physics and jargon of MRI are complex. The fundamental basis for image production is the effects induced in hydrogen protons within body tissues when placed in a strong magnetic field and pulsed by radiofrequency (RF) waves from different angles, wavelengths and time intervals ('pulse sequences'). By varying the parameters of the RF pulse, the T1 and T2 properties of the tissue are elicited. By repeating the pulse numerous times, the emitted tissue signal is progressively summated to produce a proton map recording its excitation and relaxation properties (Tables 5-14 and 5-15).

T1

- Short pulse-sequence parameters (short TR [repetition time], short TE [echo time]) highlight contrast between tissues, providing excellent depiction of anatomical detail.
- It is a short sequence, with fat being the most conspicuous normal high–signal component.
- High-signal abnormalities on T1 include lipoma, melanin, subacute hemorrhage due to methemoglobin, highly proteinaceous material and some calcified collections.
- The normal posterior pituitary is of high signal due to the presence of protein hormonal precursors.

T2

- Longer pulse sequences (long TR, long TE) allow more water to relax and contribute high signals to the image ('H_2O = T2').
- Both physiological water (e.g. CSF) and pathological water (e.g. edema) are demonstrated, with excellent anatomical detail.

Table 5-14 MRI sequences in the brain

SEQUENCE	PHYSICS	TISSUES ENHANCED	INDICATIONS	ABNORMALITIES
T1	Short TR Short TE 60–90 seconds	Fat Cystic vs solid lesions	Baseline sequence Excellent anatomical detail Pre-contrast comparison Normal and fat lesions Subacute hemorrhage	Fat—lipoma Melanin—melanoma Methemoglobin—subacute blood Protein—colloid cyst Calcium—meningioma
T2	Long TR Long TE 2–3 minutes	Water	Physiological water—CSF Pathological water—edema	Hydrocephalus Tumor, infection, inflammation
IR	Inversion pulse—fat suppression Longer TR Longer TE 3–5 minutes	Water Edema Fat suppression	STIR—edema FLAIR—edema, demyelination	Tumor, infection, inflammation Myositis Demyelination—MS, myelitis
DWI	20 seconds	Cytotoxic edema	Acute pathology	Acute infarction
GRE	Low-angled shot Can weight T1 or T2	Hemosiderin	Chronic hemorrhage Subtle previous hemorrhage	Tumors, AVM Diffuse axonal injury (DAI)
GAD	Short TR Short TE (T1) 60–90 seconds	Vessels Inflamed tissues	Subtle pathology Blood–brain barrier integrity	Tumor, infection, inflammation Surgery complications
MRA	3–5 minutes	Flowing arteries	Stroke, headache Visual disturbance	Occlusion, aneurysm, vasculitis
MRV	3–5 minutes	Cerebral veins	Headache Intracranial hypertension	Venous sinus thrombosis
CSF flow	1–3 minutes	Cerebrospinal fluid	Hydrocephalus Intracranial hypertension	Obstructive hydrocephalus Normal pressure hydrocephalus Intracranial hypertension Venous outflow obstruction
MRS	<60 seconds	Necrotic tissues	Tumor (high choline)	Tumor, abscess

AVM, arteriovenous malformation; CSF, cerebrospinal fluid; DWI, diffusion-weighted image; FLAIR, fluid-attenuated inversion recovery; GAD, post-gadolinium; GRE, gradient echo; IR, inversion recovery; MRA, magnetic resonance angiography; MRS, magnetic resonance spectroscopy; MRV, magnetic resonance venography; MS, multiple sclerosis; STIR, short T1 inversion recovery; TE, echo time; TR, repetition time.

- Both fat and water will be high signal on T2, which can be confusing with edema but can be differentiated by comparing T1—where water will not be high signal—and by selectively suppressing the fat signal with inversion recovery (STIR) or fat saturation techniques ('fat sat').

Inversion recovery (IR)

IR sequences are used widely to show both physiological water (e.g. CSF) and pathological water (e.g. edema). It is more sensitive to water than routine T2-weighted studies and has the added advantage of being able to electively suppress the signal of either fat (STIR) or water (FLAIR) to highlight more subtle pathological edema. The disadvantage is that anatomical detail is compromised.

Diffusion-weighted imaging (DWI)

DWI is a critical sequence to define, in particular, acute cerebral infarction. Ischemia impairs the cellular membrane transport mechanisms such that the cell swells due to osmosis (cytotoxic edema). Diffusion of water is then restricted across the cell membrane, and this restriction is displayed as an intense high signal.

Table 5-15 MRI basic sequences

MRI SEQUENCE	NORMAL	ABNORMAL
T1 sagittal	Excellent depiction of anatomy High signal in fat, methemoglobin, melanin Normal high signal in posterior pituitary	Glioma of the corpus callosum (arrow)
T2 axial	Cerebrospinal fluid (CSF): bright signal Gray–white matter differentiation	Pathological edema—from tumor (arrows) Compression of lateral ventricle Midline shift (arrowhead)
Inversion recovery (IR) axial	Fluid (CSF) attenuated Gray–white matter differentiation	Accentuates pathological edema—multiple sclerosis (arrows)

Table 5-15 MRI basic sequences *continued*

MRI SEQUENCE	NORMAL	ABNORMAL
Diffusion-weighted image (DWI)	Assesses movement across cell membranes	Acute restriction shows as high signal Demonstrates acute infarction (arrow)
Gradient echo (GRE)	Demonstrates hemosiderin Hemorrhagic lesions	Multiple arteriovenous malformations Low signal margins due to recurrent bleeding (arrows)
Post-gadolinium (GAD)	Contrast in vessels and choroid No parenchymal enhancement No meningeal enhancement	Multiple mass lesions (metastasis) Homogeneous enhancement (arrows)

continues

Table 5-15 MRI basic sequences *continued*

MRI SEQUENCE	NORMAL	ABNORMAL
Magnetic resonance angiography (MRA)	Flow-dependent, endoluminal flow Internal carotid (ICA), vertebral (VA), basilar (BA), anterior cerebral (ACA), middle cerebral (MCA), posterior cerebral (PCA) arteries	Occlusions, aneurysms, anomalies Acute embolic occlusion of middle cerebral artery (arrow) and internal carotid artery (arrowhead)
Magnetic resonance venography (MRV)	Flow-dependent, endoluminal flow Superior sagittal sinus (SSS), straight sinus (SS), transverse sinus (TS), sigmoid sinus (SGS), internal jugular (IJ)	Venous sinus thrombosis (arrows)

An extension of DWI is to combine the sequence with identifying the movement of molecules along the long axis of a nerve fiber, which can then be graphically displayed in three dimensions to develop brain maps (MR tractography) to show connectivity, degeneration and demyelination.

Gradient echo (GRE)

- The sequence has the advantage of being fast and using less RF power. T2 contrast is compromised and artifacts are more common.
- It is useful to identify hemosiderin content in a lesion, confirming the presence of previous hemorrhage; described as a 'blooming' effect. Hemosiderin produces signal loss, which is black and more prominent in size than on other sequences.
- It is especially useful in identifying vascular lesions, including aneurysms and arteriovenous malformations, diffuse axonal injury and bleeding tumors.

Gadolinium-enhanced (GAD)

Gadolinium is the standard IV contrast agent used in MR examinations. When placed in a magnetic field, especially with T1-weighted sequences, gadolinium exhibits strong para-magnetic effects and will emit a high signal. Fat suppression is usually applied to this T1 sequence (T1 fat sat or T1-FS), as fat has a bright signal with T1 which can be confused with enhancement.

The essential pathophysiology is that any cause for increased vascular permeability (tumor, infection, inflammation, etc.) will allow gadolinium to migrate from the intravascular compartment to the extravascular space across the blood–brain barrier.

Gadolinium-enhanced MRA (MRA-GAD) is also performed non-routinely to better show vascular anatomy, especially of the smaller vessels, such as in vasculitis.

Magnetic resonance angiography/venography (MRA, MRV)

Moving blood produces signal loss, as the blood components leave the field before they 'relax' and therefore do not emit a signal (signal void, 'black blood imaging'). Most commonly, blood is imaged with a 'time-of-flight' (TOF) method where the incoming blood is excited with a short TR allowing the emitting of a high signal ('white blood method'). Imaging of veins (MRV) uses the same methods as MRA.

MR spectroscopy (MRS)

Metabolites of neuron chemistry can provide insights into the diagnosis of tumors, infections, stroke, and metabolic and neurodegenerative diseases. The four common clinically used metabolites are choline (Cho), N-acetyl aspartate (NAA), creatine (Cr) and lactate. Water and fat signals are initially suppressed and the metabolites are then measured in very small concentrations (Table 5-16).

- Ischemic stroke induces a large amount of anaerobic glycolysis, characterized by high lactate levels.
- Choline is a marker of cell membrane breakdown, cell turnover and necrosis found in active tumors.
  - » Tumors which have been treated with radiation with complete ablation have high lactate, low NAA and creatine, but no choline.
  - » Tumor recurrence or residual tumor post-radiation will have elevated choline.
- NAA is a neuronal activity marker and decreases when any disease process reduces neuronal activity, such as Alzheimer's disease.
- Creatine provides a measure of energy stores, which are depleted in tumors.
- An abscess cavity will typically have high lactate centrally and the wall high in choline, but absent NAA.

Magnetic resonance gated intracranial cerebrospinal dynamics (MR-GILD, CSF flow study)

Quantitative measurements of CSF flow, arterial inflow and venous outflow can be made, which document disturbances in normal flow dynamics and can assist in the diagnosis particularly of normal-pressure hydrocephalus, benign intracranial hypertension and venous sinus stenoses.

PRINCIPLES OF INTERPRETATION IN BRAIN MR

Accurate interpretation of MR scans of the brain is based on knowledge of brain anatomy, key landmarks and development of a systematic approach (Box 5-15, overleaf).

Patient demographics

Name, date of study and some scanning parameters can give diagnostic clues and the clinical relevance of the study.

Technical review

Identify sequences and their anatomical planes displayed. Contrast images marked by high signal in all vessels, if available, should be identified early as these frequently show an abnormality.

Initial image review

The number of sequences and the resulting large number of images to be viewed can be rationalized using a systematic approach.

- To gain an initial overview of the case, review axial T2, then the IR and finally the axial DWIs, correlating any abnormal findings with each sequence.
- Identifying post-contrast images next can be helpful to highlight an abnormality. MRA study, when performed, needs to be surveyed to identify that all vessels are present and there is no large aneurysm or stenosis apparent.
- Any additional special MR sequence needs to be recognized.

Interpreting axial MR images can utilize a similar technique as in CT: rapid assessment, identifying the first and last scans, fast assessment of all images, and identifying normal and abnormal signal changes.

Table 5-16 MRS metabolite–pathological correlations

	NAA	CHOLINE	CREATINE	LACTATE
Stroke	Low	High	Low	High
Tumor	Low	High	Low	High
Abscess	Absent	High	Low	High
Radiation	Low	Low	Low	High

Box 5-15

**Systematic interpretation of
brain MR**

Patient demographics
- Name and other details

Technical review
- Identify sequences and anatomical planes

Initial image review
- Review T2 axial first, then IR, then DWI
- Review contrast images
- Review MRA studies for vascular disease
- Conduct fast assessment of *all* images
- Identify any gross abnormalities

Key image review
- Axial T2, IR:
  - » foramen magnum
  - » posterior fossa
  - » pituitary fossa
  - » suprasellar
  - » internal capsule—basal ganglia
  - » lateral ventricles
  - » vertex

- DWI:
  - » high signal foci of acute restricted diffusion
- Post-contrast (gadolinium)

Systematic review
- Sequential assessment of *all* images
- Correlate contrast abnormalities with non-contrast

Review areas
- Brainstem
- Cerebello-pontine angles
- Internal auditory meatus
- MRA: all vessels present
- DWI

Summary
- Comparison with previous studies
- Correlation of findings and probable diagnosis
- Need for additional imaging

DWI, diffusion-weighted image; IR, inversion recovery; MRA, magnetic resonance angiography.

Key image review

In MR studies of the brain, the axial, sagittal and coronal planes are usually displayed. To simplify the many structures and landmarks depicted on axial T2 MR images, isolation of seven key image planes can simplify interpretation (Table 5-17).

Foramen magnum

- At the skull base, the large foramen magnum is readily identifiable.
- The medulla is centrally placed, flanked by the two vertebral arteries and surrounded by high signal cerebrospinal fluid.

Posterior fossa

- The cerebellar hemispheres with the surface folia, superior cerebellar peduncle and fourth ventricle dominate the images.
- The transition from the smaller medulla to the pons is apparent.

Pituitary fossa

- The simultaneous depiction of the anterior, middle and posterior fossae produces a distinctive 'X' appearance, with the intersection at or adjacent to the pituitary fossa.

- The pituitary gland is clearly seen on sagittal T1, where the posterior lobe will be high signal due to the presence of proteinaceous hormones.

Suprasellar

- Within a few images above the sella, the high-signal CSF density of the suprasellar cistern comes into view.
- Flow voids within the circle of Willis and its major branches can be defined.

Internal capsule—basal ganglia

- At this level, the distinctive periventricular bent band of lower-signal white matter marks the internal capsule, surrounded by the higher-attenuating thalamus, lentiform and caudate nuclei.
- The Sylvian fissure delineates the temporal lobe.
- The lateral and third ventricles, cerebral aqueduct and corpus callosum dominate the midline structures.

Lateral ventricles

- The body of the lateral ventricle dominates this level.
- Additionally, the deep white matter of the corona radiata and sulci of the hemispheres are clearly visible.
- Both anterior and posterior edges of the falx, superior sagittal sinus and corpus callosum lie in the midline.

Table 5-17 MRI brain anatomy and pathological correlations

KEY IMAGE LEVEL	NORMAL	ABNORMAL
FORAMEN MAGNUM 1. Foramen magnum 2. Clivus 3. Medulla 4. Vertebral artery 5. Subarachnoid space 6. Sphenoid sinus 7. Nasal septum 8. Maxillary sinus		 Fluid-filled cyst lateral medulla Cystic astrocytoma (arrow)
POSTERIOR FOSSA 1. Cerebellum 2. Pons 3. Cerebellar tonsils 4. Internal auditory meatus 5. Temporal lobe 6. Cochlea 7. Sphenoid sinus 8. Ethmoid air cells 9. Greater wing of sphenoid		 High signal, wedge-shaped, cerebellar hemisphere infarct (arrows)
PITUITARY FOSSA 1. Transverse sinus 2. Cerebellum 3. Pons 4. Fourth ventricle 5. Basilar artery 6. Pituitary fossa 7. Internal carotid artery 8. Temporal lobe 9. Greater wing, sphenoid 10. Optic nerve 11. Globe 12. Nasal septum		 Pituitary macroadenoma (arrow)

continues

Table 5-17 MRI brain anatomy and pathological correlations *continued*

KEY IMAGE LEVEL	NORMAL	ABNORMAL
SUPRASELLAR 1. Venous confluence 2. Cerebellum, hemisphere 3. Pons 4. Middle cerebral artery 5. Optic chiasm 6. Temporal lobe 7. Temporal horn, lateral ventricle 8. Optic nerve 9. Optic foramen 10. Gyrus rectus 11. Globe		 Basilar artery aneurysm (arrow)
INTERNAL CAPSULE—BASAL GANGLIA 1. Occipital lobe 2. Posterior falx 3. Pineal gland 4. Posterior horn 5. Third ventricle 6. Septum pellucidum 7. Frontal horn, lateral ventricle 8. Corpus callosum 9. Frontal lobe 10. Head of caudate nucleus 11. Internal capsule, posterior limb 12. Lentiform nucleus 13. Sylvian fissure 14. Temporal lobe		 Colloid cyst, third ventricle (arrowhead) Obstructive hydrocephalus (arrows)
LATERAL VENTRICLES 1. Body of lateral ventricle 2. White matter, corona radiata 3. Posterior falx 4. Anterior falx 5. Frontal lobe 6. Parietal lobe		 Agenesis of the corpus callosum

Table 5-17 MRI brain anatomy and pathological correlations *continued*

KEY IMAGE LEVEL	NORMAL	ABNORMAL
VERTEX 1. Falx cerebri 2. Pre-central gyrus 3. Central sulcus 4. Post-central gyrus 5. Frontal lobe 6. Parietal lobe		Parafalcine mass, meningioma (arrow)

Vertex

High over the convexity of the hemispheres, the dominant features are the high-signal sulci and lower-signal gyri as well as the gray and white matter. Gyral edema can erase the sulci, and sulcal widening is a sign of gyral atrophy.

Systematic review

Sequential assessment of all images from base to vertex can then follow, with attention to the same and other details.

Review areas

- Anatomical regions of the brain on MR require closer scrutiny, especially the brainstem. As part of this, the cerebello-pontine angles and internal auditory meatus need to be located and reviewed for mass lesions.
- MRA images are evaluated for stenoses, occlusions and aneurysms.
- Inspection of DWIs for high-signal changes is especially relevant as a sign of acute ischemia when stroke syndromes are being investigated.

Summary

Following the systematic review, relevant positive and negative findings can be correlated and final statements made. If contrast has not been administered, its relevance for an additional study would be considered.

7. POSITRON EMISSION TOMOGRAPHY (PET)

Positron emission tomography uses various isotopes which enter into a specific biochemical pathway and accumulate where these sites are most active. One of the most commonly used is fluorine tagged with glucose (fluoro-deoxyglucose, FDG).

Once injected the isotope undergoes decay, emitting a positron which quickly encounters an electron within 3–5 mm, combines with the electron causing both to disappear ('annihilation event') and produces two gamma rays at 180° to each other. These two emitted gamma rays are detected as almost simultaneous registrations by the scanner, which allows calculation of their location in the body. The greater the number of annihilation events from a location, the brighter it will be displayed on the image. At the same time, a CT scan is performed and the PET data are co-registered into an anatomical location (PET-CT) (Figure 5-2).

The major uses are in oncology, to confirm masses with high metabolic activity as a sign of malignancy, lymphoma, staging of malignancy (especially involvement of lymph nodes), response to therapy and to document recurrence of disease.

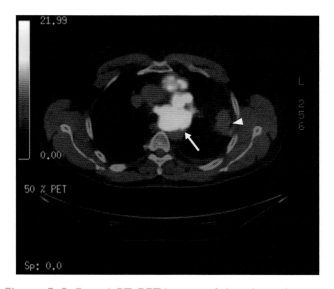

Figure 5-2 Fused CT-PET image of the chest. It shows carcinoma in the left lung (arrowhead) with extensive mediastinal lymph node metastases (arrow)

CHAPTER 6

PULMONOLOGY

David Arnold, Peter Wark, Michael Hensley, Brad Frankum
and Lucy Morgan

CHAPTER OUTLINE

1. PULMONARY MEDICINE

- **CLINICAL PRESENTATIONS OF RESPIRATORY DISEASE**

- **IMPORTANT CLINICAL CLUES**
  - Dyspnea
  - Patterns of breathing
  - Chronic cough
  - Clubbing
  - Hemoptysis
  - Solitary pulmonary nodule (coin lesion)
  - Mediastinal masses
  - Wheeze
  - Chest pain
  - Stridor

- **OVERVIEW OF THE RESPIRATORY SYSTEM AND PATHOPHYSIOLOGY**
  - Functional anatomy and physiology
  - Hypoxemia
  - Hypercapnia
  - Oxygen–hemoglobin association–dissociation curve

- **ACID–BASE DISTURBANCES FROM A PULMONARY PERSPECTIVE**
  - Respiratory acidosis
  - Respiratory alkalosis

- **MEASUREMENT OF LUNG FUNCTION**
  - Spirometry
  - Interpretation of lung volumes
  - Diffusing capacity for carbon monoxide (DLCO test)
  - Flow–volume loops
  - Interpretation of pulmonary function tests

- **CONTROL OF BREATHING**

- **RESPIRATORY TRACT DEFENSES**
  - Mechanical defenses
  - Immune system

- **GENETICS OF LUNG DISEASE**

- **PULMONARY DISORDERS**
  - Respiratory failure
  - Hypoventilation

- **DISEASES OF THE AIRWAYS**
  - Asthma
  - Allergic bronchopulmonary aspergillosis (ABPA)
  - Bronchiectasis
  - Cystic fibrosis (CF)
  - Bronchiolitis
  - Chronic obstructive pulmonary disease (COPD)
  - Interstitial lung disease (ILD)
  - Idiopathic pulmonary fibrosis
  - Occupational lung disease
  - Granulomatous ILD

1. PULMONARY MEDICINE

CLINICAL PRESENTATIONS OF RESPIRATORY DISEASE

Disorders of the respiratory system present in relatively few ways, all of which relate to the key roles of ventilation, gas exchange, maintenance of acid–base balance and protection against infection.

Failure of ventilation can occur when there is pathology at any level of the airway. Mechanical obstruction of the upper airway, damage or disease of the lower airway, impairment of the structures responsible for moving the chest wall and diaphragm, and failure of the central control mechanisms of breathing can all result in ventilatory failure (Box 6-1).

Gas exchange can fail as a result of reduced ventilation, or due to problems of perfusion. **Perfusion** of the lung can be impaired by:

- pulmonary thromboembolism
- pulmonary hypertension, either primary or secondary to other lung disease
- cardiac disease leading to pulmonary venous congestion, e.g. left ventricular failure
- Cardiac disease leading to shunting, e.g. congenital heart defects, ventricular septal defect
- pericardial disease
- hematological disorder, e.g. hyperviscosity.

Acid–base disorders can be due to primary pulmonary problems, or to renal and metabolic disorders.

- The lungs control pH through exhalation of carbon dioxide. Any fall in blood pH is a trigger for increased ventilatory drive.
- Impairment of ventilation will lead to respiratory acidosis.
- Chronic ventilatory impairment will result in renal compensation; the kidneys retain bicarbonate to compensate for CO_2 retention. Increased serum bicarbonate thus may be a sign of chronic respiratory acidosis.

Infection of the airways and parenchyma is common.

- The lung has an enormous surface area that interacts with the environment.
- Innate and adaptive immune mechanisms are under constant microbiological challenge.
- Mechanical (cough, cilia), chemical (mucus), humoral (antibodies), cellular (macrophages, neutrophils, lymphocytes) and molecular (defensins, interleukins) mechanisms are all vital in preventing tissue invasion.
- Repeated failure of these defense mechanisms should trigger investigation for immunodeficiency.

IMPORTANT CLINICAL CLUES

Dyspnea

Breathlessness or dyspnea is the most common respiratory symptom and the most important to the patient. The most accepted definition is that of the Consensus Statement from the American Thoracic Society in 1999:

Dyspnea is a term used to characterize a subjective experience of breathing discomfort that consists of qualitatively distinct sensations that vary in intensity.

The experience derives from interactions among multiple physiological, psychological, social, and environmental factors, and may induce secondary physiological and behavioral responses.

CLINICAL PEARL

The most common causes of chronic dyspnea are asthma, chronic obstructive pulmonary disease (COPD), cardiac failure and lack of fitness.

Both acute and chronic dyspnea can be due to the full range of respiratory diseases, as well as cardiac, hematologic and psychogenic causes.

The **grading** of dyspnea is essential for accurate initial assessment, and for measuring progress with and without treatment. There are a number of scales in use, such as that shown in Box 6-2.

Box 6-1

Disorders of ventilation

Upper airway pathology
- Obstructive sleep apnea
- Upper airway mechanical dysfunction, e.g. tracheal stenosis, vocal cord dysfunction
- Foreign body inhalation
- Oropharyngeal disorders, e.g. tonsillar hypertrophy, epiglottitis, malignancies

Lower airway obstructive pathology
- Reversible airways disease: asthma
- Chronic obstructive pulmonary disease: emphysema, chronic bronchitis
- Bronchiectasis
- Lobar collapse (foreign body, neoplasm, mucus plug)

Lower airway parenchymal pathology
- Infection: pneumonia
- Interstitial disease: idiopathic, pneumoconiosis, autoimmune, granulomatous, drug-induced, hypersensitivity
- Neoplasm

Chest wall and pleural abnormalities
- Pleural effusion
- Empyema
- Skeletal deformity, e.g. kyphoscoliosis, fractured ribs
- Malignancy—mesothelioma
- Pneumothorax
- Primary or secondary muscle disease, e.g. polymyositis, muscular dystrophy, drug-induced myopathy

Central control problems
- Central sleep apnea
- Sedation, e.g. due to drugs, primary cerebral disease

Box 6-2

Modified Medical Research Council (MRC) dyspnea scale

Grade/description of breathlessness

Grade 0 'I only get breathless with strenuous exercise.'

Grade 1 'I get short of breath when hurrying on the level or walking up a slight hill.'

Grade 2 'I walk slower than people of the same age on the level because of breathlessness, or have to stop for a breath when walking at my own pace on the level.'

Grade 3 'I stop for a breath after walking about 100 meters or after a few minutes on the level.'

Grade 4 'I am too breathless to leave the house, or I am breathless when dressing.'

Patterns of breathing

Tachypnea is a vital sign of respiratory illness, with respiratory rates above 30/min considered a danger sign in the context of an acute respiratory illness.

Tachypnea in the absence of clinical signs of lung disease, and with a normal chest X-ray, can be due to the following.

- Psychiatric disease (panic disorder, anxiety disorder); hyperventilation syndrome is often accompanied by peripheral paresthesiae
- Pulmonary vascular disease
  » pulmonary embolism
  » primary pulmonary hypertension
- Early stages of parenchymal lung disease
  » pulmonary edema
  » interstitial lung disease
  » lymphangitis carcinomatosis
- Neuromuscular causes
  » respiratory muscle weakness
  » brain disease, e.g. stroke, encephalitis, usually affecting the brainstem
- Miscellaneous
  » metabolic acidosis, e.g. salicylate poisoning
  » fever or pain
  » hyperthyroidism

Cheyne–Stokes respiration is rhythmical variation in ventilatory effort, which varies between hypopnea and hyperpnea.

CLINICAL PEARL

Cheyne–Stokes breathing occurs when there is dysfunction of the respiratory center in the medulla. This may be due to chronic hypoxia, metabolic disorders, or primary brain disease.

Chronic cough

Chronic cough is defined as a cough that lasts for 8 weeks or longer.

Causes

The three most common causes of chronic cough are:

1 chronic rhinosinusitis
2 asthma
3 gastroesophageal reflux.

CLINICAL PEARLS

- In the setting of chronic cough where the cause is unclear, consider performing bronchial provocation tests to diagnose an underlying airway hyper-reactivity.
- Patients may have more than one cause of cough. For example, patients with asthma will frequently be atopic and also have allergic rhinitis. Asthma may also be exacerbated by esophageal reflux.

Other causes include:

- **lung cancer**
- foreign body
- vocal cord dysfunction (also called upper airway dysfunction syndrome, UADS)
- chronic bronchitis (cough with sputum for 3 months a year, 2 years in a row)
- congestive heart failure
- bronchiectasis (usually cough with sputum daily)
- interstitial lung disease
- drugs, e.g. angiotensin-converting enzyme inhibitors (ACEIs)
- airway tumors
- tuberculosis. Everyone with chronic cough, with an unclear cause, should have an X-ray. Consider a CT, bronchial provocation testing to diagnose upper airway sensitivity and bronchoscopy.

CLINICAL PEARL

There are red flags about chronic cough:

- smoker—think lung cancer
- hemoptysis—think lung cancer or bronchiectasis
- dysphonia—think laryngeal cancer
- abnormal chest X-ray—every patient with a chronic cough must have a chest X-ray.

Clubbing

Clubbing is an important physical sign. The pathophysiology is unknown, but theories include chronic vasodilatation of digital vessels, and/or the production of growth factors such as platelet-derived growth factor in the lungs, or elsewhere (Box 6-3).

Hemoptysis

Causes of hemoptysis

- Respiratory:
  » Lung cancer
  » Chronic bronchitis, usually an acute exacerbation
  » Pulmonary infarction (from pulmonary embolism)
  » Infection:
    – bronchiectasis
    – lung abscess
    – pneumonia
    – tuberculosis
    – fungal lung disease—usually *Aspergillus*: mycetoma, invasive fungal infection
    – parasitic lung infection, e.g. fluke
  » Foreign body (aspirated)
  » Post-traumatic (lung contusion)
  » Vasculitic syndromes, e.g. Goodpasture's syndrome, anti-neutrophil cytoplasmic autoantibody (ANCA)-associated vasculitis
  » Idiopathic pulmonary hemosiderosis
  » Rupture of a mucosal vessel after vigorous coughing
  » Iatrogenic, e.g. post trans-bronchial lung biopsy (TBLB), bronchial biopsy, computed tomography (CT)-guided fine-needle aspiration biopsy (FNAB)

Box 6-3

Causes of clubbing

Common causes of clubbing

Cardiac:
- Cyanotic congenital heart disease
- Infective endocarditis

Respiratory:
- Lung carcinoma (usually not small cell)
- Suppurative lung disease:
  » bronchiectasis (cystic fibrosis and non-CF)
  » lung abscess (rare)
  » empyema (rare)
- Lung fibrosis:
  » idiopathic pulmonary fibrosis
  » other causes of interstitial fibrosis

Uncommon causes of clubbing

Familial

Respiratory:
- Tuberculosis

Gastrointestinal:
- Cirrhosis, especially biliary
- Inflammatory bowel disease
- Celiac disease

Endocrine:
- Thyrotoxicosis (thyroid acropachy)

NOT A CAUSE: COPD

- Cardiovascular:
  - » Mitral stenosis
  - » Pulmonary edema due to left heart failure
- Bleeding diathesis and airway inflammation with concomitant anticoagulation
- Spurious:
  - » Nasal bleeding
  - » Hematemesis
  - » Mouth bleeding, e.g. dental or gum disease

Causes of massive hemoptysis
- Common:
  - » Lung cancer
  - » Bronchiectasis
- Uncommon:
  - » Tuberculosis
  - » Fungus ball (mycetoma/aspergilloma)
  - » Lung abscess
  - » Pulmonary arteriovenous malformation (PAVM)

CLINICAL PEARL

In massive hemoptysis (200–600 mL in 24 hours), the cause of death is asphyxiation, not hypovolemia.

Solitary pulmonary nodule (coin lesion)

Causes

1 Primary lung cancer
2 Metastatic tumor
3 Granuloma (from past infection)
4 Hamartoma
5 Fungus ball
6 Lung abscess

Factors favoring a solitary lesion being malignant

- Smoker
- Increasing age of patient
- Previous malignancy
- Lesion that increases in size over time
- Irregular border of lesion on X-ray or CT scan

- Ground glass opacity that is partially solid is suspicious for malignancy

CLINICAL PEARLS

- A lesion in a smoker (current or ex) is malignant until proven otherwise. 1/3 new lung cancers occur in people who have never smoked. Consider lung cancer in anyone with unexplained cough.

Mediastinal masses

Mediastinal masses may present with symptoms due to pressure effects on surrounding structures, e.g. with dyspnea or dysphagia, or be found incidentally on thoracic imaging (Box 6-4). They may also be found in conjunction with symptoms of the underlying cause, e.g. in the setting of malignancy.

Wheeze

Wheeze is caused by airflow through a narrowed airway, or by high-velocity airflow.

- Expiratory wheeze is generally a sign of dynamic airway compression, and suggests pathology such as asthma or chronic obstructive pulmonary disease (COPD).
- Inspiratory wheeze is more often a sign of a fixed mechanical obstruction, such as a tumor or a foreign body in a bronchus.

CLINICAL PEARL

Lack of wheeze in the setting of obstructive airway disease due to asthma or COPD can be a sign of severity, suggesting low airflow.

Chest pain

Pleuritic chest pain is sharp, localized, and occurs on inspiration. It is a sign of disease of the parietal pleura.

Causes include infective pleurisy, pulmonary embolism with infarction, pneumothorax, malignancy, and empyema. Muscular and skeletal structures are a common cause of chest pain.

Chest pain is not an infrequent symptom in patients with asthma. It is thought to be musculoskeletal in origin in some cases, perhaps due to hyperinflation of the chest cavity.

Box 6-4
Mediastinal masses on chest X-ray

Anterior (the '5 T's')	Middle	Posterior
Thyroid	Bronchogenic cyst	Neurogenic tumor, e.g. neurofibroma
Thymoma	Pleuropericardial cyst	Aortic aneurysm
Teratoma		Paravertebral abscess
Terrible lymphoma or carcinoma		Hiatus hernia
Tortuous vessels		

Stridor

Stridor is a harsh **inspiratory** sound resulting from narrowing of the upper airway.

Causes include tracheal stenosis, upper airway foreign body, laryngeal disease, including paralysis of vocal cords and paradoxical cord movement also known as VCD, and pharyngeal disorders such as epiglottitis.

OVERVIEW OF THE RESPIRATORY SYSTEM AND PATHOPHYSIOLOGY

Functional anatomy and physiology

The respiratory system is a complex servo-control network for homeostasis of arterial oxygen, carbon dioxide and acid–base status, linked to sophisticated voluntary processes for speech, singing and other cortical functions.

The role of the lungs is to import oxygen, export carbon dioxide, and contribute to short-term control of pH while talking, whistling and singing.

The anatomy of the respiratory system defines the major disorders where problems occur, such as obstructive sleep apnea at the level of the naso/oro-pharynx, vocal cord problems, asthma and COPD, interstitial lung disease/pneumonia, pleural disease, and respiratory muscle weakness.

Gas exchange

The alveolus is the basic unit of the respiratory system.

- The matching of inspired air and venous blood in the alveolus leads to oxygen uptake and to carbon dioxide removal.
- The level or partial pressure of oxygen and carbon dioxide in each alveolus is determined by the ratio of the ventilation and the blood flow, not the absolute values.
- The ratio of alveolar ventilation to blood flow (V/Q ratio) for the whole lung is approximately 1.0 in the stable state, but the V/Q ratios vary across the lung in health, with higher ratios in the apices and lower ratios in the bases.
- The range of V/Q ratios or V/Q inequality is much greater in lung disease of all types.

Since it is too difficult to measure and identify the V/Q ratios of all 500 million or more individual alveoli, summary measures are used. The concept of the **alveolar–arterial difference for PO$_2$** (P$_{A-a}$O$_2$) is one such measure. Since the arterial PO$_2$ is influenced by the level of inspired oxygen, and the level of carbon dioxide is dependent on the alveolar ventilation, it is not possible to use arterial PO$_2$ alone.

Since it is not possible to make a single measure of alveolar oxygen pressure (P$_A$O$_2$), this is estimated using a three-compartment model of the lungs:

1. dead space (V/Q ratio = 0, P$_A$O$_2$ = inspired PO$_2$)
2. shunt (V/Q ratio = infinity; P$_A$O$_2$ = mixed venous PO$_2$)
3. ideal V/Q ratio of 1; P$_A$O$_2$ to be calculated).

Figure 6-1 shows typical values on a PO$_2$/PCO$_2$ graph.

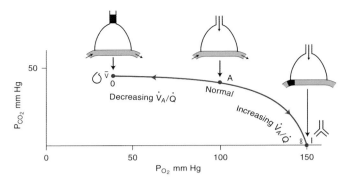

Figure 6-1 PO$_2$/PCO$_2$ graph showing the ventilation–perfusion ratio line. The PO$_2$ and PCO$_2$ values of a lung unit move along this line from the mixed venous point V to the inspired gas point I as the ventilation–perfusion ratio increases from below (V) to above (I) normal; A is located at the normal alveolar gas composition

From West JB. Respiratory physiology: the essentials, 9th ed. Philadelphia: Lippincott Williams & Wilkins, 2012.

The A–a gradient

The A–a gradient is calculated by estimating the P$_A$O$_2$ first:

$$P_AO_2 \text{ (mmHg)} = [(P_b - P_{H2O}) \times F_iO_2] - P_aCO_2[F_iO_2 + (1 - F_iO_2)]/R$$

P$_b$ is atmospheric pressure; P$_{H2O}$ is saturated water vapor pressure at 37°C; F$_i$O$_2$ is inspired fraction of oxygen (0.2093 at sea level); R is respiratory quotient, usually 0.8.

- At sea level and breathing room air at rest: P$_A$O$_2$ (mmHg) = 150 − P$_a$CO$_2$/0.8.
- For a normal P$_a$CO$_2$ of 40 mmHg, the P$_A$O$_2$ will be 100 mmHg.
- The P$_{A-a}$O$_2$ (A–a gradient) is normally 10–20 mmHg. 10 mmHg is normal for a young adult, gradually rising with age to 20 mmHg in the older adult.

CLINICAL PEARLS

- P$_{A-a}$O$_2$ (A–a gradient) is **normal** in hypoxemia due to hypoventilation, and with reduced inspired oxygen fraction such as at altitude.
- The A–a gradient is **increased** in hypoxemia due to ventilation–perfusion (V/Q) inequality, right-to-left shunting, and diffusion disorder.

V/Q inequality

CLINICAL PEARL

V/Q inequality is the most common cause of hypoxemia, and is responsible for much of the hypoxemia seen with airways disease such as COPD, and interstitial disease such as idiopathic pulmonary fibrosis.

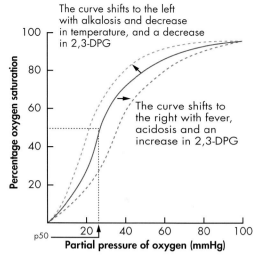

The curve shifts to the left with alkalosis and decrease in temperature, and a decrease in 2,3-DPG

The curve shifts to the right with fever, acidosis and an increase in 2,3-DPG

The avidity of hemoglobin for oxygen varies with physiological conditions as well as in pathological states.

Figure 6-2 Oxygen–hemoglobin dissociation curve. 2,3-DPG, 2,3-diphosphoglycerate

From Harward MP and Udden MM. Medical secrets, 5th ed. Philadelphia: Mosby, 2012.

The major reason that V/Q inequality causes hypoxemia is the shape of the hemoglobin–oxygen association–dissociation curve, which relates the partial pressure of oxygen in the blood to the amount of oxygen carried on hemoglobin (Figure 6-2). The areas of high V/Q ratio cannot make up for the areas of low V/Q ratio because the higher areas cannot take on extra oxygen no matter how high the local P_AO_2.

Carbon dioxide does not have the same problem; its pressure–content curve is linear, so high V/Q areas make up for the reduced output of low V/Q areas when ventilation is increased in response to chemoreceptor stimulation.

Right-to-left shunting

There are two forms of right-to-left shunting that will reduce the level of P_aO_2 below that expected from the level of P_AO_2.

An **anatomical shunt** occurs when blood flows from the right side to the left side of the circulation without any exposure to inhaled air. This may be due to:

- abnormal connections, such as
  - » atrial or ventricular septal defects
  - » direct pulmonary artery–vein anastomoses/malformations
  - » bronchial veins that drain directly into the left atrium
- a pathophysiological shunt with blood flowing past completely unventilated alveoli, such as
  - » complete atelectasis
  - » alveoli filled with liquid inflammatory material or blood, as in pulmonary edema and alveolar hemorrhage.

The $P_{A–a}O_2$ of 10–20 mmHg found in people without lung disease is due to some of the right-to-left shunts such as bronchial veins draining into the left atrium, but also includes the contribution from the effect of 'normal' V/Q inequality; this may be called a **'physiological' shunt**.

Measuring the size of a right-to-left shunt

This is estimated by measuring P_aO_2 and P_aCO_2 while breathing 100% O_2 for 15 minutes. Since the hypoxemia of hypoventilation, V/Q inequality and diffusion should be overcome by 100% oxygen, this method measures the anatomical and pathophysiologic shunts; all blood leaving low-V/Q areas will be fully oxygenated.

Normally, the shunt does not exceed 7%.

- A shunt >7% is usually due to a significant problem such as a patent foramen ovale with right-to-left flow, or a large pulmonary arteriovenous malformation.
- A 30% shunt is life-threatening.

Hypoxemia

Summary of causes

1. Ventilation–perfusion mismatch is nearly always the cause of clinically significant hypoxia (increased A–a gradient; good response to increased inspired oxygen)
2. Hypoventilation (increased P_aCO_2, normal A–a gradient)
3. Right-to-left shunt (increased A–a gradient, poor response to increased inspired oxygen)
4. Impaired diffusion (very rare)
5. Low inspired environmental O_2, e.g. high altitude

Note: Desaturation of mixed venous blood (e.g. shock) can worsen hypoxemia from other causes.

Hypercapnia

Causes

- Hypoventilation:
  - » Alveolar hypoventilation is the most common cause of hypercapnia, in keeping with the relationship between P_aCO_2 and alveolar ventilation.
  - » P_aCO_2 is inversely proportional to alveolar ventilation.
  - » If alveolar ventilation is halved, carbon dioxide pressure doubles.
- V/Q inequality:
  - » The maintenance of a normal PCO_2 in the presence of V/Q inequality depends on the level of alveolar ventilation.
  - » One example is the use of high inspired oxygen for COPD with chronic hypercapnia; since increased inspired oxygen will increase V/Q inequality by removing the homeostatic effect on V/Q of hypoxia-induced pulmonary vasoconstriction, ventilation must increase to avoid further hypercapnia. However, the increased P_aO_2 reduces the central drive to respiration, resulting in worsening hypercapnia.
- Increased inspired CO_2, for instance rebreathing during a problem with anesthetic equipment.

Oxygen–hemoglobin association–dissociation curve

Useful points to remember for the relationship between P_aO_2 and oxygen saturation:

1 P_aO_2 of 60 mmHg = saturation 90%
2 P_aO_2 of 47 mmHg = saturation 70% (normal venous blood)
3 P_aO_2 of 26 mmHg = saturation 50%.

Causes of an increased affinity for O_2

(Curve shifts to the left, i.e. better oxygen pick-up.)

1 ↑ pH
2 ↓ P_aCO_2
3 Carboxyhemoglobin, and abnormal hemoglobin, e.g. fetal
4 Methemoglobin
5 Decreased 2,3-DPG (2,3-diphosphoglycerate)
6 Hypothermia

Causes of a decreased affinity for O_2

(Curve shifts to the right, i.e. better oxygen release.)

1 ↓ pH
2 ↑ P_aCO_2
3 Fever
4 Abnormal hemoglobin, e.g. Kansas
5 Increased 2,3-DPG

ACID–BASE DISTURBANCES FROM A PULMONARY PERSPECTIVE

Respiratory acidosis

- **Acute** respiratory acidosis: reduced pH; increased P_aCO_2; normal base excess; increased HCO_3^- by approximately 1 mmol/L for every 10 mmHg increase in P_aCO_2.
- **Chronic** respiratory acidosis: HCO_3^- increases by approximately 3.5 mmol/L for every 10 mmHg increase in P_aCO_2. Associated with renal compensation to return pH toward 7.40; $HCO_3^- > 30$ mmol/L gives a clue about chronic hypercapnia.

CLINICAL PEARLS

- Base excess (BE) from the arterial blood gas machine is the BE corrected to a P_aCO_2 of 40 mmHg (i.e. normal).
- Thus, BE calculation eliminates the respiratory component of the acid–base status and shows only the metabolic component.
- Normal BE is ± 3. BE >+3 is metabolic alkalosis; BE <−3 is metabolic acidosis.

- If the HCO_3^- is **lower** than the calculated value, there is a concurrent metabolic acidosis; BE will be ↓, i.e. a negative value.
- If the HCO_3^- is **higher** than the calculated value, there is a concurrent metabolic alkalosis; BE will be ↑, i.e. a positive value.

Respiratory alkalosis

- **Acute** respiratory alkalosis: increased pH, reduced P_aCO_2, and a decrease in HCO_3^- by 2 mmol/L for every 10 mmHg decrease in P_aCO_2.
- **Chronic** respiratory alkalosis: chronic decrease in P_aCO_2 is associated with renal compensation to return pH toward 7.40. HCO_3^- should decrease 5 mmol/L for every 10 mmHg decrease in P_aCO_2.
- If the HCO_3^- is **lower** than the calculated value, there is a concurrent metabolic acidosis; BE will be a negative value.
- If the HCO_3^- is **higher** than the calculated value, there is a concurrent metabolic alkalosis; BE will be a positive value.

MEASUREMENT OF LUNG FUNCTION

The lung has four fundamental **volumes** from which lung capacities are derived:

- *residual volume* (RV)—the volume remaining after completing a full active expiration
- *expiratory reserve volume* (ERV)—the volume still available after a passive expiration
- *tidal volume* (TV)—the volume used for usual ventilation
- *inspiratory reserve volume* (IRV)—the volume available by full inspiration from the end of normal inspiration to the top of the lungs.

The **capacities** are combinations of the volumes:

- *total lung capacity* (TLC) is the sum of all four volumes
- *vital capacity* is TLC minus RV
- *functional residual capacity* (FRC) is the resting capacity RV plus ERV.

Figure 6-3 illustrates lung volumes and other measurements related to breathing mechanics.

Spirometry

Spirometry—or the forced expiratory test—is the simplest test of lung function, and is also one of the most informative and very easy to do. It should be available to all patients in every setting, similar to the measurement of blood pressure.

The **basic measurements** from the forced expiratory maneuver (Figure 6-4) are:

- the forced expiratory volume in 1 second (FEV1)
- the forced vital capacity (FVC)
- the ratio FEV1/FVC.

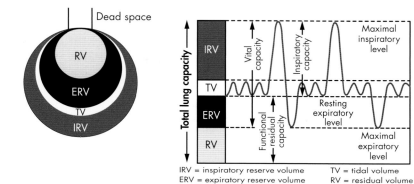

Figure 6-3 Lung volumes and some measurements related to the mechanics of breathing

Adapted from Comroe JH Jr et al. The lung: clinical physiology and pulmonary function tests 2e. Year Book, 1962.

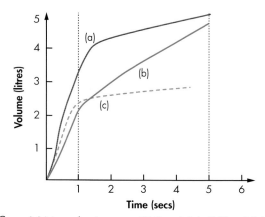

Curve (a) Normal spirometry. FEV1 = 4.2 L, FVC = 4.8 L
     (b) Obstructive defect. FEV1 = 2.2 L, FVC = 4.5 L
     (c) Restrictive defect. FEV1 = 2.4 L, FVC = 2.8 L

Figure 6-4 Example of spirometry

From Adam JG (ed). Emergency medicine: clinical essentials, 2nd ed. Philadelphia: Saunders, 2013.

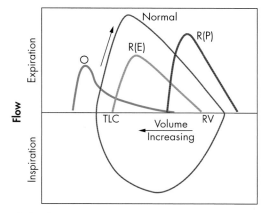

Figure 6-5 Obstructive and restrictive flow volume curves. O, obstructive disease; R(P), parenchymal restrictive disease; R(E), extraparenchymal restrictive disease with limitation in inspiration and expiration. Forced expiration is plotted in all conditions; forced inspiration is shown only for the normal curve. TLC, total lung capacity; RV, residual volume. By convention, lung volume increases to the left on the abscissa. The arrow alongside the normal curve indicates the direction of expiration from TLC to RV

From Fauci AS et al. (eds). Harrison's Principles of internal medicine, 14th ed. New York: McGraw Hill, 1998.

While other measures such as flow in the mid-part of the forced expiration can be taken, the only regular addition is to repeat the test after administration of a rapid-acting bronchodilator such as salbutamol or albuterol.

The **results** are compared with predicted normal values obtained from large surveys.

- The normal limits have been defined in the past by general rules for all age groups, such as within 80–120% of predicted for FEV1 and FVC, or >0.70 for FEV1/FVC ratio.
- Recently the lower limit of normal (LLN) has been introduced, with some changes to the interpretation of test results. For instance, a cut-off point of 0.7 overestimates the presence of airflow obstruction in the elderly, and underestimates it in young people.

Spirometry is *normal, obstructive, restrictive,* or combined *obstructive and restrictive* (Figure 6-5).

- Look at the FEV1/FVC ratio—if the ratio is below the LLN, this is obstructive.
- Look then at the FVC:
  - » If the FVC is normal, it is obstructive only.
  - » If the FVC is reduced below the LLN, it is a combined obstructive and restrictive defect on spirometry.
  - » An important point is that obstruction alone can cause a reduced FVC due to air trapping, but this cannot be measured with spirometry alone; measurement of lung volumes is required.
- If the FEV1/FVC ratio is normal, then look at the FVC.
  - » If the FVC is below the LLN, this is a restrictive defect. Restriction is best assessed by TLC, but this is not available on spirometry.
  - » If FVC is normal and FEV1/FVC ratio is normal, then spirometry is normal.

Interpretation of lung volumes

- Lung restriction is defined by reduction in TLC below the lower limit of normal.
- Hyperinflation is defined by increase in TLC to above the upper limit of normal.
- Gas trapping is characterized by an increase in RV, or more accurately by an increase in the RV/TLC ratio.
  - » In restrictive lung disease, TLC is ↓. RV is often ↓, but may be normal.
  - » In obstructive lung disease, obstruction is defined by the FEV1/FVC ratio on spirometry; RV and TLC are often increased, indicating gas trapping and hyperinflation respectively, but may be normal.

Diffusing capacity for carbon monoxide (DLCO test)

While the DLCO is called a test of 'diffusing capacity', it is really a measure of how much carbon monoxide (CO) can be picked up by the lungs over a certain period of time. This measure is also known as TLCO (transfer factor of the lung for CO).

Only very low levels of CO are required due to the exceptional affinity of hemoglobin for CO; this allows the assumption to be made that the level of CO in blood leaving the alveolus is zero.

The DLCO will depend on the volume of air in the lungs when the CO was taken in, the alveolar surface area available, pulmonary capillary volume, hemoglobin level, and pulmonary blood flow. It depends to a very minor degree, if any, on the rate of diffusion of the CO from the alveoli to the pulmonary capillary.

- DLCO is decreased in:
  - » emphysema
  - » interstitial lung disease
  - » anemia
  - » pulmonary hypertension
  - » pulmonary edema
  - » right-to-left shunts.
- DLCO is increased in:
  - » polycythemia
  - » diffuse alveolar hemorrhage
  - » left-to-right shunts.

Flow–volume loops

Flow–volume loops are a more sensitive way of detecting airway obstruction than spirometry, and may help to identify the site of obstruction (Table 6-1). Expiratory and inspiratory flows are plotted against lung volume during maximally forced inspiration and expiration (Figure 6-6).

Interpretation of pulmonary function tests

Table 6-2 summarizes characterisic changes in pulmonary function in lung disease and in the elderly.

Table 6-1 Flow–volume loops

PATTERN	EXPIRATORY PEAK	INSPIRATORY PEAK
Fixed obstruction	Plateau	Plateau
Variable intrathoracic obstruction	Plateau or concave	Preserved
Variable extrathoracic obstruction	Preserved	Plateau

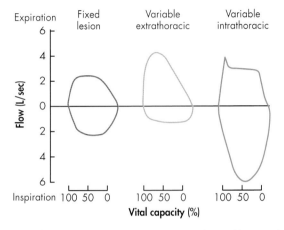

Figure 6-6 Flow–volume loops produced by major airway obstructive lesions

From Fauci AS et al. (eds). Harrison's Principles of internal medicine, 14th ed. New York: McGraw Hill, 1998.

CONTROL OF BREATHING

The system responsible for the control of breathing is summarized in Figure 6-7, which sets out the afferent and efferent aspects of the system.

The role of the upper airway in the control of breathing has been explored in the investigation of the cause and treatment of obstructive sleep apnea (OSA) and other forms of sleep-disordered breathing. The coordinated activation of upper airway muscles maintains upper airway patency in normal people and overcomes upper airway obstruction in OSA.

RESPIRATORY TRACT DEFENSES

Mechanical defenses

The **cough reflex** is responsible for clearance of airway secretions, and defense of the upper airway. The afferent limb is via a variety of receptors through the upper and lower respiratory tract. The efferent limb is through inspiratory and expiratory muscles, and laryngeal muscles.

Table 6-2 Characteristic pulmonary function changes in lung disease and in the elderly

PULMONARY FUNCTION TEST	CHRONIC OBSTRUCTIVE PULMONARY DISEASE	RESTRICTIVE LUNG DISEASE	ELDERLY COMPARED WITH THE YOUNG*
FEV1/FVC ratio	Decreased	Increased or normal	Decreased
Vital capacity (FVC)	Decreased or normal	Decreased or normal	Decreased
Residual volume (RV)	Increased or normal	Decreased or normal	
Maximum mid-expiratory flow rate (MMFR)	Decreased	Decreased or normal	Decreased
Total lung capacity (TLC)	Increased or normal	Decreased	Unchanged
DLCO	Decreased or normal	Decreased or normal	Decreased

*Less relevant when lower and upper limit of normal (LLN and ULN) are used compared with the older approach of normal being 80% or more for FEV1 and FVC, and 0.7 for the FEV1/FVC ratio.

DLCO, diffusing capacity for carbon monoxide; FEV1, forced expiratory volume in 1 second; FVC, forced vital capacity.

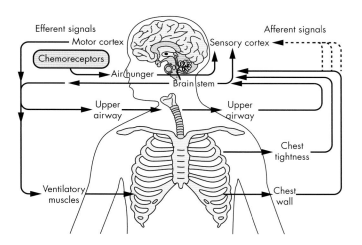

Figure 6-7 Efferent and afferent signals that contribute to the sensation of dyspnea

From Sheel AW, Foster GE and Romer LM. Exercise and its impact on dyspnea. Curr Opin Pharmacol 2011;11(3);195–203.

Mucus is responsible for clearance of micro-organisms from the airways. Its importance is reflected in cystic fibrosis, where abnormality in the CFTR gene leads to problems with electrolyte and water transport, leading to viscous, thickened mucus that facilitates chronic infection and persistent inflammation.

Airway cilia are responsible for moving mucus and its components throughout the respiratory tract. The importance of cilial function is reflected in disorders such as primary cilial dyskinesia which lead to multiple problems:

- chronic bronchitis and bronchiectasis
- otitis and rhinosinusitis

- impaired fertility
- heterotaxy and complex congenital heart disease, in a minority of cases

Immune system

The respiratory tract **innate immune system** performs the following roles:

- rapid detection and first-line defense against environmental micro-organisms
- activation of the adaptive immune system
- regulation of inflammation and homeostasis of the immune system.

Components:

- Receptors—pattern recognition receptors (PRRs) such as Toll-like receptors that recognize highly conserved pathogen-associated molecular patterns (PAMPs)
- Dendritic cells, phagocytes (monocytes, macrophages and neutrophils) and special non-B, non-T lymphocytes (natural killer or NK cells, secreting interferon-gamma and anti-microbial and pro-inflammatory cytokines)
- Enzymes, cytokines and peptides, e.g. lysozyme, IL-8 and defensins
- Systemic inflammation: C-reactive protein (CRP), complement system, lectins

The respiratory tract adaptive immune system

Lymphoid tissue is present throughout the respiratory tract, providing a strong mucosal immune system similar to that of the gastrointestinal tract, with antigen-presenting cells (macrophages and dendritic cells) to enable acquired immunity to start in the respiratory tract.

In addition to the usual roles of cell-mediated immunity and specific immunoglobulin (Ig) production through

B-lymphocyte proliferation, there are some adaptive immune roles with specific implications for lung disease:

- Airway IgA is important for mucosal immunity of the upper and lower airways in its dimeric form (monomeric in serum). Selective IgA deficiency may lead to recurrent infections of the lungs and sinuses including bronchiectasis, although this eventuates in only a minority of cases.
- The balance in lymphocyte development between the fundamental helper cell classes (Th1/Th2/Th17) may play a role in the development of diseases such as asthma where the predominance of Th2 and/or Th17 response may lead to inappropriate airway inflammation.

GENETICS OF LUNG DISEASE

Only a small number of respiratory diseases are due to single gene conditions:

- Cystic fibrosis is the most common of the single gene respiratory conditions (see details in the section below).
- Deficiency of proteinase inhibition is an autosomal recessive disorder known as either alpha-1 antitrypsin deficiency or alpha-1 proteinase inhibitor deficiency, and causes severe damage to the lungs in the form of emphysema, and in the liver as cirrhosis. About 95% of cases are due to the Z mutation (PiZZ).

PULMONARY DISORDERS

Respiratory failure

Causes of respiratory failure are classified as shown in Box 6-5.

Hypoventilation

Causes include disorders of the:

- medulla, e.g. inflammation, stroke, tumor, drugs such as narcotics
- spinal cord, e.g. trauma
- anterior horn cells—poliomyelitis, motor neuron disease

- respiratory muscle nerves—Guillain–Barré syndrome
- respiratory neuromuscular junction—myasthenia gravis
- respiratory muscles—muscular dystrophy
- chest wall—kyphoscoliosis; profound obesity
- upper airway obstruction—epiglottitis, tracheal damage, obstructive sleep apnea.

DISEASES OF THE AIRWAYS

Asthma

Definition

The Global Initiative for Asthma (GINA) 2020 states that asthma is:

> A heterogeneous disease, usually characterized by chronic airway inflammation. It is defined by the history of respiratory symptoms such as wheeze, shortness of breath, chest tightness and cough that vary over time and in intensity, together with variable expiratory airflow limitation.

Bronchial hyper-responsiveness (BHR) can be demonstrated by:

- short-term reversal of airflow obstruction, defined as a ≥12% increase *and* a ≥200 mL increase in FEV1 after administration of bronchodilator
- a ≥15% fall in FEV1 with bronchoprovocation tests (e.g. hypertonic saline, methacholine, mannitol, histamine).

Differential diagnosis

- Upper airway obstruction (inspiratory stridor usually present rather than expiratory wheeze); includes vocal cord dysfunction.
- Foreign body aspiration, tumor or bronchial stenosis (resulting in localized wheeze, often monophasic in character).
- Bronchospasm due to acute exacerbation of COPD, carcinoid syndrome, recurrent pulmonary emboli, cardiogenic pulmonary edema, systemic vasculitis, or eosinophilic pulmonary syndromes.
- Bronchospasm induced by drugs (e.g. beta-blockers, aspirin, nebulized drugs such as antibiotics).

Box 6-5

A clinical classification of causes of respiratory failure

Hypoxemia without CO$_2$ retention, clear CXR	**Hypoxemia without CO$_2$ retention, infiltrate on CXR**	**Hypoxemia, CO$_2$ retention, clear CXR**
- Pulmonary emboli	- Cardiac failure	- COPD
- Acute airway obstruction	- Interstitial disease	- Severe asthma
- Intracardiac shunt	- Pneumonia	
	- Adult respiratory distress syndrome	

COPD, chronic obstructive pulmonary disease; CXR, chest X-ray.

CLINICAL PEARL

Wheeze associated with gastroesophageal reflux may have multiple mechanisms, including vocal cord dysfunction.

Pathophysiology of asthma

Airway response to an inhaled allergen frequently involves an early bronchoconstrictive response which peaks within 30 minutes and resolves in 1–2 hours, followed by a late-phase response from 3 to 9 hours later.

- Early asthmatic responses reflect the concentration of specific IgE, and the extent of non-specific bronchial hyper-responsiveness.
- Early responses are mediated through degranulation of mast cells, and release of pre-formed and newly formed inflammatory mediators.
- Late-phase responses are characterized by the influx of inflammatory cells.
- Late-phase responses are IgE-independent, with the metabolism of mast cell membrane phospholipids such as leukotrienes, platelet-activating factor and prostaglandins being chemotactic for inflammatory cells.
- Inflammatory cells, especially eosinophils, neutrophils and T-helper cells, then release further inflammatory mediators.

Occupational exposures can induce asthma (see below).

Signs of a severe exacerbation of asthma

(after GINA 2020)

1. Talks in words
2. Sits hunched forwards
3. Agitated
4. Respiratory rate >30/min
5. Accessory muscles being used
6. Pulse rate >120 bpm
7. O_2 saturation (on air) <90%
8. PEF less than or equal to 50% predicted or best

Treatment of acute severe asthma

(after GINA, 2011 and 2020)

- Increased inspired oxygen to achieve an oxyhemoglobin saturation 93–95%
- Continuous oxygen saturation (S_aO_2) monitoring
- Continuous inhaled short-acting beta-agonist
- Inhaled anticholinergic, e.g. ipratropium bromide
- Oral or IV corticosteroids
- Consider IV magnesium sulfate
- Consider high-dose ICS
- Ventilatory support if worsening respiratory failure, initially with non-invasive ventilation (NIV) using bi-level continuous positive airway pressure (CPAP) via a mask or subsequent intubation

Management of chronic asthma

In order to formulate individualized treatment plans for asthmatics, it is necessary to characterize the pattern of disease.

- Some patients have intermittent symptoms, followed by intervening periods without any discernible symptomatology. Lung function may be normal at these asymptomatic times, or demonstrate some persistent ('subclinical') obstruction. Having an intermittent pattern does not always imply a lack of severity.
- Some intermittent asthma is predictable, e.g. exercise-induced asthma.
- Other patients have chronic daily symptoms. Again, severity of chronic symptoms will vary.

Level of symptoms is an unreliable gauge of lung function. Objective measurement via spirometry at varying times is desirable in all patients.

Treatment

- Inhaled short-acting beta-agonist therapy in combination with inhaled corticosteroid is the mainstay of treatment for **intermittent asthma**.

CLINICAL PEARLS

- The goals of asthma treatment are to control asthma symptoms and prevent exacerbations of asthma. The majority of people with asthma over the age of 6 years should be treated with a preventer that contains an inhaled corticosteroid.
- Inhaled beta-agonist drugs such as salbutamol/albuterol are used as acute symptomatic treatment ('relievers') for most people with asthma. It is now recommended they be used in combination with inhaled corticosteroids.
- Inhaled beta-agonists can be given 30 minutes before exercise to avert exercise-induced symptoms.

- **Chronic asthma** should be managed with inhaled corticosteroids.
  - » Inadequate symptom control or suboptimal lung function despite inhaled corticosteroids can be treated by the addition of long-acting beta-agonists such as salmeterol or eformoterol.
- The role of leukotriene antagonists is more clearly delineated in children, but some adults with chronic symptoms may benefit.
- Intermittent courses of oral corticosteroids will be required for acute severe exacerbations of asthma.
  - » A small minority of chronic asthmatics require long-term oral corticosteroids to allow adequacy of lung function. In these patients, steroid-sparing agents are sometimes employed, although there is limited evidence for the efficacy of drugs such as methotrexate.
- Severe forms of chronic asthma should be considered for treatment with biological agents. There is a strong evidence base for the use of anti-IgE monoclonal antibodies (e.g. omalizumab) in allergic sub-types, and anti-IL-5 monoclonal antibodies (e.g. mepolizumab,

benralizumab) or anti-IL4R monoclonal antibodies (dupilumab) in eosinophilic sub-types.

- There is strong evidence for efficacy of allergen immuno-therapy in patients with allergic sensitization to airborne allergens such as the house dust mite. This treatment must be used with caution in those with severe or unstable asthma due to the risk of anaphylaxis.

- Methylxanthines such as theophylline are rarely used due to their narrow therapeutic index and limited efficacy.

- Inhaled anticholinergics such as ipratropium and tiotropium are generally reserved for patients with COPD, but can be considered in those with chronic severe disease.

- Spacer devices should be encouraged for delivery of inhaled medication to all asthmatics. Many patients are unable to adequately coordinate the use of metered-dose inhalers.

> ### CLINICAL PEARL
>
> It is important to identify exacerbating factors for asthma in all patients.
> - Usual factors include upper respiratory tract infection, cold air, exercise, and airborne allergens such as house dust mite, animal dander, grass and tree pollens.
> - Some 10% of asthmatics will experience exacerbation after ingestion of aspirin or other cyclo-oxygenase-1 (COX-1) inhibiting drugs.
>
> All asthmatics should have:
> - routine vaccinations
> - regular review of asthma management plan and device technique

Allergic bronchopulmonary aspergillosis (ABPA)

This is an uncommon condition that can complicate asthma. Colonization of the airway by fungal elements may lead to a hypersensitivity reaction, resulting in airway inflammation, cough, dyspnea, tenacious sputum plugs, and, frequently, worsening asthma control. The plugs of resultant mucous and prolonged airway inflammation may lead to bronchiectasis. See Figure 6-8.

Diagnostic criteria

1 Asthma
2 Pulmonary infiltrates
3 Peripheral eosinophilia
4 Immediate wheal-and-flare response to *Aspergillus fumigatus*
5 Serum precipitins to *A. fumigatus*
6 Total serum IgE elevated, *Aspergillus* specific IgE elevated
7 Central bronchiectasis

Treatment

The mainstay of treatment for ABPA is systemic cortico-steroid medication. There is emerging evidence for anti-

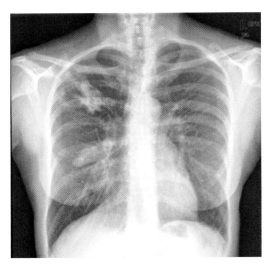

Figure 6-8 Chest X-ray of a patient with allergic bronchopulmonary aspergillosis; note the central and upper zone distribution of infiltrates

From Lazarus AA, Thilagar B and McKay SA. Allergic bronchopulmonary aspergillosis. Disease-a-Month 2008;54(8): 547–64.

fungal treatment and anti-IgE therapy as a steroid sparing strategy.

Bronchiectasis

Definition

- Pathological dilatation of the airways or bronchi presenting as recurrent or chronic airway infection.

- Presence of resistant organisms such as *Pseudomonas aeruginosa* and *Staphylococcus aureus* is a common feature.

Clinical features

- Daily cough with variable but persistent sputum production

- Varying degrees of dyspnea

- Finger clubbing often present

- Chest auscultation may be normal, or reveal wheeze, crackles, or both

- Cor pulmonale may develop in late stages

See Figure 6-9.

Causes

Inherited

1 Cystic fibrosis
2 Primary Ciliary Dyskinesia:

A genetically heterogeneous rare lung disease characterized by recurrent upper and lower respiratory tract infections that present in the neonatal period. Also associated with organ laterality defects, complex congenital heart disease and impaired fertility in both men

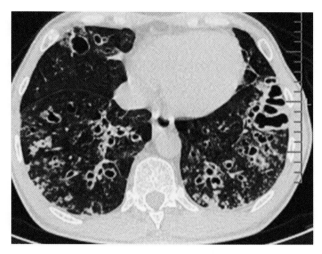

Figure 6-9 Chest computed tomography of a patient with bronchiectasis; note the dilatation of the airways with marked wall thickening. The bronchi are larger than the accompanying pulmonary arteries; this is known as the signet ring sign

From Belada D et al. Diffuse large B-cell lymphoma in a patient with hyper-IgE syndrome: successful treatment with risk-adapted rituximab-based immunochemotherapy. Leuk Res 2010;34(9): e232–e234.

(abnormal sperm motility), and women (impaired fallopian duct function).

2 Immunodeficiency (IgA deficiency, common variable immunodeficiency)

Acquired/structural

1 Post-infection, e.g. childhood respiratory tract infection including pertussis and measles; necrotizing pneumonia
2 Localized disease, e.g. bronchial adenoma, tuberculosis, foreign body
3 Airway disease and asthma, e.g. asthma, COPD, ABPA
4 Inflammatory disorders, e.g. rheumatoid arthritis, IBD, systemic lupus erythematosus (SLE)
5 Inhalation, e.g. gastro-esophageal reflux disease, recurrent pulmonary aspiration, burns, foreign body

Treatment

General Management of Bronchiectasis in Adults (see Figure 6-10)

- Airway clearance
- Influenza and pneumonia immunisations
- Pulmonary rehabilitation
- Smoking cessation
- Sputum surveillance
- Prompt treatment of exacerbations
- Treat underlying cause (specialist referral recommended)

- Inhaled corticosteroid, long-acting bronchodilators only for concomitant asthma or COPD

Cystic fibrosis (CF)

This is an autosomal recessive disorder caused by multiple mutations of a single gene on the long arm of chromosome 7.

The most common mutation is a deletion of phenylalanine at position 508, so-called ΔF508, which is responsible for about 70% of all CF. The gene codes for a multi-functional protein, cystic fibrosis trans-membrane regulator (CFTR), which is active in the membrane of epithelial cells. It operates as a chloride channel and regulates other ion channels. There are more than 1800 mutations known to reduce the function of chloride channels.

The major effects are on the lungs and pancreatic exocrine function where there are thick, tenacious secretions.

CLINICAL PEARL

Diagnosis of CF is usually made in childhood, but late presentation may occur, including with:
- recurrent respiratory tract infections
- bronchiectasis
- difficult-to-control asthma, including with ABPA
- atypical mycobacterial infections
- pancreatitis and liver disease.

Diagnostic tests

1 Gene testing
2 Sweat chloride >60 mEq/L

Pathophysiology

- Recurrent pulmonary infection, predominantly with *Haemophilus influenzae*, *Pseudomonas aeruginosa* and *Staphylococcus aureus*
- Inspissated secretions
- Bronchiectasis
- Malabsorption
- Progressive respiratory failure and cor pulmonale

Median survival is now approximately 40 years, and is increasing due to improvements in treatment.

Bronchiolitis

Definition

An inflammatory disorder of the small airways (<2 mm diameter), usually characterized by obstruction with air trapping, and usually without significant disease of the lung parenchyma. There is a wide range of causes, including the following.

1 Infection:
   a Viral—RSV (respiratory syncytial virus) and other viruses
   b Bacterial—tuberculosis (TB) and atypical TB, e.g. *Mycobacterium avium* complex

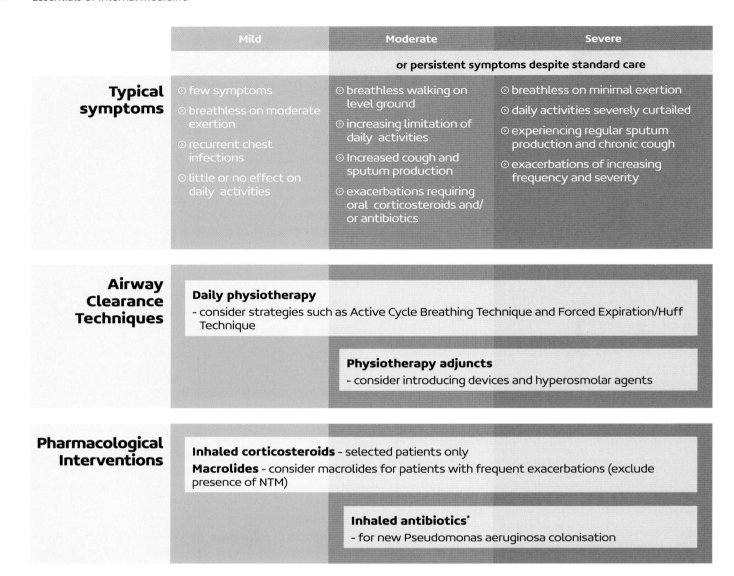

Figure 6-10 Stepwise Management of Stable Bronchiectasis
Used with permission from Lung Foundation Australia.

2 Non-infectious, often causing bronchiolitis obliterans (see below):
  a Inhalational injury
  b Connective tissue disease
  c Organ transplantation, especially lung
  d Drugs, e.g. gold, penicillamine
  e Idiopathic

Obliterative bronchiolitis/bronchiolitis obliterans

(Called bronchiolitis obliterans syndrome if it occurs in a lung transplant.)

This results from concentric narrowing of small airways due to intramural fibrotic tissue, causing scarring of bronchiolar walls and surrounding tissue, and airflow obstruction.

The pathology varies and has been divided into categories:

• *Constrictive*. This results in progressive airflow obstruction, usually following inhalational injury.

• *Proliferative*. This is the more common form, with proliferation of fibroblasts. Extension into the alveoli can occur to a varying degree. If it is extensive, it is called bronchiolitis obliterans with organizing pneumonia (BOOP; Figure 6-11) or cryptogenic organizing pneumonia (COP), and is considered an interstitial lung disease (see later section).

Treatment:

• Viral bronchiolitis is treated with respiratory support, as required.

• Other infectious causes require appropriate antimycobacterial or other antibiotic treatment.

Panbronchiolitis

This is a recently identified and uncommon disorder, initially described in Japan, with diffuse bronchiolitis presenting as cough, breathlessness and sputum production.

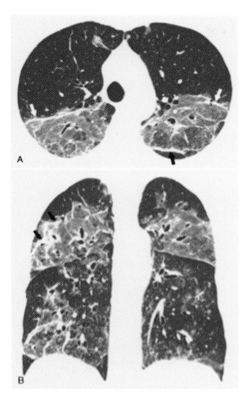

Figure 6-11 Chest computed tomography of a patient with bronchiolitis obliterans with organizing pneumonia (BOOP). Arrows indicate areas of fibrosis. Note also consolidation with air bronchograms

From Muller NL and Silva CIS (eds). Imaging of the chest. Saunders, 2008.

- There are typical high-resolution chest CT findings of diffuse, small, centrilobular nodular opacities, and a tree-in-bud pattern.
- There is often progressive decline in lung function with an obstructive defect.

It usually responds well to treatment with a macrolide, possibly due to an anti-inflammatory rather than an antibiotic mechanism.

Chronic obstructive pulmonary disease (COPD)

Definition

The GOLD (Global Initiative for Chronic Obstructive Lung Disease) definition is internationally accepted:

> *COPD is 'a common, preventable and treatable disease, characterized by persistent airflow limitation that is usually progressive, and associated with an enhanced chronic inflammatory response in the airways and the lung to noxious particles or gases. Exacerbations and comorbidities contribute to the overall severity in individual patients.'*

The usual criterion for chronic airflow limitation is a post-bronchodilator FEV1/FVC of <0.7; however, there is a change in reporting criteria to use the lower limit of normal (LLN) for the ratio since 0.7 tends to over-diagnose disease in the elderly and under-diagnose it in the young.

The chronic airflow limitation seen in COPD is due to a combination of small airways disease, equivalent to an obstructive bronchiolitis, and to loss of parenchymal support for airways due to destruction of parenchymal tissue causing emphysema. Although the most common cause of COPD is cigarette smoking, there are other causes, including an overlap with chronic asthma.

COPD is an heterogeneous disorder with a phenotype that can vary with the extent, severity and underlying pathogenesis of disease in four compartments of the lung:

- Large airways—chronic bronchitis is defined clinically as persistent cough and sputum for at least 3 months in each of 2 consecutive years.
- Small airways—damage and obstruction at the level of the bronchioles causes progressive insidious airflow limitation.
- Lung parenchyma—emphysema is defined pathologically as an abnormal enlargement in the size of the air spaces distal to the terminal bronchioles.
- Pulmonary blood vessels—increased pulmonary vascular resistance causing pulmonary hypertension, and eventually cor pulmonale from arteriolar vasoconstriction by alveolar hypoxia, and destruction of pulmonary vasculature.

Causes of emphysema

1. Cigarette smoking
2. Alpha-1-antitrypsin deficiency (emphysema/autosomal recessive)
3. Occupational exposure, e.g. coal, hematite (centrilobular emphysema), bauxite (bullous emphysema), cadmium (generalized emphysema)

Pathophysiology

- **Emphysema:** Destruction of alveolar walls by enzymes released from inflammatory cells results in loss of airway tethering, with airway obstruction, and loss of alveolar–capillary units, which is reflected by a decrease in the diffusing capacity for carbon monoxide.
- **Chronic bronchitis:** Airway obstruction results from mucous gland enlargement and smooth muscle hypertrophy, with consequent bronchial wall thickening and luminal narrowing. Recurrent bacterial infection may also be an important factor.

Differential diagnosis

1. Adult onset asthma—may be non-smoker, atopic, family history of atopic disease, and attacks may be episodic. Lung function may be near-normal between exacerbations. However, there may be overlap since long-term asthma can lead to irreversible airflow limitation.

2 Bronchiectasis—daily large-volume sputum production, clubbing, onset often in childhood, and hemoptysis common.

Treatment

(see Figure 6-12)

Complications

• Recurrent acute exacerbations, usually caused by viral infections

• Respiratory failure: acute, chronic, acute-on-chronic
• Cor pulmonale
• Spontaneous pneumothorax
• Pneumonia

Interstitial lung disease (ILD)

ILD refers to a broad group of disorders (Box 6-6, overleaf) where there is inflammation in the alveolar walls, often associated with fibrosis, that causes damage to the blood vessels in the alveolar walls and to the alveolar epithelial cells.

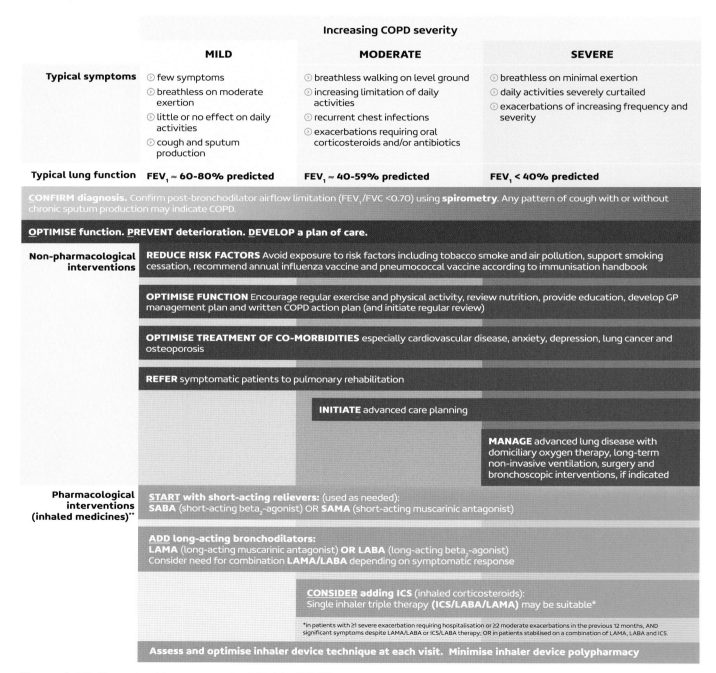

Figure 6-12 Stepwise Management of Stable COPD

Used with permission from Lung Foundation Australia.

Box 6-6
Interstitial lung disease

Interstitial lung disease limited to the lung

- Idiopathic pulmonary fibrosis
- Idiopathic interstitial types of pneumonia
  - » Usual interstitial pneumonia
  - » Cryptogenic fibrosing alveolitis
- Acute interstitial pneumonitis (Hamman–Rich syndrome)
- Familial pulmonary fibrosis
- Respiratory bronchiolitis/ desquamative interstitial pneumonitis
- Cryptogenic organizing pneumonia (COP)/bronchiolitis obliterans with organizing pneumonia (BOOP)
- Non-specific interstitial pneumonitis

Interstitial lung disease associated with connective tissue disorders

- Scleroderma/CREST
- Polymyositis/dermatomyositis
- Systemic lupus erythematosus (SLE)
- Sjögren's syndrome
- Mixed connective tissue disease
- Rheumatoid arthritis
- Ankylosing spondylitis

Interstitial lung disease secondary to known triggers
Medication
- Antibiotics, e.g. nitrofurantoin

- Antiarrhythmics, e.g. amiodarone, procainamide
- Anti-inflammatories, e.g. penicillamine, gold
- Anticonvulsants, e.g. phenytoin
- Chemotherapeutic agents, e.g. cyclophosphamide, methotrexate, busulphan, bleomycin
- Recreational: 'crack' cocaine
- Biologicals: rituximab, infliximab

Occupational and environmental causes

Inorganic:
- Silicosis
- Asbestosis
- Hard-metal pneumoconiosis
  - » Coal-worker's pneumoconiosis
  - » Berylliosis
  - » Talc pneumoconiosis
  - » Siderosis (arc welding)
  - » Stannosis (tin)

Organic:
- Hypersensitivity pneumonitis or extrinsic allergic alveolitis, e.g. bird-breeders' lung, farmer's lung

Radiation pneumonitis/fibrosis

Interstitial lung disease secondary to inflammatory autoimmune disorders
- Lymphocytic interstitial pneumonia (Sjögren's syndrome, connective tissue disease, acquired immune deficiency syndrome (AIDS), Hashimoto's thyroiditis)

- Autoimmune pulmonary fibrosis (inflammatory bowel disease, primary biliary cholangitis, idiopathic thrombocytopenic purpura, autoimmune hemolytic anemia)

Interstitial lung disease due to unclassified causes
- Sarcoidosis
- Tuberous sclerosis
- Acute respiratory distress syndrome (ARDS)
- Alveolar proteinosis
- Primary pulmonary Langerhan's cell histiocytosis (eosinophilic granuloma)
- Amyloidosis
- Pulmonary vasculitis
- Diffuse alveolar hemorrhage syndromes
- Eosinophilic pneumonia
- Piloid pneumonia
- Lymphangitic carcinomatosis
- Bronchioalveolar cell carcinoma
- Lymphangioleiomyomatosis
- Gaucher's disease
- Niemann–Pick disease
- Pulmonary lymphoma
- Hermansky–Pudlak syndrome

The mechanism of damage is as broad as the number of disorders, with some starting with diffuse injury to the gas exchange units, while in others the pathological process appears to start in the parenchyma.

Clinical clues to the etiology of diffuse pulmonary disease are:

- Raynaud's phenomenon—scleroderma, pulmonary hypertension
- Symptom onset 4–6 hours after exposure—hypersensitivity pneumonitis
- Less dyspnea than expected from chest X-ray appearance—sarcoidosis, silicosis, Langerhan's cell granulomatosis
- Erythema nodosum—sarcoidosis, histoplasmosis
- Dysphagia—scleroderma, dermatomyositis, metastatic cancer
- Hemoptysis—heart failure, bronchiectasis, Goodpasture's syndrome, idiopathic pulmonary hemosiderosis
- Clubbing—idiopathic pulmonary fibrosis, bronchiectasis, cancer (lymphangitis carcinomatosa)
- Hematuria—ANCA-associated vasculitis, Goodpasture's syndrome, systemic lupus erythematosus (SLE), polyarteritis nodosa (PAN), scleroderma.

CLINICAL PEARL

Causes of pulmonary fibrosis:

Upper lobe (mnemonic 'SCATO')
S Silicosis, sarcoidosis
C Coal miner's pneumoconiosis
A Ankylosing spondylitis, allergic bronchopulmonary aspergillosis, allergic alveolitis
T Tuberculosis
O Other: drugs, radiation, berylliosis, eosinophilic granuloma, necrobiotic nodular form of rheumatoid arthritis

Lower lobe (mnemonic 'RASHO')
R Rheumatoid arthritis
A Asbestosis
S Scleroderma
H Hamman–Rich syndrome, idiopathic pulmonary fibrosis
O Other: drugs, radiation

CLINICAL PEARL

The most common form of ILD is idiopathic pulmonary fibrosis (IPF).

Treatment

There is now good evidence of efficacy for antifibrotic drugs (nintedinib and perfenidone) in slowing the rate of decline in lung function for patients with IPF. These drugs have significant side-effects.

Scleroderma is the only CTD associated ILD where immunosuppression (cyclophosphamide and mycophenolate) has been demonstrated to provide benefit.

Idiopathic pulmonary fibrosis

This is a disease of unknown etiology, with inflammation and fibrosis of alveolar walls. Without treatment there is often an inexorable deterioration to chronic respiratory failure.

Diagnosis

There is a typical chest X-ray (CXR) and high-resolution computed tomography (HRCT) appearance of diffuse interstitial opacities (and 'honeycombing' in more advanced stages of disease), with pulmonary function tests showing reduced DLCO, arterial hypoxemia, and a restrictive ventilatory impairment suggesting the diagnosis; but a lung biopsy is necessary in most cases for definitive diagnosis, unless the HRCT shows typical changes of usual interstitial pneumonitis with predominantly lower-zone changes.

Treatment

- IPF is a progressive disease but in the last 5 years antifibrotic therapy (nintedinib and perfenidone) has been proven to be effective at slowing the rate of decline in lung function in IPF. Management of IPF would optimally be delivered by a multidisciplinary care team.

- Most patients eventually develop type I respiratory failure, and require respiratory support in the form of long-term supplemental oxygen therapy. Cor pulmonale complicates the late stages of the disease.

- Immunization to *Pneumococcus* and influenza should be kept up to date.

- Prompt treatment of superimposed respiratory infection is required.

- There is a small increase in the incidence of lung carcinoma.

- Transplantation may be appropriate in some cases.

CLINICAL PEARL

All patients with ILD require a HRCT and should be managed by a multidisciplinary team. The most common form of idiopathic pulmonary fibrosis (IPF).

Occupational lung disease

Occupational exposure to both organic and inorganic compounds can result in a variety of pulmonary conditions, including interstitial, obstructive, malignant and pleural disease.

Inorganic agents—pneumoconiosis

Asbestosis

- Asbestosis is mainly found in asbestos miners, but also in workers in the building industry, especially demolition or ship's lagging workers.

- Asbestosis is a form of diffuse interstitial fibrosis.

- Asbestos exposure can also result in pleural plaque formation (Figure 6-13), and is an important risk factor for carcinoma of the lung, and mesothelioma.

Silicosis

- Silicosis is mainly found in the mining and quarrying industries but has become a contemporary and emerging condition in people working with artificial stone products. The silica content of artificial stone is approximately 90%, far higher than natural stones (marble 3%, granite 30% on average). Artificial stone silicosis develops after a shorter exposure time and is associated with more rapid progression than silicosis secondary to natural stone dust.

- Nodular pulmonary fibrosis may progress to progressive massive fibrosis (PMF; Figure 6-14).

- Calcification of hilar nodes (eggshell pattern) occurs in 20% of cases. There is also an increased risk of tuberculosis.

- Silicosis is an interdependent risk factor for lung cancer.

Coal-worker's pneumoconiosis (CWP)

- CWP is seen in around 10% of all underground coal-miners.

- It is a form of pulmonary fibrosis.

- A small percentage also develop PMF.

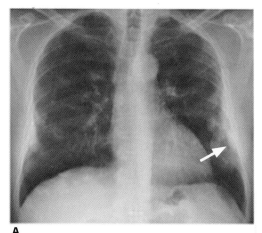

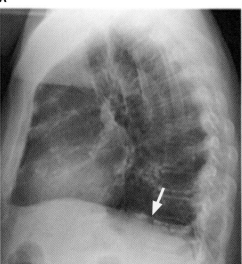

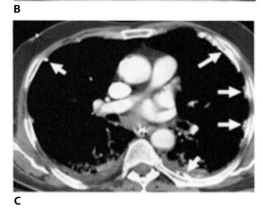

Figure 6-13 Chest X-ray and computed tomography of patient with pleural plaques (arrows)

From Müller NL and Silva CIS (eds). Imaging of the chest. Saunders, 2008.

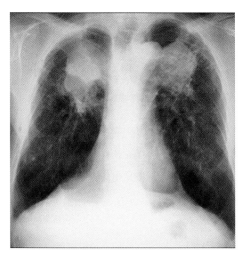

Figure 6-14 Chest X-ray of patient with progressive massive fibrosis

From Müller NL et al. Radiologic diagnosis of diseases of the chest. Philadelphia: Saunders, 2001.

Berylliosis

- Berylliosis results from exposure in the electronics, computer and ceramics industries.
- Beryllium can rarely cause an acute pneumonitis; more frequently a chronic granulomatous interstitial pneumonitis occurs.
- It is a risk factor for carcinoma of the lung, and a differential diagnosis of sarcoidosis.

Asthma

Occupational asthma can occur in:

- aluminium smelter workers
- grain and flour workers
- electronic industry workers (colophory in solder flux)
- animal workers (urinary proteins)
- paint sprayers and polyurethane workers (isocyanates)
- epoxy resin and platinum salt workers.
- hairdressers.

Organic agents—hypersensitivity pneumonitis (extrinsic allergic alveolitis)

This is a type III hypersensitivity reaction to inhaled organic dusts or animal proteins which can manifest in acute and chronic forms.

- **Acute**—4 to 6 hours after exposure a sensitized person develops dyspnea, cough, and fever without wheeze. Chest X-ray reveals nodular or reticulonodular infiltrates with apical sparing.
- **Chronic**—repeated attacks result in lung fibrosis.

Examples are:

- farmer's lung—thermophilic bacteria from moldy hay
- bird-breeder's lung—animal protein from bird droppings

- hot-tub lung—allergic response to inhaled *Mycobacterium avium* complex
- mushroom-grower's lung.

Diagnosis depends on a consistent clinical picture in association with serum precipitins to an appropriate antigen.

Pulmonary edema

Can result from irritant gas exposure, e.g. to chlorine.

Granulomatous ILD

Sarcoidosis

This is a systemic, non-caseating granulomatous disease of unknown etiology, typically with a predominant pulmonary component.

Clinical features

1 Bilateral hilar lymphadenopathy (BHL; Figure 6-15) in 80% of cases—almost always asymptomatic
2 Lung disease stages:
   0 No lung involvement
   1 BHL only (DLCO may be decreased)
   2 BHL and pulmonary infiltrate
   3 Fibrosing infiltrate (usually midzone) without lymphadenopathy
   4 End-stage pulmonary fibrosis
3 Skin—erythema nodosum (with BHL), lupus pernio, pink nodules in scars
4 Lymphadenopathy (generalized in 7%)
5 Eyes—acute uveitis, uveoparotid fever (uveitis, parotid swelling, 7th cranial nerve palsy)
6 Nervous system—cranial nerve palsy, neuropathy, myopathy
7 Liver granulomas
8 Skeletal—bone cysts, arthritis
9 Heart—heart block, cardiomyopathy
10 Hypercalcemia
11 Splenomegaly

Diagnosis

- Requires histological confirmation, usually via lung biopsy.
- Transbronchial biopsy will give a result in the majority of cases, but at times thorascopic or open lung biopsy, or biopsy of other involved tissue, is needed.
- Pulmonary function tests generally demonstrate a restrictive pattern and reduced DLCO.
- Serum ACE levels are neither sensitive enough nor specific enough to be consistently useful diagnostically. However, an elevated level in an otherwise consistent clinical picture in a patient in whom biopsy is not possible is helpful.

Treatment

- Oral corticosteroids are the mainstay of treatment, and most disease is steroid-sensitive.
- BHL alone can be treated with a wait-and-watch approach, and does not require treatment *per se*.
- Some patients will have a progressive, relentless disease which requires ongoing therapy.
- Others will go into remission, which may or may not be permanent.
- Many patients on long-term corticosteroids will require addition of a second immunosuppressive agent such as azathioprine or mycophenolate.
- Aggressiveness of immunosuppressive therapy depends on the severity and location of disease, e.g. sight-threatening ocular disease.

Cryptogenic organizing pneumonia (COP)

Also known as bronchiolitis obliterans with organizing pneumonia (BOOP).

- COP results from inflammation of the alveolar spaces, which often extends into the bronchioli causing plugging of airways by granulation tissue (see Figure 6-11).
- COP is the preferred term, as the alveolar changes are predominant while the bronchiolitis is a minor part of the condition.
- This commonly results in a restrictive pattern of abnormal lung function tests.

Causes

1 Cigarette smoking
2 Post-infectious, e.g. adenovirus, influenza, *Mycoplasma*
3 Connective tissue disease
4 Toxin inhalation (nitrogen oxides, chlorine, ammonia)
5 Chronic rejection after lung transplantation
6 Chronic graft-versus-host disease
7 Idiopathic (is the commonest cause of COP)

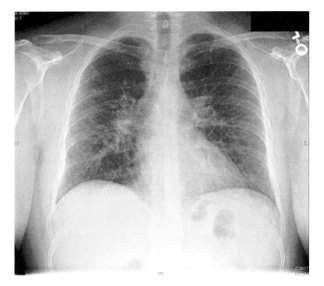

Figure 6-15 Chest X-ray of bilateral hilar lymphadenopathy due to sarcoidosis

From Mason RJ et al (eds). Murray and Nadel's Textbook of respiratory medicine, 5th ed. Philadelphia: Saunders, 2010.

Treatment

- COP/BOOP is treated with immunosuppressive drugs.
- High-dose corticosteroids are used as first-line.
- Steroid-sparing second-line agents are often required, as treatment may need to be long-term.

EOSINOPHILIC PULMONARY DISORDERS

These are rare diseases of unknown etiology and should be considered when there is incomplete response to antibiotics.

Clinical features

- Fever
- Acute hypoxemic respiratory failure
- Diffuse pulmonary (alveolar) infiltrates on CXR
- Approximately 25% eosinophils in bronchoalveolar lavage (BAL) fluid
- Peripheral blood eosinophilia (usually)

Clinical features

- Constitutional symptoms—fevers, night sweats, malaise, weight loss
- Asthma, often pre-dating the disease, in the majority of cases
- Dyspnea
- Bilateral peripheral pulmonary infiltrates, which may be fleeting
- Raised acute phase reactants
- Peripheral blood eosinophilia (usually)
- Approximately 25% eosinophils in BAL fluid

Definitive diagnosis requires lung biopsy.

Treatment

- Oral corticosteroids are used for remission induction.
- Long-term use may be required.
- Unacceptable side-effects, or inability to wean the dose, will require addition of a second agent such as azathioprine, methotrexate or mycophenolate.

CLINICAL PEARL

Pulmonary infiltrate with eosinophilia
Causes (mnemonic 'PLATE'):
P Prolonged pulmonary eosinophilia, which may be due to:
  Drugs
  Parasites
L Loeffler's syndrome—benign acute eosinophilic infiltration with few clinical manifestations
A ABPA
T Tropical, e.g. microfilaria
E Eosinophilic pneumonia
Other: vasculitis, e.g. polyarteritis nodosa, eosinophilic granulomatosis with polyangiitis

PULMONARY HEMORRHAGE

Pulmonary hemorrhage can be localized, often due to neoplastic or traumatic conditions, or secondary to diffuse alveolar hemorrhage (DAH).

- The most common causes of DAH (Box 6-7) are immune-mediated, although the differential diagnosis for DAH is broad. Of the immune-mediated causes, the ANCA-associated vasculitides are the most common.
- Diagnostic clues on imaging which suggest DAH include ground-glass opacities, rapidly changing appearance, perihilar distribution, and consolidation.

PULMONARY INFECTIONS

Bacterial

Organisms commonly implicated in community-acquired pneumonia:

- *Streptococcus pneumoniae*
- *Mycoplasma* species
- *Legionella* species
- *Haemophilus influenzae*
- *Moraxella catarrhalis*
- *Staphylococcus aureus.*

CLINICAL PEARL

Risk factors for nosocomial pneumonia:
- increasing age
- underlying chronic lung disease
- altered neurological state
- intubation
- immobilization.
- alcohol consumption.

Organisms commonly implicated in nosocomial pneumonia:

- Gram-negative bacilli
- *Staphylococcus aureus*

Box 6-7

Causes of diffuse alveolar hemorrhage

Immune-mediated causes

- Vasculitides (numerous, including ANCA-associated vasculitis, Goodpasture's syndrome)

Non-immune-mediated causes

- Toxic injury, e.g. chemical inhalation
- Coagulopathy, including anticoagulant drugs
- Increased pulmonary venous hydrostatic pressure, e.g. mitral stenosis
- Idiopathic pulmonary hemosiderosis

- anaerobic bacteria
- *Streptococcus pneumoniae.*

Causes of recurrent pneumonia (2 or more episodes in 6 months):

- Bronchial obstruction, e.g. by a lung cancer, foreign body, bronchial stenosis
- Bronchiectasis
- Recurrent pulmonary infarction
- Recurrent aspiration of gastric contents
- Hypogammaglobulinemia (congenital or acquired)
- Pulmonary eosinophilia
- HIV (human immunodeficiency virus) infection, or other immunodeficiency

CLINICAL PEARL

Causes of a slowly resolving or non-resolving pneumonia:

1. Bronchial obstruction
2. Complications of pneumonia—abscess, empyema
3. Inappropriate therapy
4. Non-adherence to therapy
5. Non-absorption of antibiotic, e.g. vomiting of tablets
6. Decreased host resistance (immunodeficiency)
7. Pneumonia mimic, e.g. cryptogenic organizing pneumonia (COP), bronchioalveolar cell cancer

Viral

Viruses which may cause pneumonia in adults:

- influenza A or B
- adenovirus
- respiratory syncytial virus
- parainfluenza
- cytomegalovirus (CMV)
- corona virus (COVID-19).

Fungal

Fungi which may cause lung infection:

- *Histoplasma capsulatum*
- *Aspergillus fumigatus*
- *Cryptococcus neoformans*
- *Blastomyces dermatiditis*
- *Coccidioides immitis*
- *Nocardia* species (bacteria)
- *Actinomyces.*

Associations with CXR findings are given in Table 6-5, those with extrapulmonary disease in Table 6-6, and morphological clues to diagnosis in Table 6-7.

Table 6-5 Chest X-ray (CXR) findings in fungal lung infection

CXR FINDINGS	ASSOCIATED FUNGAL INFECTION
Lung calcification	Histoplasmosis (spleen often also calcified)
Hilar lymphadenopathy	Histoplasmosis, blastomycosis, coccidioidomycosis
Cavitary disease	Nocardiosis, blastomycosis (thick-walled)
	Coccidioidomycosis (thin-walled)
Round opacity, with halo of translucency	Aspergilloma
Pleural effusion	Actinomycosis, nocardiosis, coccidioidomycosis

Table 6-6 Fungal infections of the lung and extrapulmonary disease

ANATOMICAL SITES	POSSIBLE FUNGAL INFECTION
Lung and skin	Blastomycosis (erythema nodosum)
	Coccidioidomycosis (erythema nodosum, morbilliform rash)
	Nocardiosis (subcutaneous abscess)
	Cryptococcosis (tiny papules, progress to ulcers)
Lung, nose, palate	Mucormycosis, aspergillosis
Lung, bone	Actinomycosis, blastomycosis, coccidioidomycosis
Lung, gut	*Candida*, histoplasmosis, *Aspergillus*, actinomycosis
Lung, urinary tract	Blastomycosis (males)

Table 6-7 Morphological clues to diagnosis of fungal infection

MORPHOLOGY	FUNGUS
45°-angled branching	*Aspergillus*
90°-angled branching and non-septate hyphae	*Nocardia*
Thick cell wall	*Cryptococcus*
Broad neck budding	*Blastomyces*
Acid-fast	*Nocardia*

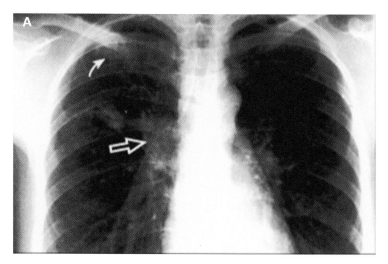
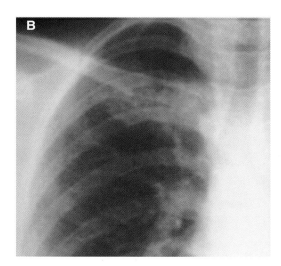

Figure 6-16 Chest X-rays showing (**A**) Ghon complex and (**B**) upper lobe tubercular lesions

From: (A) Talley NJ and O'Connor S. Clinical examination: a systematic guide to physical diagnosis, 6th ed. Sydney: Elsevier Australia, 2010. (B) Grant LE and Griffin N. Grainger & Allison's Diagnostic radiology: essentials. Elsevier, 2013.

Mycobacterial

Tuberculosis (TB)

(Infection with *Mycobacterium tuberculosis* [MTB].)

1. Primary infection—patient never previously exposed. Primary complex consists of Ghon focus in mid or lower lung zone, and hilar lymphadenopathy.
2. Secondary infection—usually reactivation of dormant infection. Lesions develop in the upper lobe or the apex of the lower lobe with minimal lymphadenopathy.
3. Extrapulmonary involvement occurs in up to 20% of patients.

Diagnosis

1. Mantoux (purified protein derivative, PPD)—an induration >10 mm signifies previous or current infection, or BCG (Bacillus Calmette-Guérin) immunization.
   a. False-negatives may occur in miliary TB, immunosuppressed patients (e.g. HIV infection, malnutrition, concurrent use of corticosteroids), elderly individuals, sarcoidosis, coexisting infection (e.g. lepromatous leprosy), or due to technical error.
   b. False-positives from non-tuberculosis mycobacteria (NTMB) may occur.
2. Interferon-gamma assay—specific for MTB, except for false-positives from the NTMB *M. kansasii, M. marinum, M. szulgai.*
3. CXR/CT (see Figure 6-16).
4. Microbiology—acid-fast staining and culture on sputum, bronchoalveolar lavage fluid, or gastric washings.

Management

1. Chemoprophylaxis with daily isoniazid for 9 months (or isoniazid and rifampicin for 3 months) is indicated if:
   a. there is conversion to a positive Mantoux test (10 mm or more >35 years of age, 15 mm or more <35 years of age) within the past 2 years
   b. patient is HIV-positive with Mantoux reaction 5 mm or more
   c. there has been recent contact with infectious patient, Mantoux 10 mm or more
   d. patient has chronic illness or is immunosuppressed, Mantoux 10 mm or more
   e. patient is in a high-incidence group, Mantoux 10 mm or more, >35 years of age (from endemic area, nursing home or institution).
2. Standard therapy:
   a. isoniazid, rifampicin, pyrazinamide and ethambutol (see Table 6-8) for 2 months (2HRZE) followed by isoniazid and rifampicin for 4 months (4HR)
   b. best outcomes are achieved with directly observed therapy, short course (DOTS).
3. Therapy for patients with drug-resistant TB (multidrug-resistant [MDR] or extensively drug-resistant [XDR]):
   a. suspect resistance in HIV-positive patients, injecting drug users, institutionalized individuals, and migrants from areas with a high prevalence of drug-resistant TB
   b. a regimen with at least four effective drugs, including an injectable drug, for an initial period that may be up to 8 months; total duration of treatment up to 24 months.

Non-tuberculous mycobacterial (NTMB) infection

Organisms

- *Mycobacterium avium* complex (MAC)—*M. avium, M. intracellulare*

Table 6-8 Drugs for tuberculosis

DRUG	SIDE-EFFECTS	COMMENTS
Isoniazid (INH)	Hepatitis (approx. 1%; fast acetylators; increased >35 years of age) Peripheral neuropathy (especially slow acetylators) Flu-like illness, fever Skin rash, purpura, arthritis, lupus phenomenon	Supplemental vitamin B_6 (pyridoxine) reduces the risk of peripheral neuropathy
Rifampicin	Hepatitis Fever Thrombocytopenia, hemolytic anemia (rare) Light-chain proteinuria Orange discoloration of urine	Increases metabolism of oral contraceptive pill, corticosteroids, warfarin, digoxin, and oral hypoglycemic agents
Ethambutol	Retrobulbar optic neuritis (reversible) Skin rash	Screen for side-effects with red–green color discrimination and visual acuity testing
Pyrazinamide	Arthralgia, gout, hepatitis	

Table 6-9 Environmental factors in pulmonary infection

ENVIRONMENTAL EXPOSURE HISTORY	INFECTIONS TO CONSIDER
Water-cooling units	*Legionella*
Military camps	*Mycoplasma*
Birds	Psittacosis, histoplasmosis, *Aspergillus*
Dogs, cats, rats, pigs, cattle	Leptospirosis
Goats, pigs, cattle	Q fever
Abattoirs, vets	Brucellosis, Q fever
Soil	Blastomycosis
Decaying wood, caves, chickens	Histoplasmosis
Potting mix	*Legionella lombaechiae*

- *M. kansasii*
- *M. Abscessus*—particularly important in CF

Clinical manifestations in non-immunosuppressed patients

- Upper lobe fibrocavitatory disease—this mimics TB. It is more common in patients with COPD
- Nodular bronchiectasis—bronchiectasis and small nodules typically in the middle lobe
- Solitary pulmonary nodule
- Hypersensitivity pneumonitis, e.g. hot-tub lung

Diagnosis

1 Culture—sputum, bronchoalveolar lavage
2 DNA probe for some species

Treatment

Prolonged combination antimycobacterial antibiotics, usually including a macrolide (azithromycin or clarithromycin), rifampicin, and ethambutol.

Other aspects

Other aspects to consider in pulmonary infections are given in Tables 6-9 to 6-11.

Table 6-10 Pneumonia: underlying diseases and common associated pathogens

DISEASE	COMMON PATHOGENS TO CONSIDER
Obstructing lung cancer	*Pneumococcus*, oral anaerobes
Chronic obstructive pulmonary disease (COPD)	*Pneumococcus, Haemophilus influenzae*
Cystic fibrosis	*Pseudomonas aeruginosa, Staphylococcus aureus*
Influenza virus	*Pneumococcus, S. aureus, H. influenzae* A and B
Alcoholism	*Klebsiella*, oral anaerobes
Alveolar proteinosis	*Nocardia*
Hypogammaglobulinemia	Encapsulated bacteria (*Pneumococcus, H. influenzae*)
Neutropenia	Gram-negative bacilli, *Aspergillus fumigatus*

Table 6-11 Atypical pneumonias

TYPE	MANIFESTATIONS	DIAGNOSIS	THERAPY
Mycoplasma	Dry cough, headache, fever, bullous myringitis, patchy pneumonitis with few chest signs in young adults, hemolysis, Guillain–Barré, hepatitis, rash, Raynaud's	CXR Cold agglutinins Specific complement fixation test Culture	Erythromycin Tetracycline Roxithromycin
Legionnaire's disease	Dry cough, pleuritic chest pain, bilateral coarse crackles with patchy pneumonitis, hyponatremia, hypophosphatemia, abnormal LFTs, fever	CXR Serology (single titer >1 : 256 suggestive, 4-fold rise at 2–6 weeks) Fluorescent antibody sputum test	Erythromycin Rifampicin (if immunocompromised) Tetracycline Roxithromycin
Q fever	Dry cough, pleuritic chest pain, headache, fever, myalgia, granulomatous hepatitis Livestock workers	Lower lobe consolidation on CXR Complement fixation test in those with hepatitis/endocarditis	Tetracycline
Psittacosis	Dry cough, pleuritic chest pain, headache, fever, patchy pneumonitis Bird-handlers	CXR Complement fixation test	Tetracycline

CXR, chest X-ray; LFT, liver function test.

Table 6-12 Pleural fluid changes in different disease states

PLEURAL FLUID ANALYSIS	ASSOCIATED DISEASE
pH <7.2	Empyema (except *Proteus* where pH >7.8), tuberculosis, neoplasm, rheumatoid arthritis, esophageal rupture
Glucose <3.3 mmol/L (<60 mg/dL)	Infection, neoplasm, rheumatoid arthritis, mesothelioma
Amylase ≥200 units/100 mL	Pancreatitis, ruptured abdominal viscera, esophageal rupture (salivary amylase)
Complement decreased	Systemic lupus erythematosus, rheumatoid arthritis
Chylous—triglycerides >1.26 mmol/L (110 mg/dL)	Tumor, thoracic duct trauma, tuberculosis, tuberous sclerosis, primary lymphoid dysplasia
Cholesterol effusion	Rheumatoid arthritis, nephrotic syndrome, old tuberculosis

PLEURAL DISEASE

The analysis of pleural fluid is a mainstay in the diagnosis of pleural disease (Table 6-12, overleaf).

Pleural effusion

Exudate

> **CLINICAL PEARL**
>
> Biochemical features of a pleural exudate:
> - protein >3 g/100 mL (30 g/L)
> - pleural/serum protein >0.5
> - lactate dehydrogenase (LDH) >200 IU/L
> - pleural/serum LDH >0.6 IU/L.

Transudate

> **CLINICAL PEARL**
>
> Biochemical features of a pleural transudate:
> - protein <3 g/100 mL (30 g/L)
> - pleural/serum protein <0.5
> - lactate dehydrogenase (LDH) <200 IU/L
> - pleural/serum LDH <0.6 IU/L.

PNEUMOTHORAX

Spontaneous causes include the following.

- **Primary**—subpleural bullae (apical) that rupture, usually in young adults.
- **Secondary:**
  - » Emphysema/COPD
  - » Rare causes:
    - – asthma
    - – eosinophilic granuloma
    - – lymphangioleiomyomatosis
    - – lung abscess
    - – carcinoma
    - – end-stage fibrosis
    - – Langerhan's cell granulomatosis
    - – Marfan's syndrome
    - – *Pneumocystis jirovecii* pneumonia.

Traumatic causes include:

- the most common traumatic cause is currently needles inserted into the chest (biopsies, central lines, drains).
- rib fracture
- penetrating injury
- high positive end-expiratory pressure (PEEP) or mechanical ventilation
- esophageal rupture.

Indications for a chest drain

1 Respiratory compromise, e.g. hypoxemia, significant breathlessness

2 Tension pneumothorax

3 Large pneumothorax, > 2 cm between lung and parietal pleura

Small bore usually, unless tension pneumothorax.

PULMONARY VASCULAR DISEASE

Pulmonary hypertension (PH)

Definition

Pulmonary hypertension exists when mean pulmonary artery pressure is ≥25 mmHg at rest, as assessed by a right heart catheter study. An estimate by echocardiography of a *pulmonary artery systolic pressure of >50 mmHg is suggestive but not diagnostic* of PH.

Irrespective of cause, all types of PH (Box 6-8) are associated with right ventricular hypertrophy, medial hypertrophy of muscular and elastic arteries, and dilatation with intimal damage to elastic pulmonary arteries.

Box 6-8

Causes of pulmonary hypertension

Primary causes
- Idiopathic
- Hereditary (rare)

Secondary causes

Lung diseases:
- Obstructive lung disease, e.g. chronic obstructive pulmonary disease
- Interstitial/parenchymal lung disease, e.g. idiopathic pulmonary fibrosis
- In association with systemic connective tissue disease, e.g. CREST syndrome
- Drug- or toxin-induced, e.g. by cocaine

Ventilatory disorders:
- Apneic syndromes, e.g. obstructive sleep apnea
- Musculoskeletal disorders, e.g. chest wall deformity

Heart disease:
- Left-sided heart disease, e.g. mitral stenosis

Pulmonary vascular disorders:
- Recurrent pulmonary thromboembolism
- Pulmonary veno-occlusive disease
- Hyperviscosity, e.g. myeloproliferative disorders

Other causes, mechanism unknown, e.g.:
- Dialysis-dependent renal failure
- Portal hypertension

Diagnosis

The management of PH depends on an accurate diagnosis of the cause of the pulmonary hypertension, in particular the assessment of left heart function, lung disease, thrombo-embolic disease, and the presence of hypoxemia from obstructive sleep apnea and any other sleep-disordered breathing.

The assessment must include an estimate of whether the degree of PH is explained by the presence of known causes or whether there is an element of what is known as Group 1 pulmonary hypertension or pulmonary artery hypertension (PAH).

- In the absence of any known cause for PAH, the term used is idiopathic PAH (IPAH).
- Where other causes are found, the terms include that cause; for instance connective tissue disease (PAH-CTD) or congenital heart disease (PAH-CHD).
- A right heart catheter with measurement of pulmonary vascular resistance and pulmonary capillary wedge pressure is an essential part of the work-up for PAH and is often required to assess progress.
- The prognosis for PAH, a rare disease with a prevalence of 15–50/million, depends initially on the severity at presentation, with 1-year survival varying from 65% to 95% and overall 5-year survival from 55% to 85%.

Treatment

The treatment algorithm for Group 1 PH (PAH) is initially based on whether, at right heart catheter, there is an immediate response to a vasodilator; if this occurs, the first-line treatment is a calcium-channel blocker.

- The initial treatment includes vaccination against influenza and pneumococcal disease, graded exercise, QUIT advice and healthy nutrition.
- Supportive therapy such as oral anticoagulants, diuretics, oxygen and digoxin.
- Specific targeted therapy is based on three pathways by which pulmonary vascular resistance can be reduced:
  » **endothelin pathway**, where endothelin receptor antagonists (ERAs) such as bosentan, ambrisentan and macitentan block the vasoconstrictor and proliferative action of endothelin
  » **nitric oxide pathway**, where stimulants of the pathway such as sildenafil and tadalafil inhibit phosphodiesterase-5 (PDE_5 I), leading to an increase in cyclic guanosine monophosphate (GMP), enhancing its vasodilator effect
  » **prostacyclin pathway**, where eproprostenol, iloprost or treprostinil promote vasodilatation systemically or by inhalation.

The sequence in which these agents are used is complex and depends on the severity of disease according to the WHO functional classification (Box 6-9), local licensing/funding arrangements, and tolerance.

When there is inadequate response to combination therapy, the alternatives include atrial septostomy and lung transplantation.

Box 6-9

World Health Organization (WHO) functional classification (FC) of pulmonary hypertension (PH)

- **Class I**—Physical activity with limitation: no undue dyspnea, fatigue or chest pain
- **Class II**—Slight limitation of physical activity: ordinary activity causes undue dyspnea, fatigue, chest pain or near syncope
- **Class III**—Marked limitation of physical activity: comfortable at rest but less than ordinary activity causes undue dyspnea, fatigue, chest pain or near syncope.
- **Class IV**—Inability to carry out any activity: dyspnea, fatigue, chest pain and near syncope even at rest.

Pulmonary embolism (PE)

CLINICAL PEARL

Pulmonary embolism is the most common cause of death found at postmortem that was not considered pre-mortem, and is found in 30–40% of autopsies.

Symptoms of PE

- Dyspnea
- Pleuritic chest pain
- Hemoptysis (uncommon)

Signs of PE

- Often minimal
- Tachycardia is the most common finding
- Pleural rub
- Signs of pulmonary hypertension or deep vein thrombosis (DVT)

Diagnosis

Before embarking on diagnostic tests, it is important to make an estimation of the **probability** of PE, using a thorough clinical evaluation with or without an objective scoring system such as the Well's Score, which includes signs/symptoms of DVT, heart rate, immobilization due to surgery, previous PE or DVT, hemoptysis, malignancy, and alternative diagnoses, to provide a *high*, *intermediate* or *low* probability of PE.

Diagnostic testing includes the following.

- Computed tomography pulmonary angiogram (CTPA) —CTPA is very sensitive at detecting centrally located thromboembolus, but may not detect smaller, peripheral clots. An advantage of CTPA is that it images the lungs and thorax and can contribute to an alternative diagnosis.

- Ventilation–perfusion (V/Q) nuclear scan—V/Q scanning is safer in patients with renal impairment who may be at risk with administration of radiocontrast media. It is less specific than CTPA when there is pre-existing lung disease, especially COPD.
- Massive PE may cause classic electrocardiographic (EKG) changes: S1, Q3, T3.
- CXR may reveal oligemia of the lung or lungs, or may show evidence of atelectasis or opacity due to infarction.
- D-dimer is sensitive but non-specific in this situation; only a negative result is of value in ruling out PE if the risk is considered low or intermediate.

Treatment

- Prompt anticoagulation.
- Consider thrombolysis if hemodynamic compromise is evident. However, the use of thrombolytic therapy is controversial, with no convincing evidence that it improves long-term outcomes.

LUNG TRANSPLANTATION

Lung transplantation is a treatment option for a range of very severe non-malignant diseases of the lungs.

- The most common disorder for which lung transplantation is used is COPD (approximately 40%), followed by idiopathic pulmonary fibrosis (about 20%), and cystic fibrosis (15–20%).
- In the past, PAH was a relatively common indication but this has reduced with the use of targeted therapy.
- The overall survival rates are: 1-year approximately 80%; 5-year approximately 50%; 10-year approximately 30%.

Table 6-13 lists selection criteria.

Complications of lung transplantation

Mortality from lung transplantation is highest in the first year, with primary graft dysfunction (PGD) and infection being the most common causes.

- PGD is the early development of radiographic evidence of pulmonary edema and hypoxia in the absence of an obvious cause such as volume overload, acute rejection, pneumonia or pulmonary venous obstruction.
  - » The cause is unknown, with an ischemic–reperfusion injury being the most likely contributor.
  - » There is no specific treatment; mortality is high and longer-term outcome is poorer.
- The most important determinant of longer-term survival after lung transplantation is the development of chronic damage to the small airways of the lungs—bronchiolitis obliterans (BOS).
  - » This involves fibroproliferative obliteration of the small airways that causes progressive airflow obstruction.
  - » BOS develops in about half of lung transplant recipients by 5 years post-transplant.

Table 6-13 Selection criteria for lung transplantation

Chronic obstructive pulmonary disease
- BODE index* of 7–10 **or** at least one of the following:
- History of hospitalization for exacerbation associated with acute hypercapnia (PCO_2 >50 mmHg)
- Pulmonary hypertension or cor pulmonale, or both, despite oxygen therapy
- FEV1 <20% of predicted and either DLCO <20% of predicted or homogenous distribution of emphysema

Idiopathic pulmonary fibrosis
- Histological or radiographic evidence of UIP **and** any of the following:
- A DLCO <39% of predicted.
- A $\geq$10% decrement in FVC during 6 months of follow-up
- A decrease in pulse oximetry to <88% during a 6MWT
- Honeycombing on HRCT (fibrosis score >2)

Cystic fibrosis
- FEV1 <30% of predicted, or rapidly declining lung function if FEV1 >30% (females and patients <18 years of age have a poorer prognosis; consider earlier listing) **and/or** any of the following:
- Increasing oxygen requirements
- Hypercapnia
- Pulmonary hypertension

Idiopathic pulmonary arterial hypertension
- Persistent NYHA class III or IV on maximal medical therapy
- Low (<350 m) or declining 6MWT
- Failing therapy with intravenous epoprostenol or equivalent
- Cardiac index <2 L/min/m^2
- Right atrial pressure >15 mmHg

Sarcoidosis
- NYHA functional class III or IV **and** any of the following:
- Hypoxemia at rest
- Pulmonary hypertension
- Elevated right atrial pressure >15 mmHg

* The BODE index is a measure that includes body mass index, degree of dyspnea, and distance walked in 6 minutes (6-minute walk test).

6MWT, 6-minute walk test; DLCO, diffusing capacity for carbon monoxide; FEV1, forced expiratory volume in 1 second; PCO_2, partial pressure of carbon dioxide.

Modified from Orens JB, Estenne M, Arcasoy S et al: International guidelines for the selection of lung transplant candidates: 2006 update. J Heart Lung Transplant 2006;25:745–55.

- » One or more episodes of acute rejection has been identified as a major risk factor for the development of BOS. Other risk factors include gastroesophageal reflux and primary graft dysfunction.
- » The prognosis is poor, with 2-year survival after onset of about 60%.
- » Macrolide therapy appears to slow progression.
- » Aggressive surgical correction of gastroesophageal reflux is favored in some centers.

RESPIRATORY SLEEP MEDICINE

Overview of sleep medicine

The starting point for understanding the breadth of sleep disorders is the International Classification of Sleep Disorders Second Edition (ICSD-2), revised in 2005 by the American Academy of Sleep Medicine:

1 Insomnia—a common symptom of problems initiating or maintaining sleep

2 Sleep-related breathing disorders—obstructive and central apneas; hypoventilation and hypoxemia

3 Hypersomnias of central origin—excessive daytime sleepiness not due to sleep restriction, disturbed sleep or circadian rhythm

4 Circadian rhythm sleep disorders—shift work; jetlag; delayed and advanced sleep phase

5 Parasomnias—sleep-walking, sleep terrors, sleep paralysis, REM (rapid eye movement) behavior disorder

6 Sleep-related movement disorders

7 Isolated symptoms and normal variants

8 Other sleep disorders.

From an internal medicine context the most important problems are those of sleep-related breathing disorders, but a sleep disorder is an important consideration in the differential diagnosis of a number of presentations, especially excessive daytime fatigue or sleepiness, chronic pain and its treatment, and the adverse effects of medications.

Important clinical clues

Snoring and apneas

- Snoring is the most frequent sleep-related symptom and often the reason why patients seek medical assessment, usually through their partners.

- Since snoring is the sound generated by airflow through a narrowed upper airway, there is great variation between people and within patients as to the loudness, duration, impact of body position, and exacerbating factors such as alcohol and nasal obstruction.

- To distinguish between 'simple' snoring and snoring that reflects significant upper airway obstruction causing apneas, hypopneas or increased respiratory effort, important clinical clues include a history of apneas, episodes of choking, obesity, a thick neck, and oropharyngeal crowding.

Excessive daytime sleepiness (EDS)

Excessive daytime sleepiness is a common symptom for which there are broadly four causes:

1 inadequate sleep or sleep restriction

2 poor-quality sleep due to a range of problems, such as sleep apnea, restless legs, and chronic pain

3 sedating medications such as benzodiazepines and narcotics

4 primary disorder of daytime vigilance such as narcolepsy–cataplexy syndrome or idiopathic hypersomnolence.

Obesity

The ongoing 'epidemic of obesity' is a major contributor to the prevalence of obstructive sleep apnea (OSA). It is the most important risk factor for OSA in middle-aged adults.

Insomnia

Insomnia is a symptom of dissatisfaction with either the quality or the quantity of sleep.

- It is exceptionally common as an acute problem, especially in response to a stressful event.

- Insomnia that lasts for more than 3 months is called chronic insomnia, and is reported by up to 10% of adults.

The patterns of insomnia include one or more of difficulty with initiation of sleep, difficulty with maintenance of sleep, or awakening too early.

For insomnia to be diagnosed it is necessary to meet three criteria:

1 adequate opportunity for sleep

2 persistent dissatisfaction with sleep

3 problems with daytime functioning.

Since mood disorders, chronic pain, and advanced disease of many organs can interfere with sleep and cause insomnia, there is great complexity in assessing and diagnosing insomnia.

Respiratory sleep disorders

Obstructive sleep apnea (OSA)

Obstructive sleep apnea is a common syndrome due to repeated episodes of obstruction of the upper airway during sleep, causing reduction in oxyhemoglobin saturation, increased respiratory effort, arousal, and sleep fragmentation. By convention the obstructions must be present for at least 10 seconds, and can be either complete obstruction (apnea) or reduced airflow (hypopnea).

Strictly speaking, OSA describes the pathophysiology and the full syndrome includes the presence of excessive daytime sleepiness (EDS; see above), as measured by subjective or objective tools.

The usual measure of severity for OSA is the Apnea–Hypopnea Index (AHI), expressing the number of events per hour of sleep:

- normal AHI: <5/hour
- mild AHI: 5–15/hour
- moderate AHI: 15–30/hour
- severe AHI: >30/hour

The consequences of OSA are related to the clinical features and to short-term and long-term impact:

- social impact of loud snoring and apneas, mainly on family members

- EDS and unrefreshing sleep, with increased risk of motor vehicle accidents, poor academic and work performance, and deterioration in personality and cognitive function

- cardiovascular impact through systemic hypertension with consequent increased risk of ischemic heart disease, stroke, and death.

The diagnosis of OSA is made by the measurement of breathing during sleep. The 'gold standard' test is an in-laboratory polysomnography (PSG) with recording of electroencephalography (EEG), electromyography (EMG), EOG (electro-oculogram), airflow, chest and abdomen movement, oxyhemoglobin saturation, pulse and limb movements.

> ### CLINICAL PEARL
>
> It is essential to identify treatable causes of OSA. These include:
> - hypothyroidism (large tongue and reduced control of breathing)
> - acromegaly (large tongue)
> - physical obstruction of the upper airway (nasal polyps, adenoids, tonsillar hypertrophy, vocal cord paralysis).

Treatment

The treatment of sleep apnea is based on abolishing the increased resistance of the upper airway during sleep.

- Prior to the availability of continuous positive airway pressure (CPAP), the only available intervention was a tracheostomy that was kept open during sleep and occluded during the daytime.

- The current treatment options for OSA include the following.
  - » Weight loss is important for patients with obesity (BMI >30), and especially for morbid obesity (BMI >40). For the latter, bariatric surgery may be an option.
  - » CPAP to keep the upper airway open through functioning as a pneumatic splint. There are technical variations that provide more sophisticated applications, but the broad principle remains the pneumatic splint. The mask may be nasal or full-face, or nasal prongs may be used. Acceptance and compliance can be a problem, with possibly only 50% using the treatment every night.
  - » A mandibular advancement splint to keep the mandible and the attached tongue forward. This increases the cross-sectional area of the pharynx; it reduces upper airway obstruction to a lesser extent than CPAP, but is better tolerated.
  - » Upper airway surgery. Evidence for the efficacy of surgical techniques such as uvulopalatoplasty is lacking.

Central sleep apnea (CSA)

Central sleep apnea is a failure of the respiratory system to generate the respiratory muscle effort to maintain adequate minute ventilation. There are two forms of CSA:

1. Hypercapnic CSA occurs in neuromuscular disease, and causes hypoventilation either only during sleep, or that is worse during sleep. Causes include amyotrophic lateral sclerosis/motor neuron disease (ALS/MND), muscular dystrophy, stroke, and syringomyelia.

2. Hypocapnic CSA seems to arise from instability of the respiratory control system through changes in the setting of chemoreceptors, and the response to those chemoreceptor outputs. The typical pattern is often Cheyne–Stokes respiration (alternating periods of hyperventilation and hypoventilation/apnea). The most common cause is congestive heart failure, but it also occurs at altitude and with use of high doses of narcotics.

Treatment

The treatment of CSA will vary with the clinical setting.

- For hypercapnic CSA the major treatment is non-invasive ventilation (NIV), using the same mask interface as OSA (see above) but with machines that deliver pressure support by having a higher pressure during inspiration than expiration.

- There are many sophisticated aspects to NIV machines that can accommodate the patient's condition, including allowance for failure to trigger a breath, and adaptive servoventilation where the machine does the opposite of Cheyne–Stokes respiration, providing ventilation during periods of hypoventilation and none during hyperventilation.

- For CSA associated with heart failure, it is important that the heart failure is under optimal treatment.

- For any potential of an obstruction component, CPAP may be used.

- In some cases, oxygen supplementation alone will be adequate.

Obesity hypoventilation syndrome (OHS)

This syndrome is being diagnosed more frequently, in severely obese people. The criteria for diagnosis include:

- obesity (BMI >30)
- chronic hypercapnic respiratory failure (P_aCO_2 >45 mmHg), in the absence of another cause such as severe COPD; an increased HCO_3^- on serum electrolytes due to metabolic compensation is a clue for the presence of chronic hypercapnia
- sleep-disordered breathing
- a sleep study may reveal OSA, as well as hypoventilation during sleep or hypoventilation alone.

The major treatment goal is weight loss, but this is often either difficult or delayed. The usual treatment is NIV, but often CPAP is tried first to overcome any contribution from upper airway obstruction.

2. CRITICAL CARE MEDICINE

The focus of critical care for internal medicine is the urgent support of acute organ failure with the aim of maintaining life, planning the definitive management of the precipitating cause, and keeping organs working while awaiting the effect of treatment and/or time. While a great deal of effort is directed to acute problems of the respiratory system, critical care medicine involves all organs at some stage.

RESUSCITATION

Cardiac arrest (CA)

Despite improvements in technology and inpatient care, there has not been a great deal of change in the outcomes for CA over time, as measured by the proportion of patients discharged from hospital. Approximately one-third of out of hospital CA patients make it to hospital, with 1 in 10 patients is eventually discharged from hospital. In-hospital CA has a similarly poor outcome, with discharge rates approximately 10-15%. The most common cause of death is hypoxic brain damage. Achieving an early return to spontaneous circulation is associated with better outcomes and earlier discharge.

> **CLINICAL PEARL**
>
> Time to defibrillation is the most important factor in the outcome of all cardiac arrests.

DIAGNOSIS AND DISEASE MANAGEMENT

Shock

Evaluation and management of shock

Shock is a pathological state defined by the abnormal physiology of reduced delivery of oxygen and other nutrients to the tissues through a reduction in systemic tissue perfusion.

- Cellular impact includes intracellular edema, acidosis, and loss of ion pumps.

- Systemic effects include lactic acidosis and stimulation of inflammatory and anti-inflammatory processes.

Initial stages of shock are reversible, but later there may be cellular death, organ damage, multisystem organ failure and death.

There are three types of shock:

1 **Hypovolemic**—inadequate intravascular volume and reduced cardiac preload, resulting from trauma and other causes of blood or fluid loss.

2 **Cardiogenic**—results from cardiac and extra-cardiac causes of reduced cardiac output, including pulmonary embolism and cardiac tamponade.

3 **Distributive**—widespread vasodilatation, reduction in systemic vascular resistance, and reduced perfusion of some tissues despite increased cardiac output, occurring due to causes such as sepsis, anaphylaxis, spinal damage, toxic shock, and neurogenic factors.

There may be combinations of the three types of shock.

Right heart catheterization in shock

Right heart catheterization, can provide valuable idiagnostic and prognostic information in a patient with shock, pulmonary edema, pulmonary hypertension, pericardial tamponade and intra-cardia shunt (let to right)(see table 6-14).

The major measurements on right heart catheterization are the vascular pressures and the oxygen saturation in each chamber/vessel. Cardiac output can be measured by either a dilution technique such as thermodilution, or the Fick method based on oxygen consumption. The measures obtained are of the three components of left heart function— preload (based on pulmonary capillary wedge pressure [PCWP], which is an estimate of left ventricular filling pressure), afterload (based on an estimate of systemic vascular resistance [SVR], from the relationship between systemic blood pressure and cardiac output), and cardiac output—and one of tissue perfusion (mixed venous oxygen saturation [S_VO_2]).

Acute respiratory distress syndrome (ARDS)

Acute respiratory distress syndrome refers to stages of acute lung damage, usually from infective or traumatic shock, that is seen in a wide range of acute illnesses. In 2012, ARDS was defined by the following:

- Bilateral pulmonary infiltrates consistent with pulmonary edema (see Figures 6-17 and 6-18)

- Acute onset

Table 6-14 Right heart catheter in shock

DISORDER/PARAMETER	PCWP (PRE-LOAD)	SVR (AFTER-LOAD)	CARDIAC OUTPUT	S_VO_2
Cardiogenic shock	increased	increased	decreased	decreased
Hypovolemic shock	decreased	increased	decreased	decreased
Distributive shock	decreased/normal	decreased	increased	increased
PWCP, pulmonary capillary wedge pressure; S_VO_2, mixed venous oxygen saturation; SVR, systemic vascular resistance.				

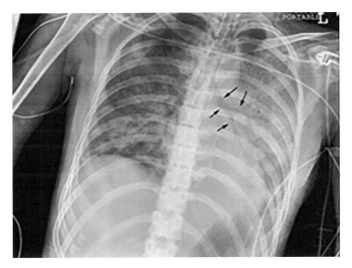

Figure 6-17 Chest radiograph showing diffuse alveolar filling in both lungs of a patient with ARDS; bilateral air bronchograms are marked by arrows, and endotracheal and nasogastric tubes can be seen

From Porté F, Basit R and Howlett D. Imaging in the intensive care unit. Surgery 2009;27(11):496–9.

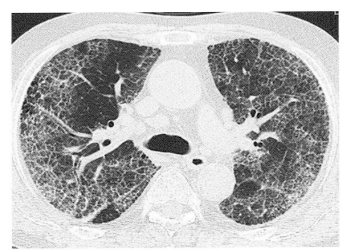

Figure 6-18 Computed tomography scan of patient with ARDS, demonstrating interlobular septal thickening and a typical 'crazy paving' pattern due to fine intralobular reticulation superimposed on ground-glass opacities

From Ichikado K. High-resolution computed tomography findings of acute respiratory distress syndrome, acute interstitial pneumonia, and acute exacerbation of idiopathic pulmonary fibrosis. Seminars in Ultrasound, CT and MRI 2014;35(1):39–46.

- No evidence of left heart failure, e.g. normal PCWP (≤18 mmHg)
- Severity is further defined by the degree of hypoxemia:
    - » mild—200 mmHg < P_aO_2/F_iO_2 ≤300 mmHg
    - » moderate—100 mmHg < P_aO_2/F_iO_2 ≤ 200 mmHg
    - » severe—P_aO_2/F_iO_2 ≤ 100 mmHg.

CLINICAL PEARL

To distinguish ARDS from pulmonary edema due to left heart failure on chest X-ray, check for pulmonary venous congestion, cardiomegaly (allowing for mobile chest X-ray), pleural effusions, and Kerley B (septal) lines. These all suggest left heart failure.

Pathophysiology of ARDS

- Diffuse alveolar damage including loss of surfactant and release of cytokines.
- Leakage of cells and protein into the alveolar space overwhelming usual lymphatic drainage.
- Three stages of pathology: exudative initially; proliferative after about 7 days; fibrosis later.
- Severity of hypoxemia is due to severe 'shunting', where there is perfusion of areas that have no ventilation due to alveoli being full of exudate.
- Pulmonary hypertension may be marked due to vasoconstriction in response to alveolar hypoxia, and other mechanisms including destruction of capillaries, microthrombi, and compression of vessels by edema and inflammation.
- There is marked reduction in lung compliance due to loss of alveoli and loss of surfactant.

Causes of ARDS

- Pneumonia e.g. Bacterial, Viral (Influenza, Sars-CoV2)
- Aspiration
- Trauma
- Sepsis
- Blood transfusion
- Adverse drug reaction
- Transplantation

Treatment of ARDS

General measures

- Aggressive treatment of underlying cause(s), including antibiotic cover for all possible organisms in sepsis.
- Maintain cardiovascular function and renal perfusion but beware of excessive fluid replacement.
- Maintain nutrition, by enteral route where possible; the parenteral route has many side-effects and complications.

Ventilatory support

- Since the major cause of severe hypoxemia is widespread occlusion of alveoli by fluid and cellular material, a mainstay of treatment is to keep the alveoli open for as long as possible during the respiratory cycle, especially in expiration (using PEEP), and to provide enough inspired oxygen to maintain a satisfactory level of arterial oxygen (P_aO2 55–80 mmHg or oxygen saturation SpO_2 88–95%).

- When ventilatory support is required, there is no evidence to support the use of non-invasive positive-pressure ventilation (NIV), but it can be used to bridge the time until expert intubation and setting up of invasive ventilation is possible.

- The major risk from mechanical ventilation is lung injury from the positive pressure, volume distension, and the repeated opening and closing cycles.
  » This is referred to as barotrauma, volutrauma, or either ventilator-associated or ventilator-induced lung injury (VALI/VILI).
  » Its acute form is pneumothorax.
  » The longer-term damage from cyclical over-distension of the alveoli is likely to affect those parts of the lungs less involved with the ARDS, as the heterogeneous loss of compliance in the lungs means that higher inspiratory pressures will over-distend the less stiff areas of the lung.
  » The principle of ventilation in this setting is to use relatively low tidal volumes (approximately 6 mL/kg ideal bodyweight), with a rate that maintains reasonable but not necessarily normal arterial P_aCO_2, and PEEP levels as required to maintain adequate arterial oxygen levels.
  » Mild respiratory acidosis through permissive hypercapnia, down to a pH of 7.30, may be accepted.

- Due to the effect of positive-pressure ventilation on venous return, maintenance of adequate cardiac output will require fluid replacement and vascular support through vasoconstrictors. However, care needs to be taken not to administer excess fluid, which can worsen pulmonary edema.

- In conditions that occur in ARDS where lung over-distension is likely to occur, tidal volumes and airway pressures should be limited, and the attendant increase in arterial CO_2 levels is considered to be acceptable trade-off to prevent lung damage. There is sufficient evidence now to suggest that lung-protective ventilation, which includes low tidal volume (approximately 6 mL/kg), and a plateau airway pressure restricted to approximately 28–30 cmH$_2$O, leads to better outcomes when compared with traditional ventilatory strategies for ARDS.

- The administration of neuromuscular blocking agents may be associated with decreased mortality when used early in the course of severe ARDS.

- In the patient with very severe ARDS in whom these measures are not adequate, there are a number of other strategies used to maintain adequate oxygenation and limit ventilation-associated lung injury. These include prone ventilation, high-frequency ventilation and extracorporeal membrane oxygenation (ECMO).

CLINICAL PEARL

In ARDS requiring mechanical ventilation, a tidal volume (TV) of 6 mL/kg is lung-protective.

Prognosis of ARDS

Initial mortality is usually due to the severity of the precipitating illness, especially if there is multi-organ failure. Subsequent mortality is more likely to be due to complications such as nosocomial infection than respiratory failure.

The duration of mechanical ventilation required and mortality if ARDS is associated with its severity. ARDS mortality is associated with severity:

While survivors may have reduced exercise ability and a number of other physical and not mental–physical and psychological problems related to prolonged intensive care, including depression/anxiety, the majority will return to work if working at the time of illness, and remain self-caring.

CLINICAL PEARL

Survivors of ARDS usually have normal lung function by 12 months, but frequently have reduced physical quality of life, and neurological complications.

MECHANICAL VENTILATION OF THE LUNGS

Mechanical ventilation is the intervention to treat severe respiratory failure. The lungs are ventilated by a machine that uses either negative or positive pressure to provide an adequate tidal and minute volume.

Respiratory failure occurs when the lungs fail to oxygenate the arterial blood and/or do not export enough carbon dioxide. Strictly speaking, respiratory failure is present when the P_aO_2 is below the lower limit of normal and/or the P_aCO_2 is above the upper limit of normal for the person's age. It is conventional to define respiratory failure as a $P_aO_2 < 60$ mmHg on room air and/or a $P_aCO_2 > 50$ mmHg.

Positive-pressure ventilation (PPV), delivered 'invasively' through either an endotracheal tube or a tracheostomy, was refined in war zones during the 1950s and 1960s. PPV via a nasal or face mask, so-called non-invasive positive-pressure ventilation (NIV), is now used widely for inpatient and home-based treatment of respiratory failure, building on the development of CPAP pumps and masks for the treatment of obstructive sleep apnea.

Mechanical ventilation can be used to treat severe respiratory failure due to disorders of gas exchange, manifested by markedly reduced arterial oxygen tension, of alveolar ventilation, manifested by hypercapnia, or both. It can be used for either acute or chronic respiratory failure.

- Arterial oxygen levels are improved by reducing shunting through opening of alveoli that have either collapsed or filled with liquid, together with the ability to provide increased levels of inspired oxygen.

- Increased alveolar ventilation is provided by the delivery of an adequate combination of tidal volume and respiratory rate.

The types of mechanical ventilation have evolved to maximize the correction of hypoxemia and hypercapnia, to minimize the risk of VALI, to minimize asynchrony between the patient and the ventilator, and to optimize the ongoing use of respiratory muscles, thereby reducing disuse atrophy.

The modes of ventilator support are known as:

- **Controlled or continuous mechanical ventilation** (CMV)—the patient is not involved in triggering or stopping inspiration or in setting the respiratory rate, and the inspiration is stopped after either a set volume or a set pressure (volume- or pressure-limited).
  - » *Assist-control* (AC) allows the patient to take some additional breaths to which the machine adds the required volume or pressure.
- **Intermittent mandatory ventilation** (IMV)—support is provided to the patient's effort as a part of a set tidal volume/pressure and rate regimen, with the patient's efforts supported to varying degrees. *Synchronized IMV* (SIMV) ensures concordance between the patient's effort and the machine.
- **Pressure-support ventilation** (PSV)—the machine provides a level of support for each inspiratory effort by the patient. Since the level of pressure support can be varied, this form of ventilation is valuable for the process of weaning off mechanical ventilation.
- **Bi-level positive airway pressure** (BPAP)—this is the mechanical ventilation provided by NIV. The usual settings are of the inspiratory positive airway pressure (IPAP), the expiratory positive airway pressure (EPAP), the rise time or inspiratory flow, and the back-up rate if a breath is not triggered. There are sophisticated versions that are used to treat central sleep apnea and Cheyne–Stokes respiration, so-called adaptive servo-ventilation (ASV).
- **Continuous positive airway pressure** (CPAP)—this is used to overcome the upper airway obstruction of obstructive sleep apnea by producing a pneumatic splint of the upper airway. It is also very effective for acute pulmonary edema, and for severe vocal cord dysfunction.

Non-invasive positive-pressure ventilation (NIV)

Successful NIV requires trained staff and appropriate equipment. It can be started in the emergency department, intensive care or high-dependency unit and wards for inpatients, and in outpatient clinics and sleep laboratories for non-inpatients. The interface between the patient and the machine for NIV may be a nasal mask, nasal cushions, a full face mask or a combination. The nasal mask provides the more physiological airflow, and allows talking and removal of secretions. The benefits of NIV have been shown to be best for acute exacerbations of COPD:

- reduced mortality
- reduced need for invasive ventilation
- reduced length of stay and complications, including nosocomial infections
- reduced re-admission to hospital.

Indications

- Acute exacerbations of COPD with respiratory acidosis (pH <7.35)
- Acute pulmonary edema where CPAP is not adequate
- Obesity hypoventilation syndrome
- Respiratory failure from neuromuscular disease
- Acute exacerbation of asthma
- Neutropenic septic patients may have a better outcome with NIV than with invasive ventilation

Contraindications

- Impaired consciousness
- Inability to cooperate
- High risk of pulmonary aspiration
- Recent esophageal or upper gastrointestinal surgery
- Facial injury or any problem that would prevent application of a mask

Invasive positive-pressure ventilation (IPPV)

Interface

- The endotracheal tube should be of a size that provides maximum cross-sectional fit.
- The cuff should be inflated to the lowest pressure that provides a seal, to minimize the risk of damage to the wall of the trachea.
- The position of the endotracheal tube should be checked clinically from the presence of breath sounds bilaterally, and with a chest X-ray.
- The timing for moving from an endotracheal tube to a tracheostomy depends on the causal problems for respiratory failure, comorbidity and the prognosis.
- A tracheostomy may be considered after 7 days if not weaned off the ventilator.

Auto-PEEP

- This can be a problem in the early stages of ventilating a patient when, due to the respiratory rate and difficulty with expiration, the breaths stack up with a gradual increase in the expiratory lung volume, causing hyperinflation.
- It is most likely to occur in patients with COPD and asthma, and carries the risk of hypotension and shock due to impedance of venous return to the right atrium.
- There is also the risk of VALI, especially pneumothorax, that can worsen or mimic the cardiovascular problem.
- The treatment includes changes in ventilator parameters to allow a longer expiratory period, and maximizing treatment of the underlying problem.

CLINICAL PEARL

Treatment of auto-PEEP may include decreasing tidal volume, decreasing respiratory rate, or increasing expiratory time.

Difficulty in weaning from IPPV

This is a relatively common problem and its potential is an important part of the discussion with a patient and/or their family prior to or just after starting IPPV, especially in someone with severe underlying cardiopulmonary or neuromuscular disease.

Causes of delayed weaning or difficulty with weaning:

- incomplete resolution of the causal illness or of a complicating illness
- reduced drive to breathe—residual sedation, metabolic alkalosis, central nervous system problems
- reduced neuromuscular strength—myopathy, malnutrition/sarcopenia, electrolyte abnormalities, neuropathy, and medication such as corticosteroids
- reduced compliance of the lungs and chest—fluid overload, fibrosis, pleural disease, obesity
- obstruction to breathing—ventilator tubing, secretions, airway inflammation and edema, bronchial muscle spasm
- increased respiratory and metabolic demand—anxiety, fever, delirium, hypoxia.

While a number of cardiac problems can complicate prolonged IPPV, cardiogenic pulmonary edema should be considered in the situation of slow or difficult weaning. The change from positive pressure to negative pressure in the lungs and pleural space as the ventilator support is reduced will lead to an increase in venous return, making Starling forces in the lung parenchyma more favorable to edema formation.

Extracorporeal membrane oxygenation (ECMO)

Extracorporeal membrane oxygenation is a term used for the process of providing oxygenation outside the body in the setting of severe lung disease, such as ARDS.

- An extracorporeal circuit directly oxygenates and removes carbon dioxide from the blood.
- To use ECMO in patients with ARDS, a cannula is placed in a central vein, and blood is withdrawn from the vein into an extracorporeal circuit by a mechanical pump and then enters an external oxygenator.
- Within the oxygenator, blood passes along one side of a membrane, which provides a blood–gas interface for the diffusion of gases.
- The oxygenated extracorporeal blood is then warmed or cooled as needed and returned to the central vein.

Box 6-10 outlines indications and contraindications for use of ECMO.

Box 6-10

Indications and contraindications for ECMO

Indications

- Severe hypoxemia (e.g. P_aO_2/F_iO_2 ratio <80) despite the application of high levels of PEEP (typically 15–20 cmH_2O) for at least 6 hours in patients with potentially reversible respiratory failure
- Uncompensated hypercapnia with respiratory acidemia (pH <7.15) despite the best accepted standard of care for management with a ventilator
- Excessively high end-inspiratory plateau pressure (>35–45 cmH_2O, according to the patient's body size) despite the best accepted standard of care for management with a ventilator

Relative contraindications

- High-pressure ventilation (end-inspiratory plateau pressure >30 cmH_2O) for >7 days
- High F_iO_2 requirements (>0.8) for >7 days
- Limited vascular access
- Any condition or organ dysfunction that would limit the likelihood of an overall benefit from ECMO

Absolute contraindications

Any condition that precludes the use of anticoagulation therapy

---

ECMO, extracorporeal membrane oxygenation; F_iO_2, fraction of inspired oxygen; P_aO_2, partial pressure of arterial oxygen; PEEP, positive end-expiratory pressure.

Modified from Brodie D and Bacchetta M. Extracorporeal membrane oxygenation for ARDS in adults. N Engl J Med 2011;365(20):1905–14.

SELF-ASSESSMENT QUESTIONS

1   A 55-year-old obese patient (body mass index = 42) complains of morning headaches and daytime sleepiness. His family reports that he snores very loudly. He has a history of systemic hypertension, and a small myocardial infarction 3 years ago with no residual cardiac dysfunction. He is a non-smoker. An overnight oximetry study shows significant hypoxemia with 20% of the night spent with an oxygen saturation below 90% and an oxygen desaturation index (3%) of 38/hour. Arterial blood gases show a pH of 7.38, P_aCO_2 of 57 mmHg, P_aO_2 66 mmHg and bicarbonate of 32 mmol/L. Which is the most likely diagnosis?

   A   Cheyne–Stokes respiration
   B   Severe obstructive sleep apnea
   C   Late-stage chronic lung disease
   D   Obesity hypoventilation syndrome
   E   Central sleep apnea

2   A 39-year-old HIV-positive male is found to have a tuberculin skin test (Mantoux) of 8 mm induration. He has no symptoms, has not had a BCG vaccination, and has had no contact with tuberculosis. Chest X-ray is normal. Which of the following treatment approaches is the most appropriate?

   A   Isoniazid treatment for latent tuberculosis for 9 months
   B   Full treatment for tuberculosis with 4 drugs for 2 months and 2 for 4 months
   C   Interferon-gamma release assay for tuberculosis (IGRA)
   D   No further action
   E   Annual chest X-rays for 3 years

3   For a 63-year-old male patient with severe COPD (FEV1 0.8 L, 32% of predicted; P_aO_2 53 mmHg), which of the following has been shown to prolong his life expectancy?

   A   Inhaled long-acting muscarinic antagonists (LAMAs)
   B   Inhaled corticosteroid therapy
   C   Pulmonary rehabilitation
   D   Domiciliary oxygen
   E   Long-term macrolide antibiotic

4   A 78-year-old man presents with chronic cough and breathlessness that has been increasing over the past 12 months. He is a lifelong non-smoker. On examination he has clubbing of the fingers and crackles over the lower half of both lungs. Lung function tests show an FVC of 75% of predicted with an FEV1/FVC ratio of 0.86; carbon monoxide transfer is 45% of predicted. A chest X-ray shows an interstitial pattern mainly in the lower lobes with a suggestion of honeycombing. A high-resolution CT of the chest shows symmetrical bilateral reticular opacities with honeycombing, predominantly in the bases of the lungs. Laboratory tests for connective tissue disease are negative. The patient wants to know what type of treatment has been shown to be of long-term benefit for his lung disease.

   A   High-dose parenteral corticosteroids
   B   Azathioprine and prednisone
   C   No current treatment
   D   Cyclophosphamide and prednisone
   E   Pirfenidone

5   A 45-year-old woman with a long history of asthma presents with gradually progressive cough and breathlessness, and with fever and mild weight loss. There is no history of rhinosinusitis, rash, or focal neurological symptoms. On examination there is bilateral wheeze; pulse oximetry is 92%. A chest X-ray shows diffuse alveolar infiltrates, predominantly peripheral. A high-resolution CT scan of the chest confirms alveolar infiltrates and mediastinal lymphadenopathy. Blood eosinophils are 5.4×10^9/mL (normal $<0.4 \times 10^9$/mL). Serum precipitins for *Aspergillus* are negative. Which of the following is the most likely diagnosis?

   A   Acute eosinophilic pneumonia
   B   Allergic bronchopulmonary aspergillosis (ABPA)
   C   Tuberculosis
   D   Chronic eosinophilic pneumonia
   E   Eosinophilic granulomatosis with polyangiitis (EGPA/Churg–Strauss syndrome)

6   A 55-year-old man suddenly collapses while cycling with friends. He has no previous medical history. The friends attempt CPR with mouth-to-mouth resuscitation, but he vomits and they are unable to effectively clear his airway. An ambulance arrives on the scene. The man is in asystole, and there is no pulse or respiratory effort. Attempts are made to continue resuscitating, but they are unsuccessful. This man's outcome may have been improved if?

   A   The bystanders were able to effectively secure his airway and prevent aspiration.
   B   Irrespective of giving mouth-to-mouth resuscitation, compression-only CPR had been carried out.
   C   Bystanders had had access to an automatic defibrillator.
   D   The ambulance had arrived sooner and established an airway and intravenous access.

7 A 60-year-old female presents to hospital with 3 days of breathlessness, cough and fevers. She has a history of asthma, but has had no prior admissions. At presentation she is diaphoretic, but her peripheries are warm. She has a pulse of 140 beats/min and sinus rhythm, blood pressure 70/40 mmHg, temperature 38.4°C. A chest X-ray shows consolidation involving the right lower and middle lobes. Electrocardiography demonstrates ST depression in leads V_3–V_5 with T wave inversion. Troponin level is elevated. Arterial blood gases demonstrate a pH of 7.29, P_aO_2 50 mmHg, and P_aCO_2 30 mmHg. Serum biochemistry reveals Na 130 mmol/L (reference range [RR] 135–145), K 4.9 mmol/L (RR 3.5–5.6), urea 11.4 mmol/L (RR 2.1–9.0), creatinine 120 micromol/L (RR 40–90), and HCO_3^- 14 mmol/L (RR 23–33). You decide that she is in shock. From your findings you should institute the following treatment based on the probable cause of her shock:

A Stabilize her, transfer her to intensive care, and place a Swan–Ganz catheter to guide resuscitation.
B Commence broad-spectrum antibiotics for community-acquired pneumonia, support circulation with intravenous fluids and commence support with non-invasive ventilation.
C Commence broad-spectrum antibiotics for community-acquired pneumonia, support circulation with intravenous fluids, and avoid vasopressors until an urgent cardiac echo can be performed.
D Commence broad-spectrum antibiotics for community-acquired pneumonia, support circulation with intravenous fluids, and use vasopressors as needed.

8 A 78-year-old ex-smoker with a history of COPD presents to the emergency room by ambulance. He has an FEV1 of 40% of predicted. He does not use home oxygen. His pulse is 120/min and regular, blood pressure 110/60 mmHg, respiratory rate 12/min, and Glasgow Coma Scale score reduced at 12. He is breathing 10 L of oxygen via a mask. Arterial blood gases (ABGs) demonstrate pH 7.21, P_aO_2 103 mmHg, P_aCO_2 90 mmHg, HCO_3^- 35 mmol/L (RR 23–33). Your approach to treatment should be:

A To reduce oxygen concentration, aiming for S_aO_2 88–92%, give nebulized bronchodilators, and commence treatment with non-invasive ventilator support via a mask
B With his reduced level of consciousness, to secure his airway and intubate
C To commence treatment with intravenous salbutamol, reduce oxygen, and repeat ABGs
D To give continuous nebulized salbutamol, intravenous hydrocortisone, and titrate oxygen to maintain S_aO_2 of 92–95%

9 A 52-year-old diabetic woman, with a background of retinopathy and hypertension, is admitted with pyelonephritis. She is febrile at 39°C, her pulse is 130/min in sinus rhythm, BP is 90/50 mmHg, respiratory rate is 18/min, and SpO2 is 93% on room air. Electrolytes demonstrate Na 130 mmol/L (reference range 135–145), K 4.3 mmol/L (RR 3.5–5.6), urea 15.6 mmol/L (RR 2.1–9.0), creatinine 224 micromol/L (RR 60–90), and blood glucose 20.3 mmol/L (RR 3.6–6.0). Urine analysis shows nitrites 2+, blood 3+, protein 3+, glucose 4+, and ketones +. Urine microscopy shows WCC>100 × 10^6/L. Blood culture isolates a Gram-negative rod. She is commenced on treatment with intravenous (IV) third-generation cephalosporin, a single dose of gentamicin, IV insulin infusion, and IV fluids. That night she becomes breathless, with pulse rate 130/min, BP 120/70 mmHg, temperature 37.8°C, respiratory rate 35/min, and SpO2 85% despite F_iO_2 0.5 via a mask. Chest X-ray shows bilateral airspace consolidation. Electrocardiography shows sinus tachycardia with no other changes. She deteriorates, is intubated and transported to intensive care. Your next action should be:

A Broaden antibiotic cover to cover community-acquired pneumonia
B Organize an urgent abdominal CT scan to determine whether she has a renal abscess that requires surgical drainage
C Continue antibiotics and a protective ventilator strategy to support, without attempting to normalize oxygenation
D Commence on dopamine and IV fluids to maintain a urine output greater than 30 mL/hour

ANSWERS

1 D.

The blood gases show chronic hypercapnic respiratory failure, as evidenced by hypercapnia and raised bicarbonate. This is a clue to the presence of the obesity hypoventilation syndrome, especially in a patient with marked obesity. This patient may also have obstructive sleep apnea in view of the loud snoring and daytime sleepiness. The lack of cardiac dysfunction makes Cheyne–Stokes less likely. The history gives no risks for central sleep apnea. The high oxygen desaturation index suggests the episodic sleep-disordered breathing of sleep apnea rather than REM-related hypoxemia seen in chronic lung disease.

2 A.

In the absence of a history of BCG vaccination, the explanation for a positive Mantoux test is previous tuberculosis (TB) infection and there is thus the risk of reactivation of latent infection, especially in a patient at risk of immunosuppression. It would be dangerous not to treat. Therefore, it is appropriate to treat with single-agent therapy for 9 months. If there were signs of active TB (e.g. abnormal chest X-ray, or productive cough), multi-drug therapy would be required. The IGRA would not give any further information in this setting.

3 D.

Unfortunately, apart from lung transplantation, the only treatment proven to prolong life in severe COPD is the use of continuous domiciliary oxygen in those with persistent hypoxemia. This is probably due to the reduction in hypoxic pulmonary vasospasm, and the consequent lessening of pulmonary hypertension. This may then delay the onset of cor pulmonale.

4   C.

This is a description of a case of idiopathic pulmonary fibrosis, for which there has been no demonstration of reduced progression of disease with the use of immunosuppressant drugs, or with the anti-fibrotic agent pirfenidone.

5   D.

EGPA is unlikely in the absence of a history of rhinosinusitis, rash or neurological symptoms. ABPA should be associated with the demonstration of both serum precipitins and specific IgE to *Aspergillus*, so negative precipitins makes this unlikely. Eosinophilic pneumonias generally cause peripheral lung infiltrates. The very high blood eosinophil count and history of asthma and fevers make one form of these the most likely diagnosis. The progressive nature of the dyspnea, and the lymphadenopathy, make chronic eosinophilic pneumonia most likely. Tuberculosis should not cause marked eosinophilia.

6   B.

Compression-only CPR is the only approach available to the bystanders in this situation that could have potentially led to successful resuscitation.

7   D.

The patient is in septic shock with evidence of a metabolic acidosis and compensatory respiratory alkalosis. This is likely to be secondary to community-acquired pneumonia. Treatment should include early empirical antibiotic therapy, and treatment to restore the circulation. There is evidence of an acute coronary syndrome, but it is unlikely to account for the cause of shock alone and is not the primary event. The aim should still be to support the circulation and resuscitate appropriately, with vasopressors as needed. Treatment guided by Swan–Ganz catheter has not been shown to improve outcomes.

8   A.

A case can be made for reducing oxygen and giving bronchodilators, then repeating ABGs before commencing NIV, but already with a reduced level of consciousness this may not be enough. It is likely that NIV has better long-term outcomes than intubation with IPPV in this setting, with equivalent acute efficacy. There is no role for continuous nebulized or intravenous salbutamol in this setting. Maintaining oxygen saturation at 92–95% is unnecessary, and is likely to promote a reduced respiratory drive with worsened hypercapnia.

9   C.

This picture is consistent with acute respiratory distress syndrome (ARDS) secondary to septic shock. There is no reason to propose another infection in this context and in this timeframe. While she is diabetic and may be at risk for ischemic heart disease, unless she has a severe myocardial infarction, acute pulmonary edema is less likely. Treatment for ARDS aims to treat the underlying cause and support respiratory function.

CHAPTER 7

CARDIOLOGY

Peter Thompson

CHAPTER OUTLINE

CLINICAL EVALUATION OF THE PATIENT

Taking the history—possible cardiac symptoms

Chest pain or discomfort

Eliciting an accurate history of chest pain or discomfort is an important skill in the evaluation of patients with suspected cardiac disease. The central challenge in the evaluation of chest discomfort (Table 7–1) is to assess whether it indicates myocardial ischemia.

- Typical angina is a central chest pain or tightness usually described as a heavy squeezing sensation, sometimes a burning, or a vague sensation of discomfort which eludes precise description. It is usually brought on with exertion and relieved with rest. Relief on resting is usually immediate, and if the discomfort persists for more than a few minutes, non-cardiac causes should be considered.
- Atypical angina can occasionally present with pain in the lower jaw, left arm, right arm, epigastrium, and occasionally in the interscapular area of the back. Eliciting a history of exacerbation by exertion and relief with rest is a very valuable clue that the pain is an atypical form of angina.
- Relief with nitroglycerin usually indicates myocardial ischemia but can occur with esophageal spasm.
- While angina can present with localized pain, finding an area of tenderness on the chest wall makes it more likely that the pain is arising from the structures of the chest wall, such as with costochondritis. Costochondritis can coexist with coronary heart disease (CHD), so finding chest wall tenderness does not exclude CHD.
- Worsening of the pain with inspiration ('pleuritic' pain) indicates a pericardial or pleural cause for the chest pain.
- The possibility of esophageal reflux or other gastrointestinal causes may be raised if the chest pain or discomfort comes on after meals or bending over.

CLINICAL PEARL

Localized chest pain with a palpable area of tenderness indicates a non-cardiac origin, but the finding does not necessarily exclude underlying coronary heart disease.

Dyspnea

- The sensation of shortness of breath (dyspnea) and its variants orthopnea (dyspnea on lying flat) and paroxysmal nocturnal dyspnea are very common, and in patients with cardiac disease usually indicate the presence of cardiac failure or significant valvular heart disease.
- Evaluating dyspnea presents a diagnostic challenge, as the same symptom can be associated with respiratory disease, anxiety or simply lack of fitness.
  - » The sudden onset of paroxysmal nocturnal dyspnea, particularly with the production of frothy sputum, is usually due to cardiac failure.
  - » Orthopnea is also usually due to cardiac failure but respiratory causes cannot be ruled out entirely.
  - » Dyspnea with wheezing can occur with cardiac failure (so-called cardiac asthma), but exacerbation with a recent respiratory infection makes respiratory disease more likely to be the cause.

Palpitations

The term 'palpitation' means different things to different people, and the term is best avoided in direct questioning. Terms such as 'irregular heart rhythm' or 'skipping of the heart beat' are much more likely to be understood by the patient. It is often helpful to distinguish regular tachycardias, ectopic beats and atrial fibrillation by having the patient tap out on their chest or on the desk how they experience the irregularity.

CLINICAL PEARL

Asking the patient to tap out the rhythm on their chest or a desktop can help elucidate the cause of palpitations.

Table 7-1 Differential diagnosis of chest discomfort

DIAGNOSIS	CHARACTER	LOCATION	COMMENT
Coronary heart disease			
Exertional angina	Heavy, squeezing pressure	Retrosternal with radiation to neck or left arm	Worse with exertion, relieved with rest; relieved rapidly with nitroglycerin
Unstable angina	Similar to above but may be more intense	Similar to above	Occurs with minimal exertion or at rest; usually responds to nitroglycerin
Acute myocardial infarction	Similar to above but more severe, and associated with sweating, clamminess, dyspnea, nausea, light-headedness	Similar to above	Sudden onset at rest, incomplete relief with nitroglycerin
Cardiovascular, non-coronary			
Pericarditis	Pleuritic, worse with inspiration	Central, parasternal	Variable with change in position; no relief with nitroglycerin; associated with pericardial rub
Aortic dissection	Severe, tearing or ripping sensation	Can be in the anterior chest but typically in the interscapular area	Occurs in patients with uncontrolled hypertension or Marfan syndrome
Pulmonary embolism	Abrupt onset, usually severe and can be pleuritic	Usually retrosternal but can be left or right chest	Marked dyspnea, tachypnea, tachycardia, and hypotension; marked oxygen desaturation
Thoracic			
Pneumonia with pleural involvement (pleurisy)	Variable, usually pleuritic	Unilateral localized, on side of infection	Dyspnea, cough, fever, crackles, pleural rub
Spontaneous pneumothorax	Sudden onset, variable severity	Lateral on side of pneumothorax	Pleuritic, dyspnea, reduced breath sounds on side of pneumothorax
Gastrointestinal			
Gastroesophageal reflux	Usually dull but can be sharp	Retrosternal, sometimes with radiation to neck or jaw	Often comes on after food or wakes people from sleep, may be relieved by antacids or proton-pump inhibitors
Cholecystitis	Dull, aching	Usually subcostal but can be retrosternal	May come on after fatty food consumption; associated with right subcostal tenderness and disordered liver function tests
Chest wall pain			
Costochondritis	Often sharp, can be dull and aching	Localized over costochondral joint	Localized chest wall tenderness; NB: does not exclude coronary heart disease
Rib fracture	Localized, pleuritic	Very localized pain over fracture	Usually after chest trauma but can occur after vigorous coughing
Herpes zoster (shingles)	Dull, disturbing, may be associated with typical blistering eruption	Unilateral in dermatome distribution	Pain is often worse before eruption of vesico-papular rash

Syncope

- A sudden episode of collapse can be a very threatening symptom, and can indicate a major bradyarrhythmia requiring urgent treatment, or a life-threatening tachy-arrhythmia such as ventricular tachycardia.
- The patient should be asked if the episode was preceded by any disturbance of the heart rhythm.
- A history of similar episodes occurring while standing or getting up from a sitting or lying position may indicate postural hypotension.
- Metabolic causes, such as hypoglycemia, should be sought by checking for recent commencement or dose change of hypoglycemic treatments.

Physical examination

General examination

- The patient's level of distress, the rate of breathing, degree of pallor, presence of sweating (diaphoresis), cyanosis, and coolness or warmth of the peripheries are all valuable observations which offer important diagnostic clues.
- Careful examination of the hands and lips can help identify the presence of cyanosis, which is traditionally classified as *central* (mainly in the lips) or *peripheral* (mainly in the extremities).

Pulse

- The *radial* pulse can give valuable clues to the regularity of the heart rhythm and rate.
- An irregularly irregular pulse is usually due to atrial fibrillation, but differentiation from frequent ectopic beats may require an electrocardiogram.
- Pulsus paradoxus (a fall in systolic blood pressure of >10 mmHg with inspiration) and pulsus alternans (alternating weak and strong beats) are often clinically evident on palpation of the *brachial* pulse, and confirmed by checking the brachial pulse with the sphygmomanometer.
- Evaluation of the pulse contour usually requires careful examination of the *carotid* pulse.
- The *femoral* pulse can be examined to detect aortofemoral delay in aortic coarctation, and may be accentuated in some patients with aortic regurgitation.

CLINICAL PEARL

Evaluate all pulses: radial pulse for rhythm, brachial for pulsus paradoxus and alternans, femoral for aorto-femoral delay, and carotid for pulse contour.

Blood pressure measurement

- Blood pressure should be measured sitting with the back supported or in a lying position.
  - » The ideal cuff should encircle at least 80% of the arm circumference.

- The systolic pressure is denoted by the 1st Korotkoff sound; there is now general agreement that the diastolic pressure is denoted by the 5th Korotkoff sound (disappearance of the sound) rather than the 4th Korotkoff sound (muffling of the sound). However, when the diastolic pressure using the 5th Korotkoff sound is very low, the 4th Korotkoff sound should be recorded, and noted as such.
- More accurate recording of blood pressure is obtained from averaging 2 or 3 readings, each about a minute apart.
- There is evidence that measurement in both arms adds to the assessment. This is rarely done as routine, but should be sought if aortic dissection with involvement of the left subclavian artery is suspected.
- Orthostatic hypotension is defined by a fall in systolic pressure >20 mmHg in response to assuming of the upright posture from a supine position within 3 minutes.

Jugular venous pulse

The jugular venous pulse (JVP) is evaluated to estimate the central venous pressure and to draw conclusions on right heart function from the pulse contour.

- An elevated JVP is a useful indicator of right heart pressure overload.
- The external jugular vein is best for measuring the height of the JVP, and the internal jugular for assessing pulsations and contour of the pulse.
- A JVP height of >4.5 cm above the angle of Louis with the patient at 45° to the horizontal, or a JVP visible above the clavicle with the patient at 45°, is considered abnormal.
- The finding of an elevated JVP on the right should always be confirmed by checking the left.
- The presence of large V waves in the neck is a reliable sign of tricuspid regurgitation.
- The normal response to inspiration is a fall in the jugular pressure; a rise or lack of fall in the JVP with inspiration is referred to as Kussmaul's sign and may be a sign of pericardial tamponade.
- Hepato- or abdomino-jugular reflux (an increase in JVP with pressure over the liver or upper abdomen) is used to elicit borderline signs of increased central venous pressure.
- Examination of the contour of the pulsations in the internal jugular vein can provide valuable information. The correlations between the jugular pulse and the phases of the cardiac cycle are shown in Figure 7-1, and the mechanism and interpretation summarized in Table 7-2.

CLINICAL PEARL

The external jugular is better for measuring the venous pressure; the internal jugular is better for measuring the venous pulse contour.

Carotid pulse

- The carotid pulse should be examined in all patients, but especially when trying to assess the severity of aortic

Table 7-2 Venous pulse contours and interpretation

VENOUS PULSE	MECHANISM	INTERPRETATION
a wave	Atrial contraction	Prominent in situations of increased atrial compliance such as COPD and pulmonary hypertension. Absent in atrial fibrillation
'Cannon' or 'giant' a wave	Right atrium contraction against a closed tricuspid valve	May indicate atrioventricular block or ventricular tachycardia
v wave	Does not represent ventricular contraction; is a reflected wave from late filling of the right atrium	Combines with c wave and is prominent with tricuspid regurgitation
c wave	Small wave, represents ventricular contraction	Usually difficult to see in clinical examination
x descent	Downward movement of the tricuspid valve during ventricular contraction; occurs between the a wave and the v wave, interrupted by the c wave	A steep x descent is said to be a sign of pericardial tamponade
y descent	Ventricular filling after opening of triscupid valve; occurs after the v wave	Steep y descent said to be typical of pericardial constriction

COPD, chronic obstructive pulmonary disease.

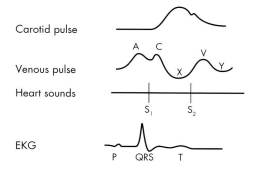

Figure 7-1 The jugular venous pressure and pulse contour

From Walker HK, Hall WD and Hurst JW, eds. Clinical methods: The history, physical, and laboratory examinations, 3rd ed. Boston: Butterworths, 1990.

stenosis. Pressure over the carotid pulse should be gentle to avoid initiating a bradycardic response, and both carotids should not be examined together.

- The clinically important carotid pulse contours are summarized in Table 7-3.

Cardiac inspection, palpation and percussion

Inspection of the precordium is often overlooked but can provide valuable clues.

- Prominent pulsations in the precordium may indicate a left ventricular aneurysm or marked right ventricular overload.
- Prominent pulsations in the suprasternal notch may indicate an aortic arch aneurysm.
- Palpation of the precordium should include documentation of the location of the *apex beat*. The location of the apex beat should be recorded with the patient lying flat, but examination in the left lateral decubitus position

Table 7-3 Summary of carotid pulse contours and their interpretation

PULSE CHARACTER	TERMINOLOGY	CAUSE
A slow-rising, low-amplitude pulse, sometimes with shuddering	Slow-rising pulse (pulsus parvus et tardus)	Severe aortic stenosis
Sharp rise and fall in the carotid pulse regurgitation	Corrigan's pulse Collapsing pulse Waterhammer pulse	Severe aortic regurgitation
A double-amplitude pulse	Bigeminal pulse (pulsus bigeminus)	Frequent ectopic beats
Prominent secondary pulsation	Bisferiens pulse (pulsus bisferiens)	Severe aortic regurgitation or hypertrophic cardiomyopathy

(patient lying half on the left side with support from the examiner's arm or a pillow) should also be performed to fully evaluate the character of the cardiac impulse.

» A diffuse apex beat may indicate marked left ventricular systolic dysfunction.

- Palpation of the left parasternal space should be routine to search for right ventricular overload.

» A systolic thrill over the left parasternal space may be felt in severe aortic stenosis, and, more rarely, a diastolic thrill may be felt in severe aortic regurgitation.

- Percussion of the precordium is occasionally helpful when trying to identify displacement of the heart or a large pericardial effusion.

» Ewart's sign is an area of dullness on percussion at the lower angle of the left scapula, indicating a large pericardial effusion.

CLINICAL PEARL

The location of the apex beat should be recorded with the patient lying supine and flat, as should the character of the cardiac pulsation in the left lateral decubitus position.

Cardiac auscultation

- Auscultation at the apex, left sternal border, right upper sternal border and right lower sternal border is essential for full evaluation.
- Abnormalities of the heart sounds give important clues to underlying pathophysiology (Table 7-4).
- Added sounds in systole or diastole can also assist to identify abnormalities in systolic and diastolic function (Table 7-5).

» The 4th heart sound indicates reduced left ventricular compliance from multiple causes, including aortic stenosis, left ventricular hypertrophy, ischemic heart disease, and restrictive cardiomyopathy. It is a valuable clue to the increasingly recognized condition of diastolic dysfunction of the left ventricle.

» A 3rd heart sound invariably indicates significant left ventricular dysfunction. It is usually low-pitched, but in the presence of a tachycardia may be of medium pitch and more readily heard. This is referred to as *gallop rhythm*.

Systolic murmurs

During auscultation, systole should be carefully examined to determine the pitch, character, timing, amplitude (loudness), location and radiation of any murmur.

- The amplitude should be recorded on a scale of 1–4 or 1–6.
- The location in which a murmur is best heard is often a guide to which valve is producing the murmur. However, careful studies comparing skilled clinicians with echocardiographic findings have shown that a murmur in the apical region can be aortic in origin and mitral regurgitation can sometimes be heard best in the 'aortic' or 'pulmonary' parasternal location.

CLINICAL PEARL

Murmurs are best described by their precise location on the chest (left sternal border/apical/right parasternal), rather than the traditional aortic/pulmonary/mitral/tricuspid locations, as these may not accurately reflect the origin of the murmur.

- The character and timing of the murmur can be described as pansystolic (holosystolic) or crescendo/decrescendo (often described as diamond-shaped from its configuration on phonocardiography).

Table 7-4 Variations in the 1st and 2nd heart sounds

SOUNDS	MECHANISM	SIGNIFICANCE
Increased amplitude of the 1st heart sound	Vigorous mitral and tricuspid valve closure	Hyperkinetic circulation or a short PR interval
Wide splitting of the 2nd heart sound	Delay in closing of the pulmonary valve or right ventricular overload	Right bundle branch block (some variation in the degree of splitting with respiration) or large atrial septal defect (fixed splitting)
Reverse splitting of the 2nd heart sound	Aortic valve closure can be so delayed that the aortic component of the sound occurs after the pulmonary component	Left bundle branch block or severe left ventricular dysfunction
Increase in amplitude of the pulmonary component of the 2nd heart sound	Vigorous pulmonary valve closure	Pulmonary hypertension
Tic-tac mechanical character	Mechanical valve closure or opening	Mechanical prosthetic valve

Table 7-5 Added sounds in systole and diastole

ADDED SOUND	MECHANISM	SIGNIFICANCE
Systole		
Early systolic click	Aortic or pulmonary valve opening; can occur alone or preceding a systolic bruit	Dilated aortic root or pulmonary artery
Mid-systolic click	Arises from the mitral valve apparatus; may be single or multiple	Usually indicates mitral valve prolapse; can occur without mitral regurgitation
Diastole		
4th heart sound—moderate- to low-pitched sound occurring just before the 1st heart sound	Atrial systole into a non-compliant left ventricle	Reduced compliance of the left ventricle
3rd heart sound—low-pitched sound in mid diastole	Abrupt deceleration of left ventricular (LV) inflow during early diastole	Indicates significant systolic dysfunction with cardiac failure
Opening snap—high-pitched sound which may precede the mid-diastolic rumble	Diastolic opening of the mitral valve	Mitral stenosis associated with mobile valve leaflets
Mid-diastolic rumble—longer and lower-pitched than the 3rd heart sound	Diastolic flow across a stenosed mitral valve	Indicative of mitral stenosis

» A **pansystolic (holosystolic) murmur** is usually an indication of mitral regurgitation, but can be due to a ventricular septal defect. If it radiates to the axilla, it favors mitral regurgitation as the cause.

» A softer pansystolic murmur heard at the left lower sternal area may indicate tricuspid regurgitation. An increase in amplitude with inspiration strengthens the evidence for tricuspid regurgitation, but this is an unreliable sign, and supportive evidence of a prominent v wave in the JVP and hepatic pulsation should be sought.

» A **crescendo/decrescendo** (ejection type, diamond-shaped) **murmur** usually indicates aortic stenosis but can represent mitral regurgitation.

- On occasions, mitral regurgitation associated with prolapse of the posterior mitral valve leaflet can be heard best in the parasternal area.
- Radiation to the neck indicates origin from the aortic valve, and radiation to the axilla indicates origin from the mitral valve.
- It is sometimes difficult to distinguish aortic valve sclerosis from stenosis on clinical grounds alone, and other features of aortic stenosis (especially a slow-rising pulse on examination of the carotid pulse) should be sought before reaching a conclusion.
- A murmur which has features of aortic stenosis and mitral regurgitation may truly reflect both conditions.
- Occasionally, hypertrophic cardiomyopathy can reproduce features of aortic stenosis from outflow tract obstruction from the septal hypertrophy, as well as

mitral regurgitation from the disruption of the mitral valve apparatus.

CLINICAL PEARLS

- A harsh mid-systolic murmur at the left sternal border with radiation to the neck indicates aortic stenosis.
- A pansystolic murmur with radiation to the axilla indicates mitral regurgitation.
- The only exception is anteriorly directed mitral regurgitation which may be heard in the left parasternal region.

Diastolic murmurs

The two main diastolic murmurs are an early diastolic murmur due to aortic regurgitation, and a mid-diastolic murmur heard in mitral stenosis.

- The **early diastolic murmur** of aortic regurgitation is high-pitched with a characteristic decrescendo character heard best at the left sternal border.
- The length, not the amplitude of the murmur, indicates the severity of the regurgitation:
  » a short early diastolic murmur indicates mild regurgitation
  » a murmur persisting to mid diastole or greater indicates severe regurgitation
  » the murmur may be enhanced by sitting the patient forward and listening in expiration.
- An early diastolic murmur heard best well to the left of the sternum may be a sign of pulmonary regurgitation.

- The **mid-diastolic murmur** of mitral stenosis has a low-pitched, rumbling character. It is heard best at the cardiac apex and must be sought with the patient in the left lateral decubitus position.
  - » As with other diastolic murmurs, the length, not the amplitude, of the mid-diastolic rumble is an index of the severity of the mitral stenosis.
  - » It needs to be distinguished from a 3rd heart sound (usually associated with other signs of cardiac failure), and from the Austin Flint murmur associated with severe aortic regurgitation (associated with other signs of aortic regurgitation such as collapsing pulse or wide pulse pressure).

CLINICAL PEARL

A diastolic rumble is usually found with other features of mitral stenosis and a 3rd heart sound with other features of cardiac failure.

Continuous murmurs

Occasionally a continuous murmur is heard. This can indicate a patent ductus arteriosus or other cause of aortic-pulmonary connection such as from infective endocarditis, trauma, or post-operative fistula.

It is important to recognize that these are rare, and a continuous-sounding murmur is more likely to be due to a more mundane cause, such as aortic stenosis and regurgitation, or a loud pericardial friction rub (see below). It may be a transmitted sound from an arteriovenous fistula in the arm in patients having hemodialysis.

Pericardial friction rubs

- A pericardial friction rub can be heard anywhere over the heart, but usually best at the left sternal border.
- Pericardial rubs vary in pitch, and usually but not always have a leathery, scratching, to-and-fro character.
- They can often vary with different positions and phases of respiration, and can be variable from hour to hour.

Respiratory examination

Chest percussion and auscultation of the chest are essential components of the clinical examination of the cardiac patient.

- **Percussion** can identify the presence and extent of a pleural effusion which may be a sign of chronic cardiac failure.
- **Auscultation** for crackles at the lung bases and for areas of dullness may reveal signs of cardiac failure.
  - » While the presence of crackles does not confirm cardiac failure, rapid resolution with diuretic treatment is a clear sign that the crackles were due to cardiac-related pulmonary congestion, and not a respiratory cause such as chest infection or pulmonary fibrosis. The extent of crackles (scattered only, extensive but confined to below mid-scapula, or throughout the whole of the lung fields) should be documented.

- » The identification of whistling or wheeze may indicate that dyspnea is more likely to be due to asthma or chronic obstructive pulmonary disease, but does not rule out the possibility of 'cardiac asthma' due to pulmonary congestion.

Abdomen

Examination of the abdomen from the cardiac perspective includes:

- palpation of the liver for pulsatile hepatomegaly indicating tricuspid regurgitation
- gentle pressure over the liver to elicit the hepatojugular reflux
- a search for ascites and free fluid which may indicate chronic right heart failure.

INVESTIGATION OF CARDIAC DISEASE

For the assessment and investigation of cardiac disease, many tests can be employed, and optimal use of testing requires an appreciation of what each test can offer. It is helpful to distinguish tests which are mainly for imaging the heart and those which test functional capacity (Table 7-6).

Electrocardiography (EKG)

The EKG is the most useful and widely used investigation for evaluating the cardiac patient. While the increasing sophistication and miniaturization of the EKG, and the readily available automated analysis, are welcome technological developments, a clear understanding of the basics of EKG interpretation remains essential (Table 7-7).

Holter (continuous EKG) monitoring

When detail is required to elucidate the cause of a patient's irregular heart rhythm, syncope, dizziness, a period of continuous monitoring of the EKG can be performed. The usual duration of monitoring is 24 hours but with recent developments in technology, longer periods of monitoring can be achieved with implanted or wearable devices.

Ambulatory blood pressure monitoring

When there is an unexplained discrepancy between home and clinic recordings (white coat hypertension), uncertainty about adequate blood pressure control, marked variation in blood pressure readings, or uncertainty if borderline blood pressure elevation warrants treatment, ambulatory blood pressure monitoring is warranted. Arm cuff devices are recommended; wrist and finger devices are not.

Exercise EKG stress testing (EST)

- The EST is a well-validated diagnostic procedure in which exercise is used to increase myocardial oxygen demand, and continuous EKG is used to detect evidence of myocardial ischemia or arrhythmia.

Table 7-6 Cardiac investigations

TEST	IMAGING	FUNCTIONAL
Electrocardiogram (EKG)	+	−
Holter (continuous EKG) monitoring	+	+
Ambulatory blood pressure monitoring	+	+
Chest X-ray	++	++
Echocardiogram	+++	+
Exercise EKG	+−	+++
Radionuclide venticulography	+	++
Stress echocardiography	++	++
Radionuclide myocardial perfusion imaging	++	++
Invasive coronary angiography	+++	+
Coronary computed tomography angiography (CTCA, CCTA)	++	+
Cardiac catheterization	+	++
Magnetic resonance imaging (MRI)	++	++
Positron emission tomography (PET)	++	++

» The exercise EKG is frequently used to evaluate a patient's risk of coronary heart disease, but is also useful to reveal residual myocardial ischemia after a coronary event or intervention.

» It can also be used to assess cardiac arrhythmias, and to assess functional capacity in patients with valvular heart disease and inform timing of intervention.

• It is widely available and relatively inexpensive.

• It is relatively safe, but death or myocardial infarction can occur in up to 5 per 100,000 tests.

» Complications can be minimized by adherence to the usual safety and quality standards, with particular emphasis on assessment of symptoms and meticulous monitoring of EKG changes.

» In modern practice, continuous monitoring of the 12-lead EKG is standard, and careful surveillance for cardiac arrhythmias and systolic blood pressure is essential.

• Exercise testing can be done with a bicycle ergometer or treadmill protocol. The most widely used protocol is the Bruce Treadmill Protocol with an increase in workload each 3 minutes.

• Drugs can affect the exercise test result. Beta-blockers affect the heart rate response to exercise, and may mask the EKG or symptomatic response to exercise. Digoxin can affect the shape of the ST segments.

EKG criteria

ST-segment depression on exercise electrocardiography can be indicative of underlying myocardial ischemia, but needs to be interpreted with care.

• The shape of the ST-segment depression can provide useful clues (see Figure 7-2). If the ST-segment depression is up-sloping, it is less significant than flat or down-sloping depression.

• The greater the extent of ST-segment depression, the greater is the likelihood of myocardial ischemia. Flat ST-segment depression of >2 mm is usually taken to be a strong indication of myocardial ischemia. If the abnormality persists for >5 minutes and occurs during recovery, this indicates more-severe disease.

• There are important caveats in interpreting ST-segment changes with exercise. Females often have more labile ST segments, and can have normal coronary arteries even with an exercise test showing >2 mm of ST-segment depression.

ST-segment elevation may indicate acute myocardial ischemia, and is an indication for immediate cessation of the test and careful post-exercise monitoring.

T wave changes with exercise are common and not usually indicative of myocardial ischemia; however, extensive deep T wave inversion, particularly if persistent, can be a marker of extensive ischemia.

Cardiac arrhythmias are common with exercise. The development of short runs of ventricular tachycardia may be of no clinical significance.

CLINICAL PEARL

Exercise EKG interpretation requires not only careful analysis of the exercise EKG, but also observation of clinical state during exercise, blood pressure response, and exercise duration.

Other clinical observations

While the EKG provides crucial diagnostic data, other observations are important in interpreting the exercise EKG.

• The patient's symptoms and their response to exercise need to be carefully recorded. The development of typical angina with exercise is diagnostic of ischemia, but other chest pains may develop from other causes, e.g. musculoskeletal pain. Careful interpretation and observation can provide valuable information.

• The blood pressure response to exercise is usually a steady rise with increasing exercise, but an exaggerated response may have adverse prognostic significance.

Table 7-7 A guide to electrocardiographic (EKG, ECG) interpretation

EKG, ECG OBSERVATION	INTERPRETATION
Quality of the tracing	Baseline stable? Minimal interference? Correct voltage standardization? Correct lead placement?
Heart rate	Heart rate: can be documented from the interpretative EKG; the simplest method is to use a heart rate ruler or to divide 300 by the number of big squares between R waves
Heart rhythm	Regular or irregular?
Frontal axis	The normal axis is −30° to +90°; left-axis deviation is < −30°, right-axis deviation is > +90°
P waves	Present? Normal morphology? Notched, tall?
PR interval	Normal = 120–200 ms
	Prolonged = 1st degree atrioventricular block
	Short = Wolff–Parkinson–White (WPW) syndrome if associated with delta wave
	Variable PR interval indicative of Wenckebach block
QRS complex	Normal duration <110 ms
	Notched but <120 ms = intraventricular conduction defect
	>120 ms = bundle branch block (BBB). Tall R in V_1: usually RBBB; no tall R wave in V_1: usually LBBB. Other causes of tall R wave in V_1: right ventricular hypertrophy, type A WPW, true posterior infarction
	Non-pathological Q waves: can occur in lateral leads, and small narrow Q waves in inferior leads. If in doubt, may need echocardiography for evaluation
	Pathological Q waves usually >25% of the R wave, and >40 ms wide
	Poor R wave progression or QS waves in anterior leads: may indicate old anterior infarction, but may be normal. Often shown to be benign on echocardiography
QT interval	Measure QT and QTc (corrected QT interval)
	Abnormal QTc in an adult male is >450 ms, and in an adult female >470 ms
ST segment	ST-segment elevation: physiological ST elevation in anterior leads and 'early repolarization' usually <2 mm
	Abnormal ST elevations:
	—ST elevation concave upwards: usually pericarditis but can indicate a normal variant of early repolarization
	—acute ST elevation in 2 contiguous leads with >1 mm elevation in the anterior leads or >2 mm in the anterior leads is indicative of ST-elevation myocardial infarction (STEMI)
	ST-segment depression: transient with myocardial ischemia; permanent with left ventricular hypertrophy, digoxin effect
T wave	Minor T wave inversion can be due to multiple causes, including electrolyte disturbances, hyperventilation, and certain drugs. The most common cause is myocardial ischemia
	Deep T wave inversion: acute myocardial ischemia, but other causes include intracerebral events, hypertrophic cardiomyopathy
	Tall peaked T waves: acute ischemia or hyperkalemia
U wave	Usually hypokalemia, but may be normal
Localization of myocardial damage	The localization of EKG abnormalities:
	—inferior: II, III and aVF
	—lateral: aVL, V_5, V_6
	—anterior: V_2–V_5

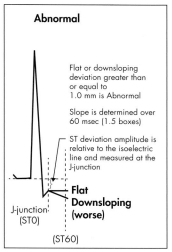

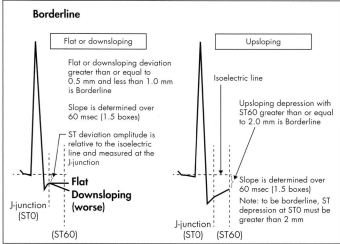

Figure 7-2 Interpretation of the exercise electrocardiogram

Modified from Fletcher GF et al. AHA Scientific Statement. Exercise standards for testing and training: a statement for healthcare professionals. Circulation. 2001;104:1694–1740.

- A drop in blood pressure of >10 mmHg can indicate extensive myocardial ischemia, and is an indication for prompt cessation of the test.
- Observation of the patient for dyspnea, pallor, cyanosis and facial expression indicating distress can all provide valuable diagnostic clues.

Sensitivity, specificity and predictive value

- The **sensitivity** (percentage of persons who have disease who will have a positive test) and **specificity** (percentage of persons who do not have disease who will have a negative test) of the exercise EKG depend largely on the type of patient undergoing the test.
- The **positive predictive value** (percentage of those with or without disease who are identified correctly) is high in patients who are likely to have coronary artery disease (CAD), e.g. those with multiple risk factors or suggestive symptoms.
- The use of the exercise EKG is not recommended as a screening test in the large number of persons at low risk in the community.
- With careful selection of patients, careful conduct of the test, and informed interpretation, the exercise EKG continues to provide valuable information despite the rapid growth of more technologically advanced procedures.

Radionuclide ventriculography

Left ventricular function can be measured by intravenous injection of radionuclide and imaging the radioisotope as it passes through the left ventricle. Because high-quality imaging requires multiple images gated to the EKG, the test is often referred to as a MUGA (multiple gated acquisition) scan. Echocardiography offers more detail and is usually preferred for assessment of left ventricular function.

Chest X-ray (CXR)

A CXR allows structural assessment of the heart in relation to the other organs within the thoracic cavity and mediastinum.

- Cardiomegaly, aortic root abnormalities, and valvular calcifications can be identified, but assessment of heart size has been largely supplanted by echocardiography in modern practice.
- Pulmonary abnormalities that are a result of cardiac dysfunction, such as acute pulmonary edema and pleural effusions, can be identified on CXR (see Figure 7-3).

CLINICAL PEARL

An important role of the chest X-ray is to identify the extent of pulmonary congestion and the response to treatment.

Echocardiography

Echocardiography is now the most widely used imaging procedure in cardiology. It has the advantage of being relatively inexpensive and readily available. With modern echocardiographic equipment, reliable imaging can be obtained at the bedside even in a critically ill patient.

Echocardiography relies on reflection and processing of ultrasound waves from the cardiac structures.

- The ultrasound probe is placed on the patient's chest, and emits and receives high-frequency ultrasound. Probes of 2 to 10 megahertz (MHz) are usually used for echocardiography; higher frequencies achieve greater definition, but with the loss of tissue penetration.
- The ultrasound waves are then processed into M mode (assessing motion in a single narrow view) or into a two-dimensional image which represents the moving cardiac structures (2D echo).

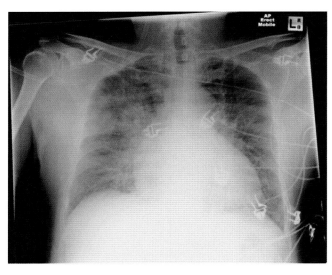 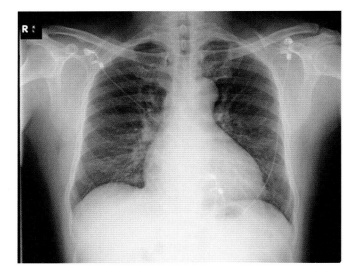

Figure 7-3 Chest X-ray in patient with pulmonary edema (left), showing shadowing and 'bat's wing' congestion appearance; and after treatment (right)

Image courtesy of Dr Angela Worthington.

- More recent processing developments have enabled the development of three-dimensional echocardiography, which can provide remarkable anatomical detail for particular views of the heart. This has been of advantage in the analysis of complex congenital heart disease, and the planning and monitoring of valve function during mitral valve surgery.

Doppler imaging is now routine during echocardiography and analysis allows the pattern of blood flow and tissue movement to be analyzed.

- The Doppler signal can be displayed as a black and white spectral image display equivalent to flow, or color-coded using the convention of motion toward the transducer = red, motion away from the transducer = blue.
- A fully optioned modern echocardiographic examination therefore uses a combination of 2D echocardiography with Doppler color-flow imaging.

CLINICAL PEARL

In viewing Doppler flow images on echocardiography, red = flow toward the transducer, blue = away from the transducer.

The usual transthoracic echocardiogram is performed with imaging from the left parasternal area, apical area, suprasternal area and subcostal area.

- The left parasternal long-axis view can provide valuable information equivalent to a sagittal section from the apex to the origin of the aorta.
- The left parasternal short-axis view can provide cross-sectional imaging of the left ventricular chamber and *en face* views of the mitral valve and aortic valve.
- Apical views are usually used to analyze the left and right ventricular shape and function.

- Subcostal views are particularly valuable for assessing pericardial disease, and suprasternal imaging is used for assessing the anatomy of the ascending aorta and aortic valve.

Transesophageal echocardiography (TEE) provides remarkably high-resolution images of the cardiac chambers, particularly of the left atrium (including left atrial appendage), mitral and aortic valves. This is of particular value in assessing left atrial appendage thrombus formation.

CLINICAL PEARL

Transesophageal echocardiography is invaluable for assessment of the mitral valve, and thrombus in the left atrial appendage.

Stress imaging with exercise or intravenous dobutamine (stress echo) can provide valuable information on wall-motion abnormalities and assess whether there is inducible ischemia as a result of the stress.

Even further miniaturization of ultrasound probes has resulted in the capacity for **intracardiac imaging** (ICE) and **intravascular imaging** (IVUS) for imaging the interior of the coronary arteries.

- Enhancement of the images can be obtained by injection of agitated saline to identify microbubbles passing across intracardiac shunts.
- The use of ultrasound contrast media can be employed for the enhancement of left ventricular endocardial borders, to better define global and regional systolic function.

Major uses of echocardiography

Analysis of systolic function of the left ventricle

- Global left ventricular function is usually expressed as the left ventricular ejection fraction (LVEF), calculated from the left ventricular end-diastolic volume (LVEDV) minus the systolic volume (LVESV), divided by the diastolic volume (LVEDV), i.e. (LVEDV − LVSEV)/LVEDV. Measurements of global longitudinal strain, based on measuring myocardial deformation, are being increasingly used to add information to serial LVEF measurements.

- Regional wall motion is graded as *normal*, *hypokinetic* (reduced systolic function), *akinetic* (no wall motion), or *dyskinetic* (paradoxical outward rather than inward motion). An akinetic segment of left ventricular wall is usually echogenic, indicating scar tissue.
- The thickness of the heart muscle can be identified (usually no greater than 1 cm in the septum and posterior walls), and the left ventricular mass overall calculated.

Left ventricular diastolic function

- On occasions, systolic function may be within normal limits but the left ventricle is pumping inefficiently because of reduced compliance or increased stiffness. This can be associated with a variant of cardiac failure (heart failure with preserved systolic function known as heart failure with preserved ejection fraction [HFPEF]). This may occur in infiltrative processes or with significant left ventricular hypertrophy.
- Measurement of diastolic dysfunction is complex; it is usually measured from the rate of inflow during mitral valve inflow.

CLINICAL PEARL

Echocardiography is an essential tool for the assessment of left ventricular function and should be performed in every patient suspected of cardiac failure.

Assessment of the right ventricle

Patients with advanced left-sided valvular heart disease or pulmonary hypertension need careful evaluation of their right ventricular function.

Intracardiac masses

Intracardiac tumors or thrombus can be readily identified and monitored on echocardiography.

Pericardial disease

Echocardiography is of particular value in assessing the presence of a pericardial effusion, and whether it is associated with cardiac tamponade.

Assessment of the cardiac valves

- **Tricuspid valve.** A minor degree of regurgitation through the tricuspid valve is physiological. Significant tricuspid regurgitation may reflect tricuspid valve abnormality, dysfunction of the right ventricle, or increased pulmonary artery pressure. It may sometimes be caused by a pacemaker or defibrillator lead as it crosses the valve to reach the right ventricle. The pulmonary artery pressure can be estimated indirectly from the flow through the tricuspid valve during regurgitation.

- **Pulmonary valve.** The pulmonary valve is well imaged with several echocardiographic views.

CLINICAL PEARL

Trivial pulmonary and tricuspid regurgitation are often seen on echocardiography and are not significant.

- **Mitral valve.** The mitral valve is well seen in transthoracic echocardiography (TTE), but even more clearly with transesophageal echocardiography (TEE). In the left parasternal long-axis view, the mitral valve apparatus and the anterior and posterior valve leaflet morphology and motion can be examined in detail.
  - » The approximate severity of mitral regurgitation can be measured by assessment of the Doppler flow signal and visualization of the color doppler flow images.
  - » Mitral stenosis can be suspected from reduced motion of the leaflets on the parasternal long-axis views, and confirmed by measures of transmitral flow and planimetry on the parasternal short-axis view.
  - » The pattern of inflow through the normal mitral valve can be calculated to estimate the degree of diastolic dysfunction.
  - » A degree of calcification in the mitral annulus is normal and increases with age.
  - » TTE with 2D and 3D imaging is frequently used before and during mitral valve surgery to assess which leaflets require repair, and to guide the surgical approach.
- **Aortic valve.** The aortic valve is well visualized in both parasternal and apical views.
  - » The degree of thickening and the mobility of the valve can be assessed with the 2D views, but the function of the valve and the extent of stenosis or regurgitation needs assessment of the Doppler color-flow images, and detailed analysis of the Doppler spectral data.
  - » The transvalvular velocities are used to calculate the peak and mean gradients, and, with consideration of the stroke volume, the valve area can be calculated.
  - » The best parameter for monitoring the progress of aortic stenosis remains undetermined, but in practice peak velocity, peak and mean gradients, valve area, and symptoms are all evaluated in deciding on the timing of intervention.
  - » The assessment of aortic regurgitation also requires careful evaluation of the 2D echo and the Doppler flow analysis. Most echo labs report the degree of regurgitation as *trivial* (minimal jet), *mild* (visible regurgitation into the ventricle), *moderate* (regurgitation reaching the mid-ventricle) or *severe* (regurgitation toward the apex of the left ventricle).

Assessment of the aorta

The parasternal and apical echo windows do not allow for assessment of more than the aortic root, coronary sinuses and the first 3–4 cm/1–1.5 in of the ascending aorta. The normal aortic root in adults should not exceed 3.6 cm/ 1.4 in. The Doppler technique can be used to assess a gradient within the aorta and may allow the diagnosis of aortic coarctation. A more detailed assessment of the ascending aorta and arch may require computed tomography (CT) or magnetic resonance imaging (MRI).

Assessment of congenital heart disease

Echocardiography has been a major advance in the evaluation of congenital heart disease.

- The most common anomaly, foramen ovale, can be recognized from careful examination of the interatrial septum. The anomaly is recognized with increasing frequency with improving technical imaging capability. It is a benign finding, but has been associated with stroke, transient ischemic attack (TIA), and migraine.
- A bicuspid aortic valve is usually recognized from a typical bicuspid appearance of the valve on the parasternal short-axis view.
- An atrial septal defect may be recognizable from identifying a defect in the interatrial septum, but requires imaging after intravenous injection with agitated saline for accurate assessment. The passage of micobubbles across the interatrial septum confirms the location and size of the defect. Evidence of right ventricular overload can further confirm the presence of a large defect.
- Ventricular septal defects, being associated with a high-velocity jet, are usually recognized from analysis of the Doppler signal, particularly in the substernal views.

Contrast echocardiography

- Contrast agents which release microbubbles on contact with the ultrasound beam can be used to enhance the blood pool, and are of particular value to enhance endocardial borders in difficult-to-image patients, including during stress echocardiography.
- Contrast agents are also used to image for specialized conditions which may not be clear on standard imaging, including left ventricular non-compaction, an apical variant of ventricular hypertrophy, or structural complications of myocardial infarction such as pseudo-aneurysm.
- Contrast echo has been of particular value in distinguishing apical shadowing suggestive of apical thrombus from physiological appearances, and for cardiac tumors.

Exercise (or pharmacological) stress echocardiography (ESE)

Exercise stress echocardiography (ESE) is a functional test that aims to detect changes in cardiac function between rest and exercise. This is usually done by displaying images simultaneously on the screen (quad screen display) to compare 'before' and 'after' images in different views.

- It is commonly used for the assessment of myocardial ischemia, but can also be used for the functional assessment of moderate aortic stenosis, diastolic function and pulmonary artery pressures.

- Standard echocardiographic images of the left ventricle are taken from different imaging windows at rest, and the patient is then exercised to peak capacity using a treadmill or bicycle. Repeat images are then taken at the peak of the patient's exercise. If pulmonary pressures, valvular gradients and diastolic parameters are of interest, these are also included in both the resting and the peak acquisition phases.
- If the patient is unable to exercise, for reasons such as orthopedic limitations, frailty or chronic illness, pharmacologic stress echo with dobutamine can be used to stimulate tachycardia.

Radionuclide myocardial perfusion imaging

Radionuclide myocardial perfusion imaging, also known as single-photon emission computerized tomography (SPECT) scan, uses technetium-99m or thallium. Both are taken up by the myocardium, and the flow through the myocardial tissue is detected by a gamma scanner which creates an image of multiple planes and segments.

- The test is conducted in two stages: a stress stage at which time the radionuclide is injected, and a post-stress stage which is usually 4 hours after stress to allow restoration of resting conditions. The stress stage employs either a treadmill/bicycle ergometer or a chemical agent, such as dipyridamole, adenosine or dobutamine, to stimulate tachycardia and thus myocardial oxygen demand.
- Radionuclide myocardial perfusion imaging is typically done when there is doubt about the interpretation of the stress EKG, to distinguish viable from non-viable myocardium, or when the functional significance of a coronary stenosis is being evaluated.
- The resting and stress images are compared to detect defects in arterial perfusion during the stress phase. Decreased perfusion during the stress phase represents arterial disease, whereas a defect at both stress and rest indicates infarcted myocardial tissue (see Figure 7-4).

Coronary angiography and cardiac catheterization

Coronary angiography is performed by the injection of radio-opaque contrast into the coronary arteries to identify their anatomy. The coronary artery nomenclature as seen in the usual projections is shown in Figure 7-5, and the appearances on angiography are seen in Figure 7-6.

- It is used for the diagnosis of CAD, and it also enables the insertion of coronary artery stents.
- When stents are inserted, the procedure is termed *percutaneous coronary intervention* (PCI).

CLINICAL PEARL

Coronary angiography is the 'gold standard' for assessing coronary artery disease. Its main limitation is that it images the lumen and cannot estimate the extent of disease in the wall of the vessel.

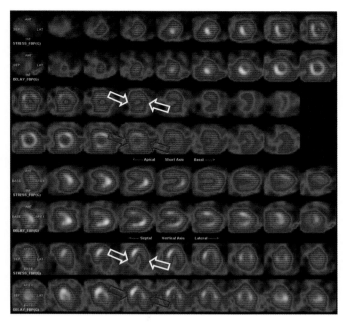

Figure 7-4 Radionuclide myocardial perfusion scans; stress images are in the upper rows and delayed images (4 hours later) in the lower rows. There are extensive anteroseptal and lateral defects (white arrows) with near-total restoration of blood flow 4 hours post exercise (red arrows). Coronary angiography confirmed severe stenoses in the left anterior descending artery, moderate disease in the mid circumflex artery, and severe disease in the distal right coronary artery

Image courtesy of Dr Geoffrey Bower, Nuclear Physician, Mount Nuclear Medicine, Perth, Australia.

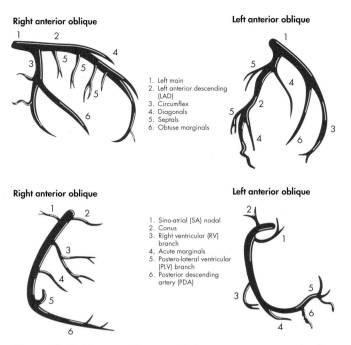

Figure 7-5 Nomenclature of the coronary arteries in the typical coronary angiography projections

From Thompson PL (ed), Coronary care manual, 2nd ed. Sydney: Elsevier Australia, 2011.

Cardiac catheterization involves insertion of catheters into the chambers of the heart or great arteries to allow pressure assessment and size analysis of these chambers.

- When catheters are placed into the left ventricle and aorta, this is called *left heart catheterization* (LHC), whereas when placed in the right ventricles and pulmonary artery it is called *right heart catheterization* (RHC).
- Bedside insertion of a right heart catheter can allow measurement of pulmonary artery pressure, by inserting the Swan–Ganz catheter into the pulmonary artery, inflating the balloon at the tip, and feeding the balloon forward until it wedges into a sub-segmental pulmonary artery. The balloon occludes any forward blood flow, obliterating the pressure from the right ventricle, and can measure the pulmonary capillary wedge pressure (PCWP).

Coronary CT angiography (CTCA, CCTA) and calcium scoring

Coronary computed tomography angiography (CTCA, CCTA) is becoming more readily available, and has a role in identifying the extent of coronary artery disease without the need for invasive catheterization (Figure 7-7). However, the technique does require injection of contrast medium and may be contraindicated in the presence of renal dysfunction or history of previous reaction to X-ray contrast.

Interpretation of the images requires a high level of skill, and limitations include perturbing of the CT image by calcification, and over-interpretation of the severity of narrowing. Nevertheless, CTCA has proven to be of assistance in the urgent assessment of patients with chest pain, and is being increasingly used as an alternative to invasive angiography to detect the presence or absence of coronary atherosclerosis.

Coronary calcification scoring has been shown to be an accurate index of prognosis, adding incremental information to the assessment of coronary risk factors. It is becoming increasingly available and favored as a reliable indication of coronary atherosclerosis and the need for active treatment and further investigation. A patient with a zero calcium score has a negligible risk of heart attack over 10 years, with gradually increasing risk to >20% with a calcium score of >400. Importantly, the risk assessment with calcium scoring has been shown to be incremental to standard methods of risk assessment, when risk factor estimation indicates an intermediate risk.

CLINICAL PEARL

A normal calcium score on CT indicates freedom from coronary disease, and is an excellent indicator of a good medium-term prognosis.

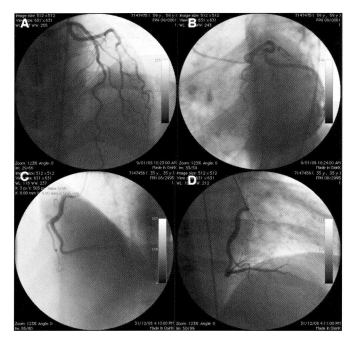

Figure 7-6 Normal coronary arteries. The left coronary artery system as seen on coronary angiography is shown in **A** and **B**. In the right anterior oblique (RAO) view (**A**) the vertebral column is to the left of the cine frame, and in the LAO view (**B**) it is to the right. In both projections, the circumflex artery is adjacent to the vertebral column; the left anterior descending artery reaches the cardiac apex. The right coronary artery system and its branches is shown in **C** and **D**

From Thompson PL (ed), Coronary care manual, 2nd ed. Sydney: Elsevier Australia, 2011.

Magnetic resonance imaging (MRI)

- Cardiac MRI performs both static and dynamic imaging of the heart, allowing precise assessment of structure and of volumes, plus very sensitive analysis of myocardial tissue.
- MRI has the advantage of avoiding the risks of ionising radiation but can interfere with some implanted cardiac devices.
- It is primarily used in the assessment of complex congenital heart disease, infiltrative heart disease, and cardiac tumors or thrombi.
- While it is capable of distinguishing *healthy* from *ischemic* from *scarred* myocardium, the complexity and cost of MRI means that it is not routinely used in the assessment of acute ischemia.
- It can be used for the assessment of myocardial viability in the context of chronic ischemia being assessed for revascularization. The injection of gadolinium-enhanced contrast is of particular use in assessing myocardial scarring, increasingly used to stratify risk in cardiomyopathies.

CLINICAL PEARL

Cardiac MRI has an important role in assessing fibrosis and prognosis in cardiomyopathies.

DYSLIPIDEMIA

The strong relationship between cholesterol levels and cardiovascular outcome has been well known for decades.

- Meta-analysis of *observational studies* has shown that each 1 mmol/L total cholesterol is associated with a higher risk of cardiovascular events: by a half for those aged in their 40s, a third for those in their 50s and a sixth for

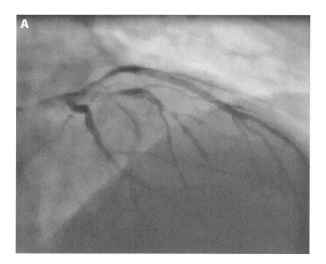
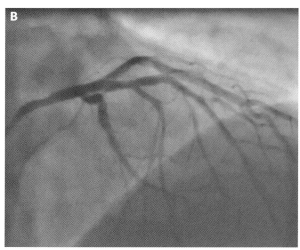

Figure 7-7 (**A**) Coronary angiogram showing severe stenoses in the left anterior descending (LAD) artery, with very poor distal flow in the artery, of a patient with an acute STEMI (ST-elevation myocardial infarction). (**B**) The same patient following balloon angioplasty and stenting of the LAD lesion

Images courtesy of Dr Angela Worthington.

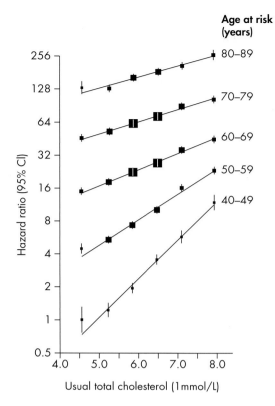

Age at risk (years)

80–89
70–79
60–69
50–59
40–49

Figure 7-8 Ischemic heart disease mortality (33,744 deaths) vs usual total cholesterol; meta-analysis of 61 observational studies. Note that the scale is log–linear, with each mark on the vertical axis indicating a doubling of risk

From Prospective Studies Collaboration, Blood cholesterol and vascular mortality by age, sex, and blood pressure: a meta-analysis of individual data from 61 prospective studies with 55,000 vascular deaths. Lancet 2007;370:1829–39.

those in their 70s and 80s. The relationship is linear, with no apparent threshold for an increase in risk in any level of cholesterol or age group (Figure 7-8).
- Meta-analysis of *clinical trials* has shown that statin therapy can safely reduce the 5-year incidence of major coronary events, coronary revascularization and stroke by, on average, about one-fifth for each mmol/L reduction in low-density lipoprotein (LDL) cholesterol.

CLINICAL PEARL

For each 1 mmol/L of LDL lowering with statin therapy, the risk of coronary events and stroke is reduced by about 20%.

Cholesterol, lipoproteins, apoproteins

- Lipid fractions vary greatly in size and density.
- They are transported by circulating **lipoproteins**.
- The protein structure that carries the lipid is referred to as the **apoprotein**. The apoproteins responsible for

Table 7-8 Circulating lipids and their related apoproteins

CIRCULATING LIPID	MAJOR APOPROTEIN
Chylomicron	B48
Chylomicron remnants	B48, E
VLDL (very-low-density lipoprotein)	B100
IDL (intermediate-density lipoprotein)	B100, E
LDL (low-density lipoprotein)	B100
HDL (high-density lipoprotein)	A-I, A-II
Lipoprotein(a)	B100, (a)

From Miller M et al. Triglycerides and cardiovascular disease: a scientific statement from the American Heart Association. Circulation 2011;123:2292–333.

each of the circulating lipoproteins are summarized in Table 7-8.

CLINICAL PEARL

Atherogenic lipoproteins are carried on ApoB, and antiatherogenic lipoproteins are carried on ApoA. A mnemonic is 'B = Bad, A = AOK'.

Which lipid should be measured?

- **Total cholesterol** predicts coronary risk in large cohorts, but the wide distribution of total cholesterol levels and variations in serial testing make individual risk stratification based on total cholesterol alone unreliable.
  » The total cholesterol level includes low-density lipoprotein (LDL) and high-density lipoprotein (HDL) cholesterol, combining atherogenic and possibly protective fractions.
- **Low-density lipoprotein (LDL) cholesterol**
  » LDL is generally regarded as the atherogenic lipid fraction. It is usually recommended for more accurate risk assessment, and is a valid predictor of coronary risk.
  » Its role in atherogenesis has been confirmed by many trials showing that lowering LDL reduces risk. The measurement of LDL-C most widely used in clinical practice is a derived measurement calculated from the Friedewald equation [LDL cholesterol = total cholesterol − HDL cholesterol − (triglyceride (mmol/L) × 0.45)]. Current recommendations no longer require a fasting sample.

» Direct measurement of the main apolipoprotein of LDL, ApoB100 (usually abbreviated to ApoB), can be a more reliable predictor of risk than indirectly measured LDL cholesterol.

- **Non-HDL cholesterol (= total cholesterol minus HDL cholesterol)** overcomes the difficulty that triglycerides can perturb the derived LDL cholesterol measurement, but despite several guidelines recommending its wider use it is not currently used as a routine replacement for estimating LDL cholesterol.

- **High-density lipoprotein (HDL) cholesterol** is related inversely and independently to risk (i.e. even after adjustment for other risk factors). Multiple studies have confirmed the inverse linear relationship to future coronary risk, including patients taking statins and with low levels of LDL cholesterol.
  » This is widely interpreted as being due to the role of HDLs in reverse cholesterol transportation, but it is increasingly appreciated that HDL cholesterol has relevant antioxidant, anti-inflammatory, and anti-thrombotic properties.
  » Despite its key role in limiting atherogenesis, drugs which significantly elevate HDL cholesterol have been tested in clinical trials and have not shown any clinical benefit. Measurement of the major apolipoprotein of HDL cholesterol, ApoA-I, may offer more specific information.

CLINICAL PEARL

Increased HDL levels are associated with an apparent protective effect, but to date it has not been possible to reduce risk by raising HDL.

- **Triglyceride** measurements correlate with cardiovascular risk, but interpretation of the role of triglycerides is confused because of multiple confounding associated risk factors, especially obesity, and other features of the metabolic syndrome and diabetes.
  » Adjustment for these confounding factors flattens the relationship between triglyceride measurements and cardiovascular disease outcomes.
  » Triglyceride itself is non-atherogenic, but the correlations between risk and triglyceride measurement may reflect atherogenic remnants of chylomicrons and VLDLs.
  » There is evidence that an elevated triglyceride level increases the risk of cardiovascular disease when associated with a low HDL cholesterol level.

Apolipoproteins

- Apolipoprotein B100 (ApoB) is the chief protein in the atherogenic VLDL, IDL and LDL particles.
- Plasma ApoB levels reflect total numbers of atherogenic particles.
- ApoA-I is the major apolipoprotein constituent of the anti-atherogenic HDLs.

- The measurement of the apolioproteins has significant advantages in more accurate prediction; it avoids the need for a fasting sample, but testing is not widely available.

Ratios

- The total cholesterol:HDL cholesterol ratio may offer a more accurate prediction of risk.
- The ratio of ApoB:ApoA-I was an excellent predictor of risk in a large international study, and the use of a non-fasting blood sample in large community studies is an obvious advantage.

CLINICAL PEARL

The ratio of ApoB:ApoA-I is a good predictor of risk and can be used without fasting.

Dyslipidemia and cardiovascular disease (CVD)

It is important to recognize that treatment decisions are not made on the basis of a single measurement of cholesterol or LDLs. The clinical setting and cardiovascular risk level need to be considered carefully. However, the higher the level of LDL cholesterol, the greater the need to institute therapy (Figure 7-9).

'Normolipidemia' in patients with established CVD

- Patients with established CVD are at very high risk of progression of atherosclerosis and future cardiovascular events irrespective of their lipid levels.
- There is convincing evidence from clinical trials that all patients with demonstrated CVD should be treated with a statin.
- The clinical trials which have guided this conclusion have shown that 'the lower the better' is probably correct, with no evidence of a 'safe' baseline level of LDL cholesterol.
- A widely used target level for significant reduction of risk is <1.8 mmol/L (<70 mg/dL), or a 50% reduction in LDL cholesterol when this target cannot be reached.

CLINICAL PEARLS

- All patients with established cardiovascular disease should be on a statin if possible.
- A widely used target for patients with coronary heart disease is to lower LDL cholesterol to <1.8 mmol/L (<70 mg/dL).

'Normolipidemia' in patients with a high risk of CVD

Treatment decisions for patients with a high absolute risk of CVD are made similarly to those with established CVD.
- Those patients with a 5-year absolute risk of CVD events of >10% (based on calculation of risk based on age, gender, cholesterol or LDL level, HDL level, systolic

Total CV risk (SCORE) %	LDL-C levels				
	<70 mg/dL <1.8 mmol/L	70 to <100 mg/dL 1.8 to <2.5 mmol/L	100 to <155 mg/dL 2.5 to <4.0 mmol/L	155 to <190 mg/dL 4.0 to <4.9 mmol/L	>190 mg/dL >4.9 mmol/L
<1	No lipid intervention	No lipid intervention	Lifestyle intervention	Lifestyle intervention	Lifestyle intervention, consider drug if uncontrolled
≥1 to <5	Lifestyle intervention	Lifestyle intervention	Lifestyle intervention, consider drug if uncontrolled	Lifestyle intervention, consider drug if uncontrolled	Lifestyle intervention, consider drug if uncontrolled
>5 to <10, or high risk	Lifestyle intervention, consider drug	Lifestyle intervention, consider drug	Lifestyle intervention, and immediate drug intervention	Lifestyle intervention, and immediate drug intervention	Lifestyle intervention, and immediate drug intervention
≥10 or very high risk	Lifestyle intervention, consider drug	Lifestyle intervention, and immediate drug intervention	Lifestyle intervention, and immediate drug intervention	Lifestyle intervention, and immediate drug intervention	Lifestyle intervention, and immediate drug intervention

Figure 7-9 Lipid treatment in patients with cardiovascular risk

Adapted from Perk et al. The Fifth Joint Task Force of the European Society of Cardiology and Other Societies on Cardiovascular Disease Prevention in Clinical Practice. ESC recommendations for treatment based on LDL. Eur Heart J 2012;33(13):1635–1701.

blood pressure and smoking habit) should be commenced on a statin, especially if they are shown to have confirmatory evidence of high risk such as a high coronary calcium score.

- The target level for high-risk patients is similar to that for patients with established CVD.
- In patients at moderate risk (5–10%), an LDL cholesterol goal of <3.0 mmol/L (less than ~115 mg/dL) should be considered.

CLINICAL PEARL

Patients at high risk (absolute 5- to 10-year risk of CVD event of >10%) should be started on a statin.

Non-CVD patients with fasting LDL >3.5 mmol/L (135 mg/dL)

- The usual causes of elevated LDL at this level are inappropriate dietary habits, polygenic hypercholesterolemia, or mixed dyslipidemia (i.e. elevated LDL with elevated triglyceride/VLDL).
- Initial treatment is with a low-fat diet, and if the LDL level remains high then statin therapy should be started.

Very high LDL cholesterol, >5.0 mmol/L (190 mg/dL)

- In these patients, a genetic disorder such as familial hypercholesterolemia is very likely.
- There may be non-vascular deposition of xanthomas or xanthelasma.
- Family testing to detect affected relatives should be routine in these patients.

Elevated triglycerides

May be caused by:
- obesity and overweight

- physical inactivity
- excess alcohol intake
- high-carbohydrate diet (>60% of energy intake)
- type 2 diabetes
- chronic renal failure
- nephrotic syndrome
- drugs (corticosteroids, estrogens, retinoids, higher doses of beta-blockers)
- genetic dyslipidemias.

Triglyceride level ranges are:
- normal <1.7 mmol/L (<150 mg/dL)
- borderline high 1.7–2.2 mmol/L (150–199 mg/dL)
- high 2.2–5.6 mmol/L (200–499 mg/dL)
- very high >5.6 mmol/L (>500 mg/dL).

CLINICAL PEARL

Markedly elevated triglycerides can often be lowered with cessation of alcohol intake and reduction of carbohydrate intake.

Low HDL cholesterol

- A low HDL cholesterol level is defined as <1.0 mmol/L (<40 mg/dL).
- It may be associated with an elevated triglyceride, due partly to biochemical interactions and partly to laboratory measurement interference.

The common causes are:
- overweight and obesity
- physical inactivity
- type 2 diabetes
- very high carbohydrate intake (>60% energy)
- drugs (some beta-blockers, high doses of diuretics, anabolic steroids, progestational agents).

Lipid-modifying treatments

Diet therapy

All guidelines on lipids encourage adherence to a low-fat diet, regular exercise, and weight reduction. While this advice is sensible and an accepted part of good medical management, the clinical trial evidence shows that the benefits are limited.

> **CLINICAL PEARL**
>
> While the trial evidence for reducing risk with diet is not strong, all patients being considered for statin therapy should have detailed dietary advice.

Statins

- The statins (HMG CoA reductase inhibitors) are the most widely used drugs for lowering LDL cholesterol.
- For each 1 mmol/L reduction in LDL cholesterol due to statin therapy, there is a significant reduction in all-cause mortality and coronary mortality.
- As a result, all guidelines recommend the liberal use of statins, not only in persons with hypercholesterolemia, but also in those with proven or a high risk of vascular disease.

Non-statin therapies

Ezetimibe

Ezetimibe inhibits the reabsorption of cholesterol by the intestine. It is well tolerated, and reduces the concentration of LDL cholesterol by 15–20% when given either as monotherapy or added to a statin. It is available in combination with simvastatin.

At present, ezetimibe remains second-line treatment for the patient who has refractory LDL elevation despite intensive statin therapy, or who has a contraindication to statins. It has been shown to improve outcomes when added to statin therapy in patients with coronary heart disease.

Fibrates

The LDL-lowering effect of fibrates (gemfibrozil, bezafibrate, fenofibrate) is relatively weak, although they have a role in the patient with hypertriglyceridemia and in the patient with the mixed dyslipidemia which accompanies the metabolic syndrome and diabetes.

> **CLINICAL PEARL**
>
> The combination of fibrates with statin therapy has been associated with an increased risk of myopathy, and close monitoring of creatine kinase is mandatory in these patients.

PCSK9 inhibitors

Monoclonal antibodies to PCSK9 (proprotein convertase subtilisin/kexin type 9) can dramatically lower LDL cholesterol, sometimes by as much as 50%. They need to be given by injection and the high cost is a limitation. They have been shown to improve outcomes when combined with statins.

Omega-3 fatty acids

Certain fish oils have high concentrations of omega-3 fatty acids, and are widely promoted for lipid control.

There is some evidence that prognosis in post-coronary patients is improved with consumption of omega-3 fatty acids, but apart from benefit shown in a single trial of a highly purified version, the effects on lipids are modest and the mechanism of the benefit remains unclear.

Lowering triglycerides

The evidence that lowering moderately elevated triglycerides is beneficial is generally lacking.

- Despite this, some guidelines, on the basis of the epidemiological association, suggest that it is reasonable to recommend a triglyceride target of <1.5 mmol/L.
- A markedly elevated triglyceride level is a significant risk factor for pancreatitis, and this itself is an indication for treatment if the triglyceride level consistently exceeds 5 mmol/L despite dietary modification and cessation of alcohol.
- Treatment of marked hypertriglyceridemia is with very-low-fat diets (≤15% of caloric intake), strict avoidance of alcohol, and early institution of an effective triglyceride-lowering drug such as a fibrate or nicotinic acid.

> **CLINICAL PEARL**
>
> Evidence for improved outcomes with all the non-statin therapies is building, but they are usually only needed for lipid control if LDL control cannot be achieved with a statin or if a patient is unable to take a statin.

CORONARY ARTERY DISEASE (CAD)

Prevalence

Coronary heart disease is one of the most common health disorders in modern life, accounting for nearly one-third of all deaths. It may be silent or may manifest as angina, acute coronary syndromes or sudden death. It is already a major cause of disability, and the World Health Organization has estimated that it will be by far the major health burden worldwide within the next two decades.

Pathophysiology

- Coronary artery disease is usually due to atherosclerosis.
- It is now well recognized that the atherosclerotic process is more complex than simple steady accretion of lipid deposits, but the unpredictable clinical course of the patient with CHD is not fully understood.
- In addition to lipid deposition, the processes of cellular infiltration, degenerative and inflammatory changes,

and associated endothelial dysfunction all have the potential for fluctuations in coronary flow.

- Interactions between multiple factors in the plaque, including a large lipid pool, thin cap, inflammatory infiltrate, and mechanical forces explain the fact that atherosclerosis is likely to increase in step-like stages, and the patient who has been stable for months or years may develop an unstable atherosclerotic plaque and progress rapidly to unstable angina, acute coronary syndromes, or sudden death.

STABLE CORONARY ARTERY DISEASE

Investigation

The approach to investigating the patient with suspected CAD with stable, minimal or absent symptoms is directed to assessing the overall cardiovascular (CVD) risk, in particular the identification of the high-risk patient who may benefit from coronary revascularization.

'Screening' asymptomatic outpatients for coronary disease is not necessary in the general population, but is justified in those in certain high-risk occupations.

> ## CLINICAL PEARL
>
> Risk stratification using standard risk factors can identify the absolute risk of cardiovascular events in the next 5–10 years with reasonable accuracy. This assessment should be done before more complex risk markers are considered.

Initial assessment of risk factors

The initial evaluation should assess the patient's risk and the need for further investigation. It includes a detailed history, including family history, physical examination, resting EKG, lipid profile and a marker of dysglycemia. From this, the patient can be categorized into a *low*, *intermediate* or *high* risk of a coronary event in the next 5–10 years.

- The most widely used risk assessment protocols categorize a patient's absolute cardiovascular risk by assessing age, gender, LDL cholesterol, HDL cholesterol, systolic blood pressure, smoking habits, and presence of diabetes or hyperglycemia.
- Other factors include a strong family or racial propensity for premature CHD, and a measure of obesity, particularly the waist circumference or waist:hip ratio.
- An example of a risk calculator (the Australian absolute risk calculator) is shown in Figure 7-10.

Further testing for identifying coronary heart disease is ideally determined by the patient's risk assessment and symptoms. Often the initial assessment is focused on identifying the small proportion of patients who may benefit from revascularization to prolong survival.

The resting EKG is helpful if signs of ischemia such as T wave inversion are identified, but the EKG is normal in the majority of patients with CHD and should never be used to rule out CHD.

Novel risk factors

A large number of alternative risk factors have been considered, but demonstrating their incremental value over the Framingham-derived risk factors has been challenging.

- Lipid subfractions have been evaluated in detail, but apart from Lp(a) they do not add predictive value to the LDL and HDL levels.
- Since the importance of inflammation in the development and destabilization of atherosclerosis has been accepted, the use of high-sensitivity C-reactive protein (hs-CRP) has been studied extensively. Despite extensive evidence that it is a valuable marker of inflammation and by itself indicates an increased risk, it has not been shown to add incremental predictive value to established risk factors. Other markers of inflammation are even less predictive than hs-CRP.
- Homocysteine is a predictive marker in some studies, but does not add incremental value to risk assessment.
- Erectile dysfunction, a sign of arterial endothelial dysfunction, is a risk factor for the development of coronary disease.

> ## CLINICAL PEARL
>
> None of the novel risk factors have been shown to add incremental risk prediction to the standard risk factors; high-sensitivity C-reactive protein is now thought to be less useful than previously thought.

Exercise EKG

- Despite the wide availability of more complex and expensive methods for assessment, the treadmill exercise test remains a very useful, widely used and relatively cost-efficient method of identifying the patient at high risk of having significant CHD.
- The role, limitations and interpretation of the exercise EKG are discussed in detail in the earlier section on investigation of cardiac disease.
- Since the exercise EKG depends on inducing myocardial ischemia, a significant obstructive lesion must be present in the coronary arteries to result in a positive test.
- The exercise EKG is not able to identify the atherosclerotic burden of non-occlusive disease, and in particular cannot recognize an unstable plaque which may be non-occlusive at the time of the test, but it is still capable of initiating an acute coronary event in the future.

Stress imaging studies (radionuclide myocardial perfusion imaging and stress echocardiography)

Stress myocardial perfusion imaging or stress echocardiography may be performed in asymptomatic patients with an

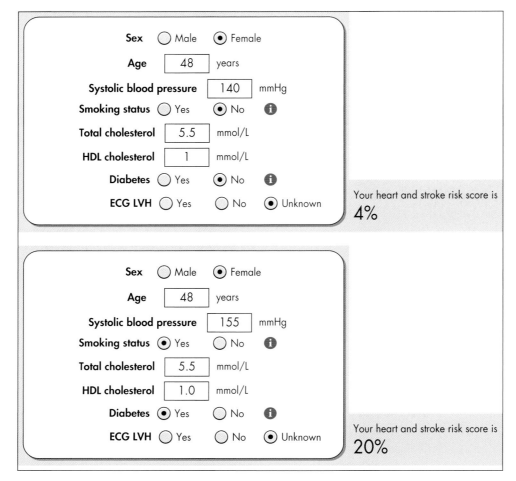

Figure 7-10 Examples of absolute risk assessment, comparing a 48-year-old female with marginal elevation of total cholesterol and normal HDL levels with and without elevated blood pressure, diabetes and smoking. The risk may be underestimated in vulnerable populations (indigenous, strong family history)

Adapted from National Vascular Disease Prevention Alliance. www.cvdcheck.org.au

intermediate risk, or an exercise score suggesting high risk. In patients not capable of exercise, pharmacological testing may be required, using adenosine or dipyridamole myocardial perfusion imaging or dobutamine stress echocardiography. (See the earlier section on investigation of cardiac disease.)

Coronary artery imaging

- Invasive coronary angiography is regarded as the 'gold standard' for the evaluation of the location and extent of coronary artery disease (see the earlier section on investigation of cardiac disease).
- Invasive coronary angiography to identify lesions suitable for revascularization is not essential for patients with a low overall risk who have been shown to have a normal exercise capacity and normal left ventricular function. Indeed, recent studies have failed to show any advantage of revascularization over medical therapy in these patients. However, if revascularization is contemplated, invasive coronary angiography is the modality of choice.

- Newer imaging technologies are being used increasingly for patients with suspected CHD. (See previous section on investigation of cardiac disease.)
- The calcium score on high-speed CT scanning has been shown to add to the Framingham risk assessment.

CLINICAL PEARL

The calcium score has been shown to add incremental value to the standard risk factors. A coronary calcium score of 0 indicates an excellent medium-term prognosis.

- Coronary CT angiography has the advantage that it is able to identify atherosclerotic deposition in the walls of the coronary arteries, and can identify soft (uncalcified) plaque as well as calcified plaque. Its value for establishing the long-term prognosis has not been established, and despite reductions in radiation exposure with modern imaging, there are still concerns about the long-term carcinogenic effect of radiation. Identification of a heavy atherosclerotic load may be an incentive for aggressive management of risk factors, including LDL lowering in a patient with a normal lipid profile.

- Magnetic resonance imaging has the advantage that it can provide additional anatomical detail, but it has not proven to be as effective as CT imaging for coronary imaging, and may be more suitable for monitoring atherosclerotic progression in larger vessels.
- Alternative imaging modalities such as intravascular ultrasound (IVUS) or optical coherence tomography (OCT) have the advantage of identifying intramural atherosclerosis, but the disadvantage that they require an invasive approach.
- Research continues using these modalities to try to identify the *vulnerable plaque* which has a thin fibrous cap and liquid lipid core. These plaques are primarily responsible for acute coronary events when they rupture or erode.

Management to improve prognosis

Risk factor management

- Weight control, regular exercise, tight blood pressure control, and cessation of smoking are mandatory for patients with stable CHD, and an improvement in the risk factor profile is likely to improve prognosis.
- A supervised exercise program improves the quality of life for patients who are prepared to persist.
- Education of the patient to report changes in the pattern of angina is essential, as risk of an acute coronary event is greatly increased when this happens.

CLINICAL PEARL

Tight control of risk factors can significantly improve prognosis and should be the basis of treatment in all patients with coronary heart disease.

Antiplatelet medications

- **Aspirin** (75–150 mg daily) should be used in all patients with coronary heart disease without contraindications.
  - » Meta-analyses have shown that the benefit for patients with known CHD is an absolute benefit of 25 fewer serious vascular events per 1000 patients treated.
  - » There is a small risk of gastrointestinal bleeding from daily aspirin and should not be used in patients at low CVD risk. Although the gastrointestinal side-effects are lower with the lower doses, daily doses below 75 mg have not been shown to be beneficial.
- **Clopidogrel** has a clear role in the patient recovering from an acute coronary syndrome or after implantation of a coronary stent, but in stable patients it delivers marginal benefits on improving cardiovascular prognosis, with an increased risk of bleeding.

CLINICAL PEARL

Low-dose aspirin can reduce vascular events by 25 per 1000 patients treated—one of the most cost-effective treatments in medicine.

- **Newer antiplatelet agents** such as prasugrel and ticagrelor have better efficacy in post-coronary patients, but with increased risks of bleeding.
- Dipyridamole has vasodilatory and antithrombotic effects, but can exacerbate angina and should not be used as an antiplatelet agent in coronary heart disease.

Beta-adrenergic blockers

- On the basis of their potentially beneficial effects on morbidity and mortality when used as secondary prevention in post-infarction patients, beta-blockers should be strongly considered as initial therapy for chronic stable angina, although their role in stable symptom-free patients has not been confirmed in clinical trials.
- $Beta_1$-selective drugs are preferred, and metoprolol and atenolol are the most widely prescribed.
- If significant left ventricular dysfunction is identified, it is preferable to use one of the beta-blockers which have been shown to be effective in cardiac failure (carvedilol, bisoprolol, nebivolol or extended-release metoprolol), commencing at a low dose and titrating to response.

Lipid-lowering agents

A large number of clinical trials have shown that reduction of LDLs with statins can decrease the risk for adverse ischemic events in patients with established coronary artery disease.

- » Meta-analysis of the trials in patients with established CHD has shown that reduction of LDL cholesterol by 2–3 mmol/L with statins reduces risk by about 40–50%.

CLINICAL PEARL

In patients with known CHD, statin therapy can reduce risk by 20% for each 1 mmol/L reduction in LDL cholesterol; the target should be to reduce the LDL level to below 1.8 mmol/L.

- » Evidence from clinical trials suggests that the benefit exists no matter what the baseline LDL level.
- » Each of the statins has been shown to be effective.
- The risks of major adverse events associated with statins are generally low, although myalgias and abnormalities of liver function are common, and usually respond to lowering the dose or cessation.
- Risks with the widespread prescribing of statins for CHD are still being monitored, but to date there is no indication of any increased risk of cancer or other adverse effects.
- Myopathy with an elevation of creatine kinase is an occasional side-effect of statins, and can be severe.

- Concerns about cognitive dysfunction with statins are widespread among patients, but there is no evidence of this from the large number of patients included in clinical trials over the past 20 years.
- Additional LDL lowering agents such as ezetemibe and PCSK9 inhibitors can be considered if target levels of LDL lowering (<1.8mmol/L) are not achieved with statins.

Angiotensin-converting enzyme inhibitors (ACEIs) and other inhibitors of the renin–angiotensin–aldosterone system (RAAS)

The role of ACEIs in improving prognosis in stable CHD patients is unclear.

- Several trials have shown that they may have a vasculoprotective benefit in high-risk patients.
- Angiotensin receptor blockers (ARBs) may be used when the patient is unable to take an ACEI.
- Aldosterone antagonists do not have a role in the asymptomatic normotensive patient who is free of cardiac failure.

Nitrates and calcium-channel blockers

- Nitrates have not been shown to improve outcomes in patients with CAD.
- Immediate-release or short-acting dihydropyridine calcium-channel blockers (nifedipine) increase adverse cardiac events, and should not be used.
- Long-acting or slow-release dihydropyridines may be prescribed for hypertension without increasing the risk.
- Non-dihydropyridines (verapamil, diltiazem) are contraindicated if there is left ventricular dysfunction.

Coronary revascularization

- In stable CHD patients, coronary revascularization with coronary artery bypass surgery (CABG) has been shown to deliver clear-cut prognostic benefits in patients with left main coronary disease or three-vessel disease with significant left ventricular dysfunction. The survival benefits of CABG in other patient groups are less clear.
- Percutaneous coronary intervention (PCI) has not been shown to deliver a prognostic benefit above optimal medical therapy. In patients with multivessel disease or diabetes who are suitable for either CABG or PCI, CABG delivers a better long-term prognosis but with a higher peri-procedural risk of stroke.

Management of symptoms in the CHD patient

Beta-adrenergic blockers

In patients experiencing angina, beta-blockers relieve symptoms by lowering the heart rate with possibly an effect on blood pressure and myocardial oxygen consumption.

- The anti-anginal effect closely correlates with the effect on lowering the heart rate at rest, and especially on exercise.
- Occasionally, patients with conduction system disease may develop high grades of atrioventricular (AV) block.

This usually responds to cessation of the beta-blocker, but may indicate the need for a pacemaker.

- Other side-effects include lethargy, reduced exercise capacity due to the slow heart rate, cold peripheries, and possible mild effects on raising of blood glucose and LDL levels.

CLINICAL PEARL

Left ventricular dysfunction is no longer considered a contraindication to beta-blockers, but caution is required at commencement to avoid bradycardia and hypotension.

Calcium-channel blockers

All calcium-channel blockers have mild coronary vasodilating effects, and can be used for symptomatic relief when beta-blockers are contraindicated, but verapamil and diltiazem should be avoided when there is associated left ventricular dysfunction.

Nitrates

- Nitrates such as glyceryl trinitrate (GTN, nitroglycerin) and isosorbide mono- and dinitrates are donors of nitric oxide (NO), the potent endothelial-derived vasodilator. The anti-ischemic effect results from reduced venous return and cardiac work, and a direct coronary vasodilating effect.
- Nitroglycerin/GTN can be taken for symptoms of angina by sublingual tablets or spray.
  - » The sublingual tablets need constant renewal as they are subject to sublimation with loss of the active ingredient over 3–4 months, especially with an open bottle or a plastic container and in bright light. The spray formulation lasts longer.
  - » Nitroglycerin/GTN should be taken immediately at the onset of angina. Relief of angina usually occurs within 30 seconds but can be accompanied by a headache.
  - » The anti-anginal effect is quite short-lived, lasting about 15 minutes.
- Nitroglycerin patches can elute GTN over 12–24 hours. The effect of isosorbide dinitrate lasts about 30 minutes, and extended-release isosorbide mononitrate (ISMN) in a dose of 30–120 mg/day has a longer duration of action—up to 12 hours or longer.
  - » All long-acting nitrates are susceptible to the induction of nitrate tolerance, with a progressive loss of the beneficial effect after 24 hours of continuous therapy. Therefore, nitroglycerin patches or ISMN must be interspersed with 'nitrate-free' periods of 10–12 hours per day.
- There is cross-tolerance between nitrates and agents with nitrate moieties such as nicorandil (see below).
- Patients should be warned that nitrates interact with cyclic GMP phosphodiesterase, and co-administration with sildenafil, vardenafil or tadalafil can result in severe hypotension.

CLINICAL PEARL

Treatment with all long-acting nitrates needs to include a nitrate-free interval of 10–12 hours in each 24-hour period.

Novel anti-anginal agents

- **Ranolazine** may reduce myocardial ischemia and angina by inhibition of the late inward sodium channel (late I_{Na}), which remains open in myocardial ischemia, and can achieve an improvement in myocardial blood flow without effects on heart rate or blood pressure. The usual oral dose is 750–1000 mg twice a day either as monotherapy or in combination with beta-adrenergic blockers, calcium-channel blockers or nitrates.
- **Nicorandil** has dual effects as an ATP-dependent potassium channel (K_{ATP}) opener with a nitrate moiety. Opening of the K_{ATP} reduces the Ca^{2+} overload associated with myocardial ischemia, as well as dilating peripheral and coronary resistance arterioles, and the nitric oxide donor action has a coronary vasodilating effect.
  - » It has been shown to reduce CHF death, non-fatal myocardial infarction, and hospital admission for angina.
  - » The dose is 10–20 mg twice daily.
- **Ivabradine** is a member of a class of selective heart-rate-lowering agents that act specifically on the sinoatrial (SA) node.
  - » It selectively inhibits the I_f, a primary SA node pacemaker current, reducing the heart rate at rest and during exercise. By this mechanism, it has been shown to be effective in reducing angina, particularly when other therapies are ineffective.
  - » It has also been shown to be effective in improving outcomes in patients with left ventricular dysfunction, particularly in patients with heart rates of 70 beats/min or more.
  - » The usual dose is 5 mg twice daily.

Coronary revascularization

In many patients in modern practice, early revascularization with percutaneous coronary intervention (PCI) or coronary artery bypass surgery (CABG) can be considered a first option for patients with angina. This can deliver immediate relief of symptoms and improved quality of life.

- The choice of revascularization technique may be determined by the coronary anatomy, patient preference, or comorbidities.
- In patients who are not initially suitable for revascularization, medical therapy may need to be maximized and then the patient reconsidered for revascularization in light of the response.
- Patients with single-vessel disease are best managed with PCI.
- Multiple-vessel disease or left main disease has been usually treated with CABG until recently, when advances in technology have allowed multiple lesions to be tackled with PCI.

CLINICAL PEARL

Multi-vessel and left main coronary disease can now be managed with PCI, but long-term outcomes are better with CABG, with reduced need for repeat procedures.

Management of refractory angina

- In patients with apparently refractory angina symptoms who are unsuitable for revascularization, a check on adherence to medications can be revealing.
  - » Errors in use of nitroglycerin/GTN and long-acting nitrates are common.
  - » A persistently high heart rate may reveal lack of adherence or misunderstanding about the dose of beta-blocker or, alternatively, undiagnosed hyperthyroidism or tachyarrhythmia.
- Adjusting the timing of nitrate administration to the period of the day when the symptoms are occurring is essential—long-acting nitrates cannot be possibly effective during the day if the angina occurs at night during the nitrate-free period.
- Encouraging the patient to use nitroglycerin/GTN spray or sublingual tablets before undertaking exercise or physical or emotional stress can help limit the frequency of distressing angina.
- Other, less common causes of persistent angina include unrecognized anemia, undiagnosed hypertrophic cardiomyopathy, severe aortic valve disease, or pulmonary hypertension.

CLINICAL PEARL

Most patients with angina can have their symptoms managed with medical therapy; failure to respond to maximal anti-anginal therapy should prompt a re-examination of the diagnosis.

- Undiagnosed cardiac failure may also cause refractory angina, and empirical treatment with a diuretic may help.
- Careful review of the patient history to ensure that the 'angina' is not arising from the chest wall, or the gastrointestinal tract, or anxiety, may be needed.
- Palliative measures with spinal cord stimulation or narcotics for pain management are rarely needed.

ACUTE CORONARY SYNDROMES

Terminology

The patient who presents with new-onset or worsening chest pain typical of myocardial ischemia is best treated

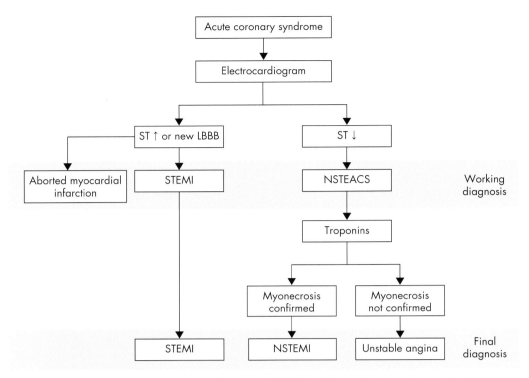

Figure 7-11 Classification of acute coronary syndromes. LBBB, left bundle branch block; NSTEACS, non-ST-elevation acute coronary syndrome; NSTEMI, non-ST-elevation myocardial infarction; STEMI, ST-elevation myocardial infarction

Adapted from White HD and Chew DP. Acute myocardial infarction. Lancet 2008;372:570–84.

as having an acute coronary syndrome until proven otherwise.

The terminology of the acute coronary syndromes is summarized in Figure 7-11. The diagnosis and subsequent categorization demands not only a brief history, but also a 12-lead EKG and a tropinin level.

- The initial working diagnosis depends on the findings on the EKG. If there is ST-segment elevation or new left bundle branch block, the patient is categorized as having an ST-elevation myocardial infarction (STEMI), which may revert to an aborted myocardial infarction after treatment.

- If the ST segments are not elevated, the patient is categorized as having a non-ST-elevation acute coronary syndrome (NSTEACS).

- Following further evaluation with troponin levels at 6 hours (normal troponin) or 3–4 hours (high-sensitivity troponin), the patient is then further categorized as having had a non-ST-elevation myocardial infarction (NSTEMI), or unstable angina.

- The rationale for the terms STEMI and NSTEACS is that these syndromes can be distinguished from each other using the initial EKG. They have different pathophysiology and require different treatments.

The definition of myocardial infarction has changed as increasingly sensitive biochemical markers for the identification of myocardial necrosis have become available (see Box 7-1).

CLINICAL PEARL

An elevated troponin level in a patient with chest pain should be assumed to indicate myocardial necrosis.

Pathophysiology of acute coronary syndromes

- It is now widely accepted that the cause of acute coronary syndromes in atherosclerotic CAD is rupture of an advanced atherosclerotic lesion with superimposed thrombus.
  - » The acceptance of the link between ruptured coronary plaque and coronary thrombosis has led to the concept of the *vulnerable plaque*, which has a large lipid pool, a thin cap separating the atheromatous material from the lumen, inflammatory infiltration, activation of matrix metalloproteinases, and reduced expression of collagen.
  - » Rupture or erosion of the plaque usually occurs at the surface of the eroded or thinned cap, or at the site of maximum strain at the junction with the vessel wall.

Box 7-1

Definition of acute myocardial infarction

The following are key points to remember from this Expert Consensus Document on the Fourth Universal Definition of Myocardial Infarction (MI):

1. The current (fourth) Universal Definition of MI Expert Consensus Document updates the definition of MI to accommodate the increased use of high-sensitivity cardiac troponin (hs-cTn).

2. Detection of an elevated cTn value above the 99th percentile upper reference limit (URL) is defined as myocardial injury. The injury is considered acute if there is a rise and/or fall of cTn values.

3. The criteria for **type 1 MI** include detection of a rise and/or fall of cTn with at least one value above the 99th percentile and with at least one of the following:
   a. Symptoms of acute myocardial ischemia;
   b. New ischemic electrocardiographic (ECG) changes;
   c. Development of pathological Q waves;
   d. Imaging evidence of new loss of viable myocardium or new regional wall motion abnormality in a pattern consistent with an ischemic etiology;
   e. Identification of a coronary thrombus by angiography including intracoronary imaging or by autopsy.

4. The criteria for **type 2 MI** include detection of a rise and/or fall of cTn with at least one value above the 99th percentile and evidence of an imbalance between myocardial oxygen supply and demand unrelated to coronary thrombosis, requiring at least one of the following:
   a. Symptoms of acute myocardial ischemia;
   b. New ischemic ECG changes;
   c. Development of pathological Q waves;
   d. Imaging evidence of new loss of viable myocardium, or new regional wall motion abnormality in a pattern consistent with an ischemic etiology.

5. Cardiac procedural myocardial injury is arbitrarily defined by increases of cTn values (>99th percentile URL) in patients with normal baseline values (≤99th percentile URL) or a rise of cTn values >20% of the baseline value when it is above the 99th percentile, but it is stable or falling.

6. Coronary intervention-related MI is arbitrarily defined by elevation of cTn values **>5** times the 99th percentile URL in patients with normal baseline values. In patients with elevated pre-procedure cTn in whom the cTn levels are stable (≤20% variation) or falling, the post-procedure cTn must rise by >20%. However, the absolute post-procedural value must still be at least five times the 99th percentile URL. In addition, one of the following elements is required:
   a. New ischemic ECG changes;
   b. Development of new pathological Q waves;
   c. Angiographic findings consistent with a procedural flow-limiting complication such as coronary dissection, occlusion of a major epicardial artery or a side branch occlusion/thrombus, disruption of collateral flow or distal embolization.

7. Coronary artery bypass grafting (CABG)-related MI is arbitrarily defined as elevation of cTn values **>10** times the 99th percentile URL in patients with normal baseline cTn values. In patients with elevated pre-procedure cTn in whom cTn levels are stable (≤20% variation) or falling, the post-procedure cTn must rise by >20%. However, the absolute post-procedural value still must be >10 times the 99th percentile URL. In addition, one of the following elements is required:
   a. Development of new pathological Q waves;
   b. Angiographic documented new graft occlusion or new native coronary artery occlusion;
   c. Imaging evidence of new loss of viable myocardium or new regional wall motion abnormality in a pattern consistent with an ischemic etiology.

8. It is increasingly recognized that there is a group of MI patients with no angiographic obstructive coronary artery disease (≥50% diameter stenosis in a major epicardial vessel), and the term 'myocardial infarction with non-obstructive coronary arteries (MINOCA)' has been coined for this entity.

9. Patients may have elevated cTn values and marked decreases in ejection fraction due to sepsis caused by endotoxin, with myocardial function recovering completely with normal ejection fraction once the sepsis is treated.

10. Arriving at a diagnosis of MI using the criteria set forth in this document requires integration of clinical findings, patterns on the ECG, laboratory data, observations from imaging procedures, and on occasion pathological findings, all viewed in the context of the time horizon over which the suspected event unfolds.

From Thygesen K, Alpert JS, Jaffe AS, et al, on behalf of the Joint European Society of Cardiology (ESC)/American College of Cardiology (ACC)/American Heart Association (AHA)/World Heart Federation (WHF) Task Force for the Universal Definition of Myocardial Infarction. Fourth Universal Definition of Myocardial Infarction (2018). J Am Coll Cardiol 2018;72(18). DOI: 10.1016/j.jacc.2018.08.1038.

» Exposure of thrombogenic atherosclerotic material in the ruptured or fissured unstable plaque initiates thrombus.
- The initially formed thrombus may fragment, leading to a variable clinical course.
- Accumulation of platelets over a ruptured site can lead to further growth of the thrombus and further impairment of flow, leading to further stenosis and thrombotic occlusion.
- Limiting the formation of thrombus in the coronary artery is a major target of modern therapy of acute coronary syndromes.
  » The effects on the myocardium from the reduction in blood flow are immediate, starting with reduced contractility.
- Cardiac arrhythmias can occur in this early stage and ventricular fibrillation, the most common cause of sudden cardiac death, may occur.
- If coronary occlusion with total myocardial ischemia persists, myocardial necrosis is inevitable.
  » Necrosis generally begins after 30–45 minutes of total ischemia, and is complete after 4–6 hours.
  » If reperfusion occurs in time to limit the amount of necrosis, the size and morphology of the infarct can be modified. Therefore, early reperfusion after coronary occlusion is a major aim of the modern treatment of STEMI.

Management of STEMI

The aim of treatment in STEMI is to achieve successful reperfusion of the totally occluded coronary artery with fibrinolytic therapy or PCI as soon as possible.

- While comparative randomized clinical trials have shown a clear superiority of PCI over fibrinolysis, due to the more certain achievement of successful reperfusion (98% in PCI versus 65% in fibrinolysis), the choice of reperfusion modality in a particular case depends on the timing of presentation and the facilities available.
- If coronary reperfusion with PCI cannot be achieved within 90 minutes after presentation by a team experienced in emergency PCI, fibrinolytic therapy is recommended to attempt early reperfusion, albeit with a lower rate of successful reperfusion. The basis for this recommendation is shown in Figure 7-12.
- Several agents are available for fibrinolysis, including streptokinase, alteplase (r-TPA), reteplase, and tenecteplase. Of these, the single-bolus administration of tenecteplase offers clear advantages.

CLINICAL PEARL

In STEMI, primary PCI is superior to fibrinolytic therapy when it can be achieved in 90 minutes from presentation; otherwise reperfusion should be started with lytic therapy.

- In hospitals offering PCI, all obstacles to delaying the door to balloon time (i.e. the time from presentation at the emergency department to successful reperfusion in the cardiac catheterization laboratory) should be removed by encouraging direct transfer to the catheter laboratory.

The choice of PCI modality depends on the clinical situation.

- It is possible to achieve excellent results with a drug-eluting stent (DES) as well as a bare metal stent (BMS).

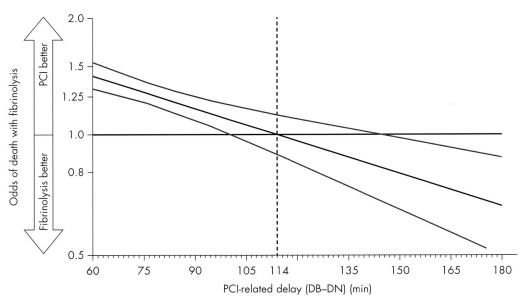

Figure 7-12 Declining superiority of percutaneous coronary intervention (PCI) with hospital delays. This study showed the benefits crossing at 114 minutes after presentation of patient to hospital and thereafter fibrinolysis achieved better outcomes. DB, door to ballon for PCI; DN, door to needle for fibrinolysis

From Pinto DS et al. Coronary heart disease hospital delays in reperfusion for ST-elevation myocardial infarction. Implications when selecting a reperfusion strategy. Circulation 2006;114:2019–25.

The risk of re-stenosis will be reduced with the use of a DES.

- Extraction of thrombus from the artery with a suction catheter is sometimes performed when there is a large burden of thrombus. However, it has not been shown to improve outcomes.
- There is still debate about whether other significant but non-occlusive lesions should be treated during the primary angioplasty procedure.

CLINICAL PEARL

Despite the urgency of the need to achieve early reperfusion, the patient's clinical situation needs to be considered particularly the risk of bleeding from lytic therapy or from antiplatelet therapy if PCI is the primary treatment.

Complications of STEMI

- If the period of total myocardial ischemia is prolonged, myocardial necrosis progresses. With extensive infarction of more than 40% of the left ventricle, cardiac failure and cardiogenic shock may occur.
  » The severity of myocardial infarction and pump failure are often graded according to the Killip classification, with an increase in case fatality from <5% in Killip class I (no signs of left ventricular dysfunction), to 30–40% for classes II (clinical or radiological signs of pulmonary congestion) and III (severe pulmonary edema), and over 80% in class IV (established cardiogenic shock without reperfusion).
  » Cardiogenic shock and severe cardiac failure as a complication of STEMI have declined with wide use of early reperfusion.
- Mechanical complications including rupture of the free wall, development of a ventricular septal defect (VSD) from rupture of the interventricular septum, and severe mitral regurgitation from rupture of a papillary muscle have also declined, but are still seen.
  » Intra-aortic balloon pumping and inotropic therapy have limited benefits on improving outcomes.

CLINICAL PEARL

Sudden development of a harsh systolic murmur may be due to severe mitral regurgitation from papillary muscle rupture or to development of a ventricular septal defect; urgent echocardiography can distinguish the two.

- Other complications of STEMI include ventricular arrhythmias, including ventricular fibrillation and ventricular tachycardia, atrial arrhythmias, and conduction disturbances.
- Apical thrombus with the potential for stroke may occur in the ventricle damaged by infarction or aneurysm.
- In the early days post-STEMI, inflammation of the epicardial surface may produce pericardial pain and a pericardial rub.
- Right ventricular infarction may occur in patients with large inferior infarction due to occlusion of the right coronary artery.

- » Subsequent to the initial injury, the infarcted tissue and the non-infarcted residual myocardium undergo a remodeling process in which the ventricular wall becomes thinner and the infarct zone lengthens.
  » Late adverse remodeling can result in dilatation of the left ventricle or localized ventricular aneurysm formation with late arrhythmias and cardiac failure. ACEIs have been shown to limit the extent of adverse remodeling.
- Dressler's syndrome is a late form of pericardial inflammation with marked elevation of inflammatory indices. It is treated with anti-inflammatory drugs, usually non-steroidal, but occasionally corticosteroids are needed.

Management of NSTEACS/NSTEMI

In NSTEACS/NSTEMI, the pathophysiology differs from STEMI and demands a different management approach.

- While the initiating event of plaque rupture is common to both STEMI and NSTEMI, in the patient presenting with a NSTEACS it is likely that the coronary occlusion will be incomplete, and the likelihood of extensive myocardial necrosis is less.
- The major aim of treatment is to ensure that the patient does not progress to total occlusion of the coronary artery. Antithrombotic therapy is therefore essential.
- Surprisingly, fibrinolysis has been shown to be ineffective or even harmful, possibly because of enhancement of thrombin activity.

CLINICAL PEARL

Counter-intuitively, fibrinolysis is not beneficial and may be harmful in NSTEACS. Other antithrombotic (antiplatelet, antithrombin) treatments are beneficial.

- The role of invasive therapy for NSTEACS has been clarified in recent years. There is now clear evidence that early coronary angiography and progression to coronary revascularization if appropriate is superior to medical management.
  » Angiography and PCI or CABG (if needed) are best done during the initial hospital admission, but there is not the same urgency as in STEMI as extensive necrosis is not occurring.
  » Patients with elevated biomarkers, persistent symptoms, variable EKG changes, and hemodynamic instability should be regarded as high risk and undergo coronary angiography as soon as possible after hospital admission.
  » Patients without these features are at lower risk and can be managed conservatively, but should be investigated further with exercise testing or stress echocardiography.
- Recent studies have shown that CT imaging of the coronary arteries may be a valuable method of distinguishing low- from high-risk patients in the emergency department.

Pharmacological therapy in acute coronary syndromes

All patients experiencing an acute coronary syndrome should receive the combination of drugs which have been shown in clinical trials to improve outcomes. These are described below.

Aspirin

In patients not already taking aspirin, treatment should commence with 300 mg followed by 100–150 mg per day. This has been shown in large clinical trials to improve short- and long-term outcomes by 20–30%.

Other antiplatelet agents

- Clopidogrel has been shown to have a benefit in patients with acute coronary syndromes. For patients likely to undergo PCI, a loading dose is required to ensure platelet inactivation. 300 mg has been standard therapy, but with increasing recognition of genetic variations in clopidogrel responsiveness, 600 mg is increasingly used.
- Prasugrel (60 mg loading dose and 10 mg daily maintenance) has been shown to be more effective than clopidogrel in patients in whom the coronary anatomy is known, without the genetic variation in response but at a higher risk of bleeding (prasugrel is no longer available on the PBS in Australia).
- Ticagrelor (90mg bd dropping to 60mg bd after 12 months) has been shown to be superior to clopidogrel and can be given in the early stages of an acute coronary syndrome before the coronary anatomy is known. It also has a higher risk of bleeding than clopidogrel.
- Dual antiplatelet therapy (aspirin with ticagrelor, prasugrel or clopidogrel) should be continued for 12 months, although the major effect is in the first 3 months, and may need to be stopped early if there is a high bleeding risk. Aspirin should be continued after the dual antiplatelet therapy has ceased.

Heparin/enoxaparin

- There is strong supportive evidence for the widespread routine use of heparin in acute coronary syndromes.
  - » Intravenous (IV) unfractionated heparin (UFH) can be given and has the advantage that it can be withheld if needed, but requires monitoring of the effect with the activated partial thromboplastin time (APTT). The ideal APTT in acute coronary syndromes has been shown to be 60–80 seconds.
- Subcutaneous enoxaparin 1 mg/kg twice daily has been shown to be equally effective and gives a more potent and consistent antithrombin effect, but may increase the risk of bleeding from invasive procedures.

CLINICAL PEARL

Switching from unfractionated heparin to enoxaparin or vice versa should be avoided because of an increased risk of bleeding.

- Many cardiac catheterization laboratories prefer to maintain IV heparin in patients who are going to the laboratory for catheterization or PCI, and there is increasing uptake of the radial approach to minimize bleeding from the groin which may occur with the femoral approach.

Beta-adrenergic blockers

- Beta-blockers given orally have been shown to improve outcomes in patients with myocardial infarction, and by extrapolation are often recommended for all patients with CHD although the evidence for this is questionable when effective coronary reperfusion has occurred.
- IV beta-blockers may have a role in patients with persistent tachycardia or hypertension, but have been shown to have adverse effects in patients who are hypotensive.
- Metoprolol and atenolol are the most widely used beta-blockers in this clinical situation.

Statins

Early administration of high-dose statins has been shown to improve outcomes. The statin shown in clinical trials to be effective is atorvastatin, given in a dose of 80 mg/day.

CLINICAL PEARL

Aspirin, beta-blockers and statins should be commenced as early as possible for all patients with STEMI or NSTEACS.

Angiotensin-converting enzyme inhibitors (ACEIs)

ACEIs may have some anti-atherosclerotic effect, but their main benefit is in patients with known left ventricular dysfunction. If ACE inhibitors are contraindicated, an angiotensin receptor blocker (ARB) can be substituted.

Nitrates

- In patients with persistent angina pain or other evidence of ongoing ischemia, intravenously infused GTN is used to reduce the frequency of ischemic episodes.
- Nitrates can also be effective in pulmonary edema, because of their venodilating effects.
- They do not have a role in routine post-coronary management.

VALVULAR HEART DISEASE

Valve disease may be of no consequence when mild, but can cause severe symptoms and adversely affect prognosis when severe.

Table 7-9 Summary of the typical murmurs of valvular heart disease

CAUSE	TYPICAL PRESENTATION
Mitral stenosis	Mid-diastolic rumble heard best at the apex with the bell or low-frequency diaphragm of the stethoscope; the longer the murmur, the more severe the stenosis
Mitral regurgitation	Usually pansystolic (holosystolic) and heard best at the cardiac apex with radiation to the axilla Murmurs of mitral valve prolapse may be mid-systolic or late systolic, and are occasionally heard better at the left sternal border than the apex
Aortic stenosis	Harsh, mid-pitch crescendo/decrescendo murmur at the left sternal border with radiation to the neck; can be loud enough to be heard at the apex
Aortic regurgitation	Early diastolic murmur heard best at the left sternal border; may require expiration or leaning forward to hear clearly; the length, not the loudness, indicates the severity of the regurgitation
Pulmonary stenosis	Soft blowing murmur heard to the left of the sternum
Pulmonary regurgitation	Short early-diastolic murmur; distinguished from aortic regurgitation because other features of right heart overload may be present
Tricuspid stenosis	Similar to mitral stenosis, but features of right heart failure are very obvious
Tricuspid regurgitation	Blowing murmur at lower left or right sternal border; increases with inspiration

The typical murmurs of valvular heart disease are summarized in Table 7-9.

MITRAL VALVE DISEASE

Mitral stenosis (MS)

The incidence of MS has declined in recent decades, but remains an important cause of disability, particularly in developing countries and low socioeconomic groups susceptible to rheumatic fever.

Etiology and pathogenesis

- Rheumatic fever is the leading cause of MS.
  - » Post-rheumatic valvular heart disease results in predominant MS in about 40% of cases, with involvement of the aortic and tricuspid valves in the remainder.
- Rarer causes include congenital MS, and encroachment onto the mitral valve orifice from mitral valvular calcification.

CLINICAL PEARL

Rheumatic heart disease is the most common cause of mitral stenosis; it is seen less commonly in developed countries.

- In rheumatic MS, progressive fibrosis and calcification of the valve leaflets leads to narrowing of the valve orifice.
  - » With further progression, involvement of the valve commissures and chordae disrupts valve function, leading to obstruction of blood flow from the left atrium to the left ventricle.
  - » Subsequent dilatation of the left atrium can predispose to development of atrial fibrillation, and thrombus formation within the left atrial appendage.
  - » On occasions, a hugely dilated left atrium can impinge on thoracic structures including the left recurrent laryngeal nerve, with dysphonia.
- Increasing left atrial pressure results in pulmonary congestion with dyspnea and reduced exercise capacity. Pulmonary hypertension may result from reactive pulmonary vascular changes, further worsening dyspnea.

Symptoms

- Sudden changes in cardiac workload or heart rate, as in pregnancy, fever and thyrotoxicosis, can bring on symptoms of MS suddenly.
- The development of atrial fibrillation can suddenly exacerbate the symptoms and lead to a rapid decline in the clinical course of a patient with MS. Sometimes a cardioembolic stroke can be the first manifestation of MS.

CLINICAL PEARL

There is usually a latent period of several decades from development of rheumatic mitral stenosis to onset of symptoms, with many patients experiencing the onset in their 40s.

Clinical signs

- A malar flush with erythema and a tendency to cyanosis over the cheeks and nose (mitral facies) is a 'classical' feature only seen in patients with severe MS.
- On auscultation, the 1st heart sound (S_1) may be prominent. The pulmonic component of the 2nd heart sound (P_2) may be accentuated if pulmonary hypertension has developed. An opening snap can be heard if the valve leaflets have not become heavily calcified and immobile.
- The typical auscultatory finding of MS is a low-pitched, rumbling, diastolic murmur, heard best at the apex with the patient in the left lateral recumbent position. Generally, the longer the murmur, the more severe the MS. In patients in sinus rhythm, the murmur may become louder with atrial systole, resulting in presystolic

accentuation of the diastolic rumble. This feature is not present in patients with atrial fibrillation.

- Clinical signs of right ventricular overload and tricuspid regurgitation may be present, with hepatomegaly, ankle edema, ascites, and pleural effusion.

CLINICAL PEARL

In mitral stenosis, the longer the murmur, the more severe the stenosis.

Investigations

- In sinus rhythm, the EKG may show features of left atrial enlargement with notching and bifid appearance, best seen in lead II. A large negative terminal component of the P wave in lead V_1 may be a confirmatory finding of left atrial enlargement. With pulmonary hypertension, right-axis deviation and right ventricular (RV) hypertrophy may be present.
- The chest X-ray may show evidence of left atrial enlargement with filling in of the gap between the aorta and left ventricle, and straightening of the upper left border of the cardiac silhouette. Evidence of pulmonary congestion may be present.
- Mitral stenosis is well visualized on echocardiography in the long-axis left parasternal views, with thickening of the leaflets, and reduced motion and doming of the leaflets during ventricular filling. The left parasternal short-axis views can visualize and measure the mitral orifice by planimetry.
- The severity of the MS is calculated from the mitral valve orifice area and transvalvular peak and mean gradients. The mean gradient is the more reliable index of severity in MS.
- Transesophageal echocardiography (TEE) is used to obtain more detail on the valve anatomy and function, to assess suitability for mitral balloon valvuloplasty, and to assess the presence of left atrial appendage thrombus.

Differential diagnosis

- A large atrial septal defect (ASD) may be associated with RV enlargement; however, the absence of radiographic evidence of pulmonary congestion, the presence of a systolic murmur over the pulmonary artery, and fixed splitting of the 2nd sound are more indicative of ASD.
- Rarely, a left atrial myxoma may obstruct the mitral valve orifice and mimic the clinical signs of MS; however, myxoma can be identified from its characteristic echocardiographic appearance.

CLINICAL PEARL

The Austin Flint murmur with severe aortic regurgitation can be confused with the murmur of mitral stenosis, but these patients have other obvious signs of aortic regurgitation.

Management

- Many patients with MS can be managed with regular clinical and echocardiographic review.
- Patients with MS frequently adjust their activity downward with the gradual progression of their symptoms, and may need to be pressed to identify a decline in physical capacity.
- The role of anticoagulants for patients in sinus rhythm is controversial. Patients with large left atrial size and spontaneous echo contrast may be at risk of thromboembolism while in sinus rhythm.

CLINICAL PEARLS

- Intervention for mitral stenosis (MS) is recommended when there are symptoms, and severe MS with valve area of <1.5 cm^2.
- Mitral balloon valvuloplasty is the preferred intervention for MS but is not suitable when there is significant mitral regurgitation.

- The timing of intervention depends on assessing symptoms and echocardiographic progression.
- Successful valvuloplasty can halve the mean gradient and double the valve area, accompanied by significant improvements in symptoms.
- Patients with extensive chordal involvement, significant mitral regurgitation, and left atrial thrombus are not considered ideal for valvuloplasty, and will need open (surgical) mitral valvuloplasty. Surgery can clear extensive calcification and improve valve function by freeing the scarred chordate and papillary muscles. Attempts are made to preserve the subvalvular mitral valve apparatus.
- In patients with atrial fibrillation, mitral valve surgery is often accompanied by a maze procedure (surgical ablation with multiple linear lesions on the atrial endocardium) to reduce the risk of atrial fibrillation, and oversewing of the left atrial appendage to reduce the risk of thromboembolic complications.

Mitral regurgitation (MR)

While mitral stenosis is usually a result of rheumatic fever with a predictable clinical course, MR has multiple causes and, because of the complex structure and function of the mitral valve, may have a variable course.

Etiology and pathogenesis

MR can result from disruption of any component of the mitral valve apparatus—mitral valve leaflets, annulus, chordae tendineae, papillary muscles, or subjacent myocardium.

- Acute MR can result from papillary muscle dysfunction or rupture in myocardial infarction, chordal rupture in myxomatous degenerative mitral valve disease, or valve destruction in endocarditis. Transient papillary muscle dysfunction may occur from papillary muscle dysfunction in myocardial ischemia.
- Chronic MR usually results from mitral valve prolapse (MVP) in younger patients, and ischemic heart

disease or extensive mitral annular calcification in older patients.

- » MVP is due to myxomatous degeneration of the mitral valve leaflets, with progressive lengthening of the mitral chordae.
- » Chronic MR in ischemic heart disease may be due to localized scarring of the papillary muscles or myocardium controlling the papillary muscles, or to generalized ischemia with functional MR as the mitral valve annulus becomes dilated with left ventricular (LV) dilatation and dysfunction. Other causes of myocardial dilatation such as cardiomyopathies have a similar effect.
- » Mitral annular calcification is an aging process exacerbated by renal dysfunction or diabetes.
- Rheumatic mitral disease, less common now than previously, results in scarring and deformity of the mitral valve leaflets and chordae.
- Dynamic, variable MR can occur in hypertrophic cardiomyopathy when there is involvement of the LV outflow tract, and results from systolic anterior motion of the anterior mitral valve leaflet into the high-velocity jet in the narrowed LV outflow tract; it varies in severity with heart rate and hemodynamic loading conditions.
- Congenital MR can occur with a cleft anterior mitral valve leaflet in ostium primum atrial septal defect.

Irrespective of the cause of the MR, the progressive enlargement of the left ventricle that accompanies MR can exacerbate the degree of regurgitation.

Symptoms

- Acute MR may present with rapid onset of dyspnea or acute pulmonary edema.
- Chronic MR may be asymptomatic for years if mild to moderate.
- Chronic, severe MR may cause fatigue, exertional dyspnea, and orthopnea. Palpitations are common and may be due to atrial ectopic beats or may indicate the onset of atrial fibrillation.
- On occasions, the presentation may be with symptoms of right heart failure with abdominal bloating due to hepatic congestion and ascites, and with peripheral edema.

Clinical signs

- The typical clinical feature of MR is a loud, harsh systolic murmur heard best at the cardiac apex. Auscultation in the left lateral decubitus position may help to clarify the features of the murmur.
- Multiple variants on the classic pansystolic (holosystolic) murmur may occur depending on the mechanism of the MR and the direction of the regurgitant jet. In patients with MVP, the murmur may be initiated with a mid-systolic click, followed by a late systolic murmur.

CLINICAL PEARL

The usual murmur of mitral regurgitation (MR) is a harsh apical pansystolic (holosystolic) murmur at the apex; the chief exception to this is posterior leaflet MR which directs the jet anteriorly and the murmur is heard at the left sternal border.

- Acute MR due to valve perforation in endocarditis, ruptured chordae, or papillary muscle rupture may cause a musical high-pitched or squeaking murmur.
- Occasionally in patients with chronic severe MR with left ventricular dysfunction, the murmur may be softer as the left atrial pressure increases to reduce the differential with the systolic left ventricular pressure.
- Differential diagnosis may include aortic stenosis (AS); the murmur of AS is typically crescendo/decrescendo in the left parasternal area but this can also be produced by MR with an anteriorly directed jet.
- In acute myocardial infarction, development of a harsh systolic murmur may indicate acute MR or possibly development of a ventricular septal defect. Urgent echocardiography may be needed to distinguish these.

Investigations

- The EKG may show left-axis deviation, a left ventricular strain pattern with T wave inversion in the lateral leads, and left atrial enlargement with P mitrale.
- MR is usually recognized readily on the echocardiogram from the Doppler flow pattern in the left parasternal long-axis and apical four-chamber views. The severity of the regurgitation can be ranked as *mild* (regurgitant jet just into the left atrium), *moderate* (regurgitant jet reaches the mid-atrium) or *severe* (regurgitant jet reaches the posterior wall). In chronic MR, enlarged left atrium or elevated pulmonary pressure may indicate greater severity. Generally, chronic mitral regurgitation cannot be considered severe until left ventricular dilatation has occurred.
- Transesophageal echocardiography (TEE) is used to identify more detail of the location of the regurgitation to assist surgical repair.

Management

- Patients with **mild MR** can be reassured that they do not need any intervention on their valves. They may require occasional clinical or echocardiographic review to monitor the progress of the MR.
- Most patients with **moderate MR** can also be monitored with clinical and echocardiographic review and do not need intervention.
- Patients with **severe MR** may present with symptoms and will require early intervention. Many patients, however, remain asymptomatic for years and can be managed conservatively. Eventually, most patients will develop symptoms of dyspnea and reduced exercise capacity, and there is now a trend to intervene earlier in

asymptomatic patients to avoid the development of left atrial enlargement, propensity for atrial fibrillation, and development of pulmonary hypertension.

- The left ventricular ejection fraction is often increased when patients have mitral regurgitation because the left ventricle unloads partly into a low resistance chamber, the left atrium. Any fall in ejection fraction, even while it remains in the normal range, is an indication of left ventricular dysfunction and need for valve surgery.
- **Acute MR** with hemodynamic deterioration requires urgent clinical stabilization of cardiac failure and early intervention.

Ideally, MR is best treated with surgical reconstruction of the valve and minimization of the MR.

- If repair of the valve is not possible, a decision has to be made between insertion of a bioprosthesis (avoiding the need for anticoagulation but with the prospect of re-operation in 10–15 years) or a mechanical valve (anticoagulation required but minimal need for re-operation). The decision-making process needs to involve cardiologist, surgeon and patient.
- Recent developments with valve-preserving operations and minimally invasive approaches, including transcatheter, percutaneous techniques to reduce regurgitation, have minimized the morbidity and improved outcomes with mitral valve surgery.
- Rapid advances have been made in non-surgical intervention for MR. Transcatheter clipping of the mitral valve leaflets is well developed and is standard therapy for reducing the severity of regurgitation in selected cases. Advances are being made in transcatheter mitral valve replacement.

Mitral valve prolapse (MVP) syndrome

- MVP syndrome is a common, occasionally familial syndrome resulting from redundant mitral leaflet tissue, associated with myxomatous degeneration of the valve.
- It is a frequent accompaniment of Marfan syndrome and may be associated with thoracic skeletal deformities.
- The posterior mitral leaflet is usually more affected than the anterior, and elongated or ruptured chordae tendineae cause or contribute to the variable clinical course of the mitral regurgitation.

Clinical features

- MVP is more common in young women.
- The clinical course is most often benign with no more than a systolic click and murmur, with mild prolapse of the posterior leaflet.
- In some patients, however, it can progress over years or decades and can worsen rapidly with chordal rupture or endocarditis.
- Palpitations and occasionally syncope can result from ventricular premature contractions and paroxysmal supraventricular and ventricular tachycardia, or atrial fibrillation.
- Sudden death has been reported in patients with severe MR and depressed LV systolic function.

- Some patients with MVP may have substernal chest pain which may occasionally resemble angina pectoris.
- Transient cerebral ischemic attacks secondary to emboli from the mitral valve have been reported.

CLINICAL PEARL

The course of mitral valve prolapse is usually benign, but syncope or major arrhythmias indicate an adverse prognosis.

- The typical finding on auscultation is a mid- or late systolic click, generated by the sudden tensing of elongated chordae tendineae or by the prolapsing mitral leaflets. Systolic clicks may be multiple and followed by a high-pitched, late systolic crescendo/decrescendo murmur at the cardiac apex.

Investigations

- The EKG may show biphasic or inverted T waves in the inferior leads.
- Echocardiography shows displacement of the mitral valve leaflets. The usual echocardiographic definition of MVP is displacement of the mitral leaflets in the parasternal long-axis view by at least 2 mm. Doppler imaging can evaluate the associated MR and estimate its severity. The jet lesion of MR due to MVP is most often eccentric, and accurate assessment of the severity of MR may be difficult.
- Transesophageal echocardiography (TEE) provides more accurate information, especially when repair or replacement is being considered.

Management

- Serial echocardiography can be used to monitor progress of MVP.
- Beta-blockers may be required if there are documented arrhythmias causing symptoms.
- The timing of intervention is usually determined by the severity of mitral regurgitation and associated symptoms.

CLINICAL PEARL

Transcatheter repair of mitral regurgitation is not ideally suitable for mitral valve prolapse because of the myxomatous degeneration of the leaflet tissue.

AORTIC VALVE DISEASE

Aortic stenosis (AS)

Etiology and pathogenesis

- Most cases of AS in younger patients result from progressive deterioration and fibrosis of the valve in patients born with a bicuspid valve.

» A bicuspid aortic valve is usually part of a more diffuse aortopathy, and coarctation and ascending aortic aneurysm are common associations.

- Calcific aortic stenosis is the usual cause in older patients. There has been controversy over whether the process of aortic valve degeneration with fibrosis and stenosis is related to atherosclerotic disease. There are similarities in the histological appearances of calcific aortic valve disease and atherosclerosis, and the two conditions share several common risk factors, but trials to delay progression with statins have generally been ineffective in calcific aortic stenosis.
- Rheumatic valve disease rarely affects the aortic valve by itself. Usually stenosis is associated with regurgitation, and occurs in association with mitral valve disease.
- Rare causes of AS include a localized sub-aortic membrane, or a supra-aortic stenosis.
- With progressive narrowing of the aortic valve there is an increase in the transvalvular pressure gradient, reduction of the valve area, and LV hypertrophy.
  » Increase in intramyocardial pressure may cause myocardial ischemia, and reduced compliance may lead to diastolic heart failure.

Symptoms

- Aortic stenosis usually remains asymptomatic until the aortic valve area is reduced below 1 cm^2.

CLINICAL PEARL

Aortic stenosis usually progresses slowly, but can accelerate in older patients and in patients with chronic kidney disease having dialysis.

- Progressive dyspnea and reduced exercise capacity may occur as the stenosis progresses.
- The development of cardiac failure is a bad prognostic sign, and indicates either that the valve stenosis is very severe or that there is associated LV dysfunction.
- Angina pectoris may develop as a result of the severity of the stenosis with LV hypertrophy, but more often indicates the presence of associated coronary disease.
- The development of syncope is also a bad prognostic sign indicating very severe stenosis, or associated conduction system disease.

Clinical signs

- A delayed upstroke and reduced amplitude in the carotid pulse are the typical pulse features of AS, but these are usually seen only in severe AS. These signs are less reliable in elderly patients who have stiff arteries.
- The murmur of AS is characteristically a crescendo/decrescendo (mid-) systolic murmur that commences shortly after the 1st heart sound, increases in intensity to reach a peak at mid-systole, and ends just before aortic valve closure.
  » It is characteristically harsh and loud, and can be high- or medium-pitched.

» It is loudest in the 2nd right intercostal space, and may be transmitted to the base of the neck or into the carotids.
» Usually a loud murmur, particularly if associated with a systolic thrill, indicates severe stenosis, but in some patients with significant left ventricular dysfunction the murmur may be relatively soft and short.

- The heart sounds are usually well heard, but the aortic component of the 2nd heart sound may be delayed, leading to a single 2nd heart sound or even reverse splitting. The latter is more likely to indicate the presence of a left bundle branch block. A 4th heart sound reflecting LV hypertrophy and reduced LV compliance may be audible at the apex.

CLINICAL PEARL

A delayed upstroke and reduced amplitude in the carotid pulse (pulsus parvus et tardus) are typical of aortic stenosis. If they are present, the stenosis is severe.

Investigations

- The EKG may show LV hypertrophy with ST–T changes in the lateral leads.
- With severe AS, the chest X-ray may show an enlarged heart, and calcification of the aortic valve and annulus is usually readily visible on a lateral projection.
- The characteristic echocardiographic appearance of calcified and immobile valve leaflets is readily seen on the left parasternal long-axis view. The calcified valve and features of a bicuspid valve are best seen '*en face*' on the parasternal short-axis view. The gradients across the valve are measured using Doppler measurements of the transaortic velocity. The valve area can be calculated from these measurements.

CLINICAL PEARL

A valve area of <1 cm^2 indicates severe aortic stenosis (AS), 1–1.5 cm^2 moderate AS, and 1.5–2 cm^2 mild AS.

- When decisions are being made about the timing of valve surgery or transcatheter intervention, and there is a discrepancy between clinical and echocardiographic assessment, there may be a need to check these valve gradients using cardiac catheterization. In modern practice this is uncommonly performed, as there are concerns that attempts to cross the valve may cause dislodgement of calcific particles. However, coronary angiography or more recently coronary CT angiography is routinely performed in older patients to assess the presence of associated coronary artery disease.

Management

- Patients with severe AS should avoid excessively heavy lifting or other isometric exercise.

- Usual treatments for cardiac failure or angina can be used, but excessive diuresis with hypovolemia should be avoided if possible as this can increase the risk of syncope.
- Statin therapy should follow usual guidelines, and has no additional benefit in AS. The timing of intervention with surgery or transcatheter intervention is determined by symptoms and the severity of the AS.
- Severe AS (mean gradient >40 mmHg) and symptoms of syncope, heart failure or angina, or an asymptomatic patient with LV dysfunction (LVEF <50%) or an adverse response to exercise, are indications for surgery or intervention.
- In patients who remain asymptomatic, serial echocardiography should follow the rate of progression of the stenosis.

CLINICAL PEARL

Patients with a biscuspid aortic valve should undergo aortic imaging with computed tomography or magnetic resonance imaging to rule out coarctation or other aortic pathology.

- Open valve replacement remains the standard for intervention in most centers.
  - » The operation can be performed with a mortality risk of about 5% depending on age and comorbidities.
  - » Recent advances in minimally invasive surgery for aortic valve replacement have reduced the morbidity and complications of surgery.
  - » Choice of valve is usually determined by age.
  - » A bioprosthetic valve will avoid the need for anticoagulants (unless there is an established indication such as atrial fibrillation). However, despite improvements in bioprosthetic valve technology, there is a high rate of failure and need for re-operation after 10–15 years. Therefore, bioprosthetic valves are usually chosen for older patients with a limited life expectancy, and mechanical valves for younger patients.
- The rapidly increasing availability of transcatheter aortic valve replacement (TAVR) has changed the indications for intervention. While the early experience with TAVR was limited to older patients too ill to safely undergo surgery, there are rapidly widening indications for this approach in younger patients with less severe AS.
- Palliation of severe AS with balloon valvuloplasty is an option in patients not suitable for surgery or TAVR, but rapid recurrence limits this as a definitive treatment.

Aortic regurgitation (AR)

Etiology and pathogenesis

Aortic regurgitation can occur as a result of primary valve disease, or from dilatation of the aortic root.

- Direct involvement of the aortic valve with regurgitation may occur from rheumatic disease, but usually in association with mitral valve disease.

- A congenital bicuspid aortic valve can progress to predominant AR, but usually with extensive thickening of the valve and associated stenosis.
- AR may result from infective endocarditis, usually on a valve previously deformed with rheumatic disease or a congenital bicuspid valve.
- Rarer causes include ankylosing spondylitis or blunt chest trauma.
- AR is often due to marked aortic dilatation; while the valve leaflets may not be involved in the primary disease process, widening of the aortic annulus and separation of the aortic leaflets may cause the AR.
- Aortic root causes of regurgitation include cystic medial degeneration of the ascending aorta, with or without Marfan's features, idiopathic dilatation of the aorta, and atherosclerotic or hypertensive degeneration of the aortic architecture with an ascending aortic aneurysm. Acute AR may occur as a result of retrograde aortic root dissection.
- In chronic AR, the regurgitation gradually leads to compensatory mechanisms which may be effective in maintaining cardiac output and preventing the development of symptoms for decades. An increase in the LV end-diastolic volume is followed by dilatation, and hypertrophy of the LV allows the heart to maintain a normal stroke volume and an apparently normal ejection fraction. Further progression leads to failure of these compensatory measures, with reduction in stroke volume and LVEF and an increase in systolic volume.
- Deterioration of LV function often precedes the development of symptoms.
- Exercise testing may unmask compensated LV dysfunction.

Symptoms

- Patients with chronic AR may remain asymptomatic for as long as 10–15 years, even when the regurgitation is hemodynamically severe on clinical examination and echocardiography.
- Subtle symptoms including an increased awareness of the heartbeat, sinus tachycardia or ventricular premature beats during exertion may be present and hardly noticed by the patient.
- Patients may present with exertional dyspnea or reduced exercise capacity.
- Chest pain suggestive of angina may occur in patients with severe AR.
- With progression of LV dysfunction, symptoms of cardiac failure may develop quite rapidly.
- In patients with acute severe AR, rapid onset of pulmonary edema and/or cardiogenic shock may be the initial presentation.

CLINICAL PEARL

Aortic regurgitation (AR) can result from pathology of the valve or the aortic root. Both should be considered when AR is detected.

Clinical signs

- The typical feature of severe AR is a prominent collapsing pulse, and an early diastolic murmur. The pulse is often described as a 'waterhammer pulse', and can manifest with several eponymous variants, including bobbing of the head (De Musset's sign), prominent carotid pulsations (Corrigan's sign), pulsation of the nail bed (Quincke's sign), pistol-shot sound (Traube's sign) or a to-and-fro murmur (Duroziez's sign) over the femoral arteries.
- There is usually a wide pulse pressure, and generally a pulse pressure of >100 mmHg indicates very severe AR.
- The murmur commences in early diastole, is best heard at the left sternal border, and is typically a high-pitched, blowing, decrescendo murmur.
  » The length of the murmur correlates with the severity of the AR, with a short murmur indicating mild AR, a murmur to mid-diastole indicating moderate AR, and a murmur filling diastole indicating severe AR.
  » The murmur is more easily heard with the diaphragm of the stethoscope, with the patient sitting forward, and auscultating in expiration.
  » The loudness of the murmur is not an indication of the severity of the regurgitation.
- In severe AR, the murmur may blend with a diastolic rumble (the Austin Flint murmur) due to vibration of the anterior leaflet of the mitral valve, and may cause confusion with mitral stenosis.

Investigations

- EKG signs of left anterior hemiblock or LV hypertrophy with T wave inversion in inferior and lateral leads may be obvious.
- On the chest X-ray, the cardiac silhouette is enlarged, the apex is displaced downward and leftward in the frontal projection, and aortic root enlargement may be visible.
- On the echocardiogram, minor degrees of AR are frequently seen when not clinically or hemodynamically relevant.
  » With more severe AR, increased LV size but normal systolic function may be seen.
  » With progression, an increase in the end-systolic dimension or a subtle deterioration of the apparently normal LVEF may be the first signs of decompensation.
- The regurgitant jet can be assessed by color-flow Doppler imaging.
- A high-frequency fluttering of the anterior mitral leaflet during diastole produced by the regurgitant jet is a characteristic finding (and the genesis of the Austin Flint murmur).
- The aortic root can be evaluated with echocardiography to assess if aortic root dilatation is the cause of the AR. However, the echocardiographic window is limited to the first 3–4 cm (1–1.5 in) of the ascending aorta, and anatomical detail of the remainder of the aorta needs to be established with cardiac CT or MRI.

Management

- Careful observation with clinical and echocardiographic surveillance is needed for patients with mild to moderate regurgitation. The rate of progression varies, with many patients remaining symptom-free without evidence of decompensation for a decade or more.
- In patients with more severe degrees of regurgitation, echocardiographic monitoring of the LV response to the regurgitation is crucial.
- In the symptom-free patient, a degree of LV dilatation may be acceptable as part of the physiological compensation, but any increase in systolic dimension needs to be carefully evaluated, as this may indicate impending decompensation.
- Control of blood pressure is important.

The development of symptoms is a late development and indicates that decompensation has already developed. Once symptoms develop, mortality in patients without surgical treatment may be as high as 10–20% per year. Symptoms of cardiac failure may need stabilization with diuretics and ACEIs, but improvement in symptoms should not be regarded as avoiding the need for surgical intervention.

- Surgery is recommended when there are symptoms of LV dysfunction (LVEF <50%), or normal LV function but marked LV dilatation with a left ventricular end-diastolic diameter of >70 mm, or left ventricular end-systolic diameter of >50 mm or >25 mm/m² body surface area.
- Surgery with a mechanical or bioprosthetic valve has been the only option until recently, but valve-sparing surgery, particularly for acute AR or in valves without extensive calcification, has been explored with success in many centers.
- When the AR is associated with marked aortic root dilatation, reconstruction of the aortic root may also be required.
- Patients with acute severe AR require early intervention with surgery.

> **CLINICAL PEARL**
>
> Surgical intervention in chronic aortic regurgitation is determined more by the response of the ventricle than by the severity of the regurgitation.

TRICUSPID VALVE DISEASE

Tricuspid stenosis (TS)

- Tricuspid stenosis is usually rheumatic in origin, and is usually associated with mitral stenosis. Rarely, isolated congenital TS can occur.
- The clinical features are those of systemic venous congestion with hepatomegaly, ascites, and edema.
  » Although a rare condition, the diagnosis may be missed if not considered in a patient showing

venous congestion in excess of that expected with their mitral valve disease.

» The jugular veins are distended, and in patients with sinus rhythm there may be giant a waves.

» A diastolic murmur of TS may be present but attributed to the murmur of mitral stenosis. However, it is generally heard best along the left lower sternal border and over the xiphoid process rather than at the apex of the heart, and may be accentuated with inspiration.

- The EKG shows features of right atrial enlargement including tall, peaked P waves in lead II, in the absence of EKG signs of right ventricular (RV) hypertrophy.
- Echocardiography shows a thickened tricuspid valve which domes in diastole.
- Treatment is with valvuloplasty or valve replacement at the same time as mitral valve surgery.

Tricuspid regurgitation (TR)

- Functional tricuspid regurgitation is due to marked dilatation of the tricuspid annulus from RV enlargement in patients with severe pulmonary hypertension.
- Other causes of RV enlargement may result in functional TR, including right ventricular infarction.
- Direct TR due to valve involvement is less common but may result from a congenitally deformed tricuspid valve, with defects of the atrioventricular canal, as well as with Ebstein's anomaly of the tricuspid valve, endocarditis or trauma or sometimes from a pacemaker or defibrillator lead.
- The clinical manifestations are those of right-sided heart failure with prominent v waves and rapid y descents in the jugular pulse, and pulsatile hepatomegaly.
- The murmur of TR is a blowing pansystolic murmur along the lower left sternal margin which is intensified during inspiration.

CLINICAL PEARL

The diagnosis of tricuspid regurgitation is usually established on the basis of the jugular venous pressure (JVP) and pulsatile hepatomegaly; the murmur may be difficult to hear.

- A trivial or mild degree of tricuspid regurgitation is a normal finding on echocardiography, but severe TR produces Doppler features of torrential regurgitation, often accompanied by hepatic-vein flow reversal. Continuous wave Doppler of the TR velocity profile is useful in estimating pulmonary arterial systolic pressure.
- Functional TR associated with heart failure may improve dramatically with control of the cardiac failure, and does not require surgical intervention. Addition of an aldosterone antagonist to diuretic therapy may help if there is secondary hyperaldosteronism from hepatic dysfunction.
- In patients in whom the TR is due to rheumatic valve disease, tricuspid valve annuloplasty at the time of surgical repair may be indicated.

PULMONARY VALVE DISEASE

- **Pulmonary stenosis** is a relatively common congenital anomaly which produces a systolic murmur at the upper left sternal border, and a characteristic doming appearance of the valve on echocardiography. It only rarely requires correction, and this can now be achieved with balloon valvuloplasty.
- Acquired pulmonary stenosis may result from the carcinoid syndrome.
- Trivial or mild **pulmonary regurgitation** is a common finding on echocardiography and does not require any further investigation.
- More severe pulmonary regurgitation may occur as a result of dilatation of the pulmonary artery due to severe pulmonary arterial hypertension, producing a high-pitched, decrescendo, diastolic blowing murmur in the 2nd left intercostal space (Graham Steell murmur).
- Moderate pulmonary regurgitation is an almost invariable result of corrected Fallot's tetralogy.

Assessing the severity of valvular heart disease and deciding on surgery

The usual indications for surgery and intervention in mitral and aortic valve disease are summarized in Table 7-10.

CARDIOMYOPATHIES

Cardiomyopathy is a chronic disease of the heart muscle (myocardium), in which the muscle is abnormally enlarged, thickened and/or stiffened. The weakened heart muscle loses the ability to pump blood effectively, resulting in increased risk of arrhythmias and heart failure.

- The cardiomyopathies are a diverse group of conditions affecting the heart muscle. The traditional classification of cardiomyopathies is into three types: *dilated*, *hypertrophic* and *restrictive* cardiomyopathies.
- New genetic and molecular biology information has shown a degree of overlap between the types, but it remains the most widely used and understood classification. Some more recently recognized cardiomyopathies do not fit into this standard classification.

Dilated cardiomyopathy (DCM)

The main causes of dilated cardiomyopathy are shown in Table 7-11.

Idiopathic dilated cardiomyopathy

- Idiopathic DCM usually presents with progressive cardiac failure or with radiographic or echocardiographic evidence of cardiac enlargement.
- Patients with this condition are at increased risk of cardiac arrhythmias and sudden death.
- Whether the etiology is due to undiscovered genetic defects in myosin, actin and other muscle proteins, to a disordered immunological response, or to a reaction

Table 7-10 Indications for surgery or transcatheter intervention in aortic and mitral valve disease

DISEASE TYPE	INDICATIONS FOR SURGERY/ INTERVENTION
Mitral stenosis	Progressive symptoms, valve area <1.5 cm² (1 cm/m² body surface area), mean gradient >10 mmHg, development of pulmonary hypertension
Mitral regurgitation	Flail leaflet, ruptured papillary muscle, large coaptation defect Symptomatic patients with LVEF >30% Asymptomatic patients with left ventricular dysfunction (LVESD ≥45 mm and/or LVEF ≤60%), development of pulmonary hypertension, or new-onset atrial fibrillation
Aortic stenosis	Severe aortic stenosis (mean gradient >40 mmHg, maximum jet velocity >4 m/s) Symptoms of syncope, heart failure, or angina Asymptomatic patients with left ventricular dysfunction (LVEF <50%) or adverse response to exercise
Aortic regurgitation	Abnormal/flail large coaptation defect Symptoms of cardiac failure or reduced exercise capacity Asymptomatic patients with left ventricular dysfunction (LVEF <50%), or normal LV function but marked LV dilatation (LVEDD >70 mm, or LVESD >50 mm or LVESD >25 mm/m² body surface area)

LVEF, left ventricular ejection fraction; LVEDD, left ventricular end-diastolic diameter; LVESD = left ventricular end-systolic diameter.

Table 7-11 Causes of dilated cardiomyopathy

DILATED CARDIOMYOPATHY	CLINICAL FEATURES
Idiopathic	Any age, usually progressive
Familial/genetic	May manifest at a young age; may be a complication of muscular dystrophy
Alcoholic	Usually with alcohol excess, but with wide individual variation
Chemotherapy	Usually anthracyclines
Viral myocarditis	Can be severe or life-threatening but may be transient with complete recovery
Parasitic infection	Chagas disease
Infiltrative disorders	Hemochromatosis, sarcoidosis
Peripartum cardiomyopathy	Usually self-limiting but can be severe

CLINICAL PEARL

The diagnosis of idiopathic dilated cardiomyopathy is made only after all correctable causes have been ruled out.

Familial/genetic cardiomyopathies

- In some families there is a pattern of early development of dilated cardiomyopathy with echocardiographic evidence of LV dysfunction and dilatation, and a propensity to early death.
- Early treatment with beta-blockers and ACEIs, and implantation of an ICD, may significantly improve the prognosis.
- A genetic susceptibility to development of dilated cardiomyopathy and viral myocarditis has long been suspected but poorly understood. A specific form of cardiomyopathy may complicate Duchenne and Becker muscular dystrophy, with the myocardial abnormality localized to the posterior wall of the left ventricle. There is a characteristic tall R wave in lead V_1 on the EKG, and hypokinesis of the posterior wall can be seen on echocardiography.
- Mitochondrial myopathies may also rarely involve the heart, with progressive cardiac failure and LV dysfunction.
- A familial form of cardiomyopathy with conduction system abnormalities may present with atrioventricular block, and symptoms of cardiac failure as a late development.

to a viral illness remains the subject of conjecture and investigation.

- The pathology varies with distorted myofibrils and varying degrees of fibrosis.
- Progressive dilatation and hypertrophy of the left ventricle leads to LV dysfunction, usually systolic.
- Echocardiography typically shows global depression of LV function, in contrast to ischemic causes which are usually regional.
- Treatment with beta-blockers, ACEIs, and aldosterone antagonists may delay progression, and can lead to significant improvements in some cases.
- Patients with marked depression of LV function are at increased risk of sudden death, and implantation of an implantable cardioverter–defibrillator (ICD) is usually recommended when the ejection fraction is consistently below 35%. Implantation of an ICD has been shown to improve prognosis significantly, especially in younger patients.

- In addition to assessment of echocardiographic left ventricular ejection fraction, MRI is helpful in identifying fibrosis, stratifying the risk of sudden death and the need for an implantable cardioverter defibrillator.

CLINICAL PEARL

Despite advances in understanding the molecular biology of cardiomyopathy, there is no advantage in genetic testing, even in families with a strong history of cardiomyopathy.

Alcoholic cardiomyopathy

- In some communities this is the most common form of dilated cardiomyopathy.
- All types of alcohol consumption can cause alcoholic cardiomyopathy, and the volume and duration of excess drinking varies greatly, but six standard drinks daily for 5–10 years is usually regarded as the dose required to damage the heart.
- It may be associated with nutritional deficiencies, which can exacerbate the severity of the cardiomyopathy, and is often associated with other alcohol-related cardiac conditions including atrial fibrillation and hypertension.

CLINICAL PEARL

Alcoholic cardiomyopathy can improve or, rarely, even resolve with complete cessation of alcohol.

Chemotherapy-induced cardiomyopathy

- Anthracyclines (most commonly doxorubicin) may directly damage the myocardium and cause clinically evident cardiac failure in 5% or more of patients treated.
  - » Lesser degrees of LV dysfunction are seen more frequently. The left ventricle may show a reduced LVEF without cardiac dilatation.
  - » Total cessation of the anthracycline can allow recovery in many cases, but permanent reduction in LV function may result.

CLINICAL PEARL

Patients having anthracycline chemotherapy should have baseline and serial echocardiography to monitor for development of cardiomyopathy.

- The monoclonal antibody trastuzumab also has some cardiotoxic effect, particularly when co-administered with anthracyclines.
- Cardiotoxicity, usually transient, can occur with very high doses of cyclophosphamide.
- 5-fluorouracil, and cisplatin, can cause coronary spasm with depressed contractility.

Viral myocarditis

- Myocarditis can present with mild cardiac failure, but on occasions can cause severe rapid-onset cardiac failure, and occasionally cardiogenic shock. In such patients with fulminant disease, urgent consideration of implantation of a left ventricular assist device is required.
  - » It often commences with a nonspecific viral illness, and there may be a latent period between the flu-like illness and the onset of the myocarditis.
  - » It can be associated with pericardial involvement.
- The typical clinical pattern with echocardiographic features of LV dysfunction usually establish the diagnosis, but MRI with gadolinium contrast is increasingly used to identify tissue edema and fibrosis.
- In some cases, the condition can progress to an established cardiomyopathy, but in many cases complete resolution can occur over a period of 3–6 months.
- Viruses implicated include coxsackievirus and Epstein–Barr virus, and cardiac involvement can be seen in HIV.

CLINICAL PEARL

In patients with probable viral myocarditis, decisions about implantation of an implantable cardioverter-defibrillator should be deferred to assess whether the LV dysfunction is permanent.

Parasitic infection

Infection with *Trypanosoma cruzi* can involve the heart in Chagas disease, resulting in LV dysfunction with a particular propensity to thromboembolic complications and cardiac arrhythmias.

Infiltrative disorders

- Hemochromatosis is a rare but important cause of cardiomyopathy. It occurs only in advanced hemochromatosis and can cause severe cardiac failure and cardiac arrhythmias, but can be reversible with venesection. Chelation with desferrioxamine has been used, but may transiently exacerbate arrhythmias and cardiac failure.
- Sarcoidosis can involve the heart, with cardiac failure and cardiac arrhythmias. MRI may demonstrate infiltration of the heart with granulomas. Occasionally positron emission tomography (PET) is used to identify the extent and localization of the granulomas. Treatment with high-dose corticosteroids may limit the extent of cardiac involvement.
- Cardiac amyloidosis is being increasingly recognized as an infiltrative cardiomyopathy. (See below under Restrictive cardiomyopathy.)

Peripartum cardiomyopathy

Cardiomyopathy in the post-partum mother, usually with mild cardiac failure, occurs in 1 in 10,000 deliveries. The cause remains poorly understood, but an inflammatory infiltrate may be seen on biopsy. With supportive measures and standard treatment of LV dysfunction, the prognosis is usually for complete recovery within several months.

Hypertrophic cardiomyopathy (HCM)

Hypertrophic cardiomyopathy is defined as marked cardiac hypertrophy in the absence of an obvious cause such as hypertension or valvular heart disease.

- Systolic function is usually normal, but diastolic dysfunction can be a significant clinical problem.
- The usual pattern is asymmetric hypertrophy with enlargement of the septum, with many cases showing obstruction of the outflow tract of the left ventricle (hence the previous terminology of hypertrophic obstructive cardiomyopathy, HOCM).
- It is now recognized that the hypertrophic pathology is generalized in the cardiac muscle, with different distribution in different patients. A variant with predominantly hypertrophy in the apical region is thought to have a more benign course.

CLINICAL PEARL

Not all patients with hypertrophic cardiomyopathy have outflow tract obstruction, hence the terminology 'HCM' rather than 'HOCM'.

Etiology and pathogenesis

- The pathological features are marked disarray of individual fibers in a characteristic whorled pattern, with fibrosis of varying degree.
- The prevalence is 1 in 500 adults, with approximately half having a distinct heritable pattern.
- Multiple genetic mutations have been identified in the sarcomeric genes, mostly in the beta-myosin heavy chain, the cardiac myosin-binding protein C, or cardiac troponin T.
- The prognosis varies between families; but at this stage, despite considerable advances in understanding the molecular biology of the condition, a specific genetic mutation to assist with targeted management of the patients at highest risk has eluded investigators.

Symptoms and clinical findings

- Common symptoms are mild dyspnea or atypical chest pain, but many patients remain asymptomatic throughout, and have the diagnosis made on incidental EKG or echocardiographic findings.
- Syncope is a rare but troubling presentation, as this can indicate a high risk for sudden death.
- Tragically, the initial presentation may be with sudden death, and this is the most common cause of sudden death in otherwise healthy young athletes.
- Typical physical findings include a systolic murmur, but this is not always present in milder cases.
- EKG anomalies include LV hypertrophy and deep T wave inversion in the anterior or inferior leads. On occasions, well-developed Q waves in the inferior leads (from activation of the hypertrophic septum) may cause confusion with inferior myocardial infarction.

CLINICAL PEARL

Deep T wave inversions and inferior-lead Q waves in the EKG of hypertrophic cardiomyopathy may (incorrectly) suggest a diagnosis of myocardial infarction.

- The echocardiogram shows features of LV hypertrophy, often with evidence of diastolic dysfunction. In the typical septal hypertrophy variant, the hypertrophy of the septum is prominent, but there is usually a degree of hypertrophy of the posterior wall as well. A gradient across the outflow tract is seen in many patients, and in more severe cases the characteristic echocardiographic finding of systolic anterior motion of the anterior leaflet of the mitral valve results from a Venturi effect in the outflow tract. This further compounds LV outflow obstruction, and contributes to disruption of the mitral valve apparatus with mitral regurgitation.
- The echocardiographic measurement of the gradient can be highly variable depending on loading conditions (reduced preload with diuretics or dehydration, reduced afterload with vasodilators) and heart rate. For these reasons, serial measurement of the outflow gradient is not a reliable method of monitoring progress. It has, however, been established that patients with a consistently high gradient have a worse prognosis than those without.
- An outflow tract gradient may develop or increase with exercise and may be revealed if the patient performs the Valsalva maneuver while having an echocardiogram.

CLINICAL PEARL

Signs of gross enlargement of the septum, a history of syncope, a family history of sudden death and high-grade arrhythmias are indicative of an adverse prognosis in hypertrophic cardiomyopathy.

- The diagnosis of a generalized hypertrophy variant may be suspected in a patient with hypertension who appears to have excessive hypertrophy for the degree of blood pressure elevation.

Management

- Many patients require no further management than serial clinical and echocardiographic review to ensure that there is no progression of their mild septal hypertrophy.
- Drug treatments have generally not been effective in slowing the rate of hypertrophy, although ACEIs have been proposed for this purpose. In patients with significant outflow tract obstruction, it may be possible to improve symptoms, particularly palpitations, with beta-blockers or calcium-channel blockers (verapamil/diltiazem).
- Patients with proven severe hypertrophy, advanced gradients and symptoms may obtain symptom relief from surgical resection of the hypertrophied septal tissue (myectomy). A valid alternative method of reducing the septal hypertrophy has been the use of alcohol ablation

by injecting alcohol in controlled doses into the septal perforator artery. While symptoms of obstruction can be improved, neither myectomy nor alcohol septal ablation have been shown to improve long-term prognosis.

- Patients with a strong family history of sudden death, a history of syncope, septal thickness in excess of 3 cm (1.2 in), or documented ventricular tachycardia should be considered for implantation of an ICD.

Restrictive cardiomyopathy

- Restrictive cardiomyopathies result from infiltration of the myocardium with a varying degree of fibrotic reaction.
- Reduced compliance of the left ventricle with abnormal diastolic function is seen, usually with only mildly depressed systolic function.
- Left atrial enlargement is common, with a propensity to atrial fibrillation.
- A mild reduction in exercise capacity is the usual presenting symptom.
- Clinical signs may show predominant right-sided heart failure with characteristic steep y descent in the jugular venous pulse. A prominent 4th heart sound in sinus rhythm reflects the reduced compliance.
- **Amyloidosis** is the most frequent cause of restrictive cardiomyopathy.
  » Cardiac amyloidosis may be due to AL (amyloid light-chain) amyloidosis with abnormal production and infiltration of immunoglobulin light chains, or transthyretin-related (TTR) amyloidosis in which the amyloid infiltrate is derived from transthyretin, a small molecule mainly produced by the liver. TTR may be due to a genetic form known as hereditary TTR amyloidosis, and a non-hereditary form called senile systemic amyloidosis (SSA). The latter has a more benign course, usually occurring in men in their 70s or 80s.
  » Waxy deposits of amyloid infiltrate the myocardium and restrict filling.
- The EKG shows typical low voltages, and the echocardiogram shows a restrictive pattern of diastolic dysfunction with a characteristic brightly speckled appearance best seen in the septum. Due to this appearance being neither sensitive nor specific, MRI is more reliable for diagnosis. Technetium pyrophosphate scans are very sensitive and quite specific for cardiac amyloidosis.

CLINICAL PEARL

Echocardiographic 'speckling' is a widely discussed sign of cardiac amyloid infiltration, but not sufficiently reliable for making a diagnosis. More reliable is a discrepancy between low voltage on the EKG and echocardiographic evidence of left ventricular hypertrophy.

- Biopsy of the abdominal fat pad may confirm the diagnosis, but the abnormal tissue may be overlooked, and cardiac biopsy may be needed to confirm the diagnosis.

- If AL amyloidosis is the likely diagnosis, a screening of the peripheral blood for light chains and bone marrow biopsy is done to assess the numbers of plasma cells, to establish the diagnosis. If there is no confirmation of AL, screening for a mutation in transthyretin may demonstrate the familial form.

The **treatment** of AL and TTR amyloidosis differs.

- The aim of treatment in AL amyloidosis is to prevent the production of light chains by the plasma cells with the use of chemotherapy, but this does not affect the cardiac prognosis.
- The prognosis in AL is often poor, due to both progressive cardiac failure and progressive involvement of other organs.
- Implantation of an ICD may improve the prognosis.
- Cardiac transplantation has been temporarily successful in some cases, but re-infiltration of the transplanted myocardium may be a limitation.
- Patients with the more common SSA variant of TTR amyloidosis often require no active treatment apart from management of their cardiac failure.
- Patients with the rarer familial TTR may need to be considered for liver transplantation as the liver is the source of the TTR. The anti-inflammatory drug tafamidis has shown promise in early trials for the treatment of TTR cardiac amyloidosis.

Other causes of restrictive cardiomyopathy

- Rare glycogen storage and other infiltrative conditions can affect the myocardium and cause a restrictive cardiomyopathy.
- Of these, Fabry's disease, due to alpha-galactosidase deficiency, is the most significant as it can be recognized with an enzyme assay to measure the level of alpha-galactosidase activity and is correctable with enzyme replacement therapy.
- In tropical countries, eosinophilic endomyocardial disease and myocardial involvement in Löffler's endocarditis can be common causes of restrictive cardiomyopathy and cardiac failure.
- Thoracic radiation therapy for breast or lung cancer can cause the late development of a restrictive cardiomyopathy.

Other cardiomyopathies

Some cardiomyopathies more recently described have not been fully characterized but do not fit the dilated/hypertrophic/restrictive classification. These are summarized in Table 7–12.

Diabetes/obesity

There is controversy as to whether the diastolic LV dysfunction which frequently complicates diabetes and obesity represents a true cardiomyopathy, or is simply fatty infiltration, but there is increasing evidence that diabetes is associated with specific changes in myocardial metabolism.

Table 7-12 Cardiomyopathies which do not fit into the classification of dilated, hypertrophic or restrictive

CARDIOMYOPATHY	FEATURES
Diabetes/obesity	More likely to cause diastolic dysfunction; may be reversible
Ventricular non-compaction	Usually benign, but arrhythmias and thromboemboli can occur
Arrhythmogenic right-ventricular cardiomyopathy	May cause ventricular tachycardia and sudden death
Takotsubo cardiomyopathy	Also known as apical ballooning or stress-induced cardiomyopathy; may mimic myocardial infarction

Ventricular non-compaction

Ventricular non-compaction was originally identified as an echocardiographic finding of prominent trabeculae at the cardiac apex. It is now recognized as a distinct form of cardiomyopathy, with an increased risk of thrombosis and major cardiac arrhythmias. Anticoagulation and implantation of an ICD may need to be considered in more severe cases.

Arrhythmogenic right-ventricular cardiomyopathy

This condition, now known as ARCM and previously known as arrhythmogenic right-ventricular dysplasia (ARVD), can be fatal and contribute to early sudden death. It is associated with fibromuscular dysplasia and fatty infiltration of the outflow tract of the right ventricle. It can be overlooked on echocardiography and requires MRI for ruling out the diagnosis in a young person with syncope and/or a family history of sudden death.

Takotsubo cardiomyopathy

This condition, recognized only recently, is associated with the sudden development of chest pain, T wave inversion in the anterior leads of the EKG, and a characteristic ballooning of the cardiac apex seen on echocardiography or ventriculography. The unusual name derives from the ventriculographic appearance of the ventricle, which is similar to a Japanese lobster pot. Coronary angiography does not show any culprit lesion and the condition is distinct from myocardial infarction. It often but not exclusively occurs in elderly females after a sudden stress, and has also been termed 'stress cardiomyopathy'. The usual pattern is for restoration of the apical ballooning to normal within several months but complications including arrhythmias and heart failure can occur.

CARDIAC ARRHYTHMIAS

Cardiac arrhythmias may vary from benign ectopic beats to incapacitating heart block and lethal ventricular arrhythmias. The assessment and planning of management requires not only a detailed examination of the EKG but also a full and detailed clinical assessment of the patient.

Sinus node disturbances

- **Sinus tachycardia** is usually defined as sinus rhythm at a rate above 100/min. Correction of the underlying abnormality, including blood loss, hyperthyroidism, anxiety, alcohol withdrawal, hypoxemia or worsening cardiac function, is usually sufficient.
- **Sinus arrhythmia** is a normal physiological response of variation of the heart rate with respiration. There is phasic variation of the P–P interval with preservation of normal P wave contour. When atrial activity arises from multiple sites, the P wave morphology and the P–P interval vary. No specific treatment is necessary. Treatment of underlying lung disease (if present) should be optimized.
- **Sinus bradycardia** is usually defined as a sinus rhythm below 50/min. It can be a normal variant and is often an indication of a high level of physical fitness. However, it can also be due to medications such as beta-blockers, calcium-channel blockers, ivabradine or digoxin, or may occur as a result of increased vagal tone. The patient's therapy should be reviewed for heart-rate-slowing medications which should be reduced or discontinued. If it is persistent and affects cardiac output or causes symptoms, atrial or dual-chamber cardiac pacing may be required.
- **Sinus arrest (or sinus pause)** (Figure 7-13) may occur as an isolated phenomenon in patients with sinus node dysfunction. If recurrent and symptomatic, especially if causing syncope, a permanent pacemaker is necessary. Drug therapy is ineffective.

CLINICAL PEARL

- Sinus tachycardia responds, usually slowly, to correction of the underlying problem.
- Supraventricular tachycardia responds rapidly to vagal maneuvers.

Sick sinus syndrome

The sick sinus syndrome is a term encompassing sinus bradycardia, chronotropic incompetence, and the tachy-brady syndrome.

- Bradycardia may be persistent and stable, or occur intermittently, particularly at the termination of supraventricular tachyarrhythmias—usually atrial fibrillation. In this situation it results from suppression of the sinus node.
- Drugs used to treat the tachyarrhythmia component of this disorder often provoke bradycardia, making back-up pacing necessary.

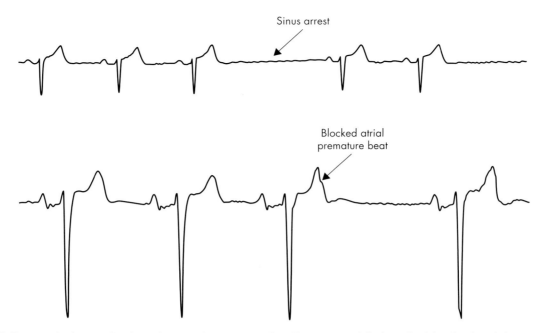

Figure 7-13 Pauses in heart rhythm due to sinus arrest (no P wave activity) and a blocked atrial premature beat (P wave, but conduction blocked)

From Thompson P (ed). Coronary care manual, 2nd ed. Sydney: Elsevier Australia, 2011.

> **CLINICAL PEARL**
>
> The 'sick sinus syndrome' includes sinus bradycardia, chronotropic incompetence, and the tachy-brady syndrome. It is the most common reason for pacemaker insertion.

Supraventricular premature complexes (ectopics)

Supraventricular ectopic beats can arise in the atria or the AV junction. They are very common and typically benign, but can be of concern if they provoke palpitations. They can be exacerbated by caffeine, tobacco and alcohol. Patients with frequent supraventricular ectopics have an increased risk of developing atrial fibrillation.

Reassurance and removal of stimulants is the best treatment for supraventricular ectopy. For highly symptomatic patients, a low-dose beta-blocker may provide relief. For intractable symptoms, antiarrhythmic drugs are occasionally used.

Supraventricular tachycardia (SVT)

- The usual clinical presentation of SVT is sudden-onset, regular, rapid palpitations. There may be associated dyspnea, pre-syncope, chest tightness or anxiety.
- SVT occurs most often in otherwise healthy individuals, and usually the resting EKG is normal.

- For some patients (with AV reciprocating tachycardia), there is evidence of ventricular pre-excitation on 12-lead EKG (Wolff–Parkinson–White syndrome). Some patients with an intra-nodal accessory pathway and SVT have a short PR interval with normal QRS complexes (Lown-Ganong-Levine syndrome).

There are three major types of SVT:

- **Atrioventricular node re-entrant tachycardia (AVNRT).** This commonest type of SVT occurs as a result of longitudinal dissociation (of conduction) within the compact AV node, or may involve a small portion of perinodal atrial myocardium.
- **Atrioventricular reciprocating (re-entrant) tachycardia (AVRT).** This occurs when there is an accessory pathway participating in the tachycardia circuit. When associated with ventricular pre-excitation on a resting 12-lead EKG, patients are described as having the Wolff–Parkinson–White syndrome. The accessory pathway may be concealed and not visible on the surface EKG when there is only retrograde conduction.
- **Atrial tachycardia (AT).** Atrial tachycardia is a focal arrhythmia arising in the atrial tissue. It may be congenital and is more often associated with underlying structural heart disease.

Supraventricular tachycardias usually have a regular, narrow, complex appearance on 12-lead EKG, but may be associated with a wide QRS complex when there is a pre-existing bundle branch block, the development of rate-related bundle branch block (aberrancy), or anterograde conduction over an accessory pathway.

CLINICAL PEARLS

- AVNRT is due to a re-entrant circuit confined to the AV node.
- AVRT uses an accessory pathway for the re-entrant circuit.
- AT is not a re-entrant tachycardia.
- Patients with WPW changes on their EKG but without episodes of tachycardia are said to have *WPW conduction*.

Management

- Immediate treatment can commence with the application of various vagal maneuvers such as the Valsalva maneuver, carotid sinus massage, breath-holding/coughing, or cold-water immersion. Carotid sinus massage is the most effective.
- If vagal maneuvers are ineffective, the treatment of choice is intravenous adenosine. An initial dose of 3 mg should be given by rapid injection into a large-bore cannula via an antecubital vein (or central access if available), then 6 mg followed by 12 mg if needed. Correctly administered adenosine will successfully terminate the majority of SVTs.
- An alternative to adenosine is intravenous verapamil given in a total dose of 5–10 mg. Verapamil should not be given as a single bolus, and is given in boluses of 1–2 mg at 1-minute intervals.
- For patients with known accessory pathways (Wolff–Parkinson–White syndrome), episodes of SVT can be treated in the same manner, although calcium-channel blockers and digoxin are best avoided as they can, rarely, accelerate conduction in the accessory pathway. Adenosine will terminate tachycardia and does not accentuate anterograde conduction in the accessory pathway.
- SVTs which do not respond to vagal maneuvers or adenosine may be due to a focal atrial tachycardia.

CLINICAL PEARL

After vagal maneuvers, intravenous adenosine is the preferred treatment. AVNRT and AVRT will respond; AT will not.

- Synchronized direct-current (DC) cardioversion with 200 joules can be used if there is hemodynamic compromise.
- Many patients with SVT can be observed long term and treated without medications.
  - » The 'pill in the pocket therapy' approach—issuing the patient with an antiarrhythmic drug to use as required—is an alternative for patients having infrequent episodes.
- Drug therapy taken on a regular basis may control recurrent episodes, but may be associated with side-effects unacceptable to the typical relatively young patient.
  - » Options include a beta-blocker or calcium-channel blocker.

- » Digoxin is an alternative, although less effective.
- » Flecainide can be used if there is clear evidence of normal LV function and no evidence of ischaemic heart disease.
- Patients with more than rare episodes of SVT should be considered for catheter ablation.
  - » Catheter ablation is the treatment of choice for patients with recurrent SVT, particularly if highly symptomatic or frequent. In patients with AVNRT, the slow pathway in the AV node is ablated. In AVRT, the target is the accessory pathway.
  - » Catheter ablation for AVNRT and AVRT is highly successful, with a cure rate exceeding 90% for experienced operators and a risk of serious complications of <1%. Focal atrial tachycardias respond less well to ablation.
- Non-paroxysmal AT ('AT with block') due to digitalis intoxication is unusual in modern practice, but requires special attention because of the potential to cause harm with inappropriate treatment. Cardioversion should be avoided.
- Chaotic (multi-focal) AT is usually seen in patients with respiratory disease, especially cor pulmonale, or infiltrative disease of the atrium. Treatments include optimization of the patient's respiratory status, and reduction of sympathomimetic bronchodilators. Amiodarone may be helpful.

Atrial flutter

- Atrial flutter usually arises in the right atrium and utilizes a re-entrant circuit in the region of tissue between the inferior vena cava and the tricuspid annulus, known as the cavotricuspid isthmus.
  - » 'Typical' atrial flutter (Figure 7-14) is usually counter-clockwise around the tricuspid valve, resulting in negative 'flutter waves' in the inferior EKG leads (II, III, aVF).
  - » Atrial flutter involving other regions of the left and right atria is called 'atypical' atrial flutter (Figure 7-14).
  - » 'Typical' atrial flutter is more readily amenable to catheter ablation therapy.
- Atrial flutter usually occurs in the presence of underlying structural heart disease such as ischemic heart disease, cardiomyopathy, or valvular heart disease. It occasionally occurs in the apparently normal heart.
- Typical atrial flutter is recognized by the presence of a 'saw-tooth' pattern of the 'flutter waves' on the 12-lead EKG. Usually there is 2:1 block of the flutter complexes at the AV node, resulting in a ventricular rate of 130–150 beats/min. There may be variable conduction through the AV node, resulting in irregular QRS complexes.

CLINICAL PEARL

The typical 'saw-tooth' pattern of atrial flutter can be exposed with carotid sinus massage.

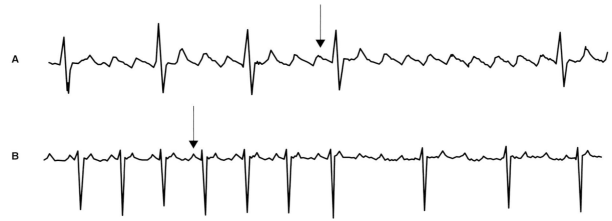

Figure 7-14 (**A**) Typical atrial flutter showing typical saw-tooth pattern in lead II and exposed by carotid sinus massage. (**B**) Atypical atrial flutter showing upright flutter waves in lead II

From Thompson P (ed). Coronary care manual, 2nd ed. Sydney: Elsevier Australia, 2011.

- The saw-tooth pattern may be obscured by the QRS complex and T wave, and therefore when assessing a patient with an unexplained tachyarrhythmia it is important to consider the possibility of atrial flutter. The typical saw-tooth pattern on the EKG can be frequently demonstrated by increasing the degree of atrioventricular block with vagal maneuvers such as carotid sinus massage.

CLINICAL PEARL

The atrial flutter pattern can be obscured by the T wave of the preceding beat; atrial flutter is a masquerader and should be considered in every case of unexplained tachycardia.

Management

- Intravenous AV nodal blocking agents may achieve slowing of the heart rate.
- Amiodarone is effective in slowing AV conduction and may achieve reversion to sinus rhythm, but the rate of reversion to sinus rhythm is variable.
- Intravenous ibutilide achieves high rates of reversion to sinus rhythm, but with a risk of inducing polymorphic ventricular tachycardia, and should be avoided in patients with structural heart disease or a long QT interval.
- If the patient is unstable, it is preferable to restore sinus rhythm as soon as possible with synchronized DC cardioversion. Alternatively, reversion of atrial flutter can be achieved with rapid overdrive atrial pacing.
- Left atrial thrombus can occur in atrial flutter, and the same precautions to avoid thromboembolism should be followed as for atrial fibrillation (see below).
- Typical atrial flutter is usually easily amenable to catheter ablation, with a success rate of approximately 90%

and a low complication rate. Atypical atrial flutter can also be treated with catheter ablation, although with a lower rate of success.

Atrial fibrillation (AF)

- Atrial fibrillation is the most common sustained cardiac arrhythmia, with a prevalence of 1–2% of the general population, 5% of patients aged 60–74 years, and approximately 10% of patients aged over 75 years.
- Atrial fibrillation can be classified as *paroxysmal* (AF terminates spontaneously or is cardioverted within 7 days), *persistent* (episodes of continuous AF that last >7 days and do not self-terminate, including episodes that are cardioverted after 7 days or more), *longstanding persistent* (AF lasting for 1 year when it is decided to adopt a rhythm control strategy) and *permanent* (when the physician and patient accept the presence of AF and stop further attempts to restore or maintain sinus rhythm). Should a rhythm–control strategy be adopted, the arrhythmia should be re-classified as 'longstanding persistent AF'.
- There have been considerable recent advances in understanding the mechanism of AF, and the recognition that the origin of AF is in the ostia of the pulmonary arteries and amenable to ablation has dramatically widened the therapeutic options.
- Atrial fibrillation is more likely to occur in patients with underlying heart disease, but 'lone' AF can also occur in patients without any demonstrable cardiac disease.
- An important consideration with AF is an increased risk of thrombus formation in the left atrial appendage and systemic thromboembolism.
  » The risk increases with increasing age, past history of stroke or transient ischemic attack (TIA), hypertension, cardiac failure and diabetes, summarized in two widely used scoring systems (see Table 7-13, below).

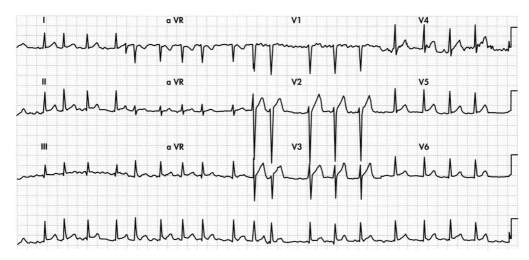

Figure 7-15 Typical example of atrial fibrillation, with rapid irregular ventricular response and absent P wave activity

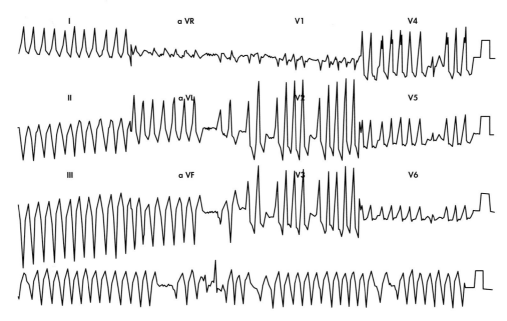

Figure 7-16 Very rapid atrial fibrillation with wide bizarre complexes in a patient with an atrioventricular accessory conduction pathway (Wolff–Parkinson–White syndrome). Digoxin can accelerate the abnormal conduction and should be avoided

- P waves are not visible on the EKG (Figure 7-15) and are replaced by fibrillation waves on the baseline. The ventricular response is usually irregular, due to varying degrees of conduction of the atrial fibrillation into the AV node.

CLINICAL PEARL

The irregularity of the ventricular response in AF is a more reliable EKG sign than attempting to see fibrillation waves.

- An important variant of AF is rapid conduction with aberration (wide QRS complexes; Figure 7-16). This may indicate AF with Wolff–Parkinson–White syndrome, indicating a high-risk situation which should not be treated with digoxin or calcium-channel blockers.

Management

- The treatment of atrial fibrillation is directed at:
  » slowing the ventricular response
  » achieving reversion to normal sinus rhythm if possible

- » reducing the frequency and hemodynamic effects of subsequent atrial fibrillation
- » preventing further episodes
- » reducing the risk of stroke.
- In recent-onset AF, a significant number of patients will revert to sinus rhythm spontaneously.
- If there is significant hemodynamic compromise, urgent DC cardioversion should be considered.
- The ventricular rate can be slowed with beta-blockers or (non-dihydropyridine) calcium-channel blockers if the increased cardiac rate is causing problems, or digoxin or amiodarone.
- If reversion to sinus rhythm does not occur when the heart rate has been slowed, cardioversion should be considered. Although there are no clear data to guide clinical practice, cardioversion is thought to have a negligible risk of thromboembolism if performed within 48 hours of onset.

CLINICAL PEARL

Synchronized cardioversion can usually be performed within 48 hours of onset of atrial fibrillation with minimal risk of thromboembolism.

- In patients not on any anticoagulants, on presentation, it is usual practice to commence anticoagulation prior to cardioversion, with intravenous heparin or subcutaneous enoxaparin, and then commence oral anticoagulation depending on thromboembolic risk.
- If more than 48 hours have passed since the onset of AF or the time since onset is uncertain, an alternative approach is to commence oral anticoagulation and arrange elective DC cardioversion after at least 3 weeks of formal anticoagulation.
  - » If it is preferable to restore sinus rhythm sooner, a transesophageal echocardiogram (TEE) can be performed to exclude thrombus in the left atrium prior to cardioversion of the fully anticoagulated patient.
  - » Due to the possibility of left atrial stasis with slow return of atrial contractility, it is currently recommended that anticoagulation be continued for at least 3 weeks after DC cardioversion.
  - » Patients with paroxysmal atrial fibrillation who revert spontaneously or with pharmacological treatment after an episode longer than 48 hours previously should also be anticoagulated for at least 3 weeks.
- For **long-term management**, the decision to use antiarrhythmic drugs and repeated cardioversion to attempt to maintain sinus rhythm ('rhythm control' approach) versus controlling the rate to minimize symptoms ('rate control' approach) requires a careful and individualized analysis of the likely risk–benefit ratio for each patient. The risk factors for recurrence of AF should be controlled if possible. These include: obesity, hypertension. obstructive sleep apnea and excess alcohol consumption.
  - » Recent studies comparing prognosis with rhythm control versus rate control concluded that rate control is equivalent in patients with minimal or no symptoms.

- » Exceptions to the rate control approach include younger symptomatic patients and those with complicated atrial fibrillation (stroke or cardiomyopathy). In these patients, rhythm control, including by catheter ablation, should be considered.

CLINICAL PEARL

The 'rate control' and 'rhythm control' approaches to managing atrial fibrillation have similar long-term prognoses.

- In addition to repeated cardioversion, drugs which may be considered for **rhythm control** include beta-blockers, calcium-channel blockers, class I antiarrhythmics (flecainide, propafenone), and class III antiarrhythmics (amiodarone, dofetilide, ibutilide).
  - » Flecainide is successful for reversion, less so for maintenance of sinus rhythm; it cannot be prescribed for patients with significant coronary heart disease or LV dysfunction.
  - » Propafenone has been used for reversion of AF but a risk of provoking ventricular arrythmias (proarrythmia) has limited its use.
  - » Amiodarone is effective in preventing recurrences, but long-term administration is fraught with a high risk of complications.
  - » Dofetilide has been used for reversion and maintenance of AF, and ibutilide for reversion of AF. Both have a risk of proarrhythmia.
  - » Sotalol is an attractive alternative, with beta-blocker and type II effects, but the development of proarrhythmia, particularly in the elderly with impaired renal function, can be a serious drawback.
- Vernakalant is a new drug with a high rate of success for reversion of acute AF, and with minimal risk of proarrhythmia.
- Drugs which may be considered for **rate control** include beta blockers (preferable), digoxin and calcium-channel blockers.
  - » Digoxin is widely used for rate control and is effective for control of the rate at rest, but is less effective with exercise and with stress. It may be preferable to combine it with a beta-blocker.

Anticoagulation decisions

The decision-making process for deciding on anticoagulation to reduce the risk of stroke with antithrombotic therapy can be challenging.

CLINICAL PEARL

Atrial fibrillation is an important cause of stroke, and all patients should be considered for anticoagulation based on their risk profile.

- Antithrombotic therapy is effective in reducing the risk of stroke, but at the expense of bleeding.
  - » Until recently, warfarin has been the most effective agent for reduction of risk of stroke.

» The recommended INR (international normalized ratio) range for warfarin therapy in non-valvular AF is 2.0–3.0.

» Recent comparisons of warfarin with novel oral anticoagulants (NOACs), including dabigatran, rivaroxaban, apixaban and edoxaban, have shown that each of the newer agents is at least equivalent to warfarin in antithrombotic effect, with lower risks of bleeding the advantage of avoiding the need for frequent INR monitoring. NOACs are now the preferred first choice for oral anticoagulation in AF, except in patients with mechanical heart valves or high-grade mitral stenosis.

- The decision to commence antithrombotic therapy is based on consideration of the risk of stroke, the likely risk of bleeding, and a range of other factors including the patient's likely adherence and comorbidities.

  » The patient's risk of stroke can be assessed from consideration of the CHA_2DS_2-VASc or CHA_2DS_2-VA scores (Table 7-13, below).

  » Patients with a CHA_2DS_2-VASc or CHA_2DS_2-VA score of ≥1 should be anticoagulated.

  » The bleeding risk should always be considered before commencing oral anticoagulation. Several bleeding risk scores have been published and validated but are not widely used in practice.

  » Increasingly, patients with coronary stents and atrial fibrillation require dual antiplatelet therapy (DAPT) with aspirin and a P2Y12 inhibitor and an oral anticoagulant (OAC). These patients have a high risk of bleeding and their exposure to the combination of DAPT and OAC (triple therapy) should be as short as possible—usually not more than 4 weeks.

» Aspirin has been shown to be less effective than warfarin in the prevention of stroke.

CLINICAL PEARL

The CHA_2DS_2-VASc and the CHA_2DS_2-VA scores are the recommended scoring systems in all modern AF guidelines.

- **Atrial appendage occlusion devices** designed to reduce the risk of thromboembolism can be inserted percutaneously to isolate the left atrial appendage. These devices are only considered in patients who are considered at high risk of thromboembolism, and who cannot tolerate anticoagulation. They can reduce the risk of stroke, but their role needs to be better defined with longer follow-up.

Ablation therapy (pulmonary vein isolation and related procedures)

Catheter ablation of the ostia of the pulmonary veins isolates the atrial fibrillation trigger, and (in selected cases) substrate modification is also performed within the atria.

- Catheter ablation is beneficial for patients with symptomatic paroxysmal or persistent AF who have not responded to antiarrhythmic drug therapy.
- In experienced centers, AF ablation can be considered as an alternative to antiarrhythmic drugs.
- AF ablation may improve prognosis in patients with combined AF and heart failure.
- Success rates of 70–85% can be expected in patients with paroxysmal AF in experienced, high-volume

Table 7-13 Comparison of the CHA_2DS_2-VA and CHA_2DS_2-VASc scores for assessing the risk of stroke in a patient with atrial fibrillation

STROKE RISK FACTOR	CHA₂DS₂-VASc SCORE	STROKE RISK FACTOR	CHA₂DS₂-VA SCORE (THE SEXLESS CHA₂DS₂VASc SCORE)
Cardiac failure	1	**C**ardiac failure	1
Hypertension	1	**H**ypertension	1
Age	1 (65–74 y) 2 (>75 y)	**A**ge	2 (>75 y)
Diabetes	1	**D**iabetes	1
Stroke/TIA, systemic embolism	2	**S**troke/TIA, systemic embolism	2
Sex	1 (female)	**S**ex	
Vascular disease	1	**V**ascular disease	1
		Age	1 (65–74 y)
Maximum score	9	**Maximum score**	9

TIA, transient ischemic attack.

Definitions for the Scores are described in detail in NHFA CSANZ Atrial Fibrillation Guideline Working Group, 2018. Heart Lung Circ. 2018;27:1209–66.

centers, but often a second or third procedure is needed to completely abolish AF.

- Persistent or permanent AF is less successfully treated with catheter ablation.
- Following ablation, most authorities recommend indefinite anticoagulation after ablation because of the risk of AF recurrence.

CLINICAL PEARL

Catheter ablation can be highly effective in abolishing atrial fibrillation, but the patient needs to be warned of the risk of recurrence, and advised that a 'course' of treatments may be needed.

Ablation of the His bundle with implantation of a permanent ventricular or biventricular pacemaker may achieve rate control of AF in patients who are highly symptomatic and intolerant of medications and not responding to AF ablation.

Lifestyle measures

There is increasing evidence that lifestyle measures including weight loss, exercise and alcohol restriction can reduce the frequency of recurrences of paroxysmal or persistent AF.

Ventricular arrhythmias

Ventricular ectopic beats (VEBs)

Ventricular ectopic beats arise from enhanced automaticity or localized re-entry circuits in the ventricles.

- Specific treatment of asymptomatic VEBs is generally not necessary. Possible contributing factors such as cardiac stimulants, electrolyte disturbance and myocardial ischemia should be corrected.
- In patients who are troubled with symptomatic VEBs, administration of oral beta-blocking drugs may be effective in reducing the frequency and the patient's awareness of the irregular heart rhythm, especially when there is associated anxiety or evidence of excess circulating catecholamines.
- Antiarrhythmic drug therapy is best avoided for this largely benign rhythm disturbance.
- Rarely, frequent VEBs (more than 5000 per day) may affect cardiac function and need to be considered for ablation of the arrhythmic focus in the myocardium.

CLINICAL PEARL

Ventricular ectopic beats are almost always benign, but can be frustratingly symptomatic and patients frequently need a lot of support. Ablation may be very effective for patients with incessantly frequent ectopics. It is definitely indicated if left ventricular dysfunction has supervened.

Ventricular tachycardia (VT)

- Ventricular tachycardia is a tachyarrhythmia arising in either the right or the left ventricle:

  » VT is usually due to a re-entrant circuit in a damaged heart. Processes such as chronic myocardial infarction, or cardiomyopathy which causes myocardial damage and scar may lead to VT.
  » VT may also occur in patients with arrhythmogenic right ventricular cardiomyopathy.
  » Accelerated idioventricular rhythm may occur due to disturbed automaticity in damaged Purkinje fibers in acute myocardial infarction.
  » VT may also occur in patients with an otherwise normal heart with congenital abnormalities of ion channels, including long QT and Brugada syndromes.

- Heart rates in VT may range from 100–300 beats/min.
- Multiple morphologies of VT and varying rates of VT commonly occur in an individual patient.
  » **Non-sustained VT** has a better prognosis than sustained VT.
  » As a general rule, salvos of a few ventricular beats are not treated as VT.
  » **Sustained VT** (lasting at least 30 seconds) is the most important form of VT, in that it usually requires prompt intervention.
- Prolongation of the QT interval may be precipitated by a variety of drugs, and torsades de pointes may occur in susceptible individuals.
- Many so-called antiarrhythmic drugs may have proarrhythmic side-effects, particularly in patients with structural heart disease.

Diagnosis

- The clinical manifestations of VT can range from asymptomatic, to syncope, to sudden death.
- The EKG features of VT (Figure 7-17) are a regular tachycardia with broad QRS complexes. Frequently, P waves can be seen dissociated from the QRS complexes and this can be a useful clue that the arrhythmia is not a conducted supraventricular arrhythmia.
- The torsades de pointes variant of ventricular tachycardia commences as an early ventricular beat during repolarization (QT interval), and is rapid, polymorphic and frequently self-reverting.
- Accelerated idioventricular rhythm is a slow, regular, wide QRS complex at a rate exceeding the sinus rate.

CLINICAL PEARL

Identifying P wave activity independent of the QRS complex can be a valuable clue that the tachyarrhythmia is ventricular tachycardia.

Management

- For **initial treatment**, patients experiencing loss of consciousness from VT require immediate resuscitation, including early DC cardioversion/defibrillation.
- Due to the risk of proarrhythmia, antiarrhythmic drugs must be used cautiously. All predisposing and triggering

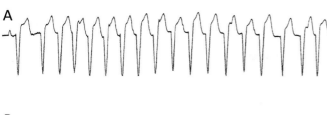

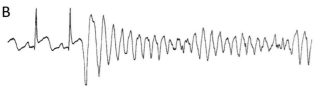

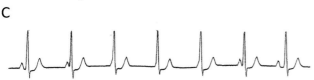

Figure 7-17 (**A**) Rapid, wide-complex tachycardia typical of ventricular tachycardia. (**B**) Torsades de pointes initiated by an ectopic beat on the T wave; has the potential to self-revert or deteriorate into ventricular fibrillation. (**C**) Accelerated idioventricular rhythm exceeding the sinus rate

From Thompson P (ed). Coronary care manual, 2nd ed. Sydney: Elsevier Australia, 2011.

factors should be addressed before considering administration of antiarrhythmic drugs.

» If antiarrhythmic drugs are needed, intravenous beta-blockers may be effective. Intravenous amiodarone (5 mg/kg) over 5–10 minutes may be used in patients with sustained VT and hemodynamic compromise if VT is refractory to DC cardioversion.

» Magnesium may be of benefit in patients with torsades de pointes, particularly if serum magnesium is low, but is not of benefit otherwise. Pacing at ~100/min may also be used to prevent torsades de pointes.

• For **long-term management**, first-line therapy for VT is implantation of an implantable cardioverter defibrillator (ICD). These devices can deliver a short burst of anti-tachycardia pacing, and have back-up defibrillation capability if there is a deterioration to ventricular fibrillation.

• Oral antiarrhythmic therapy is rarely used for maintenance treatment of VT, and usual treatment is with device therapy.

Ventricular fibrillation (VF)

Ventricular fibrillation is the usual cause of sudden death in ischemic heart disease. It is often preceded by short runs of polymorphic VT, which may spontaneously terminate; however, once VF is established, it is not self-terminating in the human heart. The patient with VF will rapidly lose consciousness. If left untreated, it will be fatal within minutes.

• The EKG shows a coarse irregular rhythm. 'Pseudo VF' patterns due to artifact, tremor, or a displaced electrode affecting the EKG should not be confused with VF, and are not associated with any change in conscious state.

• The only effective **management** is immediate, unsynchronized defibrillation with a DC shock of 200 joules (360 joules if monophasic defibrillator). If the cardiac arrest is witnessed it is reasonable to administer up to 3 maximum-energy DC shocks. If these prove ineffective, advanced cardiac life support is initiated.

CLINICAL PEARL

Ventricular fibrillation requires immediate defibrillation, even before CPR if possible.

CONDUCTION DEFECTS

Bundle branch block (BBB)

• Right and left bundle branch blocks are due to delayed conduction through the bundle branches or distal radicles of the conduction system. They can indicate underlying heart disease, but may be benign, particularly right bundle branch block.

• QRS notching and prolongation of <0.12 seconds is referred to as a *partial or incomplete* BBB if the EKG pattern is typical of right or left bundle branch block.

• Nonspecific widening of the QRS complex is referred to as an *intraventricular conduction defect* (IVCD).

• In BBB, the QRS complex is wide with duration >0.12 seconds (3 small squares) at the widest point.

» It is sometimes necessary to examine several different EKG leads to determine the maximum width of the QRS complex.

» The QRS appearances in lead V$_1$ can usually discriminate: a tall R with RSR′ pattern indicates a right bundle branch block; no tall R wave in V$_1$ indicates a left bundle branch block.

» Typical lead V$_1$ patterns are shown in Figure 7-18.

Right bundle branch block (RBBB)

• Right bundle branch block may have no prognostic significance, but may reflect right heart disease. If it is associated with left-axis deviation, it indicates more advanced conducting system disease (bifascicular block; see below).

• Right bundle branch block shows slurring and notching of the QRS, with widening >0.12 seconds, a dominant R wave in V$_1$ with a typical RSR pattern, and a slurred S wave in the lateral leads.

• Benign RBBB needs to be differentiated from the Brugada syndrome, which has a RBBB-like pattern with persistent ST-segment elevation (coved appearance) in the right precordial leads. This is associated with susceptibility to ventricular tachyarrhythmias, and sudden cardiac death.

• No **management** is necessary for RBBB except in the presence of bifascicular block and symptoms.

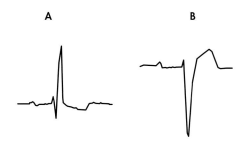

Figure 7-18 Comparison of right bundle branch and left bundle branch patterns in lead V_1. The QRS is upright with an RSR′ pattern in right bundle branch block (**A**) and downwards in left bundle branch block (**B**)

Patients with bifascicular block and syncope warrant further investigation and consideration of pacemaker implantation.

Left bundle branch block (LBBB)

- Left bundle branch block is usually associated with diffuse disease involving the left ventricle such as cardiomyopathy, ischemic heart disease, myocardial infarction or LV hypertrophy.
- On occasions it can be due to localized calcific or fibrotic disease in the conduction system and, like RBBB, can be intermittent. Sometimes it occurs at high heart rates e.g. during exercise—rate dependent LBBB.
- The QRS is prolonged, and measures >0.12 seconds. There is a small (or no) R wave in lead V_1 and slurring or notching of leads I, aVL and V_6. There is often left-axis deviation. The direction of the ST segment and T wave vectors is opposite to that of the QRS vector.

CLINICAL PEARL

The code for distinguishing RBBB from LBBB is: RSR′ in lead V_1 = RBBB.

- **Management** is directed toward the underlying cardiac problem.

Fascicular blocks (hemiblocks)

The intraventricular conduction system consists of three fascicles.

- Involvement of the anterior/superior division of the left bundle will produce a left anterior fascicular block (hemiblock).
- Involvement of the posterior/inferior division of the left bundle will produce a left posterior fascicular block (hemiblock).

Left anterior fascicular block (left anterior hemiblock)

The QRS complex may not be widened, but the main frontal axis will be directed leftward to greater than −30°, i.e. the QRS complex will be positive in lead I, negative in lead III, and predominantly negative in lead II.

Left anterior fascicular block by itself requires no treatment, but it is often associated with comorbidities and may indicate a risk of atrioventricular block if associated with RBBB (bifascicular block).

Left posterior fascicular block (left posterior hemiblock)

In left posterior hemiblock the conduction through the posterior/inferior division of the left bundle is affected. It is less common than anterior fascicular block.

Bifascicular block

- The combination of RBBB with left anterior hemiblock is referred to as *bifascicular block*. In this situation, depolarization of the left ventricle is solely via the left posterior/inferior division of the left bundle and cardiac conduction becomes less reliable.
- There is a low risk of developing high-grade atrioventricular (AV) block in a stable patient with bifascicular block, but in circumstances where further stresses on the cardiac conduction system are possible, such as myocardial ischemia, infarction, general anesthesia or surgery, cardiac pacing may be necessary.
- When bifascicular block is associated with a long PR interval this is often called *trifascicular block* and indicates more severe conduction system disease and significant risk of complete atrioventricular block.

CLINICAL PEARL

Right bundle branch block with left-axis deviation (left anterior hemiblock) indicates the presence of conduction system disease, and the risk of complete atrioventricular block.

Atrioventricular (AV) blocks

- Atrioventricular block can occur as a result of conduction delay in the AV node, bundle of His, or the bundle branches.
- Usually AV block with a narrow QRS complex indicates delay in the AV node, whereas AV block with associated bundle branch block indicates disease below the bundle of His in the ventricular conduction system.

First-degree AV block

Prolongation of the PR interval >0.2 seconds (5 small squares) constitutes first-degree AV block.

If the first-degree AV block is drug-induced, withdrawal or dosage reduction of the drug causing AV conduction delay is the only management necessary. Future administration of these drugs should be avoided.

Second-degree AV block

- Second-degree AV block can occur as a result of delay through the AV node, or in the His–Purkinje system. Delays in the AV node characteristically show the

Wenckebach phenomenon, whereas block at the level of the His–Purkinje system characteristically does not.

- The two types of second-degree AV block are referred to as *Mobitz types I and II*.
  - » **Type I block** is more commonly referred to as Wenckebach AV block; there is gradual prolongation of the PR interval, leading eventually to a dropped beat before the cycle restarts. It may be due to drugs affecting AV node function, and may be self-limiting. Permanent pacing is usually not necessary.
  - » In **type II block** there is no lengthening of the PR interval prior to the sudden loss of AV conduction. It is associated with disease of the conduction system, and requires a permanent pacemaker. The risk of developing complete AV block and syncope is high.

Third-degree (complete) AV block

In third-degree (complete) AV block there is no conduction of atrial impulses to the ventricle, which maintains its rhythm by a junctional or ventricular escape rhythm.

- The clinical features depend primarily on the rate of the ventricular escape rhythm. Rates below 40/min are frequently associated with syncope or near-syncope.
- The EKG abnormality is readily recognized, with total dissociation of the P waves and QRS complexes. The QRS complexes are usually regular. On occasion there may be partial AV conduction, producing fusion beats between the conducted QRS and the ventricular escape beat.

Patients with symptomatic AV block require cardiac pacing.

- If there is a correctable cause such as myocardial infarction or drug toxicity, temporary pacing may suffice, but usually permanent pacing is required. Transcutaneous (external) pacing can be used in an emergency.

> **CLINICAL PEARL**
>
> Pacing is the only effective treatment for symptomatic complete AV block. Drug treatments are ineffective.

CARDIAC FAILURE

Overall, cardiac failure (congestive heart failure, CHF) occurs in 1.5–2.0% of the population in Western communities, with marked racial and community differences. The incidence and prevalence rises markedly with age, with CHF occurring approximately in <1% in people aged below 60 years, 10% in people aged over 65, and >50% in people aged over 85 years in Western countries. It is one of the most common reasons for hospital admission and doctor consultation in people aged 70 and older.

Definition

The diagnosis of CHF requires both clinical features and an objective measure of abnormal ventricular function, as outlined in the definition reproduced in Box 7-2.

- **Heart Failure with reduced Ejection Fraction, HFrEF** (also known as systolic heart failure) refers to a weakened ability of the heart to contract in systole

---

> **Box 7-2**
>
> **Definition of cardiac failure**
>
> Heart failure is a complex clinical syndrome that can result from any structural or functional cardiac disorder that impairs the ability of the ventricle to fill with or eject blood.
>
> It is a syndrome in which the patients should have the following features: symptoms of heart failure, typically breathlessness or fatigue, either at rest or during exertion, or ankle swelling and objective evidence of cardiac dysfunction at rest.
>
> European Task Force on Heart Failure, 2005. Adapted from Byrne J, Davie AP and McMurray JJV. Clinical assessment and investigation of patients with suspected heart failure. In Stewart S, Moser DK and Thompson DR (eds). Caring for the heart failure patient. London: Martin Dunnitz, 2004.

and an left ventricular ejection fraction of <40% on echocardiography. It remains the most common cause of CHF but there is increasing recognition of HFpEF as a cause of CHF. This reflects the prevalence of coronary heart disease (CHD) in the Western world, although hypertension is still a significant contributor to systolic heart failure. Other important causes include cardiomyopathies.

- **Heart Failure with preserved Ejection Fraction, HFpEF** (also known as heart failure with preserved systolic function), or **diastolic heart failure**, refers to the clinical syndrome of heart failure due to impaired diastolic filling of the left ventricle, with or without impaired systolic contraction. It is more common in the elderly. Ischemia, LV hypertrophy from hypertension, age-related fibrosis, diabetes, and cardiac infiltration may all act to impair diastolic filling of the heart.

Causes

While the clinical manifestations may closely resemble each other, the causes of systolic and diastolic heart failure differ. The common, less common and uncommon causes of systolic and HFpEF heart failure are summarized in Boxes 7-3 and 7-4.

Diagnosis of congestive heart failure

Symptoms and signs

- Symptoms of cardiac failure include exertional dyspnea, orthopnea and paroxysmal nocturnal dyspnea (PND).
- A dry, irritating cough may occur, particularly at night, and this may be difficult to distinguish from asthma or bronchitis. A therapeutic trial of diuretic therapy may be useful in these patients.
- Symptoms related to fluid retention, such as abdominal distension, ascites, and sacral and peripheral edema, occur when there is associated right heart failure. Fatigue and weakness may be prominent.
- Patients with CHF may show no abnormal physical signs, as these are often a late manifestation of cardiac

Box 7-3

Causes of HFrEF (systolic heart failure)

Common
- Coronary heart disease and prior myocardial infarction

Less common
- Non-ischemic idiopathic dilated cardiomyopathy

Uncommon
- Valvular heart disease, especially mitral and aortic incompetence
- Non-ischemic dilated cardiomyopathy secondary to long-term alcohol misuse
- Inflammatory cardiomyopathy, or myocarditis
- Chronic arrhythmia
- Thyroid dysfunction (hyperthyroidism, hypothyroidism)
- HIV-related cardiomyopathy
- Drug-induced cardiomyopathy, especially anthracyclines (daunorubicin, doxorubicin)
- Peripartum cardiomyopathy

Box 7-4

Causes of HFpEF (diastolic heart failure)

Common
- Hypertension
- Coronary heart disease
- Diabetes
- Advanced age

Less common
- Valvular disease, particularly aortic stenosis

Uncommon causes
- Hypertrophic cardiomyopathy
- Restrictive cardiomyopathy, either idiopathic or infiltrative, such as amyloidosis

HFpEF, heart failure with preserved ejection fraction; HFrEF, heart failure with reduced ejection fraction.

Table 7-14 NYHA classification of cardiac failure severity

GRADE	SYMPTOMS
I	No symptoms and no limitation in ordinary physical activity, e.g. shortness of breath when walking, climbing stairs, etc.
II	Mild symptoms (mild shortness of breath and/or angina) and slight limitation during ordinary activity
III	Marked limitation in activity due to symptoms, even during less-than-ordinary activity, e.g. walking short distances (20–100 m). Comfortable only at rest
IV	Severe limitations. Experiences symptoms even while at rest. Mostly bedbound patients

The Criteria Committee of the New York Heart Association (NYHA). Nomenclature and Criteria for Diagnosis of Diseases of the Heart and Great Vessels, 9th ed. Boston, Mass: Little, Brown & Co; 1994:253–6.

CLINICAL PEARL

Clinical diagnosis of congestive heart failure may be challenging, and drug therapy can cause confusion. Beware cough which can be caused by angiotensin-converting enzyme inhibitors, edema by dihydropyridine calcium-channel blockers, and dyspnea and reduced exercise capacity by beta-blockers.

It is standard practice to grade the severity of cardiac failure using an internationally recognized grading system; the most widely used being the New York Heart Association (NYHA) grades summarized in Table 7-14.

Electrocardiogram

Abnormalities on the EKG include nonspecific ST-segment and T wave changes. Conduction abnormalities, including intraventricular conduction delays or LBBB, signs of previous infarction, or LV hypertrophy may be seen.

Chest X-ray

A normal chest X-ray does not exclude the diagnosis, but confirmatory signs of pulmonary congestion with upper lobe diversion may help to distinguish the cause of dyspnea from respiratory causes. Evidence of interstitial edema with pleural effusions or septal lines further confirms that the cause of dyspnea is due to cardiac failure.

Echocardiography

All modern guidelines for assessing patients with cardiac failure recommend that patients with suspected CHF should have an echocardiogram.
- The echocardiogram can distinguish between HFrEF and HFpEF.

failure, and on occasion the diagnosis must be made on the history alone.
- Signs of fluid retention may be present, including basal inspiratory crackles which do not clear with coughing, and increased resting respiratory rate.
- Signs of right heart failure include raised jugular venous pressure (JVP), ankle and sacral edema, ascites or tender hepatomegaly.
- On auscultation, a 3rd heart sound may be audible.
- Clinical signs of LV dysfunction or enlargement may be present, including a displaced apex beat, or a murmur may indicate underlying valvular heart disease.

» HFrEF is present when the ejection fraction is reduced. There is incomplete agreement on a cut-off for the lower level of LVEF, but a measurement below 50% makes systolic dysfunction likely, and a measurement below 40% is definite HFrEF. Patients with LVEF between 40 and 50% may be referred to as HFmEF (heart failure with mid range ejection fraction).

» LV diastolic function is diagnosed from estimation of filling pressures via transmitral and pulmonary venous pulsed-wave Doppler and tissue Doppler studies. More recently, strain measurements have made the recognition of diastolic dysfunction more reliable.

- Identification of valvular heart disease is an added benefit of echocardiography and the extent of mitral regurgitation can be measured. This is of importance in patients with advanced CHF, some of whom may respond to correction of the mitral regurgitation.

CLINICAL PEARL

All patients with cardiac failure should have echocardiography to identify the extent of systolic dysfunction, and distinguish HFrEF from HFpEF, and identify correctable valvular heart disease.

- Gated radionuclide measurement of LV function can provide a reliable estimate of LVEF, but has been largely supplanted by echocardiography for this purpose.

Hematology and biochemistry

- Mild anemia may occur in patients with CHF, and is associated with an adverse prognosis.
- Measurement of plasma urea, creatinine and electrolytes provide a simple index of renal function, and this should be performed in all patients.
- Iron deficiency, even when the Hb is normal, exacerbates heart failure and iron studies should be considered for these patients.
- In advanced CHF, dilutional hyponatremia can occur. Diuretic therapy may also affect sodium levels. Persistent hyponatremia may indicate a loss of homeostasis and indicate a poor prognosis.
- Hyperkalemia may occur with impaired renal function, especially in the presence of ACEIs, aldosterone antagonists or aggressive diuretic therapy. Hypokalemia can occur with thiazide or loop diuretics.
- Congestive hepatomegaly may cause abnormal liver function tests, and hypoalbuminemia, potentially indicating cardiac cirrhosis, may occur with longstanding CHF.

Natriuretic peptides

Plasma levels of brain-type natriuretic peptide (BNP) indicate the severity of CHF.

- Both BNP and N-terminal proBNP levels have been shown to predict all-cause mortality, including death from pump failure and sudden death; however, BNP and N-terminal proBNP levels vary with age, gender and renal function.
- Measurement of BNP or N-terminal proBNP is not recommended as routine in the diagnosis of CHF, but is particularly useful for clarifying whether dyspnea is due to CHF or to respiratory causes. A normal BNP (100 ng/L) or N-terminal proBNP (<300 ng/L) level makes the diagnosis of heart failure unlikely.
- The natriuretic peptides have not been helpful in monitoring the treatment of cardiac failure.

Treatment

The dual aims for treatment of cardiac failure are to relieve symptoms and improve prognosis.

Symptom relief

Fluid and salt management

The most prominent symptoms in cardiac failure are due to fluid retention. Careful monitoring of salt and fluid intake can be sufficient in many patients to control these symptoms without recourse to diuretics.

- For patients with mild symptoms (NYHA grade II or less), limiting sodium intake to 3 g/day assists with control of fluid balance.
- For patients with moderate to severe symptoms (NYHA grade III/IV) and requiring diuretics, a restricted sodium intake of <2 g/day should be applied.
- In most patients with cardiac failure, a fluid intake of less than 1.5 L/day is recommended. If symptomatic fluid retention is obvious, fluid intake should be restricted to <1.5 L/day.
- Fluid restrictions should be liberalized in warmer weather to avoid dehydration and hypotension.

CLINICAL PEARL

Daily weighing is an important discipline in heart failure management. A weight gain of more than 2 kg in 2 days is a reason to increase diuretic therapy.

Diuretics

Diuretics are an essential tool in managing symptoms of cardiac failure, although they have not been shown to improve survival. Diuretics increase urine sodium excretion and can rapidly decrease the symptoms and physical signs of fluid retention.

- In fluid-overloaded patients, treatment is usually initiated with a loop diuretic (e.g. furosemide 40–80 mg/day) until edema and relief of dyspnea is achieved. The diuretic dose should be decreased when symptoms and signs indicate euvolemia.
- Thiazide diuretics are an alternative in patients who find the rapid diuresis with loop diuretics unappealing.
- Occasionally loop and thiazide diuretics can be combined, but this requires careful monitoring of response to avoid hypovolemia and hypokalemia.
- Long-term use of loop and thiazide diuretics may also contribute to magnesium depletion, potentially contributing to cardiac arrhythmias.

- In patients with persistent fluid retention, especially when right heart failure and hepatic congestion and ascites are prominent, addition of an aldosterone antagonist, e.g. spironolactone, may be helpful. Aldosterone antagonists, particularly in combination with ACEIs, can increase the risk of renal dysfunction and hyperkalemia.

Angiotensin-converting enzyme inhibitors (ACEIs) and angiotensin-receptor blockers (ARBs)

These have a mild diuretic effect and can contribute to symptom relief.

Digoxin and other inotropic agents

- Oral digoxin and its digitalis predecessors have been used for more than 200 years in the symptomatic treatment of cardiac failure. In the past few decades, however, it has been established that its role in the patient in sinus rhythm is limited, and its inotropic effect may not be helpful. Despite this, low-dose digoxin may have a role in the management of the patient with advanced cardiac failure in which other therapies are not controlling symptoms.
- Other oral inotropic agents have been used, but the apparent logic of enhancing contractility of the failing heart has not translated into clinical benefit, and their use is now abandoned because of adverse effects on outcomes.
- In selected patients with severe decompensated heart failure, short-term use of intravenous inotropic agents may have a role in improving symptoms.
  » Dobutamine can be used for short-term support, and may achieve clinical stability (a dobutamine holiday).
  » Levosimendan is a calcium-sensitizing inotropic agent possibly superior to dobutamine, but its use may be limited by hypotension in some patients.

Improving prognosis in systolic heart failure

An improved understanding of the pathophysiology of the failing heart has led to substantial advances in treatment over the past 30 years. The primary paradigm of therapy has advanced from attempting to improve contractility with inotropic agents to blocking the adverse neurohumoral response to heart failure.

Renin–angiotensin–aldosterone system (RAAS) blockade

Inhibition of the RAAS and the use of angiotensin-converting enzyme inhibitors (ACEIs) or angiotensin II receptor blockers (ARBs) are central to the management of systolic heart failure.

- ACEIs have been shown in large randomized clinical trials to prolong survival and reduce the need for hospitalization in patients with moderate to severe heart failure (NYHA grades II–IV), and to moderately increase ejection fraction.
- All patients with systolic heart failure should be started on a low dose of ACEIs if tolerated, and the dose increased if possible.

- Angiotensin-receptor blockers (ARBs) are generally better tolerated and are an alternative for patients who experience ACEI-related adverse effects, such as a cough.
- ACEIs and ARBs in heart failure show similar outcomes in comparative trials. Combinations of ACEIs and ARBs have been trialed, but may have adverse effects on renal function.

CLINICAL PEARL

Multiple trials have shown that angiotensin-converting enzyme inhibitors (ACEIs) and beta-blockers are the ideal combination to improve prognosis in cardiac failure. Angiotensin-receptor blockers (ARBs) can be substituted if there is ACEI intolerance.

Beta-adrenergic blockade

- Beta-blockers inhibit the adverse effects of chronic activation of the sympathetic nervous system, and its adverse effects on the myocardium. Although the benefits of beta-blockade may be a class effect, only four beta-blockers have been shown to improve prognosis in clinical trials. The unique properties of these drugs and their usual doses are summarized in Table 7-15.
- Beta-blockers should be started cautiously, especially in patients who are hypotensive or recently decompensated. They should be started at low doses with gradual increases, to limit adverse effects of hypotension, bradycardia and reduced cardiac contractility.
- Clinical trials have shown no difference in outcomes with the order of commencing ACEIs (ARBs) and beta-blockers in heart failure.

CLINICAL PEARL

While the benefits of beta-blockade in cardiac failure may be a class effect, only carvedilol, bisoprolol, extended-release metoprolol and nebivolol have been shown to be effective in randomized clinical trials.

Mineralocorticoid receptor antagonists (MRAs)

- Aldosterone can promote fibrosis, hypertrophy and arrhythmogenesis in the failing heart, and antagonism of these effects with spironolactone provides benefit.
- Spironolactone reduces all-cause mortality and results in symptomatic improvement in patients with advanced CHF. The usual starting dose is 25 mg/day, increasing gradually to 50 mg twice a day.
  » There is a risk of hyperkalemia with higher doses, particularly in the presence of ACEIs and/or renal impairment.
  » The use of spironolactone is also limited by the development of gynecomastia.
- Eplerenone, a more selective aldosterone antagonist without feminizing effects, has been found to reduce

Table 7-15 Beta-blockers shown in clinical trials to be effective in improving outcomes in cardiac failure

DRUGS	UNIQUE PROPERTIES	USUAL DOSE
Bisoprolol	Cardio (beta-1) selective	2.5–10 mg once daily
Carvedilol	Non-cardio (beta-1) selective, vasodilating alpha-blocker effect, antioxidant	2.5–25 mg twice daily
Metoprolol	Cardio (beta 1) selective	Succinate (XL preparation) 25–100 mg once daily
Nebivolol	Non-cardioselective, vasodilating effect mediated by the endothelial nitrous oxide pathway	5 mg once daily
XL, extended-release.		

mortality in patients with LV systolic dysfunction and symptoms of heart failure.

Angiotensin receptor neprilysin inhibitor

The combination of the ARB valsartan and the neprilysin inhibitor saccubutril has been shown to improve outcomes in patients with HFrEF with persistent symptoms despite ACEI and beta-blocker therapy. This heralds a new class of heart failure drug, the angiotensin receptor neprilysin inhibitors (ARNIs).

- ARNIs are contraindicated with concomitant ACEIs and the ACEI should be stopped 48 hours before commencing an ARNI.
- The ARNI should be started at moderate dose and uptitrated by doubling the dose every 2–4 weeks, monitoring symptoms, blood pressure and renal function.

Direct sinus-node inhibition

As beta-blockers may improve heart failure outcomes with heart rate slowing, an alternative method of heart rate slowing with the sinus-node inhibitor ivabradine has been trialled and shown to reduce cardiovascular mortality and heart failure hospitalization in patients with heart rates above 70/min; this drug may be a useful alternative to beta-blockade.

Improving prognosis in heart failure with preserved ejection fraction (HFpEF)

- In contrast to the many proven treatments in systolic heart failure, there have not been any convincing drugs to improve outcomes in HFpEF (see Box 7-4, above).
- Trials of ARBs, MRAs and calcium-channel blockers have shown no benefit.

Devices

Implantable cardioverter-defibrillator (ICD)

- Patients with cardiac failure and LV dysfunction are prone to high-grade, potentially lethal arrhythmias such as ventricular tachycardia and ventricular fibrillation.
- Implantation of an ICD is associated with a 20–30% relative reduction in mortality at 1 year, with improved survival maintained over subsequent years.

- Benefits have also been shown in patients with LV dysfunction without overt cardiac failure.
- Current guidelines recommend implantation of an ICD in cardiac failure patients with LVEF <35%.
- Many patients are untroubled by the implantation of the ICD and appreciate the security of knowing that they have received a lifesaving device. However, ICDs are expensive and can worsen quality of life, particularly in patients experiencing frequent painful shocks.

Biventricular pacing—cardiac resynchronization therapy (CRT)

- Patients with symptomatic dilated heart failure may have asynchronous contraction of the left ventricle. A widened QRS complex (>120 ms) may be an electrocardiographic marker of this. There is more evidence of benefit for LBBB than RBBB and the wider the QRS the more likely there is to be benefit.
- Systolic function is improved by pacing simultaneously in the left and right ventricles (bi-ventricular pacing, not to be confused with dual chamber pacing which refers to pacing the right atrium and right ventricle). This can improve symptoms and frequency of hospitalization in patients with symptomatic dilated CHF and prolonged QRS duration, and a mortality benefit of biventricular pacing in patients with heart failure has also been shown.
- The improvement in prognosis is greater when cardiac resynchronization therapy (CRT) is combined with ICD, compared with ICD alone.

> **CLINICAL PEARL**
>
> Implantable cardioverter-defibrillator devices are indicated in patients with cardiac failure and LVEF <35%. Cardiac resynchronization therapy is beneficial when the QRS complex is widened to >120 ms.

Left ventricular assist devices (LVADs)

The use of LVADs to assist or replace LV function is now well established as a temporary bridge to cardiac transplantation.

With improving technology and the development of continuous flow devices with fewer moving parts, the prospect of LVADs as destination (permanent) therapy is feasible, but not yet widely available.

INFECTIVE ENDOCARDITIS

- The incidence of infective endocarditis varies greatly between different populations and systems of medical care, and ranges from 3 to 10 episodes/100,000 person-years.
  - » The profile of endocarditis has changed in recent years from a condition largely affecting young people with rheumatic valve disease, to now occurring more frequently in older persons, especially those with prosthetic valves or degenerative valve conditions.
  - » The changing profile has been associated with a change in the pathogenic organisms. While streptococcal endocarditis has been the most common cause in the past, there is an increasing prevalence of staphylococcal endocarditis and more exotic bacteria and fungi, particularly among immunocompromised patients and intravenous drug users.
- The infection may be confined to superficial involvement of the valve leaflets, but can erode the valve tissue and cause valve perforation, and involve the paravalvular structures with the formation of paravalvular abscesses.
- There is the potential for embolic events, with minor effects including splinter hemorrhages in the nail beds (Figure 7-19) and subconjunctival hemorrhages, or major neurological consequences with formation of intracranial mycotic aneurysms.
- There may be an immunological reaction responsible for vasculitis, Roth spots and Janeway lesions (Figure 7-19).

CLINICAL PEARL

The pattern of endocarditis has changed from predominantly viridans streptococci (strep viridans) affecting rheumatic valves to a more complex profile.

Microbiology

Streptococci and enterococci

- Oral streptococci (strep viridans or beta-hemolytic strep) form a mixed group of micro-organisms; they remain a common cause of infective endocarditis and are almost always susceptible to penicillin.
- A subgroup, members of the *Streptococcus milleri* and *S. anginosus* groups, comprises a more aggressive form with a propensity to form abscesses, and requires a longer period of treatment. Some newly classified subspecies (*Abiotrophia* and *Granulicatella*) may be tolerant to penicillin.
- Enterococci (*Enterococcus faecalis*, *E. faecium*) can also cause endocarditis and are usually sensitive to penicillin.

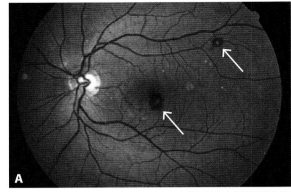
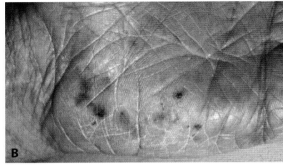
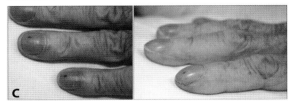

Figure 7-19 (**A**) Roth spots, (**B**) Janeway lesions, and (**C**) splinter hemorrhages

From: (A) Goldman L and Schafer AI. Goldman's Cecil medicine, 24th ed. Philadelphia: Saunders, 2012. (B) James WD, Berger T and Elston D. Andrew's Diseases of the skin: clinical dermatology, 11th ed. Saunders, 2011. (C) Baker T, Nikolic G and O'Connor S. Practical cardiology, 2nd ed. Sydney: Churchill Livingstone, 2008.

Staphylococci

Community-acquired native-valve staphylococcal infective endocarditis is usually due to *Staphylococcus aureus*, which is most often susceptible to flucloxacillin (previously methicillin). However, staphylococcal prosthetic-valve endocarditis is more frequently due to coagulase-negative staphylococci (CNS) with flucloxacillin resistance (methicillin-resistant *Staphylococcus aureus*, MRSA).

CLINICAL PEARL

Community-acquired staphylococcal endocarditis may be flucloxacillin-sensitive, but MRSA is an increasingly frequent and difficult-to-treat pathogen.

Fastidious and exotic organisms

- Initial blood cultures may be negative in endocarditis which has been previously treated with antibiotics, or is due to infections of the HACEK (*Haemophilus*, *Actinobacillus*, *Cardiobacterium*, *Eikenella* and *Kingella*) group, *Brucella*, and fungi.
- Rarely, persistently blood-culture-negative endocarditis may be due to intracellular organisms such as *Bartonella* or *Chlamydia*. In these cases, diagnosis depends on cell culture or gene amplification.
- Infections are more common in immunocompromised patients and intravenous drug users.

Diagnosis

The diagnosis of endocarditis can be challenging and requires a high level of awareness, particularly in patients with prosthetic valves or in immunocompromised patients, where missing the diagnosis even for a short time can have serious consequences.

- The traditional symptom complex of a fever and a new murmur may be a form of presentation, but is unreliable for accurate diagnosis in modern practice. There is increasing reliance on combining the findings from echocardiography and blood cultures.
- The diagnosis is confirmed if 2 major criteria, or 1 major criterion and 3 minor criteria, or 5 minor criteria are fulfilled.

The two **major criteria** are:

1 **A positive blood culture for endocarditis.**
   a Micro-organisms typical of endocarditis from 2 separate blood cultures can establish the diagnosis.
   b Organisms consistent with, but not typical of, endocarditis require at least 2 positive cultures of blood samples drawn >12 hours apart, or all of 3 or a majority of >4 separate cultures of blood with the first and last samples drawn at least 1 hour apart, to establish the diagnosis.
   c There is no justification for the practice of synchronizing blood sampling with peaks of fever.

CLINICAL PEARLS

If endocarditis is suspected, blood cultures, and if possible multiple cultures, must be taken before antibiotic treatment of any sort is begun.

2 **Echocardiographic evidence of endocardial involvement.**
   a An oscillating intracardiac mass or vegetation on a valve or supporting structure, in the path of regurgitant jets, or new partial dehiscence of prosthetic valve, or new valvular regurgitation.
   b It is important to note that an echocardiogram negative for vegetations does not exclude endocarditis.

   c Transesophageal echocardiography (TEE) may be required if there is doubt about the diagnosis on transthoracic echo, or if surgery is contemplated.

CLINICAL PEARL

The diagnostic criteria for infective endocarditis are fulfilled if there is blood culture evidence and echocardiographic evidence of mobile vegetations.

Minor criteria include:
- a predisposing heart condition
- intravenous drug use
- fever with a temperature >38°C
- vascular phenomena including major arterial emboli, septic pulmonary infarcts, mycotic aneurysm, intracranial hemorrhage, conjunctival hemorrhages, Janeway lesions
- immunological phenomena such as glomerulonephritis, Osler's nodes (painful raised spots on the palms of the hands or soles of the feet), Janeway lesions (similar distribution to Osler's nodes but painless, flat, macular and hemorrhagic), Roth spots, positive rheumatoid factor
- microbiological evidence with positive blood culture but not meeting a major criterion as noted above
- serological evidence of an active infection with an organism consistent with endocarditis

Management

- Early diagnosis is an important part of the management of infective endocarditis.
- **Antibiotic treatment** is informed by the microbiological findings with close consultation with infectious disease specialty input, and international guidelines such as the ESC Guidelines for the management of infective endocarditis (European Heart Journal. 2015 36: 3075–3123).
- Initial treatment may be necessary when the diagnosis has been established on clinical and echocardiographic criteria but the blood culture is not available. Recommended antibiotic treatments during this phase are summarized in Table 7-16.
- The standard treatment for native-valve endocarditis due to organisms fully susceptible to penicillin is penicillin 12–18 million units/day, maintained for 4 weeks.
   » Alternative regimens maintained for 4 weeks are amoxicillin 100–200 mg/kg/day IV or ceftriaxone 2 g/day IM or IV.
- 2-week regimens with these drugs supplemented with gentamicin have been used and shown to be as effective as the 4-week regimens, but need careful monitoring of the gentamicin levels.
- In beta-lactam-allergic patients, vancomycin 30 mg/kg in 2 divided doses can be used.
- Monitoring of the benefits of treatment should be undertaken with serial echocardiography and assessment

Table 7-16 Empiric treatment for infective endocarditis while awaiting definitive blood culture information

- While awaiting definitive blood culture information in the patient not sensitive to penicillin and with a native valve or prosthetic valve over a year old, treatment should commence with IV ampicillin 12 g/day in 4–6 doses, flucloxacillin 12 g/day in 6 doses, and gentamicin 3 mg/kg/day in 1 slowly administered dose per day.
- In patients with known pencillin allergy administer vancomycin 30–60 mg/kg/day i.v. in 2–3 doses and gentamicin as above.
- While awaiting definitive blood culture information in the patient with a prosthetic valve under a year old, treatment should commence with vancomycin 30 mg/kg/day in 2 doses, gentamicin 3 mg/kg/day in 1 dose, and rifampin 1200 mg/day orally in 2 doses.

of inflammatory parameters. If these are not showing convincing evidence of improvement, reassessment of antibiotic sensitivities and antibiotic regimens is needed.

CLINICAL PEARL

Following initial treatment, IV treatment should continue for 4 weeks; regimens of shorter duration have been used successfully, but require more aggressive and higher-dose antibiotics.

- **Surgery** has an important role in the management of endocarditis. It may be difficult to time the surgery, as early surgery may be complicated by operating with an active infection, whereas late surgery may allow irreversible destruction of the valve.
- Immediate surgery is indicated if there is clear evidence of valve destruction or the development of cardiac failure.

Prevention

It is important to take careful steps to prevent endocarditis in susceptible patients. In recent years, however, it has been realized that the evidence to justify the previous practice of widespread use of antibiotics for prophylaxis in all dental procedures in patients with heart murmurs was based on minimal evidence, and was exposing the community to unnecessary overuse of antibiotics. Recent guidelines have defined more carefully the high-risk patient and the situations where prophylaxis is required.

- The high-risk patient is now defined as in Box 7-5.
- The specific situations which require treatment for those identified as high-risk are defined in Box 7-6. Of note, the only procedure requiring antibiotic prophylaxis, even in the high-risk patient, is dental work with gingival or oral mucosal disruption.
- Minor dental work, respiratory, gastrointestinal or urogenital procedures do not require prophylactic antibiotics.
- The antibiotic regimens recommended for prophylaxis if it is necessary are shown in Table 7-17.

Box 7-5

Defining the high-risk patient for endocarditis prophylaxis

Antibiotic prophylaxis should only be considered for patients at highest risk of IE:

1. Patients with a prosthetic valve or a prosthetic material used for cardiac valve repair
2. Patients with previous IE
3. Patients with congenital heart disease
   a. cyanotic congenital heart disease, without surgical repair, or with residual defects, palliative shunts or conduits
   b. congenital heart disease with complete repair with prosthetic material whether placed by surgery or by percutaneous technique, up to 6 months after the procedure
   c. when a residual defect persists at the site of implantation of a prosthetic material or device by cardiac surgery or percutaneous technique

Antibiotic prophylaxis is no longer recommended in other forms of valvular or congenital heart disease

IE, infective endocarditis.

From The Task Force on the Prevention, Diagnosis, and Treatment of Infective Endocarditis of the European Society of Cardiology. Guidelines on the prevention, diagnosis, and treatment of infective endocarditis. Eur Heart J 2009;30:2369–413.

- The standard dose of amoxicillin should be taken about 1 hour before dental procedures.

PERICARDIAL DISEASES

The pericardial space is usually a thin layer of fluid. Having two surfaces (parietal and serosal), it is subject to inflammation, fluid accumulation and fibrosis.

Acute pericarditis

Etiology and pathogenesis

Acute pericarditis occurs when the serosal and parietal surfaces of the pericardium become inflamed for any reason.

- The most common cause is **viral pericarditis**. This often occurs during a viral illness, sometimes after a delay of several weeks from the onset of the flu-like illness.
  - » Viral causes include the coxsackieviruses, but other influenza and parainfluenza viruses may be implicated.
  - » The pathogenesis may involve an immunological reaction which results from the inflammatory response to the viral illness.
- There may also be associated myocardial involvement diagnosed from an elevation of the cardiac troponin level (myopericarditis).

Box 7-6

Recommendations for prophylaxis of infective endocarditis in highest-risk patients according to the type of procedure

A. Dental procedures

Antibiotic prophylaxis should only be considered for dental procedures requiring manipulation of the gingival or periapical region of the teeth or perforation of the oral mucosa.

Antibiotic prophylaxis is not recommended for local anesthetic injections in non-infected tissue, removal of sutures, dental X-rays, placement or adjustment of removable prosthodontic or orthodontic appliance or braces. Prophylaxis is also not recommended following the shedding of deciduous teeth or trauma to the lips and oral mucosa.

B. Respiratory tract procedures

Antibiotic prophylaxis is not recommended for respiratory tract procedures, including bronchoscopy or laryngoscopy, transnasal or endotracheal intubation.

C. Gastrointestinal or urogenital procedures

Antibiotic prophylaxis is not recommended for gastroscopy, colonoscopy, cystoscopy or transesophageal echocardiography.

D. Skin and soft tissue

Antibiotic prophylaxis is not recommended for any procedure.

From The Task Force on the Prevention, Diagnosis, and Treatment of Infective Endocarditis of the European Society of Cardiology. Guidelines on the prevention, diagnosis, and treatment of infective endocarditis. Eur Heart J 2009;30:2369–413.

Table 7-17 Antibiotic regimens for prophylaxis of endocarditis in high-risk patients

	ADULT DOSE	PEDIATRIC DOSE
Standard general prophylaxis		
Amoxicillin	2 g PO	50 mg/kg PO; not to exceed 2 g/dose
Unable to take oral medication		
Ampicillin	2 g IV/IM	50 mg/kg IV/IM; not to exceed 2 g/dose
Allergic to penicillin		
Clindamycin	600 mg PO	20 mg/kg PO; not to exceed 600 mg/dose
Cephalexin (cefalexin) or other first- or second-generation oral cephalosporin in equivalent dose (do not use with a history of severe penicillin hypersensitivity)	2 g PO	50 mg/kg PO; not to exceed 2 g/dose
Azithromycin or clarithromycin	500 mg PO	15 mg/kg PO; not to exceed 500 mg/dose
Allergic to penicillin and unable to take oral medication		
Clindamycin	600 mg IV	20 mg/kg IV; not to exceed 600 mg/dose
Cefazolin or ceftriaxone (do not use cephalosporins in patients with a history of severe penicillin hypersensitivity)	1 g IV/IM	50 mg/kg IV/IM; not to exceed 1 g/dose

IM, intramuscularly; IV, intravenously; PO, orally.
From Wilson W et al. American Heart Association Guideline: prevention of infective endocarditis. Circulation 2007;116:1736–54.

- The usual clinical course is benign with resolution within days or weeks, responding rapidly to anti-inflammatory medication. Some cases, however, can progress to the development of pericardial effusion or tamponade.
- Some cases can become relapsing, with multiple episodes during subsequent months, and may progress to constrictive pericarditis.

CLINICAL PEARL

Viral pericarditis is common and usually has a benign self-limiting course, but can be complicated by the development of an effusion and late development of pericardial constriction.

- Pericarditis is common after **myocardial infarction**, usually in association with extensive infarction and often associated with atrial arrhythmias.
  - » A variant of post-infarction pericarditis is Dressler's syndrome, a serositis complicating myocardial injury. It is related to post-cardiotomy syndrome, a pericardial (and occasionally pleural) inflammatory syndrome complicating cardiac surgery. Both Dressler's syndrome and post-cardiotomy syndrome are now seen less frequently.
- Pericarditis may also be a reaction to **uremia** or to **neoplastic infiltration** of the pericardium, and may occur as part of a systemic inflammatory illness such as exacerbation of rheumatoid disease or lupus.
- Rarer causes include myxedema, drugs, and tuberculosis.

Clinical features and investigations

- The typical symptom of pericarditis is an anterior chest 'pleuritic' pain which increases with inspiration. The pain is often relieved by sitting up or changing posture. It can also be a dull pain without the typical pleuritic features, and can radiate to the jaw or arms and shoulders, causing confusion with the pain of myocardial infarction.
- The characteristic clinical examination finding is a pericardial rub, usually heard best in systole, but often with a diastolic as well as a systolic component. The rub has a characteristic scratching, to-and-fro quality. It can vary from hour to hour. The rub is often accentuated by listening in expiration, or with the patient sitting forward.

CLINICAL PEARL

A pericardial rub may be transient, can be enhanced during expiration, and should be carefully sought when the diagnosis of pericarditis is suspected.

- The typical feature of the **EKG** in pericarditis is concave upwards ST-segment elevation, described as a 'Mexican saddle' appearance. It differs from the ST-elevation of myocardial infarction which is more typically (but not always) convex upward.
  - » The normal variant of 'early repolarization' may cause confusion in interpreting ST-segment elevation, but in this case the EKG remains unchanged on serial EKGs, whereas the EKG in pericarditis can change as the pericarditis evolves.
- **Echocardiography** may be normal or may show a small amount of pericardial fluid.
- **Cardiac biomarkers** may be mildly elevated if the pericarditis is associated with myocardial injury in myopericarditis, but are usually only modestly elevated in typical viral pericarditis.

Treatment

- Treatment is usually with an anti-inflammatory drug. Low-dose (0.5 mg/day) colchicine is usually effective. Occasionally, a non-steroidal anti-inflammatory drug or oral corticosteroids are necessary for symptomatic relief.
- In all patients who have had evidence of a vigorous inflammatory response accompanying the pericarditis, serial echocardiography is wise to ensure that the pericarditis is settling and a pericardial effusion is not developing.

CLINICAL PEARL

Although the echocardiogram is usually normal in acute viral pericarditis, it should be used to check that an effusion is not developing.

Pericardial effusion and tamponade

- The rate of accumulation, rather than the volume of fluid, determines the degree of cardiac compression which results from pericardial effusion.

CLINICAL PEARL

With slow build-up of pericardial fluid, stretching of the pericardium may accommodate a large effusion, but a small increase in volume can suddenly increase the intrapericardial pressure and cause tamponade.

- All of the causes of pericarditis listed above can cause pericardial effusions, but they are most commonly seen in patients who are severely uremic or with extensive neoplastic infiltration.
- **Echocardiography** is a reliable and valuable tool for the assessment of pericardial effusions. Features of tamponade on echocardiography commence with mild flattening of the right atrium, followed by compression of the right ventricle. These echocardiographic features usually occur before clinical signs of tamponade are evident.
- The classical **clinical signs** of tamponade are a rising jugular venous pressure (JVP), with Kussmaul's sign (an increase rather than a decrease in the height of the venous pulse with inspiration), and pulsus paradoxus (an increase in amplitude of the respiratory variation in pulse amplitude of >10 mmHg).

Pericardiocentesis needs to be done urgently when tamponade is present; a large effusion may need tapping if there are warning signs of tamponade developing.

- **Pericardiocentesis** for tamponade can be lifesaving. It is usually done through the subxiphoid approach, but if the echocardiogram shows a loculated effusion, alternative approaches may be used. A drainage catheter is usually left in place overnight to allow completion of drainage of the effusion. If there is rapid reaccumulation of pericardial fluid, a surgical approach with creation of a pericardial/pleural window may be needed.

CLINICAL PEARL

Pericardiocentesis is not a benign procedure. A medium-sized effusion without tamponade should not be tapped.

Chronic pericardial disease

- Constrictive pericarditis can result from progressive pericarditis.
- Tuberculosis is the classic cause, but relapsing viral pericarditis, scarring following cardiac surgery, radiotherapy and uremia are increasingly frequent causes.
- Apparently unexplained severe right heart failure is the most common presentation, and clinical signs of pericardial constriction may be subtle.
- Echocardiography with features of constriction can confirm the clinical suspicion, but CT or MRI are often required to delineate the cause.
- Surgical release of the constriction and resection of the thickened pericardium can dramatically abolish the symptomatic right heart failure.

CLINICAL PEARL

In severe unexplained right heart failure, pericardial constriction should be considered, as it is a potentially correctable cause of the right heart failure.

SELF-ASSESSMENT QUESTIONS

1   In atrial fibrillation, the A wave in the jugular venous pulse is:
    A   More prominent than usual
    B   Absent
    C   Present but cannot be seen
    D   Replaced by visible fibrillation waves

2   On the electrocardiogram, a right bundle branch block is represented by a widened QRS complex and:
    A   An 'M' shape in the lateral leads
    B   Left-axis deviation
    C   Right-axis deviation
    D   RSR' with a tall R wave in the V_1 lead

3   A patient presents with clinical features of ST-elevation myocardial infarction (STEMI). The hospital does not have facilities for percutaneous coronary intervention (PCI), and there is a 1-hour ambulance drive to the nearest PCI-capable hospital. The best treatment for this patient is:
    A   Confirm the diagnosis with an immediate and a 3-hour troponin level.
    B   Check with the PCI-capable hospital if they can receive a PCI patient in 90 minutes and transfer them there for PCI.
    C   Administer thrombolytic therapy and transfer the next morning for PCI.
    D   Check the cholesterol levels, admit to the coronary care unit and observe.

4   A 56-year-old woman presents with shortness of breath, and the clinical examination demonstrates a long, low-pitched rumbling diastolic sound in mid-diastole. The likely diagnosis is:
    A   Borborygmi
    B   Mild mitral stenosis
    C   A 3rd heart sound indicating heart failure
    D   Severe mitral stenosis

5   A 68-year-old female patient presents to the emergency department (ED) with her second episode of atrial fibrillation (AF). The episode has been going on for 18 hours, she is not distressed, and the AF reverts shortly after arrival in the ED. She has no history of hypertension, cardiac failure or diabetes.
    A   She should be reassured and sent home.
    B   She should be started on aspirin 100 mg/day.
    C   She should be started on an oral anticoagulant.
    D   She should be started on aspirin 100 mg/day and clopidogrel 75 mg/day.

6   A patient with a loud murmur and echocardiography showing moderately severe mitral regurgitation is going to see the dentist for dental extraction and requires advice on antibiotic prophylaxis. The patient is allergic to penicillin. They should be advised that they need:
    A   Amoxycillin 2 g with antihistamine cover just before the procedure
    B   Clindamycin 600 mg 1 hour before the procedure
    C   Azithromycin 500 mg just before the procedure
    D   No antibiotic cover

ANSWERS

1   B.
    The A wave in the jugular venous pulse represents atrial contraction. As atrial contraction is absent in atrial fibrillation, there is no A wave seen in the jugular venous pulse.

2   D.
    A tall R wave in lead V_1 is a reliable marker of a right bundle branch block. A simple mnemomic is 'R tall in V_1 = RBBB'. The slurred and tall R wave is due to delayed activation of the right ventricle. Other causes of a tall R wave in V_1 are right ventricular hypertrophy, true posterior infarction and type A Wolff–Parkinson–White syndrome.

3   B.
    In STEMI, 'time is muscle' and urgent reperfusion of the occluded coronary artery is the aim. If PCI can be delivered by a skilled team within 90 minutes of presentation, this is the preferable mode of reperfusion. If skilled PCI cannot be delivered in this time, reperfusion therapy should be commenced with a lytic agent.

4 D.

The severity of mitral stenosis can be determined by auscultation. In general, the longer the diastolic murmur, the more severe the mitral stenosis. For mitral stenosis to cause dyspnea, it is usually severe.

5 C.

All the recent clinical trial evidence shows that patients with atrial fibrillation, even if reverted, should be anticoagulated with warfarin or a new oral anticoagulant (NOAC) such as dabigatran, rivaroxaban or apixaban. Aspirin provides insufficient antithrombotic effect for atrial fibrillation, and the combination of aspirin and clopidogrel has been shown to be inferior to an oral anticoagulant.

6 D.

The latest guidelines recommend that antibiotic cover for valve lesions should be limited to patients at highest risk (those with prosthetic valves, patients with prior endocarditis). Mitral regurgitation is no longer regarded as sufficiently high risk for endocarditis to warrant antibiotic prophylaxis.

CHAPTER 8

HYPERTENSION

Annemarie Hennessy and Simon O'Connor

CHAPTER OUTLINE

Hypertension remains a common, widespread and increasing problem in all countries around the world. It contributes to overall cardiovascular risk, including that of stroke, cardiac disease and other vascular disease, as well as chronic kidney disease and retinopathy. It interacts strongly with diabetes, obesity, hyperlipidemia, smoking, and renal disease to accelerate the progression to irreversible organ damage.

MECHANISMS OF HYPERTENSION

The mechanisms of hypertension are best defined by the physiological processes that lead to blood pressure elevation. These mechanisms are true whether the elevated blood pressure (BP) is primary or is secondary to other conditions.

Physiological determinants of hypertension are:
- volume overload/salt overload
- increased systemic vascular resistance
- increased central drive to increase BP
- increased sympathetic nerve stimulation.

The pressure–flow–resistance relationship helps us understand that an increase both in cardiac output (CO) and in total peripheral resistance (TPR) can lead to an increase in BP.

$$BP = CO \times TPR$$

We also need to remember that cardiac output is a function of stroke volume (SV) and heart rate (HR).

$$CO = HR - SV$$

Knowing these relationships helps us understand why the pharmacological targets for hypertension include reducing the systemic vascular resistance, decreasing the heart rate, or decreasing the circulating volume.

Hypertension is considered to be **primary** if the BP is elevated due to family history, or due to lifestyle issues such as sedentary lifestyle, obesity, and dietary indiscretion (diets high in sodium and fats). The term 'essential' was coined in the 1800s when it was thought that the pressure was essential to perfuse damaged kidneys; we now know this to be the reverse, i.e. damaged kidneys cause hypertension. The term 'essential' has no place in modern medical language and the terms 'chronic hypertension' or 'primary hypertension' have better meanings. **Secondary** hypertension occurs when an underlying medical condition explains the origin of the hypertension, and there are many of these (see below).

Hypertension causes a vicious cycle of damage to the endothelium, and then the vascular smooth muscle, such that the tendency to hypertension and high shear stress within the blood vessel is reinforced with time. As a result of longstanding undertreated hypertension, a range of structural changes occur (Box 8-1).

The molecular mechanisms behind these physiological changes are divided into two categories: those acting in the periphery, and those arising from the brain (Box 8-2).

Genetic contributions to primary hypertension are the subject of much research. The search for single or multiple probable genetic explanations is important in defining mechanisms and designing new targets for treatment, but they are not widely used in everyday clinical practice. Some genetic causes, although rare, give us insight into the mechanisms of disease at a molecular level (Table 8-1).

Secondary hypertension is caused by conditions across many domains of internal medicine (Box 8-3). These are best classified as:

- endocrine
- arterial abnormalities
- renal disease
- medication-induced
- malignancy-related.

Box 8-1

Structural changes due to ongoing and progressive blood pressure elevation

Amplification:
- Vascular remodeling as a result of hypertension
- Vascular smooth muscle hypertrophy
- Increased arterial stiffness

Rarefaction:
- Loss of capillary density
- Not all antihypertensives reverse this phenomenon

Change in autoregulatory set points of the major organs, especially the kidneys:
- Potential targets of therapy

It is also seen as a direct consequence of autoimmune disease processes such as vasculitides, thyroiditis, and malignancy, with associations with parathyroid malignancies, endothelinomas, reninomas, and adrenal tumors.

Newer anticancer drugs which control the angiogenesis axis (VEGF inhibitors) are associated with hypertension.

EPIDEMIOLOGICAL EVIDENCE FOR HYPERTENSION AND ITS EFFECTS

Figure 8-1 on page 214 gives an example of the increasing prevalence of hypertension with age in Western society. These rates of chronic hypertension are similar to those seen in most developed and developing countries. There is no fundamental effect of age *per se* on increasing blood pressure outside of the effect of modern life. These increases are linked to decreasing rates of physical activity, increasing

---

Box 8-2

Mechanisms behind physiological changes in hypertension

Peripheral determinants of hypertension

Paracrine effects of local hormones:
- Endothelial derived, e.g. decreased nitric oxide, endothelin, endothelium-derived hyperpolarizing factor
- Local mitogens causing vascular smooth muscle hypertrophy, e.g. angiotensin II

Aging and structural effects on cell function:
- Prenatal imprinting—ethnic differences, reduced glomerular number, and volume
- Low birthweight—leads to increased risk of adult hypertension
- Telomere shortening—may represent early aging
- Postnatal growth patterns—growth spurts may be accompanied by increases in blood pressure, perhaps when renal growth does not match systemic growth

Central determinants of hypertension

Activation of the sympathetic nervous system:
- Alpha-1 effects include arterial constriction
- Beta-adrenergic effects include increased heart rate, cardiac contractility, and activation of the renin–angiotensin system
- Activation of the renin–angiotensin–aldosterone system results in volume expansion, and vasoconstriction

Table 8-1 Examples of genetic causes of hypertension

GENETIC DISEASE CAUSING HYPERTENSION	GENE ABNORMALITY	KEY CLINICAL FEATURES
Polycystic kidney disease	*PKD1* and *PKD2* polycystin genes	Polycystic kidneys, liver
Liddle's syndrome	Sub-units of the epithelial sodium channel *SCNN1B* and *SCNN1G* genes (gut-dominant)	Metabolic alkalosis, hypokalemia, suppressed renin and aldosterone
Multiple endocrine neoplasia type 2a	*RET* proto-oncogene	Pheochromocytoma, medullary thyroid cancer, hyperparathyroidism

---

Box 8-3

Causes of secondary hypertension

Endocrine causes
Epinephrine excess
Aldosterone excess
Thyroid disease
Pregnancy

Vascular causes
Coarctation of the aorta
Renal artery stenosis
Atherosclerosis (smokers, diabetes mellitus, advancing age)

Renal disease
Inherited
Inflammation—glomerulonephritis
Diabetes mellitus
Drug reactions
Renal tumors (renal-cell carcinoma, reninoma)

Medication-induced
NSAIDs
Corticosteroids
Analgesics
Ethanol
Cyclosporine (ciclosporin)
SSRIs
Oral contraceptives

Malignancy-related
Skin lesions such as endothelinomas
PTH- and PTHRP-producing cancers
Anti-VEGF-related cancer treatment
Adrenal tumors
Multiple endocrine neoplasia

NSAIDs, non-steroidal anti-inflammatory drugs; PTH, parathyroid hormone; PTHRP, parathyroid-hormone-related protein; SSRI, selective serotonin reuptake inhibitor; VEGF, vascular endothelial growth factor.

rates of poor dietary fruit and vegetable intake, and increasing rates of high blood cholesterol (Box 8-4).

Acute exacerbation of hypertension is seen when events of enormous stress occur, and have been associated with increased rates of cardiovascular events (e.g. the San Francisco earthquake).

Untreated malignant hypertension was in the past associated with a rapidly fatal prognosis. This was due to clear end-organ effects such as papilledema, hypertensive heart disease/cardiac failure, and nephrosclerosis, with a 79% mortality at 1 year.

There are many large-scale, modern population studies which have identified the importance of hypertension in various populations, and its association with cardiovascular disease, dementia, and death.

Box 8-4

Identified lifestyle risk factors for hypertension

Overweight and obesity

Diabetes mellitus (due to being overweight)

Sedentary lifestyle

Recreational drugs, e.g. cocaine, amphetamines

Alcohol

Contraceptive pills (estrogen, progesterone)

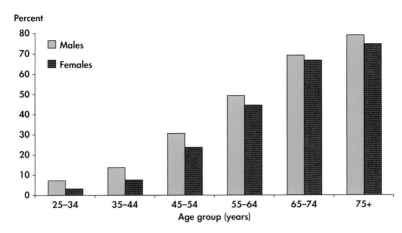

Figure 8-1 Proportion of Australians aged 25 years and over with high blood pressure, by age group, 1999–2000

Australian Institute of Health and Welfare (http://www.aihw.gov.au/prevalence-of-risk-factors-for-chronic-diseases)

DEFINITIONS OF HYPERTENSION

The mainstay of chronic hypertension management is to:

1. establish the diagnosis as primary, and treat any secondary cause
2. establish the extent of target-organ effects from the hypertension, while paying attention to
3. the importance and complications caused by additional cardiovascular risk factors and lifestyle (Figure 8-2).

Blood pressure definitions of hypertension are well supported by evidence for a continual relationship between higher blood pressures and increasing cardiovascular morbidity and mortality, as shown above. Thus, as the relationship between even moderate increases in blood pressure and stroke becomes evident, tighter BP limits and targets are set.

Current guidelines define hypertension as shown in Table 8-2.

Resistant hypertension is defined as that which is controlled with more than three medications, and **refractory hypertension** is that which cannot be controlled even on multiple medications (Box 8-5).

Establishing the validity of any single BP reading is the source of much discussion. The BP readings need to be taken reliably and repeatedly on machines that are validated for the circumstance, and by an experienced operator. Because of the potential flaws in such an approach, there is a move toward automated readings and self-taken readings, even in the physician's consulting room. Whenever the technique of the diagnostic reading is changed, it is likely that the goalposts will need to be moved in terms of classifications and targets for treatment. 24-hour BP monitoring is most useful in those with unpredictable or highly variable readings, and in those with possible white-coat hypertension.

The use of unattended surgery BP measurement in a recent clinical trial (the Systolic Blood Pressure Intervention Trial [SPRINT]) generated controversy about its relationship to standard surgery BP measurement (which has been the basis for all previous epidemiological and clinical trials

Table 8-2 Hypertension classifications

CLASSIFICATION	SYSTOLIC BP (mmHg)	DIASTOLIC BP (mmHg)
Optimal	<120	<80
Normal	120–129	and/or 80–84
High-normal (prehypertension)	130–139	and/or 85–95
Hypertension		
Stage 1	140–159	and/or 90–99
Stage 2	160–179	and/or 100–109
Stage 3	>180	and/or >110
Isolated systolic hypertension	>140	and <90

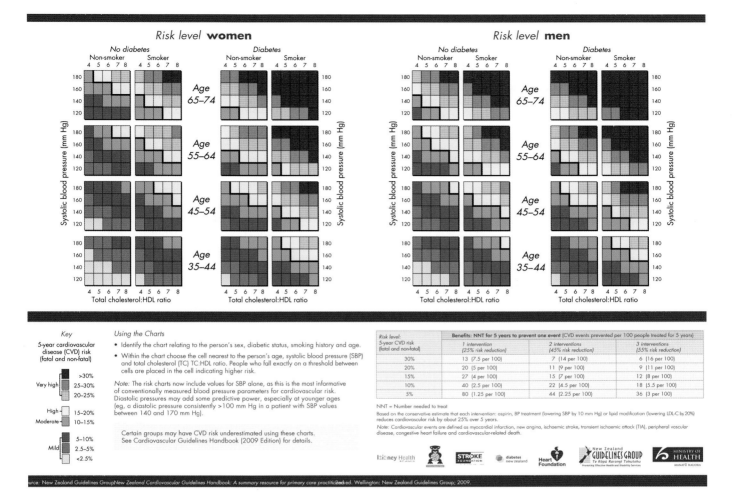

Figure 8-2 The New Zealand Risk Calculator, indicating that the risk profile for the effect of hypertension is modified by sex, age, smoking and lipid status. These sorts of risk calculator can indicate the risk of stroke in the next 5 years, and can be a powerful tool in focusing the patient on the need to reduce the risk by controlling hypertension. Blue scale: 5-year risk <2.5% up to 2.5–5%. Green scale: 5–10% and 10–15%. Yellow: 15–20%. Orange: 20–25%. Red: 25–30%. Purple >30%. In the purple category, that means that <10 are needed to be treated to prevent 1 event; and >10 cardiovascular events are prevented per 100 patients treated for 5 years

From the New Zealand Guidelines Group, http://www.nzgg.org.nz/guidelines/0035/CVD_Risk_Full.pdf

---

Box 8-5

Definition of refractory hypertension

Blood pressure that is elevated despite the use of three drugs:

- of different classes
- of which one is a diuretic
- in a patient who is adherent/compliant with their regimen, and
- where there is sustained increase in blood pressure

---

of hypertension and CV risk assessment). Its practicality in routine clinical practice has also been questioned.

Presently, the relationship between BP readings obtained with conventional office BP measurement and unattended office BP measurement is uncertain, but evidence suggests that conventional office SBP readings may be at least 5–15 mmHg higher than SBP levels obtained by unattended office BP measurements.

There is also very limited evidence on the prognostic value of unattended office BP measurements. It is not clear that they guarantee at least the same ability to predict outcomes as conventional office BP measurements.

This trial has led to a lowering of the recommended blood pressure readings that warrant drug treatment in the United States but not at this stage in Australia or Europe.

CLINICAL PRESENTATIONS AND INVESTIGATIONS

Excluding secondary causes is the mainstay of establishing the diagnosis of primary hypertension.

Given the list of secondary causes outlined above, the establishment of a diagnosis of secondary versus primary hypertension is achieved by a detailed history, and examination to identify those with diagnostic clues.

- Labile hypertension may indicate pheochromocytoma (rarely).
- Episodic hypertension associated with tachycardia and sweating could suggest a pheochromocytoma.
- Hypertension associated with recent-onset diabetes, truncal obesity, and depression should trigger investigation for corticosteroid excess.
- Radio-femoral pulse delay, a precordial systolic bruit, or a lower BP in the legs may indicate coarctation of the aorta.
- Renal enlargement is present with polycystic kidneys.
- An epigastric bruit can in some cases indicate renal artery stenosis.
- Investigations specific to a directed diagnostic possibility are more relevant than testing for all of the above. As an example, in endogenous corticosteroid excess in Cushing's syndrome, hypertension alone is rarely the presentation of this illness. Hypertension in the context of diabetes, depression and changing body shape (buffalo hump, truncal obesity, and purple striae) will lead to an appropriately directed investigation for adrenal sources of excessive corticosteroid production.
- Suspicion of hyperaldosteronism: the aldosterone:renin ratio (ARR) should be measured as a screening test. Many anti-hypertensive drugs interfere with this measurement and if the ratio is elevated the test should be repeated after 4 weeks cessation of treatment. If necessary, CCBs and alpha blockers may be used to control the blood pressure during this period.
- An abnormal result should lead to imaging using CT or MRI to look for an adrenal adenoma. Treatment of a functioning adenoma can be by laparoscopic removal or drug treatment with spironolactone or amiloride. Despite removal of the tumor, most patients continue to need anti-hypertensive treatment.
- Isolated systolic hypertension is a more likely sign in renal disease and in aldosterone excess syndrome.
- The presence of hypokalemia should be a trigger for investigating for secondary causes.

CLINICAL PEARLS

- A renal (glomerular) diagnosis is excluded by a normal urine analysis and normal renal tract ultrasound.
- There is a 60% chance that a renal bruit represents a case of renal artery stenosis.

In the absence of any symptoms or signs suggestive of secondary hypertension, some basic biochemical and radiological screening is warranted to further exclude the secondary causes.

- Serum potassium concentration: hypokalemia occurs in primary aldosteronism, renovascular disease, and corticosteroid excess syndromes.
- Serum thyroid-stimulating hormone (TSH) to exclude hyperthyroidism.
- Serum calcium to exclude primary hyperparathyroidism.
- Serum creatinine and urine dipstick to exclude glomerular disease.
- Renal ultrasound to identify renal cystic disease, renal tumors, and renal parenchymal status.

A targeted investigation for renal artery stenosis should occur when there are 'clinical clues' for renovascular disease:

- New onset of diastolic hypertension before the age of 35, or after the age of 55.
- Failure adequately to control hypertension with maximal doses of three antihypertensive agents with appropriate synergy.
- Sudden deterioration in previously well-controlled hypertension.
- Any episode of malignant hypertension.
- Acute rise in creatinine after therapy with an angiotensin-converting enzyme inhibitor (ACEI).
- Discrepancy in renal size found on ultrasonography, computed tomography (CT), or magnetic resonance imaging (MRI).
- Hypertension and papilledema.
- Presence of hypertension and aorto-iliac atherosclerosis, abdominal aortic aneurysm, or infra-inguinal peripheral arterial disease.
- Hypertension and unexplained rise in creatinine levels.
- Hypertension and multivessel coronary artery disease.

CLINICAL PEARL

Hypertension and hypokalemia should signal that this could be primary hyperaldosteronism.

Once the diagnosis of secondary hypertension has been excluded, primary hypertension (by far the most common diagnosis) is defined.

- The next step is to establish the target-organ effects of hypertension and direct treatment and expected outcome improvements accordingly.
- Initial investigation in primary hypertension includes an electrocardiogram (EKG), urine analysis, and echocardiogram if the EKG shows left ventricular hypertrophy or there is persistent or prolonged elevation of blood pressure, in order to identify target-organ effects.

TARGET-ORGAN EFFECTS OF HYPERTENSION

Blood vessels

Blood vessels themselves are the first target of hypertension:

- Vascular smooth muscle hypertrophy is evident in cardiac and renal changes with longstanding hypertension.
- Small-vessel leak is manifested as proteinuria and retinopathy.
- Hypertension contributes to atherosclerosis, and therefore myocardial ischemia, cerebrovascular disease, and peripheral vascular disease (peripheral artery occlusive disease).

Cardiac effects

- Atrial enlargement
- Left ventricular hypertrophy (Figures 8-3 and 8-4).

Retinopathy

Retinal changes from hypertension are an easily identified and important bedside test of severity (Figure 8-5, overleaf).
At their simplest, retinal arterial changes include:

- silver wiring—indicates Grade 1 hypertensive retinopathy (generalized arterial constriction).
- AV nipping—indicates Grade 2 hypertensive retinopathy (irregular constriction of the retinal vein at the point of arterial crossing).

In more severe cases there are also:

- Hemorrhages and cotton-wool spots—indicate Grade 3 hypertensive retinopathy (areas of retinal ischemia or bleeding related to vessel occlusion or rupture).
- Grade 4 changes, which are dramatic and more likely to be associated with visual loss, and increased overall patient mortality.

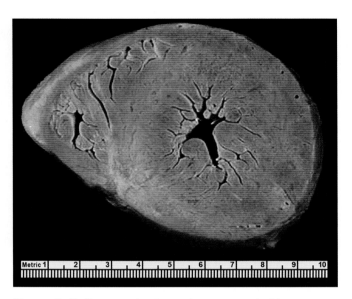

Figure 8-3 Short-axis view of an autopsied heart showing severe left ventricular hypertrophy; note the thickened wall

From Seward JB and Cassaclang-Verzosa G. Infiltrative cardiovascular diseases: cardiomyopathies that look alike. J Am Coll Cardiol 2010;55(17):1769-79

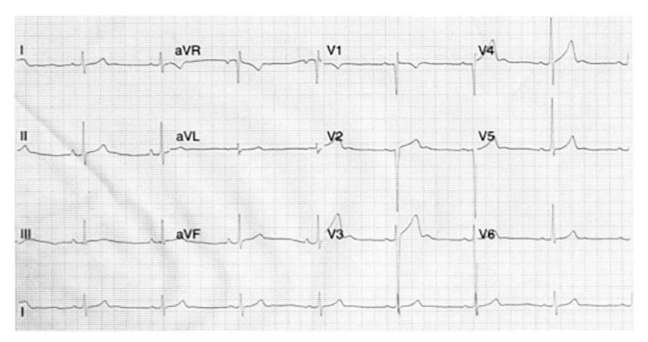

Figure 8-4 Electrocardiogram for a young professional cyclist, demonstrating sinus bradycardia, voltage criteria for left ventricular hypertrophy, and large-amplitude precordial T waves

From Saksena S and Camm AJ, eds. Electrophysiological disorders of the heart, 2nd ed. Philadelphia: Saunders, 2012.

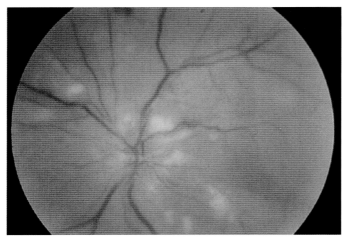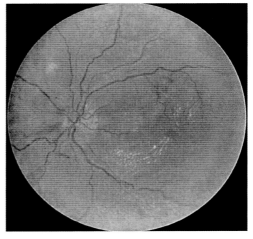

Figure 8-5 A normal retina (**left**) and a retina indicating the presence of hemorrhages, hard exudates, papilledema and cotton-wool spots in severe hypertension (**right**)

(Left) From Ralston SH, Walker BR and Colledge NR. Davidson's Principles and Practice of Medicine, 21st ed. 2010. Elsevier Ltd. (Right) Courtesy of Dr Chris Kennedy and Professor Ian Constable ©Lions Eye Institute, Perth.

- Grade 4 changes include:
  - » ischemic optic neuropathy
  - » papilledema
  - » retinal artery occlusion
  - » retinal vein occlusion
  - » retinal detachment
  - » macular damage and therefore loss of vision.

Renal changes secondary to hypertension

- Macroscopically both kidneys appear atrophic, with irregular scars, a granular subcapsular surface, and cortical thinning. This is described as 'benign nephrosclerosis', but the wisdom of the term is being questioned.

- Microscopically, there are small cortical infarcts, glomeruli show focal sclerosis, afferent arterioles show hyaline sclerosis, and small arteries show intimal proliferation and elastic re-duplication. Arteries also show fibrosis of the wall with medial hypertrophy. Larger arteries develop atheroma.

These changes all result in an increased tendency for **proteinuria**; initially as microscopic and then as manifest proteinuria.

- It may be challenging to separate proteinuria due to longstanding hypertension from that due to an underlying renal disease. The additional finding of hematuria will help make this distinction.

- The timing of hypertension relative to the development of albuminuria may give a clue. If the hypertension is present for >5 years before the onset of proteinuria, then the renal disease is unlikely to be primary. If there are markers of renal failure, hematuria or other systemic evidence of vasculitis, then the renal disease is likely to be primary.

An acute rise in serum creatinine can indicate rapidly progressive renal disease (usually glomerular) or acute kidney injury, or alternatively that malignant hypertension is occurring.

Brain

- Arterioles develop hyaline sclerosis and Charcot–Bouchard aneurysms.
- Arteries develop atheroma.
- The basal ganglia and pons show expanded perivascular spaces, small infarcts and hemorrhages.
- Dementia is linked to poorly controlled hypertension, and is likely to be due to small vessel complications.

TREATMENT AND TARGETS FOR HYPERTENSION CONTROL

The mainstay of chronic hypertension management is to:

1. Develop a plan to manage important lifestyle factors.
2. Achieve a level of appropriate BP control relative to cause, with targeted antihypertensive medication treatment, and generic antihypertensive treatment.
3. Correct correctable or secondary causes of hypertension.

It is important that **BP control** is the mainstay of all treatments, given that secondary causes are often diagnosed late, and correction of the underlying lesion is very likely not to correct the BP completely. This is especially the case if the BP has been elevated for a period of >5 years. It is also likely that the timeframe for diagnosis, given the need for metabolic testing and advanced imaging techniques, will be of the order of months, and during this time the BP should be controlled as well as possible.

Treatment strategies for hypertension require consideration of a number of factors:

1. What is the target BP?
2. How is this influenced by comorbidities?

3 Is there another diagnosis or compelling indication to use one treatment over another?

4 Is there a contraindication to the treatment being proposed?

5 What combination of therapies is appropriate, and are there additional side-effects to look out for?

6 How can these be managed with regard to managing the other cardiovascular risk factors simultaneously?

Specific targets linked to comorbid conditions

Acute hypertension or exacerbation of hypertension in a hospital setting

Often, acute medical review is required for review of acute hospital-related hypertension. Reversible factors in this setting can easily be identified through a thorough history, patient file review and physical examination.

In the first 48 hours of admission to hospital, factors such as pain and distress are important and reversible with analgesia and reassurance. Confusion about home medications (doses and timing) should also be taken into account when considering the diagnosis and the immediate need for treatment.

Iatrogenic contribution to hypertension from intravenous (IV) fluids, especially infusion of excessive normal saline (0.9%), should be treated with appropriate fluid management and perhaps a diuretic (IV furosemide), if supported by the physical examination findings.

Diabetes mellitus

In diabetes, for chronic hypertension the goal for antihypertensive treatment is a BP below 130/80 mmHg, although this depends on age. This tight target achieves a clear benefit for stroke prevention, as well as for renal protection and overall cardiovascular benefit in some age groups.

Renal disease

- In general there is evidence that a lower than usual target for proteinuria is beneficial in decreasing the risk of progressive renal disease.
    » The targets depend on the extent of the proteinuria and the age of the patient. With urinary protein excretions of <100 mg/mmol Cr, BP targets should be <140/90 mmHg; and if >100 mg/mmol Cr, the target is <130/80 mmHg.
    » These targets are very difficult to achieve in everyday clinical practice.
- There are special considerations for ACEIs or angiotensin II receptor antagonists (ATRAs)—but *not* both—as part of the therapy. Although there is a theoretical advantage of blocking the renin–angiotensin–aldosterone system (RAAS) at two locations (enzyme and receptor), there is an increased rate of potentially lethal hyperkalemia, and the combination is not recommended.
- Postural effects of increasing doses of medication need to be taken into account, especially in elderly patients, or those with autonomic neuropathy.

Pregnancy

Pregnancy is a special case for hypertension control.

- Drugs need to be category A or B in terms of fetal toxicity, need to have stood the test of time in terms of safety, and need to be flexible enough to cope with rapid changes in requirement, especially at the time of delivery and the immediate post-partum period.

CLINICAL PEARLS

- Do NOT use an angiotensin-converting enzyme inhibitor (ACEI) or an angiotensin II receptor antagonist (ATRA) in any pregnant patient.
- ACEIs or ATRAs reduce the progression of chronic kidney disease but may reduce the glomerular filtration rate in bilateral renal artery obstruction.
- ACEIs may cause hyperkalemia and cough.
- Begin treatment with a combination of a RAS inhibitor and thiazide diuretic or CCB.
- Patients with high normal blood pressure may not require drug treatment unless they have other CVS risk factors (especially known vascular disease).

- Optimal targets for control in pregnancy are uncertain.
    » Current theory suggests that very tight targets of BP control (<85 mmHg) can be associated with loss of fetal weight and birthweight.
    » This is counterbalanced by a concern that a higher target BP is associated with more episodes of severe hypertension, greater escalation to preeclampsia, and therefore greater risk of prematurity due to urgent requirement for delivery.
- There is no best suggestion for an antihypertensive agent in pregnancy.
    » The most common regimens include alpha-methyldopa, oxprenolol, clonidine, labetalol, nifedipine and hydralazine.
    » The use of pure vasodilators in the setting of hypertension in pregnancy can cause headache, which can confuse the clinical picture as headache is a diagnostic feature of preeclampsia.
- Treatment of the acute severe elevation of BP in fulminant preeclampsia (>170/110 mmHg) requires an expert team, IV medication and, usually, IV magnesium sulfate to prevent maternal seizure and maternal mortality.

TREATMENT FOR CHRONIC PRIMARY HYPERTENSION

The target for treatment and medication rests with the absolute BP, as well as the additional risk factors (cholesterol, smoking, sex and age).

Optimal or normal adult

- Systolic BP <120 mmHg and diastolic <80 mmHg.
- Recommendation is to recheck in 2 years.
- Lifestyle changes:

Table 8-3 Antihypertensive choice in the setting of cardiovascular comorbidity

COMPELLING INDICATION	DIURETIC	BB	ACEI	ATRA	CCB	ALDO ant
Heart failure	✓	✓	✓	✓		✓
Post myocardial infarction		✓	✓			✓
High risk of coronary artery disease	✓	✓	✓		✓	
Diabetes	✓	✓	✓	✓	✓	
Chronic kidney disease			✓	✓		
Recurrent stroke prevention	✓		✓			

ACEI, angiotensin-converting enyzme inhibitor; ALDO ant, aldosterone antagonist; ATRA, angiotensin II receptor antagonist; BB, beta-adrenoceptor antagonist; CCB = calcium-channel blocker.

» weight reduction
» adoption of a diet rich in vegetables and low-fat dairy products, with reduced saturated and total fats
» dietary sodium restriction—only if very-high-content fast foods are frequently consumed
» physical activity—engage in regular aerobic exercise at least 30 minutes per day
» moderation of alcohol intake.

High-normal

- Systolic BP 120–139 mmHg and diastolic 80–89 mmHg
- Recheck in 1 year.
- Assess absolute risk of cardiovascular disease.
- Lifestyle changes as above.

Stage 1 hypertension

- BP ≥140/90 mmHg.
- Lifestyle interventions.
- Identify important drug causes:
  » estrogen-containing medication
  » NSAIDs
  » illicit drug use.
- Commence medication if there are multiple risk factors or if the readings are sustained.
  » While the cheapest and most effect antihypertensive agents remain beta-blockers and diuretics, there is substantial evidence that initial treatment with an ACEI, or in fact any other antihypertensive where there is a compelling indication (Table 8-3), are reasonable choices.
- Other compelling indications might include:
  » migraine—beta-blocker or calcium-channel blocker
  » prostatism—alpha-adrenergic antagonist (e.g. prazosin)
  » anxiety disorder—beta-blocker.

Higher stages of hypertension

Stages 2 and 3 hypertension require a more aggressive approach, using the agents outlined in Table 8-3. Treatment needs to be immediate and take into account other co-morbidities and target-organ effects to achieve the required target blood pressure response. Targets are given in Box 8-6.

It is unlikely these patients will be controlled with a single agent and the current recommendations are to begin low-dose combination treatment. This is preferably with a single pill combination (SPC). Commonly this means an ACE inhibitor (or AR blocker) and thiazide diuretic or ACE-I (or ARB) with a calcium-channel blocker. Monotherapy should generally be reserved for low-risk patients with stage 1 hypertension or frail elderly patients. A three drug SPC (if available) should be tried if control is inadequate. This means a RAS inhibitor, CCB and diuretic.

Resistant hypertension is usually managed with the addition of an aldosterone antagonist (spironolactone).

Resistant hypertension may be the result of poor adherence to treatment. Careful and sympathetic questioning may help uncover this problem.

Box 8-6

Targets for hypertension management

- Control of blood pressure to a pre-set target
- Minimal medication side-effects
- Reversal of left ventricular hypertrophy over 2 years (improved echocardiogram and electrocardiogram)
- Decrease cardiovascular events, especially stroke and serious adverse events
- Decrease progressive loss of cerebral function (dementia)
- Decrease progression of renal disease

Different guidelines exist around the world with recommendations for treatment of different levels of hypertension in different target groups. Guidelines attempt to use the best available evidence to make recommendations, but all are subject to interpretation and need to be viewed in the context of treating unique individual patients with varying comorbidities. One such example is from the Eighth Joint National Committee (JNC8) (Box 8-7).

TREATMENT IN AN ACUTE SETTING

Control of hypertension acutely should take into account the relevant comorbidities and the risk of rapid decrease in BP which can occur in the setting of relative hypovolemia. Consideration should be given to:

Box 8-7
Recommendations for management of hypertension

Recommendation 1

In the general population aged ≥60 years, initiate pharmacological treatment to lower BP at SBP ≥150 mmHg or DBP ≥90 mmHg and treat to a goal SBP <150 mmHg and goal DBP <90 mmHg. (Strong Recommendation—Grade A)

Corollary recommendation: In the general population aged ≥60 years, if pharmacological treatment for high BP results in lower achieved SBP (e.g. <140 mmHg) and treatment is well tolerated and without adverse effects on health or quality of life, treatment does not need to be adjusted. (Expert Opinion—Grade E). In general consider biological age and frailty rather than chronological age.

Recommendation 2

In the general population <60 years, initiate pharmacological treatment to lower BP at DBP ≥90 mmHg and treat to a goal DBP <90 mmHg. (For ages 30–59 years, Strong Recommendation—Grade A; for ages 18–29 years, Expert Opinion—Grade E)

Recommendation 3

In the general population <60 years, initiate pharmacological treatment to lower BP at SBP ≥140 mmHg and treat to a goal SBP <140 mmHg. (Expert Opinion—Grade E)

Recommendation 4

In the population aged ≥18 years with CKD, initiate pharmacological treatment to lower BP at SBP ≥140 mmHg or DBP ≥90 mmHg and treat to a goal SBP <140 mmHg and goal DBP <90 mmHg. (Expert Opinion—Grade E)

Recommendation 5

In the population aged ≥18 years with diabetes, initiate pharmacological treatment to lower BP at SBP ≥140 mmHg or DBP ≥90 mmHg and treat to a goal SBP <140 mmHg and goal DBP <90 mmHg. (Expert Opinion—Grade E)

Recommendation 6

In the general nonblack population, including those with diabetes, initial antihypertensive treatment should include a thiazide-type diuretic, CCB, ACEI, or ARB. (Moderate Recommendation—Grade B)

Recommendation 7

In the general black population, including those with diabetes, initial antihypertensive treatment should include a thiazide-type diuretic or CCB. (For general black population: Moderate Recommendation—Grade B; for black patients with diabetes: Weak Recommendation—Grade C)

Recommendation 8

In the population aged ≥18 years with CKD, initial (or add-on) antihypertensive treatment should include an ACEI or ARB to improve kidney outcomes. This applies to all CKD patients with hypertension regardless of race or diabetes status. (Moderate Recommendation—Grade B)

Recommendation 9

The main objective of hypertension treatment is to attain and maintain goal BP. If goal BP is not reached within a month of treatment, increase the dose of the initial drug or add a second drug from one of the classes in recommendation 6 (thiazide-type diuretic, CCB, ACEI, or ARB). The clinician should continue to assess BP and adjust the treatment regimen until goal BP is reached. If goal BP cannot be reached with 2 drugs, add and titrate a third drug from the list provided. Do not use an ACEI and an ARB together in the same patient. If goal BP cannot be reached using only the drugs in recommendation 6 because of a contraindication or the need to use more than 3 drugs to reach goal BP, antihypertensive drugs from other classes can be used. Referral to a hypertension specialist may be indicated for patients in whom goal BP cannot be attained using the above strategy or for the management of complicated patients for whom additional clinical consultation is needed. (Expert Opinion—Grade E)

ACEI, angiotensin-converting enzyme inhibitor; ARB, angiotensin receptor blocker; BP, blood pressure; CCB, calcium-channel blocker; CKD, chronic kidney disease; DBP, diastolic blood pressure; SBP, systolic blood pressure.

The strength of recommendation grading system is based on the National Heart, Lung, and Blood Institute's Evidence-based Methodology Lead.

From 2014 Evidence-based guideline for the management of high blood pressure in adults: report from the panel members appointed to the Eighth Joint National Committee (JNC 8). JAMA 2014;311(5):507–20. doi:10.1001/jama.2013.284427

- age or frailty
- likelihood of postural effects
- background/previous medication choices—patients on long-acting medications, and especially ACEIs and ATRAs, are at potential risk of acute kidney injury, and hyperkalemia from hypovolemic shock.

Overall, it is advisable to use short-acting agents with minimal renal effects. Regular monitoring of BP and side-effects, and potentially frequent antihypertensive dose adjustments, will be required.

SELF-ASSESSMENT QUESTIONS

1   A 78-year-old woman presents to the hospital with acute left lower lobar pneumonia. She is noted at the time of admission to have blood pressure (BP) readings of 110/80 mmHg lying and 90/60 mmHg sitting, with a postural tachycardia. She is diagnosed appropriately and treated with intravenous (IV) antibiotics and IV fluids. At 48 hours in hospital, you are called to see her because she has a BP of 180/110 mmHg and has met the criteria for a clinical (medical) review. Your strategy after thorough review of the medical record, and physical examination demonstrating an elevated jugular venous pressure (JVP), fine bi-basal crepitations, and ankle pitting edema, should be which of the following?

   A   Continue the IV fluids and antibiotics and administer a diuretic.
   B   Withhold the IV fluids, monitor urine output and review in 4 hours.
   C   Administer an oral long-acting calcium-channel blocker (e.g. amlodipine 50 mg daily) as a regular treatment option.
   D   Reduce the IV fluids and cease the antibiotics due to the possibility of drug allergy.
   E   Treat her with IV morphine for respiratory distress and continue the treatment as prescribed by the admitting team.

2   A 65-year-old man who has had diabetes mellitus for 11 years presents for review of hypertension. You are considering which of the treatments available for blood pressure control are best indicated in his case. Which of the following would be the most appropriate treatment?

   A   He has prostate symptoms: suggest prazosin 2 mg three times daily.
   B   He has protein excretion of 0.16 mg/mmol Cr: suggest an angiotensin-converting enzyme inhibitor (ACEI) (perindopril) 10 mg daily.
   C   He has a baseline potassium of 5.8 mmol/L (reference range 3.5–5.0 mmol/L): suggest an angiotensin II receptor antagonist (ATRA) (irbesartan) 150 mg daily.
   D   He has urinary incontinence: suggest indapamide (a diuretic) 1.5 mg daily.
   E   He has intermittent asthma: suggest atenolol 50 mg daily.

3   A 55-year-old businessman presents to the emergency department with altered vision and headache. He has been told for 10 years that his blood pressure is 'borderline' and, although treatment has been suggested, he has declined medications. He drinks 6 standard alcoholic drinks per night, every night of the week. Which of the following features suggests that he has a hypertensive emergency?

   A   A reading of 180/110 mmHg
   B   The presence of retinal bleeding
   C   The presence of +protein on urine dipstick
   D   The presence of a 4th heart sound (S4) on cardiac auscultation
   E   An electrocardiogram showing atrial fibrillation

4   A 56-year-old woman presents with new-onset hypertension of 260/160 mmHg. She has never had hypertension identified in the past, but she does not like doctors. Her history reveals an alcohol intake of 1 L/day, a stressful job, and a history of childhood sexual abuse that has not previously been disclosed. She has no signs of secondary hypertension; her thyroid function is normal. You start treatment with ramipril (an angiotensin-converting enzyme inhibitor [ACEI]) and a calcium-channel blocker (amlodipine), and have sent her for addiction counseling and psychological support, which she has found valuable. She returns 3 months later and her blood pressure is still elevated, at 170/90 mmHg. What diagnosis and treatment options would you now consider?

   A   Add an angiotensin II receptor antagonist (ATRA) without any further biochemical investigation.
   B   Increase the ramipril to twice the recommended dose.
   C   Add a short-acting vasodilator (e.g. hydralazine), ensuring that her ANA (antinuclear antibody) is normal.
   D   Add a beta-blocker after ensuring that her cardiac hypertrophy has resolved.
   E   Add a diuretic after ensuring that her renal function is normal.

ANSWERS

1   **B.**

   Acute changes in BP are commonly associated with acute medical illness, in this case pneumonia. It is likely that the initial BP is a reflection of the acute illness, and her ongoing BP management needs to be considered in the context of her chronic BP state. Is she chronically hypertensive? Is she on antihypertensive medications? This might have been exacerbated by the IV fluids (including normal saline) used in her initial treatment plan. Treating the hypertension now with diuretics or calcium-channel blockers will compound the uncertainty about the IV volume and the contribution of the sepsis. Options A and C are therefore incorrect. Allergy does not usually present as hypertension, rendering option D incorrect. Controlling pain and distress are important in the setting of any hospitalization, but narcotics should be used judiciously in those with respiratory illness. Therefore, option E is incorrect.

2 A.

Compelling indications for antihypertensive use suggest that management of other symptoms, e.g. control of prostate symptoms for older men, increases the benefit of the medication, including the likely adherence. If there was a non-compelling indication, then targeting overt proteinuria or microscopic proteinuria with ACEIs or ATRAs is appropriate. For options C, D, and E there are relative contraindications for these medications.

3 B.

Absolute blood pressure readings (especially single readings) do not generally constitute an emergency. Proteinuria is an indication of an end-organ effect of chronic hypertension, rather than an acute emergency. Hypertensive heart disease is associated with an S4, but this does not usually indicate that there is imminent heart failure or other adverse cardiac event. Atrial fibrillation is also a possible consequence of chronic hypertension, not constituting an emergency. However, thyrotoxicosis should be excluded in this instance. Retinal bleeding indicates an acute blood pressure emergency and can indicate impending intracerebral bleeding, including white-matter hemorrhage. This should indicate that urgent treatment is required.

4 E.

Resistant hypertension is defined as blood pressure that is still elevated after the use of three medications at maximum doses from different classes of drugs, including a diuretic. This case assumes that the calcium-channel blocker and ACEI are at maximal doses. Therefore, a diuretic should be added. Additional dosing above the recommended dose range is associated with increased risk of side-effects (option B), but if carefully managed is sometimes used as a strategy. Use of target-organ damage to inform treatment decisions is important, but not likely to be effective in the 3-month timeframe here (option D). Short-acting medications are generally not considered to be of best adherence value in long-term management (option C). Combining an ACEI and an ATRA should not be employed due to the high risk of hyperkalemia and increased mortality (option A).

CHAPTER 9

NEPHROLOGY

Annemarie Hennessy and Randall Faull

CHAPTER OUTLINE

- TUBULO-INTERSTITIAL DISEASES
  - Acute interstitial nephritis (AIN)
  - Chronic tubulo-interstitial disease
- ELECTROLYTE DISORDERS
  - Hypernatremia
  - Hyponatremia
  - Hyperkalemia
  - Hypokalemia
- INHERITED 'CHANNELOPATHIES' ASSOCIATED WITH HYPERTENSION OR HYPER/HYPOKALEMIA
  - Hypokalemic alkalosis (with and without hypertension)
  - Renal tubular acidosis
- THE KIDNEYS IN PREGNANCY AND PREGNANCY-RELATED DISEASES
  - Normal adaptations to pregnancy
  - Underlying renal disease

INHERITED CYSTIC KIDNEY DISEASE

Autosomal dominant polycystic kidney disease (ADPCKD)

Genetics and molecular mechanisms

Autosomal dominant (AD) polycystic kidney disease (PCKD) is one of the most common inherited diseases seen in human populations.

- The medical interest in this condition arises from its classical presentation, its extrarenal manifestations, its prevalence in any dialysis population (7%), and the possibility in future that treatment could lead to a decrease in renal cyst formation, and therefore a reduction in renal parenchymal loss.
- Several randomized controlled trials testing cyst number/volume reduction strategies have been conducted, and may indicate a significant improvement in renal prognosis for affected individuals. Tolvaptan, a selective, competitive vasopressin 2 antagonist that was found to inhibit cyst growth in animal models and human trials, has recently been licensed for the treatment of polycystic kidney disease in patients at high risk of progression to end-stage kidney disease. A number of trials support the use of this agent, providing evidence that reduced rate of cyst expansion will delay need for dialysis by on average several years.

The genetic abnormalities of polycystin genes (PKD1,2,3) are mutations that lead to alterations in epithelial cell proliferation and polarization to the apical and lateral membranes.

- The unaffected gene products are transmembrane proteins localized to the primary cilia of renal epithelial cells, with extracellular domains which co-localize with other surface markers such as E-cadherin, a transmembrane protein responsible for calcium–dependent cell adhesion.
- Cysts are not present at birth due to the protective effect from the good allele (from the non–affected parent).
- With time there is somatic mutation of this protective gene, leading to cyst accumulation.
- The somatic mutation effect relates to mutation, or an environmental effect.
- The result is a clonal expansion of epithelial cells due to deficiency in cell cycle regulation.

Clinical presentations

The most usual clinical presentations occur in patients with a known family history of cystic disease, although 20% occur in individuals with no or unknown family history.

The usual **symptoms** are:

- flank pain
- back pain
- (macroscopic) hematuria.

The common **signs** are:

- gross or microscopic hematuria
- hypertension
- progressive renal failure
- increase in abdominal girth, secondary to massive renal enlargement
- associated hepatomegaly from liver cysts in some cases.

Downstream complications of hypertension also occur in this population, and include headache, left ventricular hypertrophy, retinopathy, and eventual ischemic heart disease, stroke and renal failure. Patients with PCKD are prone to renal calculus formation.

CLINICAL PEARL

The clinical sign of ballottement, which is thought to be critical in the diagnosis, is often done poorly because of too-lateral palpation. The kidneys rest in a more medial position and require that the ballotting hand sits completely under the patient at the time of ballottement.

Examination

- Physical examination should include abdominal palpation for renal enlargement.
- Tenderness is a feature of cystic disease and great care should be taken not to disrupt the cysts with physical examination.
- A right upper quadrant mass arising from the kidney can be confused with liver enlargement from hepatic involvement.
- Cystic disease in the pancreas and spleen rarely leads to demonstrable physical findings.
- **Additional clinical findings** relate to the extrarenal manifestations, including circle of Willis aneurysms

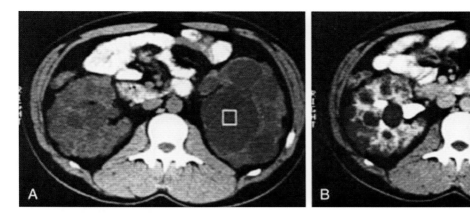

Figure 9-1 This patient (male) has autosomal dominant polycystic kidney disease, and his serum creatinine level is within the normal range. An oral contrast agent was given to highlight the intestine. (**A**) Computed tomography (CT) scan without contrast. (**B**) CT scan at the same level as A but after intravenous infusion of iodinated radiocontrast material. The cursor (box) is used to determine the relative density of cyst fluid, which in this case is equal to that of water. Contrast enhancement highlights functioning parenchyma, which here is concentrated primarily in the right kidney. The renal collecting system is also highlighted by contrast material in both kidneys

From Taal MW et al. (eds). Brenner and Rector's The kidney, 9th ed. Philadelphia: Elsevier, 2012.

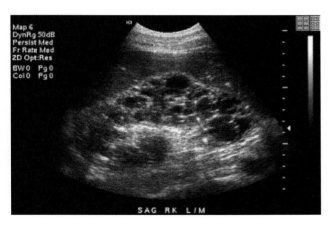

Figure 9-2 Autosomal dominant polycystic kidney disease. Sagittal scan of right kidney. Normal renal parenchyma is replaced by cysts of varying sizes

From Pretorius ES and Solomon JA (eds). Radiology secrets plus, 3rd ed. Philadelphia: Elsevier, 2011.

(visual field defects), optic atrophy, aortic stenosis, or an apical systolic murmur (mitral valve prolapse).

- Features of longstanding hypertension can include renal bruits, carotid bruits, peripheral vascular arterial stenosis, left ventricular hypertrophy with a displaced apex beat, and left or right ventricular failure.

Investigations

Ultimately, diagnosis is made by demonstrating multiple renal cysts, usually by ultrasound.

- When many bilateral cortical renal cysts are present (usually in individuals over 35 years of age), there is no doubt about the diagnosis (Figures 9-1 and 9-2).
- The defining, or minimum, number of cysts to establish the diagnosis is dependent on the age of the patient. As

an example, the presence of at least two cysts in each kidney by age 30 in a patient with a family history of the disease can confirm the diagnosis of PCKD.

- In acute episodes, the presence of cyst hemorrhage can be determined by ultrasound or computed tomography (CT) scan, but this should only be done when there is diagnostic confusion, as cyst hemorrhage is very common.
- Occasional cysts which are pendulous can cause ureteric obstruction, and this should be excluded by ultrasound examination.
- The presence of urinary tract infection complicating cystic disease is best diagnosed by urine microscopy and culture, although a walled-off collection might require blood cultures or cyst aspiration, and drainage for diagnosis.
- Progressive renal injury is reflected in a classical progression of uremic symptoms and biochemistry, and will be discussed later in the chapter.
- Genetic testing is now much more readily available as the costs have decreased dramatically. It is not generally used in routine clinical practice when family history is already present, but is being increasingly used in situations where there is uncertainty about the diagnosis (e.g. no family history), or for younger family members wishing to have more certainty for family planning purposes or if they wish to be considered as a potential live kidney donor. Interpretation of the genetic testing results requires a high level of clinical genetics expertise due to the complexity of the affected DNA and the multiple possible mutations.

Treatment and targets

While the principal burden of this disease is progressive renal failure and eventual dialysis, there is much interest currently in the mechanisms of disease and thus targets for preventing cyst development.

Box 9-1

Targets for polycystic kidney disease

- Screen for and treat urinary tract infection
- Screen for cerebral aneurysm once, and on a 5-yearly basis, in those families with a strong history of subarachnoid hemorrhage
- Monitor for deterioration in renal function
- Control hypertension to reduce progressive renal damage
- Screen for and manage proteinuria with ACEI/ATRA therapy
- Limit other nephrotoxic insults (e.g. NSAIDs) or renal vasoconstrictors (illicit drugs)
- Prepare for dialysis in progressive disease
- Provide pre-pregnancy counseling for women to reduce the risk of superimposed preeclampsia
- Treat lower tract obstruction (prostatomegaly) appropriately in older men

ACEI, angiotensin-converting enzyme inhibitor; ATRA, angiotensin II receptor antagonist; NSAID, non-steroidal anti-inflammatory drug.

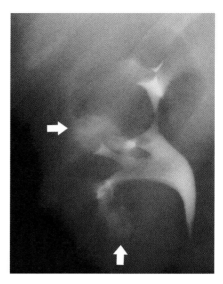

Figure 9-3 Intravenous pyelogram showing the brushlike pattern (arrows) that is indicative of medullary sponge kidney disease

From Schmitz PG and Maddukuri G. Kidneys, ureters, and bladder imaging; intravenous pyelography. Medscape Reference: Drugs, Diseases and Procedures; © 2011. http://emedicine.medscape.com/article/2165400-overview#aw2aab6b5

- Strategies designed to pharmacologically inhibit cyst growth and proliferation, as well as secondary damage such as fibrosis, are being actively studied in multiple clinical trials. Tolvaptan is the first agent of this type to be widely available, and it is hoped that other agents will become available in the next few years.
- To this end, recent trials have been undertaken in the target age group (25–45 years) to prevent cyst formation. The decrease in cyst volume was measurable, but at this time not clinically significant. It remains to be seen whether other cyst-reduction trials will be able to show improvement in parenchymal survival in the future.
- Renoprotective therapy with tight blood pressure (BP) control, usually by the use of angiotensin-converting enzyme inhibitors (ACEIs) or angiotensin II receptor antagonists (ATRAs), is warranted in patients with PCKD; these drugs should not be used together because of the risk of hyperkalemia.
- Appropriate treatment of hypercholesterolemia and timely treatment of obstruction and infections are important for preservation of functional glomerular mass and function.

Medullary sponge kidney (MSK)

Medullary sponge kidney disease is a developmental abnormality with cystic dilatation of collecting tubules. It is often an incidental diagnosis made on intravenous pyelography (IVP) (1/500).

- It is usually asymptomatic but can be discovered when investigating stone formation, nephrocalcinosis or hematuria.
- Other imaging modalities are less helpful in MSK.

  » CT may be helpful for medullary calcification, but not for tubular ectasia, as seen in the IVP.
  » Magnetic resonance imaging (MRI) is useful in those allergic to iodinated contrast medium, but is insensitive for detecting calcification.

- The typical appearance of medullary striation indicates the disease (Figure 9–3).
- MSK can be associated with renal tract infections and stone formation, but is not usually associated with hypertension or progressive renal failure.

Medullary cystic disease and autosomal recessive polycystic disease

- Medullary cystic disease is also an inherited disease, with cysts in the inner medulla. A number of gene mutations have been described, and the alternative name autosomal dominant tubulointerstitial kidney disease has now been proposed. As the disease primarily affects the tubulointerstitial compartment, symptoms are typically those of polyuria/polydipsia with normal or low blood pressure, and progressive renal function decline. The progression to renal failure is seen between 20 and 50 years of age. This is an uncommon condition.
- Other cystic diseases include autosomal recessive polycystic disease, which is rare. These cysts form *in utero*, and in the early months of life, and lead to early-life renal failure. Hepatic complications, including portal hypertension and biliary disease, are common accompaniments, and can at times be the dominant feature of this disease.

ACQUIRED KIDNEY CYSTIC DISEASE

Simple renal cysts

A common abnormality identified when investigating renal disease is a **simple renal cyst**.

- These are not inherited.
- The risk factors for simple renal cysts include age and chronic renal damage.
- Cysts generally get larger with older age, and are very rarely symptomatic.
  - » If bleeding has occurred or pain is thought to be due to size, cyst aspiration by an experienced interventional radiologist is a reasonable approach.
- There are no septa, thickenings or calcifications in a simple cyst.
  - » The presence of these abnormalities implies a complex cyst, and renal malignancy needs to be excluded.
- They are identified on ultrasound, CT and MRI scan and, as the name implies, are an even, thin-walled, spherical or elliptical fluid-filled cavity, usually in the renal cortex.

> **CLINICAL PEARL**
>
> Simple renal cysts are present in 30% of renal scans, and 50% of the 50-year-old population.

Angiomyolipomas of the kidney are benign lesions of the kidney containing fat, muscle and blood vessels. They have a cystic appearance, although with irregular features, and often need to be differentiated from more sinister renal masses.

Oncocytomas, similarly, are benign tumors arising from the intercalated cells of the collecting duct. They can be large, and require resection for diagnosis and treatment.

Renal stones/kidney stones

Metabolic environments that promote renal calculus disease

Renal calculus disease occurs in 4–20% of the population of developed countries, and 9% of that in undeveloped countries. There is also an increase in incidence in children in developed countries.

- Where infection was implicated in the past, metabolic causes are now the main concern.
- The contribution of chronic dehydration is thought to be a contributing factor in the general population, and renal calculi are more common in countries close to the equator.
- The most common cause is idiopathic, and testing for underlying causes often is normal. In a minority of cases the stones can be attributed to biochemical abnormalities such as hypercalciuria, hypocitraturia, hyperoxaluria, hypercalcemia or hyperuricemia.

- Uricosuric agents such as probenecid and sulfinpyrazone increase uric acid excretion (to reduce serum uric acid concentration). These agents therefore will increase the frequency of renal uric acid calculus disease.
  - » This is also seen with unexpected agents which have uricosuric properties such as losartan, atorvastatin, and fenofibrate.
- There is a relationship between some urinary tract pathogens and the formation of large casting (staghorn, triple-phosphate) struvite renal calculi.
- Renal calculi (Table 9-1) are seen as complications of some drug therapies (e.g. antiretroviral HIV drugs such as indinavir and atazanavir) and are also present in some of the inherited forms of renal tubular acidosis.

Clinical presentation and investigations

The classical presentation for renal stones is loin pain and hematuria.

- The pain is described as *severe*, and radiates along the upper urinary tract to the bladder.
- Symptoms of lower urinary tract irritation, frequency and dysuria may also be present.
- The key to diagnosis is imaging (Table 9-2, overleaf), ideally a CTKUB (CT scan of kidneys, ureters and bladder).
- Ultimately, the collection and analysis of the stone can provide valuable information about the likely underlying metabolic abnormality.

Diagnosis

From a physician's perspective, identifying the causes of the main metabolic derangements that lead to calculus formation is an important part of the diagnostic work-up. The most common abnormalities are hypercalcemia and hyperuricemia. Hypercalcemia has numerous causes, as listed in Box 9-2; causes of hyperuricemia are listed in Box 9-3.

Investigating for underlying causes is usually only indicated for recurrent renal calculi, due to the low yield of investigations in the absence of repeated episodes. A 24-hour-urine collection for calcium, oxalate, uric acid, citrate, phosphate, magnesium, sodium, cystine and total volume, plus a random urinary pH, with a simultaneous collection of serum for calcium concentration, uric acid, electrolytes, serum phosphate and magnesium can help determine the likely metabolic derangement. Serum hypercalcemia should be investigated, including a serum parathyroid hormone (PTH) concentration.

Treatments and targets for kidney stones

- If the stone does not pass spontaneously, treatment options include surgical stone removal (usually cystoscopic), with or without extracorporeal shock wave lithotripsy.
- The use of ureteric stents is important in patients with potential or proven obstruction and in patients undergoing lithotripsy.

A general recommendation for all patients with renal stones is to increase fluid intake to dilute the urine.

The preventative strategies for hypercalciuric stones include:

Table 9-1 Renal calculi

STONE TYPE	METABOLIC DERANGEMENT	POTENTIAL CAUSES
Calcium oxalate	Interstitial apatite plaque Low urine volume Increased urinary calcium excretion Increased urinary oxalate (dietary)	Idiopathic hypercalciuria Hypercalcemia (see Box-9-2) Renal tubular acidosis (type 1)
Calcium phosphate	Inner medullary collecting duct plaque Low urine volume Increased urinary calcium excretion	Idiopathic hypercalciuria Hypercalcemia (see Box 9-2)
Calcium carbonate	Hypercalciuria Hypercarbonaturia	Ingestion of calcium carbonate as calcium supplement (>2000 mg/day)
Cystine	Cystinuria Defective transport of cysteine and di-basic amino acids in kidney and intestine Low urinary citrate	Autosomal recessive genetic disease (incidence 1/10,000)
Struvite	Magnesium, ammonium and phosphate; alkaline urine	Infection with ammonia-producing organisms: *Proteus*, *Pseudomonas*, *Klebsiella*, *Staphylococcus* and *Mycoplasma* infections High dietary magnesium
Uric acid	Hyperuricemia	Hyperuricemia Renal tubular acidosis (types 1 and 2)
Drugs	Acyclovir, indinavir, atazanavir, triamterene	Antiviral treatment for herpes virus or HIV/AIDS; diuretics to treat heart failure

AIDS, acquired immune deficiency syndrome; HIV, human immunodeficiency virus.

Box 9-2

Causes of hypercalcemia

Parathyroid gland structure-related
- Primary hyperparathyroidism
- Parathyroid adenoma
- Parathyroid hyperplasia
- Parathyroid carcinoma (may be part of multiple endocrine neoplasia)

Parathyroid gland function-related
- Lithium use
- Calcium-sensing receptor-gene mutations causing familial hypocalciuric hypercalcemia

Vitamin D metabolic disorders
- Excessive vitamin D intake
- Sarcoidosis (elevated 1,25-dihydroxy-vitamin D)

Increased bone turnover
- Immobilization
- Excessive vitamin A intake

- Hyperthyroidism
- Paget's disease of bone

Malignancy
- Hematological malignancies
- Multiple myeloma (bone turnover)
- Osteolytic metastases: thyroid, breast, lung, renal, adrenal, prostate (release of calcitriol, or PTHrP)
- Non-small-cell lung cancer
- Renal cell carcinoma
- Pheochromocytoma

Chronic kidney disease
- Tertiary hyperparathyroidism
- Aluminium intoxication

Dietary
- Milk-alkali syndrome

PTHrP, parathyroid-hormone-related peptide.

Table 9-2 Imaging modalities for renal calculus

IMAGING MODALITY	STRENGTHS	WEAKNESSES
AXR , KUB	Good for calcium-containing stones; useful when limited radiation dose is desirable, e.g. in pregnancy Frequent X-rays useful for stone clearance/recurrence or growth assessment to reduce total radiation dose	Misses uric acid stones or matrix-component stones (non-crystalline mucoprotein), or antiretroviral-drug stones (from indinavir, atazanavir) Impaired quality in obese patients, poor differentiation from vascular calcification (phleboliths) No information regarding obstruction
Ultrasound	Safe, non-invasive High sensitivity for obstruction Better for ureteropelvic junction and ureterovesical junction stones	Operator-dependent; relies on acoustic shadowing/twinkle artifact Misses ureteric stones (<20% detected)
Non-contrast CT	Rapid, highly accurate, highly sensitive (91–100%) and specific (97–100%) for ureteric and renal stones Accurate delineation of size and location; obstruction Able to identify non-calculus causes of flank or abdominal pain; diagnoses retroperitoneal disease	Significant dose of radiation ~3 times the dose of an IVP or AXR; high fetal doses Low-dose protocols have been developed, but with reduced sensitivity and specificity
CTKUB	Combination of above	
MRI	Limited value; cannot identify calcifications Costly and time-consuming for ureteric and renal stones	T2-weighted unenhanced MRI accurate for degree and level of obstruction; gadolinium improves calculus identification
IVP	Combines calcific stone detection with function and anatomy (collecting system duplication, calyceal diverticulae), degree and level of obstruction Useful for non-calculus causes of obstruction (papillary necrosis, polyps, urothelial tumors) Limited IVP can be used in pregnancy (lower dose than a CT-based scan) when an ultrasound is inconclusive	Exposure to ionizing radiation (especially in pregnancy, and children), and contrast allergy a contraindication Study interference by overlying bowel gas Takes at least 30 minutes
Surgical—retrograde cystoscopy and ureteroscopy	Imaging associated with surgical access to the lower and upper urinary tract; diagnostic and therapeutic	Requires surgical anesthesia

AXR, abdominal X-ray; CT, computed tomography; IVP, intravenous pyelogram; KUB, X-ray of kidneys, ureters, bladder; MRI, magnetic resonance imaging.

- increasing the citrate content of the urine

- control of urinary sodium content by dietary control; increased dietary sodium concentration may increase urinary calcium excretion

- a high dietary magnesium intake can also assist with stone prevention by inhibiting calcium oxalate and calcium phosphate crystal formation, particularly in those relatively or definitively deficient in dietary magnesium

- vitamin B_6 may be warranted in those who are deficient, and this may decrease the formation of oxalate in those with excessive excretion rates.

Preventative treatment via increased fluid intake, and protein and sodium restriction in addition to thiazide diuretics is effective in idiopathic calcium oxalate and calcium phosphate stone-formers through decreasing the urine calcium concentration, as well as calcium oxalate and calcium phosphate (CaP) supersaturation, and this may also decrease plaque formation by increased proximal tubular calcium reabsorption.

Box 9-3

Causes of hyperuricemia

Increased production
- Solid-organ transplant
- Tumor lysis syndrome
- Rhabdomyolysis
- Lesch–Nyhan syndrome

Decreased excretion
- Functionally normal kidneys
  » diuretics
  » salicylates
  » pyrazinamide and ethambutol
  » nicotinic acid
  » cyclosporine (ciclosporin)-reduced glomerular filtration rate

- Associated with chronic kidney disease (CKD) stages 2–5
  » preeclampsia

Both ↑ production, and ↓ excretion
- Ethanol → lactic acid → uric acid
- Ethanol → xanthine → inhibits xanthine dehydrogenase and accelerates adenosine degradation → uric acid
- Beer → purines → uric acid
- Fructose (soft drinks) → uric acid; competes with the uric acid for transport protein in the kidney

Starvation
- Ketones compete with uric acid for excretion
- Increases conversion of purines to uric acid

- Treatment of uric acid calculi with allopurinol decreases the conversion of purines (xanthine) to uric acid, and thus decreases urinary uric acid content.
- Hyperparathyroidism should be treated with definitive treatment of the parathyroid lesion, usually by surgical excision or alcohol ablation.

KIDNEY AND URINARY TRACT INFECTION

While most urinary tract infections are intermittent and minimally troublesome, they can be a major feature of some renal diseases (e.g. vesicoureteric reflux) and at times lead to significant decline in renal function. Pyelonephritis is a particularly dangerous complication of urinary tract infections, and can result in significant renal scarring.

- Thus, awareness of the risk of infection, screening for infection, and appropriate control through treatment and prophylaxis can help with stabilizing or even improving renal function in those at risk.

Mechanisms of disease

Escherichia coli is the infecting pathogen in 85% of cases, and remaining infections are due to a range of organisms including *Staphylococcus saprophyticus* (3%) and *Proteus mirabilis*. Infections can be associated with the development of triple-phosphate (struvite) stones, as outlined above.

Risk factors
Lower tract infection/cystitis
The risk factors for lower tract infection are:
- advancing age
- dementia (it is a physical consequence of late-stage dementia)
- female, sexually active
- post-menopausal state
- persistent bacteriuria (asymptomatic)
- diabetes mellitus
- immunosuppression (e.g. post-transplantation, HIV/AIDS)
- abnormalities of the renal tract, including reflux disease
- men over 50 years, due to benign prostatic hypertrophy
- neurogenic bladder
- sickle cell disease
- instrumentation of or surgery on the renal system (e.g. cystoscopy).

Upper tract infection/pyelonephritis
Risk factors here include:
- pregnancy
- sexual intercourse (females)
- recent UTI
- diabetes mellitus
- urinary incontinence
- new sexual partner in the previous year
- recent spermicide use
- UTI history in the patient's mother
- urinary tract stents or drainage procedures.

Clinical presentation, investigation and diagnosis

CLINICAL PEARL

The presentation of lower urinary tract infection is with dysuria, urgency, stranguria, and suprapubic pain.

- Pyelonephritis (parenchymal infection) is usually unilateral, and associated with marked flank pain and systemic symptoms such as fever, sweats and rigors.

CLINICAL PEARL

10% of those with pyelonephritis develop septicemia, and show signs of septic shock as a result and require hospitalization.

The mainstay of immediate diagnosis is a urine dipstick test suggestive of infection:

- elevated urinary white cell count
- elevated urinary nitrites
- hematuria
- occasionally a small amount of urine protein (+) will be present in pyelonephritis during the acute phase only.

Treatment and targets for urinary tract infection

Treatment for UTI (Box 9-4) is straightforward and dictated by the urine culture or blood culture result, in addition to directing antibiotic treatment at the likely or proven offending organisms according to therapeutic guidelines.

Knowledge about local patterns of antibiotic resistance will assist with the choice of empirical treatment of infections in the first 24–48 hours.

INHERITED RENAL BASEMENT MEMBRANE DISEASE

Thin basement membrane disease

This is discovered on incidental urine testing finding microscopic hematuria, and can only be definitively diagnosed by measuring the basement membrane thickness on

---

Box 9-4

Targets for urinary tract infection

- Identify the offending organisms by culture of a mid-stream urine sample
- Identify the appropriate sensitivities of that organism to antibiotics
- Treat all symptoms
- Demonstrate resolution via repeat urine culture
- Screen for ongoing bacteriuria
- Reduce the risk of recurrent infection by taking an appropriate course of antibiotics, and by prophylactic antibiotics in those at greatest risk:
  - » very young children with reflux disease and >1 proven infection
  - » more than 2 infections per 6 months, or 3 per year depending on the severity

---

an electron micrograph of a renal biopsy specimen. This is usually a benign condition, although can be difficult to distinguish from the carrier state of the more serious condition of Alport syndrome.

CLINICAL PEARL

The most common cause of isolated hematuria in the community is the benign familial condition of thin basement membrane disease.

Alport syndrome

This condition is due to inherited mutations of the type IV collagen genes, leading to abnormalities in the glomerular basement membrane. The most common inheritance pattern is X-linked, which leads to a constellation of hearing loss, eye lesions including posterior subcapsular cataracts, and hematuria/proteinuria. Other inheritance patterns also exist. This is an important genetic disease in renal practice, which will frequently progress to end-stage kidney disease requiring dialysis and/or renal transplantation. The greater availability of genetic testing is proving increasingly valuable in this condition, both for establishing the diagnosis and for informing other family members.

GLOMERULONEPHRITIS (GN)

Classification

To understand glomerular disease, the challenge is to align four different classification systems in order to establish a diagnosis and develop a management plan. The classification systems are based on:

- syndrome of presentation—clinical classification
- inflammatory versus sclerosing conditions—disease mechanism
- whether the disease is primarily renal or part of a systemic disease—etiological classification
- the location of immunological deposits with respect to the basement membrane in the glomerulus—pathological classification.

Using the example of commonly known conditions, these classification systems are attempting to define diseases such as immunoglobulin A (IgA) disease, diabetic nephrosclerosis or lupus nephritis, but require the use of at least three classification systems in just these examples. A more accurate diagnosis which blends these classification systems would read something like 'nephritic syndrome from focal necrotizing crescentic glomerulonephritis complicating systemic lupus erythematosus (SLE)', rather than 'lupus nephritis'.

- The pathological system has given us the most widely accepted classification system for primary and secondary glomerular disease. This histological classification system for glomerulonephritis, the predominantly inflammatory condition, is best related to the predominant electron-microscopic features and the position of immunological deposits.

- These pathological diagnoses underpin a limited number of syndromal diagnoses which are in common use in clinical practice.
- In terms of treatment and prognosis, the etiological and disease mechanism nomenclature is the most helpful.

CLINICAL PEARL

The presence of red cell casts is common to all forms of inflammatory glomerulonephritis.

This section will concentrate on a few common glomerular diseases using elements from all four classification systems.

Primary glomerular inflammatory disease

Post-streptococcal glomerulonephritis (PSGN)

Mechanism of disease

- Post-streptococcal glomerulonephritis is the most common glomerular disease globally. This tracks with poor hygiene and poor living standards.
- It is a manifestation of usually acute but at times chronic infection, either of the skin or the upper respiratory tract (the synpharyngitic presentation).
- Although once thought to be a one-off and reversible disease, it is now clear that recurrence is common, and that repeated post-streptococcal insult can lead to progressive renal disease in a small percentage of patients.
- The mechanism is thought to be related to M and T proteins in the walls of group A beta-hemolytic streptococci that elicit the nephritogenic response.
- Significant advances have been made in terms of understanding the sequence of immunological events that lead to this type of glomerular injury, with *in situ* immunological reactions including activation of complement pathways and the capture in the membrane of circulating immune complexes.

Clinical presentation, investigation and diagnosis

CLINICAL PEARL

The usual presentation of post-streptococcal glomerulonephritis is as the nephritic syndrome with hematuria and hypertension.

- The presence of back pain and hematuria leading to oliguria or anuria has been recognized since the time of Hippocrates.
- A smaller group (<5%) present with acute azotemia and edema. Any overlap with proteinuria confers a worse long-term prognosis.
- The serological or microbiological diagnosis of streptococcal infection is required to establish the diagnosis. This is most commonly achieved with an anti-streptolysin O titer and/or an anti-DNAase test that indicates acute streptococcal infection. A throat or skin swab can also be undertaken and can assist with bacterial diagnosis and antimicrobial sensitivity.

- Non-specific tests include IgG concentrations in serum, which are elevated in 44% of patients; and hypocomplementemia, which is not universal.
- Examination of the urine reveals fragmented (dysmorphic) red blood cells, which are indicative of glomerular bleeding, and red cell casts (Figure 9-4), which are indicative of glomerular bleeding. The characterization of red cells in the urine (fragmentation) is an important indicator of passage across the filtration barrier. The identification of casts requires the careful handling of a fresh (<2 hours old) urine sample with gentle spinning and immediate microscopy. Proteinuria is also a key finding, and is quantified by either a urine protein to creatinine ratio, or by 24-hour urine protein collection.

Alternatively, a renal biopsy can be performed and shows a typical pattern.

- The light microscopy change is one of proliferation with polymorphonuclear leukocytes (PMNs) and other inflammatory cell infiltrates, in a swollen and cellular glomerulus.
- Electron microscopy shows a 'lumpy bumpy' collection of immunocomplex deposits in the subepithelial position relative to the glomerular epithelium (foot processes), and adjacent to the basement membrane. This position does not cause a basement membrane reaction, but the deposits are electron-dense and large.
- The immunofluorescent deposit pattern is also described as lumpy bumpy along the capillary walls, and dense deposits consist mostly of complement and IgG.

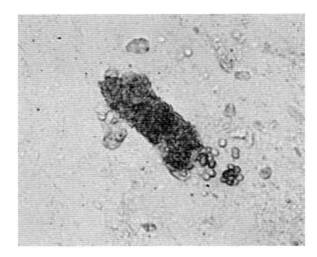

Figure 9-4 A red cell cast of urine. Red cell casts are the deposition of red cells in Tamm−Horsfall protein excreted within renal tubules, and acting as a matrix of urinary casts. These only occur in glomerular inflammation, and are quantitatively linked to severity (number of casts per high-power field)

From Zitelli BJ, McIntire S and Nowalk AJ (eds). Zitelli and Davis' Atlas of pediatric physical diagnosis, 6th ed. Philadelphia: Elsevier, 2012.

Treatment and targets

- The mainstay of treatment in the acute setting is antibiotics (preferably penicillin) for the underlying streptococcal insult.
  - » This may require longer-term antibiotics in the case of skin infection, and attention to the early treatment of repeat infections.
- Ultimately, attention to the socioeconomic determinants of poor health, and strategies that target the population at risk of post-streptococcal renal disease (low socioeconomic status, crowded housing), will decrease the incidence of this disease.

Immunoglobulin A (IgA) disease

Mechanisms

- Immunoglobulin A disease is the most common chronic glomerulonephritis seen in a population with progressive renal disease, and a common cause of acute nephritis.
- The underlying inflammatory stimulus relates to the deposition of IgA in the mesangial region of the glomerulus, and this is associated with glomerular infiltration with inflammatory cells (proliferative change), and eventual glomerular loss through sclerosis with tubulo-interstitial scarring and fibrosis.
- The male to female ratio is equal.
- Much less commonly, secondary IgA disease is seen in the context of elevated serum IgA levels due to reduced hepatic clearance in conditions such as cirrhosis.

CLINICAL PEARL

Progression to end-stage disease occurs in approximately one-third of patients with immunoglobulin A nephropathy, often over many years or even decades.

Clinical presentation, investigation and diagnosis

- Immunoglobulin A disease is suspected in asymptomatic patients with microscopic hematuria, usually with associated proteinuria.
- A classic presentation is macroscopic hematuria at the time of a throat infection (synpharyngitic haematuria).
- The typical examination findings are of hypertension and, perhaps, retinal vessel changes consistent with severe hypertension (arterial changes, and retinal hemorrhages and infarcts).
- The urine will have an increase in red cells, and red cell casts may be present.
- The presence of proteinuria is a poor prognostic sign in IgA disease, and reflects irreversible glomerular damage.
- The diagnosis can only be definitively established with a renal biopsy and with direct glomerular examination looking for typical mesangial IgA deposits and the resultant inflammatory lesions.
- The light microscopy changes are typically increased mesangial matrix and cellularity.

- Electron microscopy shows electron-dense deposits limited to the mesangial region.
- Immunofluorescence indicates that these deposits are IgA in nature.
- The prognosis can be further clarified by the degree of tubulo-interstitial scarring present on the initial biopsy.

Treatment and targets

- In less than 5% of cases, a rapidly progressive (rapidly rising serum creatinine, with glomerular crescents) form of GN can occur, which requires intensive anti-inflammatory therapy including cytotoxic agents and high-dose corticosteroids.
- The more usual treatments offered include control of blood pressure and minimizing proteinuria.
  - » Despite extensive research, no proven beneficial treatment for the actual condition has been found, although treatment with corticosteroids is favored in some parts of the world.

Membranous nephropathy

Membranous nephropathy (membranous GN) is the second most common cause of idiopathic (primary) nephrotic syndrome (proteinuria, hypoalbuminemia, hypercholesterolemia, edema) in older adults. Secondary nephrotic syndrome due to diabetes mellitus is rapidly increasing in prevalence.

- The idiopathic forms of membranous nephropathy have been associated with antibodies to M-type phospholipase A2 receptors, a highly expressed glomerular podocyte antigen.
- This results in activation of complement and other inflammatory pathways, leading to the characteristic lesion in the membrane of the glomerulus.
- The resultant proteinuria comes from destruction of the integrity of the protein barrier.
- Increased IgG excretion, HLA-DR3+/B8+, and Caucasian race have been linked to more severe disease.

Clinical presentation and investigation

This entity is clinically manifested by the gradual development of edema, malaise, foamy urine, poor appetite and weight gain. Nocturia can be a feature. This contrasts with the very rapid onset of nephrotic syndrome that is seen in minimal change disease (see below).

- Confirmation of the syndrome requires identification of hypoalbuminemia, quantification of albuminuria/proteinuria, quantification of hypercholesterolemia, and measuring edema-related weight gain.
- The identification of the type of hyperlipidemia is also helpful in directing appropriate lipid-lowering therapy.
- 70% of cases are primary idiopathic.
- The remaining secondary causes include drug-induced, bee sting (rarely), lymphoma, solid tumors (lung and colon), systemic lupus erythematosus (SLE) and other autoimmune diseases, and infections (hepatitis B, syphilis, occasionally endocarditis).
- The investigation of causes often needs to be exhaustive,

especially to exclude solid tumors as the cause in older patients.

- A standard battery of blood tests would include anti-nuclear antibodies (ANA), anti-double-stranded DNA (anti-dsDNA) antibodies, hepatitis B serology, syphilis serology, and complement levels at the onset to exclude alternative diagnoses.

Diagnosis

Diagnosis is based on histological findings and progresses through four stages based on the presence of membranous glomerular deposits:

Stage 1—intramembranous deposits; light microscopy appears normal

Stage 2—spikes grow out of the membrane

Stage 3—spikes grow together on the epithelial side to form a ladder pattern

Stage 4—disarray and gross thickening of the membrane with segmental or global glomerular sclerosis.

Treatment and targets

- Treatment trials of long-term immunosuppression for membranous nephropathy have been inconclusive. This is largely due to the natural history of spontaneous remission in one-third of cases, and lack of progression in another one-third.

- It is possible that membranous nephropathy at stage 2 or 3 is more likely to respond to immunotherapy aimed at reducing the risk of chronic disease and progression to end-stage renal disease.

- 20% of patients progress to dialysis at some time between 2 and 20 years.

- Immunosuppressive treatment may be indicated in patients with an elevated creatinine at presentation, persistent nephrotic syndrome, thromboembolism, very low serum albumin, male sex, and age over 50 years.

- Immunosuppressive regimens under consideration at present include corticosteroids, chlorambucil/cyclophosphamide, cyclosporine (ciclosporin), or mycophenolate mofetil. Rituximab can be used for severe or refractory disease.

- Treatment of secondary causes, e.g. with lamivudine for hepatitis B, is essential.

- Given the natural relapse rate, short-term studies with immunosuppression need to be viewed with some caution regarding the potential long-term benefits compared with the high rate of toxicity and side-effects.
  - » Non-specific treatment includes loop acting diuretics for control of fluid retention (usually need quite large doses), fluid/salt restriction, control of blood pressure, proteinuria reduction strategies with angiotensin converting enzyme (ACE) inhibitors or angiotensin receptor blockers (ARB), and lipid-lowering therapy.

Mesangio-capillary glomerulonephritis

Mesangio-capillary glomerulonephritis (also known as membranoproliferative GN) refers to a type of GN characterized

---

Box 9-5

Targets for membranous nephropathy

- Relieve nephrotic syndrome
- Restore and preserve renal function
- Control hypertension and hyperlipidemia
- Prevent venous thrombosis and potential pulmonary thromboembolism
- Manage long-term with minimal or no corticosteroid doses
- Screen for or instigate prophylaxis against long-term side-effects of corticosteroids (including osteoporosis, hypertension and diabetes)
- Screen for and instigate prophylaxis against opportunistic or other infection (e.g. *Pneumocystis jirovecii* pneumonia [PJP], tuberculosis, hepatitis C), and treat accordingly
- Screen for malignancy (including lung and colon cancer and lymphoma)
- Monitor for chronic kidney disease, and treat accordingly

---

by mesangial deposits and also deposits extending around the capillary loop in either a subepithelial or a subendothelial position.

- The basement membrane grows to restore its integrity and causes the appearance of a double membrane on light microscopy (double contour on silver staining).

- These lesions are more commonly seen secondary to significant and treatable conditions, such as hepatitis C with cryoglobulinemia, and SLE.

- There are subtle distinctions regarding the sites of the immune deposits within the glomerulus, with regard to the type of disease:
  - » type I has glomerular subendothelial immune deposits and duplication of the glomerular basement membrane
  - » type II has dense homogeneous deposits in the subepithelial location which expand the lamina densa of the basement membrane
  - » type III has mesangio-capillary glomerulonephritis with double contouring.

Clinical presentation, investigation and diagnosis

- The presentation is most usually with the nephritic syndrome, or mixed nephritic/nephrotic syndrome.

- A rapid decline in glomerular filtration rate (GFR) can be been in some cases, and this is usually associated with crescent formation within the glomerulus.

- Investigation includes a screen for endocarditis, vasculitis, autoimmune diseases, sarcoidosis, malignancy, hepatitis B and C, as well as lupus serology and baseline renal function.

- Renal biopsy is necessary to establish the type, to allow consideration of treatment for secondary causes, and to evaluate prognosis.

- C3 nephritic factor is also useful in determining the diagnosis.

Treatment and targets

- Treatment of mesangio-capillary GN is generally directed at the underlying cause.
- Symptomatic treatment involves close control of elevated blood pressure, diuretic use for peripheral edema and, in more aggressive cases, immunosuppression to control rapidly deteriorating renal function. This will be discussed in more detail in the sections on rapidly progressive and secondary GN.

Rapidly progressive glomerulonephritis (RPGN)

Mechanism

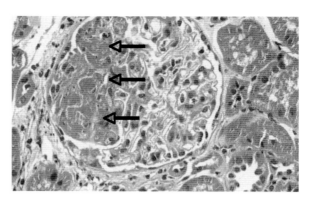

Figure 9-5 Glomeruli showing segmental necrosis with early crescent formation (arrows)

From Adkinson NF et al. (eds). Middleton's Allergy: principles and practice, 7th ed. Elsevier, 2009.

> ## CLINICAL PEARL
>
> A rapid rise in serum creatinine concentration (evidence of acute kidney injury) in the setting of abnormal urinary sediment (red cell casts, hematuria or proteinuria) defines a rapidly progressive *glomerular* disease.

- The majority of cases are vasculitides, and the first consideration will be immunosuppressive treatment; however, it is important clinically to remember that subacute and acute bacterial (infective) endocarditis can present in this fashion.
- Apart from that due to endocarditis, RPGN is more common in males, other than type 3 and 4 lupus nephritis which are more common in females.

Clinical presentation, investigation and diagnosis

The diagnosis of RPGN is a clinical one, supported by renal biopsy and urine findings consistent with acute nephritis (blood, protein, red cell casts), with rapid development of renal failure. Careful history taking will also often reveal an evolving history of ill health and nonspecific symptoms (including weight loss), but non-renal manifestations which bring the patient to hospital.

- In the case of granulomatosis with polyangiitis (GPA), the most common RPGN, it is pulmonary hemorrhage that can be the clue. The diagnosis is confirmed by typical pathological findings on the renal biopsy.
- In PAN (polyarteritis nodosa), it is abdominal pain which may be the presenting symptom; in anti-GBM (glomerular basement membrane) disease, pulmonary hemorrhage; and in microscopic polyarteritis, a leukocytoclastic vasculitic rash, although all may present as an acute nephritic syndrome with a rapidly rising creatinine. PAN can be a complication of hepatitis B infection.
  » Constitutional symptoms of fever, malaise, fatigue, anorexia and weight loss are usual. Myalgias and arthralgias or frank arthritis are occasionally present. Other inflammatory-associated conditions can also include iritis or episcleritis.
- Investigations which lead to the diagnosis include an elevated serological test (anti-neutrophil cytoplasmic

autoantibody [ANCA] or anti-GBM-antibody test), supportive tests such as an elevated erythrocyte sedimentation rate (ESR), and C reactive protein (CRP). Ultimately, the diagnostic confirmation is required for the characteristic changes of crescents in the glomeruli in a renal biopsy sample.

- Other causes of crescentic glomerular disease and RPGN include infective endocarditis, SLE-GN and at times other GNs such as IgA disease, MCGN and membranous nephropathy.
- Although preeclampsia and thrombotic thrombocytopenic purpura/haemolytic uraemic syndrome can present with rapidly progressive renal failure, these diseases are not associated with crescent formation (Figure 9-5) in the renal biopsy.

Treatment and targets for RPGN (general)

The indications for dialysis are the usual ones:

- hyperkalemia, especially in the presence of cardiac arrhythmia
- severe acidosis
- fluid overload in the presence of non-responding renal deterioration (oliguria/anuria and rising creatinine concentration)
- uremic symptoms *per se* may be a contributory indication (including uremic pericarditis).

As below, the main focus of the treatment depends on treating the underlying disease process.

Treatment and targets for infective endocarditis

- Acute kidney injury (AKI) occurs in 30% of patients with infective endocarditis, and confers a poor prognosis.
- Where renal injury has occurred, the contribution from infective emboli is as important as the inflammatory lesions.
- Immune mechanisms include circulating immune complexes and intra-glomerular formation of immune complexes, leading to glomerular inflammation with crescents.

- Culture-positive endocarditis requires treatment with predominantly bactericidal antibiotic regimens.
- Consideration of timing and dose is important with renal injury, particularly the timing and use of aminoglycosides to prevent nephrotoxicity (vancomycin toxicity can be synergistic with the aminoglycosides).
- Calculation of estimated GFR is important in determining the dose and dose interval.
- Antibiotic toxicity resulting in idiosyncratic acute interstitial nephritis needs to be considered if renal function deteriorates after the commencement of treatment.
- With appropriate long-term antibiotic therapy, the renal vasculitic lesions are reversible. Renal infarction and cortical necrosis are not.
- Other renal arterial complications such as mycotic aneurysm require specialist treatment and can potentially rupture, leading to massive blood loss and hemodynamic shock.

Treatment and targets for PAN

- Polyarteritis nodosa is a condition of granulomatous vasculitis involving any small to medium-sized blood vessel. It can be a fatal condition if not treated aggressively at the first presentation. The mortality relates to renal failure, cardiac and respiratory complications such as pulmonary hemorrhage from microaneurysms or capillaritis, and gastrointestinal complications such as bowel infarction and perforation, cholecystitis, and hepatic or pancreatic infarction.
- The mainstays of treatment are corticosteroids and alkylating agents (cytotoxic agents). This combination of treatment has improved survival dramatically.
- In hepatitis-B-related PAN, treatment will include antiviral treatment, with corticosteroids, and daily plasmapheresis for several weeks or until renal or acute extrarenal symptoms and signs resolve.

Treatment and targets for GPA (Wegener's granulomatosis)

- Whereas untreated granulomatosis with polyangiitis confers a prognosis of 95% mortality in 6 months, treatment of active disease with corticosteroids and cytotoxic chemotherapy has transformed the prognosis to 95% survival.
- The longer-term effects of malignancy and chronic infection, including with opportunistic organisms, need to be carefully considered.
- About 50% of GPA patients have a relapse at some time during the course of their illness.

Treatment doses and frequencies vary around the world.

- The more common sequence is high-dose intravenous corticosteroids for 5 days followed by high-dose oral corticosteroids. The dose is tapered off over the ensuing months, with the option of increased dose 'pulses' if symptoms recur. It may take up to 3–4 months to taper the dose, and ultimately a small dose or even a second daily dose regimen is preferred.

Box 9-6

Targets for granulomatosis with polyangiitis

- Relieve and improve pulmonary hemorrhage
- Restore renal function
- Abolish all glomerular crescents
- Monitor ANCA titer as a marker of disease activity
- Manage long-term with minimal or no corticosteroids
- Screen for long-term side-effects of corticosteroids (including osteoporosis, hypertension and diabetes)
- Limit total cytotoxic dose (e.g. cyclophosphamide to <12 g)
- Monitor for hemorrhagic cystitis and bone marrow suppression in those treated with cyclophosphamide
- Screen for and initiate prophylaxis against opportunistic or other infection (e.g. PJP, tuberculosis), and treat accordingly
- Screen for future risk of malignancy (including hematological and urological) after cytotoxic treatment

ANCA, anti-neutrophil cytoplasmic autoantibody; PJP, *Pneumocystis jirovecii* pneumonia.

- Regimens for cyclophosphamide include oral treatment, or intravenous dosing on a monthly cycle for 6 months. This is tailored to the individual patient's circumstances.
- Although a target of therapy is an optimal reduction in serum creatinine (improvement in estimated GFR, eGFR), the ANCA can sometimes be tracked as a marker of active disease, and it would not be uncommon to re-biopsy the kidney to ensure that all crescents and areas of focal necrosis are treated.
- Alternatives to cyclophosphamide such as chlorambucil have been explored over the years.
- Steroid-sparing therapy, particularly with methotrexate, mycophenolate or azathioprine, is used following completion of cyclophosphamide, and treatment during the acute phase with rituximab is also widely used.

Treatment and targets for anti-GBM disease

Anti-glomerular basement membrane disease is an autoimmune disease in which antibodies specifically attack the glomerular basement membrane, leading to aggressive glomerulonephritis.

- The mainstay of treatment for proven anti-GBM disease is immunosuppression and plasmapheresis, with a target of controlling the concentration of anti-GBM antibodies.
- Although prognosis tracks with extent of renal failure at the time of diagnosis, dialysis can often be required at diagnosis, and may be temporary if immediate immunological response is achieved.

Treatment and targets for microscopic polyangiitis

- This small-vessel vasculitis is associated with p-ANCA positivity.

Box 9-7
Targets for anti-GBM disease

- Relieve and improve pulmonary hemorrhage with plasmapheresis
- Restore renal function
- Reduce anti-GBM titers to negligible
- Abolish all glomerular crescents
- Manage long-term with minimal or no corticosteroids
- Screen for long-term side-effects of corticosteroids (including osteoporosis, hypertension and diabetes)
- Limit total cytotoxic dose (e.g. cyclophosphamide to <12 g)
- Screen for and instigate prophylaxis against opportunistic or other infection (e.g. PJP, tuberculosis), and treat accordingly
- Screen for future risk of malignancy (including hematological and urological) after cytotoxic treatment

anti-GBM, anti-glomerular-basement-membrane; PJP, *Pneumocystis jirovecii* pneumonia.

Box 9-8
Targets for microscopic polyangiitis

- Restore and preserve renal function with appropriate immunosuppression
- Treat pulmonary hemorrhage
- Reduce ANCA titer
- Abolish all glomerular crescents
- Manage long-term with minimal or no corticosteroids
- Screen for long-term side-effects of corticosteroids (including osteoporosis, hypertension and diabetes)
- Limit total cytotoxic dose (e.g. cyclophosphamide to <12 g), and monitor side-effects
- Screen for and instigate prophylaxis against opportunistic or other infection (e.g. PJP, tuberculosis), and treat accordingly
- Screen for future risk of malignancy (including hematological and urological) after cytotoxic treatment

ANCA, anti-neutrophil cytoplasmic autoantibody; PJP, *Pneumocystis jirovecii* pneumonia.

- The glomerulus can show focal and segmental necrosis and inflammation. Crescent formation is common.
- Therefore, this condition requires early aggressive immunosuppression comparable to that used for GPA to restore renal function, and to prevent rapid progression to end-stage renal disease (Box 9-8).

Minimal change disease (MCD)

- Minimal change disease, a condition with no obvious pathological changes on light microscopy but with electron microscopy changes of broad foot processes in the epithelial cells, is the most common form of nephrotic syndrome in children, but still accounts for 15% of idiopathic nephrotic syndrome in adults.
  - » The name denotes the lesion with minimal change on light microscopy, i.e. the exclusion of abnormal findings on regular magnification and staining.
- While the exact cause is not known, the typical immediate and often dramatic response to steroids points to an immunological cause.
- There is some overlap with focal sclerosing glomerulosclerosis seen in adults.
- It is thought to be a T-cell disorder, with cytokine release disrupting glomerular epithelial foot processes. This leads to a decreased synthesis of polyanions, which thereby reduce the charge barrier to albumin, allowing the leakage of albumin into urine.
- Changes in protein synaptopodin and nephrin, as well as interleukin-13, IL-18, and IL-12 have been implicated.
- The appearance of ultra-structural lesions with IgM deposits (especially in the mesangium), epithelial vacuolization, and glomerular hypertrophy are thought to confer a higher risk of progression from minimal change disease to focal sclerosing disease.
- Although usually primary, there are some secondary causes of minimal change disease such as bee sting, drugs (e.g. non-steroidal anti-inflammatory drugs, NSAIDs), and lymphoma.

Clinical presentation, investigation and diagnosis

- The diagnosis is suggested by the classical presentation of peripheral edema and proteinuria, with biochemical evidence of hypoalbuminemia and hyperlipidemia.
- The proteinuria can be extremely high (>3500 mg/1.73 m^2, >340 mg/mmol/L Cr).
- The very acute onset in adults can lead to an acute and profound hypovolemia, and there is a significant risk of acute pre-renal failure. This can also occur if diuretics are used to manage the peripheral edema in the acute phase.
- Late complications include hypertension in around 30% of adults, with increasing rates in those over 60 years old.
- Profound hypoalbuminemia is associated with an increase in prothrombotic risk. This is due in part to the urinary loss of albumin-bound clotting factors, but also to chronic hypovolemia.
- This progressive deterioration in renal function is seen in only those with the focal sclerosing end of the disease spectrum.

Treatment and targets

- The first-line treatment for MCD at any age is corticosteroids. Adult response rates are reported at 60%, and remission can take up to 16 weeks.

- Steroid-resistant disease can indicate lymphoma as a cause, and remission of the MCD relates to treatment of the underlying lymphoma.
- Steroid-sparing treatment with other immunosuppressives (including cyclophosphamide or cyclosporine) is suggested in the long term in the presence of relapsing disease, and in some circumstances when there is progression to focal sclerosing glomerulosclerosis.
  - » Management of oedema with loop acting diuretics and fluid/salt restriction is required while awaiting remission. Treatment of hyperlipidemia is not necessary as it will quickly resolve once remission occurs.

Box 9-9

Targets for minimal change disease

- Reduce edema using immunomodulatory treatment
- Reduce proteinuria using immunomodulatory treatment and ACEIs
- Monitor and treat long-term hypertension
- Treat secondary hyperlipidemia
- Manage long-term with minimal or no corticosteroids if relapse occurs
- Screen for and treat long-term side-effects of corticosteroids (including osteoporosis, hypertension and diabetes)
- Minimize side-effects of hypogammaglobulinemia (antibiotics as required)
- Minimize the risk of venous thrombosis (anticoagulation, consider if serum albumin <25 g/L)

ACEI, angiotensin-converting enzyme inhibitor.

Secondary glomerular inflammatory disease

Lupus nephritis

CLINICAL PEARL

Systemic lupus erythematosus (SLE) nephritis is the only glomerulonephritis that is more common in females than males.

- The renal manifestations of lupus glomerular disease touch on the full spectrum of glomerular disease.
- A basic understanding of the histological classification system is necessary to link to complex presentation and treatment options.
- Renal involvement in lupus occurs in 50% of affected individuals, and renal involvement confers a worse prognosis, not only because of renal involvement but also because of the impact of reduced renal function on the treatment of the extrarenal manifestations.
- The older World Health Organization classification of nephritis into five classes has been updated (since 2004) by the International Society of Nephrology (ISN) and the Renal Pathology Society (hereafter 'the ISN classification') to allow for better comparison between studies of prognosis, treatment and outcome (Table 9-3).

Clinical presentation, investigation and diagnosis

CLINICAL PEARL

Lupus nephritis can present in multiple ways: asymptomatic urinary abnormality, nephritic syndrome, nephrotic syndrome, acute kidney injury, and chronic renal disease.

Table 9-3 The spectrum of clinical presentation and histological class in lupus nephritis

CLASS	TYPICAL CLINICAL PRESENTATION	PATHOLOGICAL FINDINGS
Class I	Minimal or no proteinuria or rarely nephrotic syndrome	Minimal mesangial glomerular deposits seen on IF or EM only
Class II	Nephritic syndrome	Mesangial glomerular deposits
Class III	Nephritic syndrome and AKI	Focal proliferation (<50% of glomeruli affected); mesangio-capillary pattern; mixed-site deposits
Class IV	Nephrotic syndrome and AKI	Diffuse proliferative (>50% of glomeruli affected) Focal necrosis with crescents; mesangio-capillary pattern; mixed-site deposits
Class V	Nephrotic syndrome	Membranous deposits; diffuse thickening of the glomerular capillary wall (LM) and subepithelial deposits (IF, EM)
Class VI	Advanced sclerosing lupus nephritis	>90% glomeruli sclerosed

AKI, acute kidney injury; EM, electron microscopy; IF, immunofluorescence, LM, light microscopy.

- There is no clear correlation between nephritic syndrome, including AKI, and overall patient mortality; but in general, persistent nephrotic syndrome is linked with a worsening renal prognosis.
- Investigation of suspected lupus nephritis depends on the demonstration of acute glomerulonephritis through the presence of red cell casts in the urine.
- The ultimate diagnosis, class and prognosis are determined by histological examination of a renal biopsy.

Prognosis

- The prognosis for both the patient and renal survival is better for ISN class I and II GN than for those with ISN classes III, IV and V.
- The presence of nephrotic syndrome also influences survival, and those in whom remission is achieved have a better prognosis than those with persistent nephrotic syndrome.
- Improved survival for all patients with lupus is widely thought to be due to better supportive care, and more selective use of immunosuppressive therapy in patients with milder forms of disease.

Treatment and targets

- Patients with class I and II do not generally require any specific renal immunotherapy.
  - » The exception would be those with class I nephrotic syndrome, in whom a short course of corticosteroids may be warranted intermittently to control symptoms.
- Optimal control of blood pressure, especially with the use of ACEIs and ATRAs, or even spironolactone (aldosterone receptor antagonist) is warranted, especially in those with proteinuria.
- Treatment strategies which target the RAAS (renin–angiotensin–aldosterone system) have been shown to decrease intraglomerular pressure, lower systemic arterial pressure, reduce urinary protein excretion which is in and of itself damaging, and delay the progression of chronic renal disease to end-stage renal disease. There may even be a benefit in reducing the inflammatory component of lupus.
- Patients with class III (focal) and IV (diffuse) endocapillary disease may or may not have a sclerosing component to their disease.
  - » The most usual treatment here is an initial course of high-dose corticosteroids (intravenously) and then a high dose of oral corticosteroids tapering from 8 weeks, used in conjunction with other immunosuppressive agents.
  - » Cyclophosphamide or mycophenolate mofetil are the most commonly used and reliable treatments for this induction phase. There is some debate about oral versus intravenous (IV) therapy, but in general the monthly IV route for cyclophosphamide allows a lower cumulative dose to be used, involves less frequent cytopenias, and avoids problems of non-compliance with medication and safe home storage instructions.

  - » Combined treatment with corticosteroids has greater renal benefit but greater side-effects, including ischemic and valvular heart disease, avascular necrosis, osteoporosis and premature menopause.
  - » Major infection occurs in 45% of patients on the combination of cyclophosphamide and corticosteroids.
  - » While the higher-dose, monthly cyclophosphamide regimen is favored, a half-dose given fortnightly in association with corticosteroids has been shown to be as efficacious, with equal long-term outcomes.
  - » Mycophenolate is increasingly shown to be of benefit as a potential first-line agent in the initial phase of treatment with corticosteroids. In some of the original mycophenolate trials, there was an infection and mortality benefit from mycophenolate, but this has not been borne out by larger studies, where it is equal in effect to cyclophosphamide.
  - » Azathioprine or mycophenolate can be used as a maintenance agent.
  - » Other steroid-sparing agents include methotrexate.
  - » Rituximab (anti-CD20 monoclonal antibody) can be a useful adjuvant to the established regimen of treatment, and has not been shown to improve survival. It most likely has a role in those who are refractory and relapse from usual treatment, to prevent flares and reduce the doses of other immunosuppressives.
  - » Similarly, tacrolimus (a calcineurin inhibitor) has been trialed in the management of severe lupus nephritis.
  - » In shorter trials (up to 9 months) multi-target therapy (mycophenolate, tacrolimus and corticosteroids) has been shown to achieve high complete remission rates (up to 80%) compared with any alone. Also, adverse events were lower in the multi-target group. The longer-term benefit of these therapies is unknown.
- Class V membranous lupus requires aggressive initiation therapy, as above, when it occurs in association with diffuse or focal proliferation and mesangio-capillary involvement. In isolation, the treatment of class V targets the reduction of nephrotic syndrome, as the renal outcome is usually very good.
  - » The treatment alternatives include cyclophosphamide, cyclosporine, and corticosteroid alone (low remission rate).
  - » Mycophenolate has very similar rates of response and remission to IV cyclophosphamide.
  - » Combinations of tacrolimus, corticosteroids and mycophenolate have been tried with good effect, but show increased toxicity.
  - » As with the initiation phase of treatment, there are multiple and varied trials of appropriate agents in the maintenance phase of lupus nephritis designed to reduce relapses, maintain remission, and reduce the progression to end-stage renal disease, while at the same time reducing the net cumulative side-effect burden of immunosuppressive treatment. The most usual strategies involve low-dose continuous

or second daily dose corticosteroids and, potentially, azathioprine.

» Ocrelizumab (a fully humanized anti-CD20 monoclonal antibody), abatacept (a T-cell co-stimulator modulator) and belimumab (a soluble B-lymphocyte stimulator binding monoclonal antibody) have been trialed as add-on treatment for induction, or in refractory disease. None of them has yet replaced current standard therapeutic approaches.

» Exogenous adrenocorticotropic hormone (ACTH) is approved for refractory nephrotic syndrome and SLE (in the USA), and laquinimod (a quinolone-3-carboxamide derivative, mechanism unknown) is also undergoing clinical trials.

Box 9-10

Targets for lupus nephritis

- Relieve and improve life-threatening extrarenal manifestations of disease (neurological, cardiac and pulmonary)
- Restore and preserve renal function
- Reduce anti-dsDNA titer; improve C3/C4
- Abolish all glomerular crescents
- Manage long-term with minimal or no corticosteroids
- Minimize deleterious long-term side-effects of corticosteroids (including osteoporosis, hypertension and diabetes)
- Limit cumulative cytotoxic dose (e.g. cyclophosphamide to <12 g)
- Optimize control of blood pressure
- Screen for and actively treat urinary tract infection
- Screen for and initiate prophylaxis against opportunistic or other infection (e.g. PJP, tuberculosis), and treat accordingly
- Screen for future risk of malignancy (including hematological and urological) after cytotoxic treatment

anti-dsDNA, anti-double-stranded DNA; PJP, *Pneumocystis jirovecii* pneumonia.

Hepatitis-C-related glomerulonephritis

Mechanism of viral-induced GN

- Hepatitis C viral (HCV) infection can be associated with a range of glomerular conditions.
- The most common of these is mesangio-capillary glomerulonephritis. The mechanism is thought to be viral-induced cryoglobulinemia.
- Although immunohistochemistry has failed to reveal HCV-related antigens in the kidney biopsy samples of these patients, EM of renal tissues reveals virus-like particles in 50% and HCV RNA is often present in the cryoprecipitates (66%) or renal tissue (22%).
- The HCV-RNA positivity is linked to increased risk, and viral-derived proteins such as NS3 are located along the capillary wall and in the mesangium. Genotype 4 is sequenced in up to 70% of cases.
- Other forms of GN seen in the context of hepatitis C are membranous GN, IgA nephropathy, and amyloid nephropathy.

Clinical presentation, investigation and diagnosis

- The clinical spectrum of HCV-related glomerular injury includes microalbuminuria, nephritic syndrome, and rapidly deteriorating AKI.
- Treatment is directed at the more severe forms of renal disease.
- Renal biopsy is essential to confirm the nature of the renal lesion, the site of deposits and extent of inflammatory reaction, and to determine prognosis.
- Mesangio-capillary GN type III is associated with demonstrable cryoglobulinemia.

Treatment and targets

- Treatment of HCV-related GN focuses primarily on treatment of the hepatitis C. There has been a revolution in the treatment of this disease in recent years, with dramatic improvement in cure rate.
- In those with nephrotic-range proteinuria or rapidly progressive renal failure, immunosuppression is considered to be essential.
- Rituximab and cyclophosphamide are the first-line treatments, but caution needs to be taken with regard to a viremic flare.
- In the acute phase, plasmapheresis and pulsed high doses of corticosteroids are warranted.
- Blockade of the renin–angiotensin system is useful for control of blood pressure, renoprotection, and to reduce proteinuria.
- The eradication and control of viremia and cryglobulin production are also targets of treatment.

SCLEROSING GLOMERULAR DISEASE

Diabetes mellitus

Mechanisms of renal injury

Diabetes is a disease of enormous proportions in developing and developed countries throughout the world.

The majority of these patients will have proteinuria, either at a microalbuminuria level (<150 mg/day) or low-range albuminuria (150–1000 mg/day), or levels where symptoms start to manifest themselves (>1000 mg/day, up to nephrotic-range proteinuria and the nephrotic syndrome).

Eventually, in those susceptible, the duration and extent of hyperglycemia, the associated hypertension, and endothelial dysfunction lead to basement membrane thickening, tubular scarring and Kimmelstiel–Wilson nodules.

Clinical presentation, investigation and diagnosis of diabetic nephropathy

- The earliest manifestation of renal disease in diabetes is low-level (micro) albuminuria.
- The presence of even minute quantities of albuminuria indicates a need for tighter blood pressure control and tighter blood sugar control. The targets are well proven in the clinical trial literature, but are very hard to deliver in individual patients and in population-based interventions.
- Worldwide, there has been a steady increase in the percentage of patients on dialysis from diabetic nephropathy.

CLINICAL PEARL

40% of patients presenting with diabetes for the first time already have target-organ damage in the form of retinopathy, nephropathy, diabetic neuropathy or large-vessel atherosclerosis.

Treatment and targets for diabetic nephropathy

- Much work is being done to prevent type 2 diabetes by targeting the 'obesity epidemic' in the broader community.
- Similarly, advertising campaigns are designed to increase the early detection of diabetes and its target-organ complications.
- Treatment of early disease (Box 9-11) is focused on reduction of proteinuria and preservation of renal function.

Focal sclerosing glomerular nephropathy (FSGN)

- When focal (not global) and segmental (not diffuse) areas of progressive scarring occur without significant inflammatory change, the diagnosis of focal segmental glomerulosclerosis (FSGS) is made.
- This can be primary idiopathic or can progress from minimal change disease.
- It can also be secondary to drugs (e.g. NSAIDs or bisphosphonates), viruses (e.g. hepatitis B, HIV, parvovirus), reduced renal mass (e.g. solitary kidney, transplanted kidney, reflux nephropathy), or malignancies (e.g. lymphoma).
- The relationship with reflux nephropathy may also reflect a developmental abnormality.
- The sclerosis eventually leads to global sclerosis (all of the glomerulus) and diffuse spread (all glomeruli).

The typical sites within the glomerulus for scarring are:
- glomerular tip (at the outer 25% of the tuft, near the proximal tubule)
- perihilar variant (perihilar sclerosis)
- cellular variant (endocapillary hypercellularity)
- collapsing (associated with reduced glomerular tuft size).

Clinical presentation, investigation and diagnosis

- The most usual presentation is with proteinuria.
- This typically leads to a refractory edema that is difficult to manage.
- The additional features of hypertension and progressive renal disease are also typical.
- Progression to end-stage renal disease can occur within 4–8 years, but both rapid and slower progression is also encountered.
- Pregnancy is known to accelerate the progression to end-stage renal disease.
- The prognosis is worse in those who have rapid progression, difficult or severe hypertension, massive proteinuria, and in some ethnic groups (e.g. African-American).
- Markers of nephrotic syndrome form the basis of monitoring, as well as sequential renal function tests.

Box 9-11
Targets for diabetic nephropathy

- Reduce microalbuminuria
- Reduce frank proteinuria with ACEI or ATRA therapy
- Provide renoprotection with blockade of the RAAS (renin–angiotensin–aldosterone system)
- Monitor for deterioration in renal function
- Tightly control hypertension to reduce progressive renal damage
- Limit other nephrotoxic insults (e.g. NSAIDs) or renal vasoconstrictors (illicit drugs)

- Prepare for dialysis in progressive disease by referral to an appropriate dialysis unit and specialist nephrological care
- Pre-pregnancy counseling for women to reduce risk of superimposed preeclampsia
- Appropriate treatment of lower-tract obstruction (prostatomegaly) in older men

ACEI, angiotensin-converting enzyme inhibitor; ATRA, angiotensin II receptor antagonist; NSAID, non-steroidal anti-inflammatory drug.

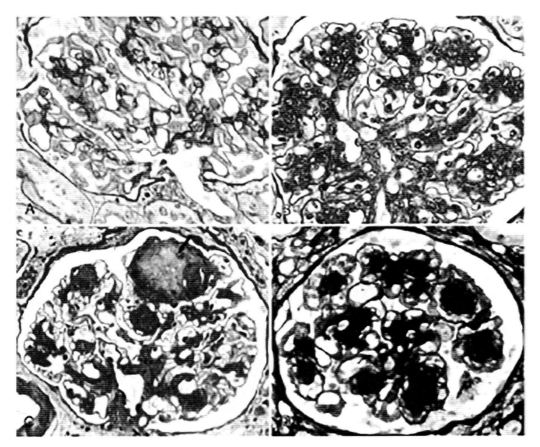

Figure 9-6 Light microscopy of structural changes in diabetic nephropathy: (**A**) normal glomerulus; (**B**) diffuse glomerular lesion demonstrated by widespread mesangial expansion; (**C**) nodular lesion as well as mesangial expansion, including a typical Kimmelstiel–Wilson nodule at the top of the glomerulus (arrow); (**D**) nodular lesion—methenamine silver staining shows the marked nodular expansion of the mesangial matrix

From Johnson RJ, Feehally J and Floege J (eds). Comprehensive clinical nephrology, 5th ed. Philadelphia: Elsevier, 2015.

- Ultimately the diagnosis is made on histopathological grounds. The nature of the lesion is also defined by the histological appearance, and can help define prognosis. The amount of glomerular involvement and the extent of tubulo-interstitial scarring are also helpful in looking at likely response to aggressive immunotherapy.
- The other complications of massive proteinuria, such as increased thrombosis risk (deep venous or renal vein thrombosis), need to be monitored, and considered whenever there is a sudden deterioration in renal function. The loss of protein S and protein C, and relative increase in fibrinogen with the massive proteinuria is part of the explanation for this increased risk. Complications and their management are outlined in Table 9-4.

Treatment and targets

- Treatment options for focal sclerosing disease have focused on proteinuria reduction with ACEIs or ATRAs.
- In some cases and on an individual basis, attempts are made to decrease disease activity with immunosuppression.
- There is no universal agreement that immunosuppression is warranted or effective, with reported response rates of 30%. This low response rate is linked to the amount of glomerular scarring but also to the extent of tubulointerstitial scarring on the renal biopsy.
- If considered worthy of a trial of treatment, prednisolone (1 mg/kg orally once daily or 2 mg/kg orally every other day for between 2 and 9 months) may be recommended in those with nephrotic-range proteinuria (>3.5 g per day) and who have rapidly deteriorating renal function.
- A trial of immunosuppressive therapy is indicated in idiopathic FSGS if proteinuria reaches the nephrotic range or if any degree of renal dysfunction is present.
- Alternatives to corticosteroids in those who respond can include cyclosporine (ciclosporin), or mycophenolate mofetil.

VASCULAR RENAL DISEASE

Renal artery stenosis

- Renal artery stenosis occurs in younger individuals (usually females) when there is a fibromuscular hyperplasia

Table 9-4 Complications of FSGN

COMPLICATION	MANAGEMENT APPROACH
Edema	Symptomatic treatment with diuretics, monitoring of renal function and blood pressure
Thrombotic risk	Monitor proteins S and C; long-term anticoagulation if albumin <20 g/L, or at any time that a documented thrombus occurs
Hyperlipidemia	Monitor and treat hypercholesterolemia and hypertriglyceridemia
Infection	Monitoring, vaccination and early aggressive treatment with antibiotics. Target: full vaccination profile to prevent infection
Hypertension	Antihypertensive and fluid management strategies. Target: BP <125/75 mmHg
Anemia	Erythropoietin replacement therapy. Targets: Hb to 110–120 g/L; ensure adequate iron stores and vitamin B_{12} and folate
Gastritis	Proton-pump inhibitor and other antacid treatment; target is reduced heartburn and nausea
Bone disorder	Calcium and vitamin D replacement. Targets: monitoring calcium concentration to within the normal range; PTH to 15–30 pmol/L
Hyperphosphatemia	Phosphate binders and appropriate dietary advice. Target: phosphate to <1.6 mmol/L
Fluid overload/hyperkalemia/uremic symptoms/acidosis	Dialysis

BP, blood pressure; FSGN, focal sclerosing glomerular nephropathy; Hb, hemoglobin; PTH, parathyroid hormone.

along the renal artery and its branches. This is a treatable form of refractory hypertension.

- In older individuals, it is due to atherosclerosis of either the aorta around the origins of the renal arteries or the renal arteries themselves, especially at the ostia.
- These are considered reversible forms of refractory hypertension.

The clinical clues for renal vascular disease include:

- past history of renovascular disease
- new onset of hypertension before age 35 or after 55 years of age
- sudden deterioration in previously well-controlled hypertension
- any episode of malignant hypertension
- a rise in serum creatinine (>30% from baseline) associated with use of ACEIs
- discrepancy in renal size
- hypertension and papilledema
- hypertension and unexplained elevated serum creatinine
- arterial bruits elsewhere (aorto-iliac, femoral vascular disease, carotid disease, coronary artery disease)
- flash pulmonary edema in the setting of uncontrolled hypertension.

Investigations include screening for arterial narrowing or differential renal function. A range of modalities is used (Figure 9-7).

Screening tools available to detect renovascular disease include duplex (Doppler), CT angiography, magnetic resonance angiography, renography, and renal vein renin concentrations or activity. Ultimately, confirmation is required by renal angiography.

Treatment of renovascular disease

- Considerable debate exists about the value of revascularization for atherosclerotic renovascular disease. In general, the requirement for antihypertensive treatment is not diminished by surgical intervention, and the effect of revascularization on saving long-term renal function is not yet known.
- Surgery (stenting or repair) is absolutely indicated in the case of renal artery aneurysms.
- Prevention of re-stenosis requires attention to the risk factors for disease, control of blood pressure and lipids, and tight glycemic control in diabetes. Antiplatelet agents can have a role in preventing re-stenosis after treatment.

THROMBOTIC THROMBOCYTOPENIC PURPURA (TTP)/HEMOLYTIC UREMIC SYNDROME (HUS)

This is an uncommon form of acute kidney injury which occurs in the setting of microthrombi in the small vessels, and endothelial injury. These conditions cause a constellation of microangiopathic hemolytic anemia, thrombocytopenia, fever, and fluctuating neurological symptoms.

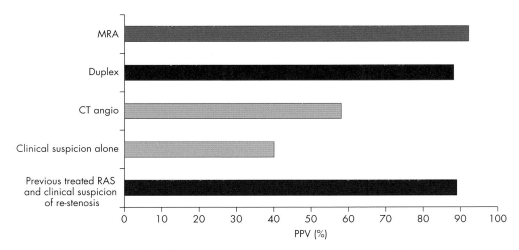

Figure 9-7 Positive predictive value (PPV) of investigations and of clinical suspicion in renal vascular disease. CT angio, computed tomography angiography; MRA, magnetic resonance angiography; RAS, renal artery stenosis; clinical suspicion refers to history of other macrovascular disease or detectable vascular bruit

From Paven G, Waugh R, Nicholson J et al. Screening tests for renal artery stenosis: a case-series from an Australian tertiary referral centre. Nephrology 2006:11;68–72.

- The renal involvement causes hematuria and proteinuria in the setting of hypertension, and a rapidly rising serum creatinine.
- The mechanism of disease is uncertain, but it occurs either as a primary abnormality (related to alterations in von Willebrand factor metabolism) or secondarily to malignancy, some medication use, and HIV infection. In some patients a genetic disorder of complement regulation is the underlying predisposing factor.
- The HUS variant is more commonly seen in children and is associated with exposure to the verotoxin (Shiga-like toxin) from *E. coli*. It has a mortality of 5–10%, with some children developing dialysis-dependent renal failure.
- Hereditary forms of both HUS and TTP have been described.
- Secondary disease can occur in association with autoimmune disease, infection, cancer, drugs, bloody diarrhea, the post-partum period, and hematopoietic stem cell transplantation.
- ADAMTS13 is a metalloproteinase which is low in patients with primary TTP.
- The treatment consists of plasma exchange, and then further immunosuppressive treatment in those who are refractory. Treatment with the monoclonal antibody eculizumab is indicated in patients with what is considered to be atypical HUS associated with complement dysregulation.

MALIGNANT HYPERTENSION

Mechanisms of renal injury in hypertension

- A sudden and dramatic increase in blood pressure (BP) to very high levels (>180/110 mmHg) can cause a dramatic vascular endothelial injury that is associated with small vessel rupture, small vessel microthrombosis, and microangiopathic hemolysis.
- This conglomerate is much less common in populations treated with modern, long-acting antihypertensives, and where the RAAS is targeted in BP-controlling treatment.
- The disease is more likely in those with a long history of poorly controlled hypertension, including due to protracted non-adherence.

Clinical presentation, investigation and diagnosis

- The presence of a rapidly rising serum creatinine concentration, severe hypertension (>180/110 mmHg), and hemolytic anemia with retinal hemorrhage would define the most urgent and aggressive form of hypertension.
- These symptoms could represent a number of the other RPGNs; however, the urine does not have red cell casts.
- Diagnosis is again made on renal biopsy, which shows duplication of the elastic lamina in medium and small vessels, marked endothelial injury, and vascular smooth muscle hypertrophy, fibrinoid necrosis, and hyaline degeneration.
- The presence of proteinuria is not a feature of the acute diagnosis, but may represent a longstanding chronic hypertensive effect prior to the onset of the accelerated hypertension syndrome.

Treatment and targets

The critical step in the management of malignant hypertension is to control the BP. Initial BP target should be to a safe level (e.g. systolic 170 mmHg), followed by more gradual reduction to long-term acceptable levels over several weeks. More rapid reduction risks cerebral hypoperfusion, with potentially fatal consequences. Initial further reduction in renal function is typical, but should stabilize and then improve with longer-term appropriate BP control.

CLINICAL PEARL

Patients with renal failure as a result of malignant hypertension may require dialysis for up to 6 months, and with excellent blood pressure control can recover sufficient renal function to come off dialysis.

SCLERODERMA KIDNEY

Mechanisms of scleroderma kidney and renal crisis

- Scleroderma is due to an accumulation of extracellular matrix protein, leading to the widespread tissue fibrosis that is the hallmark of the disease.
- The accumulation is due to activation of fibroblasts by growth factors and signaling molecules.

Clinical presentation, investigation and diagnosis

- Vascular involvement of the kidney in progressive systemic sclerosis (SSc, scleroderma) can lead to an acute deterioration in renal function, called *scleroderma renal crisis*, or slower deterioration in renal function, and proteinuria leading to chronic kidney disease.
- Scleroderma renal crisis occurs in 2–5% of patients with SSc. This occurs more frequently in patients with the diffuse cutaneous variety.
- The crisis manifests by extremely elevated BP, oligo/anuria, acute renal failure (AKI), and a high death rate (5-year mortality of 35%).
- Other associated features include microangiopathic hemolytic anemia, thrombocytopenia, and hyper-reninemia.
- The mean age at onset is 40–70 years and women are more commonly affected, as with other autoimmune diseases.
- The definitive diagnosis of scleroderma kidney can require a renal biopsy, but the fibrosing nature of the lesion makes these patients particularly prone to bleeding after the biopsy. Biopsy should only be done where there is clinical uncertainty and in a hospital large enough to cope with the likely complication of massive renal parenchymal hemorrhage.

Treatment and targets for scleroderma

- There is no consensus for the prevention of renal crisis in SSc.
- The mainstay of treatment is increasing doses of ACEIs, and addition of calcium-channel blockers if required.

- Dialysis may well be necessary, and there are case reports of renal recovery after a period of dialysis when BP control and a period of treatment on ACEIs has been observed.
- The target for treatment of SSc and of scleroderma renal crisis is a BP below 120/75 mmHg.
- The potential for treatment with serotonin receptor 2B inhibitors and other signal-controlling modifiers such as PPAR-G inhibitors and DNA methyltransferase inhibitors is under investigation at present, and may offer new treatments for the renal manifestations.

REFLUX NEPHROPATHY

- Vesico-ureteric reflux is the most common congenital abnormality of the renal tract. This is thought to be inherited in a dominant pattern involving mutations in genes controlling the development pathway of the urinary tract.
- Increasingly, this abnormality is detected by high-quality intrauterine ultrasound, allowing strategies to be put in place to monitor the infant for infection and loss of renal function.
- By the time those affected reach adulthood, the presentations are those of urinary tract infection, hypertension, proteinuria due to focal sclerosing glomerulosclerosis, and loss of renal function at an early age (mid-20s).
- Reflux is also more likely wherever there is a urinary tract abnormality such as horseshoe kidney, malrotations or ectopia of the kidneys, and ureteric duplication or bifurcation.
- Apart from the congenital variety, acquired reflux can occur in the setting of bladder outlet obstruction from enlarged prostate or bladder calculus disease.
- Reflux is a very rare complication of ureter implantation in renal transplant surgery, and is prevented by a meticulous urological approach to the surgery.

Clinical presentation, investigation and diagnosis

CLINICAL PEARL

Vesico-ureteric reflux should be suspected in adults with a history of childhood infections, particularly in the first 5 years of life.

- The organisms involved in infection are typical.
- The diagnosis is established either by a micturating cystourethrogram, whereby the active reflux of contrast-containing urine into the lower ureters is demonstrated, or by cystoscopy, revealing an open appearance of the ureteric orifices in the trigone of the bladder.
- Imaging can be used to determine the balance of renal function between the left and right kidneys (DTPA [diethylene triamine pentaacetic acid] renal scintogram or captopril renal scan).

Treatment and targets

Ureteric surgery for congenital reflux disease remains controversial. There are some instances when surgery may assist with reducing the frequency of infection, but surgery has not been shown to prevent the progression to end-stage disease, especially in those with scarring and glomerulosclerosis.

Box 9-12

Targets for reflux nephropathy

- Relieve UTIs
- Improve the risk of recurrent UTIs by prophylactic (daily) antibiotics and frequent urinary cultures
- Monitor for deterioration in renal function
- Control hypertension to reduce progressive renal damage
- Screen for and manage proteinuria with ACEI/ATRA therapy
- Limit other nephrotoxic insults (e.g. NSAIDs) or renal vasoconstrictors (illicit drugs)
- Prepare for dialysis in progressive disease
- Pre-pregnancy counseling for women to reduce risk of superimposed preeclampsia, or recurrent UTI
- Appropriate treatment of lower-tract obstruction (prostatomegaly) in older men

ACEI, angiotensin-converting enzyme inhibitor; ATRA, angiotensin II receptor antagonist; NSAID, non-steroidal anti-inflammatory drug; UTI, urinary tract infection.

CHRONIC KIDNEY DISEASE (CKD)

Classification systems and definitions

Definitions of acute and chronic renal failure have been superseded by the terminology acute kidney injury (AKI) and chronic kidney disease (CKD).

- CKD is the result of loss of glomerular mass and thereby filtration surface area, sustained over a period of at least 6 months.

CLINICAL PEARL

Chronic kidney disease can present relatively late in the progression to end-stage disease if the underlying disease process is insidious. If this is the case, the kidneys may be small and scarred at the time of presentation, and an underlying diagnosis may never be made.

- The calculation of an estimated glomerular filtration rate (eGFR) is based on the principle that there is a nonlinear relationship between serum creatinine concentration and GFR.
- The eGFR most commonly used is based on the MDRD (Modification of Diet in Renal Disease Study) formula

which takes into account age, gender, and ethnicity in some cases.

- Formulas used to derive GFR become more unreliable at the extremes of body size, extremes of age, especially very low body mass index (BMI), high (dietary supplements) or low (vegans or vegetarians) dietary intake of creatinine or creatine, patients with muscle diseases such as atrophy or amputation, and in particular ethnic groups. Calculation of the dosage of critical dose medications (e.g. aminoglycosides) should not rely on the eGFR, particularly in these examples, as the eGFR does not take into account the size of the patient.
- The conversion of serum creatinine to eGFR has been shown to be useful in targeted community screening and identification of early kidney disease in those at risk (e.g. diabetes).
- A progressive serum creatinine concentration is used when kidney disease is established to track possible disease progression (e.g. in renal transplant patients).

Early stages of CKD

- **Stage 1** kidney disease is defined as having *no* reduction in glomerular filtration rate (eGFR) despite the presence of urinary abnormalities or a diagnosis of renal disease.
  - » An example would be a nephritic lupus patient with 2.2 g of proteinuria per day, known for 18 months, with elevated serum markers of SLE, and a serum creatinine concentration of 66 micromol/L (eGFR 149 mL/min/1.73 m²). This would be graded as stage 1 CKD.
  - » The presence of hypertension here would be diagnosed as secondary hypertension.
- **Stage 2** kidney disease is defined as a reduction in eGFR to 60–89 mL/min/1.73 m² in the presence of kidney damage.
- The presence of systemic tiredness can be a feature of even very early chronic kidney disease. Other symptoms

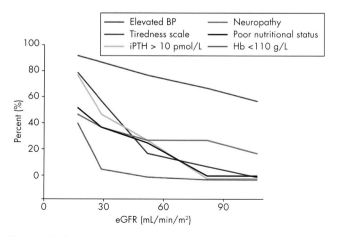

Figure 9-8 Indicative rates for complications of chronic kidney disease related to estimated glomerular filtration rate (eGFR). BP, blood pressure; Hb, hemoglobin; iPTH, intact parathyroid hormone

of progressive chronic kidney disease include weakness, muscle cramps, easy bruising, and hiccups.

Clinical presentations of stage 3 CKD

Once the eGFR has fallen below 60 mL/min/1.73 m², the early signs of chronic kidney disease are seen.

- The earliest sign may be hypertension.
- The combined contribution of hypertension and the deteriorating eGFR greatly increase the risk of cardiovascular events.
- Hyperlipidemia should be identified and defined.
- Phosphate, calcium and bone abnormalities begin to manifest at this stage.
- There are signs of poor nutritional status and weight loss with changes in protein metabolism. This is exacerbated by proteinuria if present.
- Patients are at risk of heart failure from either their underlying vascular disease or from limited renal reserves at a time of fluid challenge (e.g. postoperative management).
- The risk of infection and malignancy is increased and should be screened for.
- Neuropathy related to uremia can be identified at this level of renal dysfunction.

This group is also prone to rapidly deteriorating renal function, in the face of additional pre-renal, renal or post-renal events.

- As with earlier stages of kidney disease, observation for urinary tract stones, infection or malignancy is important in managing the risk of deteriorating renal function.
- Immunization for known infection risk and provision of advice regarding medication use, especially over-the-counter medications, NSAIDs and drugs which alter the RAAS, are important.

Clinical presentations of stages 4 and 5 CKD

Once the eGFR is below 30 mL/min/1.73 m², the patient is at stage 4 CKD.

- This is where symptoms of anemia occur, and contribute to marked tiredness and to worsening left ventricular failure if left untreated.
- At this level of eGFR, there is a further reduction in oral absorption of iron, so attention to parental iron administration, oral B_{12} and folate supplements, as well as starting erythropoietin replacement therapy (when Hb is <100 g/L) is warranted.

Once the eGFR is below 15 mL/min/1.73 m² (stage 5 CKD), the symptoms of uremia arise.

- Nausea, vomiting, tiredness and lethargy are the most common.
- As with CKD stage 3, attention to calcium, phosphate, anemia, blood pressure, and screening for events which would worsen renal function such as infection or lower tract obstruction is warranted.

End-stage renal disease (ESRD) and renal replacement therapy

- The controllable complications of ESRD include anemia, hypertension, calcium and bone disease (renal osteodystrophy) and nutritional status.
- They require frequent monitoring, and adjustment of treatment strategies at the same time as the initiation and maintenance of renal replacement therapy: dialysis or transplantation.

Dialysis

- Given time and cost constraints, more continuous or in some cases overnight dialysis is favored, and options available include peritoneal dialysis or hemodialysis (Table 9-6, overleaf).
- Ultimately, these therapies restore renal function to 20–45 mL/min/1.73 m² averaged over the week, depending on the modality chosen.
- Improvement of GFR to 50 mL/min/1.73 m² requires a well-functioning renal transplant graft.

Complications and care of the dialysis patient

The important aspects of care include each of the following:

- monitor and maintain the access for dialysis
- watch for and prevent cardiovascular complications

Table 9-5 Targets in management of chronic kidney disease

	OPTIMAL TARGETS FOR CKD STAGES 3 AND 4, AND END-STAGE RENAL FAILURE PATIENTS
Hemoglobin	110–120 g/L
Ca^{2+} × phosphate product	[Ca^{2+}] normal; [Phos] <1.6 mmol/L
PTH	<2–3 times upper limit of normal
Blood pressure	<130–139/90 mmHg, or 130/80 mmHg if proteinuria
Nutritional status	Dietary sodium <2.4 g/d (<100 mmol/d) Maintain protein at 0.8 g/kg/d (10% of calories); include fish protein Maintain BMI at or below 25 kg/m²
Cease smoking	Absolute; use nicotine replacement therapy
Immunization	Hepatitis B, influenza, *Pneumococcus*
Alcohol intake	Limited to fluid restriction
BMI, body mass index; CKD, chronic kidney disease; PTH, parathyroid hormone.	

Table 9-6 Advantages, disadvantages and dialysis prescription for end-stage renal disease

	PERITONEAL DIALYSIS	HEMODIALYSIS
Access	Abdominal wall insertion of plastic catheter into the peritoneum Limitations: swimming and bathing can be contraindicated. Previous abdominal surgery can be a contraindication; rarely, a patent pleuro-peritoneal canal exists	Arteriovenous fistula, usually in the forearm
Timing	Daily exchanges, either every 6 hours (CAPD), or attached to an overnight (continuous) cycling machine (8 hours) (CCPD); no non-dialysis days	5–7 hours every 2nd or 3rd day; in some circumstances, daily or overnight hemodialysis can be offered (e.g. pregnancy); some non-dialysis days
Complications	Peritonitis (usually staphylococcal) Poorer exchange rates over time Peritoneal sclerosis in the long term	Bleeding from insertion sites Fistula aneurysm formation Recirculation or 'steal' phenomenon Poor flow rates and technical difficulties Fistula thrombosis or infection Progressive neurological disease
Compelling indications		Pregnancy Congestive cardiac failure Unstable coronary artery disease
Other considerations	Bulky home stores	Adequate space for machines at home Adequate plumbing, good-quality water supply
2-year patient survival	77%	60–80%
2-year technique survival	64%	60–80%
CAPD, continuous ambulatory peritoneal dialysis; CCPD, continuous cycling peritoneal dialysis.		

- screen for infections and malignancy
- reach targets for optimal outcomes for those with ESRD (bone health, anemia, dietary management, and protection from chronic fluid overload).

There are several evidence-based guidelines to direct appropriate treatment and dialysis prescription (Table 9-7, overleaf).

Concerns regarding adherence to diet and fluid restrictions occur when patients present with acute pulmonary edema and recurrent hyperkalemia and hyperphosphatemia.

- The net impact on quality of life is considerable, with a requirement for very tight fluid restrictions in those who are oligo/anuric.
- The dietary restriction on potassium intake is essential to prevent repeated and malignant hyperkalemia and the risk of cardiac death. Ongoing dietary advice and monitoring are required to ensure adequate attention to dietary issues.
- Given the extremely high rate of cardiovascular disease in this population, any episode of acute pulmonary edema needs to draw attention to the risk of underlying coronary artery disease and should be fully investigated.

Formations and prescription for dialysis require a multidisciplinary team with surgeons, vascular surgeons, interventional radiologists, interventional nephrologists, general nephrologists, appropriately specialized nurse educators, dietitians and family.

Transplantation

The best alternative to restore the greatest renal functional level is a renal transplant. A well-functioning, good-quality transplant will return eGFR to close to 50%. The cost of transplantation is also considerably lower than the annual cost of dialysis treatment.

The following are considerations in any patient regarding transplantation:

- underlying diagnosis, disease progression and likely recurrence rates
- suitability of the patient for major abdominal surgery
- infective risks associated with immunosuppression
- malignancy risks associated with immunosuppression
- management of long-term medication side-effects, especially from steroid treatment
- management of long-term cardiovascular risk
- chronic allograft nephropathy (return of CKD in a transplanted kidney).

All patients on dialysis should be given consideration for a renal transplant.

- Preparation and access to the waiting list is achieved by monthly tissue-typing, regular screening for alloreactive

Table 9-7 Targets in management of the dialysis patient

MANAGEMENT OF:	TARGETS
Anemia	Hemoglobin 110–120 g/L In the setting of adequate iron stores; uremia leads to poor iron absorption, so parenteral iron is often required
Hyperphosphatemia	Phosphate <1.6 mmol/L
Calcium and PTH	Calcium: high normal range PTH: 15–30 pmol/L
Cholesterol, LDL and triglycerides	Total cholesterol: <4.5 mmol/L LDL: <2.5 mmol/L Triglcyerides: <2.0 mmol/L
Blood pressure	<140/90 mmHg
Access	Good-quality access with aseptic approach to use
Dialysis adequacy	Reasonable urea concentrations in between dialysis, controlled potassium concentration, no episodes of fluid overload and, ultimately, control of symptoms

LDL, low-density lipoprotein; PTH, parathyroid hormone.

antibodies, viral screening for CMV, HIV and hepatitis B and C, and control of regular anesthetic risk factors.

- Active malignancy is a contraindication to transplant, as is any immediate anesthetic risk (e.g. recent myocardial infarction, stroke).
- Active infection is also a contraindication to the immunosuppression associated with transplantation. This includes tuberculosis and other chronic infections which should be excluded in the relevant risk groups.

In general, on a worldwide basis the most common transplant is now the living related or non-related transplant. This has superseded the deceased donor transplant, which has seen limited availability in some countries due to lack of donation from affected families (beating-heart donation). Most deceased donor transplants come from brain dead individuals, but in recent years there has been a steady increase in donors following cardiac death.

- The acceptance of a living donor onto the transplant program is related to their underlying physical and mental fitness for the donation, and the major surgery involved.
- Tissue and cross-match compatibility directs the appropriateness of the donation, and the likely degree of immunosuppression required.

The operation of kidney transplantation involves pelvic placement of the donated kidney in the iliac blood supply circle.

- There is considerable bladder surgery to allow implantation of the ureter via a tunnel in the posterior bladder wall.

- Immediate immunosuppression is required, and is usually a multi-pronged approach with corticosteroids, calcineurin inhibition, and an antimetabolite such as mycophenolate mofetil. This blocks multiple pathways in the immunological activation cascade, antigen recognition, cell multiplication, and inter-leukocyte signaling to enhance T-cell responses.
- At times additional immunosuppression with anti–T lymphocyte antibodies is indicated, either as prophylaxis in immunologically high-risk transplants or for treatment of severe acute rejection.
- On rare occasions, additional anti–T3 and other anti-cytokine therapy is indicated.
- Considerable drug development is ensuring that new treatments are constantly evolving.
- The nonspecific effects of the current regimens, including calcineurin nephrotoxicity, limit their safety in the longer term.

Transplant is best performed in highly active units with a mutidisciplinary team approach.

Rejection

- The immediate monitoring of a renal transplant is designed to detect cellular rejection (mild interstitial and tubular lymphocyte infiltration) and vascular (severe, hemorrhagic) rejection at the earliest stages. Rejection mediated by anti-HLA or other antibodies is increasingly recognized, particularly in recipients with high levels of anti-HLA antibodies.
- This is usually identified by the clinical signs of acute renal failure in the immediate postoperative period. This includes oliguria, a rising creatinine concentration and, if severe, fever and graft tenderness.
- It is usual to biopsy the transplant in this period to determine the severity and extent of rejection, and treat accordingly. Some institutions use 'protocol' biopsies (timed post-transplant biopsies whether creatinine is elevated or not) to determine the need for rejection treatment.

The risk factors for acute rejection include:

- prolonged ischemic period (for cadaveric grafts)
- >40% panel-reactive active antibodies (sensitized recipient = 30% risk of rejection)
- cadaveric transplantation
- suboptimal immunosuppressive treatment.

Outcomes

- The immediate prognosis for the transplant itself (graft survival) is approaching 95% at 1 year.
- Patient survival with a transplant in the first 5 years is 89%, which confers a significant survival advantage over dialysis, even for those in the older age groups.
- The intermediate to long-term outcomes for renal transplantation depend in part on the progression of subsequent chronic renal damage due to chronic allograft nephropathy (Box 9-13). This entity is characterized by glomerular and tubulo-interstitial scarring, as well as multilayering of the peritubular capillaries.

Box 9-13

Risk factors for chronic allograft nephropathy

- Advanced donor age
- Delayed graft function
- Repeated acute rejection episodes
- Vascular rejection episodes
- Rejection that occurs late after transplantation

It is further contributed to by other cardiovascular risk factors such as hypertension, hyperlipidemia and prothrombotic tendency.

ACUTE RENAL FAILURE—ACUTE KIDNEY INJURY (AKI)

The usual definition of acute renal failure has been replaced by a system of determining acute kidney injury (AKI), which can be due to *de novo* renal disease but is more usually a consequence of another major, often life-threatening illness.

The RIFLE criteria classifies AKI according to urine output and/or change in serum creatinine concentration. The lowest level of injury is *Risk* and the highest is *End-stage renal disease*:

R Risk—a 1.5-fold increase in serum creatinine and oliguria <0.5 mL/kg for 6 hours

I Injury—a 2-fold increase in serum creatinine and oliguria <0.5 mL/kg for 12 hours

F Failure—a 3-fold increase in serum creatinine and oliguria (<0.3 mL/kg for 24 hours) or an absolute rise in creatinine concentration to >355 micromol/L (reference range [RR] 60–90 micromol/L)

L Loss—if these insults persist for longer than 4 weeks

E End-stage renal disease—if persisting for longer than 3 months.

This classification system is helpful in terms of tracking prognosis, i.e. length of stay in hospital, as well as hospital and intensive care unit (ICU) mortality.

- The decision to intervene with hemodialysis is determined by physiological consequences such as fluid overload, hyperkalemia and acidosis, irrespective of classification.
- The mainstay of resuscitation, including judicious fluid management, cardiac monitoring, and frequent electrolyte testing, inotropes if required, and treatment of fluid overload with loop diuretics, prevents the need for dialysis in the majority of patients.
- The association of renal injury with other serious disease confers a worse prognosis for discharge from the ICU and for full recovery.

TUBULO-INTERSTITIAL DISEASES

Acute tubular necrosis is a common consequence of protracted circulatory failure.

- In hemodynamic shock, pre-renal failure is an early manifestation of reduced renal perfusion, and when corrected rapidly, restoration of renal function occurs.
- If the pre-renal insult continues or is exacerbated by other renal toxicity, then acute tubular necrosis can ensue.
- Limited forms of acute tubular necrosis can take up to 6 weeks to recover. Dialysis may be required during this phase, and as the patient recovers renal function, dialysis is withheld.
- If renal cortical blood flow is fully compromised, bilateral cortical necrosis occurs and there is no renal recovery.
- Other acute tubular toxicity occurs with hypoperfusion, drug or contrast toxicities (e.g. aminoglycosides), and rhabdomyolysis (see Table 9-8).
  - » Rhabdomyolysis causes acute tubular injury by accumulation of myoglobin in the renal tubules, and direct toxicity to tubular epithelial cells.
- The mechanism of injury is complex, involving pre-renal insult by hypoperfusion, muscle damage and acidification of urine, and reduced filtrate volume leading to myoglobin cast formation and release of heme from the myoglobin. These lead to acute tubular necrosis, which may or may not be reversible.
- Reversibility of the decrease in renal function is best achieved by restoration of blood pressure, restoration of renal blood flow, and alkalinization of the urine.

Acute interstitial nephritis (AIN)

- Acute interstitial nephritis is an inflammation of the interstitial intertubular region of the nephron, and it may or may not be associated with a decline in renal function.

Table 9-8 Causes of rhabdomyolysis

CAUSE	PRESENTATION
Trauma	Crush Blast injury Fixed muscle position, such as with alcohol or narcotic intoxication
Exertion	Extreme physical exercise (especially with dehydration) Prolonged seizures Delirium tremens
Vascular insufficiency	Arterial embolus or thrombosis
Drugs and toxins	Statins Malignant neuroleptic syndrome (e.g. haloperidol, chlorpromazine) Serotonin syndrome (selective serotonin reuptake inhibitors, SSRIs)

- AIN has many causes, most commonly drug toxicity or autoimmune disease such as Sjögren's syndrome and systemic lupus erythematosus (SLE), or granulomatosis with polyangiitis (GPA).
- Interstitial infiltrates are seen in some forms of lymphoma, multiple myeloma, and transplant rejection.
- AIN may occur in the context of drug hypersensitivity. This is associated with fever, rash, nausea and vomiting and, usually, a reduction in urine output with a concurrent increase in serum creatinine concentration. The diagnosis is suggested by eosinophils in the urine. Ultimately the diagnosis is confirmed by analysis of a renal biopsy, with presence of eosinophils in the inflammatory infiltrate particularly characteristic.

Treatment

- The focus is on removing the toxin, or stopping the agent that is the presumed cause.
- In some cases, a short course of corticosteroids is warranted to reverse the inflammatory lesion.
- In severe cases, dialysis may be required until some level of renal function is restored.

Chronic tubulo-interstitial disease

- Although there is a strong focus on the glomerular diagnosis of disease as outlined above, the progression to end-stage kidney disease is conferred by the extent of tubulo-interstitial scarring and tubular 'drop-out'.
- Tubulo-interstitial disease frequently results in electrolyte abnormalities.
- Causes include analgesic nephropathy (now rarely seen) and some congenital diseases such as Fabry's disease, an X-linked recessive sphingolipidosis.

Clinical presentation, investigation, diagnosis and treatment of chronic interstitial nephritis

- Chronic tubulo-interstitial disease is likely to present as chronic kidney disease with a slow deterioration of the GFR, and progressive proteinuria.
- Progression toward dialysis is monitored and managed accordingly, with appropriate and timely formation of vascular access.

ELECTROLYTE DISORDERS

Hypernatremia

Hypernatremia is a concentration of sodium in the serum that exceeds the upper limit of the normal range.

- Hypernatremia is a problem of fluid volume, not salt.
- It is almost universally seen in patients who are dehydrated and where the response to conserve sodium (aldosterone) is stronger than the response to conserve water (vasopressin).

- In very rare cases it can occur from excessive salt ingestion, for example from drinking seawater.

Causes of dehydration include:

- Excessive renal water loss
  - » Diabetes insipidus
    - central decrease in vasopressin production
  - » Diabetes mellitus, glycosuria
  - » Osmotic diuretics
  - » Psychogenic polydipsia
    - reduced urinary concentrating ability
  - » Advanced age effect on renal urinary concentrating ability
- Hypovolemia from non-renal losses
  - » decreased oral intake
  - » extreme sweating/burns
  - » severe high-fluid-volume diarrhea
  - » high-volume vomiting
- Primary mineralocorticoid excess (extreme).

Clinical presentation, investigation and diagnosis

- The clinical presentation of hypernatremia is predominantly that of dehydration: low BP with a significant postural decrease, tachycardia with a postural increase, dry mucous membranes, dry skin, and poor skin turgor.
- The consequences of the hypernatremia *per se* relate to muscle weakness, neuromuscular irritability, cerebral irritability, seizure and coma.
- Extreme hypernatremia is rarely seen and is almost universally fatal.

The diagnosis of hypertnatremia is proven on routine biochemical testing. Pre-renal insult is suggested by:

- the presence of high serum osmolality
- low urinary sodium concentration (< 20 mmol/L)
- high urine osmolality (>500 mOsm/L)
- high urine/plasma creatinine ratio (>40)
- very low fractional excretion of sodium (<1%)
- low fractional excretion of urea (<35%).

Diabetes insipidus is diagnosed by:

- dilute urine (osmolality <300 mOsm/L) with a low specific gravity
- low urine sodium concentration
- elevated serum osmolality (>290 mOsml/L).

When the diagnosis is unclear, a water deprivation test will demonstrate a continued urine output of free water despite a lack of intake, weight loss (water loss), hypernatremia, and a trend to elevated serum osmolality. This is corrected with desmopressin in the second phase of the test in the case of hypothalamic causes, and not in the case of nephrogenic causes.

Treatment and targets

- Treatment is largely by treating the underlying dehydrating illness.

- Caution must be taken to give initially more water than salt, but to monitor serum sodium concentration carefully so as not to cause a dilutional hyponatremia.
- Rapid swings of serum sodium concentration are thought to be causative of central pontine myelinolysis, which is a devastating and irreversible complication of rapid sodium concentration correction.

Hyponatremia

Hyponatremia is the most common electrolyte disturbance seen both in the community and in hospital patients. This is a serum concentration of sodium below the reference range.

- It is associated with many chronic medical conditions, medication use, and aging. It has significant physical consequences, even in the milder ranges.
- It is usually a problem of excess water relative to sodium in any situation.
- The situation arises when there is a vasopressin response, either through excess or heightened vasopressin sensitivity, in comparison to the aldosterone response.

Clinical presentation, investigation and diagnosis

The easiest algorithm for hyponatremia is to confirm whether the patient is *wet*, *dry*, or *euvolemic* (Table 9-9).

Table 9-9 Causes of hyponatremia

CAUSE	PRESENTATION
Hypovolemic hyponatremia ('dry')	Vomiting/diarrhea Diuretic use
Euvolemic hyponatremia	SIADH (syndrome of inappropriate secretion of antidiuretic hormone) Pain and stress Medication use
Hypervolemic hyponatremia ('wet')	Congestive cardiac failure Chronic liver disease Chronic kidney disease

The SIADH (syndrome of inappropriate secretion of antidiuretic hormone) category includes a broad range of causes which require excellent clinical skills, history, examination and basic biochemical investigations to sort out. Causes include:

- acute head injury and subarachnoid bleed
- small cell cancer of the lung
- pneumonia, lung abscess
- brain abscess
- meningitis
- hypothyroidism
- sarcoidosis
- drugs (e.g. carbamazepine, selective serotonin reuptake inhibitors [SSRIs]).

Treatment and targets

- The initial management includes slow restoration of serum sodium concentration by 1 mmol/L per hour, or not more than 12 mmol/L every 24 hours. This is best achieved by targeting the underlying abnormality: restoration of blood volume in dehydrated states, control of fluid overload in hypervolemic states, and investigation and control of pain in the euvolemic states.

CLINICAL PEARL

The caution with rapid reversal of hyponatremia, especially in those with extreme levels or where the comorbidity includes alcoholism, is to prevent central pontine myelinolysis.

- Rapid correction is often sought when the patient has a decreased level of consciousness, and when fitting. The correction in these patients still needs to be gradual, with appropriate supportive care and airway protection.

Hyperkalemia

Serum potassium concentration is controlled within very tight limits.

- Hyperkalemia is a feature of very-late-stage CKD (end-stage) and is one of the main indicators for dialysis. This often occurs when the GFR is very reduced, but can also occur at intermediate GFR reductions, especially when ACEIs and ATRAs (particularly in combination) are being used, and when there is tissue necrosis, gastro-enterological hemorrhage, or an inflammatory collection.
- Hyperkalemia is also seen in type 4 (distal) renal tubular acidosis (RTA) due to a functional decrease in aldosterone responsiveness. This is most commonly seen in patients with diabetes mellitus.
- Similarly, low mineralocorticoid concentration (seen in Addison's disease) can lead to hyperkalemia. It also occurs as a complication of various medications including cyclosporine A and tacrolimus, ACEIs and ATRAs.
- Hyperkalemia can be a transient phenomenon seen in early acidosis, where the buffering of acid load means that potassium is released from cells. This is corrected with the treatment of the acidosis. This form of hyperkalemia/acidosis is seen in burns, tumor lysis, rhabdomyolysis and severe gastrointestinal bleeding.

Clinical presentation, investigation and diagnosis

- The usual presentation of extreme hyperkalemia for those in whom this has developed slowly over time is muscle weakness and cardiac rhythm disturbances.
- A rapid rise in serum potassium in an acute setting can cause cardiac death.
- An electrocardiograph is required to determine PR interval, peaked T waves, bradycardia, widening of the QRS complex and lengthening of the QT interval.

Box 9-14

Treatment and targets for hyperkalemia

- Diagnose and correct mineralocorticoid deficiency
- Identify tubular acidosis, especially in diabetes
- Reverse and correct any acute-on-chronic renal failure
- Monitor blockade of the RAAS
- Avoid ACEI and ATRA combination therapy; avoid potassium-sparing diuretics and NSAIDs
- Monitor for any intercurrent illness likely to increase potassium in those with limited renal reserves (e.g. pneumonia, myocardial infarction)
- Rapidly deploy potassium into cells to protect the cardiac rhythm (dextrose and insulin infusion, calcium infusion)
- Remove excess potassium from the body (oral resonium, or dialysis)

ACEI, angiotensin-converting enzyme inhibitor; ATRA, angiotensin II receptor antagonist; NSAID, non-steroidal anti-inflammatory drug; RAAS, renin–angiotensin–aldosterone system.

Treatment and targets

These are given in Box 9-14.

Hypokalemia

Hypokalaemia is the finding on biochemistry of a reduced serum potassium concentration.

- This is seen in states of fluid loss (diarrhea and vomiting, renal losses), especially those associated with alkalosis.
- It is especially important in the setting of hypertension, as this may be a marker of secondary disease.
- Secondary hypertension and hypokalemia can occur in:
  » primary aldosteronism
  » secondary aldosteronism
  » pheochromocytoma (sympathetic activation of renin)
  » renal artery stenosis (secondary aldosteronism)
  » coarctation of the aorta (secondary aldosteronism).
- The most common cause of hypokalemia is renal loss due to diuretic use. This is particularly important in the elderly.
- Hypokalemia is seen in inherited and acquired renal tubular acidosis (see below). It is also seen in rapid correction of acidosis (where hydrogen ions are removed from cells and potassium rapidly returns).
- Hypokalemia in the setting of anorexia nervosa is largely dietary, but is contributed to by secondary aldosteronism.

Clinical presentation, investigation and diagnosis

- Presentation of hypokalemia is with muscle weakness and cardiac arrhythmia (Figure 9-9).
- Lower concentrations of potassium are associated with supraventricular and ventricular ectopics, and

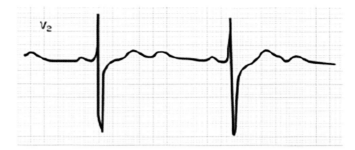
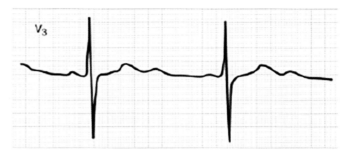
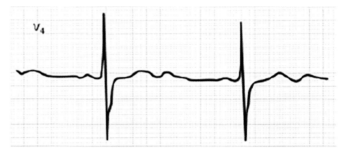

Figure 9-9 Electrocardiographic manifestations of hypokalemia: the ST segment is prolonged, primarily because of a U wave following the T wave, and the T wave is flattened

From Goldman L and Schafer AI. Goldman's Cecil medicine, 24th ed. Philadelphia: Elsevier, 2012.

tachyarrhythmias, as well as life-threatening torsades de pointes and ventricular tachycardia.

CLINICAL PEARL

Electrocardiographic changes in hypokalemia are typically an increase in amplitude and depth of the P wave, prolongation of the PR interval, T-wave flattening and ST depression, prominent U waves, and an apparent long QT due to fusion of the T and U waves.

Treatment and targets

Treatment of hypokalemia depends on treatment of the underlying condition.

- Acute management requires rapid potassium replacement, with cardiac monitoring, in a hospital environment where cardiac support can be offered.
- Where possible, particularly in chronic cases, oral potassium therapy is preferred.

INHERITED 'CHANNELOPATHIES' ASSOCIATED WITH HYPER-TENSION OR HYPO/HYPERKALEMIA

Hypokalemic alkalosis (with and without hypertension)

- This combination looks like mineralocorticoid excess, when there is hypertension.
- These conditions are a form of pseudoaldosteronism.
- In Liddle's syndrome, there is hypertension, hypokalemia and alkalosis without demonstrable aldosterone excess on repeated testing. This is due to a defect in the epithelial sodium channel (ENaC), due to an autosomal dominant inheritance. It is treated by blocking the sodium channel with a potassium-sparing diuretic (spironolactone), and control of sodium in the diet.

Similar presentations are seen in:

- the syndrome of apparent mineralocorticoid excess (autosomal recessive defect causing an increase in cortisone via 11-beta-hydroxysteroid dehydrogenase mutation, thus activating the mineralocorticoid receptor)
- glucocorticoid-remediable aldosteronism (a chimerism of the 11-hydroxylase and aldosterone synthase gene causing adrenocorticotrophic hormone [ACTH]-sensitive rises in aldosterone)
- other adrenal enzymatic disorders.

These are treated by a combination of ENaC blockade and mineralocorticoid receptor inhibition. Glucocorticoid treatment suppresses the ACTH production, and is also effective.

With sodium wasting, there is normal blood pressure. This occurs in Bartter syndrome (chloride channel defect) and Gitelman syndrome (thiazide-sensitive sodium chloride co-transporter [NCCT] in the distal convoluted tubule).

Renal tubular acidosis

The renal tubular acidoses (RTAs; Table 9-10) are a set of electrolyte and acid–base disturbances that arise from both congenital and acquired renal defects.

- The more common acquired distal (type 4) RTA is seen commonly in patients with diabetes mellitus, and features prominently in routine biochemistry in these patients.
- They are best understood by a classification system related to location within the collecting system and the presence of hyper- or hypokalemia. These are non-anion-gap acidoses, whereby the hyperchloremia and metabolic acidosis are the defining features.

Type 1 RTA

- This is the distal variety where the defect is in the cortical collecting duct of the distal nephron.
- The principal defect is one of a failure of acid secretion by the alpha-intercalated cells.
- There is also an inability to reabsorb potassium, leading to hypokalemia.

The main accompaniments of this RTA are:

- urinary calculus formation due to hypercalciuria
- low urinary citrate
- alkaline nature of the urine; there is an inability to acidify the urine to a pH of <5.3
- bone demineralization.

Acid challenge tests are used to establish the diagnosis in milder cases.

Table 9-10 Renal tubular acidosis (RTA)

TYPE	CAUSE	LOCATION	PRESENTATION	POTASSIUM STATUS
Type 1	Failure of H$^+$ secretion	Distal tubular (cortical collecting duct)	Osteomalacia Renal stones Nephrocalcinosis	Hypokalemia
Type 2	Bicarbonate wasting	Proximal tubular	Osteomalacia Uric acid stones	Hypokalemia
Type 4	Hypoaldosteronism	Distal tubular	Reduced aldosterone production or aldosterone resistance	Hyperkalemia
Mixed*	Inherited carbonic anhydrase II deficiency or early juvenile distal RTA with proximal features and high-salt diet	Combined proximal and distal	Cerebral calcification Mental retardation Osteopetrosis	

* Mixed type RTA was formerly known as type 3.

Causes

- Inherited
- Acquired:
  - » Sjögren's syndrome, SLE associations
  - » chronic urinary infection
  - » obstructive uropathy
  - » sickle cell disease
- Endocrine conditions such as:
  - » hyperparathyroidism
  - » hyperthyroidism
  - » chronic active hepatitis
  - » primary biliary cirrhosis
  - » hereditary deafness
  - » analgesic nephropathy
  - » transplant rejection
  - » renal medullary cystic disease

The disease is best understood by relating to the mechanisms of perturbed classical counter-exchange of potassium and hydrogen ions at a cellular level.

- The primary defect is either inability of the H^+ pump (proton pump) to work against the high H+ gradient, or insufficient capacity due to tubular damage. There can be back-diffusion of H^+ due to damage (seen in amphotericin B nephrotoxicity).
- Clinical presentation relates to the hypokalemia, and subsequent muscle weakness and cardiac arrhythmias.
- The inherited form in children manifests as growth retardation if not treated.

The primary **treatment** is to correct the acidosis with bicarbonate, and then correction of the hypokalemia, hypercalciuria, and salt depletion will follow.

Type 2 RTA

- Type 2 is generally easier to understand because it reflects a primary failure of main proximal tubular functions. This leads to a loss of bicarbonate in the urine, and subsequent acidemia.
- The other proximal tubular functions that may be affected result in phosphaturia, glycosuria, aminoaciduria, uricosuria and tubular proteinuria.
- This full-blown tubular loss is termed Fanconi syndrome.
- The bicarbonate loss can also be seen as an isolated defect.
- Demineralization is also seen here due to phosphate wasting.

THE KIDNEYS IN PREGNANCY AND PREGNANCY-RELATED DISEASES

Renal disease has important implications in pregnancy as the normal adaptations to pregnancy have far-reaching effects, not only on pregnancy events and outcomes *per se*, but also on the progression of underlying renal disease to end-stage kidney disease.

Normal adaptations to pregnancy

- The sequence of physiological events in pregnancy starts with a decrease in systemic vascular resistance such that there is a dramatic and persistent decrease in BP.
- This decrease in BP is resistant to the normal vascular stressors which increase BP outside of pregnancy (e.g. angiotensin II and epinephrine).
- The decrease in BP manifests as a marked increase in renal plasma flow, initiated by the decrease in renovascular resistance.
- The increase in blood flow increases the GFR dramatically, up to 40% in the 1st trimester. This is important to note, as it will lead to a dramatic decrease in the value of the serum creatinine in pregnancy, due to hyperfiltration.

Underlying renal disease

The requirement in pregnancy for massive flow adaptation means that any underlying renal disease where renal flow reserve is limited may manifest with complications in pregnancy.

- The most common of these is chronic hypertension. Of those patients with chronic hypertension and also those with renal disease, the risk of developing superimposed preeclampsia is of the order of 30% and is largely conferred by the hypertension, particularly if BP control is poor. Therefore, importance is placed on monitoring for any decline in renal function and for the fetal and maternal effects of hypertension in pregnancy.
- The effect of the pregnancy *per se* on progression of renal disease is hard to determine.
  - » It is widely held that >3 pregnancies in women in populations with higher rates of renal disease leads to a more rapid progression to CKD and eventual dialysis.
  - » There are also some kidney diseases that are worse than others in terms of progression, with FSGS and reflux nephropathy being the most aggressive. Rapid progression to end-stage kidney disease is also described in many other renal diseases.
  - » When the creatinine concentration is >140 mmol/L (RR 60–90 mmol/L), the chances of progression within the pregnancy are greatly increased. Consideration should be given to early dialysis in these circumstances, with some published data suggesting that a GFR <30 mL/min/1.73 m² should be considered for dialysis.

Management

- Both hemodialysis and continuous ambulatory peritoneal dialysis (CAPD) are options in pregnancy. The mainstay of treatment is to maintain the serum urea to <10.0 mmol/L (RR 3–8 mmol/L) in order to reduce the fetal complication of polyhydramnios (which is associated with premature delivery).
- Similarly, attempts to control BP are paramount to managing the pregnancy and improving the likely pregnancy outcome.

- Fertility is markedly reduced in women already established on dialysis. This is in part due to hyperprolactinemia, but is contributed to by the uremic milieu in women with end-stage disease.
- It is more likely that pregnancy will occur in the first 24 months on dialysis. Management requires an increase in the dialysis frequency, and targets for urea and BP control should be carefully met.
- Anemia should be carefully managed with appropriate erythropoetin (EPO) replacement.

SELF-ASSESSMENT QUESTIONS

1   A 16-year-old is brought in by her sister due to a 9-day history of periorbital and ankle edema, both of which are worse toward the end of the day. She has noticed foamy urine. She has had a sore throat in that time, but her medical history is otherwise unremarkable and she takes no medications. Her birthweight was 2350 g at 39 weeks of gestation (RR normal >2500 g) and she was born by normal vaginal delivery. Her mother consumed 1 glass of beer most days of the pregnancy. She had menarche at 13 years and has a regular cycle. On physical examination, temperature is normal, blood pressure is 160/90 mmHg, pulse rate is 60/min, and respiration rate is 12/min; body mass index is 24 kg/m^2. Fundoscopic examination shows silver wiring of the retinal arterioles. There is bilateral pedal edema to just past the knee. Urinalysis shows 4+ blood; no protein.

Laboratory studies show serum creatinine 70.7 micromol/L (RR 60–90 micromol/L), urine protein–creatinine ratio 10 mg/mmol Cr. A kidney biopsy is performed. Light microscopy of the specimen reveals diffuse inflammation within the glomerular tufts. On electron microscopy, there are subepithelial lumpy immunoglobulin deposits. Immunofluorescence testing shows widespread granular deposits. Which of the following is the most appropriate treatment for this patient?

A   Cyclophosphamide
B   Cyclosporine (ciclosporin)
C   Penicillin
D   Prednisone

2   A 35-year-old, otherwise well woman presented to the emergency department with 2 days of fever and macroscopic hematuria. She had a prodrome of a sore throat for 2 days. On examination, blood pressure was 190/90 mmHg, urine heavily bloodstained and leucocyte-positive, protein ++. She has normal heart sounds and no stigmata of bacterial endocarditis. She had had an uneventful pregnancy 12 months previously, with no hypertension or proteinuria. She is planning further children. Laboratory investigations show creatinine initially 81 micromol/L (baseline 65 micromol/L; RR 60–90 micromol/L) and rising to 109 micromol/L. Urgent renal ultrasound showed normal-sized kidneys. Urgent renal biopsy was then performed (see Figure 9-10). Which combination of treatment is most appropriate in this clinical situation?

A   Antihypertensive treatment with an angiotensin-converting enzyme (ACE) inhibitor and a course of oral penicillin
B   Antihypertensive treatment with a calcium-channel blocker and consideration of high-dose prednisone and cyclophosphamide
C   Combination antihypertensive therapy with an ACI inhibitor and an angiotensin II receptor antagonist (ATRA) with a focus on her proteinuria
D   Antihypertensive treatment with high-dose diuretics and a beta-blocker, with low-dose corticosteroids

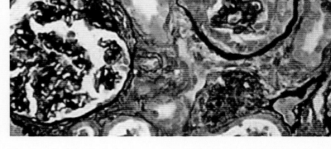

Figure 9-10 Renal biopsy results for patient in Question 2

From Lim E, Loke YK and Thompson AM (eds). Medicine and surgery: an integrated textbook. Elsevier, 2007.

3   A 29-year-old non-smoking male presents with marked lethargy and recent increased creatinine discovered on blood testing. He had had an episode of hematuria at the age of 3 years, and is known to have a duplex left ureter. A slightly elevated creatinine was noted 12 months earlier. He had a renal biopsy at that time, and had refused any treatment with steroids due to the risk of diabetes. He now presents 12 months later. Laboratory investigations show creatinine 150 micromol/L (baseline 90 micromol/L; RR 60–90 micromol/L) and rising to 553 micromol/L over the next 12 months. A renal ultrasound performed at this presentation shows small kidneys (9 cm left and 8.8 cm right). A renal biopsy performed 12 months ago showed focal glomerular sclerosis with a collapsing pattern and some mild cellular infiltration. Which of the following management approaches would be most appropriate in this situation?

A   Monitor for anemia and serum phosphate, and control any blood pressure or lipid abnormalities.
B   Commence dialysis immediately.
C   Insist on a repeat renal biopsy to determine any new pattern of glomerular injury.
D   Commence empirical treatment with steroids and cyclophosphamide.

ANSWERS

1 **C.**

This patient most likely has post-infectious/post-streptococcal glomerulonephritis (PSGN) in the setting of her recent sore throat. A combination of hypertension, hematuria and positive serology for streptococcal infection in a younger patient has a high positive predictive value for the disease. This disease is a common GN in communities of low socioeconomic status and where crowding exists; there are concerns in some disadvantaged communities that renal mass is influenced by *in utero* factors such as alcohol consumption and prematurity or low birthweight. Renal biopsy is required to confirm the diagnosis, although this is not essential in communities where PSGN is common. Empirical treatment should commence immediately. Treatment in this situation would be appropriate with antibiotics for the streptococcal infection. Despite the extent of the renal inflammation there is no indication for immunosuppressive therapy, which is generally ineffective. In those with recurrent disease and where there is progressive loss of renal function, monitoring renal function and treating infections is the mainstay of treatment.

2 **B.**

The combination of crescentic GN in the setting of immunoglobulin A (IgA) disease (mesangial IgA deposits confirm the diagnosis) is an uncommon but potentially kidney-threatening presentation of IgA disease. More commonly, IgA disease has a classic presentation of nephritic syndrome with a chronic progressive pattern. The extent of renal damage is due to the amount of progressive scarring. The presence of a crescent indicates that within 3 months all glomerular function will be lost if there is not aggressive immunosuppressive treatment. The post-sore-throat presentation is again not uncommon in IgA disease and would indicate that streptococcal disease should be excluded. Ultimately the renal biopsy is required to differentiate IgA and post-streptococcal glomerulonephritis (PSGN). The presence of crescents requires a month-long course of prednisone (1 mg/kg/day dosing) with slow tapering, and cyclophosphamide under the supervision of a nephrologist. It is usual to follow up with a repeat renal biopsy to ensure that the inflammatory component is completely resolved. Refractory lesions will require ongoing maintenance support with steroid-sparing immunosuppressive treatment (cyclosporine [ciclosporin], azathioprine or mycophenolate).

3 **A.**

He has demonstrated the rapid progression seen in about 15% of cases of focal segmental glomerulosclerosis (FSGS). Up to 50% will require dialysis in the first decade of the diagnosis. His current estimated glomerular filtration rate (eGFR) is around 13 mL/min/1.73 m^2 and this is in the category when dialysis starts to be considered. The indications for urgent dialysis are hyperkalemia uncontrolled by diet, acidosis, uremic pericarditis, fluid overload, and symptoms of nausea and vomiting. A recent study of the lifetime benefit of commencing dialysis at 15 mL/min/1.73 m^2 vs 10 mL/min/1.73 m^2 did not clearly demonstrate a survival advantage in starting early. The need for dialysis is determined by patient choice (peritoneal dialysis vs hemodialysis) and the presence of symptoms. At the time, monitoring and treating erythropoietin-deficiency anemia, controlling hyperphosphatemia with diet and binders, and managing hypertension, hyperlipidemia and other cardiovascular risk factors (smoking, weight reduction) are the important aspects of treatment.

CHAPTER 10

ENDOCRINOLOGY

David Simmons, Rohit Rajagopal, Milan K Piya, Sue Lynn Lau and Mark McLean

CHAPTER OUTLINE

SYSTEM OVERVIEW

Hormones, their transport and action

A hormone is a chemical substance released from a secretory cell that acts upon specific receptors present in another cell, to effect a physiological change in the function of the target cell. **Endocrine** action occurs in a distant organ, usually after transportation of the hormone through the circulatory system. A **paracrine** action is upon a cell adjacent to the secretory cell, and **autocrine** actions are upon receptors expressed by the hormone-secreting cell itself.

Hormonal substances fall into a number of different chemical categories:

- small peptides such as the hypothalamic-releasing factors, and glycopeptides such as thyroid-stimulating hormone and the gonadotropins
- large peptides such as insulin, glucagon and parathyroid hormone
- steroid hormones derived from cholesterol, including cortisol, aldosterone, estrogen, progesterone and androgens
- amino acid derivatives such as thyroid hormones and catecholamines
- vitamin derivatives such as the hydroxylated forms of vitamin D.

The chemical nature of different hormones dictates their sites of action and their chemical metabolism. Thyroid hormones and steroid hormones are lipid-soluble and cross cell membranes readily. Therefore, these classes of hormones are able to act on cytoplasmic receptors within the target cell.

Many hormones bind with high affinity to binding proteins in plasma. These include specific binding proteins such as thyroid-hormone-binding globulin (TBG) and cortisol-binding globulin (CBG), but there is also a substantial amount of nonspecific binding to more abundant proteins such as albumin and pre-albumin. Protein binding has an important effect on hormone function since it renders the hormone molecule biologically inactive while in the bound state, but also protects it from degradation. In this way, protein binding creates a storage pool of inactive hormone, which is in dynamic equilibrium with a smaller pool of free, biologically active hormone.

Hormone action is determined as much by receptor factors as it is by the circulating hormone concentration.

Abnormalities of receptor function or of downstream second messenger systems can cause disturbance to endocrine systems, which are not necessarily revealed by measurement of circulating hormone concentrations.

Feedback control of hormone systems

Most endocrine systems regulate the secretion of hormones through **negative feedback**. An example is the action of the hypothalamus and pituitary in regulation of the thyroid, adrenal cortex and gonads (Figure 10-1). The secretion of thyroid hormones, cortisol and sex steroids is closely regulated by pituitary release of thyroid-stimulating hormone (TSH), adrenocorticotropic hormone (ACTH) and gonadotropins, respectively. These, in turn, are regulated by hypothalamic releasing factors. The involvement of the hypothalamus allows signal input from the central nervous system (CNS) so that endocrine function can be responsive to a wide variety of stimuli. Negative feedback action occurs

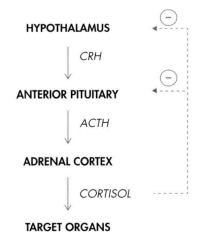

Figure 10-1 An example of a classic endocrine negative feedback loop. In this case, corticotropin-releasing hormone (CRH) from the hypothalamus stimulates adrenocorticotropic hormone (ACTH) release from the anterior pituitary, which in turn stimulates cortisol production by the adrenal gland. Cortisol provides negative feedback to the hypothalamus and pituitary to regulate its own production

when thyroid hormones, cortisol or sex steroids act upon the hypothalamus and anterior pituitary to inhibit production of stimulatory factors of each axis. This negative feedback regulation serves to stabilize the circulating hormone concentrations, while allowing the system to be responsive to external stimuli.

Hormonal systems not controlled by the pituitary also demonstrate **direct feedback** regulation. Examples include the regulation of parathyroid hormone secretion by serum calcium, control of insulin and glucagon secretion by plasma glucose concentration, and variation in antidiuretic hormone (vasopressin) in response to plasma osmolality.

Evaluating function of hormone systems

An important function of most hormone systems is to maintain a stable metabolic and physiological environment. To this end, the secretion of hormones often varies greatly in response to external stimuli. For example, in order to maintain a fairly constant plasma glucose concentration, the secretion of insulin can vary many-fold depending upon whether the individual is in a fed or a fasted state.

Further variations in hormone concentrations occur because of cyclical variation. For example, cortisol and ACTH are regulated on a diurnal cycle; in menstruating women the gonadotropins and sex steroids are regulated on a monthly cycle; still other hormonal systems are regulated upon lifetime cycles, such as those involved in the initiation of puberty. Therefore, it is often difficult to define a 'normal' hormone concentration.

CLINICAL PEARL

Always view the results of hormone measurements in the light of the physiological context. It is often appropriate to perform dynamic tests of endocrine function rather than rely on a static 'snapshot' measurement of a hormone concentration.

When excess of a hormone is suspected it is useful to undertake a suppression test, or to create a physiological circumstance in which secretion of the hormone should normally be inhibited. Conversely, when a hormone deficiency is suspected, a stimulation test will provide the most useful diagnostic information. Specific examples will be considered throughout this chapter.

Hormone measurement

Almost all laboratory measurements of hormone concentrations use forms of **immunoassay**. These laboratory techniques have high sensitivity and specificity and can be applied to a very small volume of sample. However, laboratory artifacts may occur and produce inaccurate results.

The **action of binding proteins** is a very important consideration. Most immunoassay techniques measure total hormone concentration, which includes inactive, protein-bound hormone. In the case of cortisol or thyroid hormones, less than 5% of the total hormone concentration is free and biologically active. Variations in binding-hormone

concentration (e.g. increased by pregnancy, decreased by nephrotic syndrome) greatly affect the overall measured hormone concentration, although in some circumstances it is possible to measure the free fraction of a circulating hormone (e.g. free thyroxine) to circumvent this problem.

CLINICAL PEARL

When interpreting the results of endocrine testing, a prudent physician considers the whole patient, and not just the test result. If results appear discordant with the patient's clinical condition, always recheck the test and consider potential sources of artifact.

Imaging in endocrinology

In the investigation of endocrine disorders it is important to first determine whether a hormonal abnormality is present, prior to undertaking any imaging to identify a cause.

Modern medical imaging demonstrates that 5–10% of healthy individuals harbor adenomas in the pituitary, adrenal or thyroid glands. The vast majority of these are benign and hormonally inactive. Conversely, functionally significant lesions causing, for example, hyperparathyroidism, Cushing's disease or insulinoma syndrome, may be impossible to locate by imaging procedures. It is therefore important to demonstrate that a lesion is associated with a definite hormonal abnormality before ascribing a functional diagnosis to it.

CLINICAL PEARL

Confirm the presence of a functional hormone disorder before undertaking imaging studies to locate its source. Failure to do this can cause false assumptions about the significance of incidental 'lesions' seen on imaging studies.

Pathogenic mechanisms of hormone disorders

Hormone deficiency

Endocrine hypofunction most commonly results from **primary gland dysfunction** acquired as a result of a variety of pathological processes including autoimmunity, trauma, surgery, irradiation, hemorrhage or infarction, infection or an infiltrative process. Primary glandular hypofunction can also be due to congenital agenesis of a hormone-secreting gland or a critical mutational change, which leads to reduced or absent activity of the hormone or its receptor.

In the situation of primary hypofunction there is loss of negative feedback, which may result in characteristic and diagnostic elevations of stimulating factors to the failed organ (e.g. elevated TSH secretion in response to primary hypothyroidism).

On the other hand, secondary gland hypofunction occurs when there is loss of a normal physiological stimulator of glandular function. The most common example of this is secondary dysfunction of the thyroid, adrenal cortex or gonads as a consequence of pituitary or hypothalamic disease.

CLINICAL PEARL

Secondary hypofunction can be distinguished by the lack of compensatory elevation of stimulating factors and the presence of gland hypofunction.

A final mechanism of hormonal hypofunction is **hormone resistance**, which may be relative or absolute. Resistance to hormone action in the presence of an adequate hormone concentration may be due to dysfunction of a hormone receptor or of downstream mediators of hormone action. The most common example is insulin resistance, which is a fundamental part of the pathogenesis of type 2 diabetes. Insulin resistance is usually a relative phenomenon, is multifactorial, and may be compensated by increased insulin secretion by the pancreatic beta-cell. Rarer forms of hormone resistance are associated with mutations of specific hormone receptors (e.g. thyroid hormone resistance, pseudo-hypoparathyroidism).

Hormone excess

Primary hypersecretion of hormones is most commonly due to a benign neoplasm (adenoma) within a hormone-secreting gland, which demonstrates autonomous hyperfunction and loss of normal physiological feedback inhibition. The molecular pathogenesis of most endocrine adenomas is poorly understood.

A second mechanism of primary hormone hypersecretion is autoimmune stimulation. The classic example of this is Graves' disease in which a stimulating autoantibody to the TSH receptor drives primary hyperthyroidism.

Gland hyperfunction may also rarely occur as a result of an activating mutation in a tropic hormone receptor. For example, an activating mutation of the LH receptor can cause male precocious puberty due to inappropriate secretion of testosterone (testotoxicosis).

A final cause of hormone excess, mimicking primary glandular hyperfunction, is iatrogenic administration of supraphysiological amounts of hormones as therapy. This is a particularly important consideration in the differential diagnosis of hyperthyroidism and of adrenocortical excess.

CLINICAL PEARL

A hallmark of all forms of *primary* endocrine hyperfunction is down-regulation of the physiological stimulators for that function.

Secondary hypofunction can be distinguished by the lack of compensatory elevation of stimulating factors and the presence of gland hypofunction.

Secondary hyperfunction of a hormone-secreting gland occurs when there is excessive stimulation by a physiological regulator, for example adrenal cortical hyperfunction due to ACTH hypersecretion. Primary and secondary hyperfunction will result in the same clinical syndrome but can be distinguished from each other by the fact that *secondary hyperfunction is not accompanied by negative feedback inhibition of the stimulator.*

DISORDERS OF THE PITUITARY AND HYPOTHALAMUS

Anatomy and physiology

The pituitary gland is a composite of the *adenohypophysis* (anterior pituitary) and the *neurohypophysis* (posterior pituitary), which have separate embryological origins. The adenohypophysis originates from pharyngeal epithelium and migrates into the cranial cavity in early fetal development, establishing a vascular connection to the hypothalamus (hypothalamic–pituitary portal vessels). The neurohypophysis constitutes the axonal projections of hypothalamic nerves. The important anatomical relations of the pituitary are the optic chiasm superiorly, the sphenoid bone and sphenoid air sinus inferiorly, and the structures of the venous cavernous sinuses laterally. The cavernous sinus contains the carotid arteries, venous plexus and the 3rd (oculomotor), 4th (troclear), 5th (trigeminal, ophthalmic and maxillary division) and 6th (abducens) cranial nerves (Figure 10-2). Therefore, mass lesions arising within the pituitary fossa may result in neurological symptoms from compression of these adjacent structures.

- The anterior pituitary secretes six major hormones, as well as other hormone fragments and intermediate products. Adrenocorticotropin (ACTH), thyroid-stimulating hormone (TSH), luteinizing hormone (LH), follicle-stimulating hormone (FSH), growth hormone (GH) and prolactin (PRL) are each under the control of one or more hypothalamic factors (see Table 10-1). Hypothalamic control is predominantly stimulatory, with the exception of prolactin which is predominantly regulated by inhibition. Therefore, disconnection of the anterior pituitary from the hypothalamus results in a reduction in secretion in all hormones except prolactin.

- The neurohypophysis secretes vasopressin (also known as antidiuretic hormone, ADH) and oxytocin. Hormone release occurs from nerve endings in the posterior

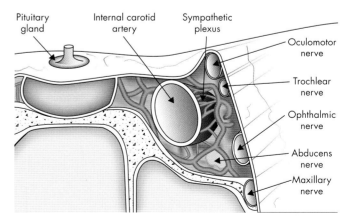

Figure 10-2 A coronal section of the right cavernous sinus showing the relationship between pituitary, cavernous sinus, vessels and nerves

From Kline LB, Acker JD and Post MJD. Computed tomographic evaluation of the cavernous sinus. Ophthalmology 1982;89:374–85.

Table 10-1 Physiological regulators of pituitary hormone secretion

HORMONE	STIMULATOR	INHIBITOR
Adrenocorticotropic hormone (ACTH)	Corticotrophin-releasing hormone (CRH)	
Thyroid-stimulating hormone (TSH)	Thyrotropin-releasing hormone (TRH)	
Luteinizing hormone/follicle-stimulating hormone [LH/FSH)	Gonadotropin-releasing hormone (GnRH)	Prolactin
Growth hormone (GH)	Growth-hormone-releasing hormone (GHRH) Ghrelin	Somatostatin
Prolactin (PRL)	TRH	Dopamine

pituitary but is controlled by the nerve bodies located in the hypothalamus.

Pituitary mass lesions

Adenomas are benign neoplasms arising from endocrine cells of the anterior pituitary and are the most common intracranial neoplasm. At autopsy, up to 20% of all adults are found to harbor a small unsuspected adenoma, mostly with no clinical significance. Pituitary adenomas are usually sporadic and their pathogenesis is poorly understood. They are classified on the basis of:

(i) size into microadenomas (<10 mm diameter) and macroadenomas (>10 mm), and

(ii) cellular origin (Figure 10-3).

The 2017 WHO classification identifies adenohypophyseal tumors as arising from corticotrope, gonadotrope or somato/lacto/thyrotrope lineage, based on the pattern of transcription factor staining on histological evaluation. Tumors without characteristic staining are termed null cell tumors. For each cell type, tumors may be termed 'functioning' or 'non-functioning', depending on their pattern of hormone secretion and consequent clinical effects. When adenohypophyseal tumors show evidence of craniospinal or associated systematic metastases, they are termed 'pituitary carcinoma'. This is a rare condition. Other disease processes may produce a mass lesion in the region of the anterior pituitary, usually causing hypopituitarism:

- non-adenomatous tumors (craniopharyngioma, germ-cell tumor)
- autoimmune inflammation (hypophysitis)
- other inflammatory disorders (sarcoidosis, histiocytosis)
- cystic lesions (Rathke's cleft cyst, arachnoid cyst)
- carotid artery aneurysm
- metastatic neoplasms.

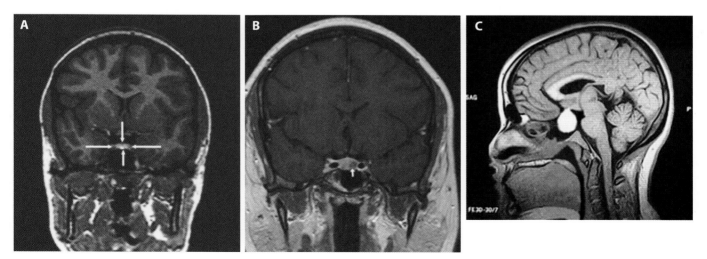

Figure 10-3 MRI images of (**A**) normal pituitary, (**B**) microadenoma, and (**C**) macroadenoma

From: (A) McMaster FP et al. Effect of antipsychotics on pituitary gland volume in treatment-naïve first-episode schizophrenia: a pilot study. Schizphr Res 2007;92(1–3):207–10. (B) Torigian DA, Li, G and Alavi A. The role of CT, MR imaging and ultrasonography in endocrinology. PET Clinics 2007;2(3):395–408. (C) Klatt EC. Robbins and Cotran Atlas of pathology, 2nd ed. Philadelphia: Elsevier, 2010.

CLINICAL PEARL

Cardinal manifestations of pituitary disorders
Abnormalities of the anterior pituitary cause three clinical problems:
- syndromes of pituitary hormone excess
- effects of a space-occupying mass
- hormone deficiencies.

All three manifestations may be present in the same patient and must be evaluated individually.

Hypopituitarism

Deficiency of anterior pituitary hormone secretion results in secondary failure of cortisol, thyroid hormone and sex steroid production. The biochemical hallmark of secondary failure is lack of a compensatory increase in pituitary hormone levels as the end organ fails (e.g. hypothyroidism *without* a rise in serum TSH). There is often a tendency for hormonal function to be lost in sequence—GH and gonadotropins first, followed by TSH, and then ACTH.

Causes of anterior pituitary failure are:

- pituitary mass lesions (as above)
- infection (bacterial, fungal, tuberculosis)
- irradiation (treatment of CNS or nasopharyngeal tumors, total body irradiation)
- trauma, surgery or vascular injury
- 'empty sella' syndrome
- congenital hypopituitarism (mutations of pituitary transcription factors)
- autoimmunity (spontaneous, or related to immune checkpoint-inhibitor therapy used in oncology).

Clinical features

The clinical effects (Table 10-2) are similar to primary adrenal, thyroid or gonadal disease. Growth failure is an important additional manifestation in children.

Diagnosis

Basal concentrations of the anterior pituitary hormones and of hormones produced by their respective target glands should be measured. Many deficiencies can be determined from a single plasma sample, best obtained in the morning. Assessment of gonadotropin function may require consideration of variations throughout the lifecycle, such as pubertal or menopausal status and stage of menstrual cycle. Function of the pituitary–adrenal axis and GH secretion may require dynamic testing:

- A 0900 plasma cortisol level <150 nmol/L (5.5 microg/dL) indicates probable ACTH deficiency; >450 nmol/L (16.5 microg/dL) indicates sufficiency; intermediate levels require clarification with a stimulation test (usually a hypoglycemia stress test, see insulin tolerance test (ITT) below).
- GH secretion is pulsatile. Normal individuals can have undetectable GH levels between pulses of secretion. Normal insulin-like growth factor 1 (IGF-1) levels

Table 10-2 Clinical effects of pituitary hormone deficiencies

HORMONE	CONTEXT	SYMPTOMS AND SIGNS
In panhypopituitarism, all are combined, although diabetes insipidus (ADH deficiency) is often absent		
ACTH	Acute	Fatigue, weakness, hypotension, weakness, vomiting
	Chronic	As in Addison's disease, except lack of pigmentation, electrolyte disturbance and hypovolemia Hypoglycemia, weight loss
TSH	Children	Growth retardation
	Adults	As for primary hypothyroidism, thyroid atrophy
GH	Children	Growth retardation, increased adiposity
	Adults	↓ Exercise capacity, ↓ lean mass, ↑ fat mass, ↑ cardiovascular risk
Gonadotropins	Children	Failure of sexual maturation, lack of pubertal growth spurt
	Men	As for primary hypogonadism, testicular atrophy, infertility
	Women	Secondary amenorrhea, infertility, osteoporosis
Prolactin	Women	Failure of lactation
Vasopressin (ADH)		Polyuria, dilute urine, thirst, nocturia, hypernatremia
ACTH, adrenocorticotropic hormone; ADH, antidiuretic hormone; GH, growth hormone, TSH, thyroid-stimulating hormone.		

suggest probable GH sufficiency. Definitive proof of GH deficiency requires failure of GH response to a stimulation test (usually an insulin tolerance test, ITT).

- An ITT is performed by administering intravenous (IV) insulin to cause hypoglycemia <2.2 mmol/L (40 mg/dL), which provokes a prompt rise in plasma cortisol and GH in normal individuals. Peak cortisol <450 nmol/L (16.5 microg/dL) or GH < 9 mU/L (3 ng/mL) is interpreted as a deficient response. Some cut-offs may vary with the assay method.

CLINICAL PEARL

Posterior pituitary function is usually preserved in cases of pituitary adenoma—even with large macroadenomas. When diabetes insipidus occurs with a pituitary mass lesion, an alternative diagnosis (inflammatory cause, non-adenomatous tumor, metastasis) should be suspected.

Pituitary hormone replacement

Hypopituitarism is usually permanent. Patients will therefore require lifelong hormone replacement therapy to replicate normal physiological hormone concentrations. With the exception of GH and ADH treatment, replacement therapy is achieved by administering target-organ hormones (glucocorticoids, thyroxine, sex steroids) rather than pituitary hormones. The dosage and administration of these hormones is identical to the treatment of primary hypoadrenalism, hypothyroidism or gonadal failure, except for the following differences:

- Treatment is monitored by measurements of the administered hormone (e.g. thyroxine), not the tropic hormone (TSH).
- There is usually no need to administer mineralocorticoid replacement as adrenal secretion of aldosterone is still regulated normally by the renin–angiotensin axis.
- To achieve fertility it is necessary to administer gonadotropins to stimulate ovulation or spermatogenesis.

CLINICAL PEARL

In treating pituitary failure, monitoring is of the administered hormone (e.g. thyroxine), not the pituitary hormone (TSH).

Syndromes of hypersecretion

Hyperprolactinemia

Prolactin-secreting adenomas (prolactinomas) are the most common functioning pituitary tumors. However, hyperprolactinemia can result from non-tumor causes because the dominant control of prolactin secretion from the pituitary is inhibitory, by dopamine release from the hypothalamus. Any interruption of dopamine release, transport or action will result in disinhibition of normal pituitary lactotropes, and the plasma prolactin concentration can increase up to sixfold above normal.

- Mild levels of hyperprolactinemia (<2 times normal range) are often transient and not related to any identifiable pathology.
- Causes of significant hyperprolactinemia (>2–3 times normal range) are:
  » prolactin-secreting pituitary adenoma (prolactinoma)
  » physiological stimulation (pregnancy, lactation, nipple stimulation, stress)
  » dopamine antagonism (antipsychotic and antiemetic drugs)
  » pituitary–hypothalamic disconnection (stalk compression, trauma, surgery).

Clinical features

Prolactin inhibits the function of the pituitary–gonadal axis at the level of gonadotropin secretion and sex steroid synthesis.

- In women:
  » abnormalities of the menstrual cycle due to anovulation or an abnormal luteal phase, presenting as amenorrhea, irregular cycles or infertility
  » loss of libido
  » galactorrhea, but only if estrogen is also present
  » if due to a prolactinoma, the tumor is most often a microadenoma.
- In men:
  » impotence, infertility, hypogonadism
  » gynecomastia, but usually no galactorrhea
  » prolactinomas are often macroadenomas and present with mass-related symptoms.

Most microadenomas do not grow, or cause mass effects or hypopituitarism.

Diagnosis

The cause of hyperprolactinemia can usually be determined by exclusion of drug-related or physiological causes, and appropriate pituitary imaging. False positive results for hyperprolactinemia can occur because of the presence of a prolactin-binding antibody (macroprolactin), which can be excluded by further laboratory analysis.

Treatment of prolactinoma

Prolactin-secreting pituitary adenomas are responsive to pharmacological suppression by dopamine agonists (e.g. bromocriptine, cabergoline, quinagolide). In >80% of cases there will be suppression of prolactin levels to close to the normal range, accompanied by reduction in tumor volume. Such medical therapy is the mainstay of treatment in most cases, and can be maintained for many years if needed.

In women desiring fertility, bromocriptine or cabergoline can be used to restore ovulatory cycles. Treatment can be ceased at conception in women with microadenomas, but should be continued in pregnancy to suppress pituitary tumor growth in women with macroadenomas.

Pituitary surgery or radiotherapy are secondary treatments for prolactinomas which do not respond well to dopamine agonists.

Acromegaly

After prolactinomas, GH-secreting tumors are the next most common functioning pituitary adenomas. In adults, the

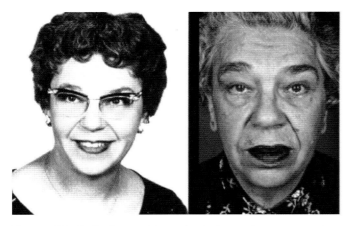

Figure 10-4 Patient with typical signs of acromegaly; note the change in the features in the photograph on the right compared with that on the left when the patient was younger

From Damjanov I. Pathology for the health-related professions, 2nd ed. Philadelphia: Elsevier, 2000.

clinical expression of GH excess is subtle and slowly evolving. Consequently, the GH excess syndrome, acromegaly, is often very advanced at the time of diagnosis. The tumors are mostly macroadenomas by the time of detection, and often present to medical attention because of mass effect rather than symptoms of GH excess. Hypopituitarism is often also present.

Clinical features of GH excess

- Facial change, jaw enlargement, frontal bone expansion (Figure 10-4, above)
- Enlargement of hands and feet, carpal tunnel syndrome
- Hypertrophic/degenerative spine or joint disease
- Excessive sweating, oily skin, skin tags
- Tongue enlargement, obstructive sleep apnea
- Impaired glucose tolerance or diabetes
- Congestive cardiac failure, hypertension, cardiomegaly

Diagnosis

GH excess cannot be reliably determined from measurement of GH levels alone, since the pulsatile release of GH in normal individuals results in a highly variable normal range.

CLINICAL PEARL

Acromegaly is diagnosed on the basis of elevated IGF-1 levels and/or failure of GH to suppress after glucose loading (oral glucose tolerance test), which completely suppresses GH secretion in normal individuals.

Imaging should then be performed to visualize the pituitary adenoma, together with testing of other pituitary hormone secretion.

Treatment

The goals of treatment of acromegaly are to control excessive GH secretion, reduce pituitary tumor mass, and preserve the normal secretion of other pituitary hormones. The treatment options are:

- Pituitary surgery, aiming to remove the adenoma. However, most tumors are macroadenomas at diagnosis and complete surgical removal is possible in only 30–40% of these. Partial tumor reduction (debulking) may still be beneficial.
- Medical therapy with long-acting somatostatin analogues (octreotide, lanreotide, pasireotide). GH and IGF-1 normalization can be achieved in 70% of cases and some reduction in tumor volume is usual.
- GH-receptor blockade using pegvisomant. Control of IGF-1 levels can be achieved in most patients, but cost is a major limiting factor. Tumor volume is not affected.
- Radiotherapy, which has a good long-term cure rate but may take many years to produce normalization of GH levels. Hypopituitarism also usually occurs.

Surgery and radiotherapy for pituitary tumors

Surgery for pituitary tumors is usually performed via the trans-nasal, trans-sphenoidal route. A trans-cranial approach may be needed for large suprasellar tumors, but is associated with much higher morbidity and mortality. Successful control of hormone-secreting adenomas is highly dependent on surgical experience and should be undertaken only in centers with considerable experience. Hormonal complications of pituitary surgery include hypopituitarism and diabetes insipidus; other occasional issues include cerebrospinal fluid (CSF) leak and infection.

External beam radiotherapy has high efficacy for control of hormone-secreting pituitary tumors. However, the effect is extremely delayed. The average delay to normalization of GH and IGF-1 levels in acromegaly is about 5 years, and to normalization of cortisol in Cushing's disease 2 years. Medical therapy can be used in the interim. In non-functioning adenomas, radiotherapy is an effective adjunct after debulking surgery and prevents tumor regrowth in over 80% of cases.

- Conventional pituitary radiotherapy is delivered at a total dose of 4500 to 5000 cGy in 25 fractional doses.
- Stereotactic radiosurgery and gamma-knife (single-dose) radiotherapy are newer techniques with practical advantages, but currently no proof of greater efficacy than conventional treatment.

Radiotherapy is damaging to normal pituitary tissue, and virtually all patients receiving pituitary irradiation will develop pituitary hormone deficiencies after a delay of 2–10 years.

Inflammatory and infiltrative disorders

These present as pituitary space-occupying masses or cause hypopituitarism, and are usually diagnosed by magnetic resonance imaging (MRI). Other features of the primary disease, or occasionally biopsy, may assist in diagnosis:

- craniopharynigiomas and Rathke's cleft tumors
- autoimmune hypophysitis—lymphocytic or granulomatous inflammation presenting as a pituitary mass and/or hypopituitarism
- immune checkpoint inhibitor therapy used in the management of several malignancies (e.g. melanoma) can induce single or multiple pituitary hormone deficiencies, related to immune dysregulation. Commonly implicated targeted therapies include the PD-1 inhibitors, CTLA4-inhibitors
- systemic inflammatory disorders frequently involve the pituitary and/or hypothalamus, causing hypopituitarism (sarcoidosis, vasculitis, Langerhans histiocytosis)
- tuberculosis, syphilis, fungal sinus disease or meningitis.

Diabetes insipidus (DI)

Diabetes insipidus is characterized by production of dilute urine in excess of 3 L/day and inability to appropriately concentrate the urine in response to dehydration. DI arises through one of two mechanisms:

1 deficiency of ADH secretion—*central DI*
2 deficiency of ADH action at the renal tubule (ADH-receptor or aquaporin defect)—*nephrogenic DI.*

An important differential diagnosis is *psychogenic polydipsia*, in which excessive water intake drives appropriate excretion of a free water load.

Patients with DI are usually well and maintain normal plasma osmolality and electrolytes, so long as they have a normal thirst mechanism and can maintain sufficient water intake to keep up with their urinary losses. Dehydration, hyperosmolality and hypernatremia quickly develop if intake of water is limited. This is the basis of the diagnostic use of a water deprivation test, in which serum and urine sodium and osmolality are measured while all fluid intake is withheld.

Central DI is usually treated using a synthetic ADH analog, desmopressin. Desmopressin is administered by intra-nasal or oral routes, twice daily. Nephrogenic DI does not respond to desmopressin treatment and partial control may be achieved using agents that affect renal water handling (e.g. thiazides, non-steroidal anti-inflammatory drugs). Excessive desmopressin treatment can result in hyponatremia.

THYROID DISORDERS

Physiology and assessment of thyroid function

The thyroid is a butterfly-shaped gland located anterior to the trachea at the level of the second and the third tracheal rings. It consists of two lobes joined by a thin band of tissue, the isthmus. The main hormones secreted by the thyroid gland, thyroxine (T_4) and triiodothyronine (T_3), are formed from iodination of the amino-acid tyrosine. The thyroid gland extracts iodine from the circulation through the sodium-iodine symporter. Thyroid stimulating hormone (TSH), secreted by the anterior pituitary, stimulates formation, storage (as thyroglobulin in colloid) and secretion of thyroid hormones, acting through a G-protein-coupled receptor. The hypothalamic–pituitary–thyroid axis is a classic negative feedback endocrine system which maintains constant concentration of circulating thyroid hormones. The relationship between TSH and thyroid hormone levels is log-linear, such that decreases in thyroid hormone secretion produce a logarithmic increase in serum TSH concentration, which is the hallmark of primary hypothyroidism. The thyroid gland also secretes calcitonin which plays a role in the regulation of serum calcium levels (see section on bone and mineral metabolism below).

T_4 and T_3 circulate in association with plasma-binding proteins (thyroxine-binding globulin, transthyretin and albumin). Less than 0.05% of T_4 and 0.5% of T_3 is free from protein binding and biologically active. The serum half-life of T_4 is approximately 7 days, and of T_3 approximately 1 day. Most (80%) of the circulating T_3 is formed in the plasma by peripheral conversion of T_4 under the action of deiodinase enzymes. Further $T4 \rightarrow T3$ conversion occurs within target cells. Thyroid hormones act by binding to nuclear thyroid-hormone receptors. These complexes bind to specific DNA sequences as heterodimers with retinoic acid X receptors (RXRs), and in this form they inhibit or stimulate gene expression.

Thyroid hormones are required for many physiological processes in the body, including skeletal growth, regulation of metabolism, organ maturation and augmentation of sympathetic nervous system responses in the cardiovascular system.

Thyroid function is traditionally tested by a measurement of circulating levels of T_4, T_3 and TSH. Assays for free thyroid hormones (fT_4 and fT_3) have replaced the older measurement of total circulating thyroid hormone levels. A matrix for interpretation of thyroid hormone levels is shown in Table 10-3. The logical approach to the evaluation of thyroid function is first to determine whether TSH is *suppressed*, *normal* or *elevated*.

- A normal TSH level effectively excludes a primary abnormality of the thyroid gland (so long as pituitary function can be assumed to be intact).
- The finding of an abnormal TSH level should be followed by measurement of fT_4 and fT_3 concentrations to confirm the diagnosis of hyperthyroidism (when TSH is suppressed) or hypothyroidism (when TSH is elevated). It is then appropriate to undertake tests to determine the etiology of the thyroid dysfunction.

In the presence of significant systemic (non-thyroidal) illness, secondary alterations in thyroid hormone levels may occur. This is known as 'sick euthyroid syndrome'. The characteristic pattern is of a low fT_3, due to inhibition of deiodinase enzymes. Plasma fT_4 and TSH vary depending upon the phase of the illness. Specific correction of the thyroid hormone abnormality is usually not required.

Thyroid imaging

Ultrasound

- Most useful for assessing thyroid size and evaluating nodules.

Table 10-3 Changes in thyroid hormone levels with disorders

DISORDER	THYROID-STIMULATING HORMONE (TSH)	fT$_4$	fT$_3$
Primary hyperthyroid	↓	↑	↑
Primary hypothyroid	↑	↓	↓
Hypopituitarism	Normal or ↓	↓	↓
Secondary hyperthyroid (TSHoma)	Normal or ↑	↑	↑
Thyroid hormone resistance	Normal or ↑	↑	↑

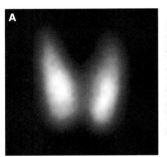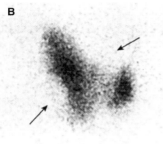

Figure 10-5 Thyroid isotope uptake scans. (**A**) Normal uptake in the thyroid lobes (seen as white on a black background). (**B**) Irregular uptake (seen as black on a white background) due to non-functioning 'cold' nodules (arrowed)

From: (A) Drakaki A, Habib M and Sweeney AT. Hypokalemic periodic paralysis due to Graves disease. Am J Med 2009;122(12):e5–e6. (B) Katz D, Math K and Groskin S. Radiology secrets. Philadelphia: Elsevier, 1998.

- No radiation exposure, can be used repeatedly for follow-up.
- Useful for differentiating solid and cystic nodules, and guiding fine-needle aspiration.
- Does *not* assess function or exclude malignancy.

Nuclear isotope scanning

- Most useful for evaluating the cause of hyperthyroidism.
- Demonstrates function (e.g. 'hot' versus 'cold' nodules; Figure 10-5).
- Not accurate for assessing size of the thyroid or individual nodules.

Computed tomography (CT) scanning

- Most useful for demonstrating the anatomy of a large goiter (e.g. retrosternal extension).
- Identifies compression of the upper airway or esophagus by an enlarged thyroid.
- Localization of nodal metastases in thyroid carcinoma.

- The use of iodine-containing contrast medium is inadvisable due to potential effects of iodine on an abnormal thyroid gland.

Thyroid autoimmunity

Thyroid autoimmunity is the most common etiology of thyroid function abnormalities.

- It has a familial tendency, is more common in females, and has an increased frequency in HLA (human leukocyte antigen) haplotypes B8 and DR3.
- Patients may have antibodies to multiple thyroid proteins (thyroid peroxidase, TSH-receptor, thyroglobulin).
- Three primary syndromes are associated with similar underlying autoimmune mechanisms:
  » Graves' disease with hyperthyroidism
  » Hashimoto's thyroiditis with euthyroidism or hyperthyroidism/euthyroidism, and
  » Hashimoto's hypothyroidism.
- An individual patient may transition from one clinical picture to another over time. The phenotypes differ according to the predominant antibody type (e.g. stimulatory versus receptor-blocking versus destructive immune responses).
- Thyroid autoimmunity may be associated with other organ-specific autoimmune syndromes (vitiligo, type 1 diabetes, Addison's disease, pernicious anemia, myasthenia gravis, premature ovarian failure, autoimmune hypophysitis).

CLINICAL PEARL

Although the presence of thyroid autoantibodies is a hallmark of autoimmune thyroid disease, their pathogenic activity is still unclear, in that such antibodies may persist for years without the patient developing a clinical disorder.

Hyperthyroidism

Clinical clues

Typical presentations

- Heat intolerance, excessive sweating

- Weight loss
- Dyspnea (even without congestive cardiac failure)
- Increase in frequency of bowel movements/diarrhea
- Weak muscles
- Emotional lability and nervousness/difficulty sleeping
- Tachycardia and/or atrial fibrillation (especially in the elderly)
- Decreased menstrual flow

Atypical presentations

- Unexplained atrial arrhythmias in the middle-aged
- Severe proximal myopathy with normal creatine phosphokinase levels
- Unexplained deterioration in cognition and functional capacity in the elderly
- Hypokalemic periodic paralysis (especially in Asian males)
- Gynecomastia
- Osteoporosis
- Chronic diarrhea

Laboratory abnormalities

- Low TSH is usually the first laboratory abnormality in primary hyperthyroidism.
- In overt hyperthyroidism there will be elevated fT_4 or fT_3 levels (usually both).

CLINICAL PEARL

In population screening studies, 2–5% of people have low TSH levels with normal fT_4 and fT_3 (termed 'subclinical hyperthyroidism'). This requires follow-up, but not necessarily treatment. There is an increased long-term risk of atrial fibrillation and osteoporotic fracture. About half will normalize their TSH levels without treatment, but 5% per year progress to overt hyperthyroidism.

Causes of hyperthyroidism

- Autonomous hormone production
  - » hot nodule (follicular adenoma)
  - » toxic multinodular goiter
  - » struma ovarii (rare)

- Excess stimulation of thyroid
  - » by immunoglobulins in Graves' disease (the most common cause)
  - » rarely, TSH-secreting pituitary adenomas
- Excess release of thyroid hormone
  - » painful subacute thyroiditis
  - » silent lymphocytic thyroiditis (e.g. initial phase of Hashimoto's, postpartum thyroiditis)
- Exogenous thyroid hormone ingestion

Causes may be distinguished by the pattern of radionucleotide uptake (Box 10-1).

Iodine load

- Iodine load may cause hyperthyroidism in the setting of pre-existing autonomous functioning thyroid tissue (hot nodule, toxic multinodular goiter). Iodine loading does not cause hyperthyroidism in most people because of suppression of iodine uptake by the thyroid (Wolff–Chaikoff effect).
- Sources of iodine load:
  - » drugs—amiodarone, cough medicines
  - » radiocontrast material
  - » surgical exposure to povidone-iodine
  - » dietary sources, e.g. seaweed.
- In the setting of previous iodine deficiency, iodine loading causing hyperthyroidism is called the Jod–Basedow phenomenon.

CLINICAL PEARL

Effects of amiodarone on the thyroid
40% of the molecular weight of amiodarone is iodine. Effects vary:
- hyperthyroidism from the high iodine load, or from thyroiditis
- hypothyroidism from chronic thyroiditis
- low plasma T_3 levels because of impaired conversion of T_4 to T_3
- nuclear thyroid scans will show no uptake of tracer because of competition from the high iodine load.

Graves' disease

- Characterized by thyroid-stimulating antibodies directed against the TSH receptor.

Box 10-1

Differentiation of causes of hyperthyroidism according to pattern of radionucleotide uptake

Reduced uptake	Generalized increased uptake	Focal increased uptake
• Thyroiditis	• Graves' disease	• Toxic multinodular goiter
• Exogenous thyroxine	• Excess thyroid-stimulating hormone stimulation	• Hyperfunctioning adenoma
• Iodine loading		
• Ectopic thyroid hormone secretion (struma ovarii)		

- The most common cause of hyperthyroidism. It is most often seen in younger women, but can occur in both sexes, and in the elderly.
- Extra-thyroidal manifestations (pretibial myxedema, ophthalmopathy, clubbing) are immune-mediated, not thyroid-hormone-related, and may be synchronous or at a different time from the onset of hyperthyroidism.
- Up to 50% of patients with hyperthyroidism due to Graves' disease may have normal thyroid size. When the thyroid is enlarged, it is usually a diffuse goiter.
- There is usually generalized increased tracer uptake on a nuclear scan.
- The condition may be characterized by spontaneous remission and relapse.

Subacute thyroiditis

- May occur after a viral illness, or sporadically, more common in women.
- Involves excess release of stored thyroid hormone from colloid.
- There is a raised erythrocyte sedimentation rate (ESR), and decreased/absent tracer uptake on a nuclear scan (suppressed by inflammation and low TSH).
- Manifests as a tender enlarged thyroid, clinical thyrotoxicosis with fever, and raised ESR lasting for months.
- Typically there is a phase of transient hypothyroidism on recovery, then return to a euthyroid state.

Treatment of hyperthyroidism

The principles are:
- block the effects of circulating thyroid hormones
- inhibit synthesis of new hormone
- consider thyroid ablation with radioactive iodine, or thyroidectomy, in persistent cases.

Note that the TSH levels may remain low in the first few months of treatment. Thyroid hormone levels should be used to determine the efficacy of treatment.

Beta-blockade

The clinical manifestations of thyrotoxicosis are mainly mediated by the sympathetic nervous system as a result of increased adrenergic hormone release and receptor expression. Beta-blockade with propranolol produces rapid improvement of tachycardia, tremor, sweating and CNS effects.

Methimazole, carbimazole and propylthiouracil

- **Mechanism:** decrease thyroid hormone synthesis by decreasing the incorporation of iodide into thyroglobulin. Propylthiouracil (PTU) also inhibits T_4 to T_3 conversion.
- These drugs have no role in the treatment of hyperthyroidism from thyroiditis as the primary defect is that of the excessive release of pre-stored hormone and not excessive hormone production.
- Remember that the half-life of thyroxine is 1 week, so there will be a delay in effect until circulating hormone is cleared.
- Anti-thyroid drugs are given in high doses until a euthyroid state is achieved, and then in smaller maintenance doses.

- **Side-effects:** fever, rash, arthralgia, myalgia, leukopenia and agranulocytosis, hepatitis, anti-neutrophil cytoplasmic autoantibody (ANCA)-associated vasculitis (PTU only).

The hyperthyroidism of Graves' disease enters spontaneous remission within a year in about 50% of patients. A trial of withdrawal of treatment may then be attempted. If relapse occurs, the patient can be re-treated, prior to definitive therapy with surgery or radioactive iodine.

Radioactive iodine (^{131}I)

- Administered as a single oral dose, after initial control of hyperthyroidism with drug therapy. Cannot be used in pregnancy or lactation.
- **Mechanism:** beta-particle emitter preferentially taken up by the thyroid, with minimal radiation effect on other organs. Onset of cell death and thyroid hypofunction is within 6–8 weeks.
- **Side-effects:** occasional acute thyrotoxicosis (7–10 days after treatment), late hypothyroidism (>50% at 10 years).
- A large goiter or active Graves' ophthalmopathy are relative **contraindications**.

CLINICAL PEARL

Treatment with ^{131}I is usually used after first relapse in Graves' disease, but as primary treatment in toxic multinodular goiter or single toxic adenoma.

Thyroidectomy

- Best treatment for patients with a large goiter, ophthalmopathy or patients unsuitable for radioactive iodine.
- Choice of total or partial thyroidectomy, depending on the individual case.
- **Risks:** hypothyroidism, hypoparathyroidism, recurrent laryngeal nerve injury.

Hypothyroidism

Clinical clues

- Weight gain
- Constipation
- Cold intolerance
- Lethargy
- Depression
- Dementia
- Hoarse voice
- Menorrhagia
- Dry skin, hair loss
- Bradycardia
- In children—growth retardation, delayed bone maturation, learning difficulty

Laboratory testing

TSH is always raised in primary hypothyroidism and is the first laboratory abnormality.

- Normal TSH excludes primary hypothyroidism (if pituitary function is intact).
- Elevated TSH in the presence of normal T_4 and T_3 levels (so-called 'subclinical hypothyroidism') is a common finding (3–7% in population screening studies, women > men).

Mildly elevated TSH levels often revert to normal without treatment, and iodine supplementation may be indicated in areas of deficiency. Commence thyroxine replacement if TSH is >10 mU/L, patient is symptomatic, an anti-thyroid antibody test is strongly positive, or there is marked hyperlipidemia.

> ## CLINICAL PEARL
>
> Because of the established connection between elevated maternal TSH during pregnancy and reduced IQ in offspring, any elevation of TSH in a woman who is pregnant or planning pregnancy is justification for thyroxine supplementation.

Causes of hypothyroidism

1. Primary

- Chronic autoimmune thyroiditis (Hashimoto's disease)
- Idiopathic atrophy
- Ablation (^{131}I, prior neck irradiation, or surgery)
- Thyroid agenesis
- Drugs (lithium, amiodarone, cancer immunotherapy e.g. ipilimumab, pembrolizumab)
- Iodine deficiency
- Inborn errors of metabolism

2. Secondary

- Pituitary or hypothalamic disease, with TSH deficiency

Hashimoto's thyroiditis

- A chronic inflammatory disease of the thyroid, often associated with goiter.
- Common in middle-aged women.
- Associated with lymphocytic infiltration of the gland.
- Usually occurs in association with positive antithyroglobulin antibodies, antithyroid peroxidase (anti-TPO) antibodies (positive in 95–98%), antimicrosomal antibodies (85%).
- Has a recognized association with other autoimmune diseases (pernicious anemia, vitiligo, celiac disease, Addison's disease, type 1 diabetes).
- Usually diagnosed by laboratory screening or because of goiter or hypothyroid symptoms.
- The patient may be diagnosed while still euthyroid, but regular follow-up shows that frank hypothyroidism develops in 80% of patients.
- It is treated with thyroxine when associated with hypothyroidism. If a symptomatic goiter occurs, this may be treated surgically.

> ## CLINICAL PEARL
>
> Subclinical hypothyroidism:
> - raised serum TSH but normal T_4 level, seen in 3–8% of the population
> - increases with age (20% of over-65-year-olds), and in women (3 : 1)
> - among them 5% per year will go on to frank hypothyroidism
> - treat if symptomatic, pregnant, TSH >10 mU/L or positive for anti-thyroid antibodies.

Thyroxine treatment (Figure 10-6)

- Hypothyroid patients usually require treatment for life.
- The full replacement dose is typically 1.6–2 microg/kg (usually 100–200 microg total) per day.
- Commence with full dose unless the patient is elderly or if there is a history of cardiac disease (then commence with half dose).
- Administration of T_3 is not needed; there is sufficient conversion from exogenous T_4.
- Thyroxine has a half-life of 7 days, so wait 4–6 weeks before reassessing thyroid function.
- Titrate the dosage to achieve a TSH level in the normal range.
- Once-daily dosing is usual, but less frequent (e.g. weekly) is also possible.
  - » Tablets need to be taken on an empty stomach at least 30 minutes before food.

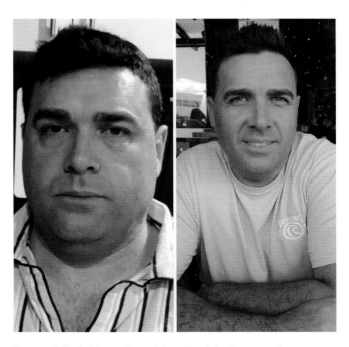

Figure 10-6 Hypothyroid patient before and following thyroxine therapy—note the improvement in the myxedematous facies, recovery of the loss of the outer third of the eyebrows and weight loss

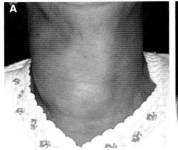
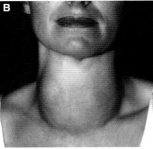

Figure 10-7 (A) Diffuse goiter; (B) multinodular goiter

From: (A) Shah JP, Patel S and Singh B. Jatin Shah's Head and neck surgery and oncology, 4th ed. Philadelphia: Mosby, 2012. (B) Quick CRG et al. Essential surgery: problems, diagnosis and management, 5th ed. Elsevier, 2014.

- Failure to respond suggests poor compliance or, rarely, malabsorption (celiac disease, co-ingestion of iron or caffeine).

Goiter and thyroid nodules

Causes of diffuse goiter

1 Idiopathic
2 Puberty
3 Pregnancy
4 Graves' disease
5 Thyroiditis
   a   Hashimoto's thyroiditis
   b   Subacute thyroiditis (tender)
6 Iodine deficiency (may be massive)
7 Goitrogens (substances which interfere with thyroidal uptake of iodine and hormone synthesis), e.g. iodine, lithium
8 Inborn errors of thyroid hormone synthesis

CLINICAL PEARL

The size of the thyroid gland does not indicate thyroid function. Most people with thyroid enlargement have normal thyroid function. Always assess thyroid *structure* and thyroid *function* as separate variables (Figure 10-7).

Management of goiter

The structure of the thyroid is best assessed by ultrasound. Nodules of >1–2 cm diameter should be evaluated by fine-needle aspiration (FNA) cytology to exclude thyroid carcinoma depending on ultrasound characteristics (see below) unless the nodules are purely cystic as these carry a very low risk of malignancy. If there is clinical evidence of retrosternal extension or thoracic inlet obstruction, this is best evaluated by CT scanning.

Thyroidectomy is the best treatment in most cases where thyroid enlargement is causing compressive or cosmetic problems. TSH suppression with thyroxine has minimal utility. Radioactive iodine may be used when surgery is contraindicated, but size reduction is modest and large doses may be required.

Thyroid nodules

Nodule formation is seen in up to 20% of all thyroid ultrasounds. The incidence increases with age. Most are asymptomatic. Nodules are not a single disease but occur as a result of different processes including adenomas, carcinomas, inflammation/scarring/regeneration, cyst formation and focal accumulation of colloid. Most nodules are hypofunctioning ('cold' on isotope scanning), although thyroid function tests should be performed to identify the minority (10%) that have autonomous hyperfunction, causing thyrotoxicosis. The main clinical issue is identification of the small proportion (<5%) of nodules that are thyroid malignancies. Ultrasound is the most useful imaging modality for nodules. It has high sensitivity, accuracy in measurement, differentiates solid from cystic lesions, and may be used to guide fine-needle aspiration biopsy. Ultrasound cannot reliably differentiate a benign thyroid nodule from a cancer. However, some ultrasonic features of a nodule are associated with an increased risk of malignancy:

- hypoechoic
- microcalcifications
- central vascularity
- irregular margins
- incomplete halo.

The risk of malignancy increases with increasing nodule size, and all nodules >1–2 cm diameter depending on the presence of the above ultrasound characteristics should be considered for FNA cytology evaluation. If FNA cytology shows atypia or suggests malignancy the patient should have a hemi- or total thyroidectomy. Nodules with normal cytology can be observed with repeat ultrasonography at 6–12 months and if no further growth occurs the follow-up can be ceased.

CLINICAL PEARL

Investigation of a thyroid nodule should include:
- thyroid function tests to detect hyperfunction
- ultrasound to assess nodule size and structure
- cytology assessment by fine-needle aspiration of lesions >10 mm diameter.

Thyroid cancer

- Usually presents as a painless thyroid nodule, sometimes associated with cervical lymphadenopathy, or as an incidental finding on ultrasound.
- Highest incidence is ages 30–60 years. The female to male ratio is 3:1.
- Commonest forms are papillary (75%) and follicular (15%). Both are well differentiated, slow-growing and take up ^{131}I, which is therefore a valuable adjunctive therapy to surgery. Hence these forms of thyroid cancer have relatively good prognosis.
- Less common is medullary thyroid cancer (5–10%), which are derived from C-cells, secretes calcitonin

and may be familial. Anaplastic cancer (1–2%) and thyroid lymphoma (2%) are highly malignant and radioiodine-resistant.

- There is a causal association with prior external beam radiotherapy to the neck (e.g. for childhood lymphoma) as well as familial forms e.g. Cowden's syndrome, MEN-2 (associated with medullary thyroid cancer).

The treatment of thyroid carcinoma is total thyroidectomy. More extensive neck dissection is performed for nodal metastases. In papillary or follicular carcinoma, adjuvant treatment with [131]I (in doses about 10-fold higher than for thyrotoxicosis) is effective, and serum thyroglobulin is a useful tumor marker. [123]I whole-body scanning and neck ultrasound can be used in follow-up to detect residual or recurrent disease and to indicate a need for further treatment with radioactive iodine. Prognosis is relatively good in well differentiated tumors, even in the presence of nodal or distant metastases. PET scanning (using 18-FDG) may detect poorly differentiated disease that is no longer iodine-avid, and guide further surgical therapy. Iodine-resistant metastatic papillary and follicular thyroid cancer may also be suitable for treatment with multi-targeted kinase inhibitors which are an emerging treatment modality that target various pathogenic pathways of the disease e.g. lenvatinib.

Thyroid in pregnancy

Thyroid disease has a high prevalence in young women, so it is relatively common in pregnancy. As maternal thyroid disease can affect the unborn child, it requires prompt diagnosis and treatment. Evaluation of thyroid function during pregnancy is made more complex by changes in maternal physiology, particularly in regard to iodine-handling and thyroid hormone production.

Hypothyroidism in pregnancy

- Thyroid hormone synthesis increases by 20–50% during normal gestation, with the increased hormone requirement partly explained by increased production of binding protein.
- Therefore, borderline hypothyroidism may decompensate during pregnancy.
- Maternal hypothyroidism impairs fetal neurological development, and therefore women should be treated with thyroxine to maintain TSH within pregnancy-specific reference ranges.
- Thyroxine replacement doses usually increase with advancing gestation, reflecting the known physiological changes.

CLINICAL PEARL

Women on thyroxine replacement should increase their dose by about 25% as soon as their pregnancy is confirmed.

Hyperthyroidism in pregnancy

- Placental human chorionic gonadotropin (hCG) has homology to TSH and weak stimulatory activity at the TSH receptor. This leads to a decrease in serum TSH in the 1st trimester, which may occasionally be quite pronounced, and is associated with elevations in T_4 and T_3. This phenomenon, known as *gestational hyperthyroidism*, is a physiological process that does not require treatment and resolves after the 1st trimester. However, it may be difficult to distinguish from true primary hyperthyroidism.
- Primary hyperthyroidism in pregnancy has been associated with increased risk of maternal complications, including miscarriage and pre-term birth. Graves' disease, in particular, may affect the fetus due to transplacental passage of thyroid-stimulating antibodies that can stimulate the fetal thyroid and cause fetal and neonatal Graves' disease.
- Antithyroid medications can be used in pregnancy if required although can be associated with an increased risk of congenital malformations when used in the 1st trimester (especially carbimazole). Anti-thyroid drugs can also cross the placenta and cause fetal hypothyroidism. Careful monitoring is therefore required. Radioactive iodine is contraindicated.

DISORDERS OF BONE AND MINERAL METABOLISM

Mineral homeostasis

The majority of calcium, phosphorus and magnesium ions in the body are located in bone, where they are essential for bone mineralization and strength. Powerful hormonal mechanisms exist to control the interchange of ions between the osseous and non-osseous compartments and to maintain extracellular concentrations within a narrow range where they are vital for cellular function throughout the body. This involves a complex interplay between gut absorption, renal excretion and bone sequestration (Figure 10-8), controlled by hormones such as parathyroid hormone (PTH), calcitriol (activated vitamin D), calcitonin, PTH-related peptide (PTHrP) and fibroblast growth factor 23 (FGF23). Sex steroids, thyroid hormones, glucocorticoids, GH and insulin may also affect bone and mineral homeostasis (Table 10-4, overleaf).

Hypercalcemia

Background

- 45% of calcium is protein-bound, predominantly to albumin; 45% is free/ionized; 10% is bound to small anions (phosphate, citrate).
- **Mild hypercalcemia** (up to 3.0 mmol/L) may be asymptomatic, or have nonspecific manifestations such as fatigue and constipation.
- **Moderate hypercalcemia** (3.0–3.5 mmol/L) is usually symptomatic if acute, but may be unrecognized if developing insidiously and chronically.
- **Severe hypercalcemia** (>3.5 mmol/L) is an emergency and may cause cardiac arrhythmia or severe obtundation/coma.

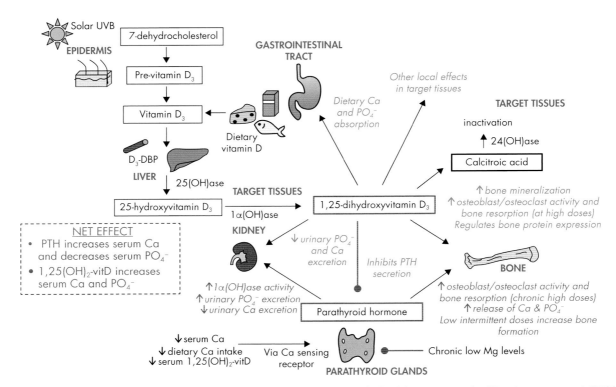

Figure 10-8 Principal regulation of calcium (Ca) and phosphate (PO$_4^-$) homeostasis. The hormones 1,25(OH)$_2$-vitamin D and parathyroid hormone (PTH) have effects on bone, kidney and the gastrointestinal tract which determine serum calcium and phosphate levels. 1,25(OH)$_2$-vitamin D is the activated form of the vitamin

Table 10-4 Hormones involved in bone and mineral metabolism

HORMONE	FEATURES
Parathyroid hormone (PTH)	Produced by the parathyroid glands Increases bone resorption, decreases urinary calcium (Ca) excretion, increases phosphate (PO$_4^-$) excretion, stimulates activation of vitamin D Net effect is to increase serum Ca and decrease PO$_4^-$
Calcitriol (1,25(OH)$_2$-vitamin D)	Produced in the kidney by 1-alpha-hydroxylation of 25-hydroxyvitamin D Increases gut absorption, decreases renal excretion of Ca and PO$_4^-$ Inhibits PTH secretion Net effect is to increase serum Ca and PO$_4^-$
Calcitonin	Produced by the thyroid parafollicular C-cells in response to high Ca levels Acts on osteoclasts to inhibit bone resorption Promotes renal PO$_4^-$ and Ca excretion Net effect is lowering of serum calcium
Fibroblast growth factor (FGF) 23	Growth factor secreted by osteocytes promotes renal PO$_4^-$ wasting Stimulated by hyperphosphatemia and calcitriol
PTH-related peptide (PTHrP)	Acts on shared PTH/PTHrP receptor; similar effects to PTH Physiological secretion by placenta and local production in breast Pathophysiological secretion by solid tumors (paraneoplastic)

Table 10-5 Symptoms and signs of hypercalcemia

	GASTROINTESTINAL	RENAL	NEUROLOGICAL/NEUROMUSCULAR	CARDIAC
Acute	Anorexia Nausea Vomiting Abdominal pain	Polyuria Dehydration Acute renal failure	Confusion Obtundation Psychosis Bone pain	Bradycardia Heart block
Chronic	Pancreatitis Dyspepsia Constipation	Kidney stones Nephrocalcinosis	Myopathy Osteoporosis Depression	Hypertension

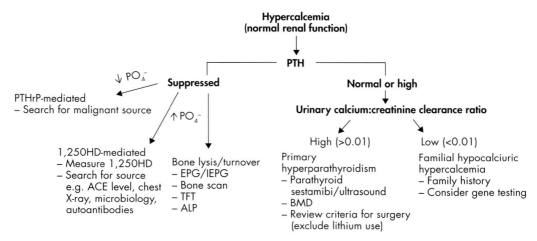

Figure 10-9 Common causes of hypercalcemia; a diagnostic algorithm. 1,25OHD, 1,25-dihydroxyvitamin D; ACE, angiotensin-converting enzyme; ALP, alkaline phosphatase; BMD, bone mineral density; EPG/IEPG, electrophoretogram/immunoelectrophoretogram; PTH, parathyroid hormone; PTHrP, PTH-related peptide; TFT, thyroid function test

CLINICAL PEARLS

- Total calcium can be corrected for serum albumin using the formula: corrected Ca (mmol/L) = measured Ca + 0.20 (40 − albumin)/10.
- In states of profound hypo- or hyperalbuminemia, the correction is less accurate.
- pH also affects Ca binding—acidosis reduces it, alkalosis enhances it. Ionized Ca is a more useful measure in such clinical situations.

CLINICAL PEARL

90% of hypercalcemia is caused by primary hyperparathyroidism or malignancy.
- Hyperparathyroidism is the common cause in the community and usually presents with mild hypercalcemia.
- Cancer is commonly the cause in hospital, and hypercalcemia may be severe.

Clinical features

Table 10-5 gives the symptoms and signs of hypercalcemia.

Diagnosis and evaluation

Figure 10-9 gives a diagnostic algorithm for common causes of hypercalcemia.

It is useful to distinguish PTH-dependent from PTH-independent causes of hypercalcemia as a first step (Box 10-2). Primary hyperparathyroidism results from overproduction of parathyroid hormone from one or more parathyroid glands, resulting in release of calcium and phosphate from bone, and urinary phosphate-wasting. If untreated, osteoporosis is a sequela. Urine calcium excretion is high, predisposing to nephrolithiasis. This distinguishes the

---

Box 10-2

Causes of hypercalcemia

PTH-dependent hypercalcemia

- Primary hyperparathyroidism—parathyroid adenoma (81%), hyperplasia (15%), carcinoma (4%), multiple endocrine neoplasia (MEN) I and IIa (<1%)
- Tertiary hyperparathyroidism—autonomous PTH secretion in chronic kidney disease
- Familial hypocalciuric hypercalcemia—inactivating mutation in calcium-sensing receptor
- Lithium-associated hypercalcemia

PTH-independent hypercalcemia

- Hypercalcemia of malignancy:
  - » paraneoplastic secretion of PTHrP (e.g. squamous cell carcinoma)
  - » osteolytic bone metastases, multiple myeloma
- Excess $1,25(OH)_2$-vitamin D:
  - » drug ingestion
  - » production in granulomatous tissue, e.g. sarcoid, tuberculosis, granulomatosis with polyangiitis, lymphoma
- Drugs—vitamin A intoxication, milk-alkali syndrome, thiazide diuretics, theophylline
- Other—thyrotoxicosis, adrenal insufficiency, renal failure, prolonged immobility (especially with Paget's disease)

PTH, parathyroid hormone; PTHrP, PTH-related peptide.

---

condition from familial hypocalciuric hypercalcemia—a benign hereditary condition not requiring treatment. Production of PTH-related peptide (PTHrP) from a tumor may mimic hyperparathyroidism. Manifestations are often more acute and severe, and PTH levels are suppressed. The PTH level will also be suppressed where hypercalcemia is the result of excess vitamin D activity (from overexpression of the vitamin D-activating enzyme, 1-alpha-hydroxylase) or direct calcium release from bone.

Management

Acute symptomatic hypercalcemia

Acute symptomatic hypercalcemia requires urgent treatment:

1. Volume expansion and diuresis—IV normal saline (4–6 L), ± loop diuretics (furosemide 40 mg) if hypervolemic.
2. Bisphosphonates, if response to saline diuresis is inadequate, to inhibit osteoclast bone resorption— e.g. pamidronate 60–90 mg IV. Onset of effect within 4–6 hours, full effect after 2–4 days, lasts 2–4 weeks. Zoledronic acid is superior to pamidronate for hypercalcemia from malignancy.
3. Denosumab—for hypercalcemia of malignancy refractory to bisphosphonates or where bisphosphonates are contraindicated e.g. acute renal failure.
4. Corticosteroids—decrease GI calcium absorption, reduce 1–hydroxylase activity. Used in high doses for granulomatous conditions, malignancy, vitamin D intoxication.
5. Calcitonin—acts more rapidly than bisphosphonates but the response is only transient.
6. Dialysis if acute, severe and life-threatening.

Primary hyperparathyroidism

1. Indications for **surgery**:
   a. moderate/severe (>0.25 mmol/L above upper limit normal) or symptomatic hypercalcemia

---

Box 10-3

Clinical features of hypocalcemia

Acute

- Delirium, anxiety, depression
- Tetany, muscle cramps, carpal spasm
- Hyper-reflexia, paresthesiae
- Positive Chvostek's and Trousseau's signs
- Laryngospasm

Chronic

- Lethargy, seizures, basal ganglia calcification, psychosis
- Prolonged QT interval on electrocardiogram
- Dry skin, abnormal dentition, cataracts

---

   b. marked hypercalciuria (>10 mmol/day), nephrolithiasis, renal impairment
   c. osteoporosis—fracture, bone mineral density T-score <–2.5, age <50 years.
2. Indications for **imaging before surgery**—distinguishing solitary adenoma from polyglandular hyperplasia, which may assist the surgical approach. Imaging techniques may include ultrasound, dual-phase 99m technetium/sestamibi nuclear scans and 4D CT scans.
3. Indications for **medical therapy** with cinacalcet (modulator of calcium-sensing receptor)—severe hypercalcemia in a patient unfit for surgery.

Hypocalcemia

Clinical features

The clinical features of hypocalcemia are listed in Box 10-3.

Diagnosis and evaluation

The commonest causes of hypocalcemia are renal failure, vitamin D deficiency, hypoparathyroidism (post-surgical,

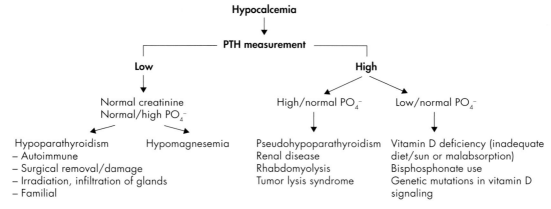

Figure 10-10 Common causes of hypocalcemia; a diagnostic algorithm

PTH, parathyroid hormone

less commonly auto immune), drugs (e.g. bisphosphonates, denosumab), hypomagnesemia and pancreatitis. PTH, creatinine, phosphate and magnesium levels assist diagnosis. A mild decrease in total calcium is often spurious; in such cases, ionized calcium is normal.

Figure 10-10 provides a diagnostic algorithm for common causes.

Management

Acute symptomatic hypocalcemia requires immediate treatment:

- IV calcium gluconate 1–2 ampoules (1 g in 10 mL) over 10 minutes, followed by continuous infusion of calcium gluconate at a rate of 4 g per 24 hours if necessary.
- Aim to raise calcium to low normal range.
- Cardiac monitoring is recommended. Infusion into a large central vein is preferred.
- It is important to correct coexisting magnesium deficiency, since this will inhibit the therapeutic response to calcium.

Chronic/persistent hypocalcemia is treated with vitamin D analogues (e.g. calcitriol) and oral calcium to maintain calcium in low normal range. This helps avoid hypercalciuria and soft-tissue calcium phosphate ($CaPO_4$) precipitation.

Osteoporosis

Features of osteoporosis include decreased bone mass and microarchitecture, leading to increased fragility and fracture risk.

Primary osteoporosis is related to the aging process and the loss of estrogen-related bone protection after menopause in women and the reduction in testosterone levels with age in men. A number of medical conditions and drugs can contribute to low bone mass (secondary osteoporosis). Risk factors are listed in Box 10-4.

Evaluation of osteoporosis

- History—height loss, kyphosis, back pain, fractures after fall from standing height, presence of risk factors.

Box 10-4
Risk factors for osteoporosis

Major

- Age
- Previous fragility fracture
- Family history of osteoporosis
- Menopause <45 years / hypogonadism
- Systemic glucocorticoids >3 months
- Prolonged immobilization
- Medical disease— malabsorption, malnutrition, Celiac disease, hyperparathyroidism, Cushing's syndrome, chronic renal failure, multiple myeloma
- Genetic e.g. osteogenesis imperfecta

Minor

- Smoking, excessive caffeine or alcohol intake
- Low dietary calcium
- Low body weight
- Chronic anticonvulsant therapy
- Chronic heparin therapy
- Medical disease— rheumatoid arthritis, previous hyperthyroidism, inflammatory bowel disease

---

- Exclusion of medical causes of osteoporosis.
- Ca, PO_4^-, PTH, 25(OH)-vitamin D, TSH, serum and urine electrophoretogram/immunoelectrophoretogram (EPG/IEPG), celiac serology, testosterone level (in men), 24-hour urine calcium.
- X-ray of thoracolumbar spine—loss of vertebral height.

The diagnosis of osteoporosis is made by assessment of bone mineral density (BMD) using dual-energy X-ray absorptiometry (DXA) scanning at the lumbar spine, femora and non-dominant forearm (in cases where the spine or hip may not be reliable or if the patient is obese or has hyperparathyroidism). Bone density is also a clinically useful tool for

Table 10-6 Osteoporosis therapies

AGENT	ADMINISTRATION	↓ RESORPTION	↑ FORMATION
Bisphosphonates	Oral/intravenous	✓	
Teriparatide (parathyroid hormone)	Subcutaneous daily		✓
Denosumab	Subcutaneous every 6 months	✓	
Raloxifene	Oral	✓	

estimating fracture risk. The result is given as a T-score or Z-score:

- Osteoporosis definition: BMD T-score −2.5 or below
- Osteopenia definition: BMD T-score between −1 and −2.5

CLINICAL PEARL

Bone mineral density test results:
- T-score = the number of standard deviations below the young adult peak
- Z-score = the number of standard deviations below the age-matched mean.

Treatment

All patients should have adequate calcium intake and vitamin D repletion. Alter modifiable risk factors—exercise, diet, smoking, medication use. Table 10-6 summarizes the currently available pharmacological therapies available to treat osteoporosis in Australia. Bisphosphonate agents which cause osteoclast death have been the mainstay of osteoporosis therapy. They are available in once daily, weekly or monthly oral formulations (alendronate, risedronate) as well as an annual intravenous formulation (zoledronic acid). They inhibit bone resorption and have proven efficacy in fracture prevention in both vertebral and non-vertebral sites. Newer agents targeting different biological pathways are also now available. They include denosumab which is an inhibitor of the RANK (Receptor Activator of Nuclear Factor kappa B) ligand pathway which is important in osteoclast formation, differentiation and survival. Teriparatide is a PTH analogue which when given intermittently enhances bone formation and causes significant increases in bone density but cost is a limiting factor in its use.

Decisions to initiate therapy should be based on estimation of fracture risk, balanced with the cost/side-effect profile of the treating agent. To assist in fracture-risk assessment, computerized algorithms are available, such as the FRAX® tool, providing a 10-year probability of hip or major osteoporotic fracture based on patient clinical data. Caution needs to be exercised, however, as estimates are imperfect and may over- or underestimate risk.

Osteomalacia and rickets

Osteomalacia is a clinical syndrome caused by impaired vitamin D activity due to deficiency or impaired action on its receptor. Impaired mineralization of bone matrix is a key feature. In children, the syndrome is referred to as 'rickets'. Osteomalacia affects only the bone, whereas rickets involves the growth plate and cartilage, leading to characteristic deformities.

Clinical features

- Osteomalacia may be silent, or may present with bone pain and fractures. Proximal myopathy is commonly associated.
- Rickets results in bowing of the long bones and widening of the cartilage of the growth plate and long bones. This is confirmed on X-ray, which demonstrates a pathognomic 'rosary' appearance at the costochondral rib junctions and wide transverse lucencies in bone (pubic rami, medial proximal femur, scapulae), at right-angles to the bone cortex, known as Looser's zones.

Etiology

Causes include vitamin D deficiency, metabolic defects in vitamin D signaling, or direct impairment of mineralization due to inadequate supply of calcium/phosphate. Underlying causes are given in Table 10-7 (overleaf).

Vitamin D deficiency

Vitamin D is predominantly obtained from sunlight exposure, and to a lesser extent from natural or fortified foods. Vitamin D deficiency is common in people with low ultraviolet (UV) exposure—institutionalized, elderly, veiled or dark-skinned populations, and those living in temperate climates during winter. Other risk factors for deficiency include fat malabsorption and obesity.

Diagnosis

Vitamin D status is best assessed by measurement of 25-hydroxyvitamin D, 25(OH)D. The recommended 'normal ranges' for vitamin D are still under debate, but a conservative approach defines *deficiency* as <25 nmol/L, *insufficiency* as 25–50 nmol/L and *sufficiency* as >50 nmol/L. Levels >75 nmol/L may be optimum.

Significant vitamin D deficiency is clearly related to hypocalcemia, hypophosphatemia, rickets, osteomalacia, osteoporosis and muscle weakness. Newer evidence suggests, however, that vitamin D may have other widespread effects throughout the body, and vitamin D has been linked to disorders including malignancy, insulin

Table 10-7 Causes of osteomalacia

MECHANISM	CAUSES
Loss of 1-alpha-hydroxylase	Loss of renal function/mass Vitamin-D-dependent rickets type 1 Renal tubular disorders (Fanconi syndrome)
Defects in vitamin-D receptor	Hereditary resistance to vitamin D
Hypophosphatemia	Familial X-linked hypophosphatemia Oncogenic osteomalacia (excess FGF23 production) Renal tubular disorders—urinary phosphate-wasting Antacids (decreased gut absorption), certain antivirals e.g. tenofovir, adefovir (cause renal phosphate wasting), iron carboxymaltose (raises FGF23 by inhibiting its breakdown)
Other mineralization defects	Hypophosphatasia (ALP gene mutation) Fluoride, older bisphosphonates (e.g. etidronate), anticonvulsants

ALP, alkaline phosphatase; FGF23, fibroblast growth factor 23.

resistance/beta-cell dysfunction, autoimmune diseases/allergy and neural function. However, evidence for a definite pathological role as opposed to a simple association, or for a beneficial effect of supplementation on these conditions, remains incomplete.

Treatment

Supplementation with cholecalciferol may be achieved with oral or intramuscular dosing. As vitamin D is a prohormone, requiring conversion to the active hormone, toxicity is rare; high-dose cholecalciferol therapy (e.g. 50,000 IU single dose) is well tolerated.

Patients with impaired 1-alpha-hydroxylation at the level of the kidney require administration of the active hormone, $1,25(OH)_2$-vitamin D (calcitriol).

Paget's disease (PD)

Paget's disease of bone is a bone remodeling disease. Increased osteoclastic resorption of bone is followed by increased osteoblastic activity, with the result being the laying down of abnormal, enlarged sections of bone.

Clinical features

- When symptomatic, the usual presentation of PD is with bone pain (typically older men). This is often described as being worse at night.
- Large bones are the usual site of disease: spine, pelvis, skull, long bones.
- Paget's disease usually progresses slowly and does not develop in new sites.
- Patients may notice deformity of their bone e.g. bowing of the legs.
- Compression neuropathy (e.g. deafness due to 8th nerve palsy when the skull is involved, or nerve root entrapment due to spinal disease), osteoarthritis due to abnormal joint mechanics in joints controlled by abnormally

shaped bones, or pathological fractures may also be the presentation.
- Asymptomatic elevation of serum alkaline phosphatase (ALP), or incidental abnormality on a radiograph, are probably the more common presentations.
- Angioid streaks may be seen in the fundi.
- High-output cardiac failure is a very rare complication.

Etiology

- The cause of PD is unknown. A viral etiology has been suspected, but never proven.
- A minority of cases are familial, and associated with a mutation of the *SQSTM1* gene in around half of these families. Sporadic mutations of this gene can also occur.
- The incidence and severity of the disease seem to be gradually decreasing in Western countries.
- Affected bones show evidence of areas of rapid bone turnover with bony lysis or sclerosis, and new bone lacking the normal lamellar pattern.

CLINICAL PEARL

In a patient with suspected Paget's disease, look for deafness, signs of basilar invagination and spinal cord compression, bowing of the femur and tibia, and localized tender swelling (possible bone sarcoma).

Diagnosis

- Elevated serum ALP is the most sensitive biomarker, and can be used to monitor both disease activity and response to treatment.
- Plain X-ray generally reveals a characteristic pattern of focal lytic lesions, bone enlargement, and loss of normal trabecular pattern.

- Bone scintigraphy can measure the extent of bony involvement.

Treatment

- Bisphosphonates are highly effective treatment for PD.
- There is evidence that intravenous zoledronate is superior to oral bisphosphonates.
- Patients need to be monitored long-term to detect evidence of relapse, and the need for re-treatment.
- There is an increased risk of osteosarcoma developing in bones affected by PD, which although rare should be borne in mind by the treating physician.

ADRENAL DISORDERS

Physiology and assessment of adrenal function

The adrenal glands are composed of two separate organs— the *adrenal cortex* (secretes steroids) and the *adrenal medulla* (secretes catecholamines). The cortex has three functional zones, each secreting a steroid type—*zona glomerulosa* (aldosterone), *zona fasciculata* (cortisol) and *zona reticularis* (androgens).

- Adrenal production of cortisol and androgens is stimulated by ACTH.
- Aldosterone production is principally regulated by the renin–angiotensin system, and catecholamine secretion by neural stimulation.
- All steroid hormones are derived from cholesterol, through multiple enzyme-stimulated steps.

Physiological cortisol production is 10–12 mg daily in humans (equivalent to 10–12 mg hydrocortisone, 2–2.5 mg prednisone), but increases by as much as 10-fold in response to stress. Diurnal variation in the activity of the hypothalamic–pituitary–adrenal (HPA; Figure 10-11) axis drive results in circadian variation of plasma cortisol from a peak of 300–500 nmol/L on wakening to <100 nmol/L overnight. This variability means that no single cut-off level can define a 'normal' plasma cortisol concentration for all circumstances. Figure 10-10 summarizes the stimulation and feedback control of cortisol production.

- A plasma cortisol concentration of >450 nmol/L in the morning, or during illness/stress, reasonably excludes deficiency of HPA axis function.
- A level <150 nmol/L in similar circumstances is highly suggestive of cortisol deficiency.
- Intermediate levels do not allow confirmation or exclusion.

CLINICAL PEARL

It is often necessary to perform dynamic testing to determine the function of the hypothalamic–pituitary–adrenal axis. If cortisol excess is suspected, perform a dexamethasone suppression test. If deficiency is suspected, stimulate with tetracosactrin (short Synacthen test) or insulin-induced hypoglycemia.

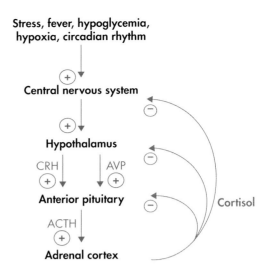

Figure 10-11 The hypothalamic–pituitary–adrenal axis: stimulation and feedback control of cortisol production. ACTH, adrenocorticotropic hormone; AVP, arginine vasopressin; CRH, corticotropin-releasing hormone

Adrenal insufficiency

Primary destruction of the adrenal cortex results in deficiency of cortisol, aldosterone and adrenal androgens. Secondary failure of the adrenal cortex can occur if pituitary or hypothalamic disease results in ACTH deficiency. In that circumstance there is deficient secretion of cortisol and androgens (which are ACTH-dependent), but not of aldosterone (which is predominantly stimulated by the renin–angiotensin axis).

Clinical clues

Cortisol deficiency

- Fatigue, weight loss
- Anorexia, nausea, vomiting
- Hypoglycemia, hypercalcemia
- Increased ACTH secretion → pigmentation

Aldosterone deficiency

- Hypotension
- Hyponatremia, hyperkalemia, acidosis
- Salt craving

Androgen deficiency

(Only relevant in women; men still have gonadal androgens.)
- Decreased axillary and pubic hair
- Loss of libido and amenorrhea in women

Features of associated autoimmune disease

- Vitiligo, other autoimmune endocrinopathies

Causes of adrenal insufficiency

1. Primary

- Autoimmune adrenal disease (80% of all cases in developed countries)
- Infection—tuberculosis, histoplasmosis, meningococcal septicemia (acute)
- Metastatic malignancy
- Lymphoma
- Bilateral adrenal hemorrhage—anticoagulation, spontaneous, trauma
  - » adrenolytic drugs—metyrapone, ketoconazole, mitotane
  - » bilateral adrenalectomy
- Congenital adrenal hyperplasia (synthetic enzyme defect) or adrenal hypoplasia

2. Secondary

- Pituitary or hypothalamic disease
- Following long-term corticosteroid therapy

Diagnosis of adrenocortical failure

1 A morning plasma cortisol level >450 nmol/L excludes adrenal insufficiency, and a level <150 nmol/L is highly predictive of cortisol deficiency. At intermediate levels a stimulation test is required.

2 Short synacthen test: 0.25 mg of synthetic ACTH (Synacthen ®) is given intramuscularly or intravenously. A normal response is a rise in plasma cortisol by >200 nmol/L (>7 mg/dL) and a peak of >450 nmol/L (>16.5 mg/dL). A normal response excludes primary adrenocortical failure but does not exclude hypothalamic-pituitary disease. Note that estrogen (e.g. through the oral contraceptive pill) influences total cortisol by increasing cortisol binding globulin (CBG) and should be ceased or higher cut-offs applied.

3 Insulin-induced hypoglycemia stress test: induction of hypoglycemia (<2.2 mmol/L) by administration of IV insulin results in a plasma cortisol level of >450 nmol/L (>16.5 mg/dL) if the hypothalamic-pituitary-adrenal (HPA) axis is intact.

4 The ACTH level allows discrimination of adrenal from hypothalamic–pituitary disease. Elevated ACTH is seen in primary adrenal insufficiency (e.g. Addison's disease).

5 Unique clinical features of Addison's disease:
   a hyperpigmentation (Figure 10-12)
   b associated autoimmune disorders such as vitiligo, autoimmune thyroid disease, pernicious anemia, type 1 diabetes mellitus, celiac disease and hypoparathyroidism are common.

Laboratory abnormalities

- Anti-adrenal antibodies (70%)
- Antithyroid antibodies (80%)

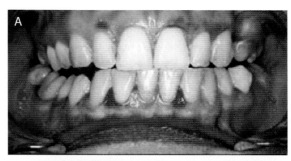
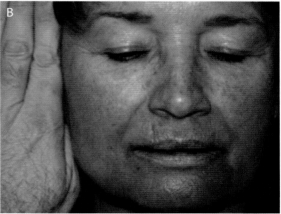

Figure 10-12 Hyperpigmentation of the gums (**A**) and face (**B**) in Addison's disease

From: (A) Gawkrodger DJ and Ardern-Jones MR. Dermatology: an illustrated colour text, 5th ed. Churchill Livingstone, 2012. (B) Bolognia JL, Jorizzo JL and Schaffer JV, eds. Dermatology, 3rd ed. Philadelphia: Elsevier, 2012.

- Hyponatremia, hyperkalemia, hyperchloremic acidosis, elevated urea
- Lymphocytosis and eosinophilia may be present
- Rarely, hypercalcemia may be present

Treatment of primary adrenocortical failure

Chronic

- Glucocorticoid replacement—hydrocortisone (10–30 mg/day in divided doses) *or* prednisone (4–5 mg each morning).
  - » Conventionally used replacement doses are in excess of physiological production and patients should be carefully monitored for clinical features of over-replacement.
  - » In children, relate the cortisol replacement dose to body surface area and monitor growth and bone maturation carefully.
- Mineralocorticoid replacement—fludrocortisone (50–100 microg daily).

Acute

- For minor illnesses or surgery in a patient with established Addison's disease, triple the dose of the usual replacement glucocorticoid.

- For severe illness or major surgery, give IV hydrocortisone 100 mg stat, then 50 mg IV every 6–8 hours.
- For adrenal crisis, give intensive saline resuscitation, and IV hydrocortisone 100 mg stat, then 50 mg IV every 6–8 hours.

An Addisonian crisis may be induced acutely by:

- an acute pituitary or hypothalamic event
- meningococcal septicemia
- bilateral adrenalectomy
- stressful situations or illness in a patient with chronic hypoadrenalism
- abrupt cessation of prolonged high-dose steroid therapy.

CLINICAL PEARL

Treatment with supra-physiological doses of glucocorticoids (>5 mg prednisone daily) for a period in excess of 4 weeks is likely to cause central suppression of the HPA axis. Subsequent abrupt withdrawal of steroid treatment may precipitate an adrenal crisis. After chronic glucocorticoid therapy, gradual steroid weaning is advisable.

Cortisol excess (Cushing's syndrome)

Cushing's *syndrome* describes the clinical manifestations of excess glucocorticoid activity, regardless of the cause. Cushing's *disease* is one specific cause of the syndrome, due to an ACTH-secreting pituitary adenoma.

Clinical clues

- Cushingoid appearance—thin skin (dorsum of hands, shins), easy bruising, moon-shaped face, facial plethora, buffalo hump, central obesity, purple striae, supraclavicular fat pads
- Weight gain
- Acne, hirsutism (adrenal androgen effect)
- Proximal muscle wasting and weakness
- Osteoporosis, pathological fractures
- Hypertension, edema, hypokalemia (mineralocorticoid effect)
- Hyperglycemia (new onset or worsening of diabetes mellitus)
- Mental changes (depression, psychosis)
- Symptoms/signs of pituitary tumor (in Cushing's disease)
- Hyperpigmentation if excess ACTH is present

CLINICAL PEARL

The classical features of Cushing's syndrome take *many months* to develop. In cases of rapid onset of hypercortisolism (ectopic ACTH syndrome, exogenous steroid administration), these may be absent and the predominant features are metabolic effects (hyperglycemia, hypokalemia, edema, hypertension) and psychiatric manifestations.

Causes of cortisol excess

- Excess administration of exogenous steroids
- ACTH-dependent causes (80% of endogenous hypercortisolism):
  - » ACTH-secreting pituitary adenoma (Cushing's disease)
  - » ectopic ACTH secretion (small-cell carcinoma of the lung/pancreas, carcinoid tumors)
- ACTH-independent causes (20%):
  - » adrenal adenoma
  - » macronodular adrenal hyperplasia (usually bilateral)
  - » adrenal carcinoma (often causes virilization)

Diagnosis

The diagnosis of Cushing's syndrome and determination of the etiology occurs in three stages:

1. Confirm the presence of excess cortisol production, *or* loss of normal diurnal regulation, *or* demonstrate failure of physiological suppression of cortisol secretion.
2. Determine whether the hypercortisolism is secondary to ACTH hypersecretion or to autonomous adrenal cortical activity.
3. Identify the source of excess ACTH or independent cortisol overproduction.

Figure 10-13 (overleaf) provides a diagnostic algorithm.

Stage 1

- 24-hour urinary free cortisol is elevated in the vast majority of those with Cushing's syndrome. However, it can also be elevated due to an intercurrent illness or stressor (therefore poor specificity in hospitalized patients), obesity, alcoholism and depression, and after trauma and surgery. In some cases, cortisol hypersecretion may occur cyclically, and 24-hour urine free cortisol levels may be 'normal' between cycles.
- Elevated midnight cortisol levels (demonstrates loss of normal diurnal regulation).
- Overnight dexamethasone suppression test: 1 mg of dexamethasone is given at midnight and an 8 a.m. plasma cortisol level is measured the next morning.
  - » In normal individuals there will be suppression of plasma cortisol to <140 nmol/L (<5 mg/dL).
  - » Patients with Cushing's syndrome usually have values >280 nmol/L (>10 mg/dL).
  - » Failure to suppress plasma cortisol can also be found in obesity, alcoholism, depression, those taking the oral contraceptive pill, and those on medications that hasten the metabolism of dexamethasone, e.g. phenytoin and barbiturates.
  - » An alternative version of this test is to administer 0.5 mg dexamethasone four times a day orally and assess plasma cortisol after 48 hours (the same cut-off values as above apply).

Stage 2

Measurement of plasma ACTH. In the presence of hypercortisolism the secretion of ACTH should normally be

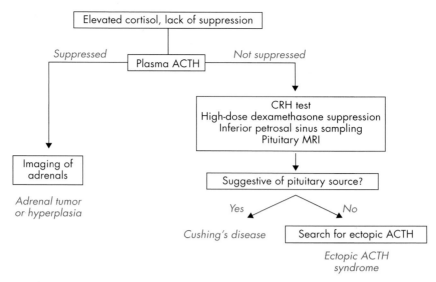

Figure 10-13 Investigation of Cushing's syndrome; a diagnostic algorithm. ACTH, adrenocorticotropic hormone; CRH, corticotropin-releasing hormone; MRI, magnetic resonance imaging

suppressed by negative feedback. Presence of a plasma ACTH level in the 'normal range' or higher demonstrates ACTH-dependent hypercortisolism.

Stage 3

Most often requires discrimination of *ectopic ACTH secretion* (usually completely autonomous) from *pituitary corticotroph adenoma* (retains some degree of physiological stimulation or inhibition). Perform stimulation of plasma cortisol with recombinant corticotropin-releasing hormone (CRH) (a positive test equals a >20% rise in plasma cortisol), or demonstrate partial inhibition (plasma cortisol to <50% baseline) with high-dose dexamethasone (single dose 8 mg overnight, or 2 mg four times a day for 48 hours). Either test, if positive, suggests a pituitary cause. Pituitary (by MRI) or adrenal (by CT) imaging may identify the causative lesion. Many cases (50% of Cushing's disease) have negative imaging. Selective petrosal sinus venous sampling for measurement of ACTH concentrations may localize the source.

Treatment options

- Definitive surgical removal of the causative lesion (transsphenoidal removal of pituitary adenoma, laparascopic removal of adrenal adenoma, resection of ectopic source of ACTH), when possible.
- Inhibition of cortisol secretion using inhibitors of steroidogenic enzymes (metyrapone, ketoconazole, aminoglutethamide, mitotane).
- Radiotherapy to the pituitary.
- Bilateral adrenalectomy (may lead to Nelson's syndrome—pituitary adenoma growth becoming aggressive after removal of inhibitory feedback from excess cortisol).

Primary hyperaldosteronism (Conn's syndrome)

Primary hyperaldosteronism refers to autonomous overproduction of aldosterone from the adrenal cortex. It may occur as a consequence of an adrenal tumor, or hyperplasia.

Aldosterone hypersecretion causes sodium and water resorption at the distal renal tubule, together with potassium and hydrogen ion loss to maintain electrical neutrality. This leads to hypokalemia, metabolic alkalosis and hypertension. High urinary potassium excretion is maintained despite the hypokalemia. Aldosterone hypersecretion continues despite feedback inhibition of the renin–angiotensin axis. Aldosterone levels are not suppressed by physiological maneuvers which normally inhibit mineralocorticoid synthesis such as salt loading or administration of fludrocortisone.

Clinical clues

- Hypertension (often refractory to treatment)
- Persistent hypokalemia (in the absence of diuretic use)
- Hypervolemia (without peripheral edema)
- Metabolic alkalosis

Causes

- Aldosterone-producing adenoma
- Idiopathic adrenal hyperplasia (may be bilateral or unilateral)
- Aldosterone-producing adrenocortical carcinoma (very rare)
- Glucocorticoid-remediable aldosteronism (GRA)
- Some subtypes of congenital adrenal hyperplasia (e.g. 11-beta-hydroxylase deficiency)

Diagnosis

In a patient with suggestive clinical and biochemical features, the best screening test is measurement of plasma aldosterone and plasma renin, expressed as a ratio. An elevated aldosterone:renin ratio supports the diagnosis of primary hyperaldosteronism. Hypokalemia should be corrected before this test is undertaken. Drugs affecting the renin–angiotensin–aldosterone axis may also need to be stopped (beta-blockers suppress renin secretion, diuretics increase aldosterone, angiotensin-converting enzyme inhibitors [ACEIs] reduce aldosterone and elevate renin). The aldosterone:renin ratio is not affected by concurrent use of slow release verapamil, prazosin or hydralazine; switching to these agents before further testing for hyperaldosteronism is prudent.

- Screen suspected hypertensive patients by measurement of plasma aldosterone:renin ratio.
- Measure 24-hour urinary aldosterone excretion.
- Demonstrate lack of normal physiological suppression of plasma aldosterone secretion after sodium loading (IV normal saline, 3-day oral salt loading) or fludrocortisone administration.
- Following confirmation of hyperaldosteronism, CT scanning can help differentiate unilateral disease (adenoma or hyperplasia) from bilateral hyperplasia.
- Adrenal vein sampling may be needed to definitively distinguish unilateral from bilateral hypersecretion, to ensure that any lesions demonstrated on CT scanning are functionally active and responsible for the aldosterone hypersecretion. The rate of incidentally found non-functioning adrenal adenomas increases with age.
- Glucocorticoid-remediable aldosteronism (GRA) is a rare autosomal dominant inherited condition in which a hybrid gene results in an ACTH-responsive aldosterone synthase enzyme. Patients with GRA have ACTH-mediated hypersecretion of aldosterone. There is usually a strong family history of hypertension and hypokalemia. Aldosterone levels are promptly suppressed by administration of dexamethasone, which suppresses ACTH release. Genetic testing is available for diagnosis.

Treatment

- Unilateral adrenal disease (adenoma or hyperplasia) can be cured by adrenalectomy, usually by a laparoscopic technique.
- Bilateral hyperplasia is treated with medical therapy. Mineralocorticoid receptor (MR) antagonists are the mainstay.
  » Spironolactone is effective but causes side-effects by also blocking androgen and progesterone receptors (gynecomastia and erectile dysfunction in men, menstrual irregularity in women).
  » Eplerenone is a newer MR antagonist with fewer side-effects but greater cost.
- If blood pressure is inadequately controlled by MR antagonists alone, addition of a potassium-sparing diuretic (amiloride, triamterene) or a dihydropyridine calcium-channel blocker is the most effective second-line treatment.

CLINICAL PEARL

ACE-inhibitors and angiotensin-receptor blockers are relatively *ineffective* antihypertensive agents in primary hyperaldosteronism because the *renin–angiotensin axis is already suppressed* by aldosterone excess.

Conditions mimicking hyperaldosteronism

As these are genetic conditions, diagnosis usually occurs in childhood.

- **Syndrome of apparent mineralocorticoid excess (SAME).** Cortisol is a natural agonist for MR but its activity is normally prevented by the presence of a cortisol-inactivating enzyme (11-beta-hydroxysteroid dehydrogenase). Genetic mutational inactivation of this enzyme allows physiological levels of cortisol to cause excessive mineralocorticoid activity in the distal renal tubule despite low plasma aldosterone levels.
- **Liddle's syndrome.** A gene mutation results in a hyperfunctioning variant of the renal epithelial sodium channel (ENaC). This results in a clinical syndrome similar to hyperaldosteronism, but the plasma aldosterone level is normal or low.
- **Bartter syndrome, Gitelman syndrome.** Involves mutations in genes encoding epithelial ion-transport proteins in the thick ascending limb of the nephron. There is marked hypokalemia and hyperaldosteronism, but hypertension is absent.

Pheochromocytoma

Pheochromocytoma is a rare catecholamine-secreting tumor derived from chromaffin cells of the sympathetic nervous system. They most commonly (90%) arise in the adrenal medulla, but may also occur at extra-adrenal sites including sympathetic neural ganglia in the abdomen, thorax or neck (also termed *paraganglioma* when occurring at these sites). Most pheochromocytomas are sporadic, but some (10–15%) occur in association with familial syndromes such as multiple endocrine neoplasia type 2 (MEN-2), neurofibromatosis, von Hippel–Lindau syndrome, and mutations of succinate dehydrogenase (SDHD, SDHB). Pheochromocytomas associated with these genetic mutations are more likely to be bilateral and occur at a younger age. Each syndrome has particular clinical features that may guide genetic testing. Most pheochromocytomas behave as benign neoplasms and the morbidity is associated with excess catecholamine secretion. A minority (10–15%) may adopt a malignant behavior and metastasize to distant sites (more common when associated with a familial syndrome, or primary lesion at an extra-adrenal location). Age of onset varies from childhood to old age. Pheochromocytoma accounts for only about 0.2% of hypertension cases.

Clinical clues

- Hypertension—50% suffer from paroxysmal hypertension, 40% have sustained elevated BP, 10% may not be hypertensive
- Classic triad or episodic symptoms: headache, palpitations/tachycardia, sweating

- Tremor, anxiety ('feeling of impending doom')
- Chest or abdominal pain
- Polyuria, dehydration, postural hypotension
- Dilated cardiomyopathy
- Hyperglycemia (especially if episodic and unexplained by dietary causes)

CLINICAL PEARL

In suspected cases of pheochromocytoma it is important to first determine whether catecholamine excess exists, before undertaking imaging studies to localize a source of catecholamine secretion.

Diagnosis

Mildly elevated catecholamine levels (less than double the upper limit of the normal range) have fairly poor specificity and are commonly seen in stress and non-adrenal illness. Catecholamine levels more than fourfold elevated above the normal range are highly predictive of pheochromocytoma.

- Confirm catecholamine excess:
  - » 24-hour urine collection for catecholamine excretion: usually free epinephrine (adrenaline), norepinephrine (noradrenaline), and their metabolites metanephrine and normetanephrine.
  - » Secretion may be intermittent. In patients with paroxysmal symptoms, have the patient commence the collection immediately after the onset of typical symptoms. Repeated collections may be necessary.
  - » Measurement of plasma metanephrine and normetanephrine have high sensitivity and specificity, but require careful observation of sampling conditions (supine, fasting, at rest, pain-free collection).
  - » The following drugs can cause false-positive urine catecholamine tests and should be avoided at the time of testing: beta-adrenergic blockers, tricyclic antidepressants, monoamine oxidase inhibitors, phenoxybenzamine, sympathomimetics, levodopa/carbidopa.
- Localization of a tumor:
  - » Imaging options are to use anatomical localization (CT or MRI) or functional imaging (^{123}I-MIBG scintigraphy). Meta-iodo-benzylguanidine (MIBG) resembles norepinephrine and is taken up by chromaffin tissue, including the adrenal medulla. Any of these approaches will identify about 95% of pheochromocytomas. Ga-68 Dotatate PET scanning is increasingly being used for imaging with its significantly greater lesion to background contrast.

Treatment

- Alpha-adrenergic blockade with phenoxybenzamine is the mainstay of medical treatment.
- Patients usually have significant plasma volume depletion and may require gradual dose escalation and/or administration of IV fluids during initiation of treatment.
- Beta-blockade is often also required for adequate blood pressure, pulse and symptom control.

- Effective pharmacological receptor blockade should be achieved before attempting surgical removal of the tumor.
- Surgery, often by laparoscopy, is the only means of definitive cure.

Malignant pheochromocytoma

Approximately 10% of pheochromocytomas demonstrate malignant behavior with evidence of metastases at the time of diagnosis, or as a postoperative recurrence. Malignancy is more common in extra-adrenal tumors, primary lesions >5 cm, and in patients with a succinate dehydrogenase complex sub-unit B (SHDB) gene mutation. The most common sites of metastasis are liver, lung and bone. Treatment options include (none are curative):

- debulking surgery
- ^{131}I-labeled MIBG therapy
- systemic cytotoxic chemotherapy
- external beam radiotherapy to localized metastases (e.g. in long bones).

New biological agents (e.g. tyrosine kinase or mTOR inhibitors) are under investigation.

Congenital adrenal hyperplasia (CAH)

All adrenal steroid hormones are synthesized from cholesterol by a multi-step pathway which requires the action of a different catalyzing enzyme at each step. Mutations in the genes coding for steroid synthetic enzymes result in impaired steroid synthesis, most commonly of cortisol. The low cortisol level causes increased ACTH drive, resulting in bilateral adrenal hyperplasia. The hyperplastic adrenal glands produce excessive quantities of steroid precursors at proximal stages of the synthesis pathway (Figure 10-14, overleaf), which may be shunted into alternative pathways (e.g. for androgen synthesis).

The resulting clinical picture, with onset in prenatal life, combines cortisol and/or aldosterone deficiency with androgen excess. In female infants this results in masculinization of the external genitals (ambiguous genitalia). Milder forms, with onset later in life, can also occur.

Each enzymatic step of steroid hormone synthesis from cholesterol can be disrupted by a genetic mutation of the relevant enzyme. The most common (95% of cases) is cytochrome P450 21-hydroxylase. This enzyme deficiency results in failure of synthesis of cortisol and aldosterone, accumulation of the precursor 17-alpha-hydroxyprogesterone, and diversion of this precursor to the androgen synthesis pathway.

Congenital adrenal hyperplasia syndromes are all inherited as autosomal recessive traits. The frequency is approximately 1:15,000 live births.

Clinical clues

In females

- Females with 'classic' CAH have ambiguous genitalia at birth due to excess adrenal androgen production in utero. The more severe forms of classic 21-hydroxylase deficiency also present with dehydration, hyponatremia

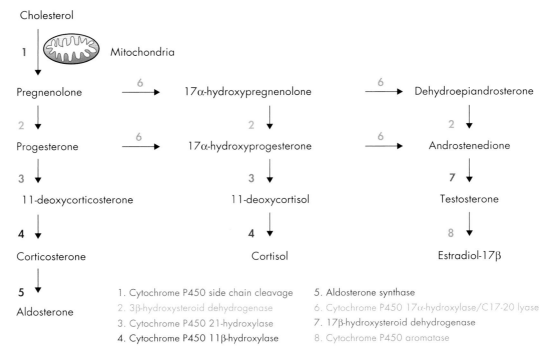

Cholesterol

1 → Mitochondria

Pregnenolone — 6 → 17α-hydroxypregnenolone — 6 → Dehydroepiandrosterone

2 ↓   2 ↓   2 ↓

Progesterone — 6 → 17α-hydroxyprogesterone — 6 → Androstenedione

3 ↓   3 ↓   7 ↓

11-deoxycorticosterone   11-deoxycortisol   Testosterone

4 ↓   4 ↓   8 ↓

Corticosterone   Cortisol   Estradiol-17β

5 ↓

Aldosterone

1. Cytochrome P450 side chain cleavage
2. 3β-hydroxysteroid dehydrogenase
3. Cytochrome P450 21-hydroxylase
4. Cytochrome P450 11β-hydroxylase
5. Aldosterone synthase
6. Cytochrome P450 17α-hydroxylase/C17-20 lyase
7. 17β-hydroxysteroid dehydrogenase
8. Cytochrome P450 aromatase

Figure 10-14 Adrenal steroid synthetic pathway

and hyperkalemia in early life due to aldosterone and glucocorticoid deficiency and are termed 'salt-wasting CAH'. Less severe forms without salt-wasting crises are called 'simple virilising CAH'. Both forms experience early adrenarche and growth spurt.

- Milder deficiencies of 21-hydroxylase or 3-beta-hydroxysteroid dehydrogenase activity may present in adolescence or adulthood with oligomenorrhea, hirsutism, acne, or infertility. This is termed 'non-classic CAH'.

In males

- Classic salt-wasting CAH in males presents in the postnatal period with failure to thrive, recurrent vomiting, dehydration, hypotension, hyponatremia, hyperkalemia, and shock.
- Males with less severe 21-hydroxylase deficiency who are not diagnosed on neonatal screening, present later in childhood with precocious puberty, accelerated growth and advanced skeletal maturation (eventual short stature).

In males and females

- In severe cases, in both genders skin hyperpigmentation may result from excessive ACTH production.

CLINICAL PEARL

Prenatal diagnosis of congenital adrenal hyperplasia may be attempted for babies who have an affected older sibling, to prevent genital abnormalities for females and life-threatening neonatal crises.

CAH in adulthood

In adulthood, even with appropriate treatment, CAH can have continuing morbidity. Adult women may have problems such as infertility or gender dysphoria. Adult men with poor compliance with steroid suppression may develop adrenal rest tissue in their testes, presenting as a scrotal mass. Excess adrenal androgen production in men can impair spermatogenesis and fertility. Careful adjustment of steroid suppressive therapy is required.

Diagnosis

- Elevated 17-hydroxyprogesterone levels
- Low cortisol levels, elevated ACTH levels, elevated adrenal androgens
- Hyponatremia, hyperkalemia, hypoglycemia
- Genetic mutation analysis

Treatment

- Classic CAH requires lifelong glucocorticoid replacement, to replace the deficient hormone and reduce the ACTH-driven production of adrenal androgens.
- Glucocorticoid management is a careful balance between adequate suppression of adrenal androgens and minimizing glucocorticoid excess.
- Higher doses of glucocorticoids are required during significant physical stress.
- Short-acting glucocorticoids are recommended in children to avoid growth suppression. Once puberty is complete, longer-acting glucocorticoids may be needed to suppress nocturnal androgen production.

- Salt supplementation and treatment with the mineralo-corticoid, fludrocortisone, is essential in salt-wasting CAH, to prevent crises. Simple-virilizing CAH may still have subclinical aldosterone deficiency, evidenced by a low aldosterone:renin ratio. Fludrocortisone may reduce glucocorticoid requirements and steroid-related side-effects.
- Non-classic CAH does not require treatment unless symptoms of androgen excess are troubling. Most men do not require daily glucocorticoids, unless they have testicular adrenal rest tissue.
- Glucocorticoids are recommended in adolescents with premature puberty, accelerated bone age or girls with virilization. They may be continued in adult women with troubling hyperandrogenism or infertility.
- Androgen blocking agents may assist in the management of virilisation, but are contra-indicated in women desiring fertility.
- Surgical correction of ambiguous genitalia in females.
- In post-pubertal females it may be necessary to give androgen-blocking agents (e.g. cyproterone acetate) to antagonize the action of excess androgens.

Incidentally found adrenal masses ('incidentaloma')

Modern abdominal imaging techniques may identify adrenal lesions in 4–5% of asymptomatic individuals, increasing to 10% in people aged >60 years (see Fig 10-15). Most are 1–4 cm diameter and are cysts, myelolipoma or non-functioning adenoma. Two important clinical questions arise:

1 **Is the lesion malignant?**
   a Diameter >4 cm makes malignancy more likely, >6 cm mandates surgical removal.
   b Benign adenomas usually have high lipid content, low CT density, rapid contrast washout.
   c Fine needle aspiration cytology is not reliable to exclude adrenal carcinoma.
   d The adrenal gland is a common site for metastatic tumor deposits. See Figure 10-15 (overleaf).
2 **Is the lesion hormonally functioning?**
   a Assess clinically for cortisol, catecholamine, aldosterone or androgen excess.
   b Measure catecholamine levels, cortisol suppressibility, plasma aldosterone:renin ratio.

Apparently non-functioning and benign lesions can simply be observed by repeat scanning to assess subsequent growth. The indications for adrenalectomy are hormonal hypersecretion, significant growth to > 4 cm diameter, or radiological indications of a high risk of malignancy.

GROWTH AND PUBERTY

Longitudinal growth depends on genetic and environmental factors. It requires constitutional good health and adequate nutrition. The most important endocrine factors are the GH–IGF1 axis (growth hormone–insulin-like growth factor axis), thyroid hormones, and gonadal steroids during the peripubertal growth spurt. It is essential to consider growth in terms of temporal development (plot progress on growth charts), the individual's genetic potential (compare with mid-parental height percentile), and the biological age (assess bone age) rather than the chronological age.

Causes of short stature

- Familial short stature
- Constitutional delay of growth
- Impaired nutrition:
  » malnutrition
  » malabsorption
  » eating disorders
- Chronic diseases of childhood (especially chronic inflammatory and infectious disorders, chronic heart disease and renal failure)
- Genetic causes:
  » Down syndrome (trisomy 21)
  » Williams syndrome
  » Turner syndrome
- Impaired GH production/action:
  » hypopituitarism
  » isolated GH deficiency
  » Laron syndrome (IGF-1 deficiency)
- Other endocrine causes:
  » hypothyroidism
  » cortisol excess
- Bone/cartilage disorders:
  » achondroplasia (dwarfism)
  » rickets

CLINICAL PEARL

The most common causes of short stature in children are familial short stature (calculate the parental height percentages) and constitutional delay (consider radiological assessment of bone age). Worldwide, the most frequent cause of growth failure is malnutrition.

Onset of puberty—physiology

Puberty is the physical process of maturation to an adult body capable of sexual reproduction. The onset of puberty marks the beginning of adolescence, the period of life during which physical, neurodevelopmental and psychosocial transition to adulthood occurs.

Puberty is characterized physically by the appearance of secondary sex characteristics, change in body composition and accelerated longitudinal growth. These changes are produced by the action of gonadal steroids (estrogen or testosterone) which are secreted as a result of activation of the hypothalamic–pituitary–gonadal axis. The earliest signs of puberty are augmentation of body fat and breast budding in females, and testicular enlargement in males. Pubertal development is classified according to the stages described by Tanner (Figure 10-16, overleaf).

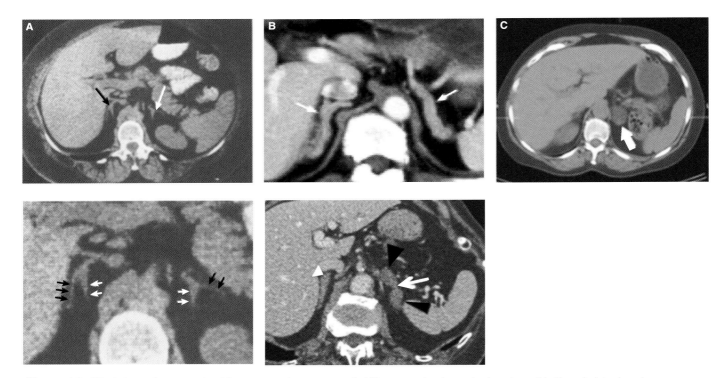

Figure 10-15 Adrenal computed tomography scans of: (**A**) normal adrenal glands, with the right gland seen as an upside-down V and the left as an upside-down Y (enlarged in the lower image); (**B**) adrenal hyperplasia, with diffuse thickening visible in the upper image and nodules (arrowheads) interspersed between normal adrenal tissue (arrow) in the lower image; and (**C**) adrenal adenoma (arrow)

From: (A, B) Haaga JR et al, eds. CT and MRI of the whole body, 5th ed. Philadelphia: Mosby, 2009. (C) Tang YZ et al. The prevalence of incidentally detected adrenal enlargement on CT. Clin Radiol 2014;69(1):e37–e42. © The Royal College of Radiologists. (D) Caolli EM et al. Differentiating adrenal adenomas from nonadenomas using ^{18}F-FDG PET/CT. Acad Radiol 2007;14(4):468–75.

Causes of delayed puberty

The most common cause is constitutional delay, for which there is often a family history. A delayed bone age and absence of a pathological cause are the clues to this. In girls, low body weight commonly delays puberty. This may be associated with eating disorders or excessive sporting activity.

Primary gonadal causes

(Elevated serum gonadotropins and low gonadal steroids.)

- Turner syndrome—45 XO (female)
- Klinefelter syndrome—47 XXY (male)
- Gonadal agenesis
- Cryptorchidism (male)
- Bilateral testicular torsion, trauma, castration (male)
- Gonadal irradiation (childhood malignancy)
- Drugs (marijuana, alcohol, chemotherapeutic agents, ketoconazole, glucocorticoid)
- Autoimmune gonadal failure
- Chronic systemic disease

Central (hypothalamic–pituitary) causes

(Low or normal gonadotropins, low gonadal steroids.)

- Constitutional delay/familial delay
- Low body weight (female)
- Kallmann syndrome—genetic isolated hypogonadotropic hypogonadism with anosmia
- Prader–Willi syndrome—disorder arising from defective paternal chromosome 15, associated with obesity and hyperphagia
- Hypopituitarism
- CNS tumors, infiltrative disorders, surgery or irradiation
- Hyperprolactinemia
- Chronic illness

Common causes of precocious puberty

Precocious puberty is the onset of puberty at an age greater than 2 to 2.5 standard deviations before the population mean, commonly before 8 years in girls and 9 years in boys. There are clear ethnic variations, and a historical trend to earlier pubertal development, perhaps related to obesity. Incidence is far higher in girls than boys. The earlier the onset, the higher likelihood of underlying pathology.

Central (gonadotropin-dependent)

- CNS tumors
- Brain injury—infection, surgery, trauma, radiation

FEMALES				
STAGE	BREASTS	PUBIC HAIR	ANNUAL HEIGHT VELOCITY	OTHER
1	Prepubertal; elevation of nipple only	Villus hair only	5.0–6.0 cm (2.0–2.4 in)	Adrenarche
2	Breast buds palpable, enlarged areola	Sparse, slightly pigmented	7.0–8.0 cm (2.8–3.2 in)	Clitoral enlargement; labial pigmentation
3	Mammary extends beyond edge of areola, no separation of contours	Coarser, darker, curled	8.0 cm (3.2 in)	Acne, underarm hair
4	Nipple mound forms secondary mound above the level of the breast	Adult type, but not beyond pubic area	< 7.0 cm (< 2.8 in)	First menstruation
5	Adult-contour breast with integral nipple mound	Adult type, spreading onto inner thigh	Final height reached at age 16	Adult genitals

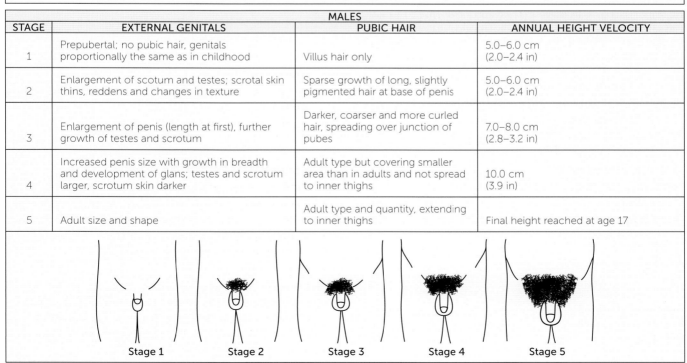

MALES			
STAGE	EXTERNAL GENITALS	PUBIC HAIR	ANNUAL HEIGHT VELOCITY
1	Prepubertal; no pubic hair, genitals proportionally the same as in childhood	Villus hair only	5.0–6.0 cm (2.0–2.4 in)
2	Enlargement of scotum and testes; scrotal skin thins, reddens and changes in texture	Sparse growth of long, slightly pigmented hair at base of penis	5.0–6.0 cm (2.0–2.4 in)
3	Enlargement of penis (length at first), further growth of testes and scrotum	Darker, coarser and more curled hair, spreading over junction of pubes	7.0–8.0 cm (2.8–3.2 in)
4	Increased penis size with growth in breadth and development of glans; testes and scrotum larger, scrotum skin darker	Adult type but covering smaller area than in adults and not spread to inner thighs	10.0 cm (3.9 in)
5	Adult size and shape	Adult type and quantity, extending to inner thighs	Final height reached at age 17

Figure 10-16 Tanner pubertal stages for males and females

Diagrams from Phelps K and Hassad C. General practice: the integrative approach. Sydney: Churchill Livingstone, 2011; based on Tanner JM. Growth at adolescence. Oxford: Blackwell Science, 1962.

Peripheral (gonadotropin-independent)

- Sex-steroid-secreting tumor (in adrenals, ovaries, testes)
- Congenital adrenal hyperplasia
- Exposure to exogenous sex steroids
- Benign, non-progressive variants also exist

MALE REPRODUCTIVE ENDOCRINOLOGY

Testicular function

The testis has two interdependent but different functions:

- testosterone synthesis by Leydig cells
- spermatogenesis by seminiferous tubules.

Leydig cell function is stimulated by luteinizing hormone (LH), and testosterone feeds back on the pituitary and hypothalamus to inhibit LH secretion. Spermatogenesis requires stimulation by FSH as well as a high local tissue concentration of testosterone from neighboring Leydig cells. Sertoli cells are specialized supporting cells in the tubules which mediate these hormonal signals, and also secrete inhibin which acts as a feedback regulator of FSH. The majority of testicular volume (90%) in the adult testis is composed of seminiferous tubules. Increase in testicular size is the first sign of onset of puberty in males.

The action of testosterone on many target cells involves conversion to dihydrotestosterone (by 5-alpha-reductase) to produce actions on androgen receptors (prostate growth, androgen sensitive hair follicles), or conversion to estradiol (by aromatase) to act on estrogen receptors (maintenance of bone mass). Circulating testosterone is predominantly (98%) protein-bound, to sex-hormone-binding globulin (SHBG) and albumin, with only about 2% circulating in the free form.

Tests of testicular function

- Serum testosterone (total testosterone assays are more reliable than those for free testosterone)
- Serum LH and FSH (distinguishes primary from secondary causes of hypogonadism)
- Testicular volume
- Semen analysis (sperm number, motility, semen volume)
- hCG stimulation test (determines capacity to synthesize testosterone)

Male hypogonadism

Clinical features of male hypogonadism

Hypogonadism with onset in infancy or childhood presents as failure to enter puberty. Onset in adult life has variable manifestations, listed below.

Symptoms

- Decreased libido

- Erectile dysfunction
- Loss of energy and muscle strength
- Hot sweats, flushing
- Mood changes, depression
- Infertility

Physical signs

- Reduced growth of body and facial hair (a late sign, indicates prolonged deficiency)
- Gynecomastia (more common with primary than secondary hypogonadism)
- Reduced muscle mass, increased body fat, bone loss
- Reduced testicular volume
- Soft facial skin with fine wrinkles

CLINICAL PEARL

Erectile dysfunction in middle-aged and older men is often an early indicator of generalized endothelial dysfunction and atherosclerosis. Drug side-effects and psychological factors are also important contributors. Endocrine causes are relatively uncommon but should be excluded as they are readily treatable.

Causes of male hypogonadism

1. Primary hypogonadism

(Low testosterone, elevated LH, FSH.)

- Gonadal dysgenesis, cryptorchidism, congenital anorchia
- Klinefelter syndrome (XXY karyotype)
- Castration or trauma
- Irradiation or chemotherapy for childhood cancer
- Excessive alcohol consumption
- Mumps orchitis
- Infiltrative disorders of the testis (hemochromatosis, amyloidosis, sarcoid)
- Androgen synthetic enzyme defects

2. Secondary (hypogonadotropic) hypogonadism

(Low testosterone, normal or low LH, FSH.)

- Pituitary or hypothalamic disease
- Trauma or irradiation (may cause selective gonadotropin deficiency with preservation of other pituitary hormones)
- Kallmann syndrome (congenital failure of GnRH production in association with anosmia)
- Hyperprolactinemia
- Drugs—marijuana, narcotics, prior anabolic steroid treatment, GnRH agonists and antagonists, steroids
- Obesity and associated syndromes—Prader–Willi syndrome, Laurence–Moon–Biedl syndrome
- Critical illness
- Chronic disease—HIV, end-stage renal failure, COPD
- Excessive exercise, eating disorder

Causes of erectile dysfunction

- Vascular causes (atherosclerosis, hypertension, trauma)
- Psychological factors
- Drug side-effects (beta-blockers, vasodilators, alcohol, opiates, marijuana, anti-androgens, antidepressants, H$_2$-receptor blockers)
- Neurogenic causes (stroke, spinal cord disorders, peripheral neuropathy)
- Hormonal causes (testosterone deficiency, prolactin excess)
- Age and systemic disease, especially diabetes (combination of above mechanisms)

Gynecomastia

> **CLINICAL PEARL**
>
> The anterior chest is a common site for fat deposition in obese men. When there is apparent enlargement of the breasts in a male it is important to distinguish by palpation between true gynecomastia (mammary ductal hyperplasia) and simple adiposity.

True gynecomastia reflects local excess of stimulatory estrogen action relative to inhibitory testosterone at the mammary ductal epithelium.

Causes of gynecomastia are:

- physiological (temporary increased estrogen)—neonatal period, puberty, old age
- estrogen excess:
  » estrogen administration
  » increased aromatase activity (thyrotoxicosis)
- cirrhosis
- increased hCG production (germ-cell tumors)
- androgen deficiency (any cause above)
- androgen blockade (spironolactone, anti-androgens used in prostate cancer, lack of 5-alpha-reductase or androgen receptor)
- hyperprolactinemia.

Medical treatment options for gynecomastia include androgens (testosterone), if the patient has hypogonadism, anti-estrogen (clomiphene citrate, tamoxifen) and aromatase inhibitors. Paradoxically, administration of testosterone can exacerbate gynecomastia especially in eugonadal men because of local aromatization of androgen to estrogen in the breast. In severe or intractable gynecomastia, it may be necessary to perform surgical mastectomy.

Androgen replacement therapy

In men with proven hypogonadism, the aim of therapy is to restore physiological levels of testosterone in the systemic circulation and to maintain normal function of androgen-responsive tissues.

- Testosterone has very poor bioavailability if administered orally, due to extensive first-pass metabolism in the liver.
- The best routes of administration are depot injection or transdermal preparations.
- Testosterone esters in oil can be given as an intramuscular depot injection. Different preparations have dosing frequency ranging from fortnightly to 3-monthly.
- Skin patches (replaced daily) or transdermal gel (applied daily) can achieve adequate serum testosterone levels.
- Serum total testosterone concentrations should be monitored to assess adequacy of replacement.
- Prostate cancer is a contraindication to testosterone treatment, and care should be exercised to avoid supraphysiological testosterone levels in older men who might have prostatic hyperplasia.
- Other adverse effects of testosterone therapy include polycythemia, worsening of obstructive sleep apnea and fluid retention leading to worsening of heart failure.
- Over-replacement and testosterone abuse are also concerns in some instances.

FEMALE REPRODUCTIVE ENDOCRINOLOGY

Anatomy and physiology

The female reproductive system is controlled by the hypothalamic–pituitary–ovarian axis. Pulsatile secretion of GnRH from the hypothalamus stimulates secretion of pituitary LH and FSH, which act in concert to control the ovary in a cyclical fashion, the primary aim being development and maturation of 1 follicle per month, ovulation, and subsequent fertilization and implantation, or menstruation. The ovarian follicle is made up of the egg and the surrounding theca and granulosa cells. LH stimulates androstenedione production in theca cells, while FSH controls estrogen production from granulosa cells. Estrogen stimulates growth of the endometrium, in preparation for pregnancy. After ovulation, the remaining follicle (corpus luteum) produces progesterone, which develops the secretory endometrium required for implantation. If pregnancy does not occur, the corpus luteum degenerates, estrogen and progesterone levels fall, and endometrial shedding results in the appearance of the menses.

The menstrual cycle

1. Early follicular phase: growth of recruited follicles
2. Late follicular phase: selection of a dominant follicle
3. Ovulatory phase: LH surge stimulates breakdown of follicle and release of mature ovum
4. Luteal phase: follicle transforms into a corpus luteum.

The hormonal changes accompanying the phases of the menstrual cycle are illustrated in Figure 10-17.

Estrogen and progesterone have effects on target reproductive organs, as well as other body systems (Box 10-5), and provide positive and negative feedback to the hypothalamic–pituitary axis.

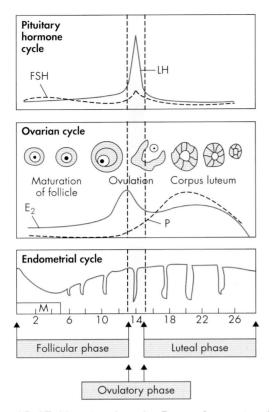

Figure 10-17 Menstrual cycle. Days of menstrual bleeding are indicated by M. E$_2$, estrogen; FSH, follicle-stimulating hormone; LH, luteinizing hormone; P, progesterone

Adapted from Rebar RW. Normal physiology of the reproductive system. In Endocrinology and Metabolism Continuing Education Program, American Association of Clinical Chemistry, November 1982. Copyright 1982 by the American Association for Clinical Chemistry; reprinted with permission.

Clinical and laboratory evaluation

Dysfunction in the reproductive axis may present as early or delayed puberty, virilization, menstrual abnormalities or altered fertility. Clinical assessment includes history and examination of secondary sexual characteristics (see Tanner staging, Figure 10-16), features of androgen excess, characterization of the menstrual cycle, and a sexual and reproductive history.

Key points in the menstrual history

- Cycle length and regularity
- Length of period, amount of bleeding
- Age of menarche/menopause
- Dysmenorrhea and other premenstrual syndromes

Laboratory tests

- Measurement of estradiol, progesterone, LH and FSH should be interpreted in relation to the timing of the menstrual cycle, or pre-pubertal or post-menopausal state.

Box 10-5

Actions of estrogen and progesterone

Estrogen actions

- Maintains uterus, endometrial proliferation
- Mammary gland—ductal epithelial proliferation
- Maintains vaginal wall and lubrication
- Reduces bone resorption, increases formation
- Increases clotting factors and platelet adhesiveness
- Increases HDLs and triglycerides, decreases LDLs
- Increases hepatic production of binding proteins
- Influences female body fat distribution (increased subcutaneous, reduced visceral fat)

Progesterone actions

- Converts endometrium to secretory stage
- Mammary gland—lobular alveolar development
- Thickens cervical mucus
- Inhibits lactation during pregnancy
- Decreases uterine contractility
- Relaxes smooth muscle

HDL, high-density lipoprotein; LDL, low-density lipoprotein

» Progesterone secretion rises during the luteal phase and indicates that ovulation has occurred during that cycle. The luteal phase lasts exactly 14 days, whilst the follicular phase may vary from 7 to 21 days. This is useful in determining the time of ovulation and interpreting a serum progesterone result.

CLINICAL PEARL

The timing of a serum progesterone test in relation to the menstrual cycle is crucial for its interpretation. In retrospect, a sample must have been taken 4–7 days prior to the next menstrual period for it to allow interpretation as to whether ovulation occurred.

- Testosterone and estradiol circulate in the bloodstream, predominantly bound to SHBG and albumin. Only the albumin-bound and the unbound (free) fraction is biologically active, therefore total testosterone and estradiol levels should be interpreted in the context of the SHBG levels. SHBG is lowered in the setting of insulin resistance (e.g. polycystic ovarian syndrome, diabetes) and hypothyroidism, and this may contribute to increased free androgen activity.
- There is poor standardization of testosterone assays. Depending on the method used, levels in normal women may be at the lower end of the assay detection range and potentially unreliable. Calculated free androgen index from testosterone and SHBG is the most clinically sensitive marker of androgen excess in women.

Hirsutism and hyperandrogenism

The definition of excess hair growth in women is subjective and varies greatly between races, as well as having variable tolerability and acceptability amongst women. It is important to differentiate true hirsutism, which is excess terminal (dark, coarse) hair growth in androgen-sensitive areas, from hypertrichosis, which is generalized excess hair growth over the body. Hypertrichosis may be related to metabolic causes such as anorexia, or drugs such as anticonvulsants, cyclosporine or minoxidil. It is also important to distinguish simple hirsutism from virilization—which includes other signs of androgen excess. Hirsutism may rarely be the first sign of virilization, but usually occurs in the context of more benign disorders, commonly, polycystic ovarian syndrome. The severity of hirsutism can be quantified using the modified Ferriman-Gallwey score. A score of >8 is considered mild hirsutism, >15 moderate-severe hirsutism. These cut-offs may differ according to ethnicity.

Simple hirsutism is often confined to the face, and drug treatment is not always necessary. Local measures and reassurance may satisfy the patient. If medical therapy is required, benefits only occur after more than 3 months, as this is the duration of a complete hair cycle. Options include estrogen (increases SHBG and androgen binding) or an anti-androgenic drug (spironolactone, cyproterone).

Virilization results from conditions that produce higher levels of androgens, including androgen-secreting tumors of the ovary or adrenal, and congenital adrenal hyperplasia. Characteristic features of virilization are a male pattern growth of androgen-dependent terminal body hair (back, chest, abdomen and face), temporal balding, clitoral enlargement, deepening of voice and acne. Clues to the diagnosis of an androgen-secreting tumor include rapid onset of signs, testosterone levels >7 nmol/L and an abdominal/pelvic mass. In severe hyperandrogenemia, localization of the source is vital and surgery is the treatment of choice.

Polycystic ovary syndrome (PCOS)

Polycystic ovary syndrome is an important cause of hyperandrogenism, ovulatory disturbance and infertility, affecting 5–15% of reproductive-age women. Its exact etiology remains uncertain, but strong genetic factors, in combination with environmental factors, lead to hormonal changes of hyperandrogenism, hyperinsulinemia and their resulting clinical features. Although obesity is more prevalent in women with PCOS and is implicated in pathogenesis, 'lean PCOS' phenotypes are also observed. There is significant heterogeneity in clinical presentation, and three different sets of diagnostic criteria have been proposed by expert committees (Rotterdam, NIH, AES), highlighting the limitations in our understanding of this condition.

Clinical features

- Onset often age 15–35 years, but manifestations continue throughout life
- Hirsutism and acne
- Menstrual disturbance (usually oligomenorrhea), subfertility, polycystic ovaries on ultrasound
- Features of insulin resistance, e.g. acanthosis nigricans, glucose intolerance or type 2 diabetes
- Features of metabolic syndrome (hypertension, dyslipidemia, abdominal adiposity) and increased cardiovascular risk
- Psychosocial implications—mood disturbance, impaired quality of life

CLINICAL PEARL

The Rotterdam criteria are commonly used in the diagnosis of PCOS, requiring two of three key features:
- oligo- or anovulation
- clinical and/or biochemical hyperandrogenism
- polycystic ovaries on ultrasound and exclusion of other causes.

Despite its name, the appearance of polycystic ovaries on ultrasound is therefore *not* an obligatory requirement for diagnosis of the syndrome. In adolescents, ultrasound is not recommended for diagnosis within 8 years of menarche and the other two criteria should be met.

Management

- Women with PCOS should be made aware of their increased risk of gestational diabetes, type 2 diabetes and other metabolic disorders such as cardiovascular disease and non-alcoholic fatty liver disease. Recommendations for a healthy lifestyle are key. Prevention of weight gain across the lifespan and weight reduction in the already overweight are first-line.
- The clinical phenotype is diverse; other management is targeted toward specific clinical presentations.
  » Hirsutism—cosmetic approaches (laser, bleaching, eflornithine cream), oral contraceptive (increases SHBG, thereby blocking androgens), anti-androgen agents (spironolactone, cyproterone).
  » Infertility—early family initiation, weight loss, clomiphene citrate, metformin (insulin sensitizer), gonadotropins, in-vitro fertilization.
  » Menstrual disturbance—oral contraceptive pill, cyclical progesterone, metformin.
  » Screen and manage other cardiovascular risk factors—including hypertension, dyslipidemia, glucose intolerance, smoking. Glycemic status should be assessed at diagnosis, prior to pregnancy, and every 1–3 years, depending on other risk factors. Long-term monitoring is key.
  » Attention to psychosocial aspects.

Female hypogonadism

Abnormal function of the hypothalamic–pituitary–ovarian axis results in impaired estrogen production. This may lead to impaired sexual development (in adolescence), or menstrual disturbance, infertility and/or symptoms of estrogen deficiency (flushing, vaginal dryness, osteoporosis in women of reproductive age). Menopause marks the end of reproductive life, when ovulation ceases and levels of estrogen and progesterone decline. Although this is a natural consequence of aging, symptoms of hypogonadism may be troubling for some women at perimenopause.

- Premature ovarian failure:
  - » Menopause before the age of 40 years
  - » Characterized by high FSH/LH and low estradiol concentrations
  - » Causes—idiopathic, genetic (Turner syndrome, galactosemia), autoimmune oophoritis, surgery, chemotherapy and irradiation.
- Hypothalamic amenorrhea:
  - » Abnormalities of GnRH pulse generation in the hypothalamus lead to low FSH/LH levels and hypoestrogenemia
  - » Causes:
    - – functional—exercise, weight loss (anorexia nervosa), low BMI, stress
    - – organic—hypothalamic lesions, genetic GnRH deficiency (Kallmann's syndrome).
- Pituitary disease.
  - » Any pituitary condition altering the cyclical production of FSH and LH in response to GnRH stimulation may lead to ovulatory failure.
  - » An important inhibitor of hypothalamic-pituitary-ovarian function is hyperprolactinemia—e.g. prolactinoma, pituitary stalk compression, drug effects.

Management

Management is largely based on replacement of ovarian hormones. Estrogen and progesterone are administered orally or transdermally. For pubertal induction, low doses of estrogen are initiated and gradually uptitrated. Progesterones are added to improve breast development and induce menses. Women with premature ovarian failure should receive estrogen replacement until the natural age of menopause to prevent premature bone loss. Progesterone is added continuously, or cyclically, to prevent endometrial hyperplasia from unopposed estrogen stimulation. Women without an intact uterus do not require progesterones. Severe menopausal symptoms during the peri-menopause may also be alleviated by judicious short-term use of ovarian hormone replacement. In hypothalamic or pituitary disorders, where fertility is desired and ovarian function remains intact, gonadotrophins are administered, to stimulate follicle development, trigger ovulation and prepare the uterus for implantation.

Endocrinology of pregnancy

Several hormonal axes are altered during pregnancy.

- **Thyroid:** increased requirement for thyroid hormone production because of increased thyroid-hormone binding protein (induced by estrogen). Impaired thyroid reserve may be unmasked during pregnancy. Beta-hCG has a stimulatory effect on TSH receptors, in some cases resulting in gestational hyperthyroidism. TSH levels are therefore lower in the 1st trimester when hCG levels are highest. Thyroid function tests in pregnancy should be interpreted according to trimester-specific reference ranges if available.

- **Hypothalamic–pituitary–adrenal axis:** there is hyperactivity of this axis during pregnancy, related to cortiocotropin production from the placenta and an estrogen-induced increase in cortisol-binding proteins. Cortisol levels may be 2–3 times the normal reference range, though pregnancy-specific reference ranges are poorly defined.
- **Prolactin:** increases 10- to 20-fold during pregnancy and lactation, in response to lactotrope expansion by estrogen. Lactotrope hypertrophy results in increased pituitary size during pregnancy.
- **Calcium:** increased renal 1-alpha-hydroxylase activity results in calcitriol production, facilitating intestinal calcium absorption and provisioning of calcium to the developing fetus. Placentally derived PTHrP may be involved in increasing calcium availability and transplacental passage.
- **Growth hormone/Insulin-like growth factor 1:** placental GH rises during pregnancy and replaces pituitary GH as the prime regulator of maternal IGFs.
- **Glucose regulation:** insulin resistance increases during pregnancy, particularly late in the 2nd trimester. This is under the influence of placental hormones and adipokines, including placental GH, cortisol and tumor necrosis factor alpha (TNF-alpha). A compensatory increase in insulin secretion normally maintains glucose tolerance. In 5–10% of women, the combination of increased insulin resistance and a failure of beta-cells to meet the demands for insulin production results in development of gestational diabetes. Testing for glucose intolerance is ideally performed around 24–28 weeks of gestation.

NEUROENDOCRINE TUMORS (NETs)

Overview

In addition to the classical organ-based endocrine system, there is a diffuse network of hormone-secreting cells spread throughout the body. Sites include:

- gastrointestinal tract—signaling gut motility, acid and fluid secretion, insulin release
- respiratory tract—signaling inflammation, toxic exposure
- skin—Merkel cells signaling physical and chemical exposure.

Neuroendocrine tumors arising from these cells are capable of secreting a variety of peptide hormones and vasoactive amines. They most commonly arise in the foregut or bronchi, and are slow-growing but have malignant potential. Histologically they are characterized by neurosecretory granules. Proteins associated with secretory vesicle function (e.g. chromogranin A) can often be used as tumor markers. Many NETs express receptors for somatostatin. Consequently, radio-labeled somatostatin is useful for diagnostic imaging, and long-acting somatostatin analogs can be effective in suppressing excessive hormone secretion and curtailing tumor growth.

Carcinoid syndrome

A clinical syndrome produced by excessive production of NET-derived vasoactive amines (serotonin, histamine, kallikrein, prostaglandins).

- Episodic symptoms—flushing, sweating, diarrhea, bronchospasm.
- Serotonin excess can induce fibrosis and scarring of right-sided cardiac valves.
- Diagnosis is by measurement of plasma serotonin, or urinary excretion of a serotonin metabolite, 5-hydroxyindoleacetic acid (5-HIAA).

Glucagonoma

- Causes insulin resistance and secondary diabetes mellitus.
- Characteristic skin rash (necrolytic migratory erythema; Figure 10-18).
- High incidence of thromboembolism.
- Diagnosis is by measurement of plasma glucagon and tumor imaging.
- Most glucagonomas are located in the pancreas.

VIPoma

- Vasoactive intestinal polypeptide (VIP) stimulates intestinal secretion of water, potassium and bicarbonate and inhibition of gastric acid secretion.

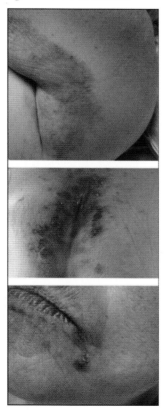

Figure 10-18 Necrolytic migratory erythema

From Compton NL and Chien AL. A rare but revealing sign: necrolytic migratory erythema. Am J Med 2013;126(5):387–9.

- VIPoma causes a syndrome of profuse watery diarrhea, hypokalemia and achlorhydria.
- Diagnose by measurement of plasma VIP and tumor imaging (most are found in the pancreas or upper gastrointestinal tract).
- It is treated by surgical excision when possible, or with somatostatin analogs.

Insulinoma

A rare NET causing hyperinsulinemia and subsequent hypoglycemia.

The cornerstone of diagnosis is deliberate provocation of hypoglycemia by a prolonged supervised fast of 48–72 hours.

- In cases of insulinoma (beta-cell tumor) or nesidioblastosis (islet-cell hyperplasia), most patients develop hypoglycemia within 18 hours of fasting.
- If hypoglycemia is provoked, samples should be obtained for measurement of plasma insulin and C-peptide while the patient is hypoglycemic.
- Imaging studies may then be undertaken to localize the source of insulin hypersecretion.

CLINICAL PEARL

Levels of C-peptide, which is co-released with insulin from pancreatic beta-cells, can be used to distinguish *endogenous hyperinsulinemia* (C-peptide high) from *exogenous insulin administration* (C-peptide low).

Insulinoma characteristics:

- insulinomas present with recurrent episodes of spontaneous hypoglycemia
- 10% are associated with multiple endocrine neoplasia type 1 (MEN-1), and up to 10% are malignant
- most commonly located in the pancreas.
- Most insulinomas are very small (<2 cm) and difficult to localize by standard imaging with CT, ultrasound or MRI.
- Endoscopic or intraoperative ultrasound and portal vein sampling for insulin may be used to localize the lesion.
- Surgery is curative in >75% of cases of localized insulinoma.
- Medical therapy with diazoxide or somatostatin analogs may be used.

Differential diagnosis of a hypoglycemic disorder

- Excessive endogenous insulin secretion/action:
  - » insulinoma
  - » nesidioblastosis (islet-cell hyperplasia)
  - » non-islet-cell tumors (secreting insulin-like growth factors)
  - » reactive hypoglycemia, alimentary hypoglycemia

- Drugs:
  - » sulphonylureas (high C-peptide and insulin levels, drug detectable in urine and plasma)
  - » insulin (including surreptitious use, will have high insulin levels but low C-peptide)
  - » ethanol
  - » beta-blockers
  - » salicylates, ACEIs, lithium
- Impaired hepatic gluconeogenesis:
  - » chronic liver disease
  - » congenital enzyme deficiencies
- Deficient counter-regulatory hormones:
  - » hypoadrenalism (cortisol)
  - » hypopituitarism (ACTH and growth hormone)
  - » pancreatic insufficiency (glucagon deficiency plus carbohydrate malabsorption)
- Autoimmune hypoglycemia (insulin antibodies, activating insulin-receptor antibodies)

CLINICAL PEARL

The classic features of a hypoglycemic disorder are termed **Whipple's triad**:
- episodes of symptoms consistent with hypoglycemia
- demonstration of low blood glucose during symptoms
- rapid amelioration of symptoms by administration of glucose.

Treatment of malignant NETS

NETs are slow-growing but may metastasize to regional lymph nodes and the liver. Many patients do not present with hormone-related symptoms until there is a substantial tumor burden, so metastases are often present at the time of diagnosis.

If curative surgery is not possible, the following options may be beneficial in palliative management. Treatment choices are individualized, and often combined with somatostatin analog therapy to suppress hormone secretion. Long-term survival is often possible, even with metastatic disease.

- Cytotoxic therapy with streptozotocin, doxorubicin or fluorouracil.
- Surgical debulking with partial hepatectomy, or liver transplantation.
- Ablation of liver metastases using chemo-embolization, radioactive sphere embolization or radiofrequency probe ablation.
- Systemic radiopharmaceutical treatment with radio-labeled somatostatin analogs.
- Multitarget tyrosine kinase inhibitors such as sunitinib show promise in this area.

DISORDERS OF MULTIPLE ENDOCRINE SYSTEMS

There are a number of rare disorders which produce endocrine dysfunction affecting multiple organs. These are predominantly familial syndromes and may be detected by screening in an asymptomatic individual with a relevant family history. The proband case in a family is usually someone diagnosed with a primary endocrine complaint who subsequently develops a second disorder.

Multiple endocrine neoplasia (MEN)

There are four MEN syndromes, all inherited as autosomal dominant traits, which produce functioning endocrine neoplasms in multiple organs.

MEN-1

- Caused by a mutation of the *MEN1* gene (11q13) which codes for a tumor suppressor protein, menin
- Most common manifestation is hyperparathyroidism (multi-gland hyperplasia), usually manifest by age 25 years
- Benign skin lesions (angiofibromas) are very common
- Pancreatic/duodenal endocrine tumors which may secrete gastrin (most common), insulin, glucagon or vasoactive intestinal peptide (VIP)
- Pituitary adenoma (any type, but prolactinoma or non-functioning most common)
- Diagnosis by *MEN-1* gene analysis
- Treatment for each tumor is similar to sporadic cases:
  - » hyperparathyroidism by surgery
  - » pancreatic tumors by surgery or somatostatin analogs
  - » pituitary adenoma by surgery, dopamine agonist (for prolactinomas) or radiotherapy
- Other rare associations are extra-pancreatic carcinoid tumors and adrenocortical tumors

---

CLINICAL PEARL

MEN-1 is characterized by the '3 Ps'—tumors/hyperplasia of:
- parathyroids
- pancreas
- pituitary.

MEN-2 and MEN-3

- Previously classified as Men-2a and Men-2b, respectively.
- Caused by a gain of function mutation of the *RET* proto-oncogene (10q11) which codes for a receptor tyrosine kinase (RTK)
- Two clinical syndromes (MEN-2 and MEN-3) differ slightly in phenotypic expression
- Earliest manifestation is usually hyperplasia of the (calcitonin-secreting) C-cells of the thyroid, with later development of medullary thyroid carcinoma (MTC) in 90%
- Pheochromocytoma (usually occurs later than the MTC) in 50%

- In MEN-2 only, parathyroid hyperplasia and adenoma formation (20–30%)
- In MEN-3 only, mucosal neuromas of lips, eyelids, tongue and Marfanoid body habitus
- Familial MTC without other manifestations also occurs with RET mutations
- Diagnosis by *RET* gene analysis
- Familial MCT without the other features of MEN-2 can be seen (also have *RET* mutation)
- Families should be screened, and total thyroidectomy is advised in childhood to prevent MTC
- Tumors are treated similarly to sporadic cases

MEN-4

- Extremely rare association of parathyroid adenoma, pituitary adenoma and reproductive organ tumors in the setting of mutations in CDKN1B gene

Other multiple endocrine tumor syndromes

Carney complex

- Autosomal dominant inheritance
- Associated with mutations in the *PRKAR1A* gene which codes for a tumor-suppressor protein
- Presents with spotty skin pigmentation and lentigines, myxomas (cardiac, skin and breast)
- There is adrenocortical hyperplasia and hyperfunction, most often causing ACTH-independent Cushing's syndrome.

McCune–Albright syndrome

- Caused by a somatic activating mutation in the gene that codes for the alpha sub-unit of the stimulatory G protein (Gs-alpha). G proteins are involved in intracellular signaling from cell-surface hormone receptors, such as the receptors for ACTH, PTH, gonadotropins, melanocyte-stimulating hormone and TSH.
- Constitutive over-stimulation of cells bearing the mutation results in clinical manifestations such as precocious puberty, skin pigmentation, fibrous dysplasia, hyperthyroidism, Cushing's syndrome, hypophosphatemia and acromegaly or gigantism.

Polyglandular autoimmunity (PGA) syndromes

In some individuals the occurrence of multiple endocrine-organ failure reflects an underlying disorder of immune regulation. Two syndromes are recognized, containing clusters of endocrinopathies together with some associated non-endocrine autoimmune disorders (Box 10-6). In both syndromes the development of endocrine organ involvement is sequential and the diagnosis is usually not realized until at least two organs are involved. The evidence for an autoimmune etiology is the presence of chronic inflammatory (lymphocytic) infiltrates in the affected organs, and the

---

> ### Box 10-6
> ### Polyglandular autoimmunity (PGA) syndromes
>
> **PGA type 1**
> - Mucocutaneous candidiasis
> - Hypoparathyroidism
> - Addison's disease
> - Celiac disease
> - Vitiligo
> - Type 1 diabetes mellitus
> - Hypogonadism
> - Autoimmune hepatitis
>
> **PGA type 2 (Schmidt syndrome)**
> - Addison's disease
> - Type 1 diabetes mellitus
> - Autoimmune thyroid disease
> - Pernicious anemia
> - Vitiligo and alopecia
> - Hypophysitis
> - Myasthenia gravis
> - Chronic biliary cirrhosis
> - Pulmonary hypertension
> - Immune thrombocytopenia

---

presence of autoantibodies to specific antigens expressed in the target tissues. The three main classes of self-antigens to which autoantibodies are produced in PGA syndromes are:

- organ-specific surface receptor molecules (e.g. TSH receptor)
- intracellular enzymes (e.g. thyroid peroxidase, adrenal 21-hydroxylase, pancreatic glutamic acid decarboxylase)
- secreted proteins (e.g. insulin).

In PGA type 1 (PGA-1) the endocrinopathies are invariably associated with coexisting mucocutaneous candidiasis. PGA type 2 is considerably more common than PGA-1 and is not associated with fungal infection. Both syndromes have a strong familial basis, and a monogenic mutation of the *AIRE* gene (autoimmune regulator) has been strongly linked to PGA-1. The genetic basis of PGA-2 has not yet been identified.

- Diagnosis is based on association of multiple disorders and positive autoantibodies.
- In individuals with Addison's disease or type 1 diabetes mellitus, it is cost-effective to screen for other endocrinopathies.
- Treatment is the same as for each individual disorder. Modulation of the underlying immune disorder is not currently possible.

CLINICAL PEARL

In a patient with type 1 diabetes mellitus, the presence of a polyglandular autoimmune syndrome is often revealed by development of *recurrent hypoglycemia* due to coexisting cortisol deficiency.

DIABETES AND METABOLISM

Overview of energy metabolism

Metabolism refers to the chemical reactions that occur inside a living cell that result in production of energy and the synthesis of new organic material to support cell growth, reproduction and survival. It consists of two processes, *catabolism* and *anabolism*. Catabolism provides the energy and the components required for anabolism (Figure 10-19).

The structural components of all living things are composed of three main classes of molecule: amino acids, carbohydrates and lipids. Catabolism of these molecules in our food provides the energy required to make new molecules for cells (biosynthesis), and carry out mechanical work and molecular transport. The energy extracted from food depends on the relative composition of molecules within that food, with fat having twice the energy density of carbohydrates and protein.

An individual's energy requirements cover the needs of basal metabolism, physical activity, and the metabolic response to food. During certain stages of the lifecycle, further energy may also be required for growth, pregnancy and lactation.

An average person consumes 2000–2400 kilocalories (8300–10,000 kJ) per day to meet energy requirements, though this is influenced by multiple factors such as age, weight, muscle mass, physical activity levels and ambient temperature. Conditions such as systemic illness, fever and endocrine disturbance can also significantly alter energy requirements. When the energy from food exceeds the body's requirements, the excess energy is stored as fat, from where it can be re-accessed at times when the daily requirement exceeds intake.

The following sections cover disturbances of the metabolic system, in particular the derangement of carbohydrate metabolism (diabetes mellitus and its complications), the consequences of long-term energy excess (overweight and obesity) and the constellation of obesity, diabetes, dyslipidemia and hypertension known as 'the metabolic syndrome'.

Carbohydrate metabolism and diabetes

Ingested carbohydrates are broken down into monosaccharides (e.g. glucose, fructose, galactose) in the small intestine and absorbed into the bloodstream. Glucose is the most important carbohydrate in animal metabolism, being used as the primary source of cellular energy.

Glucose levels are normally maintained within a tight optimum range. They both control and are controlled by the central metabolic hormone insulin (Figure 10-20). Pancreatic islet cells secrete insulin in response to food intake and rising blood glucose concentrations, resulting in glucose uptake into cells for storage and energy production. The insulin response to food is mediated by 'incretin' hormones produced by the intestine. Insulin controls lipid and amino acid metabolism, promoting anabolism. It signals to cells in the brain and bone, which further contribute to metabolism at a whole-body level.

Diabetes: definition, diagnosis and classification

Diabetes mellitus is the impairment of carbohydrate metabolism characterized by inadequate insulin secretion or action, resulting in hyperglycemia. Although the pathological consequences of sustained hyperglycemia are evident, there is no specific biological marker by which diabetes is clearly defined. Blood glucose levels (BGLs) have been used for diagnosis, but the cut-point at which 'non-diabetes' becomes 'diabetes' remains unclear. Current definitions (Table 10-8) have been reached by consensus opinion based on the BGLs at which

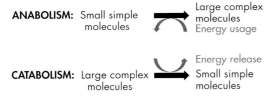

ANABOLISM: Small simple molecules → Large complex molecules — Energy usage

CATABOLISM: Large complex molecules → Small simple molecules — Energy release

Figure 10-19 Metabolism involves the complementary processes of anabolism and catabolism

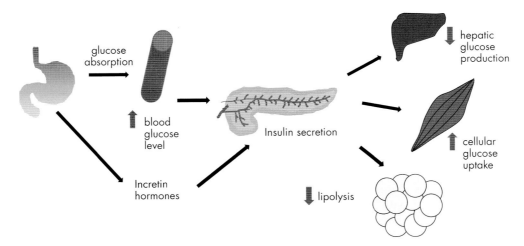

Figure 10-20 Glucose homeostasis. In response to intestinal glucose absorption and rising blood glucose levels, insulin secreted by islet cells acts on liver, muscle and fat to reduce glucose output, increase glucose uptake and prevent fat breakdown

Table 10-8 WHO criteria for diagnosis of diabetes and intermediate hyperglycemia*

DIAGNOSIS	FASTING BGL *AND/OR* 2-HOUR LEVEL ON GTT
Normal	<6.1 mmol/L *and* <7.8 mmol/L (110 mg/dL *and* 140 mg/dL)
Impaired fasting glycemia	6.1–6.9 mmol/L *and* <7.8 mmol/L (110–125 mg/dL *and* 140 mg/dL)
Impaired glucose tolerance	<7.0 mmol/L *and* 7.8–11.0 mmol/L (126 mg/dL *and* 140–199 mg/dL)
Diabetes	>7.0 mmol/L *or* >11.1 mmol/L (126 mg/dL *or* 200 mg/dL)

* Note that the American Diabetes Association (ADA) criteria use 5.6 rather than 6.1 mmol/L as the cut-off for impaired fasting glycemia. The ADA now also endorses $HbA_{1c} \geq 6.5\%$ as diagnostic of diabetes.
GTT, glucose tolerance test; WHO, World Health Organization.

the risk of complications appear to increase, and the characteristics of the BGL distribution curve in populations.

Normal levels of fasting plasma glucose are below 6.1 mmol/L (110 mg/dL). Fasting levels between 6.1 and 7.0 mmol/L (110–125 mg/dL) are borderline; termed impaired fasting glycemia (IFG). Fasting levels repeatedly at or above 7.0 mmol/L (126 mg/dL) are defined as diagnostic of diabetes. When BGL is measured in a non-fasting state, a level above 11.1 mmol/L (200 mg/dL) represents likely diabetes and levels between 7.8 and 11.0 warrant further assessment with a fasting measurement or glucose tolerance test (GTT). In a GTT, a 75 g oral glucose load is administered to a fasting patient. The BGL after 2 hours should be below 7.8 mmol/L (140 mg/dL). Levels between 7.8 and 11.1 mmol/L (140–200 mg/dL) indicate impaired glucose tolerance (IGT). Glucose levels above 11.1 mmol/L (200 mg/dL) at 2 hours confirm a diagnosis of diabetes.

The categories of intermediate hyperglycemia known as impaired glucose tolerance (IGT) and impaired fasting glucose (IFG) have been used to define a state at which the risk of complications and the risk of progression to frank diabetes is increased. The pathophysiological processes associated with diabetes are already evident, but reversion to normoglycemia is not uncommon on subsequent testing.

The underlying pathophysiology assists diabetes classification.

- Type 1A diabetes mellitus is an autoimmune condition in which inflammation of islet cells leads to destruction and subsequent deficiency of insulin secretion.
- Type 2 diabetes is characterized by resistance to the actions of insulin and by failure of islet cells to compensate for the increased secretory demand.
- Gestational diabetes is temporary carbohydrate intolerance precipitated by the hormonal changes of pregnancy.

Diabetes may develop secondary to other disease states or medications that either impair insulin secretion or action, or both (Box 10-7). Additionally, while both type 1 and type 2 diabetes mellitus are polygenic disorders with environmental influences, rare forms of diabetes result from directly inherited gene mutations that affect insulin secretion or action.

Box 10-7

Causes of secondary diabetes (or contributors to worsening glucose tolerance)

Pancreatic—insulin insufficiency
- Chronic pancreatitis
- Cystic fibrosis
- Pancreatectomy
- Fibrocalculous pancreatopathy

Pancreatic—mixed insulin insufficiency and/or impaired action
- Hemochromatosis
- Pancreatic cancer

Hormonal disorders—impaired action
- Pheochromocytoma
- Cushing's syndrome
- Glucagonoma
- Acromegaly
- Hyperthyroidism
- Somatostatinoma
- Hyperaldosteronism

Medications—insulin insufficiency or impaired action
- Antipsychotics
- Immunosuppressives, including steroids
- Antiretroviral drugs
- Pentamidine
- Beta-blockers, thiazide diuretics, oral contraceptives

Type 1 diabetes mellitus (T1DM)

Epidemiology

The prevalence and incidence of type 1A diabetes varies significantly with ethnicity and geography, being highest in white populations in Europe (Table 10-9). The incidence was increasing at a rate of 3–4% per year, particularly in the under-five age group, likely due to environmental

Table 10-9 Epidemiology of type 1A diabetes mellitus

Prevalence	<1% to 3%, depending on population
Incidence	1/100,000 per year in Japan to 41/100,000 per year in Kuwait to 63/100,000 per year in Finland Seasonal predominance in winter
Age of onset	Peak onset in puberty, but may occur at any age throughout the lifespan
Gender ratio	Equal in childhood and adolescence. Male:female ratio 1.5:1 after age 25

influences. Some countries are now leveling off, while others are increasing at 6.5% per annum (e.g. China).

Onset of disease may occur at any age, though it occurs predominantly in childhood or adolescence; hence the old term 'juvenile-onset diabetes'. In older age groups a more insidious variant known as latent autoimmune diabetes in adults (LADA) may occur.

Pathogenesis

- Cell-mediated autoimmune destruction of beta-cells leading to insulin deficiency.
- Autoantibodies (usually multiple) against islet-cell antigens (insulin, ICA512 [IA-2], GAD65, Zinc Transporter 8 antibodies (ZnT8)) are present in 85–90% of children at diagnosis.
- There is good evidence of genetic predisposition to T1DM. Concordance rates for monozygotic twins are 30–50% compared with 6–10% in dizygotic twins. More than 90% of cases have high-risk human leukocyte antigen (HLA) haplotypes.
- Environmental factors act as initiators of beta-cell autoimmunity. Possible factors include viruses (coxsackie B, mumps, cytomegalovirus, rubella), early exposure to cow's milk protein, childhood obesity or reduced exposure to the potential protective effects of breastfeeding or vitamin D.
- A small proportion of cases of T1DM have no evidence of autoimmunity, islet-cell inflammation or high-risk HLA haplotypes. Some of these will have undiagnosed monogenic diabetes.

Clinical features

Autoimmune destruction and progressive loss of beta-cell function precedes diagnosis, often by years. Symptoms (Box 10-8) do not develop until there is inadequate insulin to maintain normoglycemia. Patients with severe insulin deficiency may present with symptoms of ketoacidosis. The history may be brief, especially in young children with rapidly progressive beta-cell destruction. Adults with LADA have a more insidious onset that may resemble type 2 diabetes.

Management

Insulin therapy

Management centers around replacement of the deficient hormone, insulin, in ways that most closely resemble

---

> **Box 10-8**
>
> **Symptoms of hyperglycemia**
>
> Thirst, polyuria
>
> Weight loss
>
> Blurred vision, headache
>
> Superficial infections, especially *Candida*

---

normal physiology and to avoid hypoglycemia and hyperglycemia. In healthy individuals, basal levels of insulin are secreted to regulate glucose production from the liver and suppress lipolysis. This occurs 24 hours a day in the absence of food intake. During meals, a more rapid burst (bolus) of insulin is secreted in response to the glucose load from food. Modern insulins are manufactured with recombinant DNA technology using the human insulin gene. Alterations in the natural insulin molecule are performed to make insulin analogs, changing the pharmacokinetic properties.

The key properties of a manufactured insulin are its onset, peak and duration of action. Knowledge of an insulin's pharmacokinetics (Table 10-10) allows insulin delivery to mimic physiological patterns and be tailored to a person's diet and lifestyle. Insulin is usually administered by subcutaneous injection, often into the abdominal wall, using an injecting pen device or 'insulin pump'.

Insulin therapy in type 1 diabetes has 3 functions:

1. Providing 'background' or basal insulin to mimic the insulin secretion that occurs in the fasting state. This can be provided with:

   a. Intermediate, long-acting or ultra-long acting insulin administered once or twice daily to provide basal requirements and control fasting, before meal glucose and to avoid diabetic ketoacidosis.

   b. Basal rate insulin from subcutaneous insulin infusion therapy 'insulin pump'. This can provide many different pre-set rates to mirror any endogenous variation in background insulin requirements. The insulin pump can be linked electronically (via Bluetooth) to a glucose sensor that continuously monitors the blood glucose. Currently, feedback from the sensor can suspend the pre-set basal insulin infusion rate either when the glucose hits a pre-set 'hypoglycemic' threshold (low glucose suspend) or when the glucose is predicted to hit a pre-set threshold (predictive low glucose suspend). The newest pump technology now allows a pump to respond continuously to the glucose sensor information and change the basal rate automatically, rather than following set pre-programmed rates. This is called a hybrid closed loop system.

2. Providing rapid or ultra-fast prandial or bolus insulin to cover the carbohydrate to be eaten. Large protein meals may also require additional insulin to avoid hyperglycemia.

3. Providing rapid or ultra-fast insulin to lower the glucose level when too high (e.g. if food has contained more carbohydrate than expected, or at times of illness). This

Table 10-10 Pharmacokinetic properties of different types of insulin

INSULIN TYPE	ONSET	PEAK	DURATION	EXAMPLES
Ultra Fast acting	5 mins	30–60 mins	3 hours	FiAsp (Aspart (special formulation with niacinamide and arginine))
Rapid-acting	15 min	30–90 min	3–4 hours	Lispro, Aspart, Glulisine
Short-acting	30–60 min	2–3 hours	3–6 hours	Regular
Intermediate-acting	1–2 hours	4–14 hours	Up to 24 hrs	NPH (isophane)
Long-acting	1–2 hours	minimal	up to 24 hrs	Detemir, Glargine (100 IU/mL)
Ultra long acting	6 hours 2 hours	Minimal peak	30 hours (Toujeo) 42 hours (Ryzodeg)	Toujeo, Glargine (300 IU/mL) Degludec (as Ryzodeg—includes Aspart)

extra insulin can be provided either as a measured bolus or as a higher temporary basal rate if a pump is used.

- Insulin therapy requires substantial skill to keep the ambient glucose within a range as near to normal as possible without hypoglycemia. There are many factors that can influence the ability to keep the glucose as close to normal as possible, and achievement of the best possible glucose levels is user dependent. Glucose management therefore requires a motivated and skilled patient—best supported through structured education (e.g. the Australian form of Dose Adjustment for Normal Eating-OzDAFNE). Topics include:
  » carbohydrate counting, diet choices, physical activity, illness, stress, alcohol and drugs
  » education about correct insulin administration technique, management of hypoglycemia and sick-day management
  » specific education and management plans, including those for commercial vehicle drivers, shift-workers and women planning pregnancy
  » the aim is to tailor management to allow maintenance of a normal life.

- Real time glucose monitoring
  » through either fingerprick self-blood glucose monitoring before meals and at times during the night (to detect asymptomatic hypoglycemia) and after meals
  » through a glucose sensor with a sensor sitting within the interstitial fluid subcutaneously—this includes continuous glucose monitoring sensor (CGMS) and flash glucose sensing (intermittent–manual)
  » glucose targets are set for different times of the day, and the time within these targets ('Time in Range') is also used to guide management.

- Pumps can improve glucose control in some individuals, may improve quality of life and reduce hypoglycemia, but are expensive.

Monitoring outcomes

Efficacy of treatment is assessed by:

- home glucose monitoring results including hypoglycemia, using either fingerprick testing and meters or glucose sensing technology (continuous or Flash)

Table 10-11 Suggested HbA$_{1c}$ targets for adults with type 1 diabetes

CLINICAL SITUATION*	HbA$_{1c}$ TARGET
General target	≤7.0% (≤6.5% desirable)
Pregnancy or planning pregnancy	≤7.0% (≤6.0% desirable)
Recurrent severe hypoglycemia or hypoglycemic unawareness	≤8.0%
Time in range	70%

* Consider individual patient factors.

Adapted from Cheung NW et al. Position statement of the Australian Diabetes Society: individualisation of glycated haemoglobin targets for adults with diabetes mellitus. Med J Aust 2009;191:339–44.

- hypoglycemia awareness, where the ability to sense hypoglycemia is increasingly lost with repeated episodes of low blood glucose

- weight management

- the glycosylated hemoglobin (HbA$_{1c}$) concentration. HbA$_{1c}$ reflects average BGLs over the preceding 3 months and is closely correlated with the risk of end-organ complications.

Treatment targets are tailored to the individual's age, comorbidities and lifestyle. Appropriate HbA$_{1c}$ targets are proposed in specific situations (Table 10-11). Many parts of the world have now moved to new HbA$_{1c}$ units (mmol/mol): online conversion tools are available.

Management also focuses on minimization of cardiovascular risk by optimizing blood pressure and lipids, diet and exercise, and smoking cessation. Screening for complications of diabetes is performed regularly. T1DM is a chronic disease requiring intensive lifelong management. Depression and altered body image are significant comorbidities that warrant specific attention.

CLINICAL PEARL

Principles of type 1 diabetes mellitus management:
- insulin therapy that mimics physiological insulin secretion
- knowledge and understanding of diabetes including carbohydrate counting and lifestyle management
- glucose monitoring, appropriate HbA$_{1c}$ and glucose targets
- minimize risk and severity of hypoglycemia
- screening for complications
- minimizing cardiovascular risk
- managing psychosocial aspects of the disease.

Transplantation

Transplantation of islet cells or whole pancreas from healthy donors offers a theoretical cure, but is not yet a viable solution for most patients. In addition to the issue of reduced donor availability, the requirement for continuing immunosuppression and its side-effects currently outweigh the benefit in most individuals. Whole pancreas transplants are performed in patients with severe diabetes complications who are already undergoing renal transplantation. Islet cell transplantation is reserved for patients with severe recurrent hypoglycemia and hypoglycemic unawareness.

Immunotherapy

A variety of immunotherapies have been, and are being, trialed and are currently a research area.

Type 2 diabetes mellitus (T2DM)

Epidemiology

Type 2 diabetes (T2DM) accounts for approximately 90% of cases of diabetes. Its prevalence is increasing dramatically worldwide, in line with the rise in overweight and obesity and an aging population. In 2017, 425 million people were known to have diabetes (aged 20–79), which is projected to rise to 629 million by 2045. A huge number of patients remain undiagnosed, and often present with long-term complications on diagnosis. The prevalence is much higher in certain ethnic groups like Pima Indians, Indigenous Australians, South Pacific Islanders, Asians and those of African/Caribbean origin. It is a disease of affluence in developing countries but associated with socioeconomic disadvantage in developed countries. There is a concerning trend for increasing diagnosis in childhood and adolescence following a rise in childhood overweight/obesity.

Differentiating type 1 and type 2 diabetes

The differentiation of the type of diabetes can sometimes be difficult with the increasing prevalence of overweight and obesity and insulin resistance that may coexist in type 1 diabetes, and the younger age of onset of type 2 diabetes. Several factors may help differentiate the two (see Table 10-12).

Pathogenesis

Insulin resistance plays a major role in pathogenesis, predating the development of the disease by 10–20 years. To maintain normoglycemia, islet cells compensate for impaired insulin action by increasing insulin secretion. In genetically predisposed individuals, beta-cell reserves are insufficient to keep up with this demand for hyperinsulinemia, insulin levels cannot be sustained and progression through IGT to frank diabetes occurs.

Impaired insulin action occurs in multiple tissues, resulting in reduced glucose uptake into muscle, increased hepatic glucose production, and elevated free fatty acids. The causes of insulin resistance are multifactorial, including genetics, obesity and environmental factors such as hormones, aging, lifestyle and nutrient availability (Box 10-9). Inadequate beta-cell reserve is largely genetically determined.

Table 10-12 Differentiating type 1 and 2 diabetes mellitus

	TYPE 1 DIABETES	TYPE 2 DIABETES
Ethnic predisposition	White European	Non-white, non-European
Typical age of onset	Childhood/adolescence but may occur later in life	Adulthood (but can occur in childhood)
Typical phenotype	Lean	Overweight or obese
Family History Other features	Less likely Other autoimmune conditions co-existing e.g. Hashimoto's or celiac disease	More likely to be present Metabolic syndrome, polycystic ovary syndrome, fatty liver
Pathophysiology	Insulin deficiency	Insulin resistance with beta-cell exhaustion
Treatment	Insulin essential	Diet, lifestyle, oral hypoglycemic agents, GLP1 agonists, insulin
Diabetic ketoacidosis	Complication of insulin deficiency	Rarely develops, usually late in disease course or when on SGLT2 inhibitor therapy.
Laboratory tests	Positive antibodies, low C-peptide, susceptible Human Leukocyte Antigen (HLA) groups	Negative antibodies, high C-peptide levels (but become lower over time)

Clinical features

- Insidious onset; T2DM may be present for many years before diagnosis.
- Diagnosis is commonly made in asymptomatic individuals on routine health screening.
- Symptoms of hyperglycemia may be present.
- Delayed presentation may be with a diabetes-associated complication.
- Occasionally presents with severe hyperglycemia, dehydration with or without mental obtundation, known as hyperosmolar hyperglycemic state.

Management

In selecting from the large variety of available therapies for type 2 diabetes, consideration should be given to glycemic control, weight, risk of hypoglycemia, cardiovascular risk reduction as well as existing long-term diabetes complications. Medications with favorable side-effect profiles, long-term safety and efficacy should be chosen to achieve an HbA$_{1c}$ target, individualized to the patient. The management of diabetes includes lifestyle modification, pharmacotherapy for glycemic control, cardiovascular risk reduction, as well as screening and management of long-term complications.

Box 10-9

Risk factors for type 2 diabetes mellitus

- Age
- Obesity, especially abdominal (central) distribution
- Sedentary lifestyle
- Family history and certain ethnic groups
- Hypertension, dyslipidemia
- Personal history of gestational diabetes or intermediate hyperglycemia
- Personal history of polycystic ovary syndrome, acanthosis nigricans
- Low birth weight, child of a mother who had diabetes during pregnancy

---

Lifestyle

While age, race and genetics are unmodifiable, weight loss, increased physical activity and healthy diet target the underlying pathogenesis of type 2 diabetes. This can assist in maintenance of glycemic control and potentially slow disease progression. Weight loss improves insulin sensitivity and beta-cell capacity. Reduction in body fat (particularly central adiposity) is more important than weight loss, and is better assessed with measurements of waist circumference than body mass index.

Independent of weight loss, physical activity itself improves insulin sensitivity and lowers BGLs. 150 minutes per week of moderate-intensity exercise or 90 minutes of vigorous exercise, spread over at least 3 days of the week, is recommended. Dietary counseling advises foods with a low glycemic index and low in saturated fat foods, with modest carbohydrate intake in proportion and temporal relation to medication use.

Anti-diabetes agents

Medical therapy should be instituted in conjunction with diet and exercise, with metformin the usual first-line agent (Figure 10-21). Add-on therapy to metformin is based on the individual patient and factors including weight, hypoglycemia risk and cardiovascular risk should be taken into account, as should the individualized target HbA$_{1c}$ (Table 10-13 and Table 10-14).

CLINICAL PEARL

In older patients, or those with multiple comorbidities limiting life expectancy, the primary aim of diabetes management may be to avoid symptoms of hyperglycemia or hypoglycemia. Therefore, these patients may benefit from a higher HbA$_{1c}$ target.

Insulin therapy

Insulin may be initiated early after diagnosis, or after failure of anti-diabetes agents to maintain targets. As 'add-on' therapy, addition of once-daily basal insulin to existing anti-diabetes therapy is often used. Basal-bolus regimens may be used, as for type 1, offering greatest flexibility and glycemic

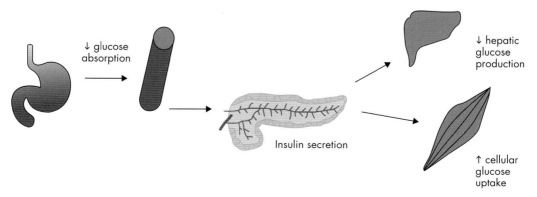

Figure 10-21 Mechanisms of action of metformin. Metformin reduces hepatic glucose production and stimulates glucose uptake into muscle, as well as reducing enteric glucose absorption

Table 10-13 HbA$_{1c}$ targets in type 2 diabetes mellitus

CLINICAL SITUATION	HbA$_{1c}$
General target	≤7.0%
Diabetes of short duration, no clinical cardiovascular disease: —requiring lifestyle modification ± metformin —requiring any anti-diabetic agents other than metformin or insulin —requiring insulin	≤6.0% ≤6.5% ≤7.0%
Pregnancy or planning pregnancy	≤6.0%
Diabetes of longer duration or clinical cardiovascular disease	≤7.0%
Recurrent severe hypoglycemia or hypoglycemic unawareness	≤8.0%

Adapted from Cheung NW et al. Position statement of the Australian Diabetes Society: individualisation of glycated haemoglobin targets for adults with diabetes mellitus. Med J Aust 2009;191:339–44.

control. Premixed insulins combine rapid- or short-acting insulin with intermediate-acting insulin in fixed proportions. These require only twice-daily injection, but provide less physiological insulin delivery and require careful adherence to dietary content and timing.

Bariatric surgery

For people with type 2 diabetes and a body mass index (BMI) >35 kg/m^2, bariatric surgery is a therapeutic option that results in significant weight loss and improvement in glycemic control. In some patients, diabetes remission can occur, especially in those recently diagnosed with T2DM. (See section on bariatric surgery in the Overweight and Obesity section, page 309.) More recent evidence has suggested that weight loss of 15 kg with low-calorie diet followed by weight maintenance in recently diagnosed diabetes may also result in diabetes remission in a significant number of patients.

Complications of diabetes

The major end-organ complications of diabetes are listed in Box 10-10.

Table 10-14 Actions of oral hypoglycemic agents

PHARMACOTHERAPY AGENT	ADVANTAGES	SIDE-EFFECTS/RISKS
Metformin	Low risk of hypoglycemia Improves lipids and fibrinolysis Weight neutral Long-term experience and safety Potential benefits for CVD and cancer	Contraindicated in renal failure Risk of lactic acidosis (rare) Gastrointestinal side-effects
Sulphonylureas	Insulin secretagogue—effective glucose lowering Long-term safety data	Late postprandial hypoglycemia Weight gain
Thiazolidinediones	↑ insulin sensitivity ↑ safe lipid storage in peripheral fat Low risk of hypoglycemia ↓ triglycerides, ↑ HDL	Weight gain, fluid retention ↑ incidence cardiac failure 1.5–2.5 × ↑ fracture risk
α-glucosidase inhibitors	Inhibits oligosaccharide breakdown at intestinal brush border ↓ postprandial glucose rise from complex carbohydrates	Gastrointestinal side-effects Low efficacy in diets already low in complex carbohydrates
DPP-4 inhibitors	↑ GLP-1 (incretin) levels—stimulate glucose dependent insulin secretion, ↓ glucagon No weight gain Low risk of hypoglycemia	Gastrointestinal side-effects
GLP-1 agonists	Stimulate glucose dependent insulin secretion so low risk of hypoglycemia Increased satiety Weight loss	Injectable therapy (subcutaneous) Gastrointestinal side-effects
SGLT2 inhibitors	Weight loss Some agents have shown cardiovascular benefit, especially in pre-existing disease Reduced risk of heart failure	Urinary tract infections Genitourinary thrush Euglycemic diabetic ketoacidosis

Box 10-10
Major complications of diabetes

Microvascular	Retinopathy, nephropathy, peripheral neuropathy, autonomic neuropathy
Macrovascular	Ischemic heart disease, cerebrovascular disease, peripheral vascular disease, renal artery stenosis
Protein glycation	Cataracts, cheiroarthropathy
Pregnancy	Maternal hypoglycemia, fetal malformations, miscarriage, stillbirth, preeclampsia, macrosomia, neonatal hypoglycemia, neonatal jaundice, respiratory distress syndrome, premature delivery, caesarean section, Neonatal Intensive Care Unit admission

Table 10-15 Stages of diabetic nephropathy

STAGE	URINE ALBUMIN EXCRETION
1. Glomerular hyperfiltration, increased kidney size	<20 microg/min or 30 mg/day
2. Early glomerular lesions	<20 microg/min or 30 mg/day
3. Microalbuminuria	20–200 microg/min or 30–300 mg/day
4. Overt nephropathy/ macroalbuminuria	>200 microg/min or >300 mg/day
5. End-stage renal disease (ESRD)	UACR >25 mg/mmol creatinine

*UACR = Urinary albumin : creatinine ratio

Hyperglycemia is the primary cause of tissue damage. The process is modified by individuals' genetic susceptibility and independent accelerating factors such as hypertension and insulin resistance. Cells which are unable to down-regulate glucose transport are vulnerable to hyperglycemic damage. These include capillary endothelial cells of the retina, mesangial cells in the glomerulus, neurons and Schwann cells, and vascular endothelium.

Diabetic eye disease triad

1. Microaneuryms formation and microhemorrhages (dot and blot hemorrhages).
2. Exudates.
3. New vessel proliferation. Hemorrhage or edema in the macula region can lead to blindness.

With regular eye screening, proliferative retinopathy and clinically significant macular edema can be identified early and treated with laser photocoagulation and intravitreal injection therapy before visual loss ensues. Diabetes also increases the risk of other eye diseases such as cataract and glaucoma.

Diabetic kidney disease

Diabetic nephropathy (Table 10-15) is the commonest cause of end-stage renal disease (ESRD) in many countries. Nephropathy is associated with a 20–40 times increase in mortality, mostly from cardiovascular disease. Urine albumin excretion reflects the stages of nephropathy.

CLINICAL PEARL

For screening and monitoring, a morning spot urine albumin:creatinine ratio is an acceptable surrogate for albumin excretion rate.

The primary management aim is to prevent the progression from normoalbuminuria to microalbuminuria and macroalbuminuria, as cardiovascular risk and risk of

Table 10-16 Manifestations of diabetic autonomic neuropathy in different organ systems

Cardiovascular	Tachycardia, orthostatic hypotension, loss of heart rate variability leading to risk of cardiac arrhythmias
Neurovascular	Anhidrosis or hyperhidrosis, altered skin blood flow
Gastrointestinal	Constipation, gastroparesis, diarrhea and incontinence
Genitourinary	Erectile dysfunction, retrograde ejaculation, neurogenic bladder
Metabolic	Hypoglycemic unawareness

ESRD increases with each stage. Optimized glycemic control, BP control (<130/80 mmHg, or <125/75 mmHg if overt nephropathy) and blockade of the renin–angiotensin–aldosterone system are key factors.

Autonomic neuropathy

Diabetic autonomic neuropathy may manifest in multiple organ systems (Table 10-16) and significantly impairs quality of life. It is a strong predictor of mortality.

Cardiovascular disease

Patients with T2DM have a 3–4-fold risk of cardiovascular disease, and atypical presentations of cardiac ischemia (e.g. silent infarcts), and have greater risk of re-occlusion after coronary revascularization. Additionally, autonomic neuropathy (poor rhythm control) and diabetic cardiomyopathy contribute to poor outcomes. Modifiable cardiac risk factors should be optimized (Box 10-11).

Box 10-11

Cardiac risk factor modification in diabetes

- Risk factor modification
  - » Cholesterol: target LDLs <2–2.5 mmol/L, HDLs >1.0 mmol/L
  - » Blood pressure: target <130/80 mmHg
  - » Weight reduction if overweight/obese, diet and lifestyle advice, smoking cessation
- Consideration of anti-platelet agents, though generally only for secondary prevention
- Consider screening for cardiac ischemia if evidence of other vascular disease elsewhere

HDL, high-density lipoprotein; LDL, low-density lipoprotein.

Diabetic foot disease

The combination of peripheral neuropathy, autonomic neuropathy, vascular disease and predisposition to infection places the diabetic foot at high risk of disease. Clinical manifestations include chronic non-healing ulcers, osteomyelitis or Charcot's neuroarthropathy. Diabetes is the leading cause of lower limb amputation in developed nations.

In addition to glycemic control and minimizing vascular risk factors, regular foot care and clinical testing for peripheral neuropathy and peripheral pulses is advised.

Pregnancy among women with pre-gestational diabetes

Women with pre-existing diabetes who become pregnant are at high risk of a range of adverse outcomes. Fetal development is very sensitive to hyperglycemia substantially increasing the chance of fetal malformations and miscarriage. Maternal hyperglycemia stimulates fetal insulin secretion and provides excess energy leading to macrosomia and increased risks of stillbirth, birth trauma, neonatal hypoglycemia, neonatal jaundice, respiratory distress syndrome, premature delivery, caesarean section, Neonatal Intensive Care Unit admission. There is also an increased risk of maternal hypoglycemia in early pregnancy due to increasing hCG production and insulin sensitivity. This may be exacerbated by hyperemesis. Management involves pregnancy planning (as close to normalization of glucose as possible for at least one month prior to conception, high-dose folic acid treatment, review of potentially teratogenic medications and complication review and management) and then close monitoring with frequent changes in insulin therapy as insulin sensitivity changes. Close obstetric monitoring and retinal review at least twice in the pregnancy are required.

Hypoglycemia

Hypoglycemia is defined as a blood sugar below 4 mmol/L (72 mg/dL). Severe hypoglycemia is when third party assistance is required to treat the low blood sugar. Normal blood glucose is maintained during fasting by the mobilization of glucose from glycogen stores (predominantly from the liver), and by activation of gluconeogenesis from various substrates including glycerol (derived from adipose stores of triglyceride) and amino acids. Gluconeogenesis is activated in the liver by the action of glucagon, and requires reduced insulin signaling. Catecholamines, cortisol and growth hormone are also potent stimulators of hepatic glucose synthesis. The release of these hormones, termed *glucose counter-regulatory hormones*, is stimulated in response to hypoglycemia.

Hypoglycemic symptoms are related to:
- activation of the sympathetic nervous system and appetite center
  - » sweating, tachycardia, tremulousness, anxiety, hunger
- brain dysfunction secondary to decreased levels of glucose
  - » confusion, impaired concentration, altered level of consciousness
  - » focal impairments (e.g. hemiplegia)
  - » seizures, coma and death
- generalized glycopenia to metabolizing tissues
  - » weakness and fatigue.

Adrenergic symptoms usually precede the neuroglycopenic symptoms and provide an early warning of hypoglycemia to the patient.

- The blood glucose threshold for onset of hypoglycemic symptoms is variable, but most people experience symptoms at <3.0 mmol/L (55 mg/dL). This threshold decreases with repeated episodes of hypoglycemia, and some patients with repeated events can have almost no symptoms until unconsciousness ensues (hypoglycemic unawareness).
- Hypoglycemic unawareness is associated with increased mortality, especially in the setting of cardiovascular disease. These patients must be managed with less stringent glycemic control to allow the return of hypoglycemia awareness.

In the context of diabetes, hypoglycemia occurs in the setting of treatment with insulin or sulphonylurea therapy and is commonly precipitated by:
- reduced dietary carbohydrate intake
- increased physical activity
- inappropriate timing of drug administration in relation to food intake
- erratic absorption of insulin due to incorrect injection technique
- impaired renal elimination of insulin/other drugs.

Diabetic emergencies

The diabetic emergencies diabetic ketoacidosis and hyperosmolar hyperglycemic state have the features given in Table 10-17. Common precipitants are listed in Box 10-12.

Diabetic ketoacidosis (DKA)

Diabetic ketoacidosis is a complication of severe insulin deficiency, resulting in hyperglycemia and generation of ketoacids. In the absence of insulin, there is a lack of glucose entry to cells. Lipolysis provides fatty acids as a substrate for production of ketones in the liver, an alternative fuel source

Table 10-17 Diabetic emergencies

DIABETIC KETOACIDOSIS	HYPEROSMOLAR HYPERGLYCEMIC STATE
Usually in type diabetes	Usually in type 2 diabetes, who are older and have several comorbidities
BGL usually >14 mmol/L	BGL often >33 mmol/L
Acidotic, pH <7.3, ketonemia	No ketonemia, may have mild ketonuria
Mortality <5%	Mortality ≥15% or greater
Acute onset	Insidious onset over days
Abdominal pain, vomiting, weight loss	Extreme dehydration, high serum osmolality >320 mosmol/kg H_2O Mental obtundation, renal failure, thrombosis
BGL, blood glucose level.	

<table>
<tr><td>

Box 10-12

Common precipitants of diabetic ketoacidosis or hyperosmolar hyperglycemic state

- Sepsis
- Acute myocardial infarction
- Stroke
- Glucose-raising medications, e.g. corticosteroids
- Alcohol abuse
- Stopping/reducing insulin (e.g. if unwell, vomiting) (usually for DKA)

</td></tr>
</table>

for energy, but also leads to the formation of ketone bodies which are toxic and acidic.

Precipitants should be sought. Management is with fluid resuscitation, insulin infusion and correction of electrolytes particularly potassium which is high on presentation and rapidly drops as insulin promotes movement into the cells.

The cardinal manifestations of DKA are:

- hyperglycemia
- ketonemia, ketonuria, acetone breath
- metabolic acidosis (with anion gap), Kussmaul respiration
- marked dehydration secondary to polyuria, vomiting
- potassium depletion, but plasma potassium may be initially high due to lack of entry into cells due to the insulin deficiency.

Hyperosmolar hyperglycemic state (HHS)

Hyperosmolar hyperglycemic state is a complication of insulin deficiency, occurring in people with T2DM. Insulin secretion is adequate to suppress ketone formation, but as a result a more insidious progression to severe hyperglycemia, hyperosmolarity and dehydration occurs. Metabolic acidosis may be present due to lactate formation, but not ketoacidosis, and is often a result of a precipitating cause and a combination of dehydration, underperfusion and renal failure.

Gestational diabetes (GDM)

Gestational diabetes mellitus (GDM) is the commonest medical disorder of pregnancy, present in 9–15% of pregnancies, though rates may vary depending on the population and the method of screening and diagnosis.

GDM is defined as any form of glucose intolerance first recognized during pregnancy. It thus includes new onset of hyperglycemia during pregnancy, as well as pre-existing hyperglycemia that was undiagnosed prior to pregnancy. The former situation is the more classic, and results from increased insulin resistance due to pregnancy-related hormones, particularly from late 2nd trimester onwards. To maintain normoglycemia, beta-cells must compensate by increasing insulin production. In situations of decreased beta-cell reserve, glucose intolerance occurs.

Diabetes in pregnancy has clinical consequences for both mother (risk of preeclampsia, obstructed labor, assisted delivery) and fetus (large for gestational age, prematurity, growth retardation, shoulder dystocia). Education, diet and exercise, intensive blood glucose control, monitoring of fetal wellbeing and pharmacotherapy where hyperglycemia persists after lifestyle change reduce the risk. Insulin is the usual therapy for GDM. Metformin is often used, with good evidence in terms of pregnancy outcomes. There is current debate over the long-term impact on the offspring of the trans-placental passage of metformin. GDM is a strong risk factor for future T2DM and cardiovascular disease in the mother and may predispose the child to later obesity and glucose intolerance.

Disorders of energy excess—overweight and obesity

Overweight/obesity is a complex chronic disease, influenced by many social, cultural, behavioral, physical and genetic factors.

Table 10-18 World Health Organization classification of overweight and obesity

CLASSIFICATION		BODY MASS INDEX (kg/m²)
Underweight		<18.5
Normal weight		18.5–24.9
Overweight		25.0–29.9
Obese	Class I	30.0–34.9
	Class II	35.0–39.9
	Class III	≥40

Definition

Overweight and obesity are defined on the basis of body mass index (BMI), according to arbitrarily determined cut-points (see Table 10-18). Irrespective of classification, morbidity and all-cause mortality increases progressively with increasing BMI above the healthy range. Abdominal fat is an independent predictor of metabolic risk (e.g. diabetes, cardiovascular disease); measurement of waist circumference (men >102 cm/40 in, women >88 cm/35 in, lower in non-Europeans) assists further risk stratification. Note that different BMI cut-offs may apply to some ethnic groups where central obesity and visceral adiposity is higher in relation to the same BMI (e.g. lower cut-offs for people of Asian ancestry).

Epidemiology

Almost 2 billion adults are overweight or obese worldwide, which is around 4 in 10 adults, and prevalence is increasing. The rate of obesity in childhood and adolescence is increasing at higher rates than in adults, and is of particular concern. This epidemic is occurring in both developed and developing nations and has huge health and economic effects.

Health consequences

Overweight and obesity increase the risk of metabolic disorder including hypertension, dyslipidemia and insulin resistance, which together contribute to the risk of coronary heart disease and stroke. It is also linked to conditions such as obstructive sleep apnea, obesity-hypoventilation, gallbladder disease, osteoarthritis and infertility. Obesity is a risk factor for breast, endometrial, prostate and colon cancer.

Reduced mobility, inability to work, stigmatization and discrimination in certain cultural contexts adds to the social cost. Depression, anxiety and eating disorders are more prevalent in obesity.

Management

Due to the complexity and multifactorial nature of obesity, the management is also complex and should be individualized. Lifestyle and pharmacotherapy measures often do not

---

> **Box 10-13**
>
> **Management of the overweight or obese patient**
>
> - **Goal-setting:** initially, 5–10% weight reduction from baseline, followed by weight maintenance, or a further attempt at weight loss after reassessment
> - **Dietary advice:** individualized plan to create 500–1000 kcal/day (2000–4000 kJ/day) deficit by reducing total/saturated fat and carbohydrates
> - **Physical activity:** most helpful in maintenance of weight loss in conjunction with caloric restriction. Aim for 30 minutes of moderate-intensity activity most days of the week
> - **Behavioral therapy:** methods to improve compliance—self-monitoring, stress management, cognitive strategies, social support
> - **Pharmacotherapy:** part of a comprehensive program, with diet and activity, for body mass index (BMI) ≥ 30 with no obesity-related comorbidities, or ≥27 if comorbidities are present
> - **Low or very low calorie diets:** short-term dietary replacement with very low (<800 Kcal/day) or low (800–1200 Kcal/day) calorie diets can allow rapid initial weight loss, that should be followed by a weight maintenance plan to avoid weight regain
> - **Bariatric surgery:** selected adults with clinically severe obesity (BMI ≥40, or ≥35 kg/m² with comorbidities) when less-invasive methods have failed and morbidity/mortality risk is high

result in significant weight loss, and weight regain is a major problem. The repeated cycles of weight loss and regain may result in reduced motivation for weight loss. Combating the problem of overweight and obesity requires prevention in the form of major changes in government policy, town planning and education, and population-based approaches to promoting healthy diet and physical activity. Several strategies and therapies exist for the management of overweight/obesity in individuals (Box 10-13), but the environment we live in predisposes us to making choices that often exacerbate weight gain. Bariatric surgery can lead to long-term sustained weight loss, and should be considered an option in severe obesity.

Pharmacotherapy is an adjunct to low-calorie diet, physical activity and behavioral therapy in patients who fail to lose weight by those measures alone and for whom the risk of obesity-related complications is high. Medications work either centrally to suppress appetite (liraglutide, bupropion/naltrexone combination, phentermine/topiramate combination, lorcaserin) or by blocking fat absorption from the gut (orlistat).

Bariatric surgery in the form of sleeve gastrectomy, gastric bypass or gastric banding can lead to substantial and sustained weight loss over many years. This may be an option in severe obesity with BMI >40 or BMI >35 with weight-related comorbidities. Although most of the procedures are done laparoscopically with relatively low risk of mortality and morbidity, operative risks must be balanced with potential benefits in this high-risk population. Long-term follow-up is required, with monitoring for nutritional deficiencies and other complications. This procedure does have good outcomes for individual patients but comes at an expense to the patient and health service, and may not be a sustainable management plan to treat the current obesity epidemic.

The metabolic syndrome

The metabolic syndrome is a cluster of modifiable factors occurring in an individual that stem from insulin resistance and increase cardiovascular risk (Box 10-14). Also known as the 'insulin resistance syndrome', the criteria were defined by the World Health Organization in 1998 and have since been revised by numerous organizations. All definitions share the common features of abdominal obesity, dyslipidemia, hyperglycemia and hypertension.

- Depending on the criteria and the population, individuals meeting the definition of the metabolic syndrome have a two- to threefold increased risk of cardiovascular morbidity and mortality.
- The syndrome is also associated with other conditions that are pathologically linked to insulin resistance—fatty liver disease, polycystic ovarian syndrome, hyperuricemia.

Pathogenesis

Patients with this cluster of risk factors have a proinflammatory and prothrombotic state. Adipose tissue, particularly visceral, is metabolically active, producing free fatty acids and inflammatory cytokines that result in impaired insulin signaling, oxidative stress, hepatic production of atherogenic lipoproteins, and endothelial dysfunction. Together, these contribute toward the genesis and progression of cardiovascular disease.

Management

Diet and lifestyle management to achieve weight loss, similar to that recommended for T2DM, is essential. Pharmacological management focuses on treating the individual components (Table 10-19). Addressing other cardiovascular risk factors such as smoking and low-density lipoprotein (LDL) cholesterol is also key.

Box 10-14

NCEP ATP III criteria for the metabolic syndrome

Any 3 or more risk factors

- **Obesity:** waist circumference ≥102 cm (40 in) for men, ≥88 cm (36 in) for women
- **Triglycerides:** ≥1.7 mmol/L (150 mg/dL), or drug treatment for elevated levels
- **HDL cholesterol:** <1.03 mmol/L (40mg/dL) in men, <1.29 mmol/L (50 mg/dL) in women, or drug treatment for low levels
- **Blood pressure:** ≥130 mmHg systolic or ≥85 mmHg diastolic, or drug treatment for hypertension
- **Fasting glucose:** ≥5.6 mmol/L (100 mg/dL), or drug treatment for diabetes

The International Diabetes Federation (IDF) criteria (2006) are similar, but use ethnic-specific cut-offs for waist circumference + 2 or more risk factors.

ATP, Adult Treatment Panel; HDL, high-density lipoprotein; NCEP, National Cholesterol Education Program.

Data from the National Institutes of Health, National Heart, Lung, and Blood Institute www.nhlbi.nih.gov/files/docs/resources/heart/atp3full.pdf

---

Table 10-19 Pharmacological management of metabolic syndrome components

Dyslipidemia	Aim to lower triglycerides and LDL cholesterol and increase HDL cholesterol
	Agents: statins, fibrates; alone or in combination, PCSK9 inhibitors
Blood pressure	Introduce therapy if BP ≥140/90 mmHg, or ≥130/80 mmHg if established diabetes
	No definitive 'best' antihypertensive agent. Drugs targeting renin–angiotensin–aldosterone system often used
Insulin resistance	Diet and lifestyle with weight loss improve insulin sensitivity.
	Metformin is sometimes used to reduce insulin resistance.

BP, blood pressure; HDL, high-density lipoprotein; LDL, low-density lipoprotein.

SELF-ASSESSMENT QUESTIONS

1 Which of the following hormones is *not* regulated by the hypothalamic–pituitary axis?
   A   Cortisol
   B   Parathyroid hormone
   C   Thyroxine
   D   Estrogen
   E   Insulin-like growth factor (IGF-1)

2 Which condition of hormonal excess is most likely to be caused by overstimulation by the pituitary tropic hormone rather than excess peripheral production?
   A   Hyperthyroidism
   B   Cushing's syndrome
   C   Conn's syndrome
   D   Hyperprolactinemia
   E   Acromegaly

3 In a patient with a toxic multinodular goiter, which of the following laboratory findings would be expected?
   A   Increased levels of thyroid-stimulating hormone (TSH) receptor and microsomal antibodies
   B   Increased TSH
   C   Decreased serum calcium
   D   Low plasma free T_3 and T_4
   E   Increased plasma free T_3 and T_4

4 A 78-year-old woman from a nursing home presents with features of hyperthyroidism. What is the *least* likely cause?
   A   Recent computed tomography scan with intravenous contrast
   B   Recent viral infection
   C   Medication error
   D   Papillary thyroid cancer
   E   Multinodular goiter

5 Which of the following hormonal conditions is *not* associated with osteoporosis?
   A   Prolactinoma
   B   Precocious puberty
   C   Hyperthyroidism
   D   Cushing's disease
   E   Hyperparathyroidism

6 In a patient with hypercalcemia, which of the following findings is consistent with a diagnosis of primary hyperparathyroidism?
   A   Low serum phosphate and an elevated urinary calcium excretion
   B   High serum phosphate and low urinary calcium excretion
   C   Soft-tissue calcification and elevated serum calcium/phosphate product
   D   Low serum vitamin D levels
   E   Elevated bone mineral density

7 Which investigations are the most appropriate for exclusion of Cushing's syndrome?
   A   8 a.m. serum adrenocorticotropic hormone (ACTH) and cortisol measurements
   B   24-hour urinary cortisol excretion and low-dose dexamethasone suppression test
   C   Serum cortisol and computed tomography scan of the adrenals
   D   Serum cortisol and magnetic resonance imaging scan of the pituitary
   E   Short Synacthen (tetracosactide) test

8 Which of the following statements regarding cortisol is *true*?
   A   Cortisol circulates in blood bound to albumin as well as a specific cortisol-binding globulin.
   B   Cortisol acts on target cells by binding to a specific cell-membrane receptor.
   C   Most of the cortisol released by the adrenals is subsequently excreted unchanged in the urine.
   D   A significant amount of cortisol secretion occurs independent of adrenocorticotropic hormone (ACTH) stimulation.
   E   Cortisol and aldosterone are both made by adrenal cortical cells and are therefore co-secreted under the influence of ACTH.

9 In a male with Addison's disease, what forms of treatment are most appropriate?
   A   Hydrocortisone and salt tablets
   B   Hydrocortisone and fludrocortisone
   C   Hydrocortisone and spironolactone
   D   Hydrocortisone and testosterone
   E   Hydrocortisone and potassium supplements

10 Which of these endocrine conditions cannot arise from autoimmune mechanisms?

    A Hypothyroidism
    B Adrenal insufficiency
    C Hypopituitarism
    D Type 1 diabetes mellitus
    E Insulinoma

11 A 58-year-old man with longstanding type 2 diabetes mellitus has poorly controlled hypertension despite taking multiple hypertensives. Which of these features would *not* be suggestive of a non-diabetes-related endocrine cause of hypertension beyond diabetes alone?

    A Significant proteinuria
    B Low serum potassium
    C Episodes of sweating and palpitations
    D Pigmented striae
    E A history of hypercalcemia

12 A 40-year-old man complains of severe fatigue, low libido and loss of muscle strength. The most appropriate investigations include:

    A Serum gonadotropins, early morning testosterone and cortisol, thyroid-stimulating hormone (TSH)
    B Early-morning luteinizing hormone (LH) and follicle-stimulating hormone (FSH), adrenocorticotropic hormone (ACTH), TSH, testicular ultrasound
    C Random testosterone, prolactin, dexamethasone suppression test, free T_3
    D 24-hour urine cortisol, pituitary magnetic resonance imaging, early-morning LH/FSH and growth hormone
    E Glucose tolerance test, 24-hour urine testosterone, short Synacthen (tetracosactide) test, prolactin

13 Which of the following is not a cause of amenorrhea/oligomenorrhea?

    A Polycystic ovarian syndrome
    B Congenital adrenal hyperplasia
    C XXY karyotype
    D Hashimoto's thyroiditis
    E Prolactinoma

14 Which of the following are characteristic of polycystic ovarian syndrome?

    A Hirsutism, insulin resistance, onset in late adulthood
    B Hyperandrogenism, insulin resistance, anovulation
    C Virilization, increased risk of type 1 diabetes mellitus, appearance of multiple peripheral ovarian cysts on ultrasound
    D Hyperandrogenism, increased risk of gestational diabetes, earlier age at menopause
    E Acne, increased risk of type 1 diabetes mellitus, anovulation

15 In which of these conditions would you expect to find low C-peptide levels?

    A Polycystic ovarian syndrome
    B Newly diagnosed type 2 diabetes mellitus
    C Insulinoma
    D Sulphonylurea overdose
    E Exogenous insulin overdose

16 A 28-year-old woman has persistent polyuria and thirst. A random laboratory blood glucose measurement is 12.2 mmol/L, and on a second occasion is 14.1 mmol/L. Which test should be done to confirm the diagnosis of diabetes mellitus?

    A Fasting blood glucose
    B Glucose tolerance test
    C Insulin tolerance test
    D Islet cell autoantibodies
    E No further tests necessary—the given results are already diagnostic.

17 What is the most sensitive investigation for detecting diabetic nephropathy?

    A Creatinine clearance rate
    B Urine microscopy
    C Urinary micro-albumin excretion
    D Urinary protein electrophoresis
    E Serum creatinine

18 Which statement is *true* regarding type 1 diabetes mellitus?

    A Early in the disease, patients may be treated with oral hypoglycemic drugs.
    B In the absence of visual symptoms, diabetic retinopathy is unlikely to be present.
    C Women with type 1 diabetes mellitus should be advised against becoming pregnant.
    D Autoimmune destruction of beta-cells precedes onset of hyperglycemia by a period of months to years.
    E All patients should aim for a target HbA_{1c} of <7%, to minimize the risk of complications.

19 Which of the following conditions is not associated with insulin resistance?
  A Pheochromocytoma
  B Diabetes insipidus
  C Cushing's syndrome
  D Acromegaly
  E Polycystic ovarian syndrome

20 Regarding obesity, which of the following statements is true?
  A Bariatric surgery is rarely recommended in severe obesity due to the increased anesthetic risk.
  B Obese diabetic patients should receive insulin therapy as first-line, as they are unlikely to respond to oral hypoglycemic agents and strict glycemic control is essential.
  C Obesity increases the risk of comorbid conditions such as cancer, osteoarthritis and cardiovascular disease.
  D The most common cause of severe obesity is an endocrinological condition such as Cushing's disease, hypothyroidism or polycystic ovarian syndrome.

ANSWERS

1 B.

Parathyroid hormone secretion is regulated by serum calcium levels acting at the calcium-sensing receptor on the surface of parathyroid cells.

2 E.

The high insulin-like growth factor (IGF-1) levels of acromegaly typically result from excess growth hormone secretion from a pituitary tumor.

3 E.

Autonomously secreting nodules within a toxic multinodular goiter secrete excess amounts of T_3 and T_4, which are not regulated by negative feedback from the pituitary.

4 D.

Most thyroid cancers are non-functional and do not secrete thyroid hormone. Exposure to excess iodine and viral infections can both result in thyroiditis and an excessive release of thyroid hormone from the thyroid gland.

5 B.

An early puberty advances bone age. Bone density is increased, appropriate for bone age. High prolactin levels increase the risk of osteoporosis by suppressing the gonadotropin–sex steroid axis. High levels of thyroid hormone, cortisol and parathyroid hormone all increase bone resorption.

6 A.

Parathyroid hormone decreases phosphate reabsorption in the proximal tubule. Although parathyroid hormone stimulates renal calcium reabsorption, the net effect of high serum calcium levels is increased urinary excretion.

7 B.

A single random cortisol measurement is generally not useful in the evaluation of excess cortisol secretion. Both 24-hour urine free cortisol and dexamethasone suppression tests are used as screening tests for Cushing's syndrome. Early-morning cortisol levels and short Synacthen test are used to evaluate adrenal insufficiency rather than excess.

8 A.

Cortisol secretion from the zona fasciculata of the adrenal cortex is stimulated by ACTH, while aldosterone secretion from the zona glomerulosa is under the control of the renin–angiotensin system. Cortisol is protein-bound in serum, but excreted as the free hormone in urine. Being a steroid hormone, it acts on intranuclear receptors.

9 B.

Addison's disease results in autoimmune destruction of the adrenal cortex. Hydrocortisone and fludrocortisone are the respective pharmacological equivalents of cortisol and aldosterone. Adrenal androgen replacement is unnecessary in males, due to testicular production of androgens (testosterone).

10 E.

Antibodies toward thyroid, adrenal, pituitary or islet cells may result in clinical deficiencies of those endocrine organs. Insulinomas are islet-cell derived tumors, unrelated to autoimmunity.

11 A.

Proteinuria may be a feature of longstanding hypertension of any cause and is a typical finding in diabetic nephropathy. Low potassium may suggest hyperaldosteronism; sweating and palpitations are associated with pheochromocytoma; and pigmented striae suggest Cushing's syndrome. Hypercalcemia has been linked to hypertension.

12 A.

Androgen deficiency is best assessed by measurement of an early-morning testosterone. Gonadotropins will be elevated if there is a primary testicular defect. Cushing's syndrome and hyperthyroidism can also produce symptoms of weakness and fatigue.

13 C.

Individuals affected by Klinefelter syndrome have an XXY karyotype and a male phenotype.

14 B.

Features of polycystic ovarian syndrome may include clinical and/or biochemical hyperandrogenism, ovulatory disturbance and insulin resistance, with increased risk of type 2 and gestational diabetes. It typically manifests in early adulthood.

15 E.

C-peptide is enzymatically cleaved from the pro-insulin molecule and co-secreted with insulin from beta cells. C-peptide is therefore elevated in conditions of high insulin secretion such as insulin resistance, insulinoma or exogenous stimulation by sulfonylureas. As exogenous insulin suppresses endogenous insulin production, C-peptide levels will be low.

16 E.

Two random blood glucose readings above 11.1 mmol/L and the presence of typical symptoms are sufficient for the diagnosis of diabetes, and a glucose tolerance test is not required for confirmation. Islet cell autoantibodies may assist in classification of the type of diabetes, but are not used for diagnosis.

17 C.

The earliest clinical evidence of diabetic nephropathy is the presence of an abnormal level of albumin in the urine. Changes in creatinine occur late.

18 D.

Ongoing autoimmune destruction of beta cells ultimately results in inadequate secretion of insulin to maintain glucose homeostasis. Target levels of glucose control should be individualized, according to clinical need. Pregnancy outcomes are good if tight glycemic control can be achieved during gestation.

19 B.

Diabetes insipidus is a disorder of water balance, unrelated to mechanisms of glucose homeostasis.

20 C.

Obesity is associated with increased risk of malignancies, including colorectal, endometrial, esophageal, pancreatic, renal and postmenopausal breast cancer. Excess weight increases mechanical stress on joints. It increases cardiovascular risk both directly and indirectly through contributing toward hypertension, dyslipidemia and insulin resistance/glucose intolerance.

CHAPTER 11

GASTROENTEROLOGY

Magnus Halland, Michael Potter, Georgia Edwards, Vimalan Ambikaipaker and Nicholas J Talley

ESOPHAGUS

Dysphagia

Difficulty swallowing is termed *dysphagia*. Patients usually report the sensation of incomplete passage or a sensation of hold-up of the swallowed bolus. Dysphagia can occur with both solids and liquids, and symptom patterns are helpful in differentiating between oropharyngeal and esophageal causes.

CLINICAL PEARL

Prominent coughing, choking and aspiration points toward oropharyngeal causes, while retrosternal pain and hold-up indicates esophageal disease.

Stroke is the most common cause of oropharyngeal dysphagia, but other neurological disorders such as Parkinson's disease, motor neuron disease, and inclusion body myositis should be considered.

It is also useful to consider whether the disease is *structural* or a *motility* disorder.

- If dysphagia is for solids and progressing, structural causes are likely. Structural causes of esophageal dysphagia include:
  » strictures (benign and malignant)
  » rings and webs
  » eosinophilic esophagitis (Figure 11-1)
  » Zenker's diverticulum (an acquired pouch in the upper esophagus due to cricopharyngeal hypertrophy).
- If dysphagia is for both solids and liquids, a motor disorder should be considered. True motor disorders of the esophagus are rare, with achalasia and pseudoachalasia the most prevalent.

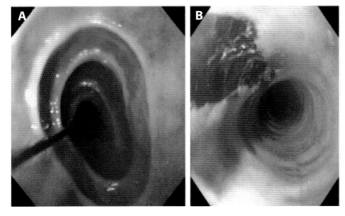

Figure 11-1 (A) Ringed esophagus in eosinophilic esophagitis. **(B)** Tear post dilatation (same case)

From Flint PW et al. Cummings Otolaryngology, 5th ed. Philadelphia: Elsevier, 2010.

CLINICAL PEARL

Generally, a narrowing in the esophagus to less than 13 mm can cause symptoms. Most endoscopes are 9 mm and can therefore miss a diffusely narrowed esophagus. An esophagram, preferably with administration of a 13 mm barium tablet, can be helpful.

The presence of pain on swallowing, *odynophagia*, generally means that esophagitis or ulcerated mucosa is present. An infectious cause or pill esophagitis is often identified in this circumstance.

Investigation

Although history and physical examination are very helpful in establishing the differential diagnosis for dysphagia and/or odynophagia, further investigation is always warranted.

- The initial test of choice is usually a barium swallow, to define the anatomy. A small risk of going straight to endoscopy is the possibility of the presence of a Zenker's diverticulum. These can be perforated during endoscopy.
- Endoscopy is indicated in nearly all patients with dysphagia for diagnosis (including biopsy) and therapy (dilatation).
- Video-fluoroscopy and nasopharyngeal laryngoscopy are also particularly helpful in patients with oropharyngeal dysphagia.
- Esophageal manometry is used when endoscopy fails to show a cause, and can differentiate between motor disorders. The characteristic finding of failure of relaxation of the lower esophageal sphincter and absence of esophageal peristalsis is found in achalasia.

CLINICAL PEARL

A rare but under-recognized cause of dysphagia is lichen planus with esophageal involvement. Examine the oral cavity of every patient with dysphagia, and ask female patients about dyspareunia as this is often present and supports the diagnosis.

Motor disorders

Achalasia

Achalasia is a rare esophageal motor disorder caused by myenteric plexus nerve degeneration. The underlying etiology remains unknown. Diagnosis is often delayed.

- Patients often present with dysphagia, which typically includes difficulty swallowing liquids as well as solids. Symptom progression is usually slow, and weight loss is common. Also suspect achalasia in heartburn unresponsive to PPI (from food fermentation) or if there is retained food in the esophagus at endoscopy.
- Typical age at diagnosis is between 25 and 60 years, and both genders are equally affected.

- No single test is diagnostic and patients should undergo triple testing as outlined below.

CLINICAL PEARLS

- Difficulties with belching and nocturnal regurgitation of ingested food in the setting of dysphagia are highly suggestive of achalasia.
- Due to the slowly progressive nature of achalasia, patients learn to adapt. Ask patients if they walk around during meals and raise their arms to facilitate passage of food.

Investigation

Triple testing should be performed:

1 *Barium swallow*—A barium study will often reveal a bird-beak-like narrowing distally with hold-up of barium above. The degree of dilatation of the esophagus is most accurately appreciated with this test.

2 *Endoscopy*—classical findings on endoscopy include a dilated esophagus with pooled saliva or food residue. Resistance to passage of the endoscopy through the gastroesohageal junction can often be appreciated.

3 *Esophageal manometry*—common manometric findings are lack of peristalsis along with a lower esophageal sphincter (LES) that fails to relax with swallowing.

4 *Endoscopic ultrasound*—helpful to identify suspected pseudoachalasia due to distal esophageal malignancy.

Treatment

Treatment aims at relieving the LES pressure, which can be achieved through pneumatic endoscopic dilatation or a myotomy. The myotomy can be performed surgically (Heller's myotomy) or endoscopically (per-oral endoscopic myotomy/POEM). Newer endoscopic techniques, in which an endoscopic myotomy is performed, are emerging as possible alternatives to surgery.

Medical therapy with calcium-channel blockers is generally ineffective, but can be trialed in patients who are unwilling or have comorbidities that prevent surgery or dilatation.

Botulinum toxin injection is short-lived (6 months), so is reserved for high-risk patients (e.g. very elderly or with severe medical comorbidities) or can be of use if the diagnosis is unclear. Repeated botulinum toxin injections should be avoided in patients who are surgical candidates as this may negatively affect surgical outcomes.

Differential diagnosis

Conditions that can mimic achalasia include tumors at the gastroesophageal junction (pseudoachalasia), which is why endoscopy is a crucial part of the diagnostic work-up. Rarely, paraneoplastic syndromes can cause a similar picture. Rapid progression of symptoms, profound weight loss and late onset (> age 60) are all red flags for possible pseudoachalasia.

Rarely, an infection with the protozoan *Trypanosoma cruzi* can mimic achalasia. This should be thought of in patients from South America or if cardiomyopathy and megacolon are also present.

Diffuse esophageal spasm (DES)

This rare condition is an esophageal motility disorder characterized by simultaneous, non-peristaltic contractions of the esophagus. Barium swallow may show a corkscrew esophagus.

The diagnosis is most commonly made in patients who undertake esophageal manometry as part of a diagnostic work-up for non-cardiac chest pain or dysphagia. The pathogenesis and natural history of DES are poorly understood, but treating gastroesophageal reflux disease improves symptoms in some patients. Patients should avoid cold liquids, as this is a precipitant.

Medical therapy with calcium-channel antagonists, tricyclic antidepressants, or sildenafil improves symptoms in some patients.

Gastroesophageal reflux disease (GERD)

Gastroesophageal reflux disease is present when the esophagus is exposed to acidic stomach contents, which may or may not lead to symptoms. Symptomatic patients notice heartburn, regurgitation or chest pain. Extra-esophageal manifestations can include:

- chronic cough
- vocal cord dysfunction
- hoarseness
- asthma.

Pathophysiologically, reflux occurs when the intra-abdominal pressure exceeds the resting LES pressure, or when inappropriate relaxations of the LES occur. Obesity is a factor.

Triggers for LES relaxation include:

- alcohol
- pregnancy
- smoking
- caffeine
- fatty foods and large meal size.

A diagnosis of GERD can be made on clinical grounds and confirmed by endoscopic evidence of reflux esophagitis. Endoscopy can also identify complications of GERD such as strictures or Barrett's metaplasia. Endoscopy is often completely normal (>70%), allowing a diagnosis of non-erosive reflux disease (NERD) to be made.

CLINICAL PEARL

Reflux symptoms in young patients who respond to therapy in the absence of alarm features do not routinely require endoscopy.

Ambulatory reflux monitoring is useful when endoscopy is normal and the diagnosis is unclear. This should be considered in patients without typical reflux symptoms, and possible extraesophageal symptoms such as hoarseness and throat discomfort. Newer techniques allow endoscopic placement of pH electrodes, avoiding the need for a nasogastric catheter. Correlation between symptoms and reflux events is crucial for determining the likely success of anti-reflux surgery in those in whom proton-pump inhibitors (PPIs) fail to improve symptoms.

Treatment

Treatment depends on the severity of symptoms and evidence of complications.

- On-demand antacids and histamine-2 receptor antagonists are appropriate for patients with mild symptoms, in conjunction with addressing lifestyle factors such as meal size reduction, avoidance of dietary triggers, and reduction in weight.
- Regular PPI therapy is required to control symptoms in most patients, and is generally effective. Patients with moderate to severe esophagitis need long-term therapy.
- A minority of patients have persistent symptoms on maximal medical therapy, and anti-reflux surgery should be considered in carefully selected patients after appropriate lifestyle modification has taken place. Esophageal manometry should be performed prior to surgery to rule out achalasia and to assess preoperative peristalsis.
- Endoscopic anti-reflux therapies, such as trans-oral incision-less fundoplication (TIF) are emerging as potential alternatives to surgery.

CLINICAL PEARL

Anti-reflux surgery is most effective at relieving regurgitation, a symptom which tends to respond poorly to medical therapy.

Barrett's esophagus (BE)

The hallmark of this condition is the metaplasia of squamous esophageal epithelium into specialized intestinal columnar type epithelium. This is a pre-malignant condition, although the progression to adenocarcinoma is low in absolute terms (0.2–0.5% per year). The greatest risk is observed in Caucasian males, obese patients, and those with longer segments of disease. Screening is generally not recommended, but can be considered in white males over 50 with longstanding (>10 years) reflux symptoms who are at highest risk. Other risk factors include smoking, abdominal adiposity and diabetes mellitus. Regular surveillance is recommended to identify patients with dysplasia or early malignancy.

Non-dysplastic Barrett's requires 3–5 yearly endoscopy with biopsies taken at 2 cm intervals in the diseased segment. Targeted biopsies should be taken from any nodular or inflamed area of Barrett's. The detection of dysplasia alters management:

- Low-grade dysplasia is more closely followed (6 months rather than annually if no progression of dysplasia occurs). Typically treated with ablation therapy, unless the patient elects close surveillance with endoscopy every 6–12 months.
- High-grade dysplasia requires treatment to prevent progression to cancer. Endoscopic ablative techniques, such as radiofrequency ablation or endoscopic mucosal resection are highly effective at eradicating dysplastic BE.

Esophagitis due to causes other than acid reflux

Eosinophilic esophagitis (EoE)

CLINICAL PEARL

Consider eosinophilic esophagitis in young patients with repeated episodes of food bolus obstruction.

Eosinophilic esophagitis is characterized by intense eosinophilic infiltration of the esophagus, leading to inflammation and submucosal fibrosis. An esophageal biopsy with an eosinophil count ≥15 eosinophils per high-power field (eos/hpf) is generally accepted as diagnostic.

The pathogenesis is incompletely understood, although chemokine eotaxin-3 is involved. The incidence is rising. The general concept is that EoE is an allergic disorder, which can respond to immune suppression or careful dietary modification to identify the offending food.

The disorder affects children and adults, and the most common symptoms are dysphagia or food impaction. In particular, a history of intermittent dysphagia or recurrent food bolus obstruction, rather than progressive symptoms, should raise suspicion. Many patients with EoE have a history of atopy and asthma. Characteristic endoscopic findings include concentric rings and longitudinal fissures, although these are present in only a minority of cases.

Treatment

- A trial of high-dose PPIs for 8 weeks is recommended as first-line therapy, as reflux can also lead to esophageal eosinophilia and some patients with true eosinophilic esophagitis respond to PPIs alone.
- Swallowed topical steroids are standard therapy when response to PPIs is inadequate. Many clinicians use a 12-week course of fluticasone (440 microg twice a day).
- A 6-food elimination diet, under guidance by a dietitian with endoscopic monitoring is successful in up to 70% of patients.
- Elimination diet e.g. milk, egg, soy, wheat, nuts, fish.

Recurrence frequently occurs after cessation of therapy. Despite medical therapy some patients require esophageal dilatation to manage their symptoms, which is safe and effective.

Esophageal infections

Bacteria, viruses and parasites all have the ability to cause esophagitis, but viral esophagitis is most commonly encountered in clinical practice. The major risk factor is immunosuppression, although herpes simplex virus type 1 can occasionally infect immunocompetent persons.

Common to most esophageal infections is the presence of chest pain, odynophagia and dysphagia. Systemic symptoms and signs of infection are often present and include fever, malaise, chills and fatigue. Peripheral blood examination often shows leukocytosis. Endoscopic findings vary from discrete small ulcers to severe esophagitis with giant, confluent ulcers. The diagnosis is confirmed by demonstrating inclusion bodies on esophageal biopsies.

Therapy is directed at the underlying viral cause (if known), and is supportive when oral intake is compromised. The most common viral causes are:

1 herpes simplex virus types 1 and 2
2 cytomegalovirus
3 varicella zoster
4 human immunodeficiency virus.

Fungal infections other than *Candida* infection are rare and usually occur in the setting of severe immunosuppression, or among those who are using topical steroid therapy in the upper aerodigestive tract. This should be considered in patients on chemotherapy who develop dysphagia.

Pill esophagitis

Many medications have the potential to cause inflammation in the esophagus if lodged there. Often another condition is present that leads to pill retention, such as achalasia or a stricture.

Oral bisphosphonates are commonly the offending agent. Other high-risk tablets include:

- tetracycline antibiotics and non-steroidal anti-inflammatory agents including aspirin
- oral potassium supplementation as well as prednisone tablets.

Correction of an underlying esophageal disorder, choice of an alternative pharmacotherapy, and medication administration advice such as ingesting tablets in the upright position with generous amounts of water can help to minimize risk.

> ### CLINICAL PEARL
>
> Ask about how patients take their tablets! Many patients admit to taking tablets with little or no water and while supine. This often causes pill retention in the esophagus and can lead to esophagitis if the tablet has erosive potential.

A rare cause of esophagitis is injury due to accidental or intentional ingestion of corrosive material. Patients who do not succumb to immediate complications such as bleeding and perforation usually develop long strictures that are difficult to dilate. Surgery may be required if endoscopic therapy fails.

Radiation

Another cause of esophagitis is radiation therapy, which is usually evident from the history. Severity is related to radiation dose and concomitant therapy with radiosensitizing medications (e.g. taxane chemotherapy). The most common symptom is odynophagia, and topical treatment (viscous lidocaine or opiates) or systemic analgesics are usually required. Development of significant strictures often occurs and dilatation is very difficult.

STOMACH

Physiology of acid secretion

Normal gastric physiology includes the ability to produce hydrochloric acid and other digestive secretions. While acid is useful in nutrient processing and absorption, the potential for inducing or potentiating gastric mucosal injury is always present.

Gastric acid secretion is closely regulated, with a small basal rate of excretion which follows a circadian pattern as well as an 'on-demand' system stimulated by a variety of factors. The main stimuli for the increased production of hydrochloric acid are summarized in Table 11-1.

The secretory activity of the parietal cell, which is responsible for hydrochloric acid production, is tightly regulated by neural and chemical messengers. The main drivers behind acid production are gastrin and histamine.

Preventing stimulation of the parietal cell is the aim of many acid-suppressing medications. PPIs directly inhibit the proton pump, while histamine antagonists reduce acid

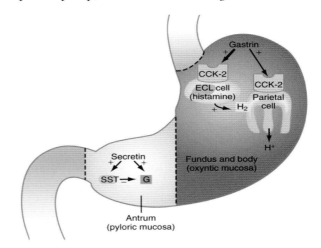

Figure 11-2 Gastric acid secretion. CCK, cholecystokinin; ECL, enterochromaffin-like cell; G, gastrin; SST, somatostatin

Table 11-1 Stimuli for gastric acid production

PHASE	RESPONSE
Cephalic	The thought, sight or smell of food increases acid production via vagal stimulation
Gastric	Distension of the stomach leads to G-cell stimulation and gastrin release. Food matter also directly leads to G-cell stimulation and gastrin release
Intestinal	Nutrient entry into the proximal small bowel also stimulates acid production. The exact mediators remain unknown

secretion by attaching to the histamine receptor and thereby blunting the response of gastrin and acetylcholine on the parietal cells.

Dyspepsia and its management

Although no consensus definition of dyspepsia exists, this usually refers to patients who suffer pain or discomfort located in the upper abdomen.

- Meal-related symptoms, such as increased discomfort after eating and the inability to tolerate a normal-sized meal, are common dyspepsia symptoms.
- No cause for symptoms can be identified in the majority of patients. In those with an organic cause, reflux esophagitis, peptic ulcer disease and malignancy are the most common explanations.

If alarm symptoms are present, prompt investigation is required. These include:

- age of onset ≥60 years
- unintentional weight loss
- dysphagia or odynophagia
- anemia or iron deficiency
- jaundice
- previous gastric surgery
- palpable abdominal mass or lymphadenopathy.

If the patient is taking aspirin or non-steroidal anti-inflammatory drugs (NSAIDs), the indication should be reviewed and alternatives sought. Screening and eradication of *Helicobacter pylori* infection should be performed in all patients. Celiac disease needs to be excluded.

For most patients an organic cause cannot be identified (functional dyspepsia), and reassurance and symptom management is important. PPIs, motility agents and tricyclic antidepressants can be trialed.

Helicobacter pylori

H. pylori infection is usually acquired in childhood, and the prevalence is falling in developing nations. All infected patients have histological gastritis. For those infected, the risk of peptic ulcers, gastric cancer and B-cell (MALT) lymphoma is increased.

Testing for *H. pylori* is well established in the following circumstances:

- all patients with current or a previous history of peptic ulcer disease (PUD)
- MALT (mucosa-associated lymphoid tissue) lymphoma
- gastric intestinal metaplasia
- patients with dyspepsia (test and treat with no endoscopy if age <60 years and no alarm features).

H. pylori testing is also considered appropriate in patients with:

- functional (non-ulcer) dyspepsia
- a family history of gastric adenocarcinoma
- the requirement for long-term non-steroidal anti-inflammatory treatment, to help prevent peptic ulcers
- unexplained iron-deficiency anemia.

How to test for H. pylori

The method of testing for *H. pylori* depends on whether the patient requires endoscopy or not.

CLINICAL PEARL

Endoscopy for the sole purpose of testing for *Helicobacter pylori* is not cost-effective and a noninvasive method should be chosen.

Invasive tests (endoscopy)

- Rapid urease tests
  - » A piece of gastric mucosa is placed in agar containing urea and a pH reagent. The presence of urease, an enzyme produced by *H. pylori*, leads to urea breakdown and a change in pH which is detected by a change in color.
  - » False-positive tests are rare, but false-negative results can occur when patients are acid-suppressed. False-negative results also occur during gastrointestinal (GI) bleeding.
- Histology
  - » This is the 'gold-standard' test for *H. pylori*, but is more expensive than rapid urease testing and not routinely performed. It is appropriate if the patient is on PPI therapy at the time of endoscopy.
- Culture
  - » This is rarely performed. Its main role lies in determining bacterial resistance patterns in patients who fail standard eradication regimens.

Noninvasive

- Urea breath testing (UBT) is a simple and reliable test provided that anti-acid therapy has ceased 1 week prior to the test. It can also be used to confirm eradication.
- Fecal antigen testing is a highly accurate test for detecting the presence and absence of *H. pylori* and is not affected by PPI therapy. It is most often used to confirm successful eradication.
- Serological testing is widely available and inexpensive, but cannot distinguish between current and past infection, and is less accurate than other tests.

CLINICAL PEARL

Urea breath testing is affected by the use of proton-pump inhibitors (PPIs), and a negative test for a patient on PPIs needs confirmation.

Treatment

All patients should initially receive triple therapy (proton-pump inhibitors and two antibiotics). See Table 11-2 for treatment options.

Table 11-2 Options for therapy for *Helicobacter pylori* infection

REGIMEN	DRUGS	DURATION	ERADICATION RATES
Triple therapy	Proton-pump inhibitor (PPI) twice daily Amoxicillin 1 g twice daily Clarithromycin 500 mg twice daily	14 days	70%
Quadruple therapy	PPI twice daily Bismuth subcitrate 525 mg four times a day Metronidazole 250 mg four times a day Tetracycline 500 mg four times a day	10–14 days	75–90%
Sequential therapy	PPI and amoxicillin 1 g twice daily for 5 days *followed by:* PPI (twice daily) plus clarithromycin (500 mg twice daily) and tinidazole (500 mg twice daily) for 5 days	10 days	>80%

Testing for eradication after therapy

Current guidelines recommend confirmation of eradication in all patients in whom therapy is prescribed, and particularly:

- peptic ulcers caused by *H. pylori*
- persistent dyspepsia after treatment
- patients with MALT lymphoma
- patients with early gastric cancer or gastric metaplasia.

Testing for eradication is best done with UBT or fecal antigen testing, but must occur at least 4 weeks after *H. pylori* therapy and preferably with the patient off PPI therapy.

Gastritis and gastropathy

Gastritis is not a clinical diagnosis, but is made by endoscopic and microscopic examination of gastric tissue. The hallmark of this disorder is the presence of inflammatory cells in the gastric mucosa. Causes include:

- infections—*H. pylori*, human immunodeficiency virus (HIV)
- autoimmune—pernicious anemia
- drug-induced—non-steroidal anti-inflammatory agents and antibiotics
- physiological stress—sepsis, admission to intensive care.

Chronic atrophic gastritis is characterized by metaplasia. Infections and autoimmune processes can lead to metaplastic changes, which are associated with increased risk of gastric adenocarcinoma. If gastric intestinal metaplasia is diagnosed, because rates of progression are low, endoscopic screening is only recommended in those with other high risk features (eg. family history of gastric cancer).

Gastropathy is present when gastric epithelial cells are damaged without the presence of inflammatory cells. It is most commonly caused by direct irritation by NSAIDs, alcohol or portal hypertension.

Peptic ulcer disease (PUD)

Peptic ulcer disease occurs most commonly in the elderly and those with comorbidities. Duodenal and gastric ulcers now occur with similar frequency. The most common cause remains infection with *H. pylori*, and those treated have a very low risk of becoming re-infected and suffering further ulcers.

The second most common cause is NSAIDs. The ulcer risk is decreased with cyclooxygenase-2 (COX-2) inhibitors, but if they are combined with low-dose aspirin the risk is identical to any NSAID!

CLINICAL PEARL

Most peptic ulcers are due to *Helicobacter pylori* or non-steroidal anti-inflammatory drugs.

Rarer causes for PUD include acid-overproduction states, most commonly due to gastrinoma (Zollinger–Ellison syndrome). Also remember that Crohn's disease can ulcerate mucosa anywhere in the GI tract, including the stomach and duodenum.

The diagnosis of PUD is often only made once complications are present (bleeding, perforation or stenosis). Asymptomatic ulcers are often found at endoscopy, and the symptoms (e.g. epigastric pain) are a poor indicator of ulcer presence. Endoscopy is the diagnostic test of choice, and is often therapeutic when complications are present by the means of epinephrine (adrenaline) injections followed by gold probe diathermy, or placement of a hemostatic clip.

CLINICAL PEARL

Remember peptic ulcer in the differential diagnosis of patients with severe abdominal pain or tenderness. Perforation is possible, and an erect abdominal X-ray examining for free intraperitoneal air should be undertaken promptly. Endoscopy is contraindicated when evidence of perforation is present.

Healing of the ulcer is successful in most cases when acid suppression is coupled with removal of the offending agent, be it infectious or medication-related. Gastric ulcers usually warrant re-endoscopy and repeat biopsy to make sure an early malignant lesion has not been missed.

Tumors

Gastrinomas/Zollinger–Ellison syndrome (ZES)

Acid hypersecretion due to a gastrinoma causing peptic ulcers and diarrhea is termed Zollinger–Ellison syndrome. It accounts for less than 1% of duodenal ulcers, and the most common presenting complaint is diarrhea and/or steatorrhea. The tumor is usually found distal to the ulcer, with most being located within an anatomical triangle bounded by the porta hepatis, mid-duodenum and head of the pancreas. Patients with ZES should be screened for multiple endocrine neoplasia (MEN) type 1 syndrome, which is present in up to 20%.

The diagnosis is often considered where there are atypical ulcers due to excessive acid despite PPI therapy or when ulcer disease is coupled with chronic diarrhea.

Most patients who are being worked up for possible ZES are already on PPI therapy. This makes interpreting serum gastrin levels difficult, as acid suppression from PPIs commonly causes hypergastrinemia, but an elevated level in a patient off PPIs is concerning. Many physicians still do a level while the patient is on PPI therapy, and if this is normal consider the diagnosis excluded. Differential diagnoses are given in Box 11-1.

Box 11-1

Differential diagnosis of elevated serum gastrin levels

Apart from proton-pump inhibitors and histamine-receptor antagonists, differential diagnosis for an elevated serum gastrin level includes:

- renal failure
- chronic atrophic gastritis
- tumors (ovarian, pheochromocytoma).

CLINICAL PEARL

To diagnose Zollinger–Ellison syndrome (ZES), a fasting serum gastrin level of >300 pg/mL in a patient off proton-pump inhibitors is suggestive, while >1000 pg/mL makes ZES likely.

Cross-sectional imaging, endoscopic ultrasound and somatostatin receptor imaging is undertaken in most patients prior to considering resection.

Treatment consists of resection of the tumor in selected patients, essentially those who are fit and have no evident metastases. Unresectable gastrinomas are treated with high-dose PPIs lifelong.

Carcinoid

Gastric carcinoids usually occur in the setting of a chronically elevated serum gastrin level due to ZES or autoimmune gastritis. The precursor cell is nearly always the enterochromaffin-like cell (ECL), which is stimulated by gastrin. Episodic flushing, often spontaneous, is common with gastric carcinoid (Figure 11-3). Most patients remain asymptomatic and the metastatic potential is low.

Gastrointestinal stromal tumors (GISTs)

Gastrointestinal stromal tumors arise from mesenchymal cells. They are often an incidental finding but can also cause bleeding. Autopsy studies as well as data from capsule endoscopy indicate that small, benign GISTs are relatively common. As they are submucosal, biopsies are often normal and fine-needle aspiration (FNA) using endoscopic ultrasound is often needed to make the diagnosis.

Some GISTs behave in an aggressive manner, leading to local invasion and metastasis. Despite this, most (80%) GISTs have mutations in the *KIT* proto-oncogene which make tyrosine kinase inhibitors an effective therapy for many patients. Prognosis is therefore better than most other metastatic malignancies in terms of survival.

Post-gastrectomy complications

Partial gastrectomy is now rarely performed, and can lead to complications depending on the size of the gastric remnant and the integrity of innervation. Many patients experience dumping syndrome:

- sweating
- tachycardia
- nausea, and
- diarrhea

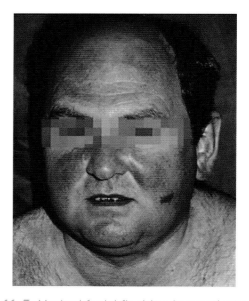

Figure 11-3 Marked facial flushing in a patient with the carcinoid syndrome

From Jayasena CN and Dhillo WS. Carcinoid syndrome and neuroendocrine tumours. Medicine 2013;41(10):566–9.

if large meals or food containing refined carbohydrates are consumed.

Dietary changes (frequent small meals, restriction of glucose and lactose) are all that are required for most patients.

Long-term vitamin B12 deficiency can arise due to lack of absorption because of absent intrinsic factor, which is produced by parietal cells in the stomach.

Bacterial overgrowth causing fat and B12 malabsorption may occur in a blind loop, and achlorhydria due to loss of acid-producing cells is a contributing factor.

Gastroparesis

Gastroparesis is the clinical syndrome that occurs due to impaired gastric emptying. Clinical clues to gastroparesis include nausea and vomiting which is usually postprandial. Early satiety and weight loss are commonly seen, along with abdominal pain. Occasionally gastroparesis is the symptom that leads to the diagnosis of diabetes mellitus. Insidious onset is common, while rapidly progressive nausea and vomiting is rarely a feature of a gastric motor disorder.

Causes of gastroparesis relate to failure of the nerves or muscles that control gastric emptying. Diabetic gastroparesis is an important cause, but rarely infiltrative processes such as amyloidosis or scleroderma produce gastroparesis. In many patients no cause is found and the disorder is labeled idiopathic.

The diagnostic work-up consists of endoscopy to rule out gastric outlet obstruction or other mucosal lesions. A gastric emptying study (usually a radioisotope-labeled meal) confirms the diagnosis. Small-bowel obstruction needs to be excluded by appropriate imaging.

Treatment

Treatment should both address the underlying cause (if identified) and the symptoms.

- Tight diabetic control is essential in halting disease progression if diabetic.
- Dietary management (small, frequent meals, split solids and liquids, low in fat, low in fiber) helps.
- Prokinetic agents and anti-nausea agents combined are the mainstay of treatment.
- Erythromycin can often help in the acute inpatient setting, but long-term efficacy is disappointing.
- Gastric electrical pacing (surgically placed) helps vomiting in refractory cases.

Currently, patients who fail medical therapy require placement of a percutaneous endoscopic gastrostomy (PEG) or jejunostomy tube to feed them.

SMALL BOWEL

Celiac disease

Celiac disease is one of the most common autoimmune diseases, with 1% of the population affected in many populations (northern Europeans have the highest incidence).

Women are more often affected than men. The immune response is directed toward gluten, which is found in wheat, barley and rye. Patients who carry HLA DQ2 or DQ8 alleles are susceptible (so those testing negative to HLA DQ2 and DQ8 can be ruled out as having celiac disease), although a substantial proportion of the population will have one of these alleles but will not necessarily have celiac disease.

The immune response triggered by gluten leads to mucosal damage in the small bowel (villous atrophy, crypt hyperplasia, epithelial lymphocytosis), and malabsorption.

The disease should be suspected in patients with:

- unexplained iron deficiency
- multiple vitamin deficiencies (vitamin D, folate, B_{12})
- abnormal liver function tests
- weight loss
- diarrhea or steatorrhea
- a positive family history
- a small bowel biopsy showing subtotal villous atrophy or epithelial lymphocytosis
- growth-delayed children.

Patients with celiac disease often have no symptoms or relatively unimpressive GI symptoms (symptoms like those of irritable bowel syndrome), dental or skeletal problems (osteoporosis or arthralgia), or infertility. The presence of dermatitis herpetiformis should raise suspicion. Celiac disease is called the great mimicker for good reason!

CLINICAL PEARL

Many patients with celiac disease are relatively asymptomatic and are found by screening for a positive family history, but their risk of long-term complications is similar to symptomatic cases, including small-bowel lymphoma and vitamin deficiencies.

Diagnosis

The 'gold standard' diagnosis is demonstration of villous atrophy on duodenal biopsies (Figure 11-4). The disease can be patchy in the duodenum, so multiple biopsies are recommended. Some patients may have intact villous architecture with only intraepithelial lymphocytosis, although this finding is less specific than villous atrophy.

Serological markers are useful and sensitive, but due to imperfect specificity the decision for a lifelong gluten-free diet should be made on biopsies. Blood tests for celiac disease are a good first step in patients with consistent symptoms or when clinical suspicion is present. The best serological tests are either tissue transglutaminase (tTG) or anti-endomysial antibodies (not anti-gliadin!).

CLINICAL PEARL

If the tissue transglutaminase (tTG) test is negative, check the total serum immunoglobulin A (IgA) level, as the tTG test measures IgA antibodies against tTG and will be negative in the 1–2% of the population with IgA deficiency.

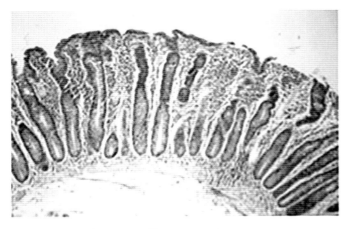

Figure 11-4 Subtotal villous atrophy

From Lo A et al. Classification of villous atrophy with enhanced magnification endoscopy in patients with celiac disease and tropical sprue. Gastrointestinal Endoscopy 2007;66(2):377–82.

Both biopsies and antibody testing are optimal if the patient is eating gluten. Making the diagnosis after a patient has commenced a gluten-free diet can be very difficult.

CLINICAL PEARL

HLA DQ2 and DQ8 testing are useful for ruling celiac disease out, owing to the high negative predictive value. (A positive test simply means 'at risk', but in no way confirms the diagnosis.)

Long-term complications

Patients with untreated celiac disease can develop long-term complications.

- Malabsorption/metabolic:
  » iron-deficiency anemia
  » metabolic bone disease (osteomalacia from vitamin D deficiency, osteoporosis)
  » vitamin deficiency
  » chronic liver disease
- Immunological:
  » functional asplenia (pathogenesis unknown, pneumococcal vaccine recommended)
- Malignancy:
  » small bowel lymphoma
- Neuropsychiatric symptoms.

Capsule endoscopy (small intestinal capsule) is useful in difficult cases to investigate anemia, weight loss or bleeding to exclude a malignancy.

CLINICAL PEARL

Patients with celiac disease may be functionally asplenic, so be aware of the increased risk of sepsis.

Box 11-2
Causes of subtotal villous atrophy

Celiac disease
Tropical sprue
Giardia
Bacterial overgrowth
Microsporidiosis
Viral infection
Hypogammaglobulinemia
Lymphoma
Zollinger–Ellison syndrome
Drugs, e.g. olmesartan, colchicine and neomycin
Radiation and ischemia

Differential diagnosis of subtotal villous atrophy

Not all flat biopsies are due to celiac disease (Box 11-2). Tropical sprue and bacterial overgrowth, in particular, are possible causes. Tropical sprue often responds to 3–6 months of tetracycline and folic acid. A travel history is important for the diagnosis of tropical sprue.

CLINICAL PEARL

If there is no response to a gluten-free diet in celiac disease:
- first consider poor diet adherence or inadvertent gluten exposure
- check the diagnosis (rule out lymphoma, diffuse ulceration, or collagenous sprue)
- consider other concurrent diseases, including lactose intolerance or pancreatic insufficiency, and treat accordingly.

Diarrhea

It is useful to categorize diarrhea into *colonic* and *small-bowel* diarrhea (Box 11-3). The duration of the diarrheal illness is important in determining the diagnosis.

Acute diarrhea

Acute diarrhea is defined as increased stool frequency (>3 loose bowel movements daily) or volume (>200 g daily) for less than 14 days.

Box 11-3
Characteristics of colonic and small bowel diarrhea

Colonic diarrhea	Small bowel diarrhea
• Typically presents with blood, mucus, tenesmus, urgency	• No blood, no mucus, no tenesmus or urgency
• Frequent, small-volume stools	• Stools are large in volume, with modest increase in stool volume

- The common causes are bacterial or viral infection, medications, and systemic illness.
- Viral infection is the most common cause, with norovirus being the most common pathogen. Bacteria are responsible for more severe acute diarrhea.
- The method of transmission most commonly implicated is fecal–oral transmission. Most cases are transmitted through contaminated water, food or direct person-to-person contact.

Diarrhea may be classified as *non-inflammatory* or *inflammatory* (Box 11-4).

The clinical history gives valuable clues to the likely causative agent in acute diarrhea (Table 11-3).

- Vomiting-predominant illness with non-bloody stools is likely to be related to viral-induced or toxin-induced food poisoning.
  » Rotavirus is a common cause of acute diarrhea in daycare centers and nurseries.
  » Norovirus is common on cruise ships, in nursing homes, schools and hospitals, and shellfish-associated outbreaks.
- If watery diarrhea is predominant, it is more likely to be due to bacterial infection with or without enterotoxin production, *Escherichia coli*, enteropathogenic *E. coli*, *Vibrio cholerae*, *V. parahaemolyticus*, *Campylobacter jejuni*, *Salmonella* spp., *Clostridium difficile*, *Yersinia enterocolitica*, *Plesiomonas* spp. or *Aeromonas* spp. (patients usually present with fever and bloody diarrhea).

- Protozoal infections are less common but are associated with chronic symptoms; causes include *Giardia*, *Cryptosporidium*, *Isospora belli* and *Cyclospora*. Bloody diarrhea occurs with *Entamoeba histolytica*, but also in *Campylobacter* and *Shigella* infection.
  » *G. lamblia* is often associated with daycare centers, travelers, and swimming pools.
  » *E. histolytica* should be considered in those who have traveled to endemic areas for more than a month, and men who have sex with men.

- Fever suggests invasive bacteria (e.g. *Salmonella*, *Shigella* or *Campylobacter*), enteric viruses or cytotoxic organisms such as *C. difficile* or *E. histolytica*.

- Systemic features of infectious diarrhea may include fever, myalgia, malaise, nausea, vomiting and anorexia. These symptoms do not help distinguish the different types of infection.

Box 11-4

Common causes of acute and chronic non-inflammatory and inflammatory diarrhea

Non-inflammatory diarrhea

- Viral disease:
  » norovirus
  » rotavirus
- Bacterial disease (toxin-mediated):
  » *Staphylococcus aureus*
  » *Bacillus cereus*
  » *Clostridium perfringens*
- Protozoal disease:
  » *Giardia lamblia*
- Medication-induced diarrhea:
  » antacid (containing magnesium)
  » colchicine
- Irritable bowel syndrome
- Dietary intolerance
- Disaccharidase deficiency, e.g. lactase

Inflammatory diarrhea

- Bacterial disease:
  » *Shigella*
  » *Salmonella*
  » *Campylobacter*
  » *Yersinia*
  » *Vibrio cholerae*
  » *Clostridium difficile*
  » Enteropathogenic *Escherichia coli*
  » Toxin-mediated—enterohemorrhagic *E. coli* (057)
- Protozoal disease:
  » *Entamoeba histolytica*
  » *Strongyloides stercoralis*
- Mesenteric ischemia
- Radiation colitis
- Inflammatory bowel disease

Table 11-3 Clinical clues to the causative agent involved in acute diarrhea

ORGANISM	INCUBATION PERIOD	FOOD
Staphylococus aureus	1–6 hours	Salads, meat and dairy foods
Bacillus cereus	1–6 hours	Rice and meat
Clostridium perfringens	8–16 hours	Meat and poultry
Escherichia coli (enteropathogenic)	1–3 days	Fecal contamination of food and water
Campylobacter spp.	2–5 days	Poultry, unpasteurized milk and water

- Women who are pregnant have a 20-fold increased risk of developing listeriosis from meat products or unpasteurized dairy products.
- In patients with AIDS, diarrhea of high volume suggests small-bowel disease. A CD4 count <200/mm³ suggests that infection is likely. If there is fever, consider cytomegalovirus (CMV), *Histoplasma*, *Cryptococcus* and *Mycobacterium*.
- Hepatitis A may occur through fecal contamination of food and water, and men who have sex with men are at higher risk.

Diagnosis

Stool culture and microscopy are helpful for making the diagnosis.

- Special culture techniques (e.g. cold enrichment for *Yersinia*, sorbitol MacConkey agar for *E. coli* O157:H7) may be needed, and ask for *C. difficile* toxin if you suspect *C. difficile*.
- About 20–40% of acute infective diarrhea cases will elude diagnosis even with appropriate cultures.
- Ova, cyst and parasite identification should be sought if traveler's diarrhea is suspected, or patients are immunocompromised, have persistent diarrhea or have traveled, or there is persistent diarrhea with exposure to infants in daycare centers.

In patients in whom bloody diarrhea does not respond to antibiotics, consideration should be given to sigmoidoscopy or colonoscopy with random biopsy to investigate the possibility of inflammatory bowel disease (IBD). Crypt abscesses are found in both infection and IBD, but crypt architectural distortion only in IBD.

Treatment

The first aim of treatment is to replace fluids and electrolytes.

- Most of the time this can be done using oral rehydration solutions.
- In patients incapable of retaining fluids, fluids should consist of glucose-based solutions as glucose facilitates the absorption of sodium and water in the face of secretory processes.
- If intravenous (IV) hydration is required, normal saline should be used. If tolerated, the normal diet should be continued, as this helps to reduce intestinal permeability induced by infection. Some patients develop lactose intolerance due to loss of brush-border enzymes. This can last up to several weeks, and these patients need lactose restrictions.

Medications:

- The combination of loperamide and antibiotics is more effective than antibiotics alone in traveler's diarrhea. However, this is not true for inflammatory diarrhea. Antimotility agents should not be used for the treatment of patients with acute diarrhea with fever or bloody stools, as this may enhance the severity of illness due to toxin retention.

- It is important to note that treatment with antibiotics for non-typhoidal *Salmonella* may actually prolong shedding of the organism. Thus, treatment is rarely required unless the host is immunocompromised or at risk for sepsis.
- The treatment of *E. coli* O157:H7 with antibiotics may induce hemolytic uremic syndrome (HUS). If *E. coli* 0157:H7 is confirmed, antibiotics are contraindicated.
- *Campylobacter* resistance to quinolones is high; an alternative is erythromycin or azithromycin as first-line treatment. If empirical therapy is warranted, treatment with fluoroquinolone for 3–5 days in the absence of enterohemorrhagic *E. coli* or *Campylobacter* infection can be considered.
- Antibiotic therapy may shorten the course of *Shigella* infection and should be considered in severe cases.

Chronic diarrhea

Chronic diarrhea is defined as the frequent passage of stools (>3/day) or loose stools >25% of the time, or more than 200–250 g/day lasting more than 1 month. At a fundamental level, the diarrhea is due to excess water in the stools because absorption of fluid from the lumen is reduced and/or secretion of fluid is increased.

Irritable bowel syndrome should be distinguished from chronic diarrhea by its clinical characteristics based on the Rome IV criteria (Box 11-5).

CLINICAL PEARLS

- High-volume diarrhea associated with persistent fasting is indicative of secretory diarrhea.
- The presence of abdominal pain and diarrhea without alarm features raises the possibility of irritable bowel syndrome.
- Diarrhea with the presence of hyperpigmentation raises the possibility of Addison's disease.

Box 11-5

Rome IV diagnostic criteria* for irritable bowel syndrome

Recurrent abdominal pain at least 1 day per week associated with 2 or more of the following:

1. Improvement or worsening with defecation
2. Associated with a change in frequency of stool
3. Associated with a change in form (appearance) of stool

---

* Criteria fulfilled for the past 3 months with symptom onset at least 6 months prior to diagnosis.

From Gastroenterology 2016;150:1257–61.

Chronic diarrhea can be categorized into the following subtypes:

- *watery* diarrhea, which is further divided into *secretory* and *osmotic* diarrhea (Table 11-4).
- *inflammatory* diarrhea
- *fatty* diarrhea.

Watery diarrhea

In normal stool, the number of cations $[Na^+]$ plus $[K^+]$ is equal to the number of anions $[Cl^-]$ plus $[HCO_3^-]$ plus other absorbable anions (e.g. short-chain fatty acids).

Normal **stool osmolality** is calculated as follows:

$$2 \times ([Na^+] + [K^+]) = 290 \text{ mOsm/L}$$

- In *secretory* diarrhea there is no osmotic gap (or it's <50 mOsm/kg), i.e. stool osmolality is normal, i.e. 290 minus $2 \times ([Na^+] + [K^+])$ stool = <50 mOsm/kg.
- In *osmotic* diarrhea there is a gap because of unmeasured/osmotically active molecules, i.e. 290 minus $2 \times ([Na^+]^\dagger + [K^+])$ = >100 mOsm/kg.

If stool osmolality is *greater* than serum osmolality, the stool collection is faulty.

Non-watery diarrhea

Forms of non-watery diarrhea are described in Box 11-6.

Box 11-6

Forms of non-watery diarrhea

Inflammatory diarrhea
- Increased white blood cells in the stool
- Stool pH is <5.6

Fatty diarrhea
- Fecal fat testing:
  » stool fat excretion >14 g/24 h suggests malabsorption or maldigestion
  » a stool fat concentration of >8% strongly suggests pancreatic insufficiency

Protein-losing enteropathy
- Should be considered in the presence of hypoalbuminemia but not nephritic syndrome or hepatic dysfunction. Confirmation via fecal clearance of alpha-1 antitrypsin (A1A)
- Elevated A1A clearance suggests excessive gastrointestinal protein loss (the positive predictive value of the test has been found to be 98% and the negative predictive value is 75%)
- Patients with protein-losing enteropathies generally have A1A clearance values >50 mL/24 h and A1A stool concentrations

---

Causes of chronic diarrhea

Common causes of chronic diarrhea are listed in Box 11-7.

Box 11-7

Common causes of chronic diarrhea by typical stool characteristics

Osmotic diarrhea
- Magnesium, PO_4^-, SO_4^- ingestion
- Carbohydrate malabsorption

Fatty diarrhea
- Short bowel syndrome
- Small bowel overgrowth
- Pancreatic exocrine insufficiency
- Post-resection diarrhea
- Mesenteric ischemia
- Severe small bowel mucosal disease (e.g. celiac disease)

Inflammatory diarrhea
- Ulcerative colitis
- Crohn's disease
- Pseudomembranous colitis
- Infective colitis
- Ischemic colitis
- Radiation colitis
- Colorectal cancer and lymphoma

Secretory diarrhea
- Laxative abuse
- Bacterial toxins
- Ileal bile acid malabsorption
- Villous adenoma
- Ulcerative colitis and Crohn's disease
- Microscopic colitis
- Vasculitis
- Diabetic autonomic neuropathy
- Hyperthyroidism
- Neuroendocrine tumors, e.g. VIPoma
- Malignancy
- Drug and poisons

Table 11-4 Secretory vs osmotic diarrhea

SECRETORY DIARRHEA	OSMOTIC DIARRHEA
High volume (>1 L/day)	<1 L/day
Stool osmolality is normal, i.e. $2 \times ([Na^+] + [K^+])$ = 290 mOsm/L No osmotic gap, i.e. <50 mOsm/kg difference	Stool osmolality is below normal, i.e. $2 \times ([Na^+] + [K^+])$ <290 mOsm/L Osmotic gap >100 mOsm/kg
Persists with fasting	Disappears with fasting
Watery diarrhea; no pus, blood or steatorrhea	Watery diarrhea

Clinical clues for making the diagnosis

- In the history:
  - » Celiac disease—history of gluten intolerance, family history of celiac disease or other autoimmune disorders
  - » Inflammatory bowel disease—rectal bleeding, abdominal pain, mucus, tenesmus, family history of inflammatory bowel disease and other autoimmune disorders
  - » Pancreatic insufficiency—history of foul-smelling stool, fat-soluble vitamin deficiency, weight loss, cystic fibrosis or chronic pancreatitis
  - » Post-surgery—blind loops leading to small-bowel bacterial overgrowth, short bowel syndrome, dumping syndrome
  - » Zollinger–Ellison syndrome—recurrent peptic ulcer disease and diarrhea
  - » Drugs—laxatives, magnesium, antacids, antibiotics, colchicine
  - » Frequent infection—immunoglobulin deficiency
  - » Milk intolerance—lactose intolerance.
- In the physical examination:
  - » Marked weight loss—consider thyrotoxicosis, cancer, malabsorption and inflammatory bowel disease
  - » Arthritis with hyperpigmentation—Whipple's disease
  - » Hyperpigmentation—Addison's disease, Cronkhite–Canada syndrome (a rare syndrome which presents with multiple polyps in the digestive tract, chronic diarrhea, protein-losing enteropathy, alopecia, abnormal atrophy of nails and skin pigmentation)
  - » Chronic lung disease—cystic fibrosis
  - » Postural hypotension—autonomic dysfunction in diabetes, Addison's disease
  - » Neuropathy—diabetes, amyloidosis
  - » Onycholysis—Cronkhite–Canada syndrome.

Treatment

Treatment of chronic diarrhea ultimately depends on the underlying condition. Therapy with anti-diarrheal drugs (e.g. loperamide) can provide symptomatic relief.

Giardia lamblia infection

Giardia lamblia is a protozoal parasite. It has been associated with epidemic and sporadic diarrheal illness (noninvasive disease).

- It is an important cause of food- or water-borne disease.
- Its incubation period is 7–14 days. The common route of transmission between individuals is fecal–oral (swimming in infected bodies of water, daycare workers or parents with young children in diapers).
- High-risk individuals include children, international travelers, immunocompromised individuals, and patients with hypochlorhydria or cystic fibrosis.

There are two morphological forms: *cysts* and *trophozoites*.

- Cysts are infectious. Once ingested, they migrate to the small bowel and trophozoites are released from the cyst. These cause malabsorption and hypersecretion.

- Trophozoites that do not adhere in the small bowel migrate to the large bowel. Here they revert back to cyst form. Once excreted in the feces, they have the potential to infect again.

About half of those infected clear the infection in the absence of clinical symptoms. 30–45% of individuals present with symptomatic infection.

- Common clinical presentations include diarrhea, malaise, abdominal cramps, bloating, vomiting, weight loss and fatty stools. Symptoms usually last 2–4 weeks. However, chronic symptoms can develop in 50% of individuals and in the absence of acute illness.
- Malabsorption can result in significant weight loss, with malabsorption of fats, sugars, carbohydrates, vitamin A, vitamin B_{12} and folate. Acquired lactose intolerance can occur in 40% of patients. Stool microscopy should be done to confirm the diagnosis.

The mainstay of treatment is oral metronidazole for 5–7 days. Alternatively, albendazole orally daily for 5 days or single-dose tinidazole can be used.

Entamoeba histolytica

The protozoan *Entamoeba histolytica* causes amebiasis, and is transmitted by the fecal–oral route (Figure 11-5). It has two forms: a *cyst* stage which is infective, and a *trophozoite* stage which is invasive. High-risk persons are from poor socio-economic groups, travelers and migrants.

E. histolytica can cause both intestinal and extraintestinal complications.

- Intestinal complications:
  - » Amebic dysentery/colitis—treatment with oral metronidazole 500–750 mg three times a day for 7–10 days, followed by a luminal agent, paromomycin, or iodoquinol
- Extraintestinal complications:
  - » Pulmonary—empyema, often secondary to liver abscess via development of an effusion, or rupture of liver abscess into the chest cavity or hematogenous spread. Factors associated with development of this complication include malnutrition, chronic alcoholism and atrial septal defect with left-to-right shunt
  - » Cardiac—pericarditis, secondary to rupture of liver abscess from left lobe of liver
  - » Brain—abscess secondary from hematogenous spread
  - » Spleen—abscess
  - » Amebic liver abscess.

Amebic liver abscess

- These patients present with fever and right upper quadrant pain with concurrent diarrhea in one-third of cases. Median incubation is about 12 weeks.
- Occasional patients can present with chronic symptoms of fever, weight loss and abdominal pain. These patients often present with anemia and hepatomegaly.
- Blood tests usually reveal leukocytosis (>10,000/mm³) without eosinophilia.

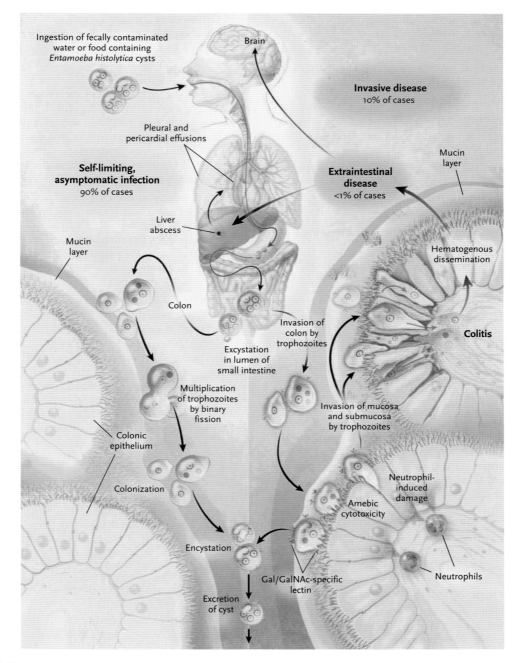

Figure 11-5 Lifecycle of *Entamoeba histolytica*

From Haque R, Huston CD, Hughes M et al. Amebiasis. N Engl
J Med 2003;348(16):1565–73.

- Liver function tests show elevation of alkaline phosphatase in 80% of cases, and hepatic transaminases may also be raised.
- Stool examination is positive in 75% of patients.
- Ultrasound, computed tomography (CT) or magnetic resonance imaging (MRI) can aid in the diagnosis of amebic liver abscess.
- Serological testing to detect antibodies is positive in 92–97% at the time of presentation, although it may be negative in the first 7 days. Indirect hemagglutination is the most sensitive method for detecting the antibodies. In some endemic areas, up to 25% of uninfected individuals have anti-amebic antibodies.

Treatment involves a tissue agent followed by a luminal agent, even if stool culture is negative.

- Use tissue amebicides to eradicate the invasive trophozoite forms in the liver.
- After completion of treatment with tissue amebicides, administer luminal amebicides for eradication of the asymptomatic colonization state.

- Failure to use luminal agents can lead to relapse of infection in approximately 10% of patients.

In general:

- metronidazole, tinidazole, emetine, and dehydroemetine are active in invaded tissues
- chloroquine is active only in the liver
- tetracycline acts on the bowel wall
- paromomycin (10 days), and iodoquinol (20 days) are luminal agents only.

The use of oral metronidazole 500–750 mg three times a day for 7–10 days results in a cure rate of 90%.

- IV treatment has no significant advantage, because metronidazole is well absorbed in the gut.
- Percutaneous drainage is not indicated for treatment, as it does not shorten recovery time.
- Asymptomatic patients with *E. histolytica* should be treated with an intraluminal agent alone.

Factitious diarrhea

CLINICAL PEARL

Think of factitious diarrhea when there is an increased fecal osmolar gap (suggesting osmotic laxatives). Urine analysis is helpful in making the diagnosis.

The most common **cause** is surreptitious laxative abuse. Ninety percent of patients with factitious diarrhea are women. These patients often seek care from many physicians and have multiple admissions.

The **key clinical features** include chronic watery diarrhea that is high in frequency and volume. About 50% of patients complain of nocturnal bowel movements. This presentation is not common in patients with irritable bowel syndrome. Other symptoms include cramping abdominal pain, weight loss and, in severe cases, cachexia. In addition, concurrent nausea and vomiting may be present in patients with anorexia and bulimia.

The **diagnosis** is confirmed by the following methods:

- Stool analysis—measurement of stool osmolality.
  - » Increase in fecal osmolar gap (> 50 mOsm/kg), indicating the presence of unmeasured solute which can be due to laxatives containing magnesium, sorbitol, lactose, lactulose or polyethylene glycol as active ingredients.
  - » Measured fecal osmolality is helpful in factitious diarrhea resulting from the addition of water in the stool; this diagnosis is suspected if the measured stool osmolality is lower than of plasma, since the colon cannot dilute stool to an osmolality which is less than that of plasma.
  - » It is important to note that if stool osmolality is higher than that of plasma, one should consider contamination with concentrated urine (particularly if there is a high sodium concentration, urea and creatinine), or stool that was not processed in a timely manner, leading to fermentation and thus an increase in osmotically active substances.

- High stool magnesium levels indicate potential abuse of magnesium-containing laxatives.
- Urine analysis—testing the urine may reveal evidence of some stimulant laxatives such as bisacodyl, but will not detect senna.
- Endoscopic appearance—melanosis coli (dark-brown discoloration of the colon with lymph follicles shining through as pale patches) occurs with anthraquinone-containing laxatives; this is not seen with osmotic or diphenolic agents. It develops within 4 months of the onset of laxative ingestion and disappears in the same timeframe when laxatives are discontinued.

Rarely, dilatation of the colon can occur as a consequence of prolonged stimulant laxative abuse, and this is termed a *cathartic colon*.

The mainstay of **treatment** involves stopping the medication and obtaining a psychiatric evaluation to help maintain abstinence from these agents.

Clostridium difficile infection (CDI)

Diarrhea associated with *C. difficile* occurs in patients infected with toxin-producing (exotoxin A and B) *C. difficile* bacteria. Toxin B is more potent.

The term 'pseudomembranous colitis' refers to the endoscopic appearance of scattered white-yellow mucosal plaques which appear in the colon (Figure 11-6). However, the presence of *C. difficile* in the colon does not always infer active infection. Asymptomatic carriage has been reported in 14% of hospitalized patients receiving antibiotics and up to 70% of healthy infants.

CLINICAL PEARLS

- *Clostridium difficile* infection is usually associated with antibiotic exposure, PPI use or hospitalization, although community-acquired infection (without recent hospitalization or antibiotic exposure) is being increasingly recognized.
- Patients with inflammatory bowel disease are at risk of *C. difficile* infection. It is important to rule this out prior to starting immunosuppressive agents.

The **risk factors** associated with the development of CDI include current or recurrent use of antibiotics, advanced age, hospitalization and comorbid illness. Inflammatory bowel disease is also a risk factor.

The **key clinical features** include the following:

- frequent semi-formed or watery non-bloody diarrhea
- patients with severe fulminant disease may develop ileus, peritoneal signs or shock
- peripheral edema or ascites has been observed due to secondary protein-losing enteropathy and hypoalbuminemia
- other clinical signs that are nonspecific include low-grade fever, diffuse abdominal tenderness and dehydration.

The **diagnosis** is usually made by detection of *C. difficile* genes on a polymerase chain reaction (PCR) assay in a patient with appropriate symptoms. Enzyme immunoassay (EIA) for toxins A and B in the stool can also be used. It

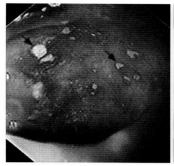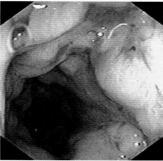

Figure 11-6 Endoscopic appearance of *Clostridium difficile*-associated pseudomembranous colitis. Plaquelike, cream-colored pseudomembranes overlie erythematous mucosa and have become confluent in the foreground

From Weidner N et al. Modern surgical pathology, 2nd ed. Philadelphia: Elsevier, 2009.

is important to note that some strains only produce exotoxin A *or* exotoxin B. The EIA test is close to 100% specific, but sensitivity is limited by the fact that the EIA does not detect small concentrations of toxins. Endoscopic findings show pseudomembranes with patchy, simple erythema, and friability with confluent ulcers, but these are found in only a small subset of patients.

Treatment

The treatment of CDI involves four main tenets, once the diagnosis is confirmed:

1 All causative antibiotics should be stopped unless absolutely required for patient care.
2 Initiate appropriate antibiotics for the treatment of CDI.
3 Monitor for signs of complications.
4 Initiate infection-control measures.

Management of *C. difficile* infection options include:

1 **First infective episode**
   a Mild-moderate: Oral vancomycin 125 mg qid for 10 days (oral metronidazole 500 mg tid if vancomycin not available)
   b Severe: Fidaxomicin 200 mg bid for 10 days
   c Fulminant disease: oral vancomycin 500 mg qid AND IV metronidazole 500 mg tid
2 **First recurrence**
   a If initially treated with metronidazole—oral vancomycin 125 mg qid for 10 days, or
   b Pulse tapered oral vancomycin, e.g. 125 mg qid for 1 week, then tid for 1 week, then bid for 1 week, then daily for 1 week, or
   c. Fidaxomicin 200 mg orally bid for 10 days
3 **Recurrent episodes**
   a Fecal microbial transplant (FMT), or pulse tapered vancomycin, or fidaxomicin, or vancomycin for 14 days followed by rifaximin for 14 days.

Most patients (>90%) will respond to treatment for 7 days with metronidazole or vancomycin after initial uncomplicated CDI. However, up to 30% will develop at least one recurrence and at least half of those will proceed to further relapses.

Fecal transplantation is now an established and highly efficacious therapy for recurrent C.Diff infection. A stool suspension from a screened donor is administered to the colon via an enema or during a colonoscopy. The treatment is highly efficacious. The aim is to restore normal fecal microbiota.

Malabsorption

Overview

Malabsorption is pathological interference with the normal physiological sequence of the *digestion* (intraluminal process), *absorption* (mucosal process) and *transport* (post-mucosal events) of nutrients. Mechanisms of intestinal malabsorption include:

- infective agents
- structural defects
- mucosal abnormality
- enzyme deficiencies
- systemic disease affecting the GI tract.

The most common causes of malabsorption are celiac disease, chronic pancreatitis, gastrectomy, Crohn's disease and a lactase deficiency. It is important in the medical history to ask the patient if they have diarrhea. If the patient admits to frequent stooling and has characteristics of steatorrhea, intestinal malabsorption is the most likely cause of weight loss.

Screening

Patients should be screened for:

- *low* albumin, iron and calcium levels
- *low* carotene and cholesterol levels, and
- a prolonged prothrombin time (PT) or international normalized ratio (INR).

If screening tests are abnormal, specific tests will be required to unravel the etiology.

Whipple's disease

This is a rare cause of malabsorption. *Tropheryma whipplei* is a Gram-positive actinomycete, most commonly causing infection in the 4th or 6th decade with a male predominance. It is more common in people involved in farm-related trades.

The clinical features include:

- diarrhea and steatorrhea, commonly
- abdominal pain, bloating, anorexia and weight loss
- migratory arthralgias or chronic polyarthritis, which is a common extraintestinal symptom and usually precedes the diagnosis
- neurological symptoms, also commonly, with dementia, paralysis of gaze and myoclonus.

Other features include pigmentation, low-grade fever, fatigue and generalized weakness.

On clinical examination, hyperpigmentation and peripheral lymphadenopathy are the most common features. Other findings include fever, peripheral arthritis, heart murmurs, pleural or pericardial friction rub, ocular abnormalities and cranial nerve involvement, and dementia.

If Whipple's disease is suspected, biopsy is essential. GI features and arthritis occur early in the disease course, whereas central nervous system (CNS) symptoms are late.

> ### CLINICAL PEARL
>
> Whipple's disease is fatal if missed. Consider Whipple's in the setting of: 1. diarrhea (malabsorption), 2. weight loss, 3. abdominal pain and 4. arthralgias (seronegative migratory polyarthritis). Other features include pigmentation, fever of unknown origin, lymphadenopathy and progressive neurological disease.

Diagnosis

- Small-intestinal mucosal biopsy is diagnostic.
- Findings of infiltration of the lamina propria of the small intestine by periodic acid–Shiff (PAS)-positive macrophages containing Gram-positive, acid-fast-negative bacilli accompanied by lymphatic dilatation is specific and diagnostic of Whipple's disease. PCR testing confirms the diagnosis.
- Differential diagnosis is lymphoma, *Mycobacterium avium* complex, and celiac disease.

There are key differences from celiac disease:

- Whipple's is caused by a pathogen and associated with occupational exposure (farm trades)
- there is no family history associated with this disorder
- malabsorption is due to obstruction of lymphatics rather than villous atrophy
- negative anti-gliadin and anti-tTG antibody
- small-bowel histology does not improve with a gluten-free diet
- small-bowel histology does improve with antibiotic treatment.

Treatment

- Treatment is trimethoprim 160 mg + sulfamethoxazole 800 mg (TMP-SMX) given twice daily for 1 year. Initial parenteral penicillin G and streptomycin for 10–14 days may be of additional benefit, resulting in a lower relapse rate.
- For patients allergic to TMP-SMX, parenteral penicillin and streptomycin for 10–14 days followed by oral penicillin V potassium or ampicillin for 1 year is a reasonable alternative.
- Repeat small-bowel biopsy following treatment is required to ensure eradication.

Relapses are common; gram-positive bacilli on electron microscopy suggest inadequate treatment. Repeated courses of antibiotics are needed in that circumstance.

Microscopic colitis

> ### CLINICAL PEARL
>
> Consider microscopic colitis in a middle-aged patient with chronic diarrhea without bleeding.

Symptoms of microscopic colitis include chronic watery diarrhea with abdominal pain. Some patients might present with mild weight loss or fecal incontinence. Colonoscopy is normal, but biopsies are diagnostic with increased intraepithelial lymphocytosis (>10–20 lymphocytes per 100 epithelial cells; normal is <5).

There are two subtypes:

- *collagenous colitis* is similar with respect to clinical and histological features, but with thickened subepithelial collagen band
- *lymphocytic colitis* has a normal collagen band.

There is an association with autoimmune conditions, e.g. celiac disease; however, there is no cancer risk associated with this condition.

Treatment

- Antidiarrheal agents (loperamide or diphenoxylate) are useful in mild cases. Bismuth subsalicylate, mesalamine or cholestyramine may be beneficial.
- Oral budesonide is highly effective but relapse is common and some patients stay on the lowest effective dose long term. Systemic corticosteroids are rarely needed.
- Disease can either be self-limiting, or follow a waxing and waning course requiring maintenance treatment.

Tropical sprue

Tropical sprue is an acquired disease of unknown etiology which occurs mainly in patients who have visited the tropics (a zone centered on the equator and limited in latitude by the tropic of Cancer in the Northern Hemisphere and the tropic of Capricorn in the Southern Hemisphere).

- It may be caused by an infection, but no organism has been identified.
- The clue to diagnosis is chronic diarrhea with recent prolonged (> 6 weeks) travel to the tropics.
- The clinical features include diarrhea, steatorrhea, abdominal pain, weight loss, fatigue, glossitis, nutritional deficiencies and anorexia. Patients often present with megaloblastic anemia (due to folate deficiency).
- The diagnosis is one of exclusion, especially of protozoa.

Tropical sprue differs from celiac disease in that:

- it is probably caused by an infective pathogen and is not immune-mediated
- there is no family history
- no gender predilection is present
- anti-gliadin and anti-tTG are negative
- the small-bowel histology is similar to that of celiac disease, but affects both proximal and distal regions (celiac disease is more proximal)

- severe folate deficiency is more common in tropical sprue, while iron-deficiency anemia is more common in celiac disease
- histology does not improve with a gluten-free diet
- histology improves with antibiotic treatment.

Treatment involves broad-spectrum antibiotics and folic acid. Tetracycline is the antibiotic of choice, for 3–6 months. Alternatively, sulfamethoxazole/trimethoprim may be used for a similar duration. Clinical response is rapid (within weeks) and complete. Relapse is common if the patient returns to or remains in the same tropical environment.

Small intestinal bacterial overgrowth (SIBO)

This is defined traditionally by the quantitative culture of aspirated juice from the proximal jejunum, or noninvasively by a glucose hydrogen breath test. More than 10^5 colony-forming units of bacteria per milliliter of aspirate (CFU/mL) is diagnostic by culture but $>10^3$ is abnormal.

The normal gut flora is maintained by five major mechanisms: gastric acid secretion, pancreatic enzyme secretion, small-intestinal motility, structural integrity of the GI tract, and an intact gut immune system.

SIBO is usually a byproduct of structural abnormalities involving the GI tract or alteration in gut motor, secretory or immunological function. A clue to the presence of bacterial overgrowth is the finding of low serum vitamin B_{12} levels and high serum folate levels (from bacterial production).

Clinical features

- Diarrhea, abdominal bloating, distension and florid malabsorption
- Nutritional deficiencies (vitamin B_{12} and fat-soluble vitamins). Megaloblastic anemia, follicular hyperkeratosis (vitamin A deficiency), and peripheral neuropathy may occur as a consequence. Serum levels of folate and vitamin K are usually normal or elevated, due to bacterial synthesis

- Diarrhea is multifactorial, with contributions from malabsorption, maldigestion, bile acid deconjugation and protein-losing enteropathy

Treatment

- Antibiotics are given to acutely decontaminate the small bowel.
  » Antibiotics should be active against aerobic and anaerobic enteric bacteria.
  » Amoxicillin and clavulanic acid, ciprofloxacin, norfloxacin, metronidazole, neomycin or doxycycline for 7–14 days are options. Rifaximin is also effective, but costly.
  » If patients have recurrent bouts of SIBO, then rotating courses of antibiotics every 4–6 weeks are effective.
- A low-carbohydrate, high-fat diet may minimize the available substrate for bacterial metabolism and is recommended.

Eosinophilic gastroenteritis (EGE)

This is a rare eosinophilic disease that can affect any part of the gut. It is subdivided into primary and secondary EGE.

- Causes of **secondary** eosinophilic gastroenteritis are hypereosinophilic syndrome, celiac disease, Crohn's disease, vasculitis (eosinophilic granulomatosis with polyangiitis, polyarteritis nodosa and scleroderma), parasites and drug hypersensitivity.
- **Primary** eosinophilic gastroenteritis is diagnosed if histopathology demonstrates predominant eosinophilic infiltration with absence of other causes of eosinophilia and no eosinophilic involvement of organs outside the GI tract. The clinical presentation is dependent on the layer of involvement (Table 11-5).

The mainstay of treatment is dietary elimination and corticosteroids. It is important to rule out *Strongyloides* before starting corticosteroids.

Relapse is common. Maintenance with dietary modification (in the form of an elemental diet) may help in difficult cases.

Table 11-5 Clinical presentation of eosinophilic gastroenteritis

LAYER OF INVOLVEMENT	DISTRIBUTION	CLINICAL FEATURES
Mucosal Most common Associated with food allergy (15%)	60%	Nausea, vomiting, abdominal pain, diarrhea Gastrointestinal hemorrhage Anemia Malabsorption Protein-losing enteropathy Failure to thrive
Muscularis propria	30%	Symptoms of bowel obstruction
Serosal	10%	Ascites (eosinophilic) High peripheral eosinophilia

Chronic idiopathic intestinal pseudo-obstruction (CIIP)

CLINICAL PEARL

Suspect the diagnosis of chronic idiopathic intestinal pseudo-obstruction in a young person with persistently dilated small or large bowel, and symptoms of bowel obstruction without an identifiable anatomical cause.

This rare syndrome is characterized by recurrent and progressive symptoms of intestinal obstruction without an identifiable anatomical cause. Affected parts of the small bowel or colon appear dilated on radiographical studies.

Causes are related to disorders of the enteric nervous system (neuropathy) or smooth muscle (myopathy), with examples being degenerative neuropathies, paraneoplastic phenomenona and genetic abnormalities. Small-bowel or colonic transit studies are the tests of choice, as specialized small-bowel or colonic manometry is not readily available. Full-thickness biopsies obtained at surgery often show abnormalities in the enteric nervous system and with the interstitial cells of Cajal.

Treatment focuses on nutritional supplementation, with cautious use of pro-motility agents. Surgery and total parenteral nutrition is often employed in severe cases. Overall the prognosis is poor.

Short bowel syndrome

CLINICAL PEARL

The presence or absence of an intact colon has a major impact on whether gut failure due to small bowel resection occurs.

Short bowel syndrome results when an inadequate length of intestine is available for nutrient absorption. In adults the most common cause is surgical resection of diseased bowel, but in children congenital abnormalities and resection following necrotizing enterocolitis predominate.

CLINICAL PEARL

The most common cause for small bowel syndrome in adults is resection due to Crohn's disease, followed by resection due to bowel obstruction with strangulation or mesenteric infarction.

Whether short bowel syndrome develops depends on several factors:
- length of the remaining small bowel
- mucosal integrity of the remaining small bowel
- presence or absence of the colon.

As a general rule, 100 cm of small bowel is sufficient to avoid short bowel syndrome if the colon is intact. Without a colon, persons with 200 cm of remaining small bowel can manage after a long period of adaptation. Total parental nutrition (TPN) is required if intestinal failure (inability to absorb sufficient nutrients) has occurred.

Remember: the length of remaining gut is a crude predictor of whether intestinal failure will occur. Measurement of plasma citrulline concentrations is a more sensitive measure of absorptive capacity and can help predict the likelihood of resuming an oral diet.

CLINICAL PEARL

Adaptation to a short gut takes years—many patients can avoid long-term parenteral nutrition if carefully managed and followed up.

Patients with short bowel syndrome need to consume frequent small meals, which should be nutrient-dense. Isotonic fluids that also contain carbohydrates are often useful, and supplemental nocturnal feeding (via nasogastric or gastrostomy tube) can help some patients avoid TPN.

It is important to know the main complications of long-term TPN:
- sepsis (bacterial and fungal) associated with IV catheters
- vascular thrombosis
- hepatic dysfunction
- small-bowel bacterial overgrowth due to stasis.

Small-bowel transplantation is an evolving treatment and is a therapeutic option in highly selected patients.

NUTRITIONAL DEFICIENCY

Vitamins are categorized as *water-soluble* or *fat-soluble*:
- fat-soluble vitamins include vitamins A, D, E and K
- water-soluble vitamins include vitamins B and C.

Clues to identifying vitamin deficiency are outlined in Table 11-6, along with treatment options.

Clinical clues to malnutrition

Clinical assessment of the severity of malnutrition:
- biochemical parameters such as low albumin or prealbumin are important clues
- malnutrition is said to be present when bodyweight is <70% of ideal or there is weight loss of >20% over 6 months
- body fat and lean muscle are estimated using anthropometric measurements
- a low triceps skinfold thickness is indicative of malnutrition
- a weak hand grip strength during physical examination can indicate malnutrition.

Nutritional assessment in end-stage liver disease

Protein energy malnutrition in end-stage liver disease is multifactorial:
- poor oral intake
- restrictive diets (overzealous sodium-restricted diets)
- altered taste sensation

Table 11-6 Clinical clues in identifying vitamin deficiency

CLINICAL FEATURES	CAUSES AND DIAGNOSIS	TREATMENT AND NOTES
Vitamin A deficiency		
Can take years to cause symptoms Xerophthalmia causing night blindness and Bitot's spots (conjunctival squamous cell proliferation and keratinization) is the earliest sign Poor bone growth Follicular hyperkeratosis Impaired immune system Conjunctival xerosis Keratomalacia	Low dietary intake (preformed vitamin A is from animals; provitamin A is found in plants) Diagnosis is made by measuring serum retinol levels	Vitamin A supplementation Daily requirement (RDA) for adult males is 3000 IU and for females is 2300 IU Vitamin A toxicity is related to chronic ingestion ($\geq$25,000 IU/d); serum retinol levels are not helpful as vitamin A is stored in the liver
Vitamin B$_{12}$ deficiency		
Can take several years to show symptoms Macrocytic anemia Smooth tongue In severe deficiency—subacute combined degeneration of the spinal cord Peripheral sensory neuropathy affecting large and small fibers Dementia	Low dietary intake Pernicious anemia Terminal ileum disease	Vitamin B$_{12}$ supplementation If both folate and vitamin B$_{12}$ deficiency are present, you must replace vitamin B$_{12}$ first to avoid subacute combined degeneration of the spinal cord
Vitamin B$_6$ (pyridoxine) deficiency		
Can take weeks to become symptomatic Glossitis Cheilosis Vomiting Seizures Scrotal dermatitis	Mainly secondary to drugs, e.g. isoniazid, cycloserine, penicillamine, phenobarbital Can measure serum levels of pyridoxal-phosphate	Vitamin supplementation Large doses can cause both impaired position and vibratory sense
Vitamin B$_2$ (riboflavin) deficiency		
Can take weeks to become symptomatic Normochromic normocytic anemia Sore throat and magenta tongue Glossitis Cheilosis Seborrheic dermatitis in perianal area, nose	Associated with phenothiazine and tricyclic antidepressants	Vitamin supplementation
Vitamin B$_1$ (thiamine) deficiency		
Can take weeks to become symptomatic Wet beriberi—heart failure secondary to cardiomyopathy Dry beriberi (neuropathy)— Wernicke encephalopathy (WE)—nystagmus, ophthalmoplegia and ataxia Peripheral neuropathy Korsakoff syndrome	Low dietary intake Alcoholic patients, chronic dialysis patients IV glucose can precipitate WE: give thiamine before glucose. Can directly measure thiamine levels in serum	Thiamine supplementation

continues

Table 11-6 Clinical clues in identifying vitamin deficiency *continued*

CLINICAL FEATURES	CAUSES AND DIAGNOSIS	TREATMENT AND NOTES
Vitamin C deficiency (scurvy)		
First symptoms are petechial hemorrhage and ecchymoses Bleeding, swollen gums (see Figure 11-7A) Hyperkeratotic papules Hemorrhagia into joints, nail beds Loosening of teeth Periosteal hemorrhages Coiled hairs Impaired wound healing Weak bones Sjögren's syndrome	Low dietary intake	Vitamin C supplementation Large doses can cause oxalate renal stones and impaired absorption of vitamin B_{12}
Iodine deficiency		
Hypothyroidism	Low dietary intake Drug and alcohol abusers	Improve dietary intake
Niacin deficiency (pellagra)		
The 3 'D's: —*dermatitis* (sun-exposed areas) —*diarrhea* —altered mental state—*depression* to dementia to psychosis Hyperpigmentation (see Figure 11-7B) Glossitis Stomatitis	Low dietary intake; tryptophan is used in the body to make niacin Carcinoid syndrome (tryptophan is used up) Isoniazid (increased excretion of tryptophan—pyroxidine supplement must be used concurrently to prevent this) Hartnup disease (autosomal recessive, cerebellar ataxia)	Replacement treatment
Zinc deficiency		
Rash (face, body: pustular, bullous, vesicular, seborrheic, acneiform; see Figure 11-7C), skin ulcers, alopecia, dysgeusia Impaired immunity Night blindness Decreased spermatogenesis Diarrhea	Low dietary intake	Zinc supplementation
Vitamin E deficiency		
Peripheral sensory and motor neuropathy Hemolytic anemia Retinal degeneration Dry skin		Vitamin E supplementation Large doses can potentiate the effects of oral anticoagulation
Vitamin K deficiency		
Bleeding tendency Easy bruisability	Low dietary intake Systemic diseases that cause fat-soluble vitamin malabsorption Can detect by checking coagulation profile (INR and PT)	Vitamin K supplementation

CLINICAL FEATURES	CAUSES AND DIAGNOSIS	TREATMENT AND NOTES
Vitamin D deficiency		
The major source of vitamin D is from sun exposure. Secondary sources are from diet or supplementation and intestinal absorption In the liver, vitamin D undergoes hydroxylation by 25-hydroxylase to 25-hydroxyvitamin D, 25 (OH)D. Further hydroxylation takes place in the kidneys to activated vitamin D (1,25-dihydroxyvitamin D). Activated vitamin D is important in bone mineralization Vitamin D deficiency leads to: —rickets in children —osteomalacia in adults —hypocalcemia —secondary hyperparathyroidism which leads to phosphaturia	Decreased exposure to the sun Decreased intestinal absorption from the intestine Renal disease Systemic diseases that cause fat malabsorption Can be directly measured by checking for serum 25(OH)D	Increase casual exposure to sunlight Vitamin D supplementation: —25(OH)D (Ostelin 1000) —activated vitamin D (calcitriol; this form should be used in renal disease) The RDA for vitamin D is 600 IU for adults Avoid excessive doses, as toxicity can cause hypercalcemia, confusion, polyuria, polydipsia, anorexia, vomiting and muscle weakness Long-term toxicity results in bone demineralization and pain

INR, international normalized ratio; RDA, recommended dietary allowance; PT, prothrombin time.

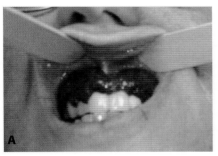 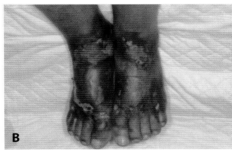 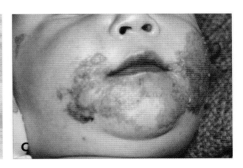

Figure 11-7 Signs of (A) scurvy, (B) pellagra and (C) zinc deficiency

From: (A) Li R, Byers K and Walvekar RR. Gingival hypertrophy: a solitary manifestation of scurvy. Am J Otolaryngol 2008;29(6):426–8. (B) Piqué-Duran E et al. Pellagra: a clinical, histopathological, and epidemiological study of 7 cases [in Spanish]. Actas Dermosifiliogr 2012;103(1):51–8. (C) Marks JG and Miller JJ. Lookingbill and Marks' Principles of dermatology, 5th ed. Elsevier, 2013.

- early satiety (gastric compression from ascites)
- portal hypertension associated with malabsorption
- insulin resistance (hyperinsulinemia and glucose intolerance)
- reduced glycogen capacity.

Weight is a poor indicator in end-stage liver disease due to the presence of ascites and/or peripheral edema. Malnutrition in cirrhotic patients is associated with an increased risk of complications. It is an independent predictor of mortality in cirrhosis.

Malnutrition should be assessed as shown in Table 11-7. Anthropometrical measurements of mid-arm circumference, triceps skinfold thickness and mid-arm muscle circumference should be performed.

Grip strength is a good reflection of protein status in these patients. Poor grip strength is associated with development of ascites, hepatic encephalopathy, hepatorenal syndrome, spontaneous bacterial peritonitis, and a longer stay

Table 11-7 Assessment of malnutrition

Weight	Weight lost in the last 6 months
Dietary intake	Adequate or not
Presence of gastrointestinal symptoms	Nausea, vomiting, diarrhea, anorexia
Functional capacity	
Metabolic demand	Harris–Benedict equation (HBE): estimation of resting energy expenditure Indirect calorimetry
Signs of micronutrient deficiencies	Vitamin deficiency, e.g. vitamin D, vitamin A, zinc

in intensive care post-transplant as well as increased risk of infection post-transplant.

Enteral and parenteral nutrition

- Enteral nutrition is generally the preferred route where possible because it sustains the digestive, absorptive and immunological barrier functions of the GI tract.
- Patients who are malnourished or at risk of malnutrition and have a non-functioning or inaccessible GI tract will need TPN.

Total parental nutrition (TPN)

The components in TPN include:

- essential and non-essential amino acids
- glucose
- fats
- electrolytes
- micronutrients.

These are given in an iso-osmotic liquid emulsion to provide an energy-rich solution.

TPN is used when required for patients in whom all avenues of oral feeding have been exhausted. Clinical scenarios where this may arise include:

- postoperative (bowel surgery, protracted recovery)
- severe acute pancreatitis
- severe inflammatory bowel disease
- selected patients with severe acute radiation enteritis or chemotherapy enteritis preventing meaningful enteral nutrition
- enterocutaneous fistula involving the small bowel
- short gut syndrome
- preoperative (severely malnourished patients only).

Complications

Access/catheter-related complications

- Pneumothorax/hemothorax from line insertion
- Cardiac arrhythmias
- Cardiac tamponade
- Venous thrombosis and pulmonary embolus
- Air embolus
- Infection (staphylococcal, enterococcal, *Candida*, *Klebsiella pneumoniae* and *Pseudomonas aeruginosa*. If catheter is in long-term, the patient is at risk of coagulase-negative *Staphylococcus*)
- Subacute bacterial endocarditis
- Chylothorax
- Thrombophlebitis

Systemic complications

Early complications:

- Hypophosphatemia (refeeding syndrome)
- Hypokalemia

- Hypomagnesemia
- Thiamine deficiency
- Volume overload and cardiac failure
- Hyperchloremic acidosis
- Hypoglycemia and hyperglycemia

Late complications:

- Azotemia and hyperosmolarity
- Liver dysfunction (hepatocellular or cholestatic and fatty liver)
- Acalculous cholecystitis
- Cholelithiasis with gallstone and gallbladder sludging (long-term treatment)
- Vitamin or mineral deficiency (rare)
- TPN-related nephropathy
- Metabolic bone disease (rare)
- Trace-mineral deficiency
- Essential fatty acid deficiency

Refeeding syndrome

Patients who have been malnourished for extended periods of time are at risk of refeeding syndrome when re-institution of nutrition occurs via either enteral nutrition or TPN. When oral nutrition is re-introduced, close monitoring of fluid and electrolyte status is mandatory.

In the starvation phase, intracellular electrolyte stores and phosphate stores are depleted. The key energy source during starvation is from fat. Upon refeeding, the body's metabolism is switched to carbohydrate as the main source of energy. The basal metabolic rate increases with increased production of insulin and further intracellular uptake of phosphate, potassium, magnesium, glucose and thiamine, causing significant deficiencies. Multi-organ involvement occurs as a consequence in refeeding syndrome.

The risk of developing refeeding syndrome is directly related to the amount of weight loss that has occurred and the rapidity of the weight restoration process.

High-risk groups

- Patients with eating disorders (anorexia nervosa/bulimia)
- Chronic malnutrition
- A prolonged fasting period
- Prolonged IV hydration therapy

Complications of refeeding syndrome

- Electrolyte disturbance
- Rhabdomyolysis, muscle weakness and tetany
- Cardiac failure and volume overload
- Cardiac arrhythmias (bradycardia) and labile blood pressure
- Respiratory failure due to muscle weakness from hypophosphatemia
- Seizures
- Coma and death

Box 11-8

Treatment of irritable bowel syndrome

Relieving constipation	**Relieving diarrhea**	**Relieving pain**
• Bulking agent (psyllium)	• Antidiarrheal (loperamide)	• Spasmolytics such as anticholinergics, peppermint oil or mebeverine
• Laxatives—try osmotic first, then bisacodyl	• Bulking agent (low dose)	
• Secretagogues e.g. linaclotide	• Bile-salt binder (e.g. cholestyramine)	• Tricyclic antidepressant (low dose)
	• Rifaximin	
	• Tricyclic antidepressant (low dose)	

LARGE BOWEL

Irritable bowel syndrome (IBS)

Irritable bowel syndrome is common, with more women than men affected. Currently no diagnostic test is useful apart from excluding other causes for symptoms. The diagnosis is based on taking the history (Rome IV criteria—see Box 11-5).

- Patients with IBS all have abdominal pain and suffer predominantly from either constipation or diarrhea, although the mixed type is also common. Symptoms are commonly made worse by eating and emotional stress, while defecation often gives relief.

CLINICAL PEARL

Irritable bowel syndrome does not cause anemia, weight loss or malnutrition.

- The discomfort can be felt anywhere in the abdomen and is often associated with bloating.

Young patients with classical features and no alarm features require few if any tests, but a full blood count, thyroid-stimulating hormone and celiac serology at baseline are often done. Onset of symptoms after the age of 50 years or abnormal baseline testing (elevated C-reactive protein, low serum albumin) is highly suggestive of alternative pathology. Patients with anemia, fever, significant weight loss, or rectal bleeding always require further evaluation. A negative fecal calprotectin (<50 microg/g) usually rules out IBD.

CLINICAL PEARL

Patients presenting with new-onset altered bowel habit after the age of 50 need a colonoscopy to exclude bowel cancer or other pathology. Patients rarely present with new-onset IBS after the age of 50.

The pathogenesis of IBS is poorly understood, but current hypotheses revolve around abnormal intestinal mobility, visceral hypersensitivity, food sensitivity, and abnormal gut microbiota, coupled with genetic and environmental triggers. Post-infectious irritable bowel can occur after an episode of gastroenteritis, and diarrhea is often the predominant symptom.

Treatment

Treatment aims at relieving the predominant symptoms (Box 11-8).

Provide reassurance, explanation and try to reduce life stressors. Whenever possible, non-pharmacological approaches should be trialed. The following treatments have robust evidence to support efficacy for improving global IBS symptoms:

- structured patient education
- moderate exercise
- adherence to an IBS specific diet or low FODMAP diet (fermentable oligosaccharides, disaccharides, monosaccharides and polyols) to identify food precipitants
- hypnotherapy and cognitive behavioral therapy.

Avoiding exacerbating foods is recommended.

Constipation

Constipation is common, and the great majority of patients affected are female. Constipation is a *symptom*, not a diagnosis.

Common symptoms:

- decreased frequency of stool (<3/week)
- excessive straining to open bowels
- hard stools
- feeling of incomplete evacuation.

Conditions causing constipation can be classified as shown in Table 11-8.

Investigations

- Basic blood tests to exclude hypothyroidism, diabetes mellitus and hypercalcemia
- History and physical examination detect most cases, but a plain abdominal X-ray is often useful, particularly if the patient cannot give a reliable history (dementia, psychiatric disease, children)

CLINICAL PEARL

In the setting of constipation, rectal examination is mandatory—fecal impaction, fissures, pelvic-floor dysfunction and rectal prolapse can readily be detected at the bedside.

Table 11-8 Classification of conditions causing constipation

CLASSIFICATION	EXAMPLE CONDITION/CAUSE
No structural abnormality	Inadequate fiber intake Constipation-predominant irritable bowel syndrome Idiopathic slow-transit constipation Pelvic-floor dyssynergia (paradoxical contraction on straining blocking defecation; rectal examination with and without straining can help identify; refer for anorectal manometry and biofeedback)
Structural abnormality	Anal fissure or stenosis Colon cancer or stricture Aganglionosis (Hirschprung, Chagas) Abnormal colonic muscle (myopathy, muscular dystrophy) Idiopathic megarectum and/or megacolon
Neurological causes	Diabetic autonomic neuropathy Spinal cord damage or disease, e.g. multiple sclerosis Parkinson's disease Anorexia nervosa (if you don't eat you don't poop)
Endocrine or metabolic causes	Hypothyroidism Hypercalcemia Pregnancy
Drug side-effects	Calcium-channel blockers Opiates Tricyclic antidepressants $5HT_3$ antagonists

Adapted from Talley NJ. Clinical gastroenterology: a practical problem-based approach. Sydney: Churchill Livingstone, 2011.

Table 11-9 Types of laxative

LAXATIVE TYPE	EXAMPLE	NOTES
Dietary fiber (bulking)	Psyllium, bran, methylcellulose	Safe, cheap, effective (unless slow colonic transit)
Osmotic	Lactulose, polyethylene glycol, sorbitol	Safe, can be used long-term
Stimulant	Senna, bisacodyl	Effective, but can cause cramps and fail to relieve constipation
Stool-softener	Docusate, poloxalkol	Safe, but less effective than osmotic laxatives

More advanced testing is reserved for patients where a simple reversible cause has not been established *and* where there has been no response to basic therapy (as described below).

- Colonic transit study—examines transit time by means of a radio-opaque marker.
- Balloon expulsion test—the ability to expel a water-filled balloon is tested. If the patient is unable to do this or it takes more than 2 minutes, this is suggestive of dyssynergic defecation.
- Anorectal manometry and balloon expulsion testing are useful tests for pelvic-floor dysfunction.
- Defecography (barium or MRI)—defines anatomy in difficult cases.

Treatment

Initially, most patients should be given a trial of a basic treatment consisting of:

- consider increased dietary intake of fiber (>30 g/daily is required)
- laxatives (preferably osmotic, e.g. polyethylene glycol) (Table 11-9).

Those not responding should undergo further investigation. If pelvic-floor dysfunction is present, biofeedback is useful in selected and motivated patients. If IBS is present, specific treatments for this condition should be trialed (see above).

For many patients constipation is a lifelong condition, and regular daily therapy is required for most.

In addition to laxatives, newer drugs are now available, but should be prescribed only when a trial of osmotic laxatives has failed and an evacuation disorder has been excluded. Newer drugs include:

- Prucalopride
  - » 5HT$_4$-receptor agonist (prokinetic)
  - » Involves direct stimulation of enterokinetic activity
  - » Nausea is the main limiting side-effect, and this drug is contraindicated in those with severe colonic inflammation (such as Crohn's disease or ulcerative colitis) or obstruction
- Lubiprostone
  - » Chloride-channel activator
  - » Increases intraluminal water contents
  - » Headaches and nausea are common side-effects, and this drug is contraindicated in those with partial or complete colonic obstruction, and in pregnancy
- Linaclotide
  - » Guanylate cyclase-C agonist—locally active
  - » Diarrhea is the main side-effect.
  - » Plecanatide—chloride channel activator—high cost.

A variety of enemas are available, mainly useful if colonic transit is normal but anorectal function is impaired (pelvic-floor dysfunction).

Constipation is a common symptom and underlying disorders *must* be sought. In many patients an easily reversible cause is not found, and a sensible management plan including lifestyle alteration and careful use of laxatives should be developed.

Diverticular disease

Diverticular disease and diverticulitis

A diverticulum is a sac-like protrusion of the colonic wall which can become symptomatic due to bleeding or inflammation (diverticulitis or segmental colitis). The incidence is rising and the condition is more common in the elderly. The cause of diverticulosis is unclear. Symptomatic diverticular disease is associated with a diet low in fiber and high in fat or red meat, obesity and smoking.

- Episodes of diverticulitis are often due to microperforations, and lead to fever and pain. Most patients will have left iliac fossa pain and tenderness. Systemic signs of infection are often present (fever, elevated white cell count). CT will be confirmatory.

Treatment of diverticulitis is conservative, with antibiotics (cover for both aerobic and anaerobic Gram-negative bacteria is needed).

- In mild disease, ambulatory treatment with ciprofloxacin and metronidazole is often sufficient.
- In more severe disease, hospitalization and broad-spectrum antibiotics are used.

Abscesses are often drained radiologically, and surgical resection of diseased bowel is indicated if conservative treatment fails.

A convalescent colonoscopic examination should be performed in all patients with an episode of acute diverticulitis 1–2 months after resolution to exclude colon cancer.

> **CLINICAL PEARL**
>
> Colonoscopy is contraindicated during an episode of diverticulitis. The air introduced at the time of the examination can turn a microperforation into a major perforation, resulting in peritonitis.

Inflammatory bowel disease (IBD)

Inflammatory bowel disease (IBD) is a chronic idiopathic inflammatory disorder that can be subdivided into *Crohn's disease* (CD) and *ulcerative colitis* (UC). In up to 10–15% of patients no subtype can be defined, and these are considered *indeterminate colitis*.

> **CLINICAL PEARLS**
>
> - Crohn's disease—chronic, transmural granulomatous inflammation characterized by 'skip lesions' typically in the colon and/or terminal ileum but anywhere from mouth to anus.
> - Ulcerative colitis—mucosal inflammation limited to the colon that occurs in a contiguous fashion from the rectum and extends proximally.

Clinical symptoms

Symptoms of IBD vary and may be a consequence of disease location, behavior and complications (Box 11-9).

Diagnosis

The diagnosis of CD and UC is based on a combination of clinical symptoms, endoscopy, imaging and histology. It should be differentiated from other causes of inflammation affecting the colon and/or small bowel (Table 11-10).

Crohn's disease (CD)

Crohn's disease is a chronic idiopathic inflammatory bowel disorder that leads to focal, asymmetric, transmural inflammation (where granuloma may be found) anywhere in the GI tract. It can occur at any age, with the highest peak incidence in the 2nd and 3rd decade and a smaller peak in the 5th to 7th decades of life. There is a slight female predominance.

Risk factors for CD include smoking, family history, genetic loci (NOD2/CARD 15), and geographical locations (colder climates). CD is becoming more common in underdeveloped countries, suggesting that Westernization of lifestyle and industrialization are possible environmental triggers for developing the disease.

CD can be classified with regard to location: *ileal* (~30%), *colonic* (~20%), *ileocolonic* (~40%), and *upper gastrointestinal* (<5%). Disease behavior can be classified into *inflammatory* (luminal), *stricturing*, and *fistulizing* (enteroenteral, enterovesical, enterovaginal, perianal). Symptoms of CD depend on the disease location, behavior (inflammatory, stricturing, and penetrating/fistulizing disease), and complications (fistulas and abscesses).

Box 11-9

Complications in ulcerative colitis (UC) and Crohn's disease (CD)

Acute/subacute

- Gastrointestinal bleeding (UC >> CD)
- Toxic megacolon (UC >> CD)
- Toxic fulminant colitis (UC >> CD)
- Perforation (CD >> UC)
- Small-bowel and colonic obstruction secondary to inflammation or strictures (CD)
- Abscesses—intra-abdominal, perianal (CD)

Long-term

- Colorectal cancer (UC > CD)
- Fistulas—enteroenteric, enterovesical, enterovaginal, perianal (CD)
- Fibrostenotic strictures—small bowel and colon (CD)
- Cholelithiasis—impaired bile acid reabsorption in the diseased terminal ileum (CD)
- Nephrolithiasis—impaired oxalate absorption (CD)
- Iron deficiency (CD and UC)
- Vitamin B_{12} deficiency (CD)

Extraintestinal

- Skin—erythema nodosum, pyoderma gangrenosum (Figure 11-8)
- Oral ulcers
- Ocular—episcleritis, scleritis, uveitis
- Primary sclerosing cholangitis
- Cholangiocarcinoma (rare)
- Autoimmune hepatitis
- Anemia
- Prothrombotic state
- Musculoskeletal—sacroiliitis, ankylosing spondylitis, peripheral (oligoarticular or polyarticular) arthritis, osteopenia, osteoporosis

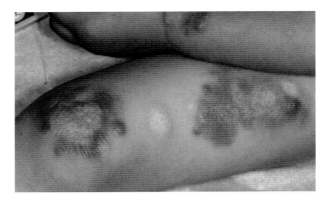

Figure 11-8 Pyoderma gangrenosum with partial response to treatment. There is persistent inflammation and evidence of healing ulcerations with residual cribriform scarring

From Paller AS and Mancini AJ. Hurwitz Clinical pediatric dermatology, 4th ed. Elsevier, 2011.

Table 11-10 Differential diagnosis of inflammatory bowel disease

Inflammatory	Collagenous colitis Lymphocytic colitis Diverticular disease Appendicitis Celiac disease
Infections	Bacteria: *Salmonella*, *Shigella*, *Escherichia coli*, *Yersinia*, *Campylobacter*, *Mycobacterium*, *Clostridium difficile* Viruses: cytomegalovirus, herpes simplex virus Parasites: amebiasis (*Entamoeba histolytica*)
Medication	Non-steroidal anti-inflammatory drugs and chemotherapy drugs
Radiation	Radiation colitis
Vascular	Ischemic colitis
Post-transplantation	Graft-versus-host disease
Eosinophilia	Eosinophilic colitis
Neoplasia	Lymphoma Carcinoid

Diagnosis

Diagnosis of CD is a combination of clinical symptoms, endoscopy, imaging and histology. *Infection should always be ruled out by checking stool studies for common bacterial pathogens and* Clostridium difficile.

- **General symptoms**
  - » Chronic diarrhea
  - » Abdominal pain
  - » Fever
  - » Weight loss
- **Specific symptoms**
  - » Perianal pain, drainage, and fevers are characteristic of perianal fistulas with or without abscesses.
  - » Hematochezia points towards colonic disease
  - » Obstructive symptoms can be seen in stricturing disease that can affect the upper and lower GI tracts.
  - » Gastric and duodenal CD is marked by epigastric pain, nausea, vomiting, or gastric outlet obstruction.
  - » Dysphagia, odynophagia or chest pain from CD are very rare.
- **Laboratory function**
  - » Raised inflammatory markers (erythrocyte sedimentation rate [ESR], C-reactive protein).
  - » Fecal calprotectin identifies active disease.

» Check a full blood count, serum iron, B$_{12}$, vitamin D levels, renal and liver function.
» Autoantibody testing in the form of pANCA (anti-neutrophil cytoplasmic autoantibodies, perinuclear pattern) and ASCA (anti-*Saccharomyces cerevisiae* antibodies)—ASCA is found in 40–80% with CD and pANCA in 20% with CD but is not useful for diagnosis.

- **Endoscopy**
  » Colonoscopy
    - abnormalities are patchy or skip, with focal inflammation adjacent to areas of normal-appearing mucosa along with polypoid mucosal changes giving a cobblestone appearance
    - ulcerations (aphthous ulcers or deep transmural ulcers)
    - strictures and fistula
  » Video-capsule endoscopy:
    - evaluates small-bowel CD that cannot be reached with upper or lower endoscopy
    - is contraindicated in stricturing CD (as the capsule can become stuck and require surgical removal)
- **Histology**—endoscopic biopsies
  » Early CD: acute inflammatory infiltrate and crypt abscesses are seen
  » Late CD: chronic inflammation, crypt distortion, crypt abscesses, and in some subjects non-caseating granulomas are seen
- **Imaging**
  » CT, MR enterography or intestinal ultrasound
    - Can assess inflammation, disease extent and complications (e.g. fistulae, abscesses, carcinoma)

Treatment

CD is a multisystem and complex disease that is not medically or surgically curable. The aim of treatment is induction and maintenance of clinical remission, with the ultimate goal of mucosal healing. The choice of medical (Table 11-11) and/or surgical treatment depends on the disease severity, location, behavior and complications.

Surgical resections, stricturoplasty, or drainage of abscesses are indicated to treat medically refractory disease or complications. Fistulizing and perianal CD are often treated with a combination of surgery and medical therapy.

In general:

- **Inflammatory CD**
  » Mild-to-moderate disease
    - *induction:* budesonide (terminal ileum and/or right colon) or corticosteroids
    - *maintenance:* immunomodulators and/or biologicals
  » Moderate-to-severe disease
    - *induction:* budesonide (terminal ileum and/or right colon) or corticosteroids or biologicals
    - *maintenance:* immunomodulators and/or biologicals
- **Stricturing CD**
  » Fibrostenotic stricture with proximal bowel dilation—surgery

» Stricture without proximal bowel dilation, possibly inflammatory stricture—trial of corticosteroids or biologicals. If no response, surgery should be considered
- **Fistulizing CD**
  » Internal fistulous tracts—biologicals and/or surgery
  » Perianal fistulizing disease—surgery, antibiotics, biologicals

Note that:
- NSAIDs can cause IBD flares and should be avoided in patients with CD.
- Smoking cessation is essential in all patients with CD, as smoking is associated with flares, more aggressive disease and an increased need for surgery.

Ulcerative colitis (UC)

Ulcerative colitis involves the colonic mucosa extending proximally from the rectum in a contiguous fashion to involve all or part of the entire colon. There is a bimodal age distribution (20s to 30s, and 50s to 60s) of disease onset, but the disease can present at any age. Males and females are equally affected. Family history and smoking cessation or smoking are risk factors. NSAIDs increase UC flares.

UC can be classified into three different phenotypes:
1 Proctitis (one-third)
2 Left-sided colitis—up to the splenic flexure (one-third)
3 Extensive colitis—past the splenic flexure (one-third).

Diagnosis

Diagnosis of UC is based on a combination of clinical symptoms, imaging, endoscopy and histology. *Infection should always be ruled out by checking stool studies for common bacterial pathogens and* Clostridium difficile.

- **Clinical symptoms**
  » Diarrhea
  » Hematochezia
  » Urgency
  » Tenesmus

Severe and fulminant UC flares require hospitalization for resuscitation, IV steroids, possible rescue therapy (infliximab or cyclosporine), and a consideration of surgery.

- *Severe UC:*
  » >6 bloody stools daily
  » Systemic symptoms: fever and tachycardia
  » Anemia
  » Elevated ESR or CRP
- *Fulminant disease:*
  » >10 bowel movements daily
  » Persistent GI bleeding
  » Systemic toxicity
  » Abdominal tenderness and distension
  » Blood transfusion requirement
  » Colonic dilatation on abdominal plain films
- **Laboratory function:**
  » Raised inflammatory markers (ESR, CRP)
  » Fecal calprotectin identifies active disease
  » Autoantibody testing—pANCA weakly associated with UC (60%) but not used routinely

Table 11-11 Medical therapy used in Crohn's disease (CD)

DRUG	RELEASE SITE	TREATMENT OF CD	SIDE-EFFECTS
Oral 5-aminosalicylates			
Sulfasalazine	Colon	Oral mesalamine for the treatment of mild CD but is at best minimally effective compared with placebo, and less effective than budesonide or corticosteroids Sulfasalazine is not useful because colonic bacteria need to cleave the drug so it is of no benefit for small intestinal disease	Rash, nausea, vomiting, headache, alopecia, and hypersensitivity reaction resulting in worsening diarrhea can occur Severe adverse events such as interstitial nephritis, pancreatitis and pneumonitis can rarely occur
Mesalamine (mesalazine)	Distal ileum, colon		
Mesalamine (mesalazine) (controlled-release)	Duodenum, jejunum, ileum, colon		
Olsalazine	Colon		
Balsalazide	Colon		
Topical 5-aminosalicylates			
Mesalamine (mesalazine) enema	Rectum, sigmoid	Topical mesalamine should only be used for distal colonic CD as adjunctive therapy to systemic therapy	
Mesalamine (mesalazine) suppository	Rectum		
Antibiotics			
Ciprofloxacin Metronidazole Amoxicillin/clavulanic acid Rifaximin	Systemic	Antibiotics are not used for the treatment of CD except for perianal CD	Ciprofloxacin: tendonitis and rupture Metronidazole: neuropathy Amoxicillin/clavulanic acid: hepatitis
Corticosteroids			
Budesonide (Entocort)	Small intestine, right colon	Induction of remission in mild-to-moderate CD involving the distal ileum and/or right colon Not used for maintenance	High first-pass metabolism More favorable side-effect profile than prednisone
Prednisone	Systemic	Induction of remission in mild-to-moderate CD Not effective for maintenance of remission	Infection, diabetes mellitus, osteoporosis, osteonecrosis, cataracts, glaucoma, and myopathy Increased risk of mortality, mood and sleep disturbance
Methylprednisolone	Systemic	Induction of remission in severe CD Not used for maintenance	As for prednisone
Immunomodulators			
6-Mercaptopurine	Systemic	Effective for maintaining a steroid-induced remission of CD Not used for induction	Allergic reactions, pancreatitis, myelosuppression, nausea, infections, hepatotoxicity, and malignancy, in particular lymphoma
Azathioprine	Systemic		
Methotrexate	Systemic	Effective at maintaining steroid-induced remission in moderate-to-severe CD Not used for induction	Rash, nausea, diarrhea, myelosuppression, hepatic fibrosis, and rarely hypersensitivity pneumonitis

DRUG	RELEASE SITE	TREATMENT OF CD	SIDE-EFFECTS
Biologicals			

Anti-TNF:
  Infliximab
  Adalimumab
  Certolizumab pegol
	Systemic
	Systemic
	Systemic (second-line, less effective)
		Have been approved for the induction and maintenance of moderate-to-severe CD
		Also used for fistulizing and perianal disease
		Combination therapy with immunomodulators is superior to monotherapy
			Infections (tuberculosis, fungal infections), autoantibody formation, psoriasis, drug-induced lupus
			Infusion reactions (infliximab), injection-site reaction (adalimumab and certolizumab), delayed hypersensitivity reaction (infliximab)
			Lymphoma (higher in combination therapy with immunomodulator)

Anti-interleukin therapy: Ustekinumab	Systemic anti-IL12/23	Second line	Nasopharyngitis (10%)
Anti-integrin therapy: Natalizumab	Systemic	Effective in the induction and maintenance of remission in moderate-to-severe CD Second-line to other biologicals due to possibly causing progressive multifocal leukoencephalopathy (PML)	Infusion reaction, hepatotoxicity, infections, and autoantibody formation
Vedolizumab	Systemic	Effective in the induction and maintenance of remission in moderate-to-severe CD	Headache, infections, abdominal pain, infusion reactions

- **Endoscopy**—colonoscopy
  » Erythema, granularity, loss of vascular pattern, friability, and ulceration
  » Changes involve the distal rectum and proceed proximally in a symmetric, continuous and circumferential pattern to involve all or part of the colon
- **Histology**—endoscopic biopsies show chronic inflammation with crypt distortion and crypt abscesses
- **Imaging**—CT or MR enterography or intestinal ultrasound
  » Used to assess for small bowel disease and rule out Crohn's disease
  » Reveals colonic bowel-wall thickening

Treatment

The goal of treatment is to induce and maintain clinical remission, with the ultimate goal of mucosal healing. Medical (Table 11-12) or surgical therapy depends on the severity of the disease and the location.

- **Distal colitis—proctosigmoiditis**
  » Oral aminosalicylates, topical mesalamine or topical steroids can be used to induce and maintain remission in mild-to-moderate distal colitis.
  » Topical mesalamine agents (enemas or suppositories) are superior to topical steroids or oral aminosalicylates. Suppositories should be used for proctitis and enemas for proctosigmoiditis.
  » Combination oral and topical aminosalicylates are more effective than either alone.

  » If refractory to the above regimens at maximum doses, budesonide extended-release or prednisone should be used for induction of remission. This is followed by thiopurines or biologicals for the maintenance of remission.
- **Left-sided ulcerative colitis and extensive colitis**
  » Induction, followed by maintenance, of mild-to-moderate extensive colitis should start with aminosalicylates in combination with topical aminosalicylates.
  » If aminosalicylates fail, oral prednisone or budesonide extended-release can be used to induce remission. This is followed by thiopurines or biologicals for maintenance.
  » Thiopurines (azathioprine and 6-mercaptopurine) are used for maintenance of remission.
  » Infliximab, adalimumab and golimumab can be used to induce and maintain remission in moderate-to-severe colitis that is steroid-refractory or not responding to thiopurines.
  » Vedolizumab has also been shown to induce and maintain remission in patients with moderate-to-severe UC.
  » Tofacitinib is an oral JAK inhibitor that can induce and maintain remission in moderate-to-severe UC.
- **Severe colitis**
  » Patients with systemic symptoms should be admitted to hospital.
  » IV methylprednisone at doses of 40–60 mg daily should be started.

Table 11-12 Medical therapy used in ulcerative colitis (UC)

DRUG	RELEASE SITE	TREATMENT OF UC	SIDE-EFFECTS
Oral 5-aminosalicylates			
Sulfasalazine	Colon	Induce and maintain remission in mild-to-moderate UC Use in combination with topical mesalamine for distal colitis	See Table 11-11. Sulfasalazine: idiosyncratic (rash, hepatitis, aplastic anemia), dose-related (nausea, hemolytic anemia, inhibits folic acid transport), oligospermia (reversible)
Mesalamine (mesalazine)	Distal ileum, colon		
Mesalamine (mesalazine) (controlled-release)	Duodenum, jejunum, ileum, colon		
Olsalazine	Colon		
Balsalazide	Colon		
Topical 5-aminosalicylates			
Mesalamine (mesalazine) enema	Rectum, sigmoid	Induce and maintain remission in mild-to-moderate distal disease Combination therapy with oral aminosalicylates are superior to monotherapy	
Mesalamine (mesalazine) suppository	Rectum		
Antibiotics			
Ciprofloxacin Metronidazole Amoxicillin/clavulanic acid Rifaximin	Systemic	Antibiotics are not used for the treatment of UC but are used for pouchitis	Ciprofloxacin: tendonitis and rupture Metronidazole: neuropathy Amoxicillin/clavulanic acid: hepatitis
Corticosteroids			
Budesonide extended-release	Colon	Induce remission in mild-to-moderate UC Should not be used for maintenance	High first-pass metabolism More favorable side-effect profile than prednisone
Prednisone	Systemic	Induce remission in mild-to-moderate and some moderate-to-severe UC flares Not used for maintenance therapy	Infection, diabetes mellitus, osteoporosis, osteonecrosis, cataracts, glaucoma, and myopathy. Increase risk of mortality
Methylprednisolone	Systemic	Induce remission in severe UC	As for prednisone
Immunomodulators			
6-Mercaptopurine	Systemic	Maintain remission in steroid-dependent, steroid-refractory, or steroid-induced-remission UC Not used to induce remission	Allergic reactions, pancreatitis, myelosuppression, nausea, infections, hepatotoxicity, and malignancy, in particular lymphoma
Azathioprine	Systemic		
Cyclosporine	Systemic	Rescue therapy to induce remission in severe UC not responding to IV methylprednisolone	Infections, hypertension, renal insufficiency, tremor, headache, hepatotoxicity

DRUG	RELEASE SITE	TREATMENT OF UC	SIDE-EFFECTS
Biologicals			
Infliximab	Systemic	Can be used to induce and maintain moderate-to-severe UC and are steroid-sparing	Infections (tuberculosis, fungal infections), autoantibody formation, psoriasis, drug-induced lupus
Adalimumab	Systemic		
Golimumab	Systemic	Infliximab is also used as a rescue therapy to induce remission in severe UC not responding to IV methylprednisolone	Infusion reactions (infliximab), injection-site reaction (adalimumab and golimumab), delayed hypersensitivity reaction (infliximab)
			Lymphoma (higher in combination therapy)
Vedolizumab	Systemic	Effective in the induction and maintenance of remission in moderate-to-severe UC	Headache, infections, abdominal pain, infusion reactions
Tofacitinib (small molecules)	Systemic	Effective in induction and maintenance	Infections (especially herpes zoster), lymphoma

» Infectious colitis should be ruled out—especially that due to *C. difficile*, CMV and common bacterial pathogens.
» Flexible sigmoidoscopy with biopsies should be performed within 48 hours of admission.
» If there is no improvement on IV steroids within 3–5 days, either colectomy or rescue therapy with IV cyclosporine (ciclosporin) or IV infliximab is indicated. Avoid cyclosporine if hypertension, renal disease or a seizure history or a low total cholesterol.
» A patient who responds to IV steroids can be switched to a tapering dose of oral corticosteroids and thiopurine or biologicals.

Indications for surgery in UC

• Severe colitis not responding to IV steroids or rescue therapy (cyclosporine or infliximab)
• Fulminant colitis with or without toxic megacolon
• Exsanguinating hemorrhage
• Perforation
• Patient unable to tolerate medication side-effects
• High-grade dysplasia (some low-grade dysplasia)
• Cancer

The most common operation performed for UC is:

• a total colectomy with formation of an ileostomy in an urgent/emergency situation
• a total proctocolectomy with ileal-pouch anal anastomosis (IPAA) in an elective setting.

Pouchitis

Patients with an IPAA are at risk of developing acute (lasting <4 weeks) or chronic (lasting >4 weeks) pouchitis. Diagnosis is made based on clinical symptoms, endoscopic appearance, and histology.

• **Clinical symptoms**—increase in stool frequency (>8–10 per day), urgency, incontinence, increase in night-time seepage, and perianal/abdominal pain.
• **Pouchoscopy**—erythema, edema, granularity, friability, loss of vascular pattern, mucous exudates, and ulcerations.
• **Histology**—inflammation with crypt distortion and crypt abscesses.
• **Stool cultures**—rule out *C. difficile*, CMV and common bacterial pathogens.

Treatment

• **Primary prophylaxis**—VSL#3 (a probiotic) daily.
• **Acute pouchitis:**
  » antibiotics for 14 days (ciprofloxacin, metronidazole, or amoxicillin/clavulanic acid)
  » VSL#3 in mild cases.
• **Chronic pouchitis:**
  » *antibiotic-dependent*—rotating antibiotics + VSL#3
  » *antibiotic-resistant*—4-week course of combination antibiotics (ciprofloxacin + metronidazole, ciprofloxacin + rifaximin).

Pouch endoscopic surveillance in those with UC every 1–3 years for pouch neoplasia is recommended.

Colon cancer screening

Patients with UC have a higher risk of colon cancer compared with patients with CD and the general population. Risk factors for colorectal cancer in UC are:

- duration of colitis
- primary sclerosing cholangitis
- extensive colitis
- backwash ileitis
- severe inflammation, pseudopolyps
- family history of colorectal cancer
- dysplasia.

The recommended screening is:

- 8–10 years after diagnosis of extensive colitis in UC or >30% colitis in CD
- 15 years after left-sided colitis
- at diagnosis of primary sclerosing cholangitis (PSC) and then every 1–2 years thereafter.

The results of screening determine the course of action.

- Flat lesions with:
  - » low-grade dysplasia—consider colectomy or close surveillance
  - » high-grade dysplasia—colectomy
- Polypoid lesions—complete removal and vigilant follow-up
- Unresectable/carpet lesions—surgery

Vaccines in IBD

All IBD patients should be vaccinated if possible, according to usual guidelines, preferably at diagnosis before they are immunosuppressed. The definition of immunosuppression in IBD is:

- treatment with corticosteroids (prednisone >20 mg/day for 2 weeks or more and within 3 months of stopping)
- treatment with azathioprine/6-mercaptopurine or discontinuation within the previous 3 months
- treatment with methotrexate or discontinuation within the previous 3 months
- treatment with anti-TNF (tumor necrosis factor) agents or discontinuation within the previous 3 months
- significant protein–calorie malnutrition.

General rules

1. Live-attenuated vaccines should be avoided for at least 3 months after finishing immunosuppressive therapy.
2. Immunosuppressive therapy should be withheld for at least 3 weeks (4–12 weeks) after a live vaccine injection.
3. It is best to vaccinate at diagnosis, before starting immunomodulator therapy.

Pregnancy in IBD

- Fertility in women with IBD without previous pelvic surgery is similar to that in the general population.
- The goal is to achieve and maintain remission at conception and during pregnancy to have favorable pregnancy outcomes.

- Smoking (for CD), discontinuation of medications, and active disease during pregnancy are risk factors for IBD flares.
- Most medications used to treat IBD are low-risk during pregnancy except for methotrexate (Table 11-13).
- Most IBD medications are safe during lactation with the exception of methotrexate, metronidazole, and cyclosporine (ciclosporin) (Table 11-13).
- The risk–benefit ratio between maintaining disease remission and possible medication side-effects should be discussed on a case-by-case basis.

Colon polyps

CLINICAL PEARLS

- Detection and removal of colonic adenomas through effective screening reduces the risk of colon cancer.

Risk factors for colon cancer include age and a history of adenomatous colon polyps (but not hyperplastic polyps). Colonic polyps may be benign (e.g. inflammatory or hyperplastic polyps) or pre-malignant/malignant (e.g. adenomas, tubulovillous adenomas, traditional serrated adenomas, sessile serrated polyps). In practice, polyps are generally removed during colonoscopy. Rectal polyps that appear consistent with hyperplastic polyps can be safely left in situ. Inflammatory polyps (often associated with IBD) are benign and don't require resection but the surrounding mucosa should be carefully inspected for dysplasia.

When adenomas or sessile serrated polyps, high-risk features (for future malignancy) include increasing number of polyps (3 or more), size (10 mm or greater), villous features or high grade dysplasia. Macroscopically flat or depressed serrated adenomas appear to have a high malignancy potential.

COLON CANCER SCREENING

Recommendations for screening and surveillance

Average risk

Persons aged between 50 and 75 years who have no symptoms of bowel cancer and no special risk factors have an average risk of bowel cancer. Those aged 50 and above should be counseled to engage in a screening program:

- There is a 15–33% reduction in mortality from bowel cancer using fecal occult blood testing (FOBT). It can miss a third of advanced cancers.
- Colonoscopy 10-yearly from age 50 is the screening procedure of choice in the USA, although many countries use an annual fecal test as the initial screening test for asymptomatic persons.

Table 11-13 Inflammatory bowel disease medications in pregnancy and breastfeeding

DRUG	FERTILITY	PREGNANCY	BREAST-FEEDING	COMMENTS
Antibiotics				
Metronidazole	✓	✓	X	Wait 12–24 hours before breastfeeding
Ciprofloxacin	✓	X	✓	
Amoxicillin/ clavulanate	✓	✓	✓	
Rifaximin	✓	(✓)	(✓)	Limited data available
Probiotics	✓	✓	✓	
Aminosalicylates				
5ASAs	✓	✓	✓	Considered safe
Sulfasalazine	✓	✓	✓	Give with folic acid 2 mg daily Reversible reduction sperm count
Corticosteroids				
Prednisone	✓	✓	✓	Low risk
Budesonide	✓	✓	✓	
Immunomodulators				
Azathioprine/ 6-mercaptopurine	✓	✓	(✓)	Continue in pregnancy if monotherapy
Methotrexate	X	X	X	Teratogenic
Cyclosporine (ciclosporin)	✓	(✓)	(✓)	If breastfeeding check infant levels
Tacrolimus	✓	✓	(✓)	If breastfeeding check infant levels
Biologicals				
Infliximab	✓	✓	✓	Considered safe
Adalimumab	✓	✓	✓	Considered safe
Certolizumab	✓	✓	✓	Considered safe but limited data
Golimumab	✓	(✓)	(✓)	Limited data available
Natalizumab	✓	(✓)	(✓)	Limited data available
Vedolizumab	?	(✓)	(✓)	Limited data available
Ustekinumab	✓	(✓)	(✓)	Limited data available
Tofacitinib	?	X	X	Teratogenic in animals. Avoid

(✓) limited data, caution
✓ relatively safe to use based on limited data
X – do *not* use

Above-average risk

Patients considered at above-average risk for colorectal cancer include those with: a prior history of colorectal cancer; family history of colorectal cancer (or certain genetic syndromes, e.g. Lynch syndrome); personal history of colonic polyps; or inflammatory bowel disease.

- In general, colonoscopy is recommended every 3–5 years.
- After polyps are found, surveillance depends on the size, number and family history.
  - » Patients with >10 adenomas should have repeat colonoscopy every 3 years. It is important to consider the possibility of an underlying familial syndrome.
  - » Patients with sessile adenomas that are removed piecemeal require repeat colonoscopy in 2–6 months to confirm complete excision.

Fecal occult blood testing (FOBT)

- There are two main types of test:
  - » guaiac test—based on the pseudoperoxidase activity of hemoglobin
  - » immunochemical test—utilizes the antibody to human hemoglobin, and is more accurate and thus preferred for population screening.
- Three stools should be sampled annually and test cards should be used at home. A single FOBT test has poor sensitivity, but this is increased by repeat testing (hence the three samples).
- Dietary restriction is highly desirable for the guaiac test (no red meat). If dietary restrictions are followed, false-positive results are uncommon (1–2%). One advantage of the immunochemical test is that dietary restriction is unnecessary.
- A person who has a positive FOBT has a 30–45% chance of having adenoma and a 3–5% chance of having cancer.
  - » FOBT is negative in up to 66% of patients with colon cancer.
  - » Positive tests should be followed up with colonoscopy.
- Fecal DNA, testing is more sensitive.
- Carcinoembryonic antigen (CEA) testing is only useful for checking for recurrence of colon cancer, and only if the levels were elevated before surgery and reduce after surgery. Other causes of CEA rise include smoking, benign biliary disease, sclerosing cholangitis and inflammatory bowel disease.

Malignant potential and surveillance

Important factors to be taken in consideration for surveillance are:

- size of polyps
- number of polyps
- histopathology.

Table 11-14 describes the malignant potential and surveillance requirements for different types of polyp.

Family history of colon cancer without genetic basis

Recommendations

- One first-degree relative with colon cancer >60 years—screening should begin at age 40, as per average risk screening recommendations.
- One first-degree relative with colon cancer younger than 60 years, or 2 or more first-degree relatives diagnosed with colon cancer at any age, should undergo colonoscopy every 5 years from age 40 or 10 years younger than the age of diagnosis of the affected relative.

Family history of colon cancer with known genetic basis

Familial adenomatosis polyposis (FAP)

- This is characterized by the presence of hundreds to thousands of colorectal adenomas that usually develop in adolescence. One in five FAP patients has new-onset mutations (no known family history of FAP). Risk of colonic cancer is 100% if not treated.
- Extracolonic features include duodenal adenomas and cancer, gastric fundic gland hyperplasia, mandibular osteomas and supernumerary teeth.
- Unless total protocolectomy is performed CRC always develops, with a mean age at diagnosis of approximately 40 years.
- Following colectomy, patients are at risk of developing duodenal cancer.
- Attenuated FAP is associated with fewer colorectal adenomas (<100) and later onset of CRC (mean age approximately 55 years).

Recommendations

- Refer for genetic counseling.
- Offer annual colonoscopy screening in the teenage years. Consider regular gastroscopy and thyroid ultrasounds.
- These patients need to be considered for protocolectomy by age 20.

Individuals who test positive for the *APC* gene mutation, or all at-risk first-degree relatives where no *APC* gene mutation has been characterized, should have annual or biennial sigmoidoscopy from 12–15 years (the exact age depending on the maturity) to 30–35 years, and less frequently to 55 years of age.

Gardner syndrome

This is a variant of FAP. There may be fewer colonic polyps than FAP, but it presents with extraintestinal manifestations (osteomas, epidermal cysts, fibromas, dental abnormalities, desmoids, tumors, etc.).

Hereditary non-polyposis colon cancer (HNPCC) or Lynch syndrome

This is the most common form of inherited colon cancer. It is an autosomal dominant disorder and caused by germ-line

Table 11-14 Malignant potential and surveillance of colonic polyps

POLYP TYPE	MORPHOLOGY	MALIGNANT POTENTIAL/ SURVEILLANCE REQUIREMENTS
Tubular adenoma	Branched tubules	<1 cm: 1% 1–2 cm: 10% >2 cm: 34% Surveillance every 5–10 years (1–2 small polyps with low-grade dysplasia after polypectomy) or every 3 years if 3–10 adenomas or one >10mm.
Villous adenoma	Frond-like pattern	<1 cm: 4% 1–2 cm: 20% >2 cm: >50% Surveillance every 3 years if 1 or more villous/ tubulovillous adenomas
Tubulovillous adenoma	Mixed pattern	<1 cm: 4% 1–2 cm: 9% >2 cm: 45% Surveillance every 3 years
Hyperplastic polyp confined to rectosigmoid	Increased glandular cells Reduced cytoplasm Nuclear atypia, stratification and hyperchromatism is absent	Small and distally located Do not appear to be associated with increased risk of colorectal cancer Surveillance every 10 years
Serrated polyps		
1. Sessile serrated polyp without dysplasia		Surveillance every 5 years if <10 mm, every 3 years if large (or dysplasia)
2. Traditional serrated adenoma with dysplasia		Surveillance every 3 years
3. Mixed: sessile serrated and tubular adenoma		Surveillance every 3 years
4. Serrated polyposis syndrome	1 cm or more, 30 or more polyps, and mixed adenomatous features have increased risk of colorectal cancer	Surveillance 1-yearly

mutations (mismatch repair genes, MMR) in *MLH1*, *MSH2*, *PMS1*, *PMS2* or *MSH6*. The most common mutations are in *MLH1* and *MSH2*.

- The median age for CRC diagnosis is 46.
- The polyps tend to be located in the more proximal colon.
- It is associated with other cancers (uterine, ovarian, genitourinary, small bowel and hepatobiliary).
- Tissue should be tested for microsatellite instability by immunohistochemistry and/or by PCR.

The Amsterdam criteria are used to help identify families likely to have Lynch syndrome:

1 At least 3 relatives with histologically confirmed colon cancer (or endometrial cancer or small-intestine cancer)

2 At least 2 successive generations

3 At least 1 colon cancer diagnosed before age 50

4 One relative should be a first-degree relative of the other two.

Recommendations

- Annual colonoscopy from age 25, or 5 years younger than the age of the earliest cancer in the family (whichever comes first).
- HNPCC-testing for microsatellite instability (MSI) and/or immunohistochemistry of the mismatch repair gene product.
- Annual screening in known mutation carriers, and biennial screening for at-risk first-degree relatives in families where the mutation is not characterized.
- Annual gynecological screening, with transvaginal ultrasound for ovarian screening and endometrial sampling,

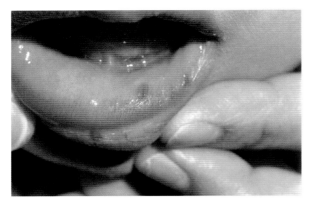

Figure 11-9 Peutz–Jeghers mucosal pigmentations

From Weston WL, Lane AT and Morelli JG. Color textbook of pediatric dermatology, 4th ed. Elsevier, 2007.

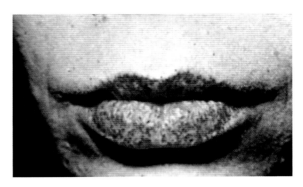

Figure 11-10 Osler–Weber–Rendu syndrome

From Feldman MD, Friedman LS and Brandt LJ (eds). Sleisenger and Fordtran's Gastrointestinal and liver disease, 9th ed. Philadelphia: Elsevier, 2010.

is recommended for pre-menopausal female gene carriers and at-risk women with family members where no mutation has been found.

- For postmenopausal women, transvaginal ultrasound to evaluate endometrial thickness, and ovarian pathology and cancer-associated antigen 125 (CA-125) is recommended.

Peutz–Jeghers (PJ) syndrome

- In this syndrome, multiple hamartomatous polyps are present in the GI tract associated with distinctive mucocutaneous pigmentations—lips and buccal mucosa, nose, perianal area, genitals and rarely in the GI tract (Figure 11-9).
- PJ syndrome is an autosomal dominant disorder, with male and females equally affected.
- The PJ gene is located on chromosome 19p13.3.

PJ syndrome is associated with an increased risk of malignancy, both GI and non-GI (gynecological—ovarian or cervical tumors; males—Sertoli cell testicular tumors), with an average age of developing malignancy of 42 years. The most common sites for cancers are colon/rectum and pancreas, and breast for non-GI cases.

GASTROINTESTINAL BLEEDING

Upper

The most common causes of upper GI bleeding are:
- bleeding peptic ulcers
- esophago-gastric varices
- ulcerative esophagitis
- Mallory–Weiss tears (physical mucosal tears due to vomiting)
- bleeding from GI vascular lesions:
  » gastric antral vascular ectasia (GAVE)
  » Dieulafoy lesion (an aberrant submucosal vessel that has eroded into the epithelial layer)

» hereditary hemorrhagic telangiectasia (Osler–Weber–Rendu syndrome: an autosomal dominant vascular disorder where epistaxis, GI bleeding and cerebral arteriovenous malformations are common; Figure 11-10).

The most common symptoms of upper GI hemorrhage are hemetemesis and melena, but some patients simply present with collapse and shock.

CLINICAL PEARL

Peptic ulcer bleeding is common in the elderly with comorbidities and use of anticoagulants. Stigmata of chronic liver disease should raise suspicion of variceal hemorrhage.

Management

Initial management is focused on management of the airway and hemodynamic resuscitation.

- The presence of tachycardia, hypotension or hematochezia indicates rapid, large-volume blood loss, and early endoscopy is indicated after resuscitation.

CLINICAL PEARL

Despite a normal supine blood pressure, hypovolemia may be present: checking for a postural drop in blood pressure is mandatory in all such patients.

- Intravenous PPI therapy should be commenced prior to endoscopy and continued depending on the pathology found.
- Placement of a nasogastric tube prior to endoscopy when upper GI hemorrhage is suspected has not been shown to improve outcomes.
- If the patient has known varices or variceal hemorrhage is suspected, vasoactive peptides (octreotide or terlipressin) should be given IV.

- All patients with suspected or confirmed variceal bleeding should receive prophylactic antibiotics. 50% of such patients have bacterial sepsis at the time of presentation, and many more develop sepsis during admission.

Peptic ulcer bleeding

In peptic ulcer bleeding, endoscopy is important for risk stratification. Larger ulcers, with visible vessels or overlying clots, are the highest risk for re-bleeding, while clean-based ulcers rarely re-bleed.

- High-dose PPI therapy helps to prevent early re-bleeding after endoscopic therapy. Few patients (2%) require surgery; the main indications are:
  - » bleeding that cannot be controlled endoscopically
  - » perforated ulcers
  - » refractory ulcers
  - » bleeding secondary to cancers.
- Appropriate investigation for and eradication of *Helicobacter pylori* should be performed in all patients with peptic ulcer bleeding.

CLINICAL PEARL

Active bleeding may lead to gastric biopsy tests being falsely negative for *Helicobacter pylori*.

Variceal bleeding

- Control of bleeding is often obtained with endoscopic banding devices or injection of sclerosing agents.
- Compression of gastric or esophageal varices with a balloon catheter (Sengstaken–Blakemore or Linton tube) or oesophageal stent is used if hemostasis cannot be achieved by other means.
- Insertion of a transjugular intrahepatic portosystemic shunt reverses portal hypertension and can be used to manage acute bleeding and also prevent re-bleeding.

Bleeding from gastrointestinal vascular lesions

Upper GI hemorrhage due to abnormal vascular lesions is not uncommon. Often the offending lesion responds well to treatment with argon plasma coagulation, which ablates the vessel. Repeated treatments are often required.

Lower

Lower GI bleeding generally includes bleeding sources below the ligament of Treitz.

Most commonly, bleeding per rectum is the presenting symptom, and the causes depend on the age of the patient and the clinical scenario. Common anorectal causes are:

- hemorrhoids
- anal fissure
- proctitis.

Colonic bleeding

Colonic bleeds are not uncommon, and the most commonly encountered pathologies are:

- diverticular bleeds
- angiodysplasia

- ischemic colitis (see below)
- cancers.

Intestinal ischemia

Inadequate blood supply to the intestines has many causes, but four distinct clinical scenarios are recognized:

1. acute mesenteric ischemia
2. chronic mesenteric ischemia
3. colonic ischemia
4. mesenteric venous thrombosis.

Acute mesenteric ischemia

Acute mesenteric ischemia is a life-threatening event. Unless revascularization (radiologically) or, more commonly, resection of the affected bowel occurs promptly, survival is poor. Embolic occlusion due to atrial fibrillation is the most common cause. It is important to recognize that prothrombotic disorders and hypercoagulability due to cancer can present like this.

CLINICAL PEARL

The presentation of acute mesenteric ischemia is nonspecific, with description of severe abdominal pain out of keeping with relatively minor abdominal tenderness on examination. The serum lactate is often high.

Clues on imaging such as pneumatosis intestinalis, thumbprinting (Figure 11-11) and bowel-wall edema are useful, but unfortunately are late signs of disease.

Chronic mesenteric ischemia

Chronic mesenteric ischemia is angina of the gut.

- It occurs due to atherosclerotic occlusion of the main mesenteric vessels (celiac, superior or inferior mesenteric arteries).
- Symptoms do not occur unless occlusion of two of the three main vessels has occurred.
- Postprandial abdominal pain (fear of eating) and weight loss are clues, and occasionally abdominal bruits may be heard.
- Investigation should be with mesenteric ultrasound Doppler and/or an angiogram.
- Endoluminal treatment is often possible, but formal bypass procedures are sometimes required.
- Any vascular risk factors need to be optimized.

CLINICAL PEARL

Postprandial pain occurring in a patient with vascular risk factors or established vascular disease should raise suspicion of intestinal angina.

Mesenteric venous thrombosis

In mesenteric venous thrombosis the outflow of blood is occluded, usually due to local swelling, infection or

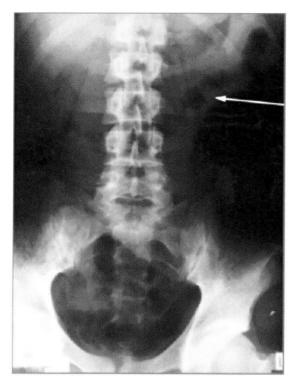

Figure 11-11 Thumbprinting of the bowel in acute mesenteric ischemia on plain abdominal X-ray

From Talley NJ. Clinical gastroenterology, 3rd ed. Sydney; Elsevier Australia, 2011.

masses, or prothrombotic states. Anticoagulation and bowel rest form standard therapy, although there are case reports of thrombolysis or thrombectomy exist.

Ischemic colitis

Ischemic colitis is more common than the conditions described above. It leads to colonic bleeding due to sloughing of necrosed mucosa. This mainly occurs from 'watershed' areas of the colon which are prone to hypoperfusion during low flow states such as dehydration or reduced cardiac output. Unlike acute mesenteric ischemia, colonic ischemia is rarely due to embolic disease.

Most patients recover without complications, but those who develop colonic gangrene and perforation have a high mortality.

Risk factors for ischemic colitis include:

- advanced age
- hemodialysis
- diabetes mellitus
- hypoalbuminemia.

The passing of maroon stools after the sudden onset of abdominal pain (most often in the left lower quadrant) is a common presentation. Colonoscopic examination with biopsies is appropriate if peritonitis is not present, and shows friable, ischemic mucosa within a distinct segment of colon.

A colonoscopic examination also helps to exclude inflammatory bowel disease or infectious causes.

Other causes of colonic bleeding are discussed below.

Diverticular bleeding

- Diverticular bleeding is often impressive in terms of blood loss, but commonly stops spontaneously and can recur days, months or years later.
- Manifestations of bleeding include bright rectal bleeding, but also red blood mixed with stool (hematochezia) or darker maroon stools.
- If colonoscopy is unhelpful, a technetium-labeled red-cell scan is often helpful for localization, and if brisk bleeding is present a CT angiogram is often diagnostic.
- Bleeding that does not cease spontaneously can be treated endoscopically, with interventional radiology or surgery.

Angiodysplasia

- Angiodysplasias are fragile, superficial blood vessels in the colon that easily bleed. They are commonly found in the cecum but can occur anywhere. Impressive bleeding can occur, particularly in the setting of anticoagulation.
- The treatment is endoscopic ablation, and repeated treatments are often required.
- Rarer causes of overt colonic bleeding include bleeding from colonic malignancies and Meckel's diverticulae.

Obscure GI bleeding

Obscure GI bleeding is a challenging clinical scenario. Often, repeat investigation of the upper or lower GI tract will reveal a cause missed by previous investigation.

- Imaging modalities such as CT angiogram and isotope-labeled red-cell scans can be helpful, but require active bleeding to be present at the time of investigation to give a positive yield.
- With the advent of video-capsule endoscopy the small bowel can now be safely investigated in most patients. The video-capsule device is ingested and takes numerous images of the GI tract. It can often identify bleeding lesions in the small bowel such as:
  » angiodysplasia
  » tumors
  » ulceration
  » stenosis.
- The main risk of video-capsule endoscopy is capsule retention, which occurs in 1% of patients. It can be asymptomatic or cause bowel obstruction.

CLINICAL PEARL

If it gets stuck, the small-bowel video-capsule is usually retained at a site of significant pathology (stenosis, tumor), and both the retained capsule and the offending lesions can be addressed surgically.

- Lesions identified by capsule endoscopy in the small bowel are often amenable to endoscopic therapy using antegrade or retrograde double-balloon enteroscopy.
- Occasionally, aorto-enteric fistulas (usually post abdominal aortic aneurysm repair) or bleeding into the biliary tract (hemobilia) will cause obscure GI bleeding.

Management of iron-deficiency anemia

Sometimes GI bleeding presents as iron-deficiency anemia without overt bleeding symptoms. Iron-deficiency anemia always warrants further investigation unless severe comorbidities lead to an unfavorable risk–benefit ratio.

Investigation of the upper and lower GI tract should be undertaken by endoscopy, with further investigation reserved for patients where no cause is found or the iron deficiency returns after adequate replacement.

PANCREAS

Acute pancreatitis

Alcohol and gallstones account for 60–75% of acute pancreatitis. Other causes include:

- trauma—after endoscopic retrograde cholangiopancreatography (ERCP), penetrating peptic ulcer or trauma
- infection (mumps, infectious mononucleosis)
- duct obstruction (carcinoma, roundworm)
- metabolic—hypercalcemia (and MEN 1), hypertriglyceridemia
- chronic kidney disease, porphyria, pregnancy
- vascular
- drugs—thiazides, steroids, contraceptive pill, tetracycline, sulfonamides, valproic acid, azathioprine
- pancreas divisum
- idiopathic.

Acute pancreatitis is a spectrum of disease.

- The milder form presents as interstitial pancreatitis with mild edema of the pancreas, with inflammation of the fat in the peripancreatic area and development of a fluid collection around the pancreas. Extra-pancreatic fluid collections can develop into a pseudocyst.
- In the more severe form, the disease is characterized by pancreatic necrosis with fat necrosis (necrotizing pancreatitis).

Mortality is dependent on the severity of the acute pancreatitis. Patients with necrotizing pancreatitis have a 10–30% mortality and a 70% risk of developing complications, whereas interstitial pancreatitis has less than 1% mortality.

Clinical features include severe abdominal pain lasting many hours. The location of the pain is frequently in the epigastric area and left upper quadrant, with radiation to the back. The character of the pain can be fluctuating and associated with nausea and vomiting.

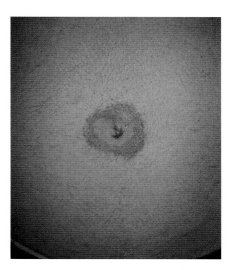

Figure 11-12 Cullen's sign

From Chauhan S et al. Cullen's and Turner's signs associated with portal hypertension. Lancet 2008;372(9632):54.

Clinical examination

Physical signs vary; therefore, look for tenderness, distention, fever, hypotension, tachypnea and hypoxemia. Cullen's and Turner's signs (caused by extravasated pancreatic exudates) should be examined for. It is important to note that these signs are not pathognomonic of acute pancreatitis.

- Cullen's sign is a faint blue discoloration around the umbilicus, indicating hemoperitoneum (Figure 11-12).
- Turner's sign is a bluish-reddish-purple or greenish brown discoloration of the flanks, resulting from retroperitoneal blood dissecting along the tissue planes (Figure 11-13).
- The differential diagnosis for both is any other cause of retroperitoneal hemorrhage.

The basic investigations that aid in the diagnosis of acute pancreatitis include pancreatic enzymes (serum amylase and lipase).

- A serum amylase level >3 times normal is indicative of a possible diagnosis of acute pancreatitis (Box 11-10). Serum amylase is elevated initially compared with lipase, and falls after 2–3 days. (Serum lipase remains elevated for longer: 7–14 days.)
- If elevated amylase persists for >10 days after acute pancreatitis, consider the possibility of leakage from a pseudocyst or, with large fluid collection, a disrupted pancreatic duct.
- It is important to note that high triglyceride levels can cause a spuriously normal amylase level. Levels of triglyceride >1000 mg/dL (11.3 mmol/L) can cause pancreatitis.
- A characteristic history with an elevated amylase/lipase is diagnostic. If there is doubt, an abdominal CT is helpful in confirming the diagnosis of acute pancreatitis (Table 11-15, overleaf).

Management

The management of high-risk patients and those with mild pancreatitis differs. The key is to determine the risk of

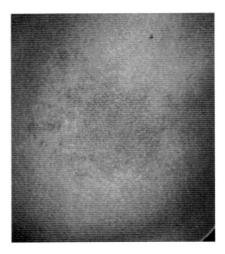

Figure 11-13 Turner's sign

From Chauhan S et al. Cullen's and Turner's signs associated with portal hypertension. Lancet 2008;372(9632):54.

Box 11-10
Differential diagnosis of hyperamylasemia

Pancreatic disease
- Chronic pancreatitis
- Pancreatic pseudocyst
- Pancreatic abscess
- Pancreatic cancer
- Trauma to the pancreas

Differential diagnosis raised lipase renal failure, cholecystitis, duodenal ulcer, celiac, type 2 diabetes, HIV, drugs, e.g. narcotics

Non-pancreatic disease
- Renal failure
- Parotitis
- Intestinal perforation
- Intestinal obstruction
- Intestinal infarction
- Ruptured ectopic pregnancy
- Drugs, e.g. morphine
- Diabetic ketoacidosis
- Burns
- Solid tumors, e.g. esophagus, lung, ovary
- Myocardial infarction
- Alcoholism

Table 11-15 CT findings and grading of acute pancreatitis (CT severity index)

GRADING BASED UPON FINDINGS ON UNENHANCED CT		
GRADE	**FINDINGS**	**SCORE**
A	Normal pancreas—normal size, sharply defined, smooth contour, homogenous enhancement, retroperitoneal peripancreatic fat without enhancement	0
B	Focal or diffuse enlargement of the pancreas; contour may show irregularity Enhancement may be inhomogeneous, but there is no peripancreatic inflammation	1
C	Peripancreatic inflammation with intrinsic pancreatic abnormalities	2
D	Intrapancreatic or extrapancreatic fluid collections	3
E	Two or more large collections of gas in the pancreas or retroperitoneum	4
NECROSIS SCORE BASED ON CONTRAST-ENHANCED CT		
NECROSIS (%)		**SCORE**
0		0
<33		2
33–50		4
≥50		6
CT SEVERITY INDEX (CTSI)		
CTSI equals unenhanced CT score plus necrosis score Maximum = 10; ≥6 = severe disease		
CT, computed tomography. Adapted from Balthazar EJ, Robinson DL, Megibow AJ, Ranson JH. Acute pancreatitis: value of CF in establishing prognosis. Radiology 1990;174(2):331–6.		

Box 11-11

Defining features of systemic inflammatory response syndrome (SIRS)

Two or more of the following conditions:

- Temperature >38.5°C or <35.0°C
- Heart rate of >90 beats/min
- Respiratory rate of >20 breaths/min or a P_ACO_2 of <32 mmHg
- WBC count of >12,000 cells/mL, <4000 cells/mL, or >10% immature (band) forms

P_ACO_2, alveolar partial pressure of carbon dioxide; WBC, white blood cell.

Data from: Annane D, Bellissant E and Cavaillon JM. Septic shock. Lancet 2005;365:63.

Table 11-16 Ranson criteria to predict severity of acute pancreatitis

MEASURE	CRITERION
0 hours	
Age	>55
White blood cell count	>16,000/mm³
Blood glucose	>200 mg/dL (11.1 mmol/L)
Lactate dehydrogenase	>350 U/L
Aspartate aminotransferase (AST)	>250 U/L
48 hours	
Hematocrit	Fall by ≥10%
Blood urea nitrogen	Increase by ≥5 mg/dL (1.8 mmol/L) despite fluids
Serum calcium	<8 mg/dL (2 mmol/L)
pO₂ (partial oxygen pressure)	<60 mmHg
Base deficit	>4 MEq/L
Fluid sequestration	>6000 mL

The presence of 1–3 criteria represents mild pancreatitis; the mortality rate rises significantly with 4 or more criteria.

Adapted from Ranson JHC, Rifkind KM, Roses DF, et al. Prognostic signs and the role of operative management in acute pancreatitis. Surg Gynecol Obstet 1974;139:69–81.

complications and identify factors that affect morbidity and mortality.

- There are a number of scoring systems used (e.g. Ranson criteria—Table 11-16, APACHE II).
  - » A limitation of the Ranson criteria is that this is only valid up to 48 hours after the onset of symptoms. The sensitivity is 73% and the criteria are 77% specific to predict mortality.
- The systemic inflammatory response syndrome (SIRS) score (based on temperature, respiratory rate, heart rate and white cell count; Box 11-11) is favored as it is simple, cheap, readily available and as accurate as any of the complex scoring systems.
- However, no single score is completely accurate. Clinical assessment of severity is important and should not be replaced by these scoring systems.
- The amylase level is not a prognostic indicator.
- Other risk factors for severity at admission include older age, comorbidity and obesity.

Complications of acute pancreatitis

Necrotizing pancreatitis

50% of patients with necrotizing necrosis will have organ failure. The remainder will have resolution of necrotizing pancreatitis as it evolves into walled-off pancreatic necrosis.

- The clinical features include intractable pain, nausea and vomiting, inability to maintain adequate weight, and low-grade fever.
  - » Abdominal pain is due to raised intra-parenchymal pressures within the walled-off pancreatic necrosis.
- Infected necrosis should be considered with necrotizing pancreatitis if the patient deteriorates, or fails to improve after a week.
- As soon as the diagnosis of necrotizing pancreatitis is made, IV antibiotics are recommended if systemic signs of sepsis are present.

  » Sterile and infected acute necrotizing pancreatitis can be difficult to distinguish clinically, as both present with fever, leukocytosis and severe abdominal pain. Gas on imaging in the necrosis suggests infection. CT-guided FNA is a safe and accurate way to confirm that infection is present.

Treatment modalities include:

1 Surgical (cystogastrectomy or Roux-en-Y cystojejunostomy with finger dissection of necrotic tissue).
2 Endoscopic technique using transgastric and transduodenal drainage catheters.
3 Less commonly, radiological percutaneous placement of a catheter to facilitate debridement.

Pancreatic abscess

This usually occurs 4–6 weeks after an acute pancreatitis attack. It can present with fever and shock. CT-guided biopsy with bacterial smear and culture helps with diagnosis.

Treatment involves immediate surgical debridement and drainage, and antibiotics. (Timing is important when the process has evolved into a walled-off necrosis.) Treatment of sterile necrosis is generally non-surgical.

Pancreatic pseudocyst

This develops in 10–15% of patients in the 2–4 weeks following an acute pancreatitis attack. Some are asymptomatic, while others can present with abdominal pain and have the potential to become infected. If the size is >5 cm and it has lasted more than 6 months, this indicates that it will not resolve spontaneously.

Treatment modalities include:

1 Surgical—cystogastrostomy or Roux-en-Y cystojejunostomy.
2 Endoscopic—endoscopic cystogastrostomy.
3 Radiological—percutaneous catheter drainage.

Chronic pancreatitis

> **CLINICAL PEARL**
>
> The classic triad of chronic pancreatitis is recurrent abdominal pain, diabetes and steatorrhea from pancreatic exocrine and endocrine dysfunction. This form of diabetes does not cause retinopathy or nephropathy.

Chronic pancreatitis is a syndrome of progressive, irreversible and destructive inflammatory changes in the pancreas, resulting in permanent structural damage and leading to impairment of the exocrine and endocrine functions.

- Unlike acute pancreatitis, serum amylase and lipase levels tend to be normal in patients with chronic pancreatitis.
- The 'gold standard' for diagnosis is tissue diagnosis, but this is invasive and rarely performed. Therefore, the diagnosis is based on a combination of clinical, radiological and functional findings.
- The hallmark of this disease is abdominal pain and exocrine dysfunction.

The most common **cause** is chronic alcohol ingestion, with a typical history of heavy alcohol (150 g) or more daily for 6 or more years. Other causes include:

- idiopathic
- hereditary pancreatitis—genetic mutations have been identified in subgroups of patients; mutations include the cationic trypsinogen gene (autosomal dominant; *PRSS1*), or the pancreatic secretory trypsin inhibitor gene (*SPINK1* [serine protease inhibitor Kazal-type 1])
- cystic fibrosis
- pancreas divisum
- tumor
- hyperparathyroidism
- autoimmune pancreatitis—rare (<1%), but important to recognize.

The **clinical presentation** involves an initial asymptomatic phase followed by recurrent abdominal pain.

- Abdominal pain can be referred to either the left or the right, or radiates to the back. If diaphragmatic involvement is present, pain may be pleuritic in nature and felt in the shoulder.
- The natural history of the disease is progressive exocrine dysfunction leading to steatorrhea and diarrhea, and endocrine dysfunction leading to diabetes.
- The classic triad of recurrent abdominal pain with pancreatic calcification, diabetes and steatorrhea increases the likelihood of the diagnosis of chronic pancreatitis.

Investigations

Blood tests are neither sensitive nor specific for the diagnosis of chronic pancreatitis. Fecal elastase is a useful screening test for moderate to severe disease. Secretin stimulation testing using a nasoduodenal tube for duodenal sampling for bicarbonate is both sensitive and specific, but not well tolerated or readily available.

Imaging modalities that help confirm the diagnosis include:

- CT abdomen to confirm the presence of calcified pancreas (Figure 11-14). The differential diagnosis of calcified pancreas includes alcoholic pancreatitis, hyperparathyroidism and hereditary pancreatitis.

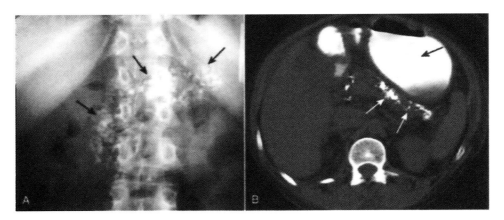

Figure 11-14 Calcified pancreas shown on computed tomography scan

From: Herring W. Learning radiology: recognizing the basics, 2nd ed. Philadelphia: Elsevier, 2012.

- Endoscopic ultrasonography (EUS) is both sensitive and specific, and may confirm the diagnosis when the CT scan is normal. However, differentiating chronic pancreatitis and pancreatic cancer is not always possible because the echoendoscopic features of lobular architecture and hypoechoic changes in pancreatic parenchyma are similar. EUS with FNA is needed to confirm the diagnosis.
- Magnetic resonance cholangiopancreatography (MRCP) can aid in the diagnosis of chronic pancreatitis and help detect stones in the common bile duct (CBD) and other biliary disease.
- ERCP is invasive and can precipitate pancreatitis. However, this approach is beneficial if CBD or pancreatic duct stones are present.

Complications

The main complications of chronic pancreatitis are related to exocrine dysfunction leading to steatorrhea and fat malabsorption, with associated fat-soluble vitamin deficiency (A, D, E or K) and low vitamin B_{12}. Endocrine dysfunction occurs when >80% of the pancreas is destroyed (late onset). Diabetes is more likely to occur when there is a family history of type 1 or type 2 diabetes.

Other complications include:

- pseudocyst (10%), secondary to ductal disruptions rather than from peripancreatic fluid accumulation as in acute pancreatitis
- duodenal and bile duct obstruction (5–10%)
- pancreatic ascites and pleural effusion, secondary to disruption of the pancreatic duct and fistula formation between the abdomen and the chest, or rupture of pseudocyst with tracking of pancreatic fluid into the peritoneal cavity
- splenic vein thrombosis secondary to inflammation of the splenic vein
- pseudoaneurysm of vessels close to the pancreas (rare).

Treatment

The treatment is directed at managing pancreatic exocrine and endocrine dysfunction, with a multidisciplinary team.

- Pancreatic enzymes are replaced by oral pancreatic enzymes (20,000–30,000 units of lipase per meal).
- A PPI is added to prevent gastric acid breaking down the enzymes.
- At present, managing the chronic pain is difficult and the potential for narcotic addiction is high. Modalities such as pancreatic enzyme supplementation, endoscopic therapy and nerve block, as well as surgery for relief of refractory pain, may be tried.

Autoimmune pancreatitis (AIP)

Autoimmune pancreatitis is a rare cause of pancreatitis (<1%). It is an important diagnosis to make, and its treatment often results in a good prognosis for the patient.

> **CLINICAL PEARL**
>
> Autoimmune pancreatitis type 1 is associated with elevated immunoglobulin G4 levels, while type 2 is associated with inflammatory bowel disease. Most patients respond to corticosteroids, but 30–40% will relapse.

- The usual clinical picture is obstructive jaundice (70%), with dramatic clinical and histopathological response to corticosteroids.
- The picture may be confused clinically with pancreatic cancer. Pancreatic cancer is much more common than autoimmune pancreatitis.
- Autoimmune pancreatitis is classified into types 1 and 2 (Box 11-12).
  - » Pancreatic histology is essential to make the definitive diagnosis of autoimmune pancreatitis. An important clinical clue to making the diagnosis is the involvement of other organs in autoimmune pancreatitis type 1.
- AIP is occasionally associated with other autoimmune diseases (most commonly Sjögren's syndrome, primary sclerosing cholangitis, systemic lupus erythematosus and ulcerative colitis).

Box 11-12

Classification of autoimmune pancreatitis (AIP)

Type 1

- Systemic IgG4-positive disease
- Peak incidence in the 6th or 7th decade (more common in Japan, Korea)
- Men are affected twice as often as women
- Associated with elevated serum immunoglobulin G4 (IgG4) levels (usually twice the upper limit of normal)
- Elevated ANA (antinuclear antibodies) may be present
- IgG4 levels have sensitivity of 95% and specificity of 97% for AIP type 1
- It characteristically involves other organs, in particular bile ducts, salivary glands, lymph nodes, kidneys and retroperitoneum synchronously or metachronously

Type 2

- Idiopathic duct-centric pancreatitis
- More commonly found in Europe
- It affects younger patients; usually 10 years earlier than AIP type 1
- There is no gender predilection
- Not associated with elevated IgG4 levels
- No systemic organ involvement
- Inflammatory bowel disease in 30%

The key **imaging modalities** to aid in the diagnosis include:

- A CT abdomen which may show a diffusely swollen, sausage-shaped pancreas with a narrowed pancreatic duct.
- EUS which may show a diffusely hypoechoic gland.
- EUS is also used as a guide to obtain a core biopsy. This is important, as the pancreatitis is not uniformly involved in the disease process. Biopsy from the major duodenal papilla has a high specificity but low sensitivity.
- ERCP or MRCP findings include a long, narrow stricture (more than one-third of the main pancreatic duct) with lack of upstream dilatation, multiple non-contiguous strictures, and stricture arising from the narrowed portion of the main pancreatic duct.

Treatment

The mainstay of treatment is corticosteroids, with improvement in morphology, biochemical and exocrine function.

- IgG4 levels can help in monitoring the response to treatment, as well as cross-sectional imaging.
- If a stent has been placed, this is usually removed at 6–8 weeks after initiation of treatment.
- 30–40% of cases have clinical, radiological, serological or histological relapse following treatment. These patients will need a prolonged course of corticosteroids. Use of azathioprine/6-mercaptopurine long-term has been only in case reports.
- All patients should be monitored for residual pancreatic exocrine and endocrine insufficiency.

Pancreatic cysts

Pancreatic cystic lesions are increasingly diagnosed with the growing use of cross-sectional imaging. Most are found incidentally in asymptomatic patients.

Many different types of lesion exist.

- No malignant potential:
  - » pseudocysts (result of inflammation, most often pancreatitis)
  - » benign (serous cystadenomas)
- Potentially malignant:
  - » intraductal papillary mucinous neoplasms (IPMNs)—main duct (high risk), branch duct (low–moderate risk)
  - » mucinous cystic neoplasms (MCNs) (females; moderate risk)
  - » solid pseudopapillary neoplasms (SPN) (moderate to high risk)
  - » obtain an MRI withh MRCP to image the cyst if not yet obtained. Refer a main duct IPMN, MCN or SPN for consideration of resection. If uncertain, but the lesion is worrying (e.g. >1.5cm), consider an endoscopic ultrasound.

CLINICAL PEARL

The larger the size of the cystic lesion, the higher the chance of malignancy. Other worrying features: a solid component, dilated main pancreatic duct, jaundice.

ACKNOWLEDGMENT

We acknowledge and thank Dr. Kara De Felice who was a contributing author to this chapter in the third edition.

SELF-ASSESSMENT QUESTIONS

1 A 74-year-old man with dyspepsia and chronic obstructive pulmonary disease (FEV$_1$ 66% of predicted), type 2 diabetes mellitus and a body mass index of 36 kg/m^2 undergoes esophagogastroduodenoscopy for an upper gastrointestinal hemorrhage. A duodenal ulcer is found and treated. At the time of endoscopy, Barrett's esophagus is suspected in a 4 cm tongue of abnormal mucosa. There are no raised lesions or nodules. Biopsies and repeat biopsies after 1 month confirm high-grade dysplasia. In this patient, the most appropriate next step is:

A High-dose proton-pump inhibitors and repeat biopsies in 3 months
B Referral for esophagectomy
C Liquid nitrogen ablation
D Endoscopic mucosal resection
E Radiofrequency ablation

2 A 34-year-old asthmatic male presents with food bolus obstruction for the third time in 6 years. He suffers mild dysphagia to solids at times, but at other times is fairly asymptomatic. He uses ibuprofen once per fortnight for muscle ache associated with exercise. He admits to smoking 5 cigarettes daily. There has been no weight loss. The most likely diagnosis is:

A Esophageal adenocarcinoma
B Achalasia
C Esophageal stricture
D Eosinophilic esophagitis
E Zenker's diverticulum

3 A 54-year-old man is hospitalized with an upper gastrointestinal hemorrhage. He takes aspirin due to a family history of heart disease. Endoscopy identified a 2 cm gastric ulcer with an overlying clot. This was treated and no further bleeding occurred. The duodenum was normal. The rapid urease test was positive, indicating likely infection with *Helicobacter pylori*. The most appropriate discharge plan is:

A Treat for *H. pylori* and schedule repeat endoscopy.
B Treat for *H. pylori* and only perform repeat endoscopy if eradication fails.
C Check fecal antigen status as an outpatient and only treat *H. pylori* if positive. Repeat endoscopy not required.
D Stop aspirin and ignore *H. pylori* positivity, as the aspirin was the likely culprit.
E Treat for *H. pylori* if urease test on repeat endoscopy remains positive.

4 A 23-year-old woman is referred to the gastroenterology outpatient clinic with bloating and alternating diarrhea and constipation. Symptoms have been present for 5 years. There is no weight loss. Stress makes her symptoms worse. She is concerned about celiac disease, and has adhered to a strict gluten-free diet for 12 months. This has improved her symptoms somewhat. Which of the following tests has the highest negative predictive value for celiac disease in this setting?

A Anti-tissue transglutaminase antibodies
B Total immunoglobulin A (IgA)
C HLA DQ2 DQ8 analysis
D Biopsies of the second part of the duodenum
E Video-capsule endoscopy

5 A 37-year-old man falls ill during a Mediterranean cruise. His symptoms are diarrhea, vomiting and crampy abdominal pain. He is febrile. He consumed shellfish the day before becoming unwell, and several other travel companions who ingested the shellfish are also sick. There is no blood or mucus in his stool. What is the most likely cause for his acute diarrheal illness?

A *Staphylococcus aureus* infection
B *Bacillus cereus* infection
C Norovirus outbreak
D *Clostridium perfringens* infection
E Enterohemorrhagic *Escherichia coli* infection

6 A 50-year-old man is hospitalized for recurrent epigastric pain, anorexia and diarrhea. He was diagnosed with diabetes mellitus 4 months ago. He describes his stools as loose, greasy and foul-smelling and difficult to flush. He has had four previous admissions with acute pancreatitis. He currently drinks 15 standard drinks of alcohol per day and has done so for a number of years. Serum amylase and lipase levels are normal. He has also noticed poor night vision lately. What is the most likely diagnosis for his recurrent abdominal pain?

A Acute pancreatitis
B Chronic pancreatitis
C Peptic ulceration
D Protein-losing enteropathy
E Gastritis

7   A 65-year-old woman with a background history of gastroesophageal reflux disease and hypertension was dehydrated with acute renal impairment due to severe diarrhea. She was recently treated with ciprofloxacin by her local physician for a urinary tract infection. She describes no recent travel or exposure to ill persons. Stool analysis confirmed the presence of *Clostridium difficile* toxin A. She was treated with IV fluids and oral metronidazole as an inpatient for 2 days. Following the resolution of her renal impairment and improvement in diarrhea, she was discharged home on oral metronidazole for 14 days in total. However, she re-presents to the hospital emergency room 2 weeks later with ongoing diarrhea and severe dehydration. What is the most appropriate next step in managing this patient?

   A   Retreatment with oral metronidazole for 14 days
   B   Oral vancomycin and intravenous metronidazole for 14 days
   C   Intravenous vancomycin for 10 days
   D   Fecal bacteriotherapy
   E   Oral rifaximin for 14 days

8   A 70-year-old asymptomatic man underwent initial screening colonoscopy 3 weeks previously for positive fecal occult blood testing and a positive family history of colorectal cancer (one first-degree relative affected at age 59). His routine blood results, including iron studies, were normal. The bowel preparation was adequate and the instrument was inserted to the cecum. No polyps were found. Which of the following is the most appropriate recommendation for colorectal cancer surveillance for this patient?

   A   Repeat colonoscopy within 6 months
   B   Repeat colonoscopy in 3 years
   C   Repeat colonoscopy in 5 years
   D   Repeat colonoscopy in 10 years
   E   No further colonoscopy required

9   A 39-year-old woman with a background of Crohn's disease presents with increased ileostomy output and upper abdominal pain. The pain is cramping and worse after meals. On clinical examination there is mild abdominal distension, but no guarding or rigidity. She is currently on methotrexate weekly. Her stool cultures are negative for *Clostridium difficile*, *Giardia* and *Cryptosporidium*. Her inflammatory markers are slightly raised. Recent gastroscopy was normal, with normal duodenal biopsies. You suspect recurrent Crohn's disease. Which of the following investigations is contraindicated in this patient?

   A   Computed tomography of the abdomen with contrast
   B   Small-bowel series with follow-through
   C   Colonoscopy
   D   Video-capsule endoscopy
   E   Magnetic resonance imaging enteroclysis

10 A 26-year-old woman has a 15-year history of ulcerative colitis. At present she is well, with only occasional diarrhea and bleeding while on mesalamine (mesalazine). She has not required corticosteroids for the past few years. Her last colonoscopy, about 12 months ago, showed mild chronic colitis in the rectum. Her liver function tests are elevated and a magnetic resonance imaging cholangiogram is highly suggestive of primary sclerosing cholangitis. Which of the following options is most appropriate for this patient to prevent colon cancer?

   A   Colonoscopy with biopsies at age 50 years and repeat at 5-yearly intervals
   B   Colonoscopy now and repeat every 12 months with biopsies
   C   Computed tomography colonography second-yearly
   D   Colonoscopy with biopsies only when patient is symptomatic or refractory to medical treatment
   E   Proceed to total colectomy

11 A 43-year-old man presents to hospital with a body mass index of 15 kg/m^2. Eight months ago he had vomiting secondary to severe NSAID-induced peptic ulcer disease leading to gastric-outlet obstruction. He subsequently underwent a Bilroth II subtotal gastroenterostomy procedure. Since his hospital discharge he has been losing weight and has developed chronic diarrhea. His fat-soluble vitamin levels are normal. Fecal elastase is normal, but his fecal alpha-1 antitrypsin is elevated. Urine analysis is normal. Gastroscopy shows post-surgical changes, and colonoscopy is normal. A small-bowel series with follow-through revealed a blind loop with slow transit of contrast. What is the most likely cause of this clinical presentation?

   A   Dumping syndrome
   B   Crohn's disease
   C   Small-bowel bacterial overgrowth
   D   Short bowel syndrome
   E   Pancreatic insufficiency

12 An 18-year-old first-year university student presents with non-bloody diarrhea for the past 8 months. She describes 5−10 bowel motions per day, which are watery. She has not been able to concentrate on her studies lately. Stool cultures were negative. Celiac serology and thyroid function tests were normal. No recent travel was noted. Gastroscopy and colonoscopy with biopsies were normal. Despite the above attempts to determine the cause, no cause was found. An inpatient work-up to quantify her diarrhea was undertaken. Stool osmolality was 13 mOsm/kg and serum osmolality was 285 mOsm/kg. Stool sodium, potassium and magnesium were within normal ranges. What is the most likely diagnosis?

A Laxative abuse
B Tropical sprue
C Whipple's disease
D Irritable bowel syndrome, diarrhea-predominant
E Factitious diarrhea

13 Which of the following vaccinations is not contraindicated while on induction therapy with anti-TNF-alpha therapy for Crohn's disease?

A Hepatitis B
B Varicella
C Polio
D Typhoid
E MMR (measles-mumps-rubella)

14 A 60-year-old man presents with a history of rectal bleeding and iron-deficiency anemia. He has a positive family history of colon cancer (adenocarcinoma). At colonoscopy there were at least 30 colonic polyps throughout his bowel, averaging 1 mm in size. Several of these polyps were excised (polypectomy). Histology showed hyperplastic polyps. Which of the following surveillance options is most appropriate for this patient?

A Colonoscopy at 5-yearly intervals
B Colonoscopy at 15-year intervals
C Colonoscopy at 10-yearly intervals
D Colonoscopy at 3-yearly intervals

15 A postmenopausal 52-year-old woman presents with vague abdominal discomfort, bloating and diarrhea. Her symptoms have been present for the past 6 months. Stress seems to worsen her symptoms, and she feels better after each evacuation. She has lost 5 kg and her family physician has mentioned that she was 'low in iron'. Her family history is negative for gastrointestinal disease. Abdominal and rectal examination is unremarkable. What is the most appropriate next step in her evaluation?

A Reassure her that her symptoms fit the criteria for irritable bowel syndrome (IBS). Ask her to try increasing her consumption of fiber and review her in 1 month.
B Proceed to endoscopic evaluation after explaining the risks and benefits to her.
C Commence iron replacement and review symptoms in 3 months.
D Perform the fecal occult blood test and only investigate further if this is positive.
E Proceed to abdomino-pelvic computed tomography studies as the first step.

16 A 39-year-old man who was admitted 5 days previously with acute alcohol-related pancreatitis is complaining of ongoing severe epigastric pain that radiates to the back, plus nausea and vomiting. He has not been able to eat or drink and has not had a bowel movement since being admitted. On physical examination he is febrile at 38.5°C, but normotensive. His heart rate is 101 beats/min. There is no scleral icterus or jaundice. The abdomen is distended and diffusely tender with hypoactive bowel sounds. His blood count reveals a leukocytosis of 12,000/mm^3. His liver function tests are deranged, and lipase remains elevated at 855 U/L. A progress computed tomography scan of the abdomen shows a diffusely edematous pancreas with a few peripancreatic fluid collections. There is no evidence of pancreatic necrosis or free gas within the abdomen. Which of the following is the most appropriate next step in the management of this patient?

A Insert a naso-jejunal feeding tube and start enteral nutrition.
B Refer to surgical opinion for consideration of necrosectomy.
C Commence broad-spectrum intravenous antibiotics.
D Oral feeding facilitated by antiemetics.
E Commence parenteral nutrition via a central venous line.

17 A 43-year-old woman has presented to hospital for the fifth time in 3 months with nausea, vomiting and dehydration. She has longstanding type 1 diabetes mellitus with suboptimal glycemic control. A gastric emptying study performed 2 years previously was consistent with gastroparesis. This has been managed with metoclopramide, but recently she developed intolerable extra-pyramidal side-effects and this medication was ceased. A trial of oral erythromycin has failed to improve her ability to tolerate even a liquid diet per mouth. She has lost 8 kg in the past 3 months. A recent blood test shows that she is not hypothyroid and identifies no other abnormality to explain her symptoms. Which of the following is the most appropriate next step in her management?

A Commence total parenteral nutrition.
B Insert a gastrostomy (PEG) tube.
C Re-commence metoclopramide.
D Commence naso-jejunal feeding.
E Repeat the gastric emptying study.

18 A 50-year-old man undergoes colonoscopy due to a positive fecal occult blood test. He has no personal or family history of colonic polyps, cancer or inflammatory bowel disease. The colonoscopy reveals large internal hemorrhoids, but no polyps or cancers. Which of the following is the most appropriate screening schedule for this patient?

A Repeat colonoscopy in 1 year
B Repeat colonoscopy in 3 years
C Repeat colonoscopy in 5 years
D Repeat colonoscopy in 10 years
E Repeat fecal occult blood test in 5 years and proceed to colonoscopy if positive

19 A 48-year-old man suffers from longstanding ulcerative colitis. Since his diagnosis 15 years ago he has had several flares, but is currently reasonably well-controlled on 6-mercaptopurine (6-MP) and oral mesalazine. He has not required corticosteroids in the past few years. He attends for a colonoscopy, which shows active proctitis but very little colonic disease activity. Random biopsies are taken and yield high-grade dysplasia in the ascending colon as well as low-grade dysplasia in the sigmoid colon. Which of the following treatment options is most appropriate?

A Total colectomy
B Right-sided colectomy with annual surveillance of the remaining colon
C Annual surveillance colonoscopy with random colonic biopsies
D Add a biological agent (TNF-alpha blocker)
E Perform a carcinoembryonic antigen (CEA) level and proceed to colectomy if this is elevated

20 A 68-year-old man presents with an upper gastrointestinal hemorrhage. He has a 2-year background of heartburn and dyspepsia. His bowel motions have also been looser than normal over this time. He takes no regular medications and denies the use of over-the-counter analgesics. Physical examination is unremarkable, but blood testing shows iron deficiency. *Helicobacter pylori* serology is negative. Endoscopy shows multiple ulcers in the stomach and the duodenum and some prominent gastric folds. One of the ulcers has a visible vessel, which is treated endoscopically. Which is the next most appropriate step?

A Somatostatin receptor scintigraphy
B Measurement of urinary 5-HIAA (5-hydroxyindoleacetic acid) levels
C Measurement of a serum gastrin level
D Computed tomography (CT) scan of the abdomen
E Urinary NSAID (non-steroidal anti-inflammatory drug) assay

21 A 70-year-old Japanese man is hospitalized because of a 2-week history of progressive jaundice, mild epigastric discomfort and anorexia. Physical examination reveals tenderness in the epigastric area and overt jaundice. Liver function tests reveal elevated bilirubin, alkaline phosphatase (ALP) and gamma-glutamyl transpeptidase (GGT). Abdominal ultrasonography reveals an intrahepatic duct and common duct dilatation without evidence of choledocholithiasis. Subsequent abdominal computed tomography (CT) shows a 5 cm pancreatic mass within the main pancreatic duct in addition to a diffusely swollen sausage-shaped pancreas with a narrowed pancreatic duct. Serum immunoglobulin G4 (IgG4) was elevated. What will be your next step in confirming the diagnosis of this patient?

A Cholecystectomy
B ERCP (endoscopic retrograde cholangiopancreatography)
C Endoscopic ultrasonography with biopsy of the pancreas and immunohistochemical staining for IgG4
D Tumor markers
E MRCP (magnetic resonance cholangiopancreatography)

ANSWERS

1 E.

For this man with many comorbidities, esophagectomy is undesirable. Repeating biopsies is unnecessary when the diagnosis is already confirmed by two biopsies. Endoscopic mucosal resection is appropriate when raised lesions are present, and liquid nitrogen ablation is currently an experimental therapy. Radiofrequency ablation has a good chance of eradicating his high-grade dysplasia and preventing progression to esophageal adenocarcinoma.

2 D.

With a history of intermittent food bolus obstruction and asthma, eosinophilic esophagitis is the most likely diagnosis. The lack of progressive symptoms makes a malignancy or motor disorder such as achalasia less likely. Zenker's diverticulum is an unlikely cause of food bolus obstruction.

3 A.

All gastric ulcers require repeat endoscopy to assess healing. The rapid urease test is reliable when positive, and *Helicobacter* eradication should be undertaken. There is no need to perform other tests to confirm *H. pylori* status, but such tests may be appropriate when the rapid urease test is negative, which it often is despite infection with *H. pylori* when blood is present.

4 C.

It is difficult to make a diagnosis of celiac disease when gluten has already been eliminated from the diet. Elimination of gluten makes histology and antibody testing unreliable. The total IgA is useful only for making sure that IgA deficiency is not causing a falsely negative anti-tissue transglutaminase antibody test. Video-capsule endoscopy has no role in this setting. The HLA test is useful if negative, as the likelihood of having celiac disease with negative DQ2 and DQ8 is less than 1%.

5 C.

The travel history and duration of onset of illness are helpful in determining the likely pathogen causing acute diarrhea and/ or vomiting. The man was on a cruise ship which served shellfish for dinner. The most likely cause of his acute diarrhea and vomiting is related to undercooked seafood. Norovirus is the most likely pathogen. *Staphylococcus aureus* infection usually presents within 6 hours of exposure and is often due to contaminated salad, dairy or meats. *Bacillus cereus* infection presents within 6 hours of exposure and is due usually to contaminated rice and meats. *Clostridium perfringens* presents within 8–16 hours after exposure to contaminated meat and poultry.

6 B.

The symptom complex of recurrent epigastric pain, anorexia and diarrhea with loose stool that is foul-smelling is in keeping with steatorrhea and fat malabsorption secondary to pancreatic insufficiency related to chronic pancreatitis. The heavy alcohol use is likely to cause chronic pancreatitis in those predisposed. Serum amylase and lipase can be normal in chronic pancreatitis and rule out acute pancreatitis. The poor night vision is indicative of vitamin A deficiency. Fat-soluble vitamins (A, D, E and K) may be low in pancreatic insufficiency. Acute pancreatitis leads to an elevated amylase and lipase level. Peptic ulcer disease does not induce diarrhea or steatorrhea (unless due to the rare Zollinger–Ellison syndrome). Gastritis does not cause this symptom complex and is usually asymptomatic. Patients with protein-losing enteropathy often have diarrhea, but usually not steatorrhea.

7 A.

The most likely cause of her ongoing symptoms is recurrent *Clostridium difficile* infection. She needs retreatment with oral metronidazole for 14 days. If this does not cure her diarrhea, then oral vancomycin 125 mg four times a day for 14 days followed by a tapering dose to ensure complete eradication of infection is appropriate. Oral vancomycin and intravenous metronidazole are often used in fulminant disease. Third-line treatments such as rifaximin should be considered when vancomycin has failed. Fecal bacteriotherapy is utilized as salvage therapy in selected patients who have failed usual management. Intravenous vancomycin does not lead to sufficient drug levels within the colon, and therefore has no role in the treatment of *C. difficile* infection.

8 C.

After a negative colonoscopy with no polyps, a patient with a family history of colorectal cancer should have a repeat procedure in 5 years (low risk). If there was no family history, 10 years would be reasonable. If a polyp was detected, then after a complete clearing colonoscopy had been accomplished after initial polypectomy, repeat colonoscopy to check for metachronous adenomas should be performed in 3 years for a patient at high risk of developing metachronous advanced adenomas. This includes those who at baseline examination have multiple (>2) adenomas, a large (>1 cm) adenoma, an adenoma with villous histology or high-grade dysplasia, or a family history of colorectal cancer. After one negative follow-up surveillance colonoscopy, subsequent surveillance may be increased to 5-yearly.

9 D.

Capsule endoscopy is contraindicated as there is likely to be subacute bowel obstruction from stricturing Crohn's disease. The small-bowel series could be helpful in determining the presence of active Crohn's disease. An MRI enteroclysis provides excellent images of the small bowel but is expensive and labor-intensive.

10 B.

The cumulative incidence of colorectal cancer is 8–18% after 20–30 years of ulcerative colitis. The cumulative incidence of colorectal cancer among patients with extensive disease (pancolitis) ranges from 6–50% after 30 years of the disease. The cumulative risk of colorectal cancer does not seem to be higher than that of the general population until 8–10 years after the diagnosis, and thereafter the increase in risk is 0.5–1% each year. This patient with a history of ulcerative colitis of more than 7 years, pancolitis and primary sclerosing cholangitis is at high risk for developing colorectal cancer. Current guidelines recommend regular colonoscopy surveillance with biopsy after 7 years of left-sided colitis or pancolitis in both ulcerative colitis and Crohn's disease. This should be done at least on a yearly basis. Patients with primary sclerosing cholangitis should begin colonoscopy surveillance immediately.

11 C.

The elevated fecal alpha-1 antitrypsin suggests protein-losing enteropathy. The small-bowel series indicates the presence of a blind loop with slow transit. The likely cause of the presentation is thus small-bowel overgrowth. Fecal elastase is low in pancreatic insufficiency. Dumping syndrome leads to characteristic symptoms of sweating and tachycardia after meals. Short bowel syndrome occurs when less than 200 cm of small bowel remains, which is not the case after a Bilroth II procedure. If his symptoms were due to Crohn's disease, the small-bowel series is likely to have been abnormal.

12 E.

The increase in the fecal osmolal gap indicates the presence of unmeasured solute, which can be due to laxatives containing magnesium, sorbitol, lactose, lactulose or polyethylene glycol as active ingredients (>50 mOsm/kg). The fecal osmolal gap is helpful in factitious diarrhea resulting from the addition of water to the stool; this diagnosis is suspected if the measured stool osmolality is lower than that of plasma, since the colon cannot dilute stool to an osmolality less than that of plasma. In irritable bowel syndrome the fecal osmolar gap is normal. Whipple's disease often results in abnormal duodenal biopsies, where PAS-positive macrophages are identified. Tropical sprue affects residents and travelers in the tropics, and usually a 4- to 6-week stay in a high-risk area is required to acquire the disease.

13 A.

All live vaccinations are contraindicated while on anti-TNF-alpha therapy. Hepatitis B vaccination does not involve a live vaccine.

14 D.

This patient has the hyperplastic polyposis syndrome, which is phenotypically defined by at least 5 histologically diagnosed hyperplastic polyps proximal to the sigmoid colon, two of which are larger than 1 cm, or any number of hyperplastic polyps occurring proximal to the sigmoid colon in an individual who has a first-degree relative with hyperplastic polyposis syndrome, or 20 hyperplastic polyps of any size but distributed throughout the colon. This condition is usually diagnosed between the ages of 40 and 60 years. The genetic basis has not yet been identified. This condition is inheritable in 5% of cases. Colorectal cancer is found synchronously in at least 50% of cases. Current guidelines recommend 1- to 3-yearly colonoscopy surveillance, and first-degree relatives over the age 40 (or 10 years earlier than the age of the index case) should be offered screening.

15 B.

Although her symptoms fit the Rome IV criteria for IBS, there are red flags present. New-onset symptoms after the age of 50, weight loss and iron deficiency are worrisome and may indicate malignancy. A diagnosis of IBS should not be made, and endoscopic evaluation is currently the 'gold standard' for ruling out bowel cancer.

16 A.

Nutrition is required for recovery, and in this clinical scenario oral nutrition is not likely to be established for some time due to pain and vomiting. Enteral feeding via the mouth will also stimulate the pancreas, which can be avoided by naso-jejunal feeding if the tip of the feeding tube is passed distally to the ligament of Treitz. Enteral feeding is preferable due to a lower risk of complications. Parenteral nutrition can lead to sepsis and is more expensive. Pancreatic debridement and intravenous antibiotics are appropriate if pancreatic necrosis is present.

17 D.

In the setting of severe gastroparesis impairing a person's nutrition, prompt action is needed. If a trial of naso-jejunal feeding is successful, a jejunostomy may allow long-term enteral feeding. A PEG tube does not bypass the stomach and is unlikely to help her symptoms. Repeating the gastric emptying study is unlikely to change management. Total parenteral nutrition is a last resort when enteral feeding is contraindicated or unsuccessful. Recommencing metoclopramide is contraindicated if extra-pyramidal (tardive) symptoms have already occurred.

18 D.

The most appropriate interval for screening is 10 years. In some countries, second-yearly fecal occult blood tests are also considered adequate. Repeated colonoscopy in 1 year is recommended if a bowel cancer was identified and resected. Patients with large adenomas (>1 cm) or more than 3 adenomas should have a colonoscopy repeated in 3 years. Patients with small (<1 cm) or only 1 or 2 adenomas can be next screened at a 5-year interval.

19 A.

This patient requires total colectomy. High-grade dysplasia in patients with ulcerative colitis has a high chance of synchronous carcinoma *in situ* or rapid progression to cancer. Adding further therapy or partially resecting the colon is therefore inappropriate. A CEA level can be useful for monitoring disease progression in a patient with confirmed colorectal cancer, but plays no role in decision-making for this patient.

20 C.

This patient probably has a gastrinoma. The diagnosis should be suspected in patients with multiple ulcers without NSAID exposure or *H. pylori* infection. An elevated gastrin level in the absence of regular proton-pump inhibitor therapy is highly suggestive. Somatostatin receptor scintigraphy is a highly sensitive test for diagnosis, but a CT is usually performed first. If gastrinoma is suspected based on the serum gastrin, a urinary NSAID assay can be ordered if occult NSAID use is suspected. Measurement of urinary 5-HIAA is a screening test for carcinoid tumor.

21 C.

The two important differential diagnoses in this case are pancreatic cancer or uncommonly autoimmune pancreatitis. CT abdomen demonstrates a diffusely swollen sausage-shaped pancreas with a narrowed pancreatic duct. This finding is more in keeping with autoimmune pancreatitis. IgG4 levels further support the diagnosis of autoimmune pancreatitis type 1. To confirm the diagnosis, EUS with core biopsy of the pancreatic mass is required with IgG4 staining.

CHAPTER 12

HEPATOLOGY

Robert Gibson, Magnus Halland and Nicholas J Talley

CHAPTER OUTLINE

- SYSTEMIC DISEASE AND THE LIVER
- PREGNANCY AND LIVER DISEASE
- GALLBLADDER AND BILIARY TREE
  – Gallstones
  – Acalculous cholecystitis

- PORPHYRIAS
  – Acute intermittent porphyria (AIP)
  – Porphyria cutanea tarda (PCT)

LIVER FUNCTION TESTS AND THEIR ABNORMALITIES

'Liver function tests' are simply serum enzyme levels:
- alanine aminotransferase (ALT), also called serum glutamic pyruvic transaminase (SGPT)
- aspartate aminotransferase (AST), also called serum glutamic oxaloacetic transaminase (SGOT)
- gamma-glutamyl transpeptidase (GGT), and
- alkaline phosphatase (ALP)

as well as tests of synthetic function:
- prothrombin time (PT)
- albumin, and
- bilirubin.

The pattern of abnormality is helpful in assessing the cause and severity of liver disease, but no pattern is specific to any given diagnosis. The serum enzymes are best thought of as either *hepatocellular* (raised transaminases) or *cholestatic* (raised GGT and ALP).

Serum enzymes

Hepatocellular enzymes

The measurement of these liver enzymes is essentially a measure of liver *damage* as opposed to liver *function*.

- ALT is a cytosolic enzyme that is more hepatospecific than AST. It is pyridoxine-dependent, which explains its relative deficiency compared with AST in alcoholic liver disease, as alcoholic patients are depleted of pyridoxine.
- AST is a mitochondrial enzyme that is not specific to hepatocellular damage. It is found, in decreasing order of concentration, in liver, myocardium, skeletal muscle, kidneys, brain, pancreas and erythrocytes.

CLINICAL PEARL

Serum transaminases (ALT, AST) don't predict dysfunction—prothrombin time, albumin, bilirubin, ascites and encephalopathy are true indicators of liver function.

Cholestatic enzymes

- ALP is not specific to the liver, being commonly found in bone and the placenta. It may be high in the rapid growth phase of adolescence and in pregnancy.
- GGT is a very sensitive marker of biliary disease, although it may also be elevated as a result of alcohol abuse and with certain medications. One important use is supporting the likelihood that an elevated ALP is from the liver.

Tests of synthetic function

Prothrombin time (PT)/international normalized ratio (INR) coagulation studies are useful for assessing liver synthesis. Vitamin K deficiency due to poor nutrition should be considered as a cause of an elevated PT, as should malabsorption due to pancreatic or biliary disease. Reversal of coagulopathy with 10 mg of parenteral vitamin K supports the conclusion that PT elongation is unrelated to synthesis.

Hypoglycemia occurs in severe liver dysfunction.

Noninvasive hepatic fibrosis assessment

While liver biopsy can offer clues to the etiology of a liver injury and quantify fibrosis, it is limited by the very small sample size and by potential complications. A more global assessment of liver fibrosis can be obtained with the use of serum markers and of transient elastography (see below).

APPROACH TO THE PATIENT WITH LIVER DISEASE

The presence of liver disease may sometimes be suggested by symptoms. These can include right upper abdominal discomfort and cholestatic symptoms (jaundice, itch, dark urine). More commonly, symptoms are nonspecific such as nausea or fatigue. Most commonly, liver disease is detected in the asymptomatic person on routine biochemical testing.

It is important to distinguish *acute* from *chronic* liver disease. Clues to the cause of liver disease (Box 12-1) are provided by a careful history and examination.

- Obesity, diabetes and dyslipidemia may suggest fatty liver. A careful alcohol history is mandatory. A commonly overlooked area is medication, including herbal and nutritional supplements, especially high-protein supplements. The history here must be meticulous and include commencement times.
- Risk factors for viral hepatitis must be sought; these include intravenous drug use, sexual behavior, especially for men who have sex with men, migration from a high-prevalence area, and blood transfusion prior to routine screening.
- Occasionally the physical examination may provide diagnostic clues.

> ## Box 12-1
> ## Clinical clues suggesting chronic liver disease
>
> ### Symptoms
>
> - Fatigue, pruritus, bleeding, abdominal pain, nausea, anorexia, myalgia, jaundice, dark urine, pale stools, fever, weight loss; may be no symptoms
>
> ### Signs
>
> *Peripheral signs of chronic liver disease with hepatocellular dysfunction:*
>
> - Spider nevi, palmar erythema, white nails, gynecomastia, body hair loss, testicular atrophy, hepatomegaly
>
> *Signs of portal hypertension:*
>
> - Splenomegaly, ascites, peripheral edema
>
> *Signs of poor hepatocellular synthetic function:*
>
> - Bruising, peripheral edema (reflecting depleted coagulation factors and albumin levels)
>
> *Signs of end-stage liver disease:*
>
> - Wasting, progressive severe fatigue, encephalopathy (asterixis, fetor, coma)

» Parotidomegaly and Dupuytren's contractures (Figure 12-1) occur in alcoholism.
» Acanthosis nigricans occurs in the metabolic syndrome and fatty liver disease (insulin resistance).
» Signs of more advanced liver diseases are palmar erythema (Figure 12-2), gynecomastia, spider nevi

(Figure 12-3), splenomegaly, jaundice, ascites and encephalopathy.

- There are many possible causes of liver enlargement (Box 12-2, overleaf).

Laboratory tests may guide you toward a hepatocellular or a cholestatic etiology. Alcohol as a cause should be increasingly suspected as the AST/ALT ratio rises above 2. At this point around 90% of patients will have alcoholic liver disease.

The magnitude of the transaminase rise may also help with finding the etiology:

- An ALT of >500 U/L is almost *never* due to alcohol alone and should prompt a search for an alternative explanation.

- Transaminases of >1000 U/L are usually due to ischemic hepatopathy, acute viral hepatitis, acetaminophen (paracetamol) toxicity, or acute biliary obstruction.

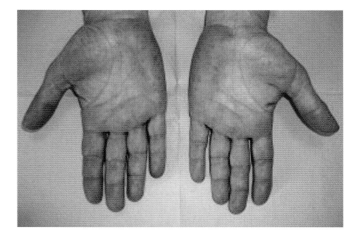

Figure 12-2 Palmar erythema

From Kluger N and Guillot B. Erythema palmare hereditarium (Lane's red palms): a forgotten entity? J Am Acad Dermatol 2010;63(2):e46.

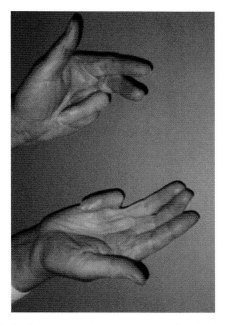

Figure 12-1 Dupuytren's contracture in the hands

From Gudmundsson KG, Jónsson T and Arngrímsson R. Guillaume Dupuytren and finger contractures. Lancet 2003;363(9378):165–8.

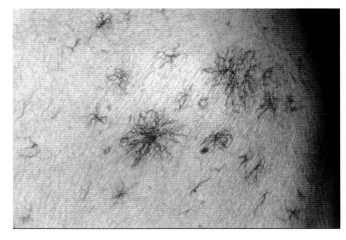

Figure 12-3 Spider nevi

From Gruber G and Hansch A. Kompaktatlas Blickdiagnosen in der Inneren Medizin, 2nd ed. Munich: Urban & Fischer/Elsevier, 2009.

Box 12-2

Causes of hepatomegaly

1. Diffusely enlarged and smooth

Massive
- Metastatic disease
- Alcoholic liver disease with fatty infiltration
- Myeloproliferative diseases (e.g. polycythemia rubra vera, myelofibrosis)

Moderate
- The above causes
- Hematological disease (e.g. chronic myeloid leukemia, lymphoma)
- Fatty liver (e.g. diabetes mellitus)
- Hemochromatosis

Mild
- The above causes
- Hepatitis (viral, drugs)
- Cirrhosis
- Biliary obstruction
- Granulomatous disorders (e.g. sarcoidosis)
- Infiltrative disorders (e.g. amyloidosis)
- Human immunodeficiency virus infection

2. Diffusely enlarged and irregular
- Metastatic disease

- Cirrhosis
- Hydatid disease
- Polycystic liver disease

3. Localized swelling
- Riedel's lobe (a normal variant—the lobe may even be palpable in the right lumbar region)
- Metastasis
- Large simple hepatic cyst
- Hydatid cyst
- Hepatoma
- Liver abscess (e.g. amebic abscess)

4. Hepatosplenomegaly
- Chronic liver disease with portal hypertension
- Hematological disease (e.g. myeloproliferative disease, lymphoma)
- Infection (e.g. acute viral hepatitis, infectious mononucleosis)
- Infiltration (e.g. amyloidosis, sarcoidosis)
- Connective tissue disease (e.g. systemic lupus erythematosus)

Medications are another common cause of this degree of hepatitis and a thorough medication history needs to be sought. Drug-induced liver injury (DILI) is a common cause of acute liver failure.

- If the transaminases are normal or near-normal but both the ALP and GGT are elevated, this suggests liver disease (cholestasis).

A history of right upper quadrant pain points toward an hepatic or biliary cause. Hepatobiliary pain can also occur in the epigastrium.

- If the pain is persistent, the liver should be considered as the cause.
- If severe and episodic, then biliary pain is suggested.

If the patient is a middle-aged woman, primary biliary cholangitis is an important consideration, and a liver ultrasound and anti-mitochondrial antibody (AMA) should be performed.

Common causes of hepatitis and cholestasis, and the specific diagnostic tests, are listed in Table 12-1.

CLINICAL PEARL

If the liver function tests suggest cholestasis (elevation of ALP and GGT), image the biliary tree but also think about drugs, and autoimmune and infiltrative disease.

An abdominal ultrasound is recommended not only to exclude extrahepatic biliary disease, but also to detect the presence of steatosis, possible cirrhosis, portal hypertension or tumors. Assessment of the splenic size as well as portal vein patency and flow adds valuable information to the assessment.

If the above strategy has been used to define the etiology of abnormal liver function tests but there is no clear diagnosis, it is most probable that the patient has non-alcoholic fatty liver disease.

CLINICAL PEARL

Celiac disease can cause a moderate elevation of alanine aminotransferase and aspartate aminotransferase, but bilirubin is usually normal.

BILIRUBIN METABOLISM AND JAUNDICE

Bilirubin is formed from the metabolism of heme, with a much lesser contribution from myoglobin and cytochromes. Its metabolism begins in the reticuloendothelial system, especially the spleen, where it is fat-soluble and is therefore bound to albumin for transport to the liver. There are three hepatic phases: *uptake*, *conjugation* and *excretion* (Figure 12-4).

- Uptake is via a large-capacity facilitated transport system.

Table 12-1 Common causes of hepatitis and cholestasis, and diagnostic tests

CAUSE	DIAGNOSTIC TESTS
Hepatitis	
Hepatitis A virus (HAV)	Anti-HAV immunoglobulin M (IgM)
Hepatitis B virus (HBV)	Surface antigen or hepatitis B IgM if acute
Hepatitis C virus (HCV)	Anti-HCV antibodies
Alcoholic liver disease	AST/ALT >2; ALT <500 U/L
NAFLD	Imaging, clinical assessment
Autoimmune hepatitis	ALT 200–2000 U/L ANA, ASMA, ALKMA Raised globulins Liver biopsy
Ischemic hepatopathy	ALT in the 1000s U/L with rapid resolution
Hemochromatosis	Serum iron studies *HFE* gene mutation
Wilson's disease	Serum copper and ceruloplasmin; urinary and liver copper levels Slit-lamp examination
Drug-induced hepatitis	Improvement off suspect culprit drug
Cholestasis	
Primary biliary cholangitis	Anti-mitochondrial antibody Liver biopsy
Primary sclerosing cholangitis	Ulcerative colitis Cholangiography
Common duct obstruction (tumor, stone, stricture)	Ultrasound Cholangiography
Infiltration (malignancy, sarcoid, amyloid)	Ultrasound, CT, liver biopsy
Drug-induced cholestasis	Resolution off suspected culprit drug

ALKMA, anti-liver-kidney microsomal antibodies; ALT, alanine aminotransferase; ANA, anti-nuclear antibodies; ASMA, anti-smooth-muscle antibodies; AST, aspartate aminotransferase; CT, computed tomography; NAFLD, non-alcoholic fatty liver disease.

- Once in the hepatocyte, bilirubin is solubilized by conjugation with glucuronide for biliary excretion. This reaction is dependent on the enzyme glucuronosyltransferase.
- The final phase of excretion into the biliary system is via multidrug-resistance-like protein 2 (MRP2).

The terms *direct* and *indirect* bilirubin correspond to conjugated and unconjugated bilirubin (Box 12-3).

- The normal levels of bilirubin are up to 1.5 mg/dL (25 micromol/L), with the conjugated portion up to 0.3 mg/dL (5 micromol/L).
- Clinical jaundice (icterus) occurs at about 2.5 mg/dL (42 micromol/L).

The first step in finding the cause of hyperbilirubinemia is reviewing the serum liver enzymes and looking for clinical and ultrasound evidence of chronic liver disease.

- If abnormal, then a search should be undertaken for a specific diagnosis. An abnormal blood film can indicate a hematological cause for the hyperbilirubinemia.
- If the serum enzymes are normal, fractionation should be done to determine the proportion of direct and indirect bilirubin. This will allow distinction between overproduction from hemolysis, and a conjugation defect or secretion problem from medication or Dubin-Johnson syndrome.

CLINICAL PEARL

Pruritus and jaundice suggest intrahepatic or posthepatic cholestasis.

Bilirubin metabolism and the causes of jaundice

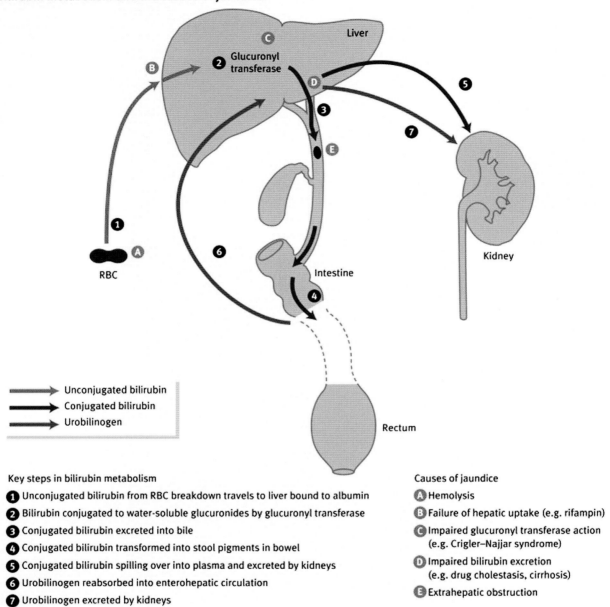

Key steps in bilirubin metabolism

1. Unconjugated bilirubin from RBC breakdown travels to liver bound to albumin
2. Bilirubin conjugated to water-soluble glucuronides by glucuronyl transferase
3. Conjugated bilirubin excreted into bile
4. Conjugated bilirubin transformed into stool pigments in bowel
5. Conjugated bilirubin spilling over into plasma and excreted by kidneys
6. Urobilinogen reabsorbed into enterohepatic circulation
7. Urobilinogen excreted by kidneys

Causes of jaundice

A Hemolysis
B Failure of hepatic uptake (e.g. rifampin)
C Impaired glucuronyl transferase action (e.g. Crigler–Najjar syndrome)
D Impaired bilirubin excretion (e.g. drug cholestasis, cirrhosis)
E Extrahepatic obstruction

Figure 12-4 Bilirubin metabolism and jaundice. Biliary excretion of conjugated bilirubin by way of MRP2 (multidrug-resistance-like protein 2) into the bile canaliculus is an energy-dependent active transport system and is the rate-limiting step in hepatic bilirubin processing. This explains why in liver failure most excess bilirubin remains conjugated

From Gilmore I and Garvey CJ. Jaundice. Medicine 2009;37(1);42–6.

Box 12-3
Classification of jaundice

Unconjugated

1 Hemolysis

2 Impaired conjugation (decreased activity of glucuronyl transferase)
   a Gilbert's syndrome (diagnosed by exclusion of hemolysis, the presence of normal liver function, and a rise in the bilirubin level after fasting)
   b Crigler–Najjar syndrome (types I and II)

Conjugated

1 Hepatocellular disease
   a Hepatitis—viral, autoimmune, alcoholic
   b Cirrhosis
   c Drugs and toxins
   d Venous obstruction

2 Cholestatic disease
   a Intrahepatic cholestasis—drugs, recurrent jaundice of pregnancy, primary biliary cholangitis, benign recurrent intrahepatic cholestasis (BRIC)
   b Extrahepatic biliary obstruction—stones, carcinoma of the pancreas or bile duct, strictures of the bile duct

3 Familial, e.g. Dubin–Johnson syndrome

Table 12-2 Distinguishing features that help to determine the cause of postoperative jaundice

ETIOLOGY	FEATURE
Hypotension	ALT >1000 U/L, LDH elevation
Drugs, e.g. halothane	No specific features
Infection	Increased white cell count, fever
Total parenteral nutrition (TPN)	Liver function test profiles rise 1–4 weeks after TPN is commenced
Hematoma resorption	Unconjugated bilirubin increase
Cardiac failure	Elevated jugular venous pressure, enlarged pulsatile liver
Hemolysis	Unconjugated bilirubin and LDH increase; haptoglobin decrease if intravascular hemolysis. Abnormal blood smear
Renal failure	Creatinine rise
Bile duct injury, retained gallstone	SAP elevation

ALT, alanine aminotransferase; LDH, lactate dehydrogenase; SAP, serum alkaline phosphatase.

Table 12-3 Common causes of jaundice in immunosuppressed patients

ETIOLOGY	EXAMPLES
Hepatitis—infectious	*Mycobacterium avium intracellulare*, tuberculosis, cytomegalovirus
Hepatitis—drugs	Isoniazid, AZT, sulfonamides
AIDS cholangiopathy	Cytomegalovirus, *Cryptosporidium*
Veno-occlusive disease	Antineoplastic drugs (e.g. busulfan)
Neoplasm	Lymphoma, Kaposi's sarcoma

AIDS, acquired immunodeficiency syndrome; AZT, azidothymidine or zidovudine.

VIRAL HEPATITIS

Hepatitis A (RNA virus)

Hepatitis A virus (HAV) is transmitted by the fecal–oral route. Immunization has decreased its incidence.

HAV is diagnosed by anti-HAV immunoglobulin M (IgM) in serum. Patients with chronic liver disease or hepatitis C should all be immunized against hepatitis A (to prevent fulminant hepatitis). The aged are also at risk of severe disease.

CLINICAL PEARL

Hepatitis A can uncommonly cause prolonged cholestasis in an adult for months (and this may lead to diagnostic confusion).

In the postoperative patient who becomes jaundiced, the differential diagnosis includes intra-operative exposures (e.g. hypotension, drugs), infection, and less common causes (Table 12-2).

A different differential diagnosis list must be considered in immunosuppressed patients (Table 12-3).

Hepatitis B (DNA virus)

Hepatitis B virus (HBV) is one of the main causes of end-stage liver disease and hepatocellular carcinoma (HCC). There are 400 million people worldwide with chronic infection, and more than 1 million people a year die from end-stage liver cirrhosis and HCC. Transmission is percutaneous, sexual and perinatal.

In active hepatitis B infection there is a lifetime risk of liver-related death of 40%. People at risk are those with multiple sexual partners, men who have sex with men, injecting drug users, those with, tattoos obtained in non-sterile environments, unscreened blood transfusions, and those being born in a high-prevalence region. There has been an 80% decline in incidence in countries with vaccination programs. As there are highly effective treatments for hepatitis B infection, those at high risk should be screened.

Prevention of hepatitis B is possible through vaccination, and ensuring that exchange of body fluids does not occur.

- The transmission rate from an e-antigen-positive mother to her child at parturition is 85%. Vaccination and administration of hepatitis B immune globulin (HBIG) reduces this by 95%, although in extremely high viral loads (>10^8 copies/mL) this may be attenuated. It is in these latter cases that the mother should receive tenofovir in the last trimester of pregnancy and the child should be vaccinated and receive HBIG administration.

- In addition, vaccination of high-risk groups is important. Among adults, hepatitis B vaccine should be offered to men having sex with men, adults with multiple sexual partners, injecting drug users, hemodialysis patients, healthcare workers, and household members of carriers.

CLINICAL PEARL

Hepatitis B maternal to fetus transmission is preventable through neonatal vaccination, HBIG administration and in mothers with very high viral loads, tenofovir in the final trimester.

Diagnosis

Viral serology (Figure 12-5) is the mainstay for diagnosis of HBV. It includes HBsAg, HBsAb, HBeAg, HBeAb and HBcAb and involves both antigen and antibody testing. HBV DNA has become an important predictor of disease progression and HCC.

Antigen testing

- Surface antigen (sAg) is a marker of viral replication and therefore infection. It is a soluble HBV-shell protein.

- e-antigen (eAg) is a marker of high-level infection and replication with high HBV DNA levels and infectivity. It is a soluble core antigen.

- Core antigen (cAg) is an insoluble core antigen. Anti-HBcAg reflects its presence. Its main use is to confirm that there has been viral exposure rather than vaccination.

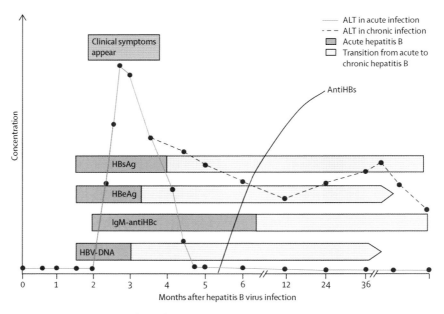

Figure 12-5 Serology of hepatitis B virus (HBV). Shaded bars indicate the duration of seropositivity in self-limited acute hepatitis B infection. Pointed bars indicate that HBV-DNA and HBeAg can become seronegative during chronic infection. Only IgG anti-HBcAg is detectable after resolution of acute hepatitis or during chronic infection. The *y*-axis is schematic concentration of serum ALT and anti-HBV antigens. ALT, alanine aminotransferase; DNA, deoxyribonucleic acid; HBcAg, hepatitis B core antigen; HBeAg, hepatitis B e-antigen; IgG, immunoglobulin G

From Liaw YF and Chu C-M. Hepatitis B virus infection. Lancet 2009;373:582–92.

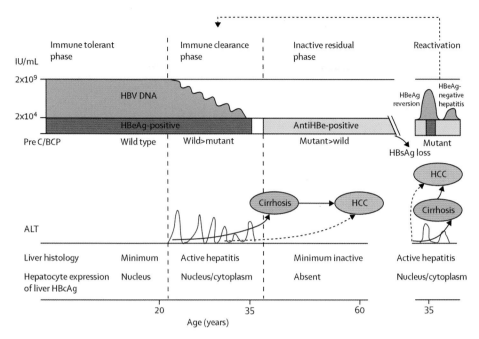

Figure 12-6 Natural history of chronic hepatitis B virus (HBV) infection acquired perinatally and during infancy. The reactivation phase is similar in every aspect to the immune-clearance phase, except for HBeAg status. Adult-acquired infection usually presents in the immune-clearance or reactivation phases (inset). The events during the immune-clearance and reactivation phases could lead to cirrhosis and hepatocellular carcinoma (HCC). ALT, serum alanine aminotransferase; anti-HBe, hepatitis B e-antigen antibody; BCP, basal core promoter; HBeAg, hepatitis B e-antigen; pre C, pre-core

From Liaw YF and Chu C-M. Hepatitis B virus infection. Lancet 2009;373:582–92.

Antibody testing

- IgM anti-HBcAb is a marker of acute HBV infection.
- IgG anti-HBcAb reflects past infection.
- Anti-HBsAg reflects exposure to the virus, immunity or vaccination.

Natural history

The natural history of HBV infection (Figure 12-6) depends on the age of the person at infection. In endemic areas characterized by vertical transmission, more than 90% of those infected progress to chronic infection (Table 12-4). In low-prevalence areas, most transmission is via high-risk sexual and injecting drug practice in adults, and only 5% progress to chronic hepatitis B infection, although these people at risk of severe acute hepatitis.

There are four phases of chronic hepatitis B infection:

1. immunotolerant
2. eAg-positive chronic hepatitis
3. eAg-negative chronic hepatitis
4. inactive carrier state.

Hepatic injury occurs during the active hepatitis phases. It is those phases that require treatment.

CLINICAL PEARL

Determine the phase of hepatitis B based on the history, e.g.:

A 23-year-old Vietnamese woman is found to have the following test results: ALT 12, HBVsAg +, HBVeAg +, HBVeAb −, and HBV-DNA 10^{10} IU/mL. There is no risk-taking behavior. Her mother had been diagnosed with hepatocellular carcinoma.

See Figure 12-6. This is the immunotolerant phase. This phase causes no active hepatitis and lasts for between 10 and 30 years. This patient should be observed for onset of the immune clearance phase, characterized by active hepatitis (eAg-positive hepatitis B).

There is a loss of e-antigen and e-antigen seroconversion at a rate of 10% per year. This can mean that one of two events has occurred:

- either the active phase has resolved into a silent carrier state (75%)
- or there has been the emergence of **core promoter or pre-core mutants**, i.e. eAg-negative chronic hepatitis B (25%).

eAg-negative chronic hepatitis B is due to the emergence of viral strains with mutations in the pre-core and core regions of the genome responsible for the soluble e-antigen and

Table 12-4 Viral and clinical features of chronic hepatitis infection

	IMMUNO-TOLERANT	eAg-POSITIVE CHB	eAg-NEGATIVE CHB	INACTIVE CARRIER	RESOLVED INFEC-TION	VACCINATION
s-antigen	Positive	Positive	Positive	Positive	Negative	Negative
e-antigen	Positive	Positive	Negative	Negative	Negative	Negative
Anti-HBe	Negative	Negative	Positive	Positive	Positive	Negative
Anti-HBs	Negative	Negative	Negative	Negative	Positive	Positive
Anti-HBc	Negative	Negative	Negative	Pos/Neg	Positive	Negative
HBV-DNA	>20,000 IU/mL (>10^5 copies/mL)	>20,000 IU/mL (>10^5 copies/mL)	>2000 IU/mL (>10^4 copies/mL)	<200 IU/mL (<10^3 copies/mL)	0	0
ALT	Normal	High	High	Normal	Normal	Normal
Histology	Normal	Hepatitis	Hepatitis	Normal	Normal	Normal

ALT, alanine aminotransferase; eAG, e-antigen; s-antigen, surface antigen; anti-HBe, antibody to hepatitis B e-antigen; anti-HBc, antibody to hepatitis B core antigen; anti-HBs, antibody to hepatitis B surface antigen; CHB, chronic hepatitis B; HBV-DNA, hepatitis B virus deoxyribonucleic acid.

nucleocapsid core antigens. Such mutants are responsible for severe and progressive hepatitis.

- Importantly, about 20% of those with eAg loss and normal ALT may reactivate, i.e. redevelop eAg positivity and a raised ALT. This mandates lifelong monitoring even in the 'silent carrier state'.
- Entry into the eAg-negative chronic hepatitis B phase leads to either persistent or fluctuating necroinflammation and a high risk of progression to advanced liver disease. This must be distinguished from the inactive carrier state. This will require monitoring of the HBV-DNA, the ALT and, at times, liver biopsy.

Chronic hepatitis can lead to cirrhosis, hepatic decompensation, HCC and death.

Hepatitis B has eight genotypes. The most significant is genotype B, having a relative early eAg seroconversion and slower progression to cirrhosis and hepatocellular carcinoma. Genotypes A and B have the highest rate of response to pegylated interferon.

CLINICAL PEARL

Patients with chronic hepatitis B require hepatocellular carcinoma (HCC) surveillance *even in the absence of cirrhosis* due to the ability of the virus to suppress tumor suppressor genes and prime tumor oncogenes.

Treatment

Indicators for commencement of treatment of chronic hepatitis B infection are as follows.

- **HBeAg-positive:**
  - » Decompensated cirrhosis
  - » Cirrhosis with HBV-DNA >2000 IU/mL or raised ALT

  - » HBV-DNA >20,000 IU/mL and hepatitis reflected by a raised ALT or on liver biopsy
- **HBeAg-negative:**
  - » HBV-DNA >2000 IU/mL and hepatitis (raised ALT or inflammatory histology)
  - » Before starting immunosuppression or chemotherapy
  - » Cirrhosis and detectable HBV-DNA

In young patients (and women wishing to become pregnant), pegylated interferon is primary therapy but only two-thirds at best obtain a complete remission at 1 year (higher in HBeAg-negative cases).

Any patient with decompensated cirrhosis should be treated with entecavir or tenofovir, rather than interferon. Referral to a transplant center should occur if the patient is transplant-eligible.

Otherwise, entecavir or tenofovir is preferred primary therapy because of high potency and low resistance, but therapy is required long term.

Vaccination

If vaccinated, HBsAb will be positive (and HBcAb negative). Vaccination is safe in pregnancy.

CLINICAL PEARL

If the HBsAg is positive in someone who otherwise appears well and has a normal ALT, consider whether the patient is a hepatitis B carrier (so neither vaccination nor hepatitis B immune globulin helps) or has early hepatitis B. The carrier state requires demonstration of very low HBV-DNA levels. It is important to note that the term 'carrier' should be avoided; it should now be termed the 'low replicative state', which while sustained is low-risk.

Close contacts of an acute hepatitis B case should be administered HBIG, then vaccinated. This includes pregnant women.

Hepatitis B mutations

There are two main clinically relevant types:
1 Mutations of the structural proteins: the core promoter and pre-core mutations result in loss of soluble core antigen (eAg). This is the cause of e-antigen chronic hepatitis. The pre-S and S mutations are responsible for vaccine escape (ineffectiveness). Other forms result in failure of HBIG immunoprophylaxis in the post-liver transplant setting.
2 Polymerase gene mutations. These relate to nucleoside resistance. The best known is the tyrosine–methionine–aspartate–aspartate (YMDD) locus.

Drug resistance

This is diagnosed in the adherent patient with rising HBV-DNA levels. Phenotypic resistance is defined as an increase in HBV-DNA by >1 log unit from the nadir on treatment or a rebound to pre-treatment levels (Figure 12-7). The hepatitis flare is the last event to occur, underpinning the requirement to monitor HBV-DNA.

> **CLINICAL PEARL**
>
> Resistance may be minimized by ensuring adherence and using the more potent nucleoside analogs such as entacavir and tenofovir.

Hepatitis C (RNA virus)

Hepatitis C virus (HCV) is a common cause of chronic liver disease. It is parenterally transmitted (injecting drug users, blood transfusions [prior to screening], needlestick injuries, unsafe tattooing). The disease is endemic in some parts of the world, e.g. Asia and the Middle East (Egypt has a 9% prevalence).

HIV is often found as a co-infection with hepatitis C (1:3), and so should always be screened for.

> **CLINICAL PEARL**
>
> Remember the rough '**rule of 2s**':
> * 2% acquire hepatitis C from a needlestick injury
> * 2% of infected cirrhotic patients develop hepatocellular carcinoma every year
> * 2% of the population is infected (based on US figures).

Diagnosis

Diagnosis is established by HCV antibody screening. Positive results must then be confirmed with HCV-RNA (for viremia).

Acute hepatitis C

This is rarely diagnosed.
* If acute hepatitis C is suspected, both HCV antibodies and HCV-RNA should be measured, and HCV-RNA then rechecked 2–4 months later to determine whether the disease is chronic (if untreated, 80% of cases become chronic).
* Once confirmed with a positive PCR (polymerase chain reaction), pegylated interferon provides viral eradication in about 90% of cases.

Chronic hepatitis C

Most chronic infection is initially asymptomatic (75%), but there is chronic hepatitis and this progresses to cirrhosis after 20 years in 25% of cases. Patients may have insidious fatigue and raised transaminases; this is variable, depending on which other risk factors for chronic liver disease are present.

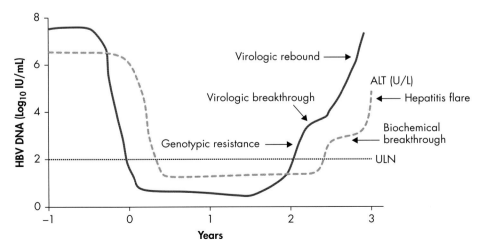

Figure 12-7 Serial changes in serum HBV-DNA. ALT, alanine aminotransferase; ULN, upper limit of normal ALT levels

From Keefe EB et al. Chronic hepatitis B: preventing, detecting and managing viral resistance. Clin Gastroenterol Hepatol 2008;6(3):268–74.

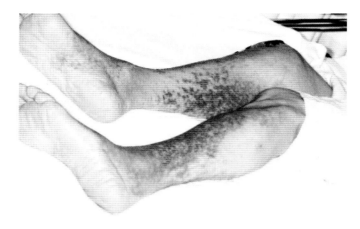

Figure 12-8 Palpable purpura

From Kitchens CS, Konkle BA and Kessler MD. Consultative hemostasis and thrombosis, 2nd ed. Philadelphia: Elsevier, 2007.

Extrahepatic manifestations of hepatitis C

These are important to remember:

- Mixed cryoglobulinemia—this has a very strong association with hepatitis C and presents with palpable purpura (Figure 12-8); this can also occur in other chronic liver diseases
- Porphyria cutanea tarda
- Polyarthralgias and polyarthritis
- Glomerulonephritis (membranoproliferative)
- Lichen planus
- Hashimoto's thyroiditis
- B-cell lymphoma.

Treatment

Successful treatment of hepatitis C (sustained virological response) reduces hepatic decompensation, liver-related death, liver transplantation and HCC, particularly in those with more advanced fibrosis (bridging fibrosis or cirrhosis).

General management

General management includes:

- vaccinating against hepatitis A and B, if not immune
- managing chronic liver disease, if present
- advising against dangerous alcohol consumption
- aiming at a healthy bodyweight
- regular surveillance for HCC in those with cirrhosis (by ultrasound every 6 months; alpha-fetoprotein testing may add little extra value, but some recommend it).

Specific antiviral therapy

With the event of direct-acting antiviral drugs (DAA) most people can be treated with relatively few side-effects. This now includes those with prior contraindications such as decompensated liver cirrhosis and chronic kidney disease.

DAAs have effectively replaced the interferon and ribavirin containing combination therapies. Most regimens are now pan-genotypic and contain simple orally taken drugs over either 8 or 12 weeks. Success rates are over 95% as defined by a qualitative polymerase chain reaction (PCR) taken 3 months after the end of therapy. The first-generation protease inhibitors telaprevir, boceprevir and simeprevir have become obsolete and should not be considered.

General regimens

The 3 classes of drugs used are now in general use

1. NS5B polymerase inhibitor (sofosbuvir)
2. NS5A inhibitors (velpatasvir, elbasvir and pibrentasvir)
3. Protease inhibitors (glecaprevir, grazoprevir and voxilaprevir)

Use these as follows.

Sofosbuvir/velpatasvir for 12 weeks in any genotype but to be avoided in patients with chronic kidney disease (GFR < 30) due to sofosbuvir's renal excretion.

Elbasvir/grazoprevir in genotypes 1, 4 or 6 for 12 weeks though as grazoprevir is a protease inhibitor, it must be avoided in decompensated cirrhosis.

Glecaprevir/pibrentasvir for 8-12 weeks for any genotype though as pibrentasvir is a protease inhibitor, it must be avoided in decompensated cirrhosis.

Special groups

Decompensated Cirrhosis. These patients may be successfully treated. They often achieve recompensation and MELD score improvement. They should be linked with a liver transplant unit if they are transplant candidates. The only treatment available in this case is the sofosbuvir/velpatasvir combination given with ribavirin. Avoid protease inhibitors as their use will result in deteriorating liver function.

Renal Impairment. Elbasvir/grazoprevir or glecaprevir/pibrentasvir are safe, even in dialysis patients. Sofosbuvir is to be avoided as it is renally excreted.

DAA Failures. The best option is the sofosbuvir/velpatasvir/voxilaprevir combination. However, it is not able to be used in those with chronic kidney disease or decompensated cirrhosis. If resistance to sofosbuvir has been proven then glecaprevir/pibrentasvir for 16 weeks may be used.

Hepatitis D, E and G

- **Hepatitis D (RNA virus)**—infection only occurs with hepatitis B virus surface-antigen positivity, and the risk factors are similar. Superinfection in a hepatitis B carrier can lead to severe disease and death. Successful hepatitis B vaccination or immunity is protective.
- **Hepatitis E (RNA virus)**—this should be considered in a traveler from the developing world with acute hepatitis and negative serology for hepatitis A and B. In the third trimester of pregnancy, this is particularly dangerous with a high risk of fatal fulminant hepatitis.

- **Hepatitis G**—this is a rare cause of hepatitis, and not a cause of chronic liver disease. There are two types: hepatitis G and GB virus type C. GBV-C may protect against HIV replication in co-infected patients.

Other viruses causing hepatitis

Tests for other viruses causing acute hepatitis are listed in Table 12-5.

Noninvasive assessment of liver fibrosis

Liver fibrosis is a dynamic process that gradually increases and decreases over the classic histological metavir staging scores of F0, F1 (minimal fibrosis), F2, F3 (advanced fibrosis) and F4 (cirrhosis). While liver biopsy is a useful method of assessing fibrosis and overall histology, it is limited by small sample size and its often painful invasive nature. Standard imaging tests such as ultrasound, CT and MRI are very insensitive to the presence of fibrosis. Noninvasive assessment of liver fibrosis involves either serological tests or measurement of liver stiffness. It is important to note that these 2 modalities complement one another and the overall clinical impression. Most noninvasive tests of liver fibrosis allow reasonable assessment of minimal versus advanced fibrosis (F0, F1 versus F2–F4) and lack the accuracy in differentiating small increments of fibrosis, such as between fibrosis scores F2–F3.

Serum biomarkers

The most common are APRI, fibrotest and NFS.

APRI = AST to platelet ratio. (AST/AST upper limit of normal)/(platelet count $\times 10^9$/L) $\times 100$. This is most useful in helping to exclude significant fibrosis. An APRI < 1 makes cirrhosis unlikely and under 0.7 lessens the likelihood of significant fibrosis (F2–4).

Fibrotest. This is a patented test using Alpha-2-macroglobulin, haptoglobin, gamma-globulin, apolipoprotein-A1, GGT and total bilirubin. Its sensitivity and specificity for the detection of significant fibrosis (F2–F4) is around 70% and 85%, respectively.

NFS = NAFLD fibrosis score. This uses the age, BMI, blood glucose, transaminases, platelets and albumin. A high score over 0.676 is very suggestive of F3–F4. A score under −1.455 makes significant fibrosis unlikely.

Elastography

Elastography uses ultrasound or MRI to measure the speed of a mechanical disturbance through the liver. This speed is related to the stiffness of the liver which in turn correlates with the amount of fibrosis.

Transient elastography (fibroscan) uses ultrasound to measure the velocity of a shear wave propagating through the liver. The speed of the shear wave correlates with the liver stiffness in kPa. It has the benefit of being a painless, fast, bedside test with high inter-observer reproducibility. It assesses a cylinder of the liver 4 cm long and 1 cm in diameter, vastly more than a biopsy. It is the most studied and best validated noninvasive technique for liver fibrosis assessment. It performs very well at detecting either minimal or advanced fibrosis. A stiffness of 13 kPa (11–14) or above is accepted as reflecting cirrhosis. Obesity and a narrow intercostal space may result in scan failure and the presence of ascites makes the test impossible.

MR elastography has the advantage of being able to provide a full morphological scan at the same time and provides a fibrosis assessment on the entire liver. It has similar accuracy to a fibroscan.

CIRRHOSIS

Cirrhosis is a histological diagnosis characterized by advanced (bridging) fibrosis, and architectural (nodule formation) and microvascular distortion. Its clinical features relate to loss of synthetic function, portal hypertension and HCC.

Cirrhosis represents a disease generally associated with a reduced life expectancy, particularly if there are features of synthetic dysfunction or portal hypertension (decompensation). The dominant causes in the Western world are non-alcoholic fatty liver disease, alcohol and viral hepatitis, although in developing nations hepatitis B is the major etiology.

Table 12-5 Tests for other viruses causing acute hepatitis

TEST	MEANING OF A POSITIVE RESULT	COMMENT
Cytomegalovirus (CMV) IgM	Recent acquisition of CMV	Acute hepatitis illness is likely to be due to CMV
Epstein–Barr virus (EBV) IgM	Recent acquisition of EBV	Acute hepatitis illness is likely to be due to EBV
Anti-HIV	HIV-AIDS	Opportunistic hepatobiliary infections
Toxoplasmosis serology	Consider toxoplasmosis	Adenopathy with hepatosplenomegaly characteristic
Q fever serology	Consider Q fever	Think of this in pneumonia with hepatitis
AIDS, acquired immunodeficiency syndrome; HIV, human immunodeficiency virus; IgM, immunoglobulin M.		

Clinical features are:

- Leukonychia, palmar erythema, spider angiomata, loss of male-pattern body-hair distribution, and gynecomastia.
- Signs of decompensation are jaundice, asterixis (together with impaired mentation) and hepatic fetor.
- Examination of the abdomen may reveal a firm irregular liver, splenomegaly, caput medusa and ascites. In advanced disease, muscle wasting is usually present.
- Signs that may direct one to a particular diagnosis are parotidomegaly in alcoholic cirrhosis, hypogonadism in alcohol- and hemochromatosis-related cirrhosis, and xanthelasma in primary biliary cholangitis (PBC).

Useful investigations

- Abdominal ultrasound may show a small, irregular liver or splenomegaly. Ultrasound may identify complications such as ascites, portal vein thrombosis or HCC.
- Computed tomography (CT) and magnetic resonance imaging (MRI) are reserved for diagnosis of HCC and for confirming suspected portal vein thrombosis.
- Most imaging modalities are insensitive for advanced fibrosis. Fibroscan (elastography) in a cirrhotic patient is useful, as a liver stiffness of less than 21 kPa has a high negative predictive value for complications of portal hypertension over the following 2 years.
- Serological fibrosis tests.

Blood tests are not diagnostic but are supportive of cirrhosis; in particular, thrombocytopenia has been validated as a reasonable serum marker of advanced fibrosis. In the presence of clinical suspicion, normal serum enzymes are *not* reassuring, as up to 15% of biopsy-proven cirrhosis is accompanied by normal transaminases.

Once a diagnosis of cirrhosis is established, it is inevitable that decompensation will occur. This involves development of any of the following: ascites, hepatic encephalopathy (portosystemic encephalopathy, PSE), jaundice, coagulopathy or variceal bleeding. A search for a precipitant must be made (Box 12-4).

CLINICAL PEARL

Suspect cirrhosis based on the history and physical examination findings. Look for thrombocytopenia. The transaminases can sometimes be normal in cirrhosis.

Prognosis

Prognosis is dependent on the presence or absence of decompensation as well as the presence of an ongoing insult such as alcohol or untreated viral hepatitis. The frequency of decompensation is about 4% per year in hepatitis C and 10% per year in active hepatitis B infection. It is higher with severe alcohol excess. Once decompensation has occurred, mortality is as high as 85% over 5 years.

The Childs–Pugh–Turcotte score is predictive of survival (Table 12-6). The Model for End-Stage Liver Disease (MELD) score was established initially as a predictive

---

Box 12-4

Causes of hepatic decompensation in cirrhosis

Infection

UTI, SBP, pneumonia, primary bacteremia, cellulitis

Metabolic

Renal failure, hyponatremia, uremia, volume depletion (variceal bleed)

Drugs

Alcohol, acetaminophen (paracetamol) especially

Also NSAIDs, diuretics, benzodiazepines, opiates, phenothiazines, anticonvulsants

Viral infection

Hepatitis A, B, C, D; cytomegalovirus, Epstein–Barr virus

Malignancy

Hepatocellular carcinoma (HCC), cholangiocarcinoma, metastasis

Vascular

Portal vein thrombosis, Budd–Chiari syndrome

HCC, hepatocellular carcinoma; NSAIDs, non-steroidal anti-inflammatory drugs; SBP, spontaneous bacterial peritonitis; UTI, urinary tract infection.

---

tool of survival post transjugular intrahepatic portosystemic shunting (TIPS). This was adapted to predict survival on transplant waiting lists. It utilizes the predictive variables of INR, bilirubin and, importantly, creatinine. This is the best predictor of survival as well as selection of patients for liver transplant.

$$MELD = [0.957 \log_e(\text{creatinine, micromol/L}) + 0.378 \log_e(\text{bilirubin, micromol/L}) + 1.12 \log_e(\text{INR}) + 0.643] \times 10$$

Management

Management should be directed at the underlying cause, and in particular alcohol cessation is mandatory.

- Treatment of viral hepatitis needs consideration. In the compensated state, hepatitis C infection should be treated if present. Treatment of hepatitis C may be undertaken in the decompensated state with sofosbuvir/velpatasvir though liver transplant should be considered in those eligible. A nucleoside analog should be used if active hepatitis B is present.
- Any possible offending medication should be ceased.
- Specific management of autoimmune liver disease, Wilson's disease and hemochromatosis should be commenced.

Table 12-6 Childs–Pugh–Turcotte (CPT) score for survival in cirrhosis

	1 POINT	2 POINTS	3 POINTS
Encephalopathy	Absent	Medically controlled	Poorly controlled
Ascites	Absent	'Medically controlled' (for consistency)	Poorly controlled
Bilirubin mcmol/L (mg/dL)	<34.2 (<2)	34.2–51.3 (2–3)	>50.3 (>3)
Albumin (g/L)	>35	28–35	<28
INR	<1.7	1.7–2.3	>2.3

Classification:

CPT CLASS	LIFE EXPECTANCY (YEARS)	PERIOPERATIVE MORTALITY (ABDOMINAL SURGERY)
A (5–6 points)	15–20	10%
B (7–9 points)	4–14	30%
C (10–15 points)	1–3	80%

INR, international normalized ratio.
Adapted from Schuppan D and Afdhal NH. Liver cirrhosis. Lancet 2008;371(9615):838–51.

- General factors such as a high-energy and high-protein diet as well as moderate exercise should also be encouraged. A high-energy meal prior to bed-time helps prevent catabolism leading to muscle loss (sarcopenia).
- Nutritional deficiencies if suspected should be corrected, particularly vitamin D and thiamine.

The **complications** of cirrhosis are ascites, hepatorenal syndrome, PSE, portal hypertensive bleeding, portopulmonary hypertension, hepatopulmonary syndrome and cirrhotic cardiomyopathy. Hepatocellular carcinoma is covered elsewhere. Table 12-7 summarises the specific management of the most common complications.

CLINICAL PEARL

A diagnostic tap looking for spontaneous bacterial peritonitis needs to be performed at the first episode of ascites and in every subsequent presentation in which the clinical condition of the patient with ascites has deteriorated.

ASCITES

Ascites and hepatorenal syndrome are a part of the same pathophysiological spectrum. They are a manifestation of hepatic resistance to blood flow, splanchnic vasodilatation and portosystemic shunt formation, with release of systemic vasodilators leading to activation of the renin–angiotensin–aldosterone axis and the sympathetic nervous system. This leads to compensatory sodium and therefore water retention. As refractory ascites (and type 2 hepatorenal syndrome)

occurs, progressive renal vasoconstriction results. There is marked impairment of excretion of sodium and often free water, the latter being largely responsible for hyponatremia in end-stage cirrhosis.

Once ascites is diagnosed, a cause must be found (Table 12-8, overleaf). A diagnostic paracentesis should always be performed when new-onset ascites is detected.

- The most useful measure for ascites is the serum ascites to albumin gradient (SAAG; a difference, not a ratio). If the SAAG is over 11 g/L, then the ascites is almost always due to portal hypertension.
- On initial fluid analysis, fluid should be tested for infection and cytology. Fluid protein, lactate dehydrogenase (LDH), microscopy, and culture and cytology should be performed.

Management

- Initially, management of ascites due to cirrhosis is simple: either a no-added-sodium diet or initiation of diuretics. The aim is to achieve a negative sodium balance.
- Inevitably a diuretic becomes necessary. Spironolactone 100 mg, often combined with furosemide 40 mg, is a common regimen. Serum biochemistry must be monitored.
  » A response is noted by a fall in extravascular fluid, best measured by weight, and an increase in urinary sodium excretion (well over 20 mmol/L).
  » In those with edema, weight loss may be 1 kg/day; if no edema, 0.5 kg/day.

As liver disease progresses, sodium and therefore water excretion diminishes, leading to **refractory ascites**.

Table 12-7 Prevention and treatment of complications of cirrhosis

	PREVENTION	TREATMENT
Variceal bleeding	Non-selective beta-blockers* Variceal band ligation	*Acute:* —resuscitation —vasoconstrictors† —sclerotherapy —band ligation —TIPS —surgical shunts *Chronic:* —variceal obliteration —TIPS —surgical shunts
Ascites	Low-sodium diet	Low-sodium diet Diuretics Large-volume paracentesis Peritoneovenous shunt
Renal failure	Avoid hypovolemia	Discontinue diuretics Rehydration Albumin infusion Hepatorenal syndrome: add terlipressin or midodrine (noradrenaline) and somatostatin (octreotide)

Encephalopathy	Avoid precipitants	Treat precipitating factors:
		  Infection
		  Bleeding
		  Electrolyte imbalance
		  Sedatives
		  High protein intake
		Lactulose
		Neomycin, metronidazole, rifaximin

Spontaneous bacterial peritonitis	Treat ascites	Early diagnosic paracentesis, >250 neutrophils/mL: intravenous antibiotics (plus albumin) Secondary prophlaxis with oral antibiotics such as levofloxacin

* Nadolol, propranolol.

† Vasopressin, octeotride (somatostatin), terlipressin.

TIPS, transjugular intrahepatic portosystemic shunt.

Reprinted from Schuppan D and Afdhal NH. Liver cirrhosis. Lancet 2008;371(9615):838–51.

- Initially, increased diuretics are required until either maximal doses are reached or more commonly complications of these drugs occur. These are renal impairment, hypotension, electrolyte imbalance and often hepatic encephalopathy.

- The presence of dietary sodium excess must be sought. If the patient is excreting more than 78 mmol/day or the spot urine Na/K is >1, it is likely that dietary sodium excess is present. The use of non-steroidal anti-inflammatory agents must be excluded.

- The options are then large-volume paracentesis, transjugular intrahepatic portosystemic shunt (TIPS) or liver transplant.

» Large-volume paracentesis in the outpatient setting is safe and widely accepted. IV albumin should be given at a dose of 8 g for every litre of ascites removed. This helps prevent orthostatic hypotension and renal failure resulting from fluid shifts.

» TIPS is an option. Ascites improves at a cost of increased hepatic encephalopathy. It is essential that patients have an echocardiogram to ensure that the left ventricular ejection fraction is greater than 60%, to minimize the risk of shunt-induced congestive cardiac failure.

» As 6-month mortality in those with refractory ascites is 20%, consideration should be given to liver transplantation if the patient is otherwise eligible.

Table 12-8 Diagnosis of ascites

CLASSIFICATION OF ASCITES BY SERUM ASCITES–ALBUMIN GRADIENT (SAAG)	
SAAG HIGH (≥11 g/L)	**SAAG LOW (<11 g/L)**
Cirrhosis Alcoholic hepatitis Cardiac ascites Massive liver metastases Fulminant hepatic failure Cirrhosis plus another cause	Peritoneal carcinomatosis Tuberculous peritonitis Pancreatic ascites Bile leak

CHARACTERISTICS OF PARACENTESIS FLUID						
ETIOLOGY	COLOR	SAAG (g/L)	RBCs	WBCs (CELLS/ MICROL)	CYTOLOGY	OTHER
Cirrhosis	Straw	≥11	Few	<250		Protein <25 g/L
Infected ascites	Straw	≥11	Few	≥250 poly-morphs or >500 cells		Positive culture
Neoplastic	Straw/ hemorrhagic/ mucinous	<11	Variable	Variable	Malignant cells	Protein >25 g/L
Tuberculosis	Clear/turbid/ hemorrhagic	<11	High	>1000, 70% lymphocytes		Acid-fast bacilli + culture Protein >25 g/L
Cardiac failure	Straw	≥11	0	<250		Protein >25 g/L
Pancreatic	Turbid/ hemorrhagic	<11	Variable	Variable		Amylase increased
Lymphatic obstruction or disruption	White	<11	0	0		Fat globules on staining
RBC, red blood cell; WBC = white blood cell.						

HEPATORENAL SYNDROME (HRS)

There are two clinical types of hepatorenal syndrome:

- **Type 1 hepatorenal syndrome**—rapidly progressive reduction of renal function as defined by doubling of the initial serum creatinine to a level of >2.5 mg/dL (226 micromol/L) in less than 2 weeks.
  - » Clinical pattern: acute renal failure (acute kidney injury).
- **Type 2 hepatorenal syndrome**—moderate renal failure (serum creatinine ranging from 1.25 to 2.5 mg/dL or 113–226 micromol/L) with a steady or slowly progressive course.
  - » Clinical pattern: refractory ascites.

HRS is a marker of decompensated cirrhosis, requiring the presence of ascites. It is characterized by a rising creatinine level in the absence of other causes of renal failure.

- Pre-renal failure, obstructive renal failure and renal parenchymal disorders must be excluded.

- It is common to find a precipitant, most commonly bacterial infection and in particular spontaneous bacterial peritonitis (SBP), GI hemorrhage and occasionally large-volume paracentesis.

- HRS types 1 and 2 are separated mainly by prognosis and rate of deterioration of renal function. Type 1 HRS has a median survival of 2 weeks, while type 2 HRS has a median survival of 4–6 months.

Diagnosis should lead to diuretic cessation, volume expansion and adequate treatment of infection, as well as exclusion of renal parenchymal disease and renal tract obstruction. All patients require full septic screen including diagnostic paracentesis.

Management

- Management of type 2 HRS is avoidance of nephrotoxins, cessation of diuretics, and a low-sodium diet. Terlipressin will often reverse this, although it has no survival benefit. Liver transplantation is the only treatment that can lead to long-term survival in those eligible.

- Type 1 HRS is rapidly lethal. If survival is the aim, then liver transplant is usually required.
  - » The management is the same as for type 2 HRS, although liver transplantation must be strongly considered and discussion with a liver transplant center must take place immediately.
  - » The use of vasoconstrictors is also indicated. Providing splanchnic and systemic vasoconstriction allows for improved renal perfusion and correction of HRS in 50% of patients. Terlipressin, a vasopressin analog, should be administered if available. Midodrine with octreotide is a reasonable alternative. Albumin infusion given with terlipressin improves efficacy. There is a short-term survival benefit with vasoconstrictor therapy; however, it must be emphasized that liver transplant must be strongly considered.
  - » TIPS may be considered if vasoconstrictor therapy fails and there are no contraindications. TIPS has been shown to improve renal function in HRS type 1.

CLINICAL PEARL

The most common cause for acute renal failure in end-stage liver disease with ascites is not hepatorenal syndrome but pre-renal failure (40%) and acute tubular necrosis (40%).

HYPONATREMIA

Hyponatremia is a common problem in end-stage cirrhosis. It is due to impaired free-water excretion from increased antidiuretic hormone secretion. Hyponatremia is a marker of poor prognosis both before and after liver transplant.

Treatment should be considered once the sodium is below 130 mmol/L. The patient must be assessed as *hypovolemic* or *hypervolemic*.

- If the patient is hypovolemic, then correction of the cause and volume replacement is the treatment. Most commonly this will involve diuretic cessation.

- If hypervolemic with ascites and edema, fluid restriction is the initial management. This becomes difficult for patients to tolerate once fluid restrictions is less than 1200 mL/day.

Vaptans (e.g. tolvaptan) block V_2 vasopressin (ADH) receptors, increasing free water excretion. These agents improve serum sodium, urine volume and free water clearance.

- Vaptans where available should be considered in patients with a sodium level of 125 mmol/L or less, particularly if liver transplantation is an option.

- Great care must be taken not to reverse hyponatremia too quickly because of the risk of osmotic demyelination syndrome. The rate of correction must be no more than 3–5 mmol/day.

- Because of the risk of rapid osmotic reversal, these agents need to be commenced only on inpatients with a normal mentation and who can access water. Side-effects include thirst, hypernatremia, renal impairment and dehydration.

CLINICAL PEARL

Do *not* correct hyponatremia too quickly or you will risk osmotic demyelination syndrome (central pontine myelinolysis).

SPONTANEOUS BACTERIAL PERITONITIS (SBP)

Spontaneous bacterial peritonitis is common and is a high-risk problem in cirrhotic patients with ascites. Presentation may be with abdominal pain and signs of peritonitis, although more commonly patients present with deteriorating liver function, encephalopathy, renal failure or shock. Up to 30% develop HRS (see above).

SBP may be asymptomatic. A diagnosis is made only by ascitic fluid analysis. A positive diagnosis is made by any one of the following:

- neutrophil (PMN) count >250 cells/microL
- white cell count >500 cells/microL
- positive ascitic fluid culture.

Culture alone has a sensitivity of only 40%, so the neutrophil count is the most important indicator. Bacterial yield is increased by sending a sample in blood culture bottles. The most common organisms are Gram-negative rods, particularly *Escherichia coli*, and streptococci, particularly *Enterococcus*.

A secondary cause for peritonitis (e.g. bowel perforation) is more likely when there are localizing peritoneal signs or a polymicrobial ascitic fluid culture has been obtained.

Treatment

Empirical treatment with cefotaxime or ceftriaxone should be commenced and adjusted according to sensitivities when these are available.

- Treatment should be culture- and sensitivity-based, as 30% of Gram-negative rods are quinolone-resistant.

- Nephrotoxic agents such as aminoglycosides must be avoided.

- Antibiotics must continue for 7 days, although if there is rapid patient improvement, IV antibiotics may be ceased and an oral preparation such as ciprofloxacin or amoxicillin/clavulanic acid commenced.

- If there are concerns about patient improvement, a repeat paracentesis after 2 days should take place. If the ascitic fluid neutrophil count has not dropped to 25% of the original count, a resistant organism should be suspected and the antibiotics changed.
- To reduce the risk of hepatorenal syndrome, IV albumin infusion should be given for at least 3 days.
- General management of shock, portal hypertensive bleeding, encephalopathy and renal dysfunction must continue.

Antibiotic prophylaxis should be given to all patients with ascites who have a high risk of SBP, including:
- those with past SBP, and
- those with active variceal bleeding (see section below).

Those with a past episode of SBP have a 70% chance of recurrence within 12 months and a poor prognosis. Secondary prophylaxis with norfloxacin should be considered, although ciprofloxacin or co-trimoxazole are reasonable alternatives. This strategy is effective in infection prevention, although a survival benefit has not been demonstrated.

Those with no prior episodes of SBP should receive primary prophylaxis with norfloxacin 400 mg daily if they have a fluid protein content of under 10 g/L or have a bilirubin >2.5 mg/dL. This improves short-term survival and reduces the risk of HRS.

PORTAL HYPERTENSIVE BLEEDING

This may occur from esophageal, gastric or rarely duodenal and small-intestinal varices. Another common finding is portal hypertensive gastropathy; this tends to present with anemia rather than obvious GI hemorrhage.

The risk of bleeding relates to a portal pressure of 12 mmHg or above. The measurement of portal pressure is not routine, so clinical features are the mainstay of risk assessment. This relates to stage of liver disease and endoscopic features.

- The higher the Childs–Pugh–Turcotte score (Table 12-6), the more likely the patient is to have varices.
- The endoscopic features indicating higher risk are the size and presence of red wale signs (a red streak overlying a varix that suggests recent bleeding).

Large varices have a risk of bleeding of 30% over 2 years, and must therefore be considered for primary prophylaxis (Figure 12-9).

- The best-proven medical treatment for this is a beta-blocker such as propanolol. An alternative is carvedilol.
- There is much debate over the use of endoscopic band ligation as a primary preventative measure.
- In high-risk varices, both medical and endoscopic prophylaxis should be attempted. The likelihood of developing high-risk esophageal varices is about 9% over 3 years.
- All patients with definite or suspected cirrhosis should have upper endoscopy performed to look for esophageal varices. If normal, this should be repeated every 2 years.

Management

Management of acute variceal bleeding has two components: the acute phase and the secondary prophylaxis phase.

The **acute phase** involves:
- General measures, including volume resuscitation and blood transfusion.
- Correction of coagulopathy and thrombocytopenia if severe.
- Management of alcohol withdrawal.
- Management of comorbid conditions such as chronic obstructive pulmonary disease.
- If there is a large GI bleed, activation of a massive transfusion protocol and intensive care admission should

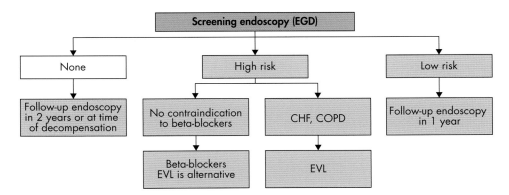

Figure 12-9 An algorithm for the primary prophylaxis of variceal hemorrhage. CHF, congestive heart failure; COPD, chronic obstructive pulmonary disease; EGD, esophagogastroduodenoscopy; EVL, endoscopic variceal ligation; MAP, mean arterial pressure

Redrawn from Sanyal AJ et al. Portal hypertension and its complications. Gastroenterology 2008;134(6):1715–28.

occur. The most likely problems to arise will be sepsis, hepatic encephalopathy and acute kidney injury.

- Empirical antibiotics such as ceftriaxone or norfloxacin are given as prophylaxis. This improves outcomes.
- Some centers advocate endotracheal intubation to prevent aspiration.
- Careful volume management, resolving active bleeding, and prevention and early aggressive management of infection are the keys to the renal management.
  - » The bleeding requires specific management with a somatostatin analog such as octreotide, or a vasopressin analog such as terlipressin.
  - » However, upper endoscopy is indicated urgently to provide endoscopic band ligation of high-risk varices (those bleeding or with fibrin clot or red wale signs).
  - » If the above measures fail to control bleeding, endoscopy should be reattempted, reserving balloon tamponade or TIPS for endoscopic failure. It is becoming apparent that in a center that has TIPS available, control of bleeding is more reliable and complications are fewer if TIPS is used. It should be considered for first-line management.

Secondary prophylaxis includes an aggressive variceal banding regimen to obliteration, and propanolol.

Gastric varices tend to bleed less often but more dramatically. They are more likely to be associated with non-cirrhotic portal hypertension.

Portal hypertensive gastropathy (PHG) most often presents with anemia or low-grade bleeding. If there is evidence of bleeding, the patient requires propanolol. If ineffective, then TIPS should be considered.

PORTOSYSTEMIC ENCEPHALOPATHY (PSE)

Portosystemic encephalopathy refers to the neurological and psychiatric dysfunction that occurs in individuals with significant hepatic dysfunction and with portosystemic shunts. It presents as a spectrum varying from subtle neuropsychiatric symptoms to deep coma.

It is usual to find a reversible precipitant in overt encephalopathy. There are three forms of PSE in portal hypertension: *precipitant-induced PSE*, *persistent PSE* and *minimal PSE*.

Diagnosis relies on objective clinical findings in the context of cirrhosis. They are confusion and drowsiness and, in extreme cases, coma. Asterixis and hepatic fetor are supportive signs, although their absence does not exclude PSE. An

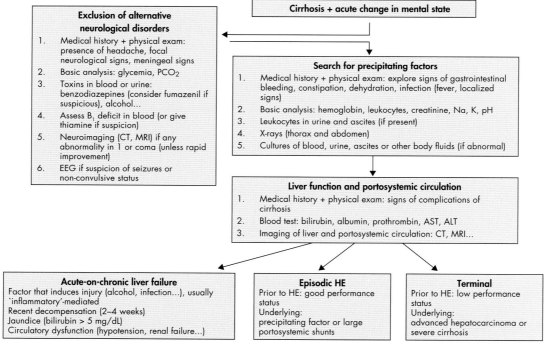

Figure 12-10 Evaluation of a patient with cirrhosis and an acute change in mental status should be initiated by excluding toxic, metabolic and structural encephalopathies. In parallel, the patient should be assessed following a protocol to investigate precipitating factors and should undergo blood tests and imaging studies to evaluate liver function and portal–systemic circulation. According to the results, patients are classified as episodic HE (hepatic encephalopathy), acute-on-chronic liver failure, or terminal liver disease, and are managed accordingly. ALT, alanine aminotransferase; AST, aspartate aminotransferase; CT, computed tomography; EEG, electroencephalograpy; MRI, magnetic resonance imaging; PCO₂, partial pressure of carbon dioxide

From Córdoba J. New assessment of hepatic encephalopathy. J Hepatol 2011;54:1030–40.

Table 12-9 Managing precipitants of portosystemic encephalopathy

PRECIPITANT	MANAGEMENT
Volume depletion	Commonly from diuretics. Correct with IV albumin and stop diuretics
Infection	Treat specific infection. If SBP, give antibiotics and IV albumin
Renal failure and electrolyte imbalance	Identify cause and correct
Alcohol	Cease and manage withdrawal
Sedatives	Cease
Portosystemic shunt (TIPS)	Lactulose or rifaximin
Hepatocellular carcinoma	Specific management; see section on liver tumors
Protein load, including GI bleed	Endoscopy and management of portal hypertensive bleed. Dietary protein restriction is rarely required and should not be chronically commenced to avoid malnutrition
Constipation	Lactulose

GI, gastrointestinal. IV, intravenous; SBP, spontaneous bacterial peritonitis; TIPS, transjugular intrahepatic portosystemic shunt.

> **Box 12-5**
>
> **Encephalopathy grading**
>
> - Grade 1—Minor lack of awareness, euphoria, shortened attention span, impaired performance of addition or subtraction
> - Grade 2—Lethargy or apathy, minor disorientation to time or place, personality changes and inappropriate behavior
> - Grade 3—Drowsiness, remaining responsive to verbal stimuli; gross confusion and disorientation
> - Grade 4—Coma (unresponsive to all stimuli)

approach is outlined in Figure 12-10. Grading of encephalophathy (Box 12-5) does not include minimal hepatic encephalopathy.

Precipitant-induced PSE

- Removal of precipitating factors will often resolve the episode (Table 12-9).
- Once PSE has occurred, lactulose should be given as secondary prophylaxis. The dose should be titrated to cause 2–3 semi-formed stools per day. An alternative is rifaximin (a non-absorbable antibiotic).
- Dietary protein avoidance is not recommended, as it makes no difference to outcome and will jeopardise the already tenuous nutrition in those with decompensated cirrhosis.
- Supplementation with branched-chain amino acids should be considered, although robust evidence for its benefits is lacking.

Persistent PSE

- This may be due to the presence of a large dominant portosystemic shunt, which can be closed radiologically if liver function is well preserved (normal bilirubin) and more conservative measures fail.
- More commonly, a dominant shunt is not present and medical treatment is indicated. This addresses the known mechanisms of PSE.
  - » Ammonia is one of the leading candidates as the culprit substance in the blood leading to PSE.
  - » Non-absorbable disaccharides (lactulose) are first-line treatment in persistent PSE. They work by acidifying the colon, reducing the absorbable ammonia load and reducing cerebral water content.
  - » Rifaximin should be commenced in any patient whose encephalopathy does not resolve with adequate lactulose or any patient who is intolerant of lactulose.
  - » Gamma-aminobutyric acid (GABA)-receptor blockade with flumazenil may help reverse deep encephalopathy, although it is not available for chronic use.

Minimal encephalopathy

This consists of subtle cognitive dysfunction without the features of overt PSE. It is not noted by the physician, usually being detected by close family members and work colleagues. Its prevalence is 15% in Childs A cirrhosis and 50% in Childs C cirrhosis.

Investigation requires psychometric testing, and should not be routinely sought as there is little benefit to be gained from treatment.

- Investigation is indicated if a patient or family member wishes this to be done on the basis of declining work performance or for symptoms such as forgetfulness or a perception of confusion.

- Those at risk of accidents, such as truck drivers or those responsible for dangerous machinery, should also be screened.
- There is no consensus on the best diagnostic tests.

While this may be treated with lactulose or rifaximin, the evidence for a benefit remains unclear, although these medications can improve driving performance in a driving simulator.

PORTOPULMONARY HYPERTENSION (POPH)

This condition is defined as the presence of pulmonary arterial hypertension (PAH) in the presence of portal hypertension once other secondary causes have been excluded. It is present in 6% of people with cirrhosis; those at highest risk are females and those with autoimmune hepatitis. The condition is associated with high perioperative mortality, including during liver transplantations.

- Presenting symptoms are breathlessness on exertion, fatigue, and occasionally chest pain and palpitations. Clinical features are of right heart strain and failure.
- Other causes of pulmonary hypertension need to be excluded. They are left heart disease, chronic obstructive pulmonary disease, sleep apnea, pulmonary thromboembolism and connective tissue disease such as scleroderma.
- The initial investigation is echocardiography, and confirmation is by right heart catheterization.

The success of liver transplantation is dependent on response to medical pulmonary vasodilator therapy, and should be reserved for responders only. Treatment attempts with vasodilators such as prostaglandins and phosphodiesterase-5 inhibitors are indicated. Other agents to be considered are bosentan or other endothelin antagonists.

HEPATOPULMONARY SYNDROME (HPS)

This is a syndrome of increased pulmonary perfusion without an increase in ventilation, leading to hypoxemia. Pulmonary vascular dilatation and the opening of vascular channels between pulmonary arteriole and vein lead to increases in blood flow (lower transit time) beyond the capacity of the alveoli to oxygenate.

- HPS is a risk factor for death after adjustments for severity of liver disease. Prevalence is around 5% in those with cirrhosis.
- HPS should be suspected if there is severe hypoxemia (pO$_2$ <60 mmHg) in the presence of chronic liver disease. Dyspnea on exertion and at rest is the most common symptom. Due to increasing ventilation–perfusion mismatch, dyspnea may deteriorate in the upright position (platypnea). This phenomenon should be

accompanied by a fall in partial arterial oxygen pressure (P$_A$O$_2$) of at least 4 mmHg (orthodeoxia).

- There are no specific findings, although clubbing, cyanosis and the stigmata of chronic liver disease, particularly spider nevi, are usually present.

Diagnosis is made by demonstrating intrapulmonary vascular shunts. Qualitative echocardiography is the least invasive and most sensitive test. The echo is performed while microbubbles are injected in a peripheral vein. These are detected in the left atrium 3–6 cardiac cycles after the right atrium, thus detecting a shunt as these bubbles would not flow through normal pulmonary vasculature.

There is no proven **treatment** other than liver transplantation. This should be considered in those with proven HPS and an arterial pO$_2$ below 60 mmHg.

CLINICAL PEARL

- Suspect HPS in a patient who has cirrhosis and becomes hypoxemic. Ask if dyspnea deteriorates in the upright position (platypnea), and look for a fall in partial arterial oxygen pressure of at least 4 mmHg (orthodeoxia). Look for a shunt on echo.
- Consider POPH in cirrhosis and progressive dyspnea on exertion. Confirm with right heart catheterization.

CIRRHOTIC CARDIOMYOPATHY

In cirrhotic cardiomyopathy there is evidence of systolic dysfunction, diastolic dysfunction and QT prolongation in cirrhotic patients.

- The systolic function is usually normal at rest, with dysfunction becoming apparent with stress. There is a link between systolic dysfunction and the development of hepatorenal syndrome.
- As cirrhosis becomes more advanced, diastolic dysfunction becomes more prominent. The clinical relevance of this is particularly related to increases in preload occurring after TIPS, with the cirrhotic heart unable to accommodate increases in flow. The presence of measurable diastolic dysfunction is predictive of death after TIPS.
- QT prolongation is present in 50% of cirrhotic patients and is unrelated to etiology. In alcohol-related cirrhosis this is related to sudden cardiac death, although probably not in cirrhosis with other etiologies. In those cirrhotic patients with a prolonged QT interval there is a prolonged mechanical systole, i.e. an altered excitation–contraction association that contributes to systolic dysfunction.

The main clinical relevance is the contribution to HRS, post-TIPS cardiac failure and death, and perioperative performance in liver transplantation. The cardiac changes largely resolve post liver transplant.

Treatment is relatively undefined, although it should include diuretics, particularly spironolactone, and nonselective beta-blockers such as propranolol or carvedilol. Angiotensin-converting enzyme inhibitors (ACEIs) and angiotensin–receptor blockers should be avoided because of the risk of HRS.

ACUTE LIVER FAILURE (ALF)

ALF is a frightening and often rapidly lethal disease caused by loss of hepatocellular function. It is characterized by the development of coagulopathy and altered mentation in a patient with no known chronic liver disease.

- The usual causes are drug-induced liver injury (DILI), acetaminophen (paracetamol) overdose, mushroom poisoning (*Amanita phalloides*) and viral hepatitis.
- Rarer causes such as Wilson's disease, Budd–Chiari syndrome, autoimmune hepatitis and ischemic hepatopathy may require consideration.

A meticulous medication review is required (Box 12-6). About 15% of cases do not receive a causal diagnosis.

CLINICAL PEARL

Acute liver failure is a clinical syndrome defined by altered mentation due to cerebral edema and/or encephalopathy in the setting of jaundice and coagulopathy. The serum enzymes are not part of this diagnosis, although are usually abnormal. Management should be carried out in a liver transplant unit.

Management is supportive, with aggressive diagnosis and treatment of infection. Death is commonly due to raised intracerebral pressure, which may require hyperventilation or mannitol. Liver transplantation is often required. It is important to treat specific etiologies if detected. They are:

- acetaminophen (paracetamol) overdose—*N*-acetylcysteine
- mushroom poisoning—*N*-acetylcysteine and penicillin G
- acute hepatitis B—nucleoside analog
- autoimmune hepatitis—prednisolone or other corticosteroid.

However, delaying transplantation while waiting for specific treatment to occur is unwise in the deteriorating patient.

CLINICAL PEARLS

- If acetaminophen (paracetamol) toxicity is suspected, give *N*-acetylcysteine immediately.
- If the arterial pH is <7.3 in acetaminophen-induced acute liver failure (ALF) or the international normalized ratio (INR) is >6.5 in ALF of another cause, the patient needs an urgent liver transplant (King's College criteria).

LIVER TRANSPLANTATION

- **Disease-specific indications** for transplantation include: end-stage cirrhosis (any cause), primary sclerosing cholangitis, Caroli disease (intrahepatic biliary tree with multiple cystic dilatations), Budd–Chiari syndrome, and fulminant hepatic failure.
  - » Hepatitis C patients do as well as others despite the fact that recurrent infection in the graft is usual.
  - » In active hepatitis B, graft survival is reduced by up to 20% but prophylactic HBIG increases the success rate, as does pre-treatment with a nucleoside analog such as lamivudine.
- **Absolute contradictions** include: active sepsis outside the biliary tract, metastatic hepatobiliary malignancy, HIV infection and advanced cardiopulmonary disease.

Box 12-6

Initial laboratory testing for acute liver failure (ALF)

- Prothrombin time/international normalized ratio
- Chemistries:
  - » sodium, potassium, chloride, bicarbonate, calcium, magnesium, phosphate, glucose
  - » AST, ALT, ALP, GGT, total bilirubin, albumin creatinine, blood urea nitrogen
- Arterial blood gases
- Arterial lactate
- Full blood count
- Blood type and screen
- Acetaminophen (paracetamol) level
- Toxicology screen
- Viral hepatitis serologies:
  - » anti-HAV IgM, HBsAg, anti-HBc IgM, anti-HEV*, anti-HCV, HCV-RNA[#], HSV1 IgM, VZV
- Ceruloplasmin level[‡]
- Pregnancy test (females)
- Iron studies for haemochromatosis, HLH
- Ammonia (arterial if possible)
- Autoimmune markers:
  - » ANA, ASMA, immunoglobulin levels
- HIV-1, HIV-2 [§]
- Amylase and lipase

---

* If clinically indicated.

[#] Done to recognize potential underlying infection.

[‡] Done only if Wilson's disease is a consideration (e.g. in patients younger than 40 years without another obvious explanation for ALF); in this case uric acid level and bilirubin to alkaline phosphatase ratio may be helpful as well.

[§] Has implications for potential liver transplantation.

ALP, alkaline phosphatase; ALT, alanine aminotransferase; ANA, antinuclear antibodies; ASMA, anti-smooth-muscle antibodies; AST, aspartate aminotransferase; GGT, gamma-glutamyl transpeptidase; HAV, hepatitis A virus; HCV, hepatitis C virus; HEV, hepatitis E virus; HIV, human immunodeficiency virus; IgM, immunoglobulin M; RNA, ribonucleic acid; VZV, varicella zoster virus.

From Lee WM, Larson AM and Stravitz RT. AASLD Position Paper. The management of acute liver failure: update 2011. Baltimore, MD: American Association for the Study of Liver Diseases; 2011 Sep 26.

- **Relative contradictions** include: older age (>60 years), biliary infection, unreformed alcoholism, a blocked portal vein, previous major upper abdominal surgery, major renal impairment, and other medical disease (e.g. poorly controlled diabetes).

Figure 12-11 provides an algorithm for treatment decisions, and post-transplant complications are outlined in Figure 12-12.

DRUGS AND THE LIVER

Drugs are an important cause of liver disease (Table 12-10).

CLINICAL PEARLS

- Very few diagnoses cause transaminase levels above 1000 U/L—think about drug/toxin reactions (not alcohol), acute biliary obstruction, acute viral hepatitis and ischemic hepatopathy.
- In a patient with arrhythmias on therapy and liver test abnormalities, consider amiodarone toxicity.

The contraceptive pill can cause or stimulate the growth of hepatic adenoma (and very rarely hepatocellular carcinoma); it can also cause focal nodular hyperplasia (FNH) and peliosis hepatitis, although the association with FNH is very vague. Other associations include Budd–Chiari syndrome, cholestasis, cholesterol gallstones, and unmasking Dubin–Johnson syndrome.

Acetaminophen (paracetamol) and acute liver disease

The liver's cytochrome P450 system oxidizes 5% of acetaminophen, producing the potent hepatotoxin N-acetyl-p-benzoquinoneimine (NAPQI). Glutathione protects the liver from this toxin. In its absence, the result is severe hepatic necrosis, liver failure (fulminant hepatitis) and death unless transplantation is performed.

Acetaminophen is dangerous in the following settings:

- Overdose, where glutathione is overwhelmed.
- Chronic moderate alcohol use or a binge, a risk factor for acetaminophen–induced liver failure at therapeutic dosages. Alcohol reduces the amount of liver glutathione,

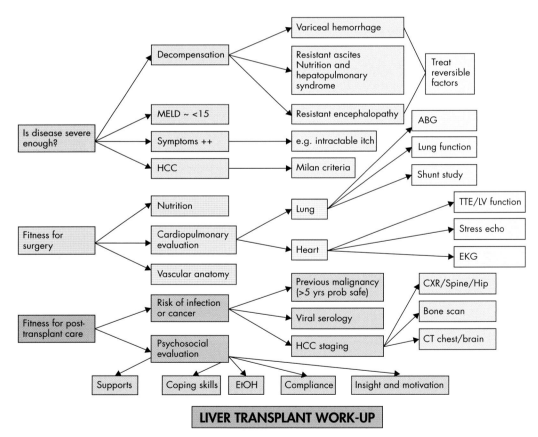

Figure 12-11 Work-up for liver ABG, arterial blood gases; CT, computed tomography; CXR, chest X-ray; EKG, electrocardiography; EtOH, alcohol; HCC, hepatocellular carcinoma; LV, left ventricular; MELD, model for end-stage liver disease; TTE, trans-thoracic echocardiogram

Redrawn from an original figure created by Dr Gokulan Pavendranathan, Central Clinical School, AW Morrow Gastroenterology and Liver Centre, NSW, Australia.

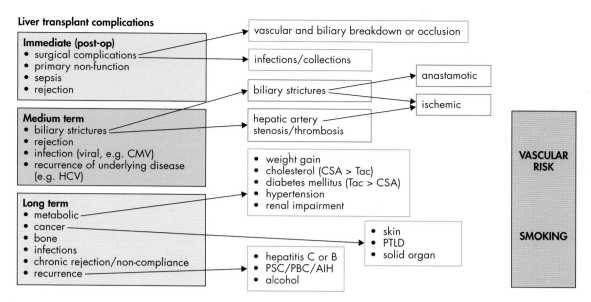

Figure 12-12 Complications post-liver transplant . AIH, autoimmune hepatitis; CSA, cyclosporine A (ciclosporin A); PBC, primary biliary cirrhosis; PSC, primary sclerosing cholangitis; PTLD, post-transplant lymphoproliferative disorder; Tac, tacrolimus

Redrawn from an original figure created by Dr Gokulan Pavendranathan, Central Clinical School, AW Morrow Gastroenterology and Liver Centre, NSW, Australia.

Table 12-10 Drugs and the liver

LIVER DISEASE	DRUG EXAMPLES
Acute hepatitis	Halothane, phenytoin, chlorothiazide
Cholestasis	Hypersensitivity reaction:* chlorpromazine, other phenothiazines, sulfonamides, sulfonylureas, rifampin, nitrofurantoin, erythromycin
	Dose-related:† anabolic steroids, contraceptive pill
Mixed cholestasis/hepatitis	Amoxicillin/clavulanic acid‡
Fatty liver	Tetracycline, valproic acid, salicylate, amiodarone, vitamin A, zidovudine (microvesicular); methotrexate, alcohol, corticosteroids, cisplatin (macrovesicular)
Peliosis hepatitis (large blood-filled cavities)	Anabolic steroids, contraceptive pill, tamoxifen
Cytotoxic (liver cell necrosis)	Acetaminophen (paracetamol), carbon tetrachloride (zone 3)
Angiosarcoma	Vinyl chloride, thorotrast, arsenic

* Canalicular bile plugs ± portal tract inflammatory infiltrate with eosinophils.

† No inflammatory infiltrate or necrosis.

‡ Amoxicillin/clavulanic acid can cause acute cholestatic hepatitis.

plus it turns on the cytochrome P450 system leading to more NAPQI—double jeopardy!

- Little or no eating (malnutrition, dieting) which leads to glutathione deficiency.

ALCOHOL AND THE LIVER

CLINICAL PEARL

A high AST/ALT ratio suggests alcoholic liver disease in the absence of cirrhosis.

The key facts to remember are:

- Distinguishing alcoholic liver disease from non-alcoholic fatty liver disease can be challenging. An AST/ALT ratio over 2 and a disproportionally raised GGT can occur in both, but is much more typical of alcohol.
- Acute alcoholic hepatitis is treated by alcohol withdrawal, supportive care and nutritional supplementation; if severe (based on the prothrombin time and bilirubin—Maddrey score), corticosteroids are indicated (prednisolone for 4 weeks, then a tapered dose).
- Acetaminophen (paracetamol) is dangerous even in therapeutic doses in alcoholics, who not only may be drinking heavily but also may be malnourished.

Complications of alcoholism are given in Box 12-7.

SPECIFIC LIVER DISEASES

Budd–Chiari syndrome (BCS)

This is a varied group of disorders with the common link of hepatic outflow obstruction. This may occur at varying levels, including hepatic sinusoids, venules, veins, vena cava and right atrium.

The clinical presentation depends on the rate of thrombus formation. It may be classified as *fulminant*, *acute*, *subacute* and *chronic*.

- Fulminant BCS presents with severe necrosis and jaundice, with hepatic encephalopathy developing within 8 weeks.
- In acute BCS the development of collaterals has not occurred, so pain, hepatic necrosis and ascites dominate the clinical picture.
- With a subacute (most common) and chronic BCS, collaterals have developed so hepatic necrosis is minimal. Presentation of subacute BSC is with unexplained splenomegaly or varices.
- Chronic BCS presents as decompensated cirrhosis.

CLINICAL PEARL

Suspect Budd–Chiari syndrome in a younger patient (more often female) presenting with acute-onset abdominal pain, hepatomegaly and ascites.

Box 12-7

Complications of alcoholism

Gastrointestinal tract
1 Chronic liver disease (alcoholic hepatitis, cirrhosis)
2 Hepatomegaly (fatty liver, chronic liver disease)
3 Diarrhea (watery due to alcohol), or steatorrhea due to chronic alcoholic pancreatitis or rarely liver disease
4 Pancreatitis (although acute attacks occur, usually there is underlying chronic disease)
5 Acute gastritis (erosions)
6 Parotitis/parotidomegaly

Cardiovascular system
1 Hypertension
2 Cardiomyopathy
3 Arrhythmias

Nervous system
1 Nutrition-related problems: Wernicke encephalopathy, Korsakoff syndrome (thiamine deficiency), pellagra (dermatitis, diarrhea, dementia due to niacin deficiency)
2 Withdrawal syndromes: tremor, hallucinations, 'rum fits', delirium tremens
3 Dementia (cerebral atrophy and Marchiafava–Bignami disease [corpus callosum demyelination])

4 Cerebellar degeneration
5 Central pontine myelinosis (causing pseudobulbar palsies, spastic quadriparesis)
6 Autonomic neuropathy
7 Proximal myopathy
8 Acute intoxication

Hematological system
1 Megaloblastic anemia (dietary folate deficiency, rarely B_{12} deficiency due to chronic pancreatitis with failure to cleave B_{12}–R-protein complex)
2 Iron-deficiency anemia due to bleeding erosions or portal hypertension
3 Aplastic anemia (direct toxic effect on the bone marrow)
4 Thrombocytopenia (bone marrow suppression, hypersplenism)

Metabolic abnormalities
1 Acidosis (lactic, ketoacidosis)
2 Hypoglycemia
3 Hypocalcemia, hypomagnesemia
4 Hypertriglyceridemia, hyperuricemia

Causes

The cause is usually a hypercoagulable state (Box 12-8), although rarely an inferior vena caval web is responsible.

Diagnosis

Diagnosis depends on demonstration of impaired hepatic outflow.

- The best test is Doppler ultrasonography, although CT and MRI are of value and may also find associated malignancy.
- If the suspicion is high and tests remain negative, then hepatic venography should be performed; this may also reveal a caval web.

The ALT is elevated in fulminant and acute BCS, but may be near normal or normal in the chronic form.

Treatment

This includes management of ascites with diuretics, sodium restriction and, if required, large-volume paracentesis. Management of complications of cirrhosis (encephalopathy, HRS) should occur as previously outlined. Lifelong anticoagulation is generally accepted as necessary.

Treatment of acute forms of Budd–Chiari syndrome should be directed at reperfusion treatment or liver transplantation.

Non-alcoholic fatty liver disease (NAFLD) and non-alcoholic steatohepatitis (NASH)

These are the most common causes of chronic liver disease in the developed world. Fatty liver disease represents a spectrum from excess fat to inflammation. A subset of 5–20% of patients progress to cirrhosis. These tend to have inflammatory histology (NASH) rather than bland steatosis.

- Clinical features are those of the metabolic syndrome. Patients are usually asymptomatic, although dull right upper quadrant discomfort may be present. Hepatomegaly is common. Signs of cirrhosis and portal hypertension may be present.
- The diagnosis is usually clinically based, with abnormal transaminases in the right clinical setting (e.g. obesity, diabetes mellitus or hyperlipidemia); other causes for liver disease are excluded, especially alcohol, but also viral hepatitis, medication and iron overload.
- The abdominal ultrasound is usually consistent with the diagnosis, although it may be normal in 10% of cases.

Other causes of hepatic steatosis are given in Box 12-9.

CLINICAL PEARL

Cardiovascular disease and malignancy remain the most common cause of morbidity and mortality in non-alcoholic fatty liver disease. Management must include preventative measures for these diseases.

The **treatment** should address insulin resistance. This includes the following:

- Diet and weight loss—a low-glycemic-index and low-fat diet should be adopted, and a goal of 10% total body-weight loss over 6 months should be adopted. This has been shown to improve liver function and histology.
- Exercise—exercise alone has been shown to improve liver function.
- The use of insulin-sensitizing drugs in selected patients. However, the insulin-sensitizing drug therapy evidence is very borderline. Metformin is the only drug that is used at this stage. The role of thiazolidinediones is controversial.
- Alcohol must be stopped.

Box 12-8

Causes of Budd–Chiari syndrome

Think: hypercoagulable states

Inherited
- Factor V Leiden mutation

Antithrombin III deficiency
- Protein C deficiency
- Protein S deficiency
- Prothrombin mutation

Acquired hypercoagulable state
- Pregnancy
- Oral contraceptives

Myeloproliferative disorders
- Paroxysmal nocturnal hemoglobinuria (PNH)

Other
- Antiphospholipid syndrome
- Cancer

Box 12-9

Other causes of hepatic steatosis

1 Protein-calorie malnutrition or starvation*
2 Total parenteral nutrition*
3 Drugs, e.g. glucocorticoids*, estrogens*, aspirin‡, calcium-channel blockers*, amiodarone, tamoxifen*, tetracycline‡, methotrexate*, valproic acid‡, cocaine‡, antivirals (e.g. zidovudine*)
4 Lipodystrophy*
5 Acute fatty liver of pregnancy‡
6 Inflammatory bowel disease*

---

* Causes macrovesicular steatosis.
‡ Causes microvesicular steatosis.

Wilson's disease (hepatolenticular degeneration)

This is a rare but important autosomal recessive disease of copper excess secondary to mutation in the *ATP7B* copper transport gene.

- The disease presents in young adult life (usually up to age 35; it is extremely rare over 40, so those above this age with unexplained liver disease would not normally be screened for Wilson's disease).
- Wilson's disease may present with liver disease, neurological disease (e.g. parkinsonian features, psychiatric disease), or both. Those with neurological disease usually have detectable liver disease if it is sought.
  » Liver disease from Wilson's disease is highly variable. It may be that of an uncomplicated chronic hepatitis, decompensated cirrhosis, or acute liver failure. It should be suspected in a young patient with hemolysis and acute liver failure.
  » Neurological signs (e.g. tremor, rigidity) are present in one-third of cases.
  » Kayser–Fleisher (K-F) rings are present in almost all Wilson's patients with neurological disease, and about half with hepatic disease (Figure 12-13).

CLINICAL PEARL

A young patient with neurological symptoms and liver disease—exclude Wilson's disease!

Diagnosis depends on combination testing: slit-lamp exam (for K-F rings), serum ceruloplasmin (reduced) and 24-hour urine copper (excess). It is unusual for all screening tests to be positive. Liver biopsy is required for definitive diagnosis.

CLINICAL PEARL

Ceruloplasmin is an acute-phase reactant, and may be elevated falsely in hepatitis and depressed in cirrhosis with impaired synthetic function. Diagnosis of Wilson's disease relies on combination testing.

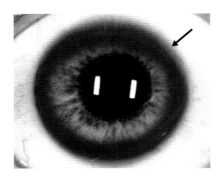

Figure 12-13 Kayser–Fleischer (K–F) ring

From Goldman L and Schafer AI. Goldman's Cecil medicine, 24th ed. Philadelphia: Elsevier, 2012.

Treatment is with penicillamine (plus pyridoxine), which promotes urinary copper excretion and inhibits GI copper absorption, or with trientine and/or oral zinc, which are chelators. There is growing evidence that trientine is as effective and better tolerated than penicillamine and may be considered as first-line therapy.

Liver transplant is indicated in fulminant disease and is curative.

Alpha-1 anti-trypsin deficiency

This is an autosomal recessive disease and can present in adults. Diagnosis is with serum electrophoresis (A1AT phenotype). Transplantation in end-stage liver disease is curative (of liver disease).

Hemochromatosis

This is an important and relatively common disease of iron overload. There are two types:

1. **Hereditary** (autosomal recessive)—affecting 1 in 250 Caucasians. The genetic defect leads to abnormal iron absorption. The gene is *HFE* and there are two well-known mutations—*C282Y* and *H63D*. Most patients with this disease are homozygous for *C282Y*. Only a few cases are compound heterozygotes (*C282Y* and *H63D*). Homozygotes for *H63D* probably have no risk of hemachromatosis. There are rare cases with no known mutations.
2. **Acquired**—secondary to multiple blood transfusions, or secondary erythropoiesis (e.g. thalassemia or sideroblastic anemia).

Most patients with hereditary hemochromatosis present in the asymptomatic phase, as a result of iron studies being found to be abnormal for other reasons.

Men are much more likely to present with clinical features, as women are protected by menses until the menopause. Classical clinical features in advanced disease (Figure 12-14) include:

- hepatomegaly (from iron deposition; most cases)
- diabetes mellitus (in two-thirds)
- pigmentation ('bronzed diabetes' is a classic but rare finding in a subgroup of patients)
- arthropathy ('big knuckles'; 2nd and 3rd metacarpophalangeal (MCP) joints) (in two-fifths)
- cardiomyopathy (dilated) (in one-sixth)
- erectile dysfunction (secondary to pituitary iron overload).

CLINICAL PEARL

In a patient with diabetes mellitus and evidence of liver disease, screen for hemochromatosis with iron studies.

Screening is by looking for an increased fasting transferrin saturation of >62% in men and >50% in women, and a raised ferritin level of which >300 microg/mL in men and >200 microg/mL in women is suggestive, and >1000 microg/mL very suggestive.

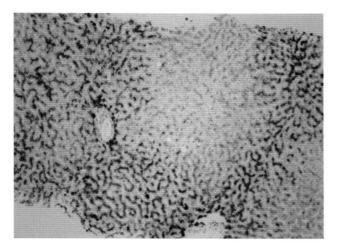

Figure 12-14 Hemochromatosis: this liver biopsy reveals increased iron stores (blue-green staining)

From Goldman L and Schafer AI. Goldman's Cecil medicine, 24th ed. Philadelphia: Elsevier, 2012.

- It should be noted that the ferritin can be raised as an acute-phase reactant in any inflammatory process, including NASH, alcoholic liver disease and chronic viral hepatitis. An important feature that helps distinguish between reactive causes and true iron overload is the progression of the ferritin, with fluctuation in reactive cases and a progressive rise in hemochromatosis.
- Hemochromatosis often remains undiagnosed in women until after the menopause.

If the diagnosis is suspected on iron studies, genetic testing is helpful to confirm the disease in most cases. MRI is indicated if the ferritin is above 1000 microg/mL, to estimate. If non-diagnostic or uncertain, liver biopsy and chemical iron staining should be performed to determine the hepatic iron index (usually >1.9).

> ### CLINICAL PEARL
> Beware of hemochomatosis patients who stops requiring venesection—they may need investigation for gastrointestinal blood loss.

Treatment includes the following:
- Avoidance of excess alcohol.
- Regular venesection (weekly initially and with monitoring of iron studies until iron is depleted to a normal ferritin level, then third-monthly). This should be modified according to response. Arthropathy and endocrine changes do not respond to venesection, as the organs are irreparably damaged.
- Screening for HCC should occur 6-monthly if there is underlying cirrhosis. If there is no cirrhosis, the HCC risk is not increased once the patient is venesected and iron-depleted.

AUTOIMMUNE LIVER DISEASES

These include autoimmune hepatitis (AIH), primary biliary cholangitis (PBC) and primary sclerosing cholangitis (PSC). Overlap syndromes may also occur. Diagnosis relies on a combination of clinical assessment, liver enzyme pattern and autoantibodies. Histology and cholangiography are required in most patients.

Autoimmune hepatitis (AIH)

Autoimmune hepatitis is an idiopathic necroinflammatory liver disease that is characterized by the presence of auto-antibodies, elevated globulins and interface hepatitis on liver biopsy. Presentation is varied.

- It can be diagnosed in the investigation of the well patient with abnormal liver enzymes, or present as either decompensated cirrhosis or acute liver failure.
- Fatigue and arthralgia are common complaints. If advanced, jaundice, splenomegaly and ascites may be present.
- The globulins are typically elevated and autoantibodies are present. These include anti-nuclear antibodies (ANA), anti-smooth muscle antibodies (ASMA) (type 1 AIH) and anti-liver-kidney microsomal antibodies (ALKMA) (type 2 AIH).

Diagnosis is made based on the presence of these features and the exclusion of other causes of liver disease. Liver biopsy is recommended in suspected cases. The histological hallmark is interface hepatitis with a prominent plasma cell infiltrate.

Treatment of AIH is based on immune suppression, initially with prednisone and often with the addition of an immunosuppressant such as azathioprine. Management of decompensated liver disease is the same as for any other etiology and may include liver transplantation.

Primary biliary cholangitis (PBC) and primary sclerosing cholangitis (PSC)

It is important to distinguish between PBC and PSC (Table 12-11).

- Both are cholestatic liver diseases and can cause jaundice and pruritis, and the alkaline phosphatase (ALP) will be elevated.
- PBC affects middle-aged women, causing fatigue and pruritus.
- PSC typically affects men who have ulcerative colitis.

Diagnosis is based on serum liver enzymes and auto-antibodies.

- Cholangiography is required in the case of PSC. MRCP is the modality of choice, with endoscopic retrograde cholangiopancreatography (ERCP) reserved for cases with non-diagnostic MR cholangiography where the index of suspicion remains high. ERCP can also treat dominant strictures, and allows for biliary brushing and biopsy for suspected cholangiocarcinoma or a dominant stricture. Liver biopsy has a role in the setting of diagnostic uncertainty.

Table 12-11 Primary sclerosing cholangitis (PSC) vs primary biliary cholangitis (PBC)

FEATURE	PSC	PBC
Age	Young	Middle-aged and elderly
Sex	Typically men (70%)	Typically women (90%)
Clinical	Pain Cholangitis Hepatosplenomegaly ALP elevated	Pruritus Xanthomas, xanthelasma Hyperpigmentation Hepatosplenomegaly ALP elevated
Liver function tests	Bilirubin fluctuates	
Antimitochondrial antibody	Negative	Positive in 90% (also elevated in chronic hepatitis, connective tissue disease)
pANCA	Positive (up to 80%)	Negative
MRCP	Irregular and beaded ducts	Pruned ducts
Associated diseases	Ulcerative colitis (70%) Crohn's disease (rare) Sjögren's syndrome (rare) Thyroiditis (rare) Hypothyroidism (rare) Pancreatitis (rare) Retro-orbital and retroperitoneal fibrosis (rare)	CREST syndrome Sjögren's syndrome Thyroiditis Renal tubular acidosis
Complications	Portal hypertension Liver failure Bile duct carcinoma	Osteomalacia Steatorrhea (due to bile acid deficiency, associated pancreatic insufficiency or coexisting celiac disease) Portal hypertension, liver failure (late)
Treatment	Ursodeoxycholic acid Liver transplant	Liver transplant

ALP, serum alkaline phosphatase; CREST, calcinosis, Raynaud's syndrome, esophageal dysmotility, sclerodactyly and telangiectasia; MRCP, magnetic resonance cholangiopancreatography; pANCA, peri-nuclear anti-neutrophil cytoplasmic antibody.

- Antimicrobial antibody (AMA) is positive in 95% of cases of PBC. Liver biopsy is required to diagnose and stage PBC.

Treatment:

- There is no proven treatment for PSC, although ERCP with biliary stenting may be required to relieve cholestatic symptoms if there is a dominant stricture.

- Ursodeoxycholic acid at 15 mg/kg/day is the recommended treatment for PBC.

- Both PSC and PBC may progress to cirrhosis, which when complicated requires specific therapy. Surveillance for esophageal varices and hepatocellular carcinoma should occur once cirrhosis is diagnosed.

- Management of osteopenia and osteoporosis is important in both diseases.

- Measurement and replacement of vitamin D should be undertaken.

PSC may be complicated by cholangiocarcinoma and intermittent cholangitits. These must be sought if there is a rapid change in the liver function tests.

SYSTEMIC DISEASE AND THE LIVER

Remember that a number of diseases may affect not just the liver, but also other organs. Some diagnostic hints to remember are presented in Box 12-10.

PREGNANCY AND LIVER DISEASE

It is important to recognize both the specific liver diseases that occur in pregnancy and the effects in pregnancy of other liver diseases (Table 12-12).

GALLBLADDER AND BILIARY TREE

The major diseases to consider are gallstones, cholangitis (infection of the bile secondary to obstruction, usually from

Box 12-10

Diagnostic hints: liver and other systemic disease

1 Liver and cardiac disease—consider underlying cardiac failure, constrictive pericarditis, hemochromatosis, alcoholism, amyloidosis, amiodarone

2 Liver and lung disease—consider underlying alpha-1 antitrypsin deficiency

3 Liver and neurological disease—consider underlying Wilson's disease, hepatic encephalopathy or alcohol

4 Liver disease and photosensitivity—consider underlying porphyria cutanea tarda and hepatitis C

5 Liver and renal disease—consider hepatorenal syndrome, but carefully consider acute tubular necrosis or pre-renal failure

a stone or tumor) and cholestasis (obstructive, e.g. stone or tumor; or hepatocellular, see above).

Gallstones

Most gallstones are asymptomatic. Gallstones can cause biliary pain (severe, constant pain in the epigastrium or right upper quadrant lasting at least 30 minutes that occurs in discreet episodes and is unpredictable).

Natural history of asymptomatic gallstones:

- 80% remain asymptomatic, and cholecystectomy is not recommended unless symptoms occur.
- Fewer than 20% who experience symptoms will develop complications, but cholecystectomy is indicated.

Associated with an increased incidence of cholesterol gallstones are:

- increasing age
- female gender, estrogen therapy, the contraceptive pill (more lithogenic bile)
- race, e.g. Native Americans
- obesity (lithogenic bile)
- intrahepatic cholestasis of pregnancy
- pancreatitis
- drugs, e.g. clofibrate (lithogenic bile), ceftriaxone (biliary sludge).

Associated with an increased incidence of calcium bilirubinate (pigment) stones are:

- chronic hemolysis
- ileal disease, e.g. Crohn's disease
- cirrhosis
- biliary infection.

At increased risk of complications are the elderly, diabetics, those with large stones, and those with a non-functioning or calcified gallbladder.

Diagnosis of gallstones

- An ultrasound, rather than a CT scan, is the first-line test.
- If the liver function tests and ultrasound are normal, a common duct stone is unlikely.
- If a common duct stone is a consideration (e.g. persistent pain and abnormal liver function tests), an MRCP should be performed. ERCP is used to remove the stone.

Table 12-12 Liver disease in pregnancy

DISEASE	CAUSE	COMMENT
Incidental to pregnancy	Viral hepatitis	Most common cause of liver disease in pregnancy
	Alcohol-related	
	Autoimmune chronic hepatitis	Most prevalent in females of reproductive age
Related to pregnancy (possibly influenced by hormones present in pregnancy)	Complicated gallstone disease	Bile ducts enlarge in pregnancy, tend to regress after delivery
	Hepatic adenoma	May enlarge and bleed, rare
	Focal nodular hyperplasia	Unclear whether enlargement of nodules is promoted in pregnancy
	Budd–Chiari syndrome	Hepatic venous outflow obstruction
Specific to pregnancy	Intrahepatic cholestasis	Pruritus, jaundice in third trimester
	Acute fatty liver of pregnancy (AFLP)	Vomiting, pain, jaundice, liver failure—deliver immediately
	HELLP (hemolysis, elevated liver enzymes, low platelets)	In preeclampsia Can be confused with AFLP Deliver immediately

- Hepatobiliary iminodiacetic acid (HIDA) scanning is useful in the diagnosis of acute cholecystitis (acute cystic duct obstruction).

CLINICAL PEARL

Charcot's triad—right upper quadrant pain, fever and jaundice—suggests cholangitis, but patients may just present initially with mental status change or hypotension.

Acalculous cholecystitis

This should be considered in a very ill patient where the gallbladder is enlarged on imaging. If the patient is too ill for a cholecytectomy, cholecystostomy is lifesaving.

A palpable gallbladder (Box 12-11) usually indicates longstanding biliary obstruction or gallbladder cancer rather than gallstones.

CLINICAL PEARL

If an X-ray shows a calcified gallbladder outline ('porcelain gallbladder'), operate—as this is likely to be cancer.

PORPHYRIAS

There are several major porphyria syndromes in adults (which are all autosomal dominant).

Acute intermittent porphyria (AIP)

In AIP the defect is a partial deficiency of porphobilinogen deaminase.

Clinical features (similar to lead poisoning)

- Abdominal pain, vomiting, constipation
- Peripheral neuropathy (motor)
- The skin is *never* affected

Attacks may be precipitated by drugs (alcohol, barbiturates, sulfonamides, and the contraceptive pill).

Investigation

- Acute attacks—increased urinary porphobilinogen (PBG) and delta-aminolevulinic acid (ALA), thus the urine is dark; fecal porphyrins are normal.
- Between acute attacks, the findings are the same i.e. PBG and ALA remain elevated for days to weeks and may remain elevated for months-years.
- DNA testing confirms the diagnosis.

Box 12-11
Causes of a palpable gallbladder

With jaundice

1. Carcinoma of the head of the pancreas
2. Carcinoma of the ampulla of Vater
3. Mucocele of the gallbladder due to a stone in Hartmann's pouch and a stone in the common bile duct (rare)

Without jaundice

1. Mucocele of the gallbladder
2. Carcinoma of the gallbladder

Treatment

- Stop alcohol and medications that are known to be unsafe, e.g. estrogens, carbemazepine, non–steroidal anti–inflammatory drugs (NSAIDs).
- Treat any intercurrent infection.
- Manage SIADH (syndrome of inappropriate secretion of antidiuretic hormone) if present.
- Monitor vital capacity (bulbar paralysis).
- Intravenous hemin (intravenous glucose only if mild).
- RNA interference therapy given subcutaneously.

Porphyria cutanea tarda (PCT)

In PCT, the defect is uroporphyrinogen decarboxylase deficiency. Iron overload is a determinant of the clinical expression.

Clinical features

- There are no acute attacks in PCT and they are not usually drug-related.
- The skin shows bullae and hyperpigmentation on exposed areas.
- Underlying hepatitis C is common; alcoholic liver disease may be present.

Investigations

- Normal PBG and ALA in urine, and normal porphyrins in stools.
- Greatly increased uroporphyrin in urine, causing red urine.

Treatment

Phlebotomies are performed to reduce serum ferritin.

SELF-ASSESSMENT QUESTIONS

1 A 35-year-old man presents with a 4-day history of jaundice, dark urine and upper abdominal pain. Over the past 3 months he has noted a 6 kg weight loss and his appetite has also decreased. He has been on mesalamine for 8 years for the treatment of ulcerative colitis. He has not had any recent flare. He drinks about 60 g/day of alcohol and he is a type 2 diabetic on metformin and insulin. On clinical examination he is obese and jaundiced. Abdominal examination shows only a previous laparoscopic cholecystectomy scar. His family physician had noted slightly deranged liver function tests over the past few years, and it was thought to be related to fatty liver disease. During his present inpatient stay, an abdominal ultrasound showed dilated intrahepatic ducts and common hepatic duct, and no features of fatty liver were noted. The common bile duct was not dilated. The following are his liver function tests: bilirubin 100 micromol/L (reference range [RR] 3–15), alkaline phosphatase 820 U/L (RR 30–115), alanine aminotransferase 2800 U/L (RR 1–40), aspartate aminotransferase 240 U/L (RR 1–30). Which of the following is the most appropriate next step?

A Endoscopic retrograde cholangiopancreatography (ERCP)
B Magnetic resonance cholangiopancreatography (MRCP)
C Tumor markers:Ca19.9, CEA and AFP
D Endoscopic ultrasonography with fine-needle aspiration biopsy
E Start ursodeoxycholic acid

2 A 29-year-old man presents with hematemesis after ingesting 150 g of alcohol the previous night. He denies retching prior to the episode of hematemesis. Despite his young age, stigmata of chronic liver disease are present. His blood pressure is 70/40 mmHg and his heart rate is 128 beats/min. He appears pale. Rectal examination is normal. He continues to vomit blood in the emergency room. An artificial airway is placed and fluid resuscitation commenced. Emergency endoscopy is likely to show:

A Gastric ulcer
B Duodenal ulcer
C Mallory–Weiss tear
D Gastric antral vascular lesion
E Esophageal varices

3 A 54-year-old man is noted to be anemic (hemoglobin 74 g/L). He has no clinical signs of end-organ dysfunction, but feels fatigued after exercise. His iron studies show:

Ferritin	3.5 ng/mL (normal range 40–200)
Transferrin saturation	5% (normal range 20–50)
Serum iron	4 mmol/L (normal range 10–27)
Total iron binding capacity (TIBC)	78 micromol/L (normal range 48–80)

Vitamin B_{12} and folate studies are normal. His red cells are hypochromic and microcytic. In addition to undertaking investigations for his iron deficiency, the most appropriate initial action in terms of managing his iron deficiency is:

A Await investigations prior to commencing iron replacement.
B Infuse 1 g iron sucrose intravenously.
C Infuse 1 g iron polymaltose intravenously.
D Commence oral iron replacement.

4 A 32-year-old woman is referred by her family physician with joint aches, jaundice and fatigue. Her liver function tests are abnormal, showing an elevated bilirubin and transaminases three times the upper limit of normal. Alkaline phosphatase and gamma-GT are just above normal. She has no significant medical background and has not recently traveled overseas. She takes no regular medications, but occasionally takes fish oil and a multivitamin. She drinks 20–30 g of alcohol every 2nd weekend. Her family history is positive for maternal hypothyroidism. On examination, her observations are within normal limits. Scleral icterus and jaundice are present. No signs of chronic liver disease can be found. Further blood tests show:

Antinuclear antibody (ANA)	1:40
Anti-smooth-muscle antibody (ASMA)	1:640
Anti-mitochondrial antibody (AMA)	Not detected
Hepatitis B and C serology	Negative

Which of the following is the most likely diagnosis?

A Hepatitis associated with lupus
B Autoimmune hepatitis
C Primary biliary cirrhosis
D Primary sclerosing cholangitis
E Drug-induced liver injury

5   A 60-year-old businessman is referred with abnormal liver function tests for investigation. His past medical history is positive for diabetes, hypercholesterolemia and osteoarthritis. His current medications include long-acting insulin, rosuvastatin, acetaminophen (paracetamol) and occasional use of non-steroidal anti-inflammatory drugs (NSAIDs). He denies illicit drug use, and states that he drinks 10–20 g of alcohol less than once a month. He was adopted and has no knowledge of any family history. He has three adult sons. He has no tattoos and has not traveled overseas recently. Physical examination shows a normotensive but slightly overweight man. His cardiorespiratory examination is unremarkable. He has palmar erythema, but no spider nevi or hepatosplenomegaly. There are no signs of hepatic encephalopathy. His blood tests reveal:

Hemoglobin	144 g/L (reference range [RR] 138–172)
Glucose (fasting)	8.0 mmol/L (RR 3.6–6.0)
Bilirubin (total)	18 micromol/L (RR 3–15)
Aspartate aminotransferase (AST)	68 U/L (RR 1–30)
Alanine aminotransferase (ALT)	82 U/L (RR 1–40)
Alkaline phosphatase (ALP)	134 U/L (RR 30–115)
Albumin	42 g/L (RR 36–47)
Ferritin	1267 ng/mL (RR 40–200)
Transferrin saturation	85% (RR 20–50)

Which of the following is the next most appropriate step?
A   Commence immediate venesection.
B   Start oral deferoxamine therapy.
C   Cease all alcohol intake and repeat iron studies in 3 months.
D   Perform genetic testing mutations in the HFE gene.
E   Perform a liver biopsy with separate core for iron staining.

6   A 23-year-old woman is referred by her family physician with a 3-week history of jaundice, fatigue and anorexia. She is an injecting drug user who also consumes 60–100 g of alcohol on weekends. There is no personal or family history of liver disease. On examination she has scleral icterus and jaundice. Her cardiorespiratory examination is normal. Abdominal examination reveals tender hepatomegaly, but no splenomegaly. There are no signs of chronic liver disease. Her blood tests reveal:

Bilirubin	68 micromol/L (reference range [RR] 3–15)
Aspartate aminotransferase (AST)	420 U/L (RR 1–30)
Alanine aminotransferase (ALT)	680 U/L (RR 1–40)
Alkaline phosphatase (ALP)	134 U/L (RR 30–115)
Gamma-glutamyl transpeptidase (GGT)	222 U/L (RR 0–30)
Albumin	36 g/L (RR 36–47)
Coagulation profile	Normal
Hepatitis B surface antigen	Negative
Hepatitis C antibody	Negative
Hepatitis A IgG and IgM	Negative

An ultrasound confirms hepatomegaly, but shows no masses or intra- or extrahepatic duct dilatation. Which of the following is the most appropriate next diagnostic test?
A   Liver biopsy
B   Hepatitis C RNA
C   Hepatitis B DNA
D   Hepatitis delta serology
E   Observe and repeat hepatitis serology in 6 weeks

7 A 42-year-old woman is referred with uncomfortable abdominal fullness which has been present for 6 weeks. She is alcohol-dependent, drinking 100 g of alcohol on a daily basis for the past 12 years. Her background medical history is positive for diabetes mellitus and thyroid disease, and she takes metformin as well as thyroxine. She has no significant family history and denies intravenous drug use. On examination her blood pressure is 110/80 mmHg with a pulse rate of 80 beats/min. She has scleral icterus and spider nevi across the precordium. The abdomen is distended, with 8 cm shifting dullness. There is no palpable hepatomegaly or splenomegaly. Blood tests reveal thrombocytopenia and an elevated bilirubin level of 76 micromol/L (reference range [RR] 3–15). Her coagulation profile is abnormal with an INR (international normalized ratio) of 2.0. There is mild transaminitis. The creatinine is 280 micromol/L (RR 45–85). An abdominal ultrasound confirms the presence of ascites. The liver has increased echotexture and is small. No portal or hepatic vein obstruction is seen. What is the next most appropriate step in management?

A   Perform a diagnostic paracentesis.
B   Commence ceftriaxone intravenously and give intravenous albumin.
C   Commence fluid restriction along with furosemide and spironolactone.
D   Perform urinary electrolyte analysis.
E   Arrange transjugular intrahepatic shunting (TIPS).

8 A 64-year-old man is referred with abnormal iron studies. He has no diagnosed medical conditions, but appears mildly obese. He works as a truck driver, and was adopted as a child and hence is unaware of any family history of illnesses. He has drunk 60–80 g of alcohol on a daily basis since his teenage years. He smokes 40 cigarettes daily. He takes no regular medications nor any over-the-counter or herbal preparations. Examination shows a ruddy complexion of the face, along with central adiposity without palpable organomegaly. Spider nevi and palmar erythema are present. His iron studies show:

Ferritin	678 ng/mL (normal range 40–200)
Iron	25 mmol/L (normal range 10–27)
Total iron binding capacity (TIBC)	54 micromol/L (normal range 48–80)
Transferrin saturation	34% (normal range 20–50)

His hemoglobin is 165 g/L and both mean cell volume (MCV) and mean cell hemoglobin (MCH) are elevated. Which of the following is the most likely cause for his elevated ferritin?

A   *C282Y* homozygote
B   *C282Y* heterozygote
C   Alcohol
D   *H63D* homozygote
E   *H63D* heterozygote

9 A 54-year-old diabetic man is referred with abnormal liver function tests. He has previously suffered a myocardial infarction, and commenced statin therapy for hypercholesterolemia 6 months ago. He also receives insulin therapy along with 'baby-dose' aspirin. He drinks 1–2 standard drinks most days of the week. He denies overseas travel, has no tattoos and has never used intravenous drugs. He did receive a blood transfusion in 2003 after a motor vehicle accident. Physical examination is unremarkable apart from a body mass index of 34 kg/m². His liver function tests are as follows:

Alkaline phosphatase (ALP)	125 U/L (normal range 30–115)
Gamma-glutamyl transpeptidase (GGT)	160 U/L (normal range (0–30)
Alanine aminotransferase (ALT)	60 U/L (normal range 1–40)
Aspartate aminotransferase (AST)	45 U/L (normal range 1–30)

His albumin and coagulation profile are normal. His platelet count is normal. You proceed to liver biopsy. Which of the following is the most likely abnormality on the liver biopsy?

A   Hepatic steatosis
B   Normal liver histology
C   Chronic inflammation consistent with viral hepatitis
D   Advanced fibrosis
E   Drug-induced liver injury from statin therapy

ANSWERS

1 A.

This patient most likely has primary sclerosing cholangitis on a background of ulcerative colitis. ERCP is most helpful as a diagnostic and therapeutic tool, allowing stent placement to help with drainage of bile. MRCP would also probably provide the diagnosis, but this patient needs biliary drainage. Tumor markers are often elevated in the setting of biliary obstruction and would not help guide management in this scenario. An endoscopic ultrasound would give excellent images of the pancreatic and biliary ducts, but a biliary stent needs to be placed in this patient. Ursodeoxycholic acid is useful in many cholestatic liver diseases, but should not be commenced in the setting of obstructive jaundice.

2 E.

The most likely cause of this significant upper gastrointestinal hemorrhage is esophageal varices due to portal hypertension. Young patients often suffer Mallory–Weiss tears associated with retching and vomiting, but the history and severity of bleeding makes this less likely here. Although bleeding gastric or duodenal ulcers could present like this, they are uncommon in the young without comorbidities.

3 D.

Commence oral iron replacement. There is no reason to delay replacement, although clearly further investigations are needed. Intravenous iron does lead to a more rapid hemoglobin response as iron stores take longer to restore with oral therapy, but in this case there is no urgency as the patient is not compromised, and oral replacement is less hazardous. Intramuscular injections should be avoided and only used if other treatment methods are not available.

4 B.

The most likely scenario here is autoimmune liver disease. Young females are often affected. A personal or family history of autoimmune disease is often present. Lupus can cause liver function test abnormalities, but the ANA is strongly positive in the majority of cases. Primary biliary cirrhosis usually presents later in life (age 40–60 years), and typically the AMA is positive. Primary sclerosing cholangitis leads to a markedly elevated alkaline phosphatase and is often associated with ulcerative colitis. Drug-induced liver injury could present in this manner, but multivitamins and fish oil are not usual causes.

5 D.

Although the first-line treatment of genetic hemochromatosis is venesection, the diagnosis needs to be confirmed first. This will also facilitate genetic counseling and potential testing of offspring. Iron-chelation therapy is reserved for patients who are anemic and cannot tolerate regular venesection. His alcohol consumption is a very unlikely explanation for the abnormalities observed. A liver biopy is likely to confirm iron deposition, but is not the next appropriate step.

6 B.

The most appropriate step is to determine whether this is acute hepatitis C, as seroconversion can take 2 months. In the setting of abnormal liver function tests and negative hepatitis B antibodies, the presence of hepatitis B is very unlikely (seroconversion occurs prior to clinical disease in most patients). A liver biopsy could be considered if the noninvasive liver screens were negative. The hepatitis delta virus is a defective virus which requires the presence of hepatitis B infection to survive.

7 A.

This patient requires a diagnostic paracentesis. With new-onset ascites it is important to exclude spontaneous bacterial peritonitis (SBP). This also gives an opportunity to measure the serum ascites–albumin gradient (SAAG), which if above 11 g/L usually indicates ascites from portal hypertension. Intravenous ceftriaxone is appropriate treatment for SBP, but a diagnostic paracentesis is the first step. Fluid restriction along with diuretics is inappropriate in the setting of an elevated creatinine level. It may precipitate or worsen hepatorenal syndrome. TIPS is not first-line therapy for new-onset ascites. Urinary electrolytes are helpful in identifying sodium retention due to renin–angiotensin system activation, and to guide diuretic therapy.

8 C.

This man's abnormal liver function tests and iron studies are likely to be due to alcohol. His ferritin is elevated, which does occur in hemochromatosis as well. However, the most sensitive marker in iron studies for hemochromatosis is the iron saturation, which almost universally is elevated. *C282* homozygosity certainly confers risk for iron overload, while heterozygotes are generally unaffected carriers. Compound heterozygotes (*C282Y* and *H63D*) are also at risk. *H63D* homozygotes can rarely develop iron overload.

9 A.

The most likely scenario here is fatty liver disease. He has no risk factors for viral hepatitis, and transmission via blood transfusion is extremely unlikely after 1992. Advanced fibrosis and cirrhosis is unlikely, given that there are no signs of chronic liver disease on physical examination and the platelet count is normal. Drug-induced liver injury from statin therapy is possible, but this usually presents with an acute hepatocellular picture (high AST and ALT). Completely normal liver histology is unlikely in an obese diabetic with abnormal liver function tests.

HEMATOLOGY

Stephen James Fuller

- Staging
- Risk stratification
- Treatment
- PLASMA CELL DISORDERS
  - Monoclonal gammopathy of uncertain significance (MGUS)
  - Asymptomatic myeloma
  - Symptomatic myeloma
  - Prognostic markers in myeloma
  - Treatment of myeloma
  - Differential diagnosis

- ANEMIA
  - Mechanisms of anemia
  - Common laboratory tests used for diagnostic work-up
  - Approach to iron-deficiency anemia
  - Management of iron deficiency
  - Anemia of chronic disease
  - Thalassemias
  - Sideroblastic anemias
  - Macrocytic anemias
  - Hemolytic anemias
  - Drug-induced hemolysis
  - Non-immune acquired hemolytic anemias

HEMOSTASIS

Essential concepts

Interaction between coagulation, inflammation and immunity

Coagulation and innate immunity have co-evolved to provide a multifaceted attack to repel infections.

- Neutrophils and platelets form extracellular traps that kill bacteria.
- There are close interactions between the cellular and soluble components of the hemostatic and immune systems. For example, thrombin—the key enzyme that generates fibrin—also activates platelets and complement proteins C3 and C5. Activated C5a can in turn stimulate neutrophils and endothelial cells.
- Endothelial cells and platelets must be sufficiently activated past a threshold for a clot to form.

While the hemostatic processes are primarily designed to be protective, their unrestricted activity can also be detrimental, e.g. thrombotic thrombocytopenic purpura (TTP) and disseminated intravascular coagulation (DIC). Hence, there is a very efficient and prompt counterbalance provided by coagulation-inhibitory systems.

Components of the hemostatic system

Platelets

Steps in platelet activation and aggregation

In undisturbed vasculature, platelets may roll along endothelial surfaces without any significant interaction, and platelets circulate in close proximity to fibrinogen and von Willebrand factor (vWF) without demonstrating spontaneous activation and aggregation. A sufficient threshold of stimulation has to be crossed before platelets proceed through the sequential steps of:

1 adhesion
2 activation
3 aggregation.

Platelet adhesion

Injury to the protective endothelial surface exposes major matrix proteins such as collagen, vWF and other proteins including thrombospondin, laminin and fibronectin, all of which can interact with platelet integrin receptors.

Interaction of platelets with damaged endothelium proceeds through the steps of:

1 tethering
2 rolling
3 activation
4 firm adhesion.

In veins and large arteries, collagen is the principal platelet-adhesive macromolecule. Platelet receptors glycoprotein VI and $\alpha2\beta1$ are the principal contacts with collagen. In small arteries and areas of atherosclerosis and stenosis, the interaction of vWF with the platelet receptor glycoprotein Ibα (GPIbα) is critical for platelet recruitment. GPIbα is a part of a large receptor complex that includes integrins GPIbβ, GPIX and GPV.

Interaction between the coagulation pathways and primary hemostasis is exemplified by the role of thrombin as an important platelet activator. Inactive precursor zymogen prothrombin is converted to its active form, thrombin, by both intrinsic and tissue factor (TF)-initiated clotting pathways (see below). In addition to its role in generating fibrin from fibrinogen, thrombin is a potent activator of platelets by signaling via the protease-activated receptors 1 and 4 (PAR1 and PAR4).

Platelet activation

Interaction of platelet integrin receptors GPVI and GPIbα to their ligands, collagen and vWF respectively, initiates intracellular signaling cascades that involve activation of:

- Src kinases
- phospholipase Cγ2 (PLCγ2), which leads to an increase in cytosolic Ca^{2+} and generation of diacylglycerol (DAG).

The final step in platelet activation is the 'inside-out' activation of the fibrinogen receptor.

Platelet integrin αIIbβ3 is the most abundant integrin on the platelet surface (up to 80,000 copies per cell) and, in resting platelets, exhibits an 'inactive' conformation that does not recognize fibrinogen. Following platelet activation, raised cytosolic Ca^{2+} and DAG lead to a sequence of events that result in a transformation of αIIbβ3 from a bent inactive form to an extended active form that permits interaction with fibrinogen, and under high shear stress, vWF.

Amplification of platelet activation

Platelets contain three types of granules:

1 alpha granules (contain vWF, fibrinogen and chemokines)
2 dense granules (contain Ca^{2+} ions, nucleotides such as adenosine diphosphate [ADP], histamine and serotonin)
3 lysosomes (containing a variety of enzymes).

Platelet activation leads to a release of granule contents in the proximity of the endothelial–platelet milieu.

This initiates signaling via several pathways that serve to amplify platelet activation. ADP released from activated platelets in turn interacts with the purinergic G protein-coupled receptors, P2Y1 and P2Y12. The importance of the contribution of ADP is confirmed by the efficacy of the thienopyridine class of antiplatelet agents that include ticlopidine, clopidogrel and prasugrel.

Increased Ca^{2+} leads to activation of phospholipase A_2, followed by the release of arachidonic acid from fatty acids. Arachidonic acid in turn forms a substrate for cyclo-oxygenase and is converted to cyclic endoperoxides; which, in turn, are converted to thromboxane A_2 (TXA_2) by the action of thromboxane synthase. TXA_2 provides a positive feedback loop; and interacts with the thromboxane receptor (TP) to initiate signaling that further consolidates platelet activation.

Platelet aggregation

Platelet activation culminates in the unfolding of the αIIbβ3 receptor, which then interacts with fibrinogen.

- Fibrinogen has multiple platelet interaction sites, resulting in a stable aggregate mesh of platelets and fibrinogen on injured endothelium.
- Raised cytosolic Ca^{2+} generated in the process of platelet activation triggers platelet membrane reorganization, with exposure of negatively charged phosphatidylserine (PS)

on the surface. PS together with Ca^{2+} ions forms a procoagulant surface for the binding and activation of clotting factors, leading to thrombin and fibrin generation.

- Thrombin amplifies platelet activation via the PAR1 and PAR4 receptors.

Coagulation

The depiction of coagulation as part of an intrinsic or an extrinsic pathway, and the series of activation events as a 'cascade', has been replaced by a model that explains the cell-surface-dependency of the clotting process.

The new model takes into account the concentration of coagulation factors at the site of a developing thrombus, and explains the place of fVIII and fIX, which are deficient in hemophilia A and B respectively. It also lends itself to the understanding of the processes that restrict clotting to the physiological need.

The new cell-based model describes four overlapping phases (Figure 13-1):

1 **Initiation.** This occurs on the surface of a TF-bearing cell. A break in the vessel wall permits subendothelial TF to come into contact with fVII in the plasma. The TF/fVIIa complex can then activate both fX and fIX; the fXa (activated factor X) thus produced generates a small amount of thrombin. This initial thrombin accelerates the process by activating platelets (via PAR1 and PAR4), and the procofactors fV and fVIII.

2 **Amplification.** Amplification of coagulation is stimulated by the small amount of thrombin generated in the first step. Thrombin activates more platelets, fVIII and fXI, each of which plays an important role in the maintenance of the coagulation process. Activated platelets release fV and expose a negatively charged phosphatidylserine (PS)-containing surface. The platelets' integrin receptor binds vWF and makes it accessible for activation by thrombin. Activated platelets also display high-affinity binding sites for fIXa, fXa and fXI. Thus, a perfect clot-promoting surface is created with the presence of fVIIIa, fVa and assembly of the coagulation proteases.

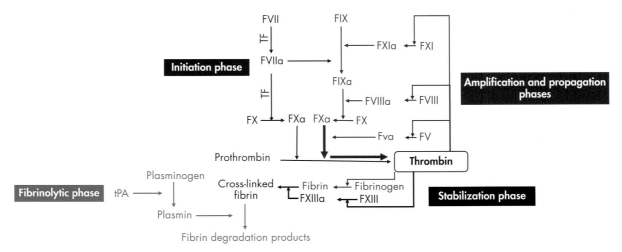

Figure 13-1 Coagulation and fibrinolysis. TF, tissue factor; tPA, tissue plasminogen activator

3 **Propagation.** In this phase, efficient assembly of the 'tenase' (fVIIIa/fIXa/Ca^{2+}), leading to the generation of fXa and subsequent 'prothrombinase' (fXa/fVa/Ca^{2+}), results in significant generation of thrombin (fIIa), more than can be achieved in the initiation phase. Thrombin converts fibrinogen to fibrin monomers.

4 **Stabilization.** Thrombin activates the generation of fXIIIa, which cross-links fibrin monomers to form a stable hemostatic plug.

The fibrinolytic system

The fibrinolytic system is designed to restrict the fibrin clot to the area of injury. Key components of this pathway are:

- plasminogen (PLG)
- tissue plasminogen activator (tPA).

Both are associated with the developing fibrin clot, and thus clot dissolution is finely tuned to clot formation.

PLG binds to the lysine (Lys) residues on cross-linked fibrin, and this creates an optimal environment for PLG to be activated by tPA, which is also fibrin-bound.

PLG and tPA form a self-activation loop, wherein PLG cleaves tPA and enables it to bind fibrin with higher affinity, and this increases the ability of tPA to cleave PLG to form active plasmin.

CLINICAL PEARL

Fibrin is proteolyzed by plasmin to form a number of fibrin degradation products (FDPs), of which the disulfide-linked fragment D (D-dimer) is detected in a commonly used laboratory assay and incorporated in a clinical algorithm to predict venous thrombosis.

Inhibitory control of coagulation

The coagulation pathway activated by injury must be restricted to hemostatic need. There are two groups of inhibitors operational in the coagulation pathways:

1 serine protease inhibitors
2 inhibitors of coagulation cofactors fVa and fVIIIa.

The critical role of these inhibitors is underscored by the observation that haplo-insufficiency with activity between 50% and 70% of normal levels is associated with an increased risk of thrombosis. Homozygous deficiencies either cause embryonic mortality, or cause devastating thrombosis in early life.

Tissue factor pathway inhibitor (TFPI)

This is a Kunitz-type protease inhibitor that inactivates fXa and fVIIa. Almost 85% of TFPI is associated with endothelial cells, in part by binding to glycosaminoglycans. TFPI in the circulation is bound to lipoproteins and has greatly reduced activity. Hence, quantification of TFPI in plasma is of doubtful value.

Serine protease inhibitors (serpins)

Antithrombin and heparin cofactor II (HCII) are two serpins active in clotting. Antithrombin forms a 1:1 complex with thrombin and fXa, and to a lesser extent with fIXa and fXIa.

- Unfractionated heparin interacts with antithrombin as well as thrombin, and improves the capacity to inhibit thrombin and fXa 2000-fold.
- Heparin inactivates thrombin by acting as a template that brings antithrombin together. Heparin also induces a confrontational change in antithrombin making it more accessible to fXa.
- Low-molecular-weight heparins can only potentiate the inhibition of fXa, as they are not of adequate length to interact with both antithrombin and thrombin.
- Homozygous antithrombin deficiency in mice causes embryonic death from thrombosis, and antithrombin deficiency in humans is an important risk factor for familial thrombophilia.

HCII inhibits only thrombin and has no effect on fXa. Heparin also increases the ability of HCII to inhibit thrombin; however, this effect is less prominent when compared with the activity of antithrombin in the presence of heparin.

Protein C pathway and inhibition of fVa and fVIIIa

Protein C (PC) is converted to activated protein C (APC) by thrombin-mediated proteolysis. This process is considerably facilitated when thrombin is in complex with thrombomodulin, an endothelial protein.

- APC inhibits fVa and fVIIIa bound to the procoagulant phospholipid surface of platelets, and this inhibition is facilitated by the interaction of APC with cofactor protein S (PS).
- As fVa and fVIIIa are essential cofactors for the procoagulant 'thrombinase' and 'tenase' complexes, respectively, their inactivation is a potent inhibitor of the coagulation pathway. The important role played by this pathway is demonstrated by the factor V Leiden mutation (Arg506Gln). This mutation alters the protease cleavage site of fVa, rendering it less susceptible to inactivation by APC. Thus in the presence of factor V Leiden, there is reduced inhibition of the 'thrombinase' complex and this is associated with a threefold increased risk of venous thrombosis for the heterozygous state.
- Reduced levels of protein C (and to a lesser extent protein S) are important in the etiology of familial thrombophilia. PC and PS are both vitamin K-dependent proteins that are produced in the liver. Protein C is subject to the effect of warfarin more rapidly than factors II, VII, IX and X. Hence, patients commencing warfarin are simultaneously treated with heparin to prevent a relative prothrombotic state.

VENOUS THROMBOSIS

Predisposition to venous thrombosis

Thrombosis follows the perturbation of one or more arms of Virchow's triad:

1 reduced or turbulent blood flow
2 changes to blood that are prothrombotic and/or inhibit fibrinolysis
3 vascular wall injury.

Up to 50% of all episodes of venous thromboembolism (VTE) may be 'provoked' (hospitalization, trauma, surgery), while the remaining are spontaneous, possibly in part due to thrombophilia. The current panel of thrombophilia tests fails to identify the underlying predisposition to venous thrombosis in almost 25% of cases.

Prothombotic risk factors are listed in Box 13-1.

Two or more thrombophilic factors may synergize to increase the risks of thrombosis; for example the oral contraceptive pill in the presence of factor V Leiden is associated with increased risk of venous thrombosis compared with that contributed by the individual risk factors (Table 13-1). Testing for thrombophilia should not be performed in most patients. It should be considered only if there is a positive family history, in patients with thrombosis at unusual sites, recurrent idiopathic thromboses, patients <45 years

with unprovoked thrombosis, and patients with warfarin-induced skin necrosis (PC deficiency).

Diagnosis of venous thrombosis

Clinical suspicion

Lower limb deep vein thrombosis (DVT) typically presents with calf swelling and pain, and redness. Previous venous thrombosis, immobilization and thrombophilia risk factors, in particular cancer, should be assessed.

Laboratory diagnosis

Fibrinolysis of the venous thrombus releases D-dimers. However, elevated D-dimers are not specific for VTE as they can occur with recent surgery, pregnancy, infection, trauma and with increasing age. The best use for a D-dimer assay is in the algorithm to exclude VTE. A negative D-dimer assay has a >90% negative predictive value in patients with a low clinical pre-test probability using validated prediction rules such as the Wells criteria for DVT.

Diagnostic imaging of DVT

- Compression ultrasound is the most commonly used modality to diagnose DVT, with a sensitivity and specificity of over 95% for the diagnosis of symptomatic proximal (popliteal vein and above) DVT.
- Compression ultrasound has 70% sensitivity in the diagnosis of calf vein DVT with a positive predictive value of 80%.

Box 13-1

Prothrombotic risk factors

Hematological conditions and genetic factors
- Factor V Leiden mutation
- Prothrombin gene mutation
- Deficiencies of endogenous anticoagulants—antithrombin, protein C and protein S
- Dysfibrinogenemia
- Increased levels of coagulation factors VIII, IX, XI
- Hyperhomocysteinemia
- Myeloproliferative disorders
- Antiphospholipid syndrome
- Paroxysmal nocturnal hemoglobinuria

Patient factors
- Increasing age
- Obesity
- Smoking
- Hormonal supplementation (oral contraceptive pills, hormone replacement therapy)
- Varicose veins
- Pregnancy/puerperium
- Long-distance air travel (>4–5 hours)

Medical factors
- Congestive cardiac failure
- Myocardial infarction
- Stroke
- Active cancer
- Inflammatory bowel disease
- Acute respiratory disease
- Vasculitis, e.g. granulomatosis with polyangiitis

Surgical factors
- Major lower limb surgery, including joint replacement
- Abdominal or pelvic surgery, particularly for cancer
- Trauma and immobilization
- Lower limb casts/splints after surgery or injury

Adapted from Colledge NR, Walker BR and Ralston SH (eds). Davidson's Principles and practice of medicine, 21st ed. Churchill Livingstone, 2010.

Table 13-1 Increased predisposition to venous thrombosis with coexisting risk factors

THROMBOTIC FACTOR	RELATIVE RISK (%)
OCP use	2–4
Hyperhomocysteinemia	2.5
FVL heterozygous	3–10
FVL heterozygous + HRT	15
FVL heterozygous + OCP use	30–40
FVL heterozygous + pregnancy	35
FVL homozygous	79
FVL homozygous + OCP use	100
Prothrombin gene mutation	1–5
Prothrombin gene mutation + FVL	6–10
Prothrombin gene mutation + OCP use	16
Protein C, S, ATIII deficiencies + OCP use	10

ATIII, antithrombin III; FVL, factor V Leiden; HRT, hormone replacement therapy; OCP, oral contraceptive pill.

Treatment of venous thromboembolism (VTE)

- Direct oral anticoagulants (DOACs) and warfarin are equally effective for the treatment of VTE. However, these agents (rivaroxaban, apixaban, and dabigatran) have not been validated for use in patients with cancer-associated thrombosis, prothrombotic disorders and prosthetic valves, and are contraindicated in pregnancy and severe renal or hepatic failure. Patients with active cancer are better treated with LMWH.
- Low-molecular-weight heparin (LMWH) is usually administered as a daily dose (e.g. enoxaparin 1.5 mg/kg daily or 1 mg/kg twice a day subcutaneously). LMWH dosing should be reduced in patients with severe renal impairment.
- Warfarin is commenced concomitantly with LMWH.
- At least 5 days of initial heparin therapy is recommended, and heparin should be continued until the international normalized ratio (INR) has been in the target range for 2 days.
- DOACs can be used as sole agents without the need for initial heparin therapy. These new anticoagulants do not need regular monitoring with INR testing.
- Generally, 3-6 months of anticoagulation with warfarin (target INR 2.0–3.0) is recommended for proximal DVT.
- Extended therapeutic anticoagulation is reserved for patients presenting with multiple spontaneous thrombotic events (2 or more unprovoked), the presence of strong thrombophilia, thrombosis at unusual sites (see below) or when thrombosis has occurred in the presence of ongoing cancer.
- Extended low intensity anticoagulation (rivaroxaban 10 mg daily or apixaban 2.5 mg twice daily) beyond 3-6 months should be considered for first unprovoked or non-surgically provoked VT.
- Thrombolytic therapy is reserved for the very rare presentations with impending venous gangrene.

CLINICAL PEARL

LMWH dosing should be reduced in patients with severe renal impairment.

Inferior vena cava filters

Inferior vena cava filters will reduce the incidence of pulmonary embolism in the first 2 weeks of DVT. Their use is reserved for clinical situations where anticoagulant therapy is contraindicated due to bleeding risk or the need for frequent surgery (e.g. multi-trauma).

- Most of the filters in use now can be successfully removed, usually within 2–3 weeks of placement, when the contraindication to anticoagulation is resolved.
- The purpose of the filter is to make suspension of anticoagulation safer.
- Anticoagulation is commenced as soon as it is safe to do so, especially if filters are to remain *in situ* for the longer term.

Recurrence of DVT after the first episode

- The overall risk of recurrence of DVT after a spontaneous episode is 5–10% per year, with a lifetime risk of up to 30%.
- Persistent thrombosis after 6 months of therapeutic anticoagulation in combination with a raised D-dimer 30 days after cessation of warfarin therapy may confer an increased risk of recurrence.

Post-thrombotic syndrome (PTS)

- Thrombus that is not promptly resolved by the action of the fibrinolytic system and scavenger cells adheres to the vessel wall, and will eventually destroy venous valves during the repair process.
- This can lead to gravity-assisted stasis in the lower limbs, extravasation of tissue fluid, chronic edema, skin discoloration, atrophy and venous ulceration.
- Symptoms of PTS may occur in up to 30% of patients with proximal DVT. The best prevention is by:
  » strictly maintaining the INR in the therapeutic range
  » prolonged use of well-fitting, graduated compression stockings.

ANTIPHOSPHOLIPID SYNDROME (APS)

Antiphospholipid syndrome (APS) is an autoimmune disease characterized by the presence of antibodies that react with proteins that bind negatively charged phospholipids, and are collectively called antiphospholipid antibodies.

A large number of protein and phospholipid targets have been identified *in vitro* and some of them have been demonstrated to be relevant *in vivo* in mouse models.

Currently the most accepted explanation is that pathogenic antiphospholipid antibodies:

- recognize beta$_2$-glycoprotein-1 (B2-GPI), a naturally occurring five-domain protein with weak anticoagulant function that exists in a circular conformation
- bind to phospholipids on the cell surface, changing the conformation of B2-GPI to an 'open' structure that exposes new epitopes that react with antiphospholipid antibodies.

Antibody-stabilized B2-GPI subsequently interacts with a number of cell-surface proteins, and triggers signaling pathways on placental trophoblasts, endothelial cells and monocytes to cause generation of a pro-coagulant and pro-inflammatory environment.

Second messenger systems altered by the B2-GPI-antibody complexes include:

- activation of the complement cascade
- inhibition of the normal protective function of annexin 5
- activation of Toll-like receptors
- inhibition of the protein C and fibrinolytic pathways.

Antiphospholipid antibodies are conventionally detected either in:

- a clotting assay containing phospholipid (lupus anticoagulant, LA)

- or solid-phase enzyme-linked immunosorbent assay (ELISA) of immobilized anti-cardiolipin and B2-GPI.

LA is an *in vitro* phenomenon, as it competes with coagulation factors for binding to the phospholipid reagent and thereby prolongs the clotting time.

Correlation of clinical disease activity with antibody titres suggests that in acitve disease the following features are seen

- antiphospholipid antibodies with LA activity
- anti-B2-GPI antibodies of immunoglobulin G (IgG) isotype present in medium or high-titer
- low-titer anti-cardiolipin antibodies without LA activity and without B2-GPI positivity.

Coagulation tests with limited availability of phospholipid increase the sensitivity of LA detection. LA is confirmed by the demonstration of phospholipid-dependent shortening of the clotting time with addition of excess phospholipid.

Clinically, APS is associated with venous and/or arterial thrombosis and the occurrence of miscarriages and pregnancy complications. Thrombotic events are characteristically recurrent in the same vascular bed.

Treatment

- Anticoagulation with warfarin (INR target 2.0–3.0) is standard therapy. The duration of therapy is usually indefinite, or at least until antiphospholipid antibodies are undetectable.
  - » A higher target INR (2.5–3.5) may be necessary for recurrent events.
- Arterial thromboses are treated with warfarin and aspirin or clopidogrel.
- Pregnancy related morbidity can be managed with a combination of LMWH and low-dose aspirin.

Catastrophic APS, a more intense disease with multi-organ involvement and small vessel thrombosis, requires intensive anticoagulation together with plasmapharesis and immunosuppression e.g. corticosteroids, cyclophosphamide, rituximab or IVIg.

THROMBOSIS AT UNUSUAL SITES

Cerebral vein thrombosis (CVT)

Cerebral vein thrombosis is a rare condition that affects large central venous sinuses and may extend into the cortical veins.

- Symptoms and signs may range from those attributable to intracranial hypertension (headache, photophobia) to those due to cortical infarction (hemiparesis, aphasia).
- Magnetic resonance imaging (MRI) and computed tomography (CT) venography have replaced cerebral angiography as the diagnostic tests of choice, with MRI documented to have a sensitivity and specificity between 75% and 100%.
- CVT is more frequently seen in young women, due to the prothrombotic association of the oral contraceptive pill and pregnancy.

- Genetic or acquired thrombophilia, head trauma, and infections of surrounding sites (e.g. ear infections, meningitis) play a contributory role.

If there is no/small hemorrhagic infarction, LMWH followed by oral anticoagulation therapy of the same duration as for lower limb DVT (3 months if provoked, 6 months if unprovoked and consideration of extended low-intensity anticoagulation, or lifelong in the presence of recurrence or markers of severe thrombophilia). If there is a large hemorrhagic infarction, anticoagulation is delayed until a stabilization or reduction of hemorrhage is documented.

Portal vein thrombosis (PVT)

Portal vein thrombosis results from a combination of local and systemic prothrombotic factors.

- The most common local precipitant is hepatic cirrhosis. Other risk factors are hepatic cancer, abdominal inflammatory conditions (diverticulitis, appendicitis, pancreatitis), and injury to the abdominal veins (splenectomy, cholecystectomy).
- Myeloproliferative disorders are now considered to be the major etiology for 'idiopathic' PVT, manifestations of which can pre-date clinical hematological disease.
- Mutations in the Janus kinase 2 (JAK2) gene are the hallmark of almost all patients with polycythemia vera and in approximately 50% of patients with essential thrombocythemia and myelofibrosis. The JAK2 mutation may be seen in ~30% of patients with PVT without overt evidence of myeloproliferative disease.

Patients with acute PVT present with abdominal pain, while chronic disease may be accompanied by signs and symptoms of portal hypertension. Diagnosis is generally made with Doppler ultrasonography.

- Anticoagulation is most effective in acute PVT without concomitant cirrhosis, and long-term anticoagulation should be considered in patients with a hypercoagulable state including myeloproliferative disease.

CLINICAL PEARL

When portal vein thrombosis (PVT) is identified in cirrhosis, treat the underlying liver disease as indicated *without* anticoagulation for the PVT.

CANCER AND THROMBOSIS

Patients with active cancers are predisposed to venous thrombosis as a consequence of:

- the procoagulant milieu generated by cancer cells (examples are the expression of TF and the liberation of mucins that activate leukocytes and platelets)
- the effects of chemotherapy (examples include thalidomide, lenalidomide and bevacizumab)
- stasis created by bed rest and surgery
- endothelial irritation by the placement of central lines.

Primary thromboprophylaxis in ambulatory patients is generally not recommended; exceptions include selected malignancies such as pancreatic adenocarcinoma.

Patients with myeloma will benefit from aspirin when treated with thalidomide or lenalidomide alone, and heparin is recommended in combination with high-dose steroids or chemotherapy.

Primary thromboprophylaxis for central lines is not routinely recommended.

CLINICAL PEARL

Low-molecular-weight heparins have higher efficacy than warfarin in the treatment of patients with venous thromboembolism in the context of cancer.

BLEEDING DISORDERS

Suspicion of the presence of a bleeding disorder is raised by a clinical presentation with unusual bruising or bleeding, either spontaneously or after minimal trauma or post-operatively. Prolongation of prothrombin time (PT) and activated partial thromboplastin time (APTT) on routine 'coagulation screen' tests also prompts investigation.

The history and clinical presentation (Table 13-2) can easily separate bleeding disorders from a failure in hemostasis:

- primary (platelet function defect)
- secondary (coagulation defect).

While von Willebrand disease and hemophilia A or B (Figure 13-2) are the most common congenital bleeding disorders, acquired etiologies are common causes of excessive bleeding in hospitalized patients (Box 13-2) and need to be considered while planning diagnostic tests.

Von Willebrand disease (vWD)

Von Willebrand factor is:

- encoded by a gene on chromosome 12
- produced as a single-chain pro-vWF monomer; two monomers dimerize via the C-terminal domain in the endoplasmic reticulum and the dimer is exported to the Golgi apparatus. Dimers undergo N-terminal association via formation of disulfide bonds to form multimers ranging from 1000 to 20,000 kDa. vWF is heavily

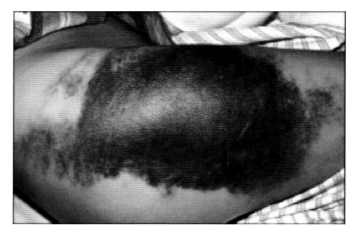

Figure 13-2 Ecchymoses and hemarthrosis in a male with hemophilia

From Little JW et al. Dental management of the medically compromised patient, 7th ed. St Louis: Mosby Elsevier, 2008.

Box 13-2

Causes of excessive bleeding

Congenital

- Hemophilia A and B (X-linked)
- Von Willebrand disease (autosomal)
- Individual or combined deficiencies of clotting factors (other than fVIII and fIX) (autosomal) and of fibrinogen (autosomal)

Acquired

- Liver disease (impaired synthesis, platelet sequestration in hypersplenism)
- Disseminated intravascular coagulation
- Acquired hemophilia and coagulation factor inhibitors

Drug-induced

- Antiplatelet therapy (e.g. aspirin, dipyridamole, clopidogrel, etc.)
- Warfarin, heparins, rivaroxaban, dabigatran, apixaban

Table 13-2 Primary and secondary bleeding disorders

	PLATELET DISORDERS—PRIMARY	COAGULATION DISORDERS—SECONDARY
Petechiae	Characteristic	Rare
Superficial ecchymoses	Small, multiple	Large, solitary
Hematoma	Rare	Characteristic
Hemarthrosis	Rare	Characteristic
Late bleed	Rare	Common
Gender	More prevalent in females	Mainly in males
Family history	Variable	Common

glycosylated, and N-linked glycans undergo further processing with the addition of an ABO blood group antigen as determined by the ABO genotype

- primarily formed in endothelial cells
- also synthesized to a much smaller extent in megakaryocytes
- released constitutively as a steady state concentration, or rapidly released after stimulation by a number of agonists including thrombin, epinephrine (adrenaline) and vasopressin.

vWF serves two principal functions:

- **Primary hemostasis:** vWF binds to collagen at the site of vascular injury and to the platelet integrin receptors GPIb and αIIbβ3, which also function as the fibrinogen receptor. vWF therefore recruits platelets to the sites of vascular injury; this function is maximal with high-molecular-weight multimers. The role of vWF is most prominent in small arterioles and in areas of vascular plaque, where shear stress uncoils vWF multimers that adhere to and activate platelets.
- **Secondary hemostasis:** vWF interacts with fVIII in the circulation and protects fVIII from proteolysis. This interaction also serves to enrich fVIII at the site of a developing thrombus.

Classification

Von Willebrand disease is described in terms of a quantitative deficiency or qualitative defects, with either reduction in high-molecular-weight multimers or abnormalities in the capacity of vWF to interact with platelets or to bind fVIII (Table 13-3).

Clinical features

Clinical presentation is typically with easy bruising, epistaxis, menorrhagia, or excessive bleeding after trauma,

dental extraction or surgery. The severity of symptoms depends on the extent of vWF deficiency. Type 3 vWD, with complete absence of vWF and fVIII activity of 1–2%, may present with clinical features resembling hemophilia.

Diagnosis

Common investigations are full blood examination (FBE) (for thrombocytopenia), vWF quantification (ELISA), capacity to agglutinate platelets (ristocetin cofactor activity) and fVIII activity. Sub-classification of type 2 vWD requires an estimation of multimers (either by gel analysis or by the ability to bind collagen) and demonstration of an increased capacity to bind platelets (type 2B) by ristocetin-induced platelet agglutination.

Treatment

- Tranexamic acid is useful for mucosal bleeding and menorrhagia.
- Desmopressin (1-desamino-8-D-arginine vasopressin, DDAVP) is useful in type 1 disease through stimulating release of vWF and fVIII from endothelial stores. Frequent administration can be less effective until vWF is re-synthesized.
- DDAVP is ineffective in type 3 vWD and should not be given in type 2B because it induces platelet aggregation.
- Coagulation factor concentrates containing vWF and fVIII are necessary to treat type 3 and type 2B vWD.

CLINICAL PEARL

DDAVP is contraindicated in type 2B von Willebrand disease, as enhanced release of abnormal vWF with increased platelet binding will cause thrombocytopenia.

Table 13-3 Classification of von Willebrand disease

CLASSIFICA-TION	vWF DEFICIENCY	vWF FUNCTION	vWF MULTIMERS	vWF ASSOCIATION WITH PLATELETS	fVIII-BINDING CAPACITY
Type 1	Quantitative	Normal	Normal	Normal	Normal*
Type 2A	Qualitative	Abnormal	Reduced	Reduced	Normal*
Type 2B	Qualitative	Abnormal	Reduced	Increased	Normal*
Type 2M	Qualitative	Abnormal	Normal	Decreased	Normal*
Type 2N	Qualitative	Abnormal	Normal	Normal	Markedly reduced
Type 3	Quantitative	vWF undetectable	vWF undetectable	vWF undetectable	vWF undetectable

* Common finding.

vWF, von Willebrand factor.

Adapted from: Sadler JE, Budde U, Eikenboom CJ et al. The Working Party on von Willebrand Disease Classification. Update on the pathophysiology and classification of von Willebrand disease: a report of the Subcommittee on von Willebrand Factor. J Thromb Haemost 2006;4:2103–14; and Federici AB. Diagnosis and classification of von Willebrand disease. Hematol Meeting Rep 2007;1:6–19.

Hemophilia A

In the propagation phase of the clotting cascade, fVIII and fIX are essential for forming the 'tenase' leading to the generation of fXa, and consequently the amplification of the clotting cascade.

- Genes for both fVIII and fIX are located on the long arm of the X chromosome.
- Deficiencies in fVIII and fIX cause hemophilia A and hemophilia B, respectively.

fVIII is synthesized primarily in the liver, and to a minor extent in vascular endothelial cells. After release from the liver, most of the fVIII circulates bound to vWF. fVIII is activated and released from vWF by thrombin-mediated cleavage. The procoagulant actions of fVIIIa are controlled by activated protein C (APC), which inactivates fVIII by proteolysis.

Hemophilia-causing alterations of the fVIII gene comprise mutations (missense, nonsense, frame-shift, splicing) in virtually all cases. One-third of cases are due to inversion of intron 22, which results in the production of 2 shortened mRNA transcripts (exons 1-22 and exons 23-26) and severe deficiency in the production of contiguous fVIII protein. Inversion of intron 22 contributes to almost 50% of the cases of severe hemophilia.

Clinical features

- Almost all patients are male, with the disease rarely occurring in females (see below).
- The severity of symptoms depends on the level of residual fVIII (Table 13-4), with spontaneous bleeding predominantly occurring only when fVIII activity is <1 U/dL.
- Spontaneous mucosal bleeding is rare in this disease.
- Spontaneous central nervous system (CNS) bleeding is uncommon. However, minor head trauma can have devastating consequences.
- Bleeding is common in load-bearing joints and in load-bearing muscle groups (in the thigh, calf, iliopsoas and posterior abdominal wall). Hemarthrosis causes an inflammatory response in the synovium, leading to synovial proliferation, friability and further cycles of bleeding and proliferation. Blood components are also toxic to the joint cartilage and chondrocytes, leading to degenerative arthropathy.

- The consequences of recurrent hemarthrosis and muscle bleeds are joint ankylosis, muscle contractures and wasting.

There is no family history in almost one-third of cases because of occurrence of new mutations. The disease may manifest after interventions such as circumcision or when an infant starts to walk and is prone to minor injuries.

Investigation

Mild hemophilia manifesting as a bleeding disorder in later life or acquired hemophilia (see below) may be suspected during work-up of a prolonged APTT.

- Diagnosis in all cases is confirmed by a quantitative assessment of fVIII activity.
- In a woman known to be at risk of being a carrier, chorionic venous sampling or cord blood sampling will help to verify fetal genotype and fVIII level with a view to genetic counseling.
- During the course of treatment with fVIII, up to 25% of patients develop inhibitors necessitating quantification of inhibitor activity, as this reduces the efficacy of supplemental fVIII.

Treatment

Recombinant FVIII (rFVIII) concentrates are the treatment of choice for hemophilia A. Donor-derived products should only be used for urgent treatment in cases where recombinant products are not available.

- Donor-derived fVIII is screened for hepatitis B, hepatitis C and HIV and undergoes viral elimination processing.
- Recombinant fVIII was made possible by cloning of the fVIII gene, and recombinant proteins are produced either as full-length molecules or with domain deletions. Recombinant fVIII is now produced to reduce inhibitor development and to prolong in vivo half-life of fVIII.

Factor VIII replacement can be either on-demand, in the situation of bleeding, or as prophylaxis in young boys to reduce the incidence of hemarthrosis and muscle bleeds. Therapeutic fVIII in response to a bleed is administered 2–3 times daily to maintain fVIII levels at 30–100%, dependent on the severity and site of bleeding (hemarthrosis 30–50%; surgery and CNS bleed 50–100%).

Table 13-4 Severity of hemophilia symptoms

fVIII OR fIX LEVEL (U/dL)	CLINICAL PICTURE	INCIDENCE IN HEMOPHILIA A	INCIDENCE IN HEMOPHILIA B
<1	Severe spontaneous bleeding	70%	50%
1–5	Moderate bleeding with minimal trauma or surgery	15%	30%
5–30	Mild bleeding with trauma or surgery	15%	20%

Development of inhibitors and management

Some 25–30% of patients with severe hemophilia will develop inhibitors to fVIII due to an immune response to donor fVIII.

- Inhibitors may be transient and with low-level inhibitory activity; however, high-activity inhibitors occur in 10–15% of cases.
- Most inhibitors develop during childhood with initial exposure to fVIII.

> **CLINICAL PEARL**
>
> The propensity for inhibitor development correlates with the type of mutation in the fVIII gene. Large deletions are particularly susceptible to inhibitor development, and approximately 25% of patients with intron 22 inversion develop inhibitors.

- Porcine fVIII is biologically functional in humans, and its activity is neutralized to a lesser extent by inhibitors. Recombinant porcine fVIII is currently undergoing clinical development.

The most effective therapy to combat bleeding in patients with inhibitors is to administer coagulation activity that will bypass the inhibitor effect.

- The most common method is administration of recombinant activated fVII (fVIIa).
- An alternative is the plasma-derived prothrombin complex concentrate containing activated coagulation factors.
- Immune-tolerance induction regimens are in use and are most useful in younger patients.

Management of high-activity inhibitors may also require immunosuppressive therapy and plasmapharesis.

Hemophilia in females

- As females possess two X chromosomes which undergo random inactivation, carriers of hemophilia display approximately 50% activity.
- Skewed inactivation of the normal X chromosome can produce a mild hemophilia phenotype.
- A new mutation in the sperm of the father will generate a female carrier without prior family history.

> **CLINICAL PEARL**
>
> Von Willebrand disease is the most common differential diagnosis in females with low fVIII activity.

Hemophilia B

Mutations in the fIX gene, also located on the long arm of the X chromosome, cause hemophilia B. The clinical features correlate with residual fIX activity.

Recombinant fIX is available for the treatment of hemophilia B. Plasma-derived products should only be used in these patient groups for urgent treatment in cases where recombinant products are not available. As fIX has a longer half-life, once-daily administration will generally suffice during episodes of bleeding, and twice-weekly prophylaxis is adequate.

Development of inhibitors occurs uncommonly (~3%) in patients with severe hemophilia B, and situations of bleeding are managed similarly to hemophilia A.

Bleeding disorders due to deficiencies of other coagulation factors

Inherited deficiencies of the coagulation factors II, V, VII, X, XI and XIII are uncommon and are grouped as 'rare bleeding disorders' (RBDs). Studies in mice have confirmed the pivotal role played by these proteins in the maintenance of normal hemostasis.

- Homozygous deficiency of fII, fV, fVII and fX is incompatible with life. Similarly, complete deficiency of enzymes participating in the vitamin K pathway (gamma-glutamyl carboxylase and vitamin K epoxide reductase complex subunit-1) leads to life-threatening bleeding. Diagnosis of individual deficiencies relies on quantification of coagulation factor activities and family studies.
- Combined deficiencies of fV and fVIII occur at an incidence of 1 in 1 million and are due to abnormalities in the LMAN1 and MCFD2 genes, which encode proteins that regulate the folding and intracellular transport of fV and fVIII.
- fXI deficiency differs from hemophilia A and B, as bleeding frequency does not correlate with factor levels. Both mild and severe deficiencies exhibit similar incidences of bleeding. Spontaneous bleeding is rare; bleeding occurs preferentially in sites with high fibrinolytic activity such as the oral cavity and urogenital tract.
- Deficiency of fXII is commonly detected during a work-up for prolongation of APTT, and does not lead to a bleeding phenotype.
- fXIII is critical for cross-linking of fibrin monomers to form a stable clot; the enzyme activity is delivered by a complex of two catalytic and two carrier subunits. Patients with fXIII deficiency have a severe bleeding tendency and also demonstrate slow healing. fXIII has a very long *in vivo* half-life (11–14 days) and management is by administration of fXIII (cryoprecipitate, concentrates or recombinant protein) at 3- to 4-weekly intervals.

PLATELET DISORDERS

Idiopathic thrombocytopenic purpura (ITP)

Pathophysiology

- An autoimmune disorder with platelet destruction mediated by autoantibodies and also cell-mediated immunity.
- Enhanced clearance of antibody-bound platelets is commonly recognized as the basis of the disease.

- There is also evidence of suppression of thrombopoiesis, leading to the use of thrombopoiesis-stimulating drugs as an adjunct to immunosuppressive therapies.
- May be a truly 'idiopathic' primary disorder, a feature of other autoimmune diseases (e.g. SLE), or related to chronic infections such as HIV, hepatitis C, and possibly *Helicobacter pylori*.
- Adult ITP is more frequent in young females, with no gender preponderance in older adults.

Diagnosis

Diagnosis requires exclusion of recognizable causes such as:

- medication effects
- infections
- autoimmune diseases
- disseminated coagulopathy
- portal hypertension.

Other blood parameters, including hemoglobin, white cell count and blood film, should remain normal. Characterization of anti-platelet antibodies is not essential. Bone marrow biopsies are usually restricted to patients over 60 years, or if there is suspicion of myelodysplasia or bone-marrow–infiltrative disorders, and prior to splenectomy.

Treatment

The need for treatment is dictated by platelet count and comorbidities.

- Generally, no intervention is necessary for a platelet count >30 × 10^9/L. Coexisting conditions that may need higher platelet counts to ensure hemostasis, such as menorrhagia, concomitant anti-platelet therapy, history of peptic ulcer, or impending major surgery, may trigger intervention at a higher count.
- First-line therapy is usually with corticosteroid regimens such as prednisolone 1 mg/kg/day for 2–4 weeks followed by tapering, or dexamethasone 40 mg/day for 4 days repeated 2- to 4-weekly for 2–4 cycles.
- Emergency therapy for very severe thrombocytopenia with evidence of bleeding is intravenous immunoglobulin (IVIG) 1 g/kg/day for 1–2 days.
- Platelet transfusions are ineffective and are not used unless there are extenuating circumstances.
- Second-line therapies are indicated to minimize corticosteroid exposure and to improve response. These include immunosuppressive drugs such as azathioprine, cyclosporine (ciclosporin) and rituximab, and danazol.
- Splenectomy is considered to be the standard of care for patients not responding to prednisolone or other immunosuppressive therapies or in the presence of unacceptable side-effects. Almost two-thirds of patients achieve and maintain durable responses.
- Two thrombopoietin receptor agonists (TRAs), romiplostin and eltrombopag, are now available for patients not responding to corticosteroids and are generally reserved for use after splenectomy, unless surgery is contraindicated. TRAs bind the thrombopoietin receptor and initiate signaling in hemopoietic stem cells and

progenitors, stimulating platelet production. TRAs must be taken continuously to prevent relapse.

Thrombotic thrombocytopenic purpura and hemolytic uremic syndrome

Thrombotic thrombocytopenic purpura (TTP) and hemolytic uremic syndrome (HUS) share the common pathophysiological features of:

- consumption thrombocytopenia
- microvascular thrombosis
- microangiopathic hemolytic anemia.

Clear separation between the two diagnoses can sometimes be difficult.

- Identification of the presence of ultra-large vWF multimers with an enhanced ability to bind with platelet integrin GPIb and initiate aggregation and consequent thrombosis in the microcirculation provides an explanation for the findings of multi-organ ischemia and thrombocytopenia in the absence of overt coagulopathy.
- An explanation for the persistence of the high-molecular-weight multimers in TTP is provided by the identification of a deficiency of ADAMTS-13, a vWF-cleaving protease that normally functions to regulate the abundance of vWF multimers to physiological need.
- While TTP is characterized by an inherited or acquired deficiency of ADAMTS-13, the enzyme levels are mostly normal in HUS; hence, while the spectrum of pathological alterations shows significant overlap, differences remain between the two diseases.

Thrombotic thrombocytopenic purpura (TTP)

Thrombotic thrombocytopenic purpura occurs as an inherited form due to mutations in the ADAMTS-13 gene (autosomal recessive), or as an acquired form with deficiency of ADAMTS-13 due to autoantibodies or to release of large quantities of ultra-large vWF multimers due to endothelial activation.

- **Congenital TTP** is a rare disease due to homozygous or double heterozygous mutations of the ADAMTS-13 gene located on chromosome 9. Most mutations are missense and lead to decreased production or reduced function of the protease.
  - » There is a considerable heterogeneity in the presentation, varying from occasional episodes to frequent manifestations. Also, the same genetic defect can lead to a very different spectrum of the disease within families.
- **Autoimmune TTP** is more common, and is due to the presence of antibodies that either impair activity of the ADAMTS-13 protease or enhance its clearance. The antibodies are directed to epitopes that are important for enzyme activity as well as binding to vWF.
- Drug-induced TTP can be caused by ticlopidine, quinine, cyclosporine, gemcitabine and bevacizumab.

TTP is a clinical diagnosis. Patients may be febrile and demonstrate the presence of severe thrombocytopenia, red cell fragmentation (schistocytes), high lactate dehydrogenase (LDH) levels and end-organ ischemia typically associated with renal impairment and a myriad of neurological symptoms (stroke, seizures, other focal deficits and fluctuating consciousness).

CLINICAL PEARLS

- Thrombotic thrombocytopenic purpura classically presents with a pentad of signs: remember with FAT RN—fever, anemia, thrombocytopenia, renal failure and neurological signs.
- Hemolytic uremic syndrome is clinically similar, but renal rather than neurological features predominate.

Laboratory diagnosis

The diagnosis of TTP is strongly suggested with

- schistocytes and
- thrombocytopenia

in the absence of coagulopathy.

Confirmation of the diagnosis is dependent on the demonstration of:

- reduction in ADAMTS-13 protease activity in the plasma. A level of <10% supports the diagnosis, and if >50%, an alternate diagnosis should be considered.
- the presence of autoantibodies to ADAMTS-13, either by ELISA or immunoblotting.

Box 13-3 gives the differential diagnosis of TTP.

Box 13-3

Differential diagnosis of thrombotic thrombocytopenic purpura and thrombotic microangiopathies

- Disseminated intravascular coagulation
- Catastrophic antiphospholipid syndrome
- Heparin-induced thrombocytopenia
- Disseminated malignancy
- HELLP syndrome (**H**emolysis, **E**levated **L**iver enzymes and **L**ow **P**latelets) and preeclampsia

---

Management

The cornerstone of treatment is plasma exchange with cryoprecipitate-depleted plasma or fresh frozen plasma (FFP). Daily exchanges should continue until features related to organ involvement have resolved, the platelet count has stably recovered, and hemolysis has ceased.

In the absence of facilities to deliver plasma exchange, prompt infusion of FFP is recommended. Additional therapies found to be useful include corticosteroids and immunoglobulin. Resistant disease may benefit from chemotherapy (cyclophosphamide, vincristine) and rituximab (anti-CD20).

CLINICAL PEARL

Treatment of thrombotic thrombocytopenic purpura should not be delayed until the availability of ADAMTS-13 assays.

Hemolytic uremic syndrome (HUS)

The most common form of HUS is associated with gastrointestinal (GI) infection with toxin-producing bacteria (*Escherichia coli* 0157:H7 and *Shigella dysenteriae*).

- Toxin produced by the bacteria is absorbed into the circulation and causes activation and desquamation of glomerular capillary endothelial cells, with consequent renal impairment.
- There is systemic endothelial activation, with fibrin deposition and evidence of compensated coagulopathy.
- The presence of ultra-large vWF multimers is less common as compared to TTP, and ADAMTS-13 levels are normal or only mildly reduced.

Most cases of diarrhea-associated HUS remit without recurrence. Temporary renal support with dialysis is often necessary, although permanent renal failure can occur in up to one-third of cases.

CLINICAL PEARL

In the setting of *Escherichia coli* O157:H7, do *not* prescribe antibiotics as this may precipitate HUS.

Atypical HUS (aHUS) occurs as a familial form with mutations of complement proteins (C3) and complement regulatory proteins (factor H, factor I, MCP [membrane cofactor protein] and factor B), with consequent unrestricted complement activation and endothelial toxicity. In addition, some patients with aHUS have mutations in molecules not directly linked to the complement system, including diacylglycerol kinase, plasminogen, factor XIII, and thrombomodulin. Eculizumab, a monoclonal antibody that inhibits the production of the terminal complement components and the membrane attack complex by binding to complement C5, is used to treat aHUS. Eculizumab is effective in treating acute hemolysis, thrombocytopenia, and stabilizing renal function. Severe aHUS can be maintained in remission using a long-term maintenance dose every 2 weeks.

DISSEMINATED INTRAVASCULAR COAGULATION (DIC)

Coagulation is a tightly regulated homeostatic system which limits physiological clotting to the site of need and for the duration of injury; any failure of the regulatory process will result in clot formation that is in vast excess of need ('disseminated') and causes consumption of platelets and coagulation proteins.

The main 'driver' of clotting is the generation of thrombin, most commonly by the TF-mediated extrinsic pathway.

Thrombin activates platelets and the intrinsic pathway to amplify clotting, and simultaneously initiates fibrinolysis by plasminogen conversion to plasmin and generates activated protein C that functions to inactivate f V and f VIII.

Various disease processes that are associated with DIC (Box 13-4) share the common feature of excessive TF exposure, leading to deregulation of thrombin activity. Other pathological processes that commonly contribute to DIC are endothelial activation (platelet aggregation, TF expression) and inflammation (cytokines and interleukins lead to accumulation of neutrophils, activation of complement cascade and coagulation).

Diagnosis

Establishing the diagnosis of DIC requires clinical suspicion and:

- PT (prolonged)
- APTT (prolonged)
- thrombin time (prolonged)
- D-dimers (raised due to formation and breakdown of disseminated clotting)
- fibrinogen quantification (reduced due to consumption)
- FBE (thrombocytopenia due to consumption, and leukocytosis secondary to sepsis or inflammation).

The International Society on Thrombosis and Haemostasis has proposed a scoring system for the diagnosis of DIC, to be used in patients with an underlying disorder known to be associated with DIC (Table 13-5).

Treatment

Treatment of DIC is complicated by the dual risks of bleeding from platelet and clotting factor deficiency, and the risk of thrombosis.

- Platelet transfusion should be reserved for patients who are actively bleeding or at high risk of bleeding and are thrombocytopenic with a platelet count $<50 \times 10^9$/L.
- FFP can be used for patients who are bleeding or at high risk of bleeding and have prolonged coagulation times.

- Evidence of thrombosis should be treated with therapeutic doses of intravenous unfractionated heparin.
- Treatment of the underlying cause of the DIC (e.g. sepsis, pregnancy complications) is essential.

Box 13-4

Diseases associated with disseminated intravascular coagulation

Sepsis
- Typically Gram-negative bacteria containing lipopolysaccharide in their cell membranes, but can be seen with any micro-organism

Pregnancy and obstetric complications
- Preeclampsia
- Placental abruption
- Amniotic fluid embolism

Malignancy
- Acute promyelocytic leukemia (characteristic feature)
- Solid tumors

Trauma
- Burns
- Fat embolism
- Severe trauma

Envenomation and immunological reactions
- ABO-incompatible red cell transfusion
- Snake bite

Miscellaneous
- Severe pancreatitis
- Giant hemangiomas

Table 13-5 Scoring system for diagnosis of disseminated intravascular coagulation (DIC)

SCORE	PLATELET COUNT (× 10⁹/L)	FDPs OR D-DIMERS	PROLONGATION OF PT (s)	FIBRINOGEN (g/L)
0	>100	No increase	<3	>1
1	<100	–	>3 and <6	<1
2	<50	Moderate increase	>6	
3		Strong increase		
A score ≥5 is compatible with DIC				
FDPs, fibrin degradation products; PT, prothrombin time. Proposed by the International Society on Thrombosis and Haemostasis (www.isth.org).				

COAGULOPATHY IN INTENSIVE CARE PATIENTS

Abnormalities in coagulation tests are commonly observed in patients in intensive care. The etiology is multifactorial, and a thorough history of anticoagulant or antiplatelet therapy is essential in the interpretation of tests. Abnormalities in the commonly used coagulation tests are described in Table 13-6.

MYELOPROLIFERATIVE DISORDERS

These myeloproliferative neoplasms (MPN) are characterized by proliferation of components of myeloid, erythroid, or megakaryocyte lineages. There is overlap amongst these clonal disorders, and multiple cell lines are usually elevated. Based on the type of MPN, patients are at risk of hepatosplenomegaly, thrombosis, and progression to myelofibrosis or acute myeloid leukemia. There are 4 MPNs defined:

- polycythemia vera
- essential thrombocythemia
- primary myelofibrosis.
- Chronic myeloid leukemia is classified as a myeloproliferative disorder; however, this condition will be discussed in the section on chronic leukemias.

Polycythemia vera (PV)

The pathogenetic hallmark of PV is the demonstration of the proliferative autonomy of erythroid precursors in agar cultures without the need for exogenous erythropoietin stimulation.

In most cases (>98%), the Val617Phe mutation of the JAK2 gene can be identified on molecular testing. JAK2 is a cytoplasmic tyrosine kinase that mediates signal transduction downstream of the erythropoietin receptor (EpoR). Binding of erythropoietin (Epo) to its receptor initiates a signaling cascade involving the recruitment of JAK2 to the EpoR and subsequent phosphorylation of downstream targets, including the transcription factor STAT3. The Val617Phe mutation renders JAK2 constitutively active, leading to erythroid hyperplasia in the absence of erythropoietin.

Erythropoietin levels are suppressed in PV by a negative feedback mechanism. Patients with PV and an absence of the Val-617Phe mutation display somatic gain-of-function mutations affecting exon 12 of JAK2 serving the same proliferative effect.

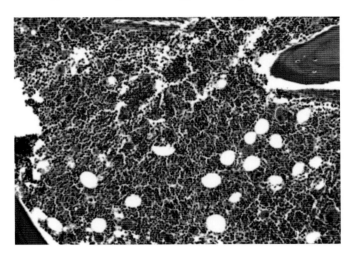

Figure 13-3 Bone marrow trephine showing increase in erythroid precursors in polycythemia vera

From Aster JC, Podznyakova O and Kutok JL (eds). Hematopathology: a volume in the High Yield Pathology Series. Philadelphia: Elsevier, 2013.

Table 13-6 Typical laboratory findings for coagulation disorders in intensive care patients

CONDITION	PLATELET COUNT	APTT	PT	FIBRINOGEN	D-DIMER	THROMBIN TIME
DIC[a]	↓	↑	↑	↓[b]	↑	↑
Liver failure	↓/N	↑	↑	↓/N	N	↑
Vitamin K deficiency	N	↑/N[c]	↑	N	N	N
Acquired hemophilia	N	↑	N	N	N	N
Heparin effect	N	↑	↑/N	N	N	↑
Abnormal platelet function	N	N	N	N	N	N

[a] Differential diagnosis is TTP (usually normal coagulation and high levels of schistocytes).

[b] Fibrinogen level may be normal in compensated DIC.

[c] In early or mild vitamin K deficiency, only PT is prolonged. In more severe deficiency, APTT is also prolonged.

APTT, activated partial thromboplastin time; DIC, disseminated intravascular coagulopathy; N, normal; PT, prothrombin time; TTP, thrombotic thrombocytopenic purpura.

Table modified from: Shander A, Walsh CE and Cromwell C. Acquired hemophilia: a rare but life-threatening potential cause of bleeding in the intensive care unit. Intensive Care Med 2011;37:1240–9.

Clinical features

- Patients may appear plethoric, with symptoms of erythromelalgia (derived from three Greek words: *erythros* red, *melos* extremities, and *algos* pain).
- Pruritus, particularly after a warm shower, is also a common feature.
- Palpable splenomegaly may be identified in approximately 30% of patients, although splenomegaly by radiological criteria is more frequent.
- Some patients may present with thrombosis as the disease-identifying illness.
- Arterial occlusive diseases (ischemic heart disease and stroke) can occur with uncontrolled hematocrit.
- Increasingly, myeloproliferative disorders are suspected on the basis of abnormalities on incidental blood tests and patients may be asymptomatic.

CLINICAL PEARLS

- Patients with polycythemia vera (PV) may present with microcytosis and low ferritin, and inadvertent iron supplementation leads to a rapid increase in hemoglobin with increased risk of thrombotic events.
- A high proportion of patients with splanchnic vein thrombosis display the JAK2 mutation without evidence of overt PV.

- It is essential that patients are commenced on aspirin as antiplatelet therapy. PV also predisposes to venous thrombosis at uncommon sites.

Diagnosis

Figure 13-4 outlines criteria for diagnosis of PV.

Treatment

- Venesection is the treatment modality in the absence of thrombocytosis, where the intention is to deplete iron stores so that the hematocrit is maintained at <0.45.
- The presence of thrombocytosis and constitutional symptoms will need cytoreductive therapy.
  » The most common drug is hydroxyurea at the dose of 0.5–2.0 g daily. Careful monitoring is required to prevent leukopenia and, rarely, thrombocytopenia. Hydroxyurea is generally well tolerated. A rare but significant complication is leg ulcers, which is a contraindication for ongoing use. While there is concern that hydroxyurea is potentially leukemogenic, the probability is very low when it is used as a single agent.
  » The leukemogenic effects are higher for busulfan, which is often used in older patients. The advantage of busulfan is that, unlike hydroxyurea, it can be given intermittently and doses can be several months apart.

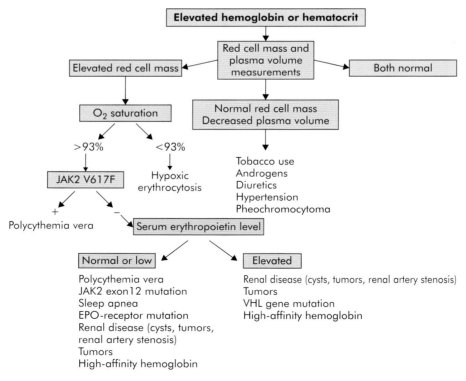

Figure 13-4 World Health Organization criteria for the diagnosis of polycythemia vera

From Spivak JL and Silver RT. The revised World Health Organization diagnostic criteria for polycythemia vera, essential thrombocytosis, and primary myelofibrosis. Blood 2008;112:231–9.

» An alternative to hydroxyurea in younger patients is interferon-alpha, usually at the dose of 3 million units three times a week. Interferon is effective in controlling the hematocrit as well as thrombocytosis. Its use is restricted by cost and the side-effects of fatigue, myalgia (resembling influenza) and depression.

» Anagrelide is an effective therapy for patients with PV who have thrombocytosis that works by inhibiting megakaryocytic differentiation. It is, however, expensive and the common side-effects are headache, fluid retention and palpitations.

Recommendations for the management of PV are given in Box 13-5.

Long-term complications

Increased reticulin in the bone marrow may be identified in about 15% of patients at the time of diagnosis; overt myelofibrosis occurs in 10–15% after a period of observation of 15 years.

The probability of leukemic transformation is determined by therapy; the risk is very small (1–3%) in patients treated only with hydroxyurea, and rises significantly if radioactive phosphorus, irradiation and other chemotherapeutic agents are used in the treatment.

Differential diagnosis of erythrocytosis

Polycythemia vera causes primary erythrocytosis, but secondary causes are more common and need to be considered (Box 13-6).

Box 13-5

BCSH recommendations for management of polycythemia vera

- Venesection to maintain the hematocrit to <0.45
- Aspirin 75 mg/day unless contraindicated
- Cytoreduction should be considered if there is:
  » poor tolerance of venesection
  » symptomatic or progressive splenomegaly
  » other evidence of disease progression, e.g. weight loss, night sweats
  » thrombocytosis

BCSH, British Committee for Standards in Haematology.

From McMullin MF et al. and the General Haematology Task Force of the British Committee for Standards in Haematology. Guidelines for the diagnosis, investigation and management of polycythaemia/erythrocytosis. Br J Haematol 2005;130:174–95. Blackwell Publishing Ltd.

Essential thrombocythemia (ET)

Essential thrombocythemia should be diagnosed only after elimination of secondary (reactive) etiology (Box 13-7, overleaf).

- ET is a clonal disorder, with up to 55% of patients demonstrating the presence of the Val617Phe mutation in the JAK2 gene.

Box 13-6

Classification of erythrocytosis

Primary erythrocytosis

Polycythemia vera

Secondary erythrocytosis

Congenital
- High-oxygen-affinity hemoglobin
- 2,3-Biphosphoglycerate mutase deficiency
- Erythropoeitin receptor-mediated
- Chuvash erythrocytosis (*VHL* mutation)

Acquired

EPO-mediated
- Hypoxia-driven
  » Central hypoxic process
    - chronic lung disease
    - right-to-left cardiopulmonary vascular shunts
    - carbon monoxide poisoning
    - smoker's erythrocytosis
    - hypoventilation syndromes including sleep apnea (high-altitude habitat)

- Hypoxia-driven (continued)
  » Local renal hypoxia
    - renal artery stenosis
    - end-stage renal disease
    - hydronephrosis
    - renal cysts (polycystic kidney disease)
- Pathological EPO production
  » Tumors
    - hepatocellular carcinoma
    - renal cell cancer
    - cerebellar hemangioblastoma
    - parathyroid carcinoma/adenomas
    - uterine leiomyomas
    - pheochromocytoma
    - meningioma
- Exogenous EPO
  » Drug-associated
    - treatment with androgen preparations
    - postrenal transplant erythrocytosis
    - idiopathic erythrocytosis

EPO, erythropoietin.

From McMullin MF et al. and the General Haematology Task Force of the British Committee for Standards in Haematology. Guidelines for the diagnosis, investigation and management of polycythaemia/erythrocytosis. Br J Haematol 2005;130:174–95. Blackwell Publishing Ltd.

Box 13-7

Causes of thrombocytosis

Primary	Secondary	Spurious
Essential thrombocythemia	Infection	Microspherocytes (e.g. severe burns)
Polycythemia vera	Inflammation	Cryoglobulinemia
Primary myelofibrosis	Tissue damage	Neoplastic cell cytoplasmic fragments
Myelodysplasia with del(5q)	Hyposplenism	Schistocytes
Refractory anemia with ring sideroblasts associated with marked thrombocytosis	Postoperative	Bacteria
	Hemorrhage	Pappenheimer bodies
Chronic myeloid leukemia	Iron deficiency	
Chronic myelomonocytic leukemia	Malignancy	
Atypical chronic myeloid leukemia	Hemolysis	
MDS/MPN-U	Drug therapy (e.g. corticosteroids, epinephrine)	
	Cytokine administration (e.g. thrombopoietin)	
	Rebound following myelosuppressive chemotherapy	

MDS/MPN-U, myelodysplastic/myeloproliferative neoplasms, unclassifiable.

From Harrison CN et al. and the British Committee for Standards in Haematology. Guideline for investigation and management of adults and children presenting with a thrombocytosis. Br J Haematol 2010;149:352–75. Blackwell Publishing Ltd.

CLINICAL PEARL

The combination of high Hb and thrombocytosis in the presence of JAK2 mutation is more likely to be polycythemia vera than essential thrombocythemia. Homozygous mutations of the JAK2 gene are uncommon in ET, in contrast to PV.

- Leukocytosis may occur in ET, and it has clinical implications (see below).

- Mutations in the thrombopoietin receptor gene *MPL* are noted in 4–8% of patients with ET, 15–30% have a CALR mutation, while 10–20% of the patients do not express any one of the three mutations (triple-negative).

Clinical features

Patients with JAK2 mutations and ET demonstrate:
- more bone marrow hypercellularity
- a higher likelihood of leukocytosis
- a higher risk of thrombotic events

Table 13-7 Proposed diagnostic criteria for essential thrombocythemia

Diagnosis requires A1–A3 or A1 + A3–A5	
A1	Sustained platelet count >450 × 10^9/L
A2	Presence of an acquired pathogenetic mutation (e.g. in the JAK2 CALR, or MPL genes)
A3	No other myeloid malignancy, especially PV,* PMF,[†] CML[‡] or MDS[§]
A4	No reactive cause for thrombocytosis and normal iron stores
A5	Bone marrow aspirate and trephine biopsy showing increased megakaryocyte numbers displaying a spectrum of morphology with predominant large megakaryocytes with hyperlobated nuclei and abundant cytoplasm. Reticulin is generally not increased (grades 0–2/4 or grade 0/3)

* Excluded by a normal hematocrit in an iron-replete patient; PV, polycythemia vera.

[†] Indicated by presence of significant marrow bone marrow fibrosis (greater than or equal to 2/3 or 3/4 reticulin) AND palpable splenomegaly, blood film abnormalities (circulating progenitors and tear-drop cells) or unexplained anemia PMF, primary myelofibrosis.

[‡] Excluded by absence of *BCR-ABL1* fusion from bone marrow or peripheral blood; CML, chronic myeloid leukemia.

[§] Excluded by absence of dysplasia on examination of blood film and bone marrow aspirate; MDS, myelodysplastic syndrome.

These criteria are modified from WHO diagnostic criteria.

From Harrison CN et al. and the British Committee for Standards in Haematology. Guideline for investigation and management of adults and children presenting with a thrombocytosis. Br J Haematol 2010;149:352–75. Blackwell Publishing Ltd.

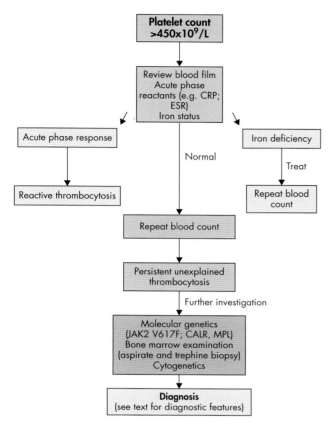

Figure 13-5 Diagnostic pathway for the investigation of thrombocytosis. CRP, C-reactive protein; ESR, erythrocyte sedimentation rate

From Harrison CN et al. and the British Committee for Standards in Haematology. Guideline for investigation and management of adults and children presenting with a thrombocytosis. Br J Haematol 2010;149:352–75. Blackwell Publishing Ltd.

- more likelihood of progressive myelofibrosis
- a greater possibility of transformation to leukemia.

Proposed diagnostic criteria are given in Table 13-7 and a diagnostic pathway in Figure 13-5.

CLINICAL PEARL

The presence of JAK2 mutation in essential thrombocytosis suggests a higher risk of thrombotic events, progression to myelofibrosis, and transformation to leukemia, although the risk is lower than in patients with polycythemia vera.

Management

Elevated platelet count on its own is not an indication for intervention. Management is based on the level of risk.

High-risk patients:

- are >60 years of age with JAK2 or MPL mutation or
- history of thrombotic events (arterial or venous)

Patients with a history of arterial thrombosis should be treated with a combination of hydroxyurea and aspirin while those who have had a venous thrombosis should be treated with hydroxyurea and systemic anticoagulation, and if JAK2 or MPL positive, aspirin should be added.

- Interferon-alpha should be considered for younger patients, and is the preferred treatment in pregnancy, as hydroxyurea and anagrelide are associated with teratogenic potential.
- Anagrelide is not usually first-line therapy, and the combination of anagrelide and aspirin is associated with more thrombotic and myelofibrotic events than hydroxyurea and aspirin.

Intermediate-risk patients (age >60 years, JAK2/MPL unmutated, no thrombosis, no cardiovascular risk factors: either aspirin alone or with hydroxyurea. Cardiovascular risk factors present: hydroxyurea and aspirin) should receive aspirin. In this group the decision for cytoreduction is individualized.

Low-risk patients are <60 years, no history of thrombosis, JAK2/MPL positive. If no cardiovascular risk factors present, once-daily aspirin; if cardiovascular risk factors present, twice daily aspirin.

Very low-risk: <60 years, no thrombosis, JAK2/MPL negative. If no cardiovascular risk factor, observation alone, if cardiovascular risk factors, once-daily aspirin.

Patients with platelet counts >1000 × 10⁹/L are at risk of bleeding and should be treated with hydroxyurea.

Primary myelofibrosis (PMF)

- This is a clonal hemopoietic stem cell disorder characterized by the proliferation of hemopoietic lineages accompanied by bone marrow fibrosis.
- Approximately 50% of patients exhibit the JAK2 Val617Phe mutation, indicating an overlap with PV and ET.
- While myelofibrotic transformation is a longer-term consequence for a limited number of patients with ET and PV, primary myelofibrosis occurs without overt preceding myeloproliferative disorder and carries the worst prognosis of the MPNs.

Clinical features

Splenomegaly is characteristic of the disease, and PMF should be considered as a differential diagnosis in the evaluation of massive splenomegaly. Splenic infarcts are common sequelae of splenomegaly. Splenomegaly is a consequence of extramedullary hemopoiesis and blood pooling.

Systemic symptoms of:

- fever
- weight loss, and
- night sweats

are a consequence of a hypercatabolic state and imply worse prognosis.

Leukemic transformation occurs in up to one-third of cases and has a poor prognosis.

Diagnosis

Box 13-8 (overleaf) lists diagnostic criteria.

Characteristic blood film findings are of a 'leukoerythroblastic picture' (the presence of immature myeloid cells

---

Box 13-8

Diagnostic criteria for primary myelofibrosis

- Leukoerythroblastic blood picture
- Increased marrow reticulin in the absence of an infiltrative or granulomatous process
- Splenomegaly
- JAK2 V617F assay (peripheral blood; expression establishes the presence of an MPD but not its type; PV is always a consideration; absence does not exclude an MPD)
- Increased circulating CD34+ cells (>15 × 10^6/L) and no increase in marrow CD34+ cells by *in situ* immunohistochemistry
- Characteristic cytogenetic abnormalities (peripheral blood: del(13q), 9p, del(20q), del(12p), partial trisomy1q, trisomy 8, and trisomy 9)
- Absence of BCR-ABL, AML, or MDS cytogenetic abnormalities by FISH (peripheral blood)

AML acute myeloid leukemia; FISH, fluorescence *in situ* hybridization; MDS, myelodysplastic syndrome; MPD, myeloproliferative disorder; PV, polycythemia vera.

From Spivak JL and Silver RT. The revised World Health Organization diagnostic criteria for polycythemia vera, essential thrombocytosis, and primary myelofibrosis: an alternative proposal. Blood 2008;112:231–39.

---

including occasional blasts, nucleated red cells and tear-drop red cells). Pancytopenia is common in later stages of the disease.

Treatment

- Cytoreductive therapy, most commonly hydroxyurea, will assist in the control of systemic symptoms.
- Splenectomy or splenic irradiation may be considered. Splenectomy is only performed in patients with debilitating symptoms who are not candidates for transplantation.

Ruxolitinib, a JAK inhibitor with selectivity for subtypes JAK1 and JAK2, improves hypermetabolic symptoms and splenomegaly, and activity is independent of JAK2 mutational status. It does not prevent transformation to acute myeloid leukemia.

Allogeneic bone marrow transplantation should be considered for patients up to 55 years with features of rapid progression. Conventional myeloablative transplantation is associated with significant transplantation-related mortality and morbidity. Reduced-intensity myeloablation (conditioning) may expand the availability of allogeneic transplantation to older patients, although it remains to be established for this disease.

LEUKEMIA

Acute myeloid leukemia (AML)

Acute myeloid leukemia is one of the most common hematological malignancies and is increasing in frequency due to an aging population. The peak incidence is in the 7th decade, but it occurs in all age groups.

AML is a clonal disorder with the leukemic transforming event having occurred in the hemopoietic stem cells.

- The transformed cells retain a proliferative advantage and demonstrate an associated failure of differentiation into mature cells, thus leading to an accumulation of the leukemic 'blast' cells.
- This replaces bone marrow with blasts, and pancytopenia ensues with the clinical presentation being fatigue, bruising or infection.
- Lymphadenopathy is uncommon, and tissue infiltration with blasts is noted in certain subtypes (e.g. gum hypertrophy in acute monocytic and acute myelomonocytic leukemias).
- Acute promyelocytic leukemia uniquely presents with disseminated intravascular coagulation (DIC).

While radiation and chemical exposure may play a role, the causative agent is not identified in the vast majority of cases.

Classification of subtypes

In the World Health Organization (WHO) classification, the presence of 20% or more blasts in the peripheral blood or bone marrow is considered to be:

- AML when it occurs *de novo*
- evolution to AML when it occurs in the setting of a previously diagnosed myelodysplastic syndrome (MDS) or myelodysplastic/myeloproliferative neoplasm (MDS/MPN)
- blast transformation in a previously diagnosed myeloproliferative neoplasm (MPN).

Prognostic variables determining outcome in AML

Age

Increasing age and poor performance status at diagnosis adversely affect prognosis. Older patients tolerate the complications of chemotherapy poorly, with a significant risk of death during induction chemotherapy.

The impact of age on the overall survival of children and adults treated in successive AML trials is shown in Figure 13-6.

Tumor burden

Poor prognosis is associated with:

- high blast count
- organomegaly
- raised LDH.

Cytogenetic abnormalities

Genetic events identified at diagnosis are one of the most important predictors of outcome, and are incorporated in the WHO classification of AML (Table 13-8).

Molecular mutations and overexpression

These are point mutations—small genetic modifications or overexpression of genes that are not identifiable by conventional

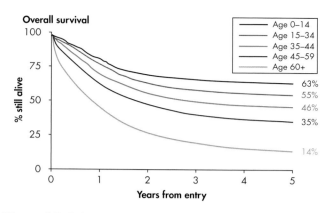

Figure 13-6 Impact of age on overall survival of children and adults (*n* = 11,421) treated in successive Medical Research Council (MRC-UK) AML trials

Adapted from Smith ML, Hills RK and Grimwade D. Independent prognostic variables in acute myeloid leukaemia. Blood Rev 2011;25:39–51.

cytogenetics but have an impact on the outcomes, particularly in cytogenetically defined intermediate-risk patients.

1 ***FLT3*** **mutation:** *FLT3* is a member of the class III receptor tyrosine kinase (RTK) family and is expressed on hematopoietic progenitors. Mutations are seen in approximately one-third of patients, resulting in constitutive activation of the receptor and adverse prognosis.

2 ***KIT:*** *KIT* (CD117) is the receptor for stem cell factor (SCF) (*KIT* ligand), and is expressed on stem cells. *KIT* mutations have an adverse impact on prognosis.

3 Molecular markers of overexpression of genes: overexpression of the Brain and Acute Leukemia, Cytoplasmic (*BAALC*) gene and the ETS-related gene (*ERG1*) are further independent adverse factors in normal-karyotype AML. The mechanisms underlying the overexpression remain to be understood.

4 ***NPM1:*** a variety of mutations have been identified within the *NPM1* gene and predict improved CR and reduced risk of relapse.

Table 13-8 Acute myeloid leukemia risk stratification by cytogenetic abnormalities found at diagnosis

ADULT		PEDIATRIC	
CYTOGENETIC ABNORMALITY	INCIDENCE	CYTOGENETIC ABNORMALITY	INCIDENCE
Favorable risk[a]			
t(15;17)(q24;q21)	5–13%	t(15;17)(q24;q21)	8–11%
t(8;21)(q22;q22)	5–7%	t(8;21)(q22;q22)	11–13%
inv(16)(p13.1q22)/t(16;16)(p13.1;q22)	5–8%	inv(16)(p13.1q22)/t(16;16)(p13.1;q22)	3–6%
		t(1;11)(q21;q23)	3%
Intermediate risk			
t(9;11)(p21;q23)	2%	t(9;11)(p21;q23)	10%
Normal karyotype	40–45%	t(1;22)(p13;q13)	2–3%
–Y	3%	Normal karyotype	20–25%
+8	10%	<3 abnormalities	6–7%
Adverse risk[b]			
inv(3)(q21q26)/t(3;3)(q21;q26)	1–2%	inv(3)(q21q26)/t(3;3)(q21;q26)	1–2%
–5/del(5q)/ add(5q)	4–12%	–5/del(5q)/ add(5q)	5–6%
–7/del(7q)/ add(7q)	8%	–7/del(7q)/ add(7q)	1–2%
t(8;16)(p11;p13)	<1%	t(11q23) [excluding t(9;11)]	18–22%
t(11q23) [excluding t(9;11)]	3–4%	t(6;9)(p23;q34)	1%
t(6;9)(p23;q34)	1–2%	t(9;22)(q34;q11.2)	1%
t(9;22)(q34;q11.2)	1%	–17/abn(17p)	2%
–17/abn(17p)	5%	Complex (≥3 unrelated abnormalities)	10%
Complex (≥3 unrelated abnormalities)	6%–14%		

[a] Irrespective of additional cytogenetic abnormalities.

[b] Excluding favorable cytogenetic abnormalities.

Adapted from Morrissette J and Bagg A. Acute myeloid leukemia: conventional cytogenetics, FISH, and moleculocentric methodologies. Clin Lab Med 2011;31:659–86.

5 **CEPBA:** encodes the transcription factor CCAAT enhancer binding protein alpha (C/EBPα), which is important in the regulation of myeloid differentiation. *CEBPA* mutations are now recognized as a good prognosis factor.

Treatment

The goals of treatment need to be individualized to patients, particularly with reference to age and performance status.

- In younger, fit patients the goal is to induce complete remission and consolidate gain.

- Further options such as allogeneic stem cell transplantation depend on stratification to *intermediate* and *poor* risk categories. Young patients with a high risk of relapse will benefit from allogeneic bone marrow or stem cell transplantation from a matched sibling or unrelated donor. The advantage in improvement in disease-free survival must be balanced against transplant-related mortality and morbidity from infections and acute and chronic graft-versus-host disease.

- **Induction treatment** consists of 1–2 cycles of an anthracycline (daunorubicin, doxorubicin), cytosine arabinoside (intermediate or high doses) and occasionally a third drug. Achievement of response is confirmed by bone marrow morphology, immunophenotyping, and cytogenetic studies to confirm the resolution of any genetic abnormality detected at diagnosis.

- **Consolidation therapy** consists of 2–3 courses of combination chemotherapy using cytosine arabinoside, anthracyclines, etoposide or *m*-amsacrine. Midostaurin, a multi-targeted protein kinase inhibitor, is used for patients who are positive for internal tandem duplication (ITD) or tyrosine kinase domain (TKD) FMS tyrosine kinase 3 (FLT3) mutation positive. It is given orally following induction and consolidation chemotherapy courses.

With advancing age and frailty, the plan should be toward supportive care and maintenance of the quality of life.

Therapy-related AML (t-AML)

Therapy-related acute myeloid leukemia is a complication of the cytotoxic therapy used for primary cancer treatment and accounts for 10–20% of myeloid neoplasms.

- t-AML is observed after ionizing radiation as well as conventional chemotherapy including alkylating agents, topoisomerase–II inhibitors and antimetabolites.

- t-AML may appear *de novo* or progress through an intermediate stage of myelodysplastic syndrome.

- Some differences between t-AML arising after alkylating agents and after topoisomerase inhibitors are shown in Table 13-9.

- Achievement of complete response is low in t-AML, and patients should be recommended for stem cell transplantation or experimental therapies.

Acute promyelocytic leukemia (APML)

Acute promyelocytic leukemia is characterized by specific chromosomal translocations that always involve the retinoic acid receptor alpha (RARA) gene on chromosome 17 to create a variety of X–RARA fusions. The most common is the t(15;17) translocation encoding the PML–RARA fusion gene, which is associated with >98% of cases. The PML-RARA fusion protein exhibits a dominant negative activity, disrupting the role of retinoic acid (RA) in the differentiation of multiple progenitors as well as myeloid cells; it also disrupts PML nuclear bodies.

- Patients often present with overt DIC or display laboratory abnormalities consistent with subclinical DIC.

- Morphological features are typical, with abundance of abnormal promyelocytes with increased granulation and

Table 13-9 Therapy-related acute myeloid leukemia: associations with different therapeutic agents

THERAPY	ABNORMALITY	FREQUENCY	MDS PHASE	APPROXIMATE TIME FROM EXPOSURE
Alkylating agents—70% (e.g. melphalan, cyclophosphamide, chlorambucil) Ionizing radiation therapy	5q deletion/ monosomy 5[a]	70%[b]	Common	Long latency (5–10 years)
	7q deletion/ monosomy 7[a]			
Topoisomerase inhibitors—30% (e.g. etoposide, daunorubicin, mitoxantrone)	*MLL* rearrangements	3–32%	Rare	Short latency (1–5 years)
	RUNX1 rearrangements	2.5–4.5%		
	t(15;17)	2%		
	inv(16)/t(16;16)	2%		
	Others	15–20%		

[a] Often associated with additional cytogenetic abnormalities [del(13q), del(20q), del(11q), del(3p), −17, −18, −21, +8].

[b] Of abnormalities of chromosome 5, 7, or both.

MDS, myelodysplastic syndrome.

Adapted from Morrissette J and Bagg A. Acute myeloid leukemia: conventional cytogenetics, FISH, and moleculocentric methodologies. Clin Lab Med 2011;31:659–86.

clusters of Auer rods. Microgranular variants are less common.

- Complete remission can be induced in over 90% of cases and cure in >80%, using all-trans retinoic acid and anthracyclines. The addition of arsenic trioxide enables the therapeutic approach of rationally targeted frontline protocols with minimal or no traditional cytotoxic chemotherapy.
- Patients are at a significant risk of DIC during the induction phase and require significant blood product support.
- A unique complication of treatment in APML is the 'differentiation syndrome', characterized by pulmonary infiltration by differentiating APML blasts. It requires treatment with steroids at the earliest symptom or sign.
- Quantitative PCR for the fusion PML-RARA transcript is useful in monitoring for minimal residual disease and relapse.

Acute lymphoblastic leukemia (ALL)

Acute lymphoblastic leukemia is characterized by the accumulation of malignant immature lymphoid cells in the bone marrow.

- It is the most common malignancy in children, representing one-third of pediatric cancers.
- It has an age-adjusted incidence rate of 1.6 per 100,000 per year, and follows a bimodal distribution with a peak between the ages of 4 and 10 years and a second peak after the age of 50 years.

Clinical presentation in adults is generally with:

- nonspecific constitutional symptoms
- features of pancytopenia.
- Bone pain, splenomegaly and lymphadenopathy are common.

Diagnosis is established on the basis of morphology and immunophenotype. Cytogenetic analysis and molecular studies are essential at diagnosis, especially the detection of t(9;22) translocation (Philadelphia chromosome) by fluorescence *in situ* hybridization (FISH) and PCR so that tyrosine kinase therapy (imatinib, nilotinib and dasatinib) can be incorporated into the treatment.

Poor **prognosis** on clinical grounds correlates with:

- age (>35 years)
- elevated white blood cell count at the time of diagnosis ($\geq 100 \times 10^9$/L for T lineage and $\geq 30 \times 10^9$/L for B lineage)
- CNS involvement at presentation
- achievement of complete remission >28 days after the initiation of induction therapy.

Cytogenetic abnormalities are independent determinants of prognosis.

Treatment of adult ALL

The aim of therapy is to obtain complete remission. Effective chemotherapy drugs include:

- L-asparaginase anthracyclines (especially in young people)
- corticosteroids
- vincristine

- cytosine arabinoside
- cyclophosphamide.

Achievement of complete remission is followed by consolidation and maintenance therapy.

- CNS prophylaxis is important to prevent relapse, and consists of cytosine arabinoside and methotrexate given intrathecally and systemically.

CLINICAL PEARL

Because of the high incidence of relapse, adult patients in first remission of acute lymphoblastic leukemia should be considered for allogeneic transplantation.

- Philadelphia-positive ALL constitutes a poor prognostic group. However, the recent incorporation of tyrosine kinase inhibitors (including imatinib and ponatinib if expressing the T315I mutation) has considerably improved prognosis.
- Detection of minimal residual disease by sensitive techniques (PCR, FISH, immunophenotype) is associated with poorer outcomes in adults and children, and serves to identify patients who need further treatment intensification, allogeneic transplantation or use of novel agents. CAR T-cell therapy for relapsed/refractory ALL, in addition to relapsed/refractory diffuse large cell lymphoma, and bi-specific T-cell engager therapy (blinatumomab) directed against CD19 on B-ALL cells.

Myelodysplastic syndrome (MDS)

Myelodysplastic syndromes are clonal stem cell disorders characterized by the presence of peripheral blood cytopenias due to impaired production from a dysplastic bone marrow.

The most common peripheral blood abnormalities are:

- macrocytic anemia, occurring in more than 80% of patients
- thrombocytopenia, noted in 30–45% of MDS cases
- neutropenia, a feature in approximately 40% of patients.

MDS is a disease of the elderly, with more than 60% of patients over the age of 70 years at the time of diagnosis. There is an increased risk of leukemic transformation.

Etiology

- MDS may appear *de novo* or following exposure to chemotherapy (alkylating agents, topoisomerase inhibitors, nucleoside analogs).
- Aplastic anemia and paroxysmal nocturnal hemoglobinuria (PNH) show an increased risk of progression to MDS.
- Constitutional genetic disorders (trisomy 21, trisomy 8 mosaicism, familial monosomy 7) and DNA repair deficiencies (e.g. Fanconi anemia) also increase the risk of developing MDS.

Classification

The WHO system incorporates cytogenetics and recognizes the importance of mono- and bi-cytopenias.

Prognosis stratification

The Revised International Prognostic Scoring System (IPSS-R; Table 13-10) separates patients into discrete survival subgroups (related to the risk of progression to AML) using:

- the percentage of bone marrow blasts
- cytogenetic abnormalities
- the number of cytopenias.

Very low-risk patients with scores of 1.5 or less have a median survival of 8.8 years, while very high-risk patients with a score of more than 6 have a median survival of only 0.8 years.

Management

The principal point of stratification is to determine suitability for allogeneic stem cell transplantation.

- Younger patients with an intermediate (> 3–4.5) or high-risk IPSS score should be considered for transplantation. Low-risk subtypes may be managed conservatively.
- Patients with del5q and symptomatic anemia respond to thalidomide and lenalidomide.
- Intermediate (> 3–4.5) or high-risk MDS patients not suitable for allogeneic transplantation should be considered for the use of hypomethylating agents.
  - » Azacitidine and decitabine are cytosine nucleoside analogs that inhibit methyltransferase activity, leading to hypomethylation of DNA. This results in restoration of normal growth control and differentiation to mature hematopoietic cells. The response to hypomethylating agents is slow, and first response may be delayed until the 6th cycle.
- Hypoplastic MDS, especially with the presence of PNH clones, responds to immunosuppressive therapy.
- Supportive care with blood and platelet transfusions and management of infections is central to the management of MDS.

- There is emerging evidence for iron chelation, particularly for patients in low-risk IPSS categories.

Chronic myeloid leukemia (CML)

Chronic myeloid leukemia results from a specific genetic event: the Philadelphia (Ph) chromosome, a reciprocal translocation of long-arm segments between chromosomes 9 and 22, t(9;22)(q34;q11).

- The long arm of chromosome 9 contains ABL1, a non-receptor tyrosine kinase, and the 'breakpoint cluster region' (BCR) is on 22q, the function of which is less clear.
- The translocation generates the Ph chromosome (*BCR-ABL1*) and the derivative 9q+ (*ABL1-BCR*). *BCR-ABL1* is functionally a tyrosine kinase with deregulation of its activity which initiates a number of signaling events that are responsible for the malignant phenotype (see below).
- An important corollary is that selective inhibition of *BCR-ABL1* tyrosine kinase activity by targeted drugs such as imatinib have the capacity to induce remission.

CLINICAL PEARL

BCR-ABL1 is also present in almost 30% cases of adult acute lymphoblastic leukemia (Ph+ ALL).

Cell biology

The pivotal oncogenic role of the dysregulated tyrosine kinase activity of *BCR-ABL1* is confirmed by the observation that tyrosine kinase inhibitors as single agents are able to induce morphological and molecular remission. *BCR-ABL1* phosphorylates a number of proteins that participate in downstream oncogenic events such as cell proliferation, survival and escape from apoptosis.

Table 13-10 Revised International Prognostic Scoring System (IPSS-R) for myelodysplastic syndromes

IPSS-R PROGNOSTIC VARIABLE	SCORE VALUE						
	0	0.5	1	1.5	2	3	4
Cytogenetics	Very good	-*	Good	-	Intermediate	Poor	Very poor
BM blast, %	≤ 2	-	> 2% - < 5%	-	5 – 10%	>10%	-
Hemoglobin (g/dL)	≥ 10	-	8 - < 10	< 8	-	-	-
Platelets (x 10⁹/L)	≥ 100	50 - < 100	< 50	-	-	-	-
Absolute neutrophil count (x 10⁹/L)	≥ 0.8	< 0.8	-	-	-	-	-

*indicates not applicable
IPSS-R risk score groups
Very low = ≤ 1.5
Low = > 1.5 - 3
Intermediate = > 3 – 4.5
High = > 4.5 - 6
Very high = > 6

Data from Greenberg P et al. Revised international prognostic scoring system for myelodysplastic syndromes. Blood 2012; 120: 2454–65

Clinical features

Untreated CML progresses through the following phases:

- *Chronic phase*—peripheral blood blasts fewer than 10% in the blood and bone marrow.
- *Accelerated phase*
  - » myeloblasts are 10–19% in the blood or bone marrow
  - » >20% basophils in the blood or bone marrow
  - » persistent thrombocytopenia ($<100 \times 10^9$/L) unrelated to therapy, or persistent thrombocytosis ($>1000 \times 10^9$/L) unresponsive to therapy
  - » increasing white blood cells and spleen size unresponsive to therapy
  - » cytogenetic evidence of clonal evolution with new abnormalities in addition to the Philadelphia chromosome.
- *Blast crisis*
  - » myeloblasts or lymphoblasts ≥20% in the blood or bone marrow
  - » extramedullary blast proliferation (chloroma)
  - » large foci or clusters of blasts on bone marrow biopsy.

Symptoms and signs correlate with the stage of disease at presentation.

- Fatigue, increased sweating, easy bruising and presence of splenomegaly are features of advanced disease.
- Lymphadenopathy is rare, and helps to clinically separate lymphoma from CML.
- Testicular swelling, headaches and meningeal irritation should alert clinicians to the development of a leukemic phase, particularly ALL.

Most patients are now identified on the basis of abnormalities on incidental full blood count tests.

CLINICAL PEARL

Lymphadenopathy is rare in chronic myeloid leukemia, and helps to distinguish it clinically from lymphoma.

Diagnosis

Typically, FBE identifies leukocytosis with left shift and the presence of basophilia. While myelocytes are commonly present, blasts are rare in the chronic phase of CML.

Diagnosis is confirmed by the typical morphological features of increased cellularity and myeloid proliferation with a left shift and eosinophilia and basophilia; megakaryocytes are commonly small in size and monolobular. Increase in blast presence in the peripheral blood or bone marrow is indicative of accelerated and blastic transformation.

Staging and prognosis

Several prognostic algorithms (Sokol and Hasford indices) have been developed to predict prognosis and response to therapy. These take into account:

- age
- leukocytosis

- platelet, eosinophil, basophil and blast counts
- spleen size.

Treatment

Neither hydroxyurea nor busulfan decrease the cells expressing Ph+ chromosome. Hydroxyurea is only used now to decrease the count while awaiting commencement of specific therapy. Occasionally, leukapharesis may be necessary for patients presenting with very high white cell counts.

Tyrosine kinase inhibitors (TKIs)

Development of specific tyrosine kinase inhibitors has dramatically changed the treatment algorithm and prognosis.

- Imatinib used as initial therapy (400 mg daily) for chronic-phase CML generates a complete cytogenetic response in 83% of patients, with an overall survival rate at 96 months of 85% and an event-free survival rate of 81%.
  - » Recent studies have confirmed that initial treatment with higher doses (600 mg or 800 mg daily) translate to improved molecular response; however, the higher doses are not well tolerated.
  - » Side-effects include fatigue, skin rash and fluid retention, which are treated symptomatically.
  - » Myelotoxicity is a feature more commonly noted in the first 2–3 months of therapy. Dose reduction should be avoided, and temporary support with granulocyte colony-stimulating factors (G-CSFs) may be used.

Therapy is continued indefinitely. Recent evidence suggests that it may be possible to cease therapy after 2 years of complete molecular response with the benefit preserved in approximately 50% of patients. Vigilance by quantitative polymerase chain reaction (Q-PCR) monitoring is essential, and re-institution of imatinib on the basis of increasing Q-PCR will re-establish response.

2nd-generation inhibitors

Dasatinib and nilotinib are two of the most widely available 2nd-generation TKIs. Their use is now recommended for first-line treatment. Trials have provided evidence that use of these drugs as first-line therapy is more efficacious than imatinib in achieving molecular response, with lower rates of progression to accelerated and blast phases.

- Dasatinib has a different structure to imatinib; it can inhibit the Src family of kinases in addition to *BCR-ABL1*. This extended repertoire of enzyme activity may contribute to its improved effectiveness, but also to the side-effect profile which may include pleural effusions and myelosuppression.
- Nilotinib is based on the structure of imatinib with modifications to improve potency, generating an improved cytogenetic response. Common side-effects include myelosuppression and elevation of hepatic and pancreatic enzymes.

Role of interferon-alpha and chemotherapy

Interferon-alpha can induce a complete hematological response in 70–80% of patients with CML, and there is some degree of cytogenetic response in approximately 50% of patients, which is complete in up to 20–25%.

Achievement of complete response translates to an improved survival (10-year survival rate of 75% or more for complete response, compared with <40% for those having a partial response and <30% for individuals having a smaller or no response).

Combination of interferon-alpha with cytarabine improves the response rate.

Monitoring

Monitoring the response to CML therapy begins at diagnosis and carries on serially throughout the entire course of the disease.

- Complete morphological remission is an easily achievable goal with tyrosine kinase inhibitor therapy and significant advances in technologies to detect BCR–ABL positive cells have now refocused therapeutic goals on cytogenetic and molecular endpoints.
- Cytogenetic and molecular responses provide a measure of minimal residual disease, guide treatment choices and predict long-term outcome.
- Complete cytogenetic response (CCyR) is achieved when no Ph+ metaphases are detectable in the bone marrow.
- Karyotyping or FISH studies are not routinely indicated for disease monitoring, but have a place to monitor development of additional genetic changes that may herald poor prognosis.
- Response to therapy is now monitored by quantification of peripheral blood BCR-ABL1 transcript by quantitative reverse transcriptase PCR (RT-PCR). Major molecular response (MMR) occurs when there is ≥3-log reduction of BCR-ABL mRNA, and complete molecular response (CMR) is defined as BCR-ABL mRNA undetectable by RT-PCR.

Treatment failure on imatinib

The most frequently identified mechanism of resistance to imatinib is the development of mutations at the ABL kinase domain.

- Rising BCR-ABL1 levels in patients compliant with imatinib therapy is an indication to sequence for BCR-ABL1 mutations.
- Mutations are identified in 40–60% of patients with imatinib resistance, with the most frequent occurring in the P-loop that prevents access of the drug to the catalytic site.
- Not all mutations confer the same level of resistance to imatinib, and some may be overcome by increased concentrations of imatinib. The decision to change therapy and the choice of 2nd-generation inhibitors are guided by the specific mutations.

CML with T315I mutation

1st- and 2nd-generation TKIs are not effective against this mutation. A 3rd-generation inhibitor, ponatinib, is approved for use in the T315I mutation, and a protein translation inhibitor, omacetaxine (homoharringtonine), has been approved for use by the FDA.

Younger patients with T315I mutation should be considered for allogeneic bone marrow transplantation.

Role of allogeneic transplantation in CML

Allogeneic bone marrow transplantation (BMT) was the cornerstone of therapy in young patients with CML who had compatible donors. This modality of treatment is potentially curative, although transplant-related mortality and morbidity from graft-versus-host disease have to be considered. With the availability of TKI therapy, allogeneic BMT is now restricted to patients with disease failure to 2nd- or 3rd-generation TKIs.

Chronic lymphocytic leukemia and other B-cell disorders

Chronic lymphocytic leukemia (CLL)

This is increasingly diagnosed early in asymptomatic patients with a mild lymphocytosis found incidentally when a full blood examination is done for another reason.

- CLL is the most common of all leukemias in adults over the age of 50 years, with a male:female ratio of 2:1. The median age of presentation is 65–70 years.
- 8–10% of patients have a family history, although no single causative gene has been found. Some association has been seen with interferon regulatory factor 4 (IRF4), a key regulator of lymphocyte maturation and proliferation.
- Approximately 50% of CLL cases retain an unmutated immunoglobulin heavy chain. There is also preferential use of a restricted set of B-cell receptors and variable heavy-chain genes. It is hypothesized that CLL proliferates due to stimulation by yet unknown antigens. There is emerging evidence that chemokines secreted by bone-marrow stromal cells can activate signaling pathways in CLL cells, leading to survival signals.

Diagnosis

The diagnosis of CLL requires the presence of ≥5 × 10⁹/L B-lymphocytes in the peripheral blood for at least 3 months, with monoclonality confirmed by flow cytometry.

- CLL cells typically co-express the T-cell antigen CD5 and the B-cell surface antigens CD19, CD20 and CD23.
- Peripheral blood film reveals characteristic 'smear' cells.
- Bone marrow examination is generally not required for the diagnosis of CLL.
- Coexisting cytopenias directly related to leukemia-cell infiltration of the marrow may be present.
- Serum LDH and beta-2 microglobulin are important measures for prognostication.

Other tests that predict prognosis at the time of diagnosis include assessment of the mutational status of the immunoglobulin heavy chain, phosphorylation of the B-cell signaling messenger Zap70, and cell-surface expression of CD38; however, these tests are not widely available and are usually performed in a research setting. Karyotype abnormalities common in CLL include deletions of 17p (loss of the tumor suppressor p53), 11q and 13q.

Prognostic factors

Poor outcomes correlate with:

- unmutated immunoglobulin heavy chain
- high beta-2 microglobulin levels
- non-responsiveness to fludarabine
- 11q and 17p deletions
- p53 mutations.

Clinical staging

The Rai and Binet scores are the two most widely accepted staging systems, of which the Rai score is described here. It has three prognostic categories:

1 Low-risk disease is defined by the presence of lymphocytosis only.
2 Intermediate-stage disease includes lymphocytosis, lymphadenopathy at any site, and splenomegaly and/or hepatomegaly.
3 High-risk disease includes patients with disease-related anemia (Hb < 110 g/L) or thrombocytopenia (platelet count <100 × 10⁹/L).

Treatment

1 Early-stage patients without symptoms do not need treatment, as there is no survival benefit.
2 Patients with intermediate-stage and high-risk disease will benefit from treatment. Treatment options include:
   a An alkylating drug such as chlorambucil is very well tolerated and is preferred in the elderly; the complete remission rate is very low when chlorambucil is used as the sole agent and it is usually used in combination with rituximab or the latest anti-CD20 antibody, obinutuzumab.
   b In patients <65, fludarabine is frequently combined with cyclophosphamide and the anti-CD20 antibody rituximab as the 'FCR' regimen. This combination should be considered as a first-line option in physically fit patients, as it delivers overall response rates in excess of 90%, complete remission in approximately 50% of patients and 3-year survival in more than 80%.
   c In relapsed/refractory patients, ibrutinib, a Bruton's tyrosine kinase inhibitor, is used. This agent has activity in p53-deleted CLL cases and may in future be used as first-line therapy. A second agent used in relapsed/refractory disease is the BCL-2 inhibitor, venetoclax. This agent is used in combination with rituximab, and in heavily pre-treated patients and those with p53 deletion, over 75% of patients respond, including over 20% complete responders.
3 Patients with del17p (lacking the tumor suppressor protein p53) are considered as high-risk and do not respond satisfactorily to FCR. In this cohort, a promising strategy is the use of ibrutinib or venetoclax. Non-myeloablative allogeneic peripheral blood stem cell transplantation currently remains a relevant treatment option. However, patient selection and timing for transplantation have become more difficult because novel compounds offer a chance of long-term remission in patients with TP53-deficient CLL.

Richter transformation in CLL

Large-cell transformation (the Richter syndrome) may occur in one or several lymph nodes. This is accompanied by systemic symptoms of weight loss and night sweats, and laboratory tests demonstrate raised LDH levels. The histology resembles diffuse, large B-cell lymphoma and intensive treatment is necessary in common with large cell lymphoma.

Monoclonal B-cell lymphocytosis (MBL)

This condition is defined as <5 × 10⁹/L monoclonal B-lymphocytes in the peripheral blood with an immunophenotype identical with CLL. There is absence of lymphadenopathy, splenomegaly, cytopenias or symptoms related to the disease. MBL may progress to CLL at a rate of 1–2% per year. No specific intervention is necessary.

Prolymphocytic leukemia

Patients present with high peripheral blood lymphocyte counts and splenomegaly. Anemia and thrombocytopenia are also common. The typical appearance on a film is of large cells with abundant cytoplasm and a prominent nucleolus. Treatment includes intensive chemotherapy, radiotherapy and sometimes splenectomy.

Hairy cell leukemia

- Hairy cell leukemia (HCL) is more prevalent in males (male:female ratio is 4:1).
- Patients present with splenomegaly and neutropenia. Anemia and thrombocytopenia may occur due to bone marrow infiltration and splenic sequestration.
- Diagnosis is established by the presence of large lymphocytes with abundant cytoplasm and 'hairy' villous projections (Figure 13-7, overleaf).
- Bone marrow biopsy reveals diffuse infiltration with a clear zone around each cell. The immunophenotype is typically CD5–, FMC7+, CD25+ and CD123+.
- Differential diagnosis includes HCL variant, characterized by a high lymphocyte count and splenomegaly, and splenic lymphoma with villous lymphocytes (SLVL). Neither HCL variant nor SLVL express CD25 and CD123.

Splenectomy and interferon-alpha are well-established treatments but have been replaced by the use of the purine nucleoside analogs cladribine and pentostatin.

- These drugs achieve an overall complete remission rate of over 80% and median relapse-free survival in excess of 15 years.
- Relapsing patients respond to retreatment and addition of rituximab (monoclonal antibody against CD20).

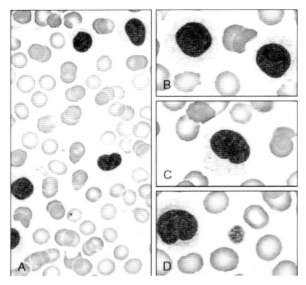

Figure 13-7 Blood film of hairy cell leukemia; note the large lymphocytes with abundant cytoplasm

From Hoffbrand AV, Pettit JE and Vyas P. Color atlas of clinical hematology, 4th edn. Philadelphia: Elsevier, 2010.

Patients commonly experience fever and neutropenia in the immediate period following nucleoside analogs, and need supportive care. Prophylaxis with co-trimoxazole and acyclovir (aciclovir) is also suggested.

NON-HODGKIN LYMPHOMAS

These comprise a diverse group encompassing malignancies arising from clonal B cells or T cells and with a clinical spectrum extending from indolent low-grade disease to an aggressive phenotype.

Certain viruses are implicated in the pathogenesis of some of the lymphomas:

- Kaposi sarcoma–associated herpesvirus/human herpesvirus 8 in primary effusion lymphoma, post-transplant lymphoproliferative disease and multicentric Castleman disease
- hepatitis C virus in splenic marginal zone lymphoma and essential mixed cryoglobulinemia
- human T-cell lymphotropic virus type I (HTLV-I) in adult T-cell leukemia/lymphoma (ATLL)
- Epstein–Barr virus in endemic Burkitt's lymphoma, HIV-associated lymphoma and post-transplant lymphoproliferative disease.

Localized chronic antigenic stimulation by *Helicobacter pylori* is implicated in the development of mucosa-associated lymphoid tissue (MALT) lymphoma.

A number of recurrent genetic alterations have implicated oncogenes in the pathogenesis of non–Hodgkin lymphomas.

Diagnosis

- Adequate tissue sample from a core biopsy or an excision biopsy is required. The tissue sample is processed for histology, including immunochemistry for proteins specific to each disease.
- *In situ* hybridization is also performed, as required, to detect viral integration (e.g. Epstein–Barr virus in aggressive diffuse large B-cell and Burkitt lymphoma) and gene alterations (e.g. cyclin D1 in mantle cell lymphoma).
- Tissue samples should be collected in the absence of fixative, and immunophenotyped by flow cytometry.

Staging

Full blood count, electrolytes, creatinine, liver function tests, LDH and bone marrow biopsy are commonly performed.

Anatomical staging is conventionally done with CT tomography and described using the Ann Arbor system (Table 13-11). An FDG-PET-CT is now a standard staging test for FDG-avid lymphomas, including Hodgkin lymphoma, diffuse large B-cell lymphoma, and follicular lymphoma.

Diffuse large B-cell lymphoma (DLBCL)

Management of DLBCL is individualized based on performance status, age, stage and the International Prognostic Index risk group (Box 13-9), which is still a valid predictor of prognosis in the era of rituximab therapy.

Table 13-11 Ann Arbor staging system (with Cotswold modifications A, B, E and X)

Stage I	Involvement of a single lymph-node region or extralymphatic site
Stage II	Involvement of two or more lymph-node regions on the same side of the diaphragm; localized contiguous involvement of only one extralymphatic site and lymph-node region (IIE)
Stage III	Involvement of lymph-node regions or lymphoid structures on both sides of the diaphragm
Stage IV	Disseminated involvement of one or more extralymphatic organs with or without lymph-node involvement Any involvement of liver or bone marrow
A	No symptoms
B	Unexplained weight loss of >10% of bodyweight during the 6 months before staging investigation Unexplained, persistent, or recurrent fever with temperatures >38°C during the previous month Recurrent drenching night sweats during the previous month
E	Localized, solitary involvement of extralymphatic tissue, excluding liver and bone marrow
X	Largest deposit is >10 cm ('bulky disease'), or the mediastinum is wider than one-third of the chest on a chest X-ray

Box 13-9

International Prognostic Index for aggressive lymphoma

Prognostic factors: one point awarded to each if present
- Age >60 years
- Ann Arbor stage III or IV
- Raised serum lactase dehydrogenase
- ECOG* performance score 2 or higher
- Involvement of more than one extranodal site

Scoring
- 0, 1 prognostic factors: 3-year survival 91%
- 2 prognostic factors: 3-year survival 80%
- 3 prognostic factors: 3-year survival 55%
- 4, 5 prognostic factors: 3-year survival 59%

* ECOG, Eastern Cooperative Oncology Group scale (now the World Health Organization Performance Scale), in which 0 indicates that the patient has no symptoms; 1 indicates that the patient has symptoms but is ambulatory; 2 indicates that the patient is bedridden less than half the day; 3 indicates that the patient is bedridden half the day or longer; and 4 indicates that the patient is chronically bedridden and requires assistance with the activities of daily living.

Data from Standard International Prognostic Index Remains a Valid Predictor of Outcome for Patients With Aggressive CD20+ B-Cell Lymphoma in the Rituximab Era. J Clin Oncol (2010) 28:2373-2380.

Treatment

- Younger (<60 years), with favorable IPI (0, 1) and non-bulky localized disease (stage I): dual modality therapy comprising 4 cycles of R-CHOP (rituximab, cyclophosphamide, adriamycin, vincristine and prednisolone) and involved-field radiotherapy are generally adequate and confer a 5-year overall survival of above 90%.

- Older patients with any stage and younger patients with stages II–IV are best managed with 6–8 courses of R-CHOP with additional radiotherapy to any site of bulky disease (>10 cm). Relapse requires intensive 'salvage' therapy followed by stem cell collection and transplantation.

'Cell of origin' classification of DLBCL

- Immunohistochemistry algorithms classify DLBCL into germinal center B-cell (GCB)-like subtype and the activated B-cell (ABC)-like subtype.

- Patients with the ABC disease subtype have significantly poorer outcomes to standard up-front rituximab containing chemoimmunotherapy programs compared to GCB disease.

'Double-hit' (DH) and 'triple-hit' (TH) lymphomas

- Double-hit lymphomas are defined by a chromosomal breakpoint affecting the *MYC*/8q24 locus in combination with another recurrent breakpoint, mainly a t(14;18)(q32;q21) involving *BCL2*. Triple-hit lymphomas have genetic rearrangements of MYC, BCL2 and BCL6.

- DH and TH lymphomas often have a complex karyotype with many additional genetic alterations.

- The prognosis is generally poor, with a median overall survival of only 0.2–1.5 years. Prospective data are needed to inform an optimal induction regimen, and studies are actively enrolling patients with DH/THL.

Burkitt lymphoma

Burkitt lymphoma is aggressive. There are three subtypes:

1 The endemic variant occurs mainly in Africa and Epstein–Barr virus (EBV) is found in almost all cases; the variant comprises about half of all cancers diagnosed in childhood.

2 The sporadic type occurs in the rest of the world, being mainly predominant in North America and Europe. It is has a peak incidence at 11 years of age in pediatric patients, and 30 years of age in adults; and is associated with EBV only 10% to 20% of the time.

3 The immunodeficiency-related type is seen most often in patients with HIV infection. Less than 40% of US and European cases are associated with EBV.

Patients with endemic Burkitt lymphoma most frequently present with jaw or periorbital swellings, or abdominal involvement. The most common presentation of sporadic BL is as an abdominal mass followed by lymphadenopathy in the neck, and involvement of tonsils and sinuses.

Diagnosis

Diagnosis is made by the observation of intermediate-size cells containing coarse chromatin and prominent basophilic nucleoli. Macrophages ingesting apoptotic cells against a deep basophilic cellular background give the appearance of a 'starry sky'.

Diagnosis is confirmed by immunophenotype and demonstration of translocations involving the *MYC* gene and heavy [t(8;14)] or light [t(2;8) or t(8;22)] chains of immunoglobulin genes.

Treatment

BL has an excellent cure rate in children and adults, with the use of intensive multi-agent chemotherapy, although survival is inferior in older patients usually as a result of increased therapy-related toxicity. Combinations such as such as R-CODOX-M/R-IVAC (rituximab, cyclophosphamide, vincristine, doxorubicin and methotrexate, alternating with rituximab, ifosfamide, mesna, etoposide and cytarabine) are frequently used in adults.

Follicular lymphoma (FL)

Follicular lymphoma is generally an indolent B-cell lymphoproliferative disorder of transformed follicular-center B cells.

- The median age of presentation is 55–60 years.

- FL is characterized by diffuse lymphadenopathy and bone marrow involvement is common.

- In general, cytopenias can occur but constitutional symptoms of fever, night sweats and weight loss are uncommon.

Diagnosis is based on histology of an excision or core biopsy of a lymph node.

- Immunohistochemical staining is positive in virtually all cases for cell-surface CD19, CD20, CD10 and monoclonal immunoglobulin, as well as cytoplasmic expression of Bcl-2 protein.
- The overwhelming majority of cases have the characteristic t(14;18) translocation involving the *IGH* and *BCL2* genes.

The Follicular Lymphoma International Prognostic Index 2 (FLIPI-2) prognostic model uses five independent predictors of inferior survival:

1. age >60 years
2. hemoglobin <12 g/dL
3. beta-2 microglobulin > normal
4. bone marrow involvement
5. bulky disease > 6 cm

The presence of 0, 1–2, and 3–5 adverse factors defines low, intermediate and high-risk disease respectively.

The 5-year overall survival in the rituximab era are approximately 95, 70 and 80%, respectively.

Treatment

- Low-volume asymptomatic disease requires monitoring only.
- Localized stage I disease responds well to involved-field radiotherapy.
- Advanced-stage lymphoma is now treated with rituximab plus chemotherapy including CVP (cyclophosphamide, vincristine and prednisolone) or bendamustine. Addition of maintenance rituximab has demonstrated improved duration of remission.
- Autologous stem cell transplant and allogeneic stem cell transplant should be considered in suitable patients with relapsing or refractory disease.

Mantle cell lymphoma (MCL)

Patients with MCL have a median age in their 60s and male predominance (3:1). Patients generally have stage III/IV disease and present with:

- extensive lymphadenopathy
- blood and bone marrow involvement
- splenomegaly.

Approximately 50% have gastrointestinal involvement.

Morphological appearance is typically of monomorphic small to medium-sized lymphoid cells with irregular nuclear contours.

The hallmark chromosomal translocation t(11;14) identifies MCL. The oncogene on chromosome 11 is *CCND1* that encodes a Cyclin-D1, a protein involved in cell-cycle control.

Treatment

Mantle cell responds to conventional chemotherapy and newer treatments; however, relapses are frequent. A minor subset of patients have indolent disease. In patients requiring treatment:

- Younger patients need aggressive treatment.

- The most widely used regimens include R–HyperCVAD (rituximbab, cyclophosphamide, vincristine, doxorubicin and dexamethasone) with high-dose cytarabine (± methotrexate) or R–CHOP (rituximab–CHOP) alternating with R-DHAP (R-dexamethasone, cytarabine, and cisplatin) followed by autologous stem cell transplant.
- Rituximab combined with bendamustine is used in older patients and those ineligible for stem cell transplant.
- The median duration of remission is 1.5–3 years and the median overall survival is 3–6 years with standard chemotherapy.
- As standard therapy does not cure patients with MCL, a 'watch and wait' strategy is appropriate for elderly patients with asymptomatic disease.

Cutaneous lymphomas

Primary cutaneous lymphomas are a heterogeneous group of extranodal non-Hodgkin lymphomas.

- In contrast to nodal non-Hodgkin lymphoma, most of which are B-cell-derived, approximately 75% of primary cutaneous lymphomas are T-cell-derived (cutaneous T-cell lymphoma, CTCL). The two major types of CTCL are *mycosis fungoides* (MF) and *Sézary syndrome* (SS).
- The incidence of CTCL increases significantly with age, with a median age at diagnosis in the mid-50s and a fourfold increase in incidence in patients over 70 years.
- The cell of origin in:
  » SS is the central memory T cell
  » MF is the effector memory T cell.
- MF is frequently characterized by clinical stages of cutaneous disease comprising patch/plaques, tumors and erythroderma with extensive skin involvement.
  » Patch/plaque lesions develop in a 'bathing suit' distribution and vary in size, shape and color. These lesions are frequently large (>5 cm), pruritic and multifocal.
- SS is defined as a leukemic form of CTCL associated with erythroderma.

Staging

Staging by TNMB (tumor, node, metastasis and blood) remains an important prognostic factor in MF and SS.

- Patients with only patches and plaques have:
  » stage IA (<10% body surface area involved, or T1)
  » stage IB (≥10% body surface area involved, or T2).
  » For practical purposes, the area of one hand (including both palm and digits) represents approximately 1% of body surface area.
- Further stages depend on:
  » lymph node involvement
  » erythroderma
  » leukemic involvement.
  » visceral involvement

Treatment

- Early-stage disease is managed with topical therapy (steroids, nitrogen-mustard, carmustine) and with PUVA (psoralen with ultraviolet radiation), narrow-band ultraviolet A (NB-UVA) and localized radiotherapy.

- Systemic chemotherapy is reserved for advanced-stage disease, using methotrexate, doxorubicin, retinoids, bexarotene combined with denileukin diftitox (immunotoxin), extracorporeal phototherapy, and for suitable patients, allogeneic stem cell transplant.

HODGKIN LYMPHOMA (HL)

Hodgkin lymphoma most frequently affects young adults in the age group 15–29 years. The incidence is about 3 per 100,000 in resource-rich countries. A previously reported second peak of incidence in older adults is probably due to misclassification of non-Hodgkin lymphomas.

Familial HL represents 4.5% of all newly diagnosed cases. HLA associations have been described in familial HL, including *HLA A1, B5, B18, DPB1, DRB1, DQA1* and *DQB1*.

Histological subtypes and cell biology

Based on cellular composition, HL can be divided into classic HL, which is the most common (95%), and nodular lymphocyte-predominant HL (NLPHL). It is important to distinguish between the two categories, since they differ in prognosis and treatment options.

Sub-classification of classic HL is described in Box 13-10.

In classic HL, the tumor cells are designated Hodgkin and Reed–Sternberg (HRS) cells, while in NLPHL they are now called LP (lymphocyte-predominant) cells.

- Detection of clonally rearranged immunoglobulin V (IgV) heavy chain and light chain genes confirm the origin of HRS cells from mature B cells at a germinal center (GC) or post-GC stage of differentiation. However, several of the classic cell-surface markers and transcription factors that are present in B cells are not detectable in HRS cells, and the molecular basis for re-programming of B cells to the HRS phenotype remains unclear.

- Molecular profiling of LP cells suggests that they resemble GC B cells but have already acquired features of memory B cells, indicating that these cells may derive from late-GC B cells at the transition to memory B cells.

- HRS cells thrive in a microenvironment that is enriched for B and T cells, plasma cells, eosinophils and plasma cells. HL is unique among all cancers because malignant cells are greatly outnumbered by reactive cells in the tumor microenvironment and make up only approximately 1% of the tumor.

Box 13-10

World Health Organization classification of Hodgkin lymphoma

- Nodular lymphocyte-predominant Hodgkin lymphoma (NLPHL) (5%)
- Classic Hodgkin lymphoma (95%)
  - » Nodular sclerosis
  - » Mixed cellularity
  - » Lymphocyte-rich
  - » Lymphocyte-depleted

- Expression of a variety of cytokines and chemokines by the HRS and LP cells is believed to be the driving force for an abnormal immune response, inflammatory environment, and the maintenance of a malignant phenotype.

- Epstein–Barr virus DNA and peptides can be identified in 20–100% of HRS cells, and EBV is probably implicated in the disease process.

- Immunosuppressive states such as HIV increase the risk of developing HL; however, the risk surprisingly does not correlate with low CD4 count, and the incidence of HL has actually increased with the introduction of highly active antiretroviral therapy and improvement in CD4 cell counts. HIV-associated HL is usually mixed cellularity or lymphocyte-depleted, is of advanced stage at diagnosis, and has a near-universal association with EBV infection.

Immunophenotype

The presence of CD30 and CD15 identify HRS from LP cells (where these markers are usually absent).

- In classic HL, a minority of HRS cells express CD20 to a variable intensity. EBV antigens (EBNA, LMP1) can be detected in HRS cells.

- In contrast, LP cells exhibit their B-cell origin more prominently than HRS by the expression of several B-cell markers, including CD20 and Ig.

Staging

The Cotswold modification maintains the original four-stage clinical and pathological staging framework of the Ann Arbor staging system, but also adds information regarding the prognostic significance of bulky disease (denoted by an X) and regions of lymph-node involvement (denoted by an E)—see Table 13-11. The A and B designations denote the absence or presence of symptoms, respectively; the presence of symptoms correlates with treatment response. The importance of imaging modalities, such as computed tomography (CT and FDG-PET-CT) scanning, is also underscored.

Risk stratification

Based on the clinical scenario, staging and degree of end-organ damage, patients with HL can be categorized into the following three groups:

1. early-stage favorable
2. early-stage unfavorable (bulky and non-bulky)
3. advanced stage.

This classification affects treatment selection and so must be performed carefully in every patient with HL.

Patients with advanced disease are further risk-stratified using the International Prognostic Score (IPS), which includes the following risk factors. For each factor present, the patient receives 1 point.

- Albumin <4 g/dL (<40 g/L)
- Hemoglobin <10.5 g/dL (105 g/L)
- Male
- Age ≥45 years
- Stage IV disease

- Leukocytosis: white blood cell (WBC) count > 15,000/microL
- Lymphopenia: lymphocyte count <8% of WBC count and/or absolute lymphocyte count <600 cells/microL

Based on the IPS score, patients with advanced disease can be categorized as follows:

- good risk—IPS 0–1
- fair risk—IPS 2–3
- poor risk—IPS 4–7.

Treatment

Treatment options for classic HL

Good-risk classic HL is now a curable disease in most patients. Treatment options are determined by stage (early/advanced) and risk factors.

- Early-stage disease with favorable risk factors is managed with 2 cycles of chemotherapy (most commonly the combination of doxorubicin, bleomycin, vinblastine and dacarbazine, 'ABVD') with involved-field radiotherapy (up to 30 Gy).
- Advanced-stage disease with a poor risk score needs intensive chemotherapy. Common regimens include 'ABVD' and 'BEACOPP' (bleomycin, etoposide, doxorubicin, cyclophosphamide, vincristine, procarbazine and prednisolone given as 'standard dose' or with dose escalation). Bulky sites (>10 cm in diameter) need supplementation with radiotherapy.
- Relapsed disease needs intensive salvage chemotherapy, mobilization of peripheral blood stem cells, followed by autologous stem cell transplantation. Options for relapsed/refractory disease following autologous stem cell transplantation include the anti-CD30 antibody, brentuximab vedotin, and the anti-PD1 antibody pembrolizumab.

Treatment options for nodular lymphocyte-predominant HL

This entity is different from classic HL in terms of its biology and prognosis, and has a better prognosis than classic HL. Patients commonly present early with limited-stage disease and the natural history is that of an indolent, relapsing nature. Less aggressive approaches are preferred.

- Localized disease may need radiotherapy to the involved region.
- Advanced disease requires combination chemotherapy, either ABVD or CHOP, with the inclusion of rituximab (anti-CD20 antibody).

PLASMA CELL DISORDERS

The characteristic feature is the proliferation of a single clone of plasma cells that produces a monoclonal protein (M-protein). The disease spectrum extends between monoclonal gammopathy of uncertain significance, asymptomatic myeloma, symptomatic multiple myeloma, and plasma cell leukemia. Prognosis and initiation of therapy depend on the disease category.

Monoclonal gammopathy of uncertain significance (MGUS)

Also known as benign monoclonal gammopathy, MGUS increases in frequency with advancing age and has a prevalence of approximately 5% at the age of 70 years. It is defined by the presence of:

- serum M-protein of <30 g/L
- <10% plasma cells in the bone marrow
- absence of organ damage caused either by proliferation of plasma cells or by toxicity of M-protein (related-organ tissue injury, ROTI)
- no evidence of any other B-lymphoproliferative disorder.

MGUS is a benign disease with an annual rate of progression to myeloma of approximately 1%. There is no need to treat, and management is usually 6- to 12-monthly review with quantification of M-protein, renal function and other tests for organ damage.

Asymptomatic myeloma

Also known as smoldering myeloma, this is an intermediate stage defined by:

- M-protein >30 g/L, and/or
- 10% or more plasma cell infiltration in the bone marrow
- without evidence of ROTI.

Treatment decisions need to be individualized; close monitoring alone is acceptable based on the level of M-protein and the degree of plasma cell infiltration in the bone marrow.

Symptomatic myeloma

This stage is defined by the presence of ROTI (Table 13-12), including:

- Pancytopenia due to extensive plasma-cell proliferation
- Nephrotoxicity
  » cast nephropathy due to accumulation of excreted light chains in the renal tubules

Table 13-12 Related-organ tissue injury (ROTI) in myeloma

Increased calcium level	Corrected serum calcium >0.25 mmol/L above the upper limit of normal, or >2.75 mmol/L
Renal insufficiency	Creatinine >173 micromol/L
Anemia	Hemoglobin <100 g/L, or 20 g/L below the lower limit of normal
Bone lesions	Lytic lesions, or osteoporosis with compression fractures on magnetic resonance imaging or computed tomography
Other	Symptomatic hyperviscosity, amyloidosis, recurrent bacterial infections (>2 episodes in 12 months)

» glomerular deposition of immunoglobulin (light and/or heavy chains)
» osteolysis causing hypercalcemia
- Hyperviscosity (secondary to M-protein)
- Immune-deficiency states due to the suppression of normal immunoglobulin production

Skeletal involvement is a particularly common feature, including:

- osteoporosis
- discrete osteolytic lesions.

An important pathogenetic mechanism for osteolysis is the secretion of RANK-L (receptor activator of NF-kappaB ligand), a potent activator of osteoclast activity.

Almost one-third of patients with myeloma are anemic at presentation; neutropenia and thrombocytopenia are less frequent. The etiology of anemia includes:

- extensive bone-marrow infiltration with plasma cells
- renal impairment.

Box 13-11 outlines the initial diagnostic work-up.

Prognostic markers in myeloma

Prognostic markers at diagnosis identify high-risk patients for stratification to more intensive therapy, while sparing those who may do well without intensification.

The International Prognostic Index model utilizes serum beta$_2$ microglobulin (B2M) and albumin. This can create three prognostic groups:

- Stage I includes those with serum B2M <3.5 mg/L and serum albumin >35 g/L. Median survival is 62 months.

Box 13-11

Initial diagnostic work-up in myeloma

- Full blood count and blood film examination
- Biochemistry including electrolytes, renal function, calcium, phosphate, lactate dehydrogenase, liver function tests
- Beta$_2$ microglobulin
- Serum protein electrophoresis (SPEP) and immunofixation electrophoresis (IFE)
- 24-hour urine collection—protein excretion, creatinine clearance, Bence–Jones protein
- Serum free light chain (SFLC)
- Bone marrow aspirate and trephine
- Cytogenetics (if percentage of plasma cells in the aspirate is >15%)
- FISH for: t(4;14), t(14;16), 17p del, 1q21 amplification
- Skeletal imaging by whole-body low-dose CT scan or MRI (in selected cases with back pain, suspected vertebral fractures or solitary plasmacytoma)
- Bone densitometry (in selected cases with suspicion of osteoporosis)

FISH, fluorescence *in situ* hybridization; MIBI, methoxyisobutylisonitrile; MRI, magnetic resonance imaging.

- Stage II is the intermediate category when criteria for stages I and III are not met. Median survival is 45 months.
- Stage III contains patients with serum B2M >5.5 mg/L. Median survival is 29 months.

Chromosomal abnormalities, including deletion (del) 17p and t(4;14) and t(14;16), also carry poor prognosis.

Treatment of myeloma

Myeloma is incurable. The therapeutic aim is to maintain response and avoid complications of the disease and treatment.

Treatment is indicated only for symptomatic myeloma with evidence of ROTI. Patients needing treatment are stratified based on the feasibility of autologous stem cell transplantation.

- The best outcome in patients eligible for autologous transplant is with induction therapy to achieve as deep a remission as possible, followed by high-dose therapy and autologous stem cell transplant. This approach maximizes the progression-free survival and overall survival.
  » Induction therapy includes steroids, cyclophosphamide, thalidomide and newer drugs such as lenalidomide and bortezomib (a proteasome inhibitor). Peripheral blood stem cells are collected after mobilization with granulocyte-colony stimulating factor, followed by high-dose melphalan and stem-cell re-infusion.
  » Post-transplant, single-agent lenalidomide, thalidomide or bortezomib maintenance therapy can be used to prolong progression-free survival and overall survival.
- A number of options exist for initial therapy in patients who are not fit for autologous transplantation, including thalidomide, bortezomib, combined with cyclophosphamide and dexamethasone, carfilzomib combined with dexamethasone, and lenalidomide combined with dexamethazone. Relapsed myeloma can be treated with drugs such as pomalidomide, and the anti-CD38 antibody, daratumumab.
- Other modalities of treatment include radiotherapy for osteolytic areas and spinal cord compression, and surgical fixation of pathological fractures.

Allogeneic stem cell transplantation is an option for a very select group of relapsed patients.

Supportive therapy

- Bisphosphonates have demonstrated benefit in:
  » reducing bone pain
  » reducing the number and delaying the onset of fractures
  » reducing hypercalcemia.

Differential diagnosis

1 Benign monoclonal gammopathy.
2 Waldenstrom's macroglobulinemia, a lymphoplasmacytic lymphoma resulting in overproduction of IgM, characterized by:
   a monoclonal IgM peak on the electrophoretogram
   b splenomegaly and anemia
   c frequently, hyperviscosity.

ANEMIA

Anemia is defined as reduction in hemoglobin levels below the normal range appropriate for age and gender. While the diagnosis of anemia is made on laboratory criteria, the impact of the condition is modified by clinical parameters: for example mild anemia may cause more symptoms when coexistent with coronary artery disease or lung disease. Most anemias can be diagnosed by a combination of history, physical examination and the common laboratory parameters of:

- mean red cell volume
- red cell morphology (Figure 13-8)
- reticulocyte count.

Mechanisms of anemia

Etiological descriptors of anemias comprise the following.

1. Disorder of production:
   a. Bone-marrow failure, e.g. aplastic anemia, red cell aplasia
   b. Decreased erythropoietin, e.g. chronic renal impairment
2. Disorder of maturation:
   a. Nuclear maturation defects: B_{12} or folate deficiency, myelodysplasias
   b. Cytoplasmic maturation defects, e.g. iron deficiency, thalassemias
3. Decreased survival:
   a. Inherited defects, e.g. spherocytosis, G6PD deficiency, sickle-cell anemia
   b. Acquired defects, e.g. autoimmune hemolysis, malaria, DIC, TTP
4. Sequestration in spleen: e.g. hypersplenism
5. Blood loss: e.g. gastrointestinal hemorrhage, perioperative bleeding

Common laboratory tests used for diagnostic work-up

Full blood examination (FBE) is used to ascertain the following:

- Hb: indicates the severity of the anemia
- mean cell volume (MCV): demonstrates microcytosis, macrocytosis or normocytosis
- WBC count and platelets: indicate whether anemia is a part of pancytopenia or other primary bone-marrow conditions including leukemia, or an infiltrative disorder
- blood film: typical appearances of red cells give clues to the diagnosis, e.g. sickle cells
- reticulocyte count: indicates the presence of compensatory erythropoiesis
- hemolytic parameters—serum LDH, haptoglobin, bilirubin
- direct antiglobulin test (DAT): to detect autoimmune hemolysis
- Hb electrophoresis: for diagnosis of thalassemia.

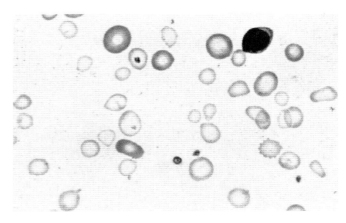

Figure 13-8 Blood film of iron-deficiency anemia; note the pale, small cells and variability in cell size (anisocytosis) and shape (poikilocytosis)

From Bain BJ et al. Dacie and Lewis Practical Haematology, 11th ed. Elsevier, 2012.

The full work-up for anemia diagnosis is given in Table 13-13, and differential diagnosis is outlined in Table 13-14.

Approach to iron-deficiency anemia

- The etiology of iron-deficiency anemia in a female of childbearing age is usually a combination of diet, multiparity in quick succession, and menstrual blood loss. Occasionally, malabsorption syndromes may be present. Management usually requires just the replenishment of iron stores.
- Iron deficiency in an older person should be regarded as a sign of another underlying disease; in resource-rich countries, particular attention should be made to exclude a source of gastrointestinal bleeding.

Causes of iron deficiency are listed in Box 13-12 (overleaf).

Stages of iron deficiency

Anemia occurs only after persistent depletion of iron stores. The preceding events sequentially progress through:

- biochemical depletion of iron stores (normal Hb and MCV, reduced ferritin)
- iron-deficient erythropoiesis (normal Hb, with fall in transferrin saturation, MCV reduced or normal, and low ferritin)
- iron-deficiency anemia (microcytic and hypochromic red cells with falling Hb, increased transferrin, decreased transferrin saturation and low ferritin).

Systemic effects of iron deficiency

Persistent and severe iron deficiency may result in extra-hemopoietic manifestations, which include:

- brittle and ridged nails (koilonychia)
- angular stomatitis
- thinning hair
- glossitis
- pharyngeal webs with dysphagia (Paterson–Kelly syndrome).

Table 13-13 Anemia work-up

	PARAMETERS	INTERPRETATION
History	Diet (meat and green vegetables)	Risk of malnutrition if lacking: suggests susceptibility to iron and folic acid deficiency
	Blood loss	Obvious gastrointestinal bleeding Chronic subclinical blood loss, e.g. NSAIDs, colon polyps, hereditary telangiectasias, menorrhagia
	Gastrointestinal surgery	Gastrectomy or ileal resection: vitamin B_{12} deficiency Small-bowel resections: iron, folate deficiency
	Comorbidity	Chronic infections and inflammatory disorders suggest risk of anemia of chronic disease
Examination	Pallor	Severity of anemia
	Icterus	May suggest hemolysis
	Lymphadenopathy, hepatomegaly, splenomegaly, bone tenderness	Coexistence of another primary hematological disorder
	Evidence of portal hypertension	Hypersplenism and potential for variceal bleed
Red cell size and hemoglobinization	Microcytic hypochromic	Iron deficiency Thalassemia Anemia of chronic disease Sideroblastic anemia
	Normocytic	Acute bleeding Bone-marrow infiltration Aplastic anemia Renal failure
	Macrocytic	Vitamin B_{12}/folate deficiencies Myelodysplasia Medication effects Other medical conditions: hypothyroidism, liver impairment

NSAIDs, non-steroidal anti-inflammatory drugs.

Table 13-14 Differential diagnosis of microcytic hypochromic anemia

PARAMETER	IRON-DEFICIENCY ANEMIA	ANEMIA OF CHRONIC DISEASE	THALASSEMIAS	SIDEROBLASTIC ANEMIA
MCV	↓	↓ / N	↓	↓ / N
Serum iron	↓	↓	N	↑
Transferrin saturation	↓	↓ /N	N	↑
TIBC	↓	↓ / N	N	N
Serum transferrin receptor	↑	↓	N	N / ↑
Serum ferritin	↓	↑/ N	N	↑
Serum hepcidin	↓	↑	N / ↓	↓
Bone-marrow iron stores	↓	↑/ N	↑/ N	↑/ N Ring sideroblasts

MCV, mean cell volume; N, normal; TIBC, total iron-binding capacity

> ## Box 13-12
> ## Causes of iron deficiency
>
> **Inadequate intake**
> - Veganism, dietary choices
>
> **Inadequate absorption**
> - High gastric pH or antacid therapy
> - Excess tannins and phytates in diet
> - Bowel resection
> - Celiac disease
> - Inflammatory bowel disease
>
> **Increased physiological requirement**
> - Pregnancy and breastfeeding
> - Infancy, puberty
>
> **Increased loss**
> - Gastrointestinal blood loss
> - Genitourinary blood loss
> - Menorrhagia
> - Operative blood loss
> - Parasitosis
> - Trauma
> - Excessive phlebotomy

Impairment of bacterial killing by neutrophils and impaired cell-mediated immunity can also occur.

Management of iron deficiency

- Oral iron supplementation is the most convenient treatment if the patient is adherent and there are no ongoing losses. All iron preparations are similarly absorbed, and the usual dose is 105 mg/day elemental iron or 325 mg/day ferrous sulfate. Higher doses often cause gastrointestinal intolerance, which may limit adherence.

- Parenteral iron preparations should be reserved for patients who are intolerant of oral supplements, those with malabsorption syndromes, and for patients with ongoing losses and large store deficits. Iron polymaltose is available as a deep intramuscular injection. Particular attention to the injection technique is essential, as leakage under the skin leads to prolonged discoloration.

- Iron carboxymaltose and iron sucrose preparations are available for intravenous infusions. Potential side-effects of intravenous preparations include allergic reactions that may extend to anaphylaxis, so should only be administered under close medical supervision.

Anemia of chronic disease

The underlying pathogenesis of the anemia of chronic disease is the suppression of erythropoiesis by a variety of mechanisms in the context of prolonged systemic illness or inflammation. Commonly associated conditions are:

- infections
- cancers
- autoimmune disease
- the chronic inflammatory state that contributes to the anemia of aging.

The main pathogenetic mechanisms include the suppression of erythropoiesis by:

- inflammatory cytokines (tumor necrosis factor alpha, interleukin-1)
- reduced erythropoietin production as a response to anemia
- a relative inhibition of the proliferative capacity of the erythron in response to the available erythropoietin.

Hepcidin is now considered to be the key mediator of this condition. Hepcidin levels are increased as a consequence of inflammatory signaling, and hepcidin leads to inhibition of iron export by the enterocytes and sequestration of iron within these cells, hepatocytes and macrophages.

Diagnosis is suggested by the presence of:

- microcytic hypochromic indices
- elevation of inflammatory markers (e.g. C-reactive protein)
- raised ferritin levels.

Two advances to improve diagnostic specificity include:

- the measurement of soluble transferrin receptor (sTFR). An sTFR/ferritin ratio of <1 makes anemia of chronic disease likely
- quantification of hepcidin levels, which are elevated in this condition and reduced in iron-deficiency anemia.

Treatment should be directed toward correction of the underlying condition. Iron supplementation is generally without effect. Erythropoiesis-stimulating agents should be used with caution, as increased cardiovascular events and thrombotic episodes have been observed. There is also concern about tumor progression when used in patients with active malignancy.

Thalassemias

The thalassemias are a group of hereditary anemias due to impairment in the synthesis of one of the polypeptide globin chains, alpha and beta, resulting in alpha-thalassemia and beta-thalassemia.

Each Hb molecule in adults (HbA) contains two alpha and two beta chains, denoted $\alpha 2\beta 2$. Stable HbA requires the presence of α- and β-globin dimers which combine to form a tetramer. Imbalances in the proportion of α- or β-globins results in unstable combinations of globin chains.

- There are two genes for α-globin on each chromosome 16, giving four genes in total as autosomes exist as pairs. The globin product from each gene is identical, and thus each gene contributes to one-quarter of the product.

- The β-globin locus on chromosome 11 contains several genes that are sequentially arranged and synthesize globin chains during specific stages of development.

The ϵ gene is expressed in early embryogenesis, followed by the γ gene during fetal development. Thus fetal Hb (HbF) is $\alpha 2\gamma 2$. Just prior to birth there is a progressive switch to synthesis of β-globins, and γ-globin synthesis reciprocally diminishes. However, γ-globin synthesis is not completely lost and most adults contain traces (<0.6%) of HbF. Persistence of HbF in some patients with beta-thalassemia has the capacity to ameliorate the severity of the phenotype.

Alpha-thalassemias

- Deletion of one out of the four α-globin genes does not lead to a hematological abnormality; this is a silent carrier state.

- Deletion of two genes causes mild microcytic anemia. Southeast Asian populations with two-gene deletion often carry both deleted genes on the same chromosome. There is increased risk of the occurrence of severe alpha-thalassemia syndrome (HbH disease) with coinheritance from the other parent of a single gene deletion, and of hydrops fetalis with coinheritance of a two-gene deletion.

- HbH disease (three-gene deletion) is manifested as moderately severe microcytic anemia. Excess β-globins cause Hb instability and precipitate, leading to removal by the spleen and hemolysis.

- Deletion of four genes causes hydrops fetalis, with stillbirth or death in the early postnatal period.

Beta-thalassemias

Mutations may either completely block β-globin production or may dampen it.

- Loss of one β-globin gene leads to *thalassemia trait*, presenting as mild microcytic hypochromic anemia.

- *Thalassemia major* results from the deletion of both β-globin genes. The fetus and newborn infant are normal, as γ-globin synthesis is unaffected and HbF contains α2γ2. As the postnatal switch from γ-chains to β-chains occurs, there is development of severe anemia with symptoms of pallor, growth retardation and hepatosplenomegaly due to extramedullary hematopoiesis. Typical morphology includes:
  - » microcytosis
  - » target cells
  - » poikilocytosis
  - » precipitation of excess α-globin aggregates visible on supravital stain
  - » the presence of nucleated red cells.

Diagnosis and treatment

Additional laboratory tests for the work-up of thalassemia include the quantification of HbF, HbA2 (α2δ2), Barts Hb (γ4) and HbH (β4) on Hb electrophoresis. Supravital stain demonstrates precipitated excess β-globin in HbH disease and hydrops fetalis, and excess α-globin in beta-thalassemia major.

Treatment of the thalassemias involves a red cell transfusion program and iron chelation.

Sideroblastic anemias

This group of disorders is characterized by the presence of at least 15% ring sideroblasts, which are erythroblasts that contain 5 or more perinuclear iron granules covering one-third or more of the nuclear circumference.

These anemias occur as inherited or acquired forms.

- Inherited sideroblastic anemias are either X-linked due to mutations in the delta-aminolevulinate synthase 2 (delta-ALAS2) locus or to mutation in the ATP-binding cassette transporter gene (*ABCB7*), or autosomal.

> ### CLINICAL PEARL
>
> Delta-aminolevulinate synthase 2 (delta-ALAS2) catalyzes heme biosynthesis and utilizes pyridoxal phosphate as a cofactor; hence anemia due to mutations in delta-ALAS2 is responsive to dietary supplementation with pyridoxine (vitamin B_6).

- » *ABCB7* mutations cause anemia and non-progressive cerebellar ataxia due to iron toxicity to neuronal mitochondria.
  - » Autosomal sideroblastic anemias result from mutations of several genes important in mitochondrial heme synthesis. One of the mutations is in the gene *SLC19A2* that encodes a thiamine transporter, and the anemia can respond to supplementation with excess thiamine.

- Refractory anemia with ring sideroblasts is an acquired sideroblastic anemia and a form of myelodysplasia. Causes of secondary sideroblastic anemias include:
  - » drugs (isoniazid, chloramphenicol)
  - » lead poisoning
  - » alcoholism with malnutrition.

Macrocytic anemias

Macrocytic anemias occur with or without features of abnormal megaloblastic maturation. The diagnosis of megaloblastic differentiation can only be made after visualization of erythroid precursors on a bone marrow biopsy, or in peripheral blood in the case of a leukoerythroblastic phenotype. Megaloblastic anemias are often due to cobalamin (vitamin B_{12}) and folate deficiencies; other causes of macrocytic anemia without megaloblastosis are hypothyroidism, liver disease, alcoholism, and myelodysplasia.

Peripheral blood findings in megaloblastic anemias (Figure 13-9, overleaf) are:

- ovalomacrocytes with MCV >100 f L

- considerable anisocytosis

- characteristic hypersegmentation of neutrophils (more than 5 lobes).

Leukopenia, thrombocytopenia and leukoerythroblastic appearance (Figure 13-10, overleaf) may also be noted.

Cobalamin (vitamin B_{12}) deficiency

Cobalamin deficiency results in neurological disturbances as well as hematological abnormalities, which distinguishes it from folate deficiency which has no neurological deficits. Neurological and hematological disturbances do not necessarily occur together, and patients may display neurological

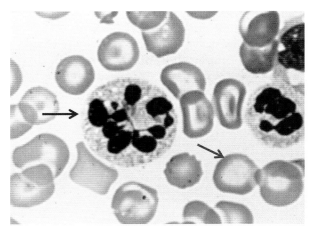

Figure 13-9 Blood film of megaloblastic anemia. The red arrow identifies a macrocyte and the blue arrow indicates hypersegmentation of a neutrophil

Teaching collection of Vicky Smith, ASH Image Bank 2014; 2014-16885. © 2014 American Society of Hematology

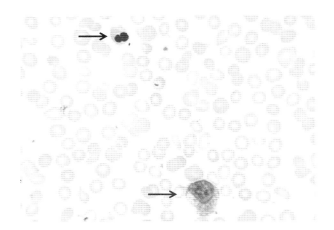

Figure 13-10 Blood film showing leukoerythroblastic features. The red arrow identifies a myelocyte and the blue arrow a nucleated red cell

Hussain Said Baden, ASH Image Bank 2011; 2011-3926. © 2011 American Society of Hematology.

manifestations in the absence of anemia. The physical examination and pathological findings include:

- peripheral neuropathy
- demyelination of the posterior columns and pyramidal tracts
- optic atrophy
- impaired cognition.

Typical symptoms include paresthesiae, weakness and gait disturbance.

Cobalamin metabolism

The obligatory requirement of cobalamin is 2.4 microg/day. The body stores 2–3 mg which is adequate for 3–4 years even if intake ceases. Vegetables and fruits do not contain cobalamin and the only available source is from food of animal origin. The highest concentration of cobalamin is in liver and kidney, and to a lesser extent in muscle meats and shellfish.

Cobalamin absorption proceeds through a number of discrete steps involving the requirement of cofactors and a functioning stomach and terminal ileum.

- Almost all cobalamin is actively absorbed via the terminal ileum in conjugation with intrinsic factor (IF). Passive absorption of oral cobalamin through the gastro-intestinal tract is less than 1%.
- The stomach is vital to cobalamin absorption through the secretion of free acid, pepsin and IF. Gastric acidity facilitates the release of cobalamin from food complexes, and free cobalamin binds with the 'R binder' secreted in the saliva. Pepsin produced in the stomach and duodenum releases cobalamin from the R-binder, and this conjugates with IF that is released by the parietal cells of the stomach.
- IF-bound cobalamin transits through the intestine. Epithelial cells in the terminal ileum contain receptors for IF–cobalamin complex that mediate transfer to the plasma, where it binds to the transport protein transcobalamin II (TCII). The TC–cobalamin complex binds to specific receptors present on the surface of target cells and is taken up into the lysosome; cobalamin is then released from TCII and transferred into the cytoplasm.

Cobalamin participates in two distinct cellular pathways, in the mitochondria and in the cytoplasm proper.

1. Within the mitochondria, cobalamin catalyzes the conversion of methylmalonyl-coenzyme A (CoA) to succinyl-CoA, which is an important intermediate in the Kreb's cycle for energy production.
2. In the cytoplasm, cobalamin is essential for the synthesis of homocysteine to methionine and the conversion of 5-methyl-tetrahydrofolate to tetrahydrofolate (THF). THF is then converted to 5,10-methylene-THF, which is important in DNA synthesis.

Bone marrow morphology in cobalamin deficiency

During normal erythroid development, nuclear maturation is seen as progressive condensation of the nucleus and then loss of the nucleus as the cytoplasm of the erythroid progenitors acquire Hb and differentiate to ultimately form reticulocytes that exit the bone marrow. The characteristic finding in cobalamin deficiency is dissociation between nuclear and cytoplasmic maturation in the erythroid progenitors. Nuclear maturation is delayed and the nucleus displays fine, dispersed chromatin ('open chromatin'), while cytoplasmic maturation and hemoglobinization proceed normally.

Other lineages are also affected, explaining the occurrence of pancytopenia. Metamyelocytes are typically large and abnormal, and megakaryocytes are also large and hyperpolyploid. Severe megaloblastic changes may be confused with acute erythroleukemia.

Etiology of cobalamin deficiency

Dietary cobalamin deficiency only occurs in strict vegans. Cobalamin deficiency in a non-vegetarian diet is almost always due to perturbations in the absorption process.

Pernicious anemia

This is an autoimmune disease in which autoantibodies directed against gastric parietal cells cause chronic atrophic gastritis and reduced secretion of IF, while anti-IF antibodies block IF function in B_{12} absorption. A familial predisposition exists for this condition.

Pernicious anemia may occur in association with other endocrine diseases such as Hashimoto's thyroiditis, vitiligo and Addison's disease. Pernicious anemia results in cobalamin deficiency by the process of neutralization of IF by autoantibodies, decreased IF production by gastric parietal cells, and atrophic gastritis produces gastric achlorhydria which impairs the release of dietary cobalamin from food complexes.

Chronic atrophic gastritis

This condition causes patchy gastritis extending from the antrum. The main consequence is decreased acid and pepsin production, which impairs the release of cobalamin from food complexes and also R-binder. There is no impairment of IF production.

Structural defects in the gastrointestinal tract

Partial or total gastrectomy, or resection of the terminal ileum, interrupts the cobalamin absorption pathway. Blind loops of bowel result in bacterial overgrowth and high cobalamin demand. Crohn's disease affecting the terminal ileum impairs IF–cobalamin absorption.

Tests for cobalamin deficiency

Once reduced levels of vitamin B_{12} are detected, quantification in the serum of autoantibodies toward parietal cells (present in almost 90% patients, but less specific for pernicious anemia) and IF (noted in approximately 55% cases, but more specific for pernicious anemia) should be performed. This will detect the vast majority of autoimmune cases of cobalamin deficiency.

Treatment of cobalamin deficiency

Parenteral (intramuscular) replacement is effective. Tissue stores are replenished with the administration of 250–1000 microgram of cobalamin on alternate days for 1–2 weeks and then 250 microgram weekly until blood counts are normal. Maintenance may require lifelong supplementation of 1000 microgram every 2–3 months.

Folate deficiency

Folate deficiency results in megaloblastic anemia but without the neurological complications seen with cobalamin deficiency. Treatment of cobalamin deficiency with folate supplementation only may transiently improve the blood parameters but neurological deficits will continue to worsen.

The daily folate requirement is about 100 microgram, with total body stores being 10 mg. Hence, malnutrition that causes folate deficiency occurs far earlier than cobalamin deficiency.

- Fresh fruit and vegetables are a good source of folate, but cooking can destroy biologically active folate.
- Folates are absorbed through the small bowel, with the upper jejunum demonstrating the most capacity.

Folate is needed for synthesis of thymidine (a DNA nucleotide). Drugs such as methotrexate inhibit dihydrofolate reductase and disrupt the role of folate in thymidine synthesis.

Etiology of folate deficiency

Common causes include:

- *Nutritional*—total cessation of folate intake will deplete stores within 3–6 months, and poor diet is a common precipitant of folate deficiency. Fresh food is relatively expensive, and the poor and aged are particularly susceptible. Other at-risk groups are those with poor dentition and alcoholics.
- *Malabsorption*—celiac disease, tropical sprue, Crohn's disease, extensive jejunal resection.
- *Increased demand*—pregnancy, prematurity, chronic hemolysis (folate is not completely re-utilized and is lost in excretion).
- *Anti-folate drugs*—methotrexate, trimethoprim, phenytoin, barbiturates.

Investigation of folate deficiency

This requires measurement of serum and red cell folate. Serum folate levels are altered by recent diet and blood should be drawn for testing before nutritional correction.

CLINICAL PEARL

Red cell folate reflects tissue stores better than serum folate and is not altered by recent diet.

Treatment of folate deficiency

Oral supplementation with 5 mg folic acid daily for 4 months is effective.

Hemolytic anemias

Hemolytic anemias are classifiable as *hereditary* or *acquired*, and also as *extracorpuscular* or *intracorpuscular*, based on the site of the lesion (Table 13-15, overleaf).

Features of hemolysis

- In hemolytic anemias due to membrane defects, hemolysis is extravascular and takes place in the liver and spleen, mediated by the reticuloendothelial tissues.
- During intravascular hemolysis, free Hb is released into the plasma that is filtered by the urine as hemoglobinuria and hemosiderinuria. A portion is bound to plasma albumin as methemalbuminemia.

Anemias due to enzyme defects

- Red cells need to generate energy to maintain the integrity of the cell membrane and for the proper functioning

Table 13-15 Classification of hemolytic anemias

Intracorpuscular	1. Abnormalities within cytoplasm	Hereditary
	—Enzyme defects	
	—Hemoglobinopathies	
	2. Cell membrane abnormalities (extravascular)	
	—Hereditary spherocytosis	
	—Paroxysmal nocturnal hemoglobinuria	Acquired
Extracorpuscular	—Spur cell anemia	
	3. Extrinsic causes	
	—Immune hemolysis	
	—Microangiopathic hemolysis	
	—Hypersplenism	

of the ion channels. Red cells can only produce ATP by anerobic glycolysis, as they lack mitochondria.

- A reducing capacity is also necessary to counteract oxidative stress and to reduce methemoglobin to deoxy-hemoglobin with the capacity to bind oxygen.

Reduced nicotinamide adenine dinucleotide (NADH) produced from NAD as a part of the glycolytic pathway reduces methemoglobin. The pentose phosphate pathway and the glutathione cycle linked with the glycolytic pathway generates reduced nicotinamide adenine dinucleotide phosphate (NADPH) and glutathione (GSH) to provide the reducing capacity to detoxify free oxygen radicals and hydrogen peroxide.

Pyruvate kinase deficiency

Pyruvate kinase (PK) catalyzes the conversion of phospho-enolpyruvate to pyruvate, associated with the generation of ATP. There are two genes which produce four types of PK in different tissues (e.g. PKR in red cells).

- PK deficiency presents as an autosomal recessive disorder with a prevalence of 50 per million.
- It leads to impairment of ATP production and accumulation of upstream intermediates such as 2,3-diphosphoglycerate (2,3-DPG). The increased concentration of 2,3-DPG reduces the oxygen affinity of Hb, thereby permitting greater delivery of oxygen to the metabolizing tissues even in the presence of anemia.
- The severity of the phenotype and the age of onset of manifestation varies.

The common phenotype is chronic non-spherocytic hemolysis.

- Jaundice may be noted, gallstones are frequent, and spleen size correlates with severity of hemolysis.
- Laboratory features are anemia in the absence of spherocytes, reticulocytosis and crenated cells. Typical features of spur cells and acanthocytes become prominent post splenectomy. Demonstration of low red cell PK

establishes the diagnosis. Elevated levels of 2,3-DPG can be indicative.

Anemia can be well tolerated due to the shift in oxygen affinity of Hb. Chronic and symptomatic hemolysis may be managed with splenectomy. Folic acid supplementation is recommended to compensate for the increased requirement.

Glucose-6-phosphate dehydrogenase deficiency

Glucose-6-phosphate dehydrogenase (G6PD) catalyzes the conversion of glucose-6-phosphate to 6-phosphogluconate with the generation of NADPH and, subsequently, glutathione (GSH).

- G6PD is an essential component of all cells, although deficiency causes only a red cell phenotype with a rare abnormality of leukocyte function.
- There are more than 100 mutants known, and the most common consequence is an alteration in RNA stability. As a result, reticulocytes have high amounts of G6PD, which decrease with red cell aging.
- G6PD deficiency is prevalent in the Mediterranean areas, Africa, the Middle East, Southeast Asia and the Indian subcontinent. The high prevalence of mutations correlates with regions where *Plasmodium falciparum* is endemic, as G6PD deficiency offers protection from lethal malaria.

Clinical presentation

Glucose-6-phosphate dehydrogenase deficiency is an X-linked disease with manifestation in males. Heterozygous females remain susceptible to oxidative stress. Patients with G6PD may present with four syndromes:

1. neonatal jaundice
2. favism—hemolysis is precipitated by exposure to fava (broad) beans
3. chronic non-spherocytic hemolytic anemia
4. drug-induced hemolysis.

Table 13-16 World Health Organization classification of G6PD deficiency

CLASS	ENZYME ACTIVITY (% OF NORMAL)	CLINICAL CHARACTERISTICS
I	<2	Chronic non-spherocytic hemolytic anemia
II	<10	Favism Severe episodic drug-induced hemolysis Neonatal jaundice
III	10–60	Episodic drug-induced hemolysis Neonatal jaundice
IV	100	None
G6PD, glucose-6-phosphate dehydrogenase.		

Table 13-17 Agents that precipitate hemolysis in G6PD deficiency*

CLASS	AGENTS
Antimalarials	Primaquine, chloroquine, mepacrine
Antibiotics	Sulfonamides, co-trimoxazole, dapsone, chloramphenicol, nitrofurantoin, naladixic acid
Antihelminths	B-naphthol, stibophan, niridazole
Analgesics	Aspirin, phenacetin
Other drugs	Sulfasalazine, phenothiazines, vitamin K, vitamin C (high doses), hydralazine, procainamide
Chemicals	Naphthalene (mothballs), methylene blue
Foods	Raw fava beans (broad beans)

*The drugs listed are representative examples and not a complete list. Many other drugs produce hemolysis in particular individuals.
G6PD, glucose-6-phosphate dehydrogenase.

G6PD deficiency is classified as shown in Table 13–16, and agents that precipitate hemolysis are described in Table 13–17.

Diagnosis

Blood films reveal 'ghost', 'blister' or 'bite' cells, with evidence of biochemical parameters of hemolysis. Quantification of G6PD enzyme activity establishes the diagnosis. Older red cells are more susceptible to oxidative stress.

CLINICAL PEARL

Reticulocytes contain higher levels of glucose-6-phosphate dehydrogenase, and testing for this enzyme may yield false-normal results if the test is done during the early period of recovery when reticulocyte counts are high.

Structural hemoglobin variants causing hemolysis

Unstable hemoglobins

These are a result of mutations that cause structural changes in the hemoglobin molecule that lead to intracellular precipitation and spleen-mediated removal of affected red cells.

- The clinical presentation is that of chronic hemolytic anemia with splenomegaly.
- Heinz bodies are present.
- Testing for instability at high temperatures confirms diagnosis.
- Splenectomy and blood transfusions may be needed in severe cases.

Sickle cell disease

This is the first disorder to be characterized at the molecular level.

- It results from a single substitution of valine for glutamic acid in the 6th amino acid position of the β-globin hemoglobin chain; the resultant hemoglobin is denoted by HbS.
- Deoxygenated HbS leads to exposure of a hydrophobic area on the β-globin surface that binds to hydrophobic patches on other β-globin molecules, ultimately causing polymerization.
- Acidosis and elevated 2,3-DPG levels promote polymerization by reducing the affinity for oxygen binding. The presence of HbA and HbF inhibits polymerization by diluting the HbS, and also because of amino acid differences between HbS and HbF.

Sickle cell disease has a high prevalence in regions endemic for *Plasmodium falciparum*, including Africa, Mediterranean countries, Saudi Arabia and India.

Clinical manifestations

Clinical syndromes associated with HbS are:

- anemia
- vaso–occlusive crisis

- impaired growth and development
- infections (pneumococcal, *Haemophilus*, *Salmonella*)
- neurological events (cerebral infarction and hemorrhage)
- acute chest syndrome (due to vaso-occlusion, infection and fat embolization)
- renal complications (papillary necrosis, loss of concentration capacity)
- priapism (vaso-occlusion of the corpora cavernosa)
- bone complications (bone infarction, avascular necrosis)
- leg ulcers
- ocular complications (vaso-occlusion is typical in the variant HbSC disease).

Diagnosis

Peripheral blood reveals:

- polychromasia
- nucleated red cells
- Howell–Jolly bodies
- sickled red cells.

Diagnosis is established by hemoglobin electrophoresis. Prenatal diagnosis is available by direct detection of the mutation in fetal cells.

Management

Good care involves a multidisciplinary approach in a specialized center. The cornerstones of care include:

- blood transfusion
- rapid treatment of infections
- pain relief.

CLINICAL PEARLS

- In sickle cell disease, hydroxyurea therapy increases HbF levels and leads to a significant reduction in acute chest syndrome, vaso-occlusive crises, and transfusion requirements.
- Hemopoietic stem cell transplantation using a matched sibling donor is used for subgroups with high risk of severe disease.

Variants of sickle cell syndromes

1 **Sickle cell trait**—generally there is no hematological manifestation; impairment of urine-concentrating function and splenic infarction (at high altitudes) can occur. Sickling and vaso-occlusive crisis can be precipitated in young athletes.

2 **HbSC disease**—a compound heterozygous state in African patients due to high prevalence of HbC. Proliferative retinopathy is present at very high incidences. Vaso-occlusive crises and splenic infarctions also occur.

3 **Sickle cell beta-thalassemia**—a compound heterozygote state with a mild phenotype that correlates with the relative amounts of HbA and HbS.

4 **Sickle cell hereditary persistence of HbF**—elevated HbF levels inhibit HbS polymerization and the clinical course is benign.

Anemias with hereditary red cell membrane abnormalities

The red cell membrane is a lipid bilayer in close association with cellular proteins. There are two types of membrane–protein interactions:

1 membrane-integral proteins such as ion channels (band 3), which interact with each other and also with the second group of proteins

2 proteins that form the cytoskeleton (α- and β-spectrin).

Ankyrin is a protein that bridges β-spectrin to band 3. Mutations of the integral proteins usually result in spherocytosis, while abnormalities of the cytoskeletal proteins cause elliptocytosis and other abnormalities. Gallstones (pigment stones) are also frequent and cause episodes of cholecystitis and biliary colic.

Hereditary spherocytosis

This is a chronic hemolytic anemia with an autosomal dominant inheritance.

- It is characterized by the presence of spherocytes on peripheral blood examination and evidence of jaundice.
- The clinical phenotype may vary, and anemia is exacerbated by coincident viral or bacterial infections. Parvovirus infections can precipitate severe anemia due to marked inhibition of erythropoiesis.
- Splenomegaly is common, since the spleen is the site for the removal of spherocytes.

Diagnosis is made by family history, blood film examination (Figure 13-11) and the eosin-5′-maleimide (EMA) binding test, which is a flow cytometric test. EMA binds to plasma

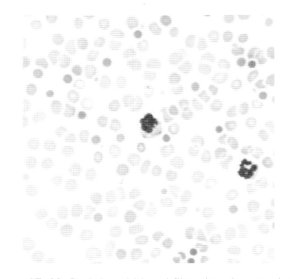

Figure 13-11 Peripheral blood film showing marked spherocytosis, including microspherocytic cells

From Hoffbrand AV, Pettit JE and Vyas P. Color atlas of clinical hematology, 4th edn. Philadelphia: Elsevier, 2010.

membrane proteins of red blood cells, mainly to band 3 protein. In hereditary spherocytosis, the mean fluorescence of EMA-stained RBCs is lower when compared with control RBCs due to the decreased amount of target proteins.

Splenectomy is indicated for chronic symptomatic hemolysis but carries an early risk of precipitating thrombosis and a long-term risk of sepsis with encapsulated microorganisms. Folate supplementation is also recommended to keep up with the increased requirements in chronic hemolysis.

Hereditary elliptocytosis and pyropoikilocytosis

These are less common than hereditary spherocytosis. Diagnosis is suspected on the basis of distinct red cell morphology. Folate supplementation and splenectomy are useful in severe cases.

Immune hemolytic anemias

In this group of disorders, antibodies recognize and bind to antigens on the surface of red cells.

The site of hemolysis is mainly extravascular:

- splenic macrophages bear receptors for the Fc portion of the IgG and bind and opsonize IgG–coated red cells
- complement-coated red cells are mainly destroyed in the liver, as liver macrophages recognize the complement component C3b.

Hemolysis can be intravascular if the antibodies fix complement avidly and generate the membrane attack complex. Antibodies are defined as *autoantibodies* when formed by the patient and directed against self-antigens, or *alloantibodies* when produced by the patient to recognize antigens on foreign cells. Hemolysis after incompatible blood transfusion is an example of an alloantibody destroying transfused donor red cells.

Autoimmune hemolytic anemia (AIHA)

Autoimmune hemolytic anemia may be:

- idiopathic or
- secondary to:
  - » another immune disease (e.g. SLE)
  - » hematological malignancies (e.g. CLL)
  - » drug exposure.

Antibodies are classified based on the optimal temperature at which they recognize the antigen (37°C, warm; 4°C, cold), and on whether IgG or IgM is involved.

Diagnosis of AIHA

- Biochemical evidence of hemolysis
- Peripheral blood film reveals spherocytes and polychromasia (reticulocytosis)
- Nucleated red cells may be noted if the hemolysis is particularly brisk

Additional disease-specific features may be present (e.g. lymphocytosis in CLL, or lymphoma cells in circulation; Table 13-18). A key diagnostic aid is the DAT (also called the Coombs test). This test detects antibody and/or complement components that are already present on red cell surfaces. The

Table 13-18 Etiology of autoimmune hemolytic anemia

ETIOLOGY	DISEASES
Idiopathic	None
Autoimmune	Systemic lupus erythematosus (SLE), rheumatoid arthritis, ulcerative colitis
Lymphoproliferative disorders	Lymphoma, chronic lymphocytic leukemia (CLL)
Infections	Hepatitis C, human immunodeficiency virus
Drugs	Cephalosporins, methyldopa

indirect Coombs test is used in blood cross-matching, as it detects antibodies in recipient serum that have the capacity to recognize donor red cells.

Warm-type AIHA

- Antibodies are usually polyclonal, of the IgG subtype, and react at 37°C. Antibodies are 'pan-reactive', i.e. react with nonspecific antigen specificity. Rhesus antigen-specific antibodies are noted in 10–15% of cases.
- Approximately 30% cases of warm AIHA are idiopathic.
- The highest frequency is in early childhood, with a second peak in the 3rd decade.
- The tempo of presentation may vary, but it is often insidious.
  - » Tiredness and dark urine may be the only symptoms. Pallor, jaundice and mild splenomegaly are often the only signs in idiopathic AIHA.
  - » Hemolysis secondary to other diseases may be accompanied by signs specific to that condition (e.g. lymphadenopathy in CLL, or arthritis and rash with SLE).
- Corticosteroids are first-line treatment in warm AIHA. Most patients respond initially, but only 15–20% may remain in long-term remission. Steroids should be tapered off slowly to prevent relapse.
  - » Azathioprine and cyclophosphamide are added as steroid-sparing drugs. Other immunomodulators include cyclosporin (ciclosporin) and mycophenolate mofetil.
- Splenectomy is an option for resistant cases and those dependent on high-dose steroids. One-third of patients remain in remission; in another third the dose of steroids can be significantly reduced, with the remaining third showing transient or no response.

Cold-type AIHA

These disorders are etiologically grouped as:

1 **Cold hemagglutinin disease (CHAD).** Idiopathic CHAD comprises 15% of cases and is due to a IgM

antibody directed against 'I' antigen. Hemolysis worsens at cold temperatures. Typically, there is acrocyanosis due to sluggish circulation in the extremities, caused by red cell agglutination. Blood films reveal gross hemagglutination. DAT is positive only for complement, as IgM elutes from the cell surface leaving C3d behind.

2 **Secondary cold agglutinin syndromes.** May be associated with lymphoproliferative disorders (monoclonal IgM or IgG against antigen 'I' or 'i'), or with infections such as *Mycoplasma pneumoniae* and infectious mononucleosis (polyclonal against 'I'). Antibodies are produced as a consequence of the infection and cross-react against red cells.

3 **Paroxysmal cold hemoglobinuria.** This is a disease of children following viral infections. The presentation is acute with abdominal pain, pallor and dark urine. The disease occurs when a polyclonal antibody reacts against 'P' antigen. The antibody is biphasic, binding red cells at 20°C, and fixing complement and causing complement-mediated hemolysis at 37°C. The disease is usually self-limiting; it is important to maintain warmth.

Treatment of idiopathic and secondary cold agglutinin disease is difficult; remaining in a warm environment is important.

- Corticosteroids are generally ineffective.
- Chlorambucil may be useful in the setting of lymphoproliferative disorder. Idiopathic CHAD is particularly resistant to treatment and chlorambucil is commonly ineffective.
- Blood transfusions should only be given using an in-line blood warmer.
- Rituximab therapy has shown promise in early studies.

CLINICAL PEARL

Splenectomy in secondary cold agglutinin syndromes is ineffective, as hemolysis takes place in the liver via recognition of C3d on red cells.

Drug-induced hemolysis

There are four pathogenetic mechanisms underlying drug-induced hemolysis.

1 **Drug adsorption.** The typical drug implicated is penicillin; in high doses, penicillin adsorbs on the surface of red cells by nonspecific interaction with membrane proteins. Patients may develop high-titer anti-penicillin IgG antibodies that bind to red cell surfaces and cause extravascular hemolysis.

2 **Immune-complex mechanism.** This is seen with 3rd-generation cephalosporins and rifampin (rifampicin). The drugs interact with plasma proteins, and antibodies are formed against the hapten–carrier complex. Hemolysis typically occurs after the second or third drug exposure.

3 **Membrane-modification mechanism.** Cephalosporins and carboplatin are examples of drugs that bind to red cell membranes and modify them so that immunoglobulins, complement components and plasma proteins bind nonspecifically. Hemolysis is uncommon.

4 **Autoimmune mechanism.** This is typically seen with methyldopa after 6 weeks. IgG antibodies are raised, causing extravascular hemolysis.

Non-immune acquired hemolytic anemias (DAT negative)

These occur secondary to diverse conditions that include:

1 **Infections:** malaria (intracellular organism causing hemolysis), meningococcal sepsis (toxin-mediated DIC), mycobacteria (activation of hemophagocytosis).

2 **Mechanical fragmentation:** thrombotic thrombocytopenic purpura (shear in fibrin-occluded microcirculation), perivalvular leak (due to shear), march hemoglobinuria (mechanical shearing).

3 **Acquired membrane modifications:** paroxysmal nocturnal hemoglobinuria (somatic mutation causing failure of complement-regulatory mechanisms, leading to sensitivity to complement-mediated lysis by formation of a membrane attack complex), liver disease (acanthocytes due to modification of red cell membrane by lipids and cholesterol changes).

4 **Chemicals and physical agents:** drugs (oxidative damage), drowning (osmotic stress), burns (heat trauma).

ACKNOWLEDGMENT

We acknowledge and thank Dr. Harshal Nandurkar who was a contributing author to this chapter in the third edition.

SELF-ASSESSMENT QUESTIONS

1   A 70-year-old woman presents to her family physician for an annual health check. Routine full blood count reveals hemoglobin 125 g/L (reference range [RR] 115–165), white cell count 23.5×10^9/L (RR 4.0–11.0) with differential of neutrophils 7.0×10^9/L (RR 2.0–7.5), lymphocytes 15.0×10^9/L (RR 1.5–4.0), normal numbers of monocytes, eosinophils and basophils, and platelets 395×10^9/L (RR 150–400). Blood film findings report the presence of 'smear cells'. She has no particular symptoms. Clinical examination does not identify any lymphadenopathy or hepatosplenomegaly. Routine biochemical tests, including lactate dehydrogenase, are within normal limits. Which of the following is the best next step in her management?

   A   Request serological evidence for infectious mononucleosis.
   B   Arrange for bone marrow biopsy to confirm lymphoma/leukemia.
   C   Verify the presence of abdominal lymphadenopathy by computed tomography (CT).
   D   Request peripheral blood flow cytometry.
   E   Arrange a time to discuss chemotherapy options.

2   A 78-year-old male of Italian descent complains of fatigue that has developed over the past few months. On inquiry, he admits to 'some' weight loss but his diet has not been optimal in the past 3–4 months. He takes low-dose aspirin for previous ischemic heart disease and occasional naproxen 500 mg tablets for arthralgia. He has no complaints of dyspepsia. The patient has commenced taking laxatives to maintain bowel regularity. Preliminary tests by his family physician reveal hemoglobin (Hb) 70 g/L (reference range [RR] 130–180), mean cell volume 68 fL (RR 80–98), with normal white cell count and platelet numbers. Blood film comments are of 'hypochromia, microcytosis and pencil cells'. Urea and electrolytes are not perturbed but liver function tests reveal elevation in gamma-glutamyl transpeptidase (GGT) and alkaline phosphatase (ALP) to three times the upper limit of the normal range. The full blood examination and biochemical parameters were normal when last tested 4 years previously as a part of a general check-up. Which of the following is the best next step?

   A   Correct anemia with oral iron supplementation or intravenous iron infusion, followed by regular follow-up to confirm improvement.
   B   Anemia is due to aspirin and naproxen use and these should be discontinued and proton-pump inhibitors commenced.
   C   Refer him for gastroscopy and colonoscopy.
   D   His Mediterranean heritage and hypochromic microcytic anemia are suggestive of thalassemia and should be confirmed with Hb electrophoresis.
   E   Anemia is due to liver abnormalities, so patient should be advised to cease alcohol intake.

3   A 24-year-old woman is experiencing heavy menstrual bleeding and easy bruising. Her younger sister and mother also give similar histories. She is constantly tired and this is interfering with her training for a triathlon. Her medications include the oral contraceptive pill, an iron supplement, non-steroidal anti-inflammatory drugs (NSAIDs) 2–3 times per week for musculoskeletal pain from endurance training, and over-the-counter multivitamin preparations. She has developed a ligament tear after a fall from her bike and knee arthroscopy needs to be performed. A coagulation screen prior to arthroscopy reveals activated partial thromboplastin time (APTT) 50 seconds (reference range [RR] 27–38), international normalized ratio (INR) 1.2 (RR 0.8–1.2), and normal thrombin time and plasma fibrinogen levels. Further preoperative coagulation tests are performed. Mixing with normal plasma corrects APTT and the factor VIII level is 35% (RR 50–150). Factors IX, XI and XII are normal. The patient wishes to proceed with the arthroscopy and ligament repair as soon as possible. Which of the following is the most correct statement?

   A   Menorrhagia and prolonged APTT are because of the anti-platelet effects of NSAIDs. Arthroscopy should proceed after suspension of NSAIDs for 1 week.
   B   The most likely interpretation is the presence of lupus anticoagulant causing coagulopathy leading to menorrhagia and prolongation of APTT.
   C   She should be investigated for von Willebrand's disease.
   D   Low factor VIII levels make mild hemophilia A the likely diagnosis, and arthroscopy can proceed with factor VIII supplementation.
   E   Coagulopathy will always remain a contraindication to arthroscopy.

4   A 70-year-old man is on warfarin for non-valvular atrial fibrillation as his $CHADS_2$ score is 4. He is brought to the emergency department with bruising over his right hip after a fall from a three-step ladder. There is some suspicion of head trauma from the fall, although there is no obvious scalp discoloration or tenderness and no symptoms of any change in consciousness. There is no clinical suspicion of deep-tissue hematoma or anatomical derangement of the affected hip. He is otherwise well and has no other complaints. He adheres to his warfarin intake, and frequency of international normalized ratio (INR) monitoring is once every 4 weeks. Tests in the emergency department reveal INR 5.0 (reference range 0.8–1.2), consistent with warfarin effect. The best approach to correct the coagulopathy will be:

   A   Withhold next dose of warfarin and recommence at a lower dose.
   B   Warfarin continuation will be contraindicated in the future due to this fall.
   C   Aspirin is the preferred drug to prevent stroke in his case, as he is at high risk of warfarin-associated bleeding.
   D   Warfarin effect should be reversed with vitamin K.
   E   Warfarin effect should be reversed with prothrombin complex concentrates.

5 A 68-year-old man presents with pleuritic chest pain and shortness of breath developing after a 90-minute flight. He has symptoms of dry cough and runny nose without fevers in the preceding 3 days. He had partial colectomy for cancer 2 years ago and is currently on chemotherapy for new hepatic metastasis. He has complained of a sore right calf for the past week but attributed it to his cycling sessions on a stationary bike at home which he has commenced to remain fit while on chemotherapy. He is known to have prior smoking-related chronic obstructive pulmonary disease (COPD) requiring bronchodilator therapy. Clinical examination reveals a swollen right calf with mild pedal edema, mild wheeze, a pulse rate of 100/min (regular) and normal blood pressure. Which of the following is the most correct statement?

A Pulmonary embolism is likely, caused by his plane flight.
B Pulmonary embolism is likely, provoked by his malignancy.
C Pneumothorax is likely, due to the COPD and the plane flight.
D Respiratory tract infection is the most likely explanation for his pleuritic pain and preceding cough.
E Pre-test probability for venous thromboembolism is low, and another diagnosis such as lung metastasis should be considered.

6 A 30-year-old male presents with fatigue and unexplained weight loss of 2−3 kg over 4 months. Full blood examination reveals white cell count 68×10^9/L (reference range [RR] 4.0−11.0), hemoglobin 160 g/L (RR 130−180) and platelets 600×10^9/L (RR 150−400). Blood film reveals a left shift with the presence of numerous myelocytes, metamyelocytes and basophils. Blasts were not present. Clinical examination reveals palpable splenomegaly, 1 cm below the costal margin. Subsequent cytogenetic studies reveal the presence of the Philadelphia chromosome. Which of the following is the most correct statement?

A The most likely diagnosis is essential thrombocytosis as evidenced by the high platelet count.
B Philadelphia chromosome is detected on karyotypic analysis as the t(15;17) translocation.
C Philadelphia chromosome leads to the generation of an aberrant *BCR-ABL* fusion protein.
D Philadelphia chromosome leads to over-expression of the ABL tyrosine kinase by the promoter effects of the *BCR* gene.
E The patient will require regular bone marrow biopsies for the karyotype assessment of the Philadelphia chromosome to monitor response to therapy.

7 A 72-year-old woman is noted to have comments of 'rouleaux' on a blood film performed as part of a routine check-up. Further investigations reveal normal full blood examination, electrolytes, renal function and calcium levels. A monoclonal IgG (kappa) paraprotein of 5.5 g/L is noted on serum electrophoresis. There is no immune paresis, and serum free light chains were absent. She is asymptomatic. Which of the following is the most correct statement?

A Bone marrow biopsy should be organized to consider a diagnosis of myeloma.
B Magnetic resonance imaging of the spine is indicated to look for bone lesions.
C Bisphosphonate therapy should be commenced for protection from bone fractures.
D She is at an increased risk of recurrent infections.
E The risk of progression is low, approximately 1% annually.

8 A 28-year-old female presents with symptoms of hallucinations, fever and rash developing over 5 days. Examination reveals bruises at multiple sites. There is no arthritis. Tests reveal hemoglobin 99 g/L (reference range [RR] 115−165), normal mean cell volume, normal white cell count and platelets 80×10^9/L (RR 150−400). A blood film reveals schistocytes. Biochemical tests indicate acute renal failure. International normalized ratio, activated partial prothrombin time, fibrinogen and liver function tests are normal. The most likely diagnosis is:

A Thrombotic thrombocytopenic purpura
B Idiopathic thrombocytopenic purpura
C Disseminated intravascular coagulation
D HELLP syndrome
E IgA vasculitis (Henoch-Schönlein purpura)

9 A 55-year-old woman presents with tiredness. She is jaundiced on examination and there is no lymphadenopathy or hepatosplenomegaly. Full blood examination (FBE) reveals hemoglobin 80 g/L (reference range [RR] 115−165), mean cell volume 101 fL (RR 80−98), and normal white cell count and platelets. A blood film reveals the presence of spherocytes and polychromasia. Coagulation tests are normal. She has recently returned from a trip to India and took malarial prophylaxis. An incidental FBE 5 years ago was completely normal. The most correct of the following statements is:

A A direct antiglobulin test (DAT, also known as a direct Coombs test) should be performed.
B The presence of anemia and the history of a trip to India makes malaria very likely despite prophylaxis.
C The most likely diagnosis is hereditary spherocytosis.
D Drug-induced oxidative hemolysis secondary to malaria prophylaxis is most likely.
E Reticulocytopenia is an expected finding.

10 A 60-year-old male is admitted with pneumonia and sepsis requiring intravenous antibiotics. During admission he develops an acute coronary syndrome and is commenced on an unfractionated heparin infusion. Development of thrombocytopenia is noted 2 days after the commencement of heparin. Platelet nadir is 80×10^9/L, from a previously normal platelet count of 280×10^9/L (reference range 150−400). The patient develops deep vein thrombosis (DVT) despite the heparin infusion. He discloses a history of unfractionated heparin given for thromboprophylaxis three weeks ago for an elective arthroscopy. Which of the following statements is the most correct?

A   Thrombocytopenia is due to idiopathic thrombocytopenic purpura (ITP).
B   Unfractionated heparin should be immediately replaced by low-molecular-weight heparin (LMWH).
C   Drug-induced thrombocytopenia secondary to antibiotics is the most likely explanation.
D   The presence of DVT requires commencement of warfarin anticoagulation as soon as possible.
E   Heparin-induced thrombocytopenia (HIT) is likely despite the thrombocytopenia developing only 2 days after heparin therapy.

11 A 32-year-old female presents with a headache and right upper quadrant abdominal pain at 36 weeks gestation. This is her first pregnancy and she is taking folic acid supplementation. On examination, the blood pressure is 150/100 and pulse rate 100 bpm. She is afebrile and the respiratory rate is 18. The neurological examination is normal. There is bilateral lower limb pitting edema. Laboratory studies show: hemoglobin 110 g/L (reference range [RR] 115−165), white cell count 13.5 × 10^9/L (RR 4.0−11.0 × 10^9/L), platelets 50 × 10^9/L (RR 150−400), alanine aminotransferase 60 U/L (RR 0−35 U/L), aspartate aminotransferase 65 U/L (RR 0−35 U/L), creatinine 100 micromol/L (RR 61.9−115 micromol/L) and urinalysis shows 3+ protein. The peripheral blood film shows the presence of schistocytes. Which of the following is the most appropriate management?

A   Plasma exchange
B   Eculizumab
C   Emergency delivery
D   Intravenous immunoglobulin
E   Dexamethasone

12 A 25-year-old male presents to the emergency department with a 3-day history of mild shortness of breath and right-sided chest pain. He takes no medications and is otherwise well apart from anxiety related to upcoming university examinations. On examination, the respiratory rate is 14 breaths per minute and pulse rate 65 beats per minute. The oxygen saturation is 99% on room air, the chest X-ray is clear, and an ECG and full blood count are both normal. The pulmonary embolism rule-out criteria (PERC) for pulmonary embolism is zero.

Which of the following is the most appropriate diagnostic step?

A   CT pulmonary angiogram
B   Ventilation-perfusion scan
C   No further testing required
D   D-dimer
E   Echocardiogram

13 A 76-year-old woman taking dabigatran for prevention of systemic embolism from non-valvular atrial fibrillation presents with a 48-hour history of macroscopic hematuria. Her last dose of dabigatran was about 4 hours before presentation. On examination, the blood pressure was 130/85 with no postural drop and pulse rate 80 bpm. The urine sample shows blood. The activated partial thromboplastin time is 60 s (RR 27−38 s); prothrombin time 13 s (RR 11−13 s); hemoglobin 125 g/L (RR 115−165); creatinine 90 micromol/L and urinalysis shows pH 5.5; 4+ blood; no protein, no casts and no dysmorphic erythrocytes. You cease the dabigatran.

Which of the following is the most appropriate next management step?

A   Fresh frozen plasma
B   Observation
C   Idarucizumab
D   Prothrombinex
E   Andexanet alfa

14 A 70-year-old man presents to the emergency department with progressive shortness of breath and hypoxia 1 week after undergoing surgery for adenocarcinoma of the colon. He has liver metastases and is due for adjuvant chemotherapy. On examination, his pulse rate is 100 bpm and his oxygen saturation is 90% on room air. A CT pulmonary angiogram shows a right lower lobe pulmonary embolus. Which of the following is the most appropriate treatment?

A   Rivaroxaban
B   Dabigatran
C   Apixaban
D   Warfarin
E   Enoxaparin

15 A 25-year-old man with a background history of sickle cell disease presents to the emergency department with a 3-day history of increasing shortness of breath and fatigue. His current medications are hydroxyurea and folic acid. On examination, he is afebrile, the pulse rate is 120 beats per minute and the respiratory rate is 28 breaths per minute. The spleen is not palpable. The oxygen saturation is 95% and CXR normal. Laboratory studies show: hemoglobin 35 g/L (RR 130−180 g/L), white cell count 12 × 10^9/L (RR 4.0−11.0 × 10^9/L), platelet count 450 × 10^9/L (RR 150−400), reticulocyte count 0.1% (0.5−1.5%).

The most likely diagnosis is:

A   Hemolytic crisis
B   Aplastic anemia
C   Acute sequestration crisis
D   Parvovirus B19 infection
E   Vaso-occlusive crisis

16 A 72-year-old female presents to your clinic for follow-up 1 week after discharge from hospital with a stroke. She has a past medical history of hypercholesterolemia and type 2 diabetes mellitus. Her current medications are aspirin, metformin and atorvastatin. A full blood count showed: hemoglobin 120 g/L ([RR 115−165), white cell count 10.5 × 10⁹/L (RR 4.0−11.0 × 10⁹/L), platelets 850 × 10⁹/L (RR 150−400). Mutation testing of JAK2, MPL and CALR genes was negative and BCR-ABL transcripts were negative. A bone marrow biopsy showed increased numbers of large megakaryocytes, some in clumps. Iron stores were normal.

Which of the following is the most appropriate management?

A Hydroxyurea
B Clopidogrel
C No change
D Change aspirin to clopidogrel
E Anagrelide

17 A 29-year-old female presents to the emergency department with nausea, menorrhagia and vomiting. She had been previously well. On examination, she was afebrile and the blood pressure was 170/120. Laboratory studies showed: hemoglobin 70 g/L (RR 110−150), platelets 75 × 10⁹/L (RR 150−400), reticulocytes 4.8% (RR 0.5−1.5%), lactate dehydrogenase 1646 U/L (RR 120−250), direct antiglobulin test negative, creatinine 350 micromol/L (RR 61.9−115 micromol/L), ADAMTS13 level 78% (RR 40−130), and stool Shiga toxin negative. The peripheral blood film showed schistocytes.

Which of the following is the most appropriate management?

A Plasma exchange
B High-dose corticosteroids
C Rituximab
D Eculizumab
E Cyclophosphamide

18 A 33-year-old female presents to the emergency department with fever and easy bruising. She has been feeling generally unwell for a few weeks with malaise and anorexia; however, over the last 48 hours she has developed fever and rigors. She takes no regular medications. On examination, the temperature is 39°C, blood pressure 100/60, pulse rate 100 beats per minute, and respiratory rate 28 breaths per minute. There are bruises over the abdomen and limbs, and petechiae on both legs. There is no lymphadenopathy and no hepatomegaly or splenomegaly. Laboratory studies show: hemoglobin 90 g/L (RR 110−150), white cell count 3 × 10⁹/L (RR 4.0−11.0 × 10⁹/L), with 30% neutrophils, 30% lymphocytes, 15% monocytes, 5% band neutrophils, and 20% atypical cells. The platelet count is 20 × 10⁹/L (RR 150−400), activated partial thromboplastin time 58 s (RR 27−38 s); prothrombin time 20 s (RR 11−13 s); and fibrinogen 0.5 g/L (RR 1.5−3.5 g/L). The peripheral blood film shows immature white cells with cytoplasmic granules.

The most likely diagnosis is:

A Acute lymphoblastic leukemia
B Chronic myeloid leukemia
C Acute promyelocytic leukemia
D Chronic lymphocytic leukemia
E Immune thrombocytopenic purpura

19 A 62-year-old man presents to the clinic for follow-up of chronic lymphocytic leukemia 2 years after receiving treatment with 6 cycles of fludarabine, cyclophosphamide and rituximab. He reports weight loss, night sweats and fevers for the past 6 weeks. On examination, the spleen is palpable 4 cm below the left costal margin. Laboratory studies show: hemoglobin 90 g/L (RR 130−180), white cell count 150 × 10⁹/L (RR 4.0−11.0 × 10⁹/L), lymphocytes 140 × 10⁹/L (RR 1.5−4), and platelets 80 × 10⁹/L (RR 150−400). The lactate dehydrogenase is 200 U/L (RR 120−250). Bone marrow biopsy FISH shows TP53 deletion.

Which of the following is the most appropriate management?

A Repeat fludarabine, cyclophosphamide and rituximab
B Ibrutinib
C Obinutuzumab and chlorambucil
D Bendamustine and rituximab
E Allogeneic stem cell transplant

20 A 20-year-old female is referred for investigation of chronic anemia. She has no significant past medical history and her only current medication is the oral contraceptive pill. Her mother also has a mild anemia. On examination, there is no lymphadenopathy, splenomegaly or hepatomegaly. Laboratory studies show: hemoglobin 100 g/L (RR 110−150 g/L), mean corpuscular volume 67 fL (RR 80−100 fL), serum iron 25 micromoll/L (RR 11−29), ferritin 200 microg/L (15−200 microg/L), total iron-binding capacity 50 micromol/L (RR 45−82 micromol/L). Hemoglobin electrophoresis shows normal migration of HbA, and normal levels of HbA2 and HbF.

Which of the following is the most likely diagnosis?

A Alpha-thalassemia trait
B Beta-thalassemia trait
C Anemia of inflammation
D Beta-thalassemia intermedia
E Alpha-thalassemia silent carrier

ANSWERS

1   D.

The most likely diagnosis is chronic lymphocytic leukemia (CLL). This is commonly identified by mild lymphocytosis in routine blood films. The presence of 'smear cells' is a typical finding. Flow cytometry will confirm the diagnosis and exclude the possibility of other lymphoproliferative disorders. Routine CT scans or bone-marrow biopsies are not necessary. Early introduction of therapy is not indicated, as there is no improvement in survival. Routine full blood examination and clinical examination is adequate for early-stage CLL.

2   C.

Although this patient is of Italian ethnicity, a previously normal full blood examination will exclude thalassemia trait significant enough to cause anemia. Anemia is most likely due to iron deficiency and should be confirmed by assessment of iron stores. While iron supplementation will be necessary, it is vital to exclude gastrointestinal blood loss in a person of his age. Non-steroidal anti-inflammatory drug (NSAID)-induced chronic low-volume blood loss can be the cause, but it will be incorrect to assume this and not investigate further. Gastroscopy and colonoscopy should be arranged. The description of weight loss and constipation raises significant concerns of colon cancer. Abnormalities in GGT and ALP suggest the possibility of liver metastasis, but this is not the typical appearance of anemia associated with liver disease.

3   C.

The close family history of menorrhagia and bruising make von Willebrand's disease (vWD) the most likely differential diagnosis. Inherited platelet function defects are possible but are much less common than vWD. Moreover, coagulation test abnormalities do not occur with platelet function defects. NSAIDs can contribute to bruising and menorrhagia but do not account for prolonged APTT and low factor VIII, and are less likely to be the culprit in this setting. A factor VIII level of 35% is consistent with vWD, as von Willebrand's factor (vWF) protects factor VIII from proteolysis. Quantification of vWF and assessment of vWF multimers is the next most logical step. Hemophilia A or vWD is not an absolute contraindication to surgery provided that an appropriate plan is in place for perioperative correction of factor deficiencies.

4   A.

In the absence of bleeding, it is preferable to miss a warfarin dose and recommence at a lower dose. It is also important to verify the reason for the unexpectedly high INR. Factors such as dietary changes and new medications should be considered. This fall was after a known event (climbing a ladder) and is not a reason to contraindicate warfarin. The patient's risk of stroke is considerable and there is extensive evidence that warfarin will reduce the risk and that aspirin is inadequate. Vitamin K is not indicated at an INR of 5.0 and will make re-introduction of warfarin difficult. When vitamin K is used in the absence of bleeding, a low dose of 1–3 mg is preferred. Prothrombin complex concentrates are only indicated in the context of bleeding while on warfarin.

5   B.

The pre-test probability for venous thromboembolism (VTE) is high, and pulmonary embolism is the most likely and significant diagnosis for this patient's symptoms of pleuritic chest pain. Generally, plane flights of more than 4–5 hours are associated with an increased risk of VTE. In this case, metastatic cancer is the most likely precipitant. Respiratory tract infection, pneumothorax and pulmonary metastasis are possible, but are unlikely to be the main diagnosis given the coexistent unilateral calf pain and swelling.

6   C.

The full blood examination findings are typical of chronic myeloid leukemia, which is confirmed by the presence of the Philadelphia chromosome. This is a reciprocal translocation between chromosomes 9 and 22, leading to the generation of an aberrant *BCR-ABL* fusion protein with dysregulated tyrosine kinase activity. Patients are treated with tyrosine kinase inhibitors (imatinib, nilotinib, dasatinib) and monitored by quantitative polymerase chain reaction (PCR) of the *BCR-ABL* mRNA using peripheral blood.

7   E.

The diagnosis is monoclonal gammopathy of undetermined significance (MGUS). Rouleaux result from red blood cells stacking together in the presence of elevated serum protein levels, in this case a paraprotein. The risk of progression is very low, and monitoring of paraprotein with clinical review suffices. Normal calcium levels, preserved renal function, absence of anemia, and bone involvement is mandatory to make a diagnosis of MGUS. Magnetic resonance imaging of the spine is not indicated in MGUS unless the patient has symptoms. Bisphosphonate therapy is not necessary in MGUS.

8   A.

The pentad criteria for thrombotic thrombocytopenic purpura are present: thrombocytopenia, microangiopathic hemolysis (indicated by anemia and schistocytes on blood film), neurological symptoms, renal impairment and fever. Disseminated intravascular coagulation is excluded by normal coagulation tests. IgA vasculitis is associated with arthritis, and renal impairment may be present but without red cell fragmentation. Normal liver function tests make the HELLP syndrome unlikely. ITP would not cause fever, anemia, renal impairment and neurological symptoms.

9 A.

The diagnosis is most likely to be autoimmune hemolytic anemia as evidenced by the presence of spherocytes and polychromasia. A DAT will confirm the presence of immunoglobulin or complement proteins adherent on red cell surfaces. Hereditary spherocytosis is unlikely as FBE was normal previously. Oxidative hemolysis typically shows 'bite cells' on blood film. Reticulocytosis, indicated by polychromasia, is an expected finding. Malaria is unlikely if appropriate prophylaxis was taken, and in the absence of fever. Reticulocytosis rather than reticulocytopenia is expected in the setting of autoimmune hemolysis.

10 E.

Thrombocytopenia in HIT typically develops between 5 and 10 days after heparin exposure, but can occur earlier if there has been prior exposure within 30 days. Pathogenic antibodies (directed against platelet factor 4 and heparin complex) can cross-react with LMWH. Development of DVT is highly suggestive of HIT. Drug-induced thrombocytopenia is always possible, but less likely in this setting. Immediate initiation of warfarin can cause skin necrosis. The clinical scenario of temporal relationship to unfractionated heparin and development of DVT is a better fit with HIT than ITP.

11 C.

The most appropriate management of this patient with HELLP (hemolysis, elevated liver enzymes and low platelet) syndrome is emergency delivery. The patient has pre-eclampsia with hypertension (systolic BP >140 mmHg or diastolic BP >90 mmHg), edema, proteinuria, and features of a microangiopathic hemolytic anemia (MAHA) with thrombocytopenia. Although she has features of MAHA, the elevated blood pressure and proteinuria make pre-eclampsia more likely than TTP, and plasma exchange is not appropriate. Atypical hemolytic uremic syndrome is the most common HUS in pregnancy; however, the normal creatinine is not consistent with aHUS and treatment with eculizumab is not indicated. ITP in pregnancy occurs as an isolated low platelet count and intravenous immunoglobulin or dexamethasone are not indicated.

12 C.

This patient with a low pre-test probability of PE requires no further testing. The PERC are: 1. Age <50 years; 2. Pulse rate <100 bpm; 3. SaO_2 >95%; 4. No hemoptysis; 5. No hormone use; 6. No prior VTE; 7. No unilateral leg swelling and; 8. No trauma or surgery within 4 weeks. The patient has 0 criteria and the risk of PE is <2%. In patients with any criteria, a D-dimer should be performed. Negative D-dimer rules out PE; if the D-dimer is positive, a CTPA is recommended.

13 B.

Minor bleeding in a patient taking a direct oral anticoagulant can be managed by discontinuation of the treatment alone. Neither fresh frozen plasma nor prothrombinex will reverse the anticoagulant effect of dabigatran. Idarucizumab is a humanized monoclonal antibody that is a specific reversal agent for dabigatran. Idarucizumab is used in patients when rapid reversal of the anticoagulant effects of dabigatran is required, specifically for emergency surgery/urgent procedures and in life-threatening or uncontrolled bleeding. This patient does not have life-threatening or uncontrolled bleeding and therefore idarucizumab is not indicated. Andexanet alfa is used for the reversal of rivaroxaban and apixaban, not dabigatran.

14 E.

The most appropriate treatment for malignancy-associated venous thromboembolism is enoxaparin. Active cancer or cancer being treated with chemotherapy or radiotherapy increases VTE risk by approximately 5 times, although risk is not increased in those who have been cured following treatment. This patient has been diagnosed with metastatic carcinoma of the colon and is due for adjuvant therapy; however, in the meantime he has developed a PE. The CLOT trial showed LMWH is superior to warfarin in patients with malignancy and VTE. Extended therapy with enoxaparin is indicated while the cancer remains active; however, the benefit should be weighed against the risk of bleeding, quality of life, and life expectancy. There are no data for treatment of malignancy-associated VTE with DOACs although trials are currently underway and standard of care may change in the future.

15 D.

This patient with sickle cell anemia presents with pure red cell aplasia secondary to parvovirus B19 infection. The patient's low reticulocyte count is consistent with PRCA, which in adults is usually asymptomatic. The low reticulocyte count is not consistent with hemolytic crisis and aplastic anemia is unlikely with no other cytopenias. Acute splenic sequestration causes a sudden painful enlargement of the spleen and anemia. The lack of a painful, enlarged spleen and low reticulocyte count are not consistent with the diagnosis of acute splenic sequestration. Patients with a vaso-occlusive crisis can present with an acute chest syndrome which occurs as a result of infarction of the lung parenchyma. The absence of pain (dactylitis, priapism, or abdominal pain) makes this diagnosis unlikely.

16 A.

This patient has essential thrombocythemia with the presence of increased numbers of large megakaryocytes in clumps. Although molecular testing for JAK2, MPL and CALR mutations were negative, 10–20% of patients do not have known gene mutations. There is no evidence of other causes of raised platelets, including iron deficiency, inflammation or malignancy. The patient's age (>60 years) and previous stroke increases her risk of another thrombosis and a platelet-lowering therapy such as hydroxyurea should be added to aspirin. Anagrelide is registered by the Therapeutic Goods Administration for the treatment of essential thrombocythemia but is not listed on the Pharmaceutical Benefits Scheme.

17 D.

This patient has atypical hemolytic uremic syndrome (aHUS), with severe hypertension, hemolytic anemia, thrombocytopenia, acute kidney injury, and stool culture negative for Shiga toxin. The normal ADAMTS13 level excludes thrombotic thrombocytopenic purpura. Eculizumab is the treatment of choice for aHUS. Eculizumab is a humanized monoclonal antibody that inhibits the production of the terminal complement components, C5a and the membrane attack complex (C5b-9) by binding to complement protein C5a. TTP is treated with plasma exchange, corticosteroids and rituximab.

18 C.

The combination of pancytopenia, disseminated intravascular coagulation, and peripheral blood film showing immature leukocytes with features consistent with promyelocytes makes acute promyelocytic leukemia the most likely diagnosis. Aplastic anemia presents with pancytopenia; however, these patients would not have circulating immature leukocytes or DIC. Immune thrombocytopenia purpura presents with bleeding and low platelets; however, these patients do not have DIC or pancytopenia. Chronic myeloid leukemia and chronic lymphocytic leukemia both present with a raised white cell count. Approximately 10% of patients with ALL have DIC at the time of diagnosis; however, findings on the peripheral blood film makes APML the more likely diagnosis.

19 B.

This patient is considered unsuitable for retreatment with fludarabine having had a progression-free interval of less than 3 years from treatment with FCR and the presence of the TP53 deletion. Multiple clinical trials have confirmed the efficacy and safety of ibrutinib in relapsed CLL, among patients with and without TP53 disruption. If the patient progresses on ibrutinib, then an allogeneic transplant or other cellular therapy would be considered. Obinutuzumab and chlorambucil can be used in older patients as first-line therapy, and bendamustine and rituximab is less effective as a first-line therapy compared to FCR.

20 A.

In this patient with a microcytic anemia, the most likely diagnosis is alpha thalassemia trait. Patients with alpha-thalassemia trait have 2 copies of the alpha-globin gene (α - / α – or $\alpha\alpha$ / - -). There is no increase in HbA2 or HbF. Patients who are silent carriers for alpha thalassemia have a defect/loss of one alpha gene and have a normal hemoglobin and MCV. Patients with beta-thalassemia minor have a microcytic anemia, a normal electrophoretic pattern for HbA, but increased amounts of HbA2. Anemia of inflammation is characterized by a low serum iron level, and reduced iron-binding capacity.

CHAPTER 14

ONCOLOGY

Victoria Bray, Wei Chua, Christos S Karapetis and Melissa Moore

- LUNG CAN CER
  - Clinical presentation
  - Risk factors
  - Epidemiology and pathology
  - Non-small-cell lung cancer (NSCLC)
  - Molecular profiling
  - Monoclonal antibodies
  - Anaplastic lymphoma kinase gene rearrangement as a treatment target
  - ROS-1 and other targets
  - Small-cell lung cancer (SCLC)
- RENAL CANCER
  - Background
  - Diagnosis and staging
  - Treatment
  - Prognosis
- TUMORS OF THE PELVIS, URETER AND BLADDER
  - Epidemiology
  - Risk factors
  - Clinical presentation
  - Investigation and diagnosis
  - Treatment
- PROSTATE CANCER
  - Epidemiology
  - Screening
  - Staging
  - Management
- TESTIS CANCER
  - Epidemiology and risk
  - Pathology
  - Diagnosis
  - Prognostic factors in stage I NSGCT
  - Treatment
  - Post-chemotherapy residual masses
  - Relapsed disease
  - High-dose chemotherapy (HDCT)
- HEAD AND NECK CANCER
  - Early-stage disease
  - Advanced-stage disease
  - Human papillomavirus (HPV) infection
- ESOPHAGEAL CANCER
  - Pathology and epidemiology
  - Clinical presentation
  - Diagnosis and screening
  - Management
- GASTRIC CANCER
  - Epidemiology
  - Clinical presentation
  - Diagnosis
  - Treatment
  - Gastric MALT lymphoma

- COLORECTAL CANCER
  - Pathology and epidemiology
  - Diagnosis and staging
  - Management
  - Future directions
- PANCREATIC CANCER
  - Key points
  - Epidemiology
  - Diagnosis
  - Management
- HEPATOCELLULAR CARCINOMA (HCC)
  - Key points
  - Risk factors
  - Prognosis
  - Treatment
- BRAIN TUMORS
  - Low-grade glioma (astrocytoma and oligodendroglioma)
  - Glioblastoma multiforme (GBM)
- LYMPHOMA—SEE CHAPTER 13
- MELANOMA
  - Pathology and epidemiology
  - Diagnosis and staging
  - Management
- NON-MELANOMA SKIN CANCER
  - Risk factors
  - Management
- SARCOMA
  - Clinical presentation
  - Diagnosis
  - Treatment
- BREAST CANCER
  - Epidemiology
  - Risk factors
  - Pathology
  - Screening
  - Diagnosis and staging
  - Management
  - Recent research and future directions
- OVARIAN CANCER
  - Key points
  - Pathology and epidemiology
  - Diagnosis
  - Management
  - Future directions
- ENDOMETRIAL CANCER
  - Pathology and epidemiology
  - Diagnosis
  - Management
- CANCER SURVIVORSHIP

WHAT IS CANCER?

Regulation of cell growth is complex, but is vital for survival. A cancer is a cell or group of cells that develops and progresses without regard to all the physiological checkpoints and controls that regulate cell growth. This defective cell growth is usually initiated by a series of changes or mutations in the genes of the cancer cell.

DNA and genes

All cellular processes are controlled through the DNA inside each cell. DNA (deoxyribonucleic acid) is a self-replicating material present in nearly all cells and is the main constituent of chromosomes. Each DNA molecule consists of two strands coiled around each other to form a double helix. All the genetic information of a cell is coded in this helix in the form of chemical groups called *bases*—the purines adenine and guanine, and the pyrimidines thymine and cytosine—that form specific sequences and pairs across the two adjoining strands. Adenine pairs with thymine; cytosine pairs with guanine; in RNA, uracil replaces thymine.

Specific segments of the building blocks form discrete *genes* from which proteins are produced by a process of gene transcription and translation. DNA integrity needs to be maintained by each cell, and this is an active process. The DNA replication process is not always exact, and replication errors can occur. DNA is constantly repaired; or, failing that, the cell is set on a path of programmed cell death.

Apoptosis

In essence, all of the cells that make up the human body have a defined function and lifespan. The death of the cell is programmed through a process called *apoptosis*.

The cancer cell is one that has developed a gene mutation or multiple mutations that affect gene function, and this subsequently has an impact on the growth and survival characteristics of the cell. A failure of apoptotic mechanisms develops and the cancer cells grow, form clusters, interact with the surrounding tissue environment, and develop aberrant blood supply. The cells can migrate via lymphatic channels and blood vessels and settle in other sites, forming metastases. Ultimately, as the cancer grows it affects on the function of the regions it involves, leading to possible organ failure. The cancer can also produce systemic adverse effects such as anorexia, weight loss, fatigue and malaise.

Gene mutations

The genetic aberrations that lead to cancers can be inherited, although most are acquired. Gene mutations can take the form of gene rearrangement, translocation, deletion, insertion or amplification. Genetic damage may arise directly from exposure to certain carcinogens (such as ionizing radiation or tobacco).

Basic elements of cancer biology

- *Clonality*—cancers are derived from a single cell line.
- *Autonomy*—cancers are not responsive to normal physiological control mechanisms in the cell cycle.
- *Anaplasia*—cancer cells differ from normal cells in appearance.
- *Invasion/metastases*—most cancer cells have the ability to grow at sites other than the primary site, either by direct invasion or by spread via blood or lymph. Different cancer types have different propensities to metastasize.

Essential elements of cancer diagnosis and treatment

Cancer survival is strongly correlated with the stage of the cancer at diagnosis, so in most cases the earlier that a cancer is diagnosed, the better the chance of a cure or a positive outcome.

When a cancer cannot be cured, doctors should be able to counsel patients, their families and carers, appropriately. Optimal measures for symptom control should be applied. The supportive care of patients through their cancer treatments is also very important.

Figure 14-1 demonstrates the rate of growth of cancer, which follows what is called a Gompertzian curve. It shows that:

- the cancer growth rate slows down as the cancer gets bigger
- there may be a large number of cancer cells present that cannot be clinically detected.

Figure 14-2 (overleaf) illustrates cell kill and cell regrowth per treatment cycle; it shows why it is important to have a sufficient number of treatment cycles even if the cancer is no longer clinically apparent.

PREVENTION

It has been estimated that at least one-third of all cancers are preventable. The following strategies have been shown to be useful preventative measures.

- Cessation of smoking
- Reduction or cessation of alcohol consumption
- Education about a healthy diet

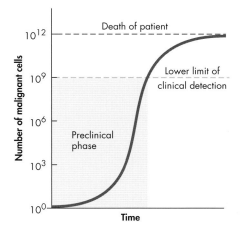

Figure 14-1 Rate of growth of cancer (Gompertzian curve)

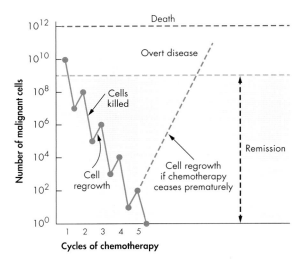

Figure 14-2 Logarithm of cells killed (log cell kill) and cell regrowth per treatment cycle

- Weight-reduction initiatives in those who are obese or overweight
- Chemotherapy prevention:
  » tamoxifen or exemestane, for breast cancer
  » vaccines (e.g. human papillomavirus vaccine to prevent cervical cancer, hepatitis B vaccine to reduce the risk of hepatocellular carcinoma)
  » aspirin to reduce colonic polyp development
  » antiviral treatment of hepatitis C to prevent hepatocellular cancer.
- Minimizing exposure to ultraviolet light (protection from sun)
- Screening for pre-cancerous conditions:
  » endoscopy in Barrett's esophagus
  » Papanicolaou (Pap) tests—for cervical dysplasia
  » colonoscopy—for polyps
  » mammographic screening for precancerous lesions (ductal carcinoma *in situ*)
- Surgery—e.g. prophylactic mastectomy or oophorectomy in women with specific familial risk factors.

DIAGNOSIS

Screening

Screening for cancer involves the process of investigating people who are otherwise well and have no symptoms or signs of cancer, with the aim of detecting cancer at a pre-clinical stage.

Examples of positive results through screening, usually measured as improved overall disease-specific survival rates in the screened population, include:

- breast cancer screening with bilateral mammography from age 50
- cervical cancer screening with Pap smears from the onset of sexual activity
- colorectal cancer screening with fecal occult blood tests from age 50.

Other cancers where screening is being investigated include non-small-cell lung cancer (low-dose computed tomography in high-risk smokers) and prostate cancer (prostate-specific antigen [PSA]). These tests have not been universally accepted and established.

Signs and symptoms

The signs and symptoms of cancer are not specific, but persistence of any of the following should always raise concern about the possibility of cancer.

- Anorexia—loss of appetite usually associated with weight loss
- Weight loss—unexplained
- Unexplained pain, including headache
- Lumps—e.g. breast lump, testicular lump, swollen lymph gland
- Bleeding from the bowel, bladder, vagina or lung
- Difficulty swallowing
- Skin rash or pigmented skin lesions
- Seizures (new onset).

Specific clinical signs and syndromes

These include:

- Horner's syndrome—partial ptosis of one eye, which reflects infiltration of the sympathetic nerves as they ascend through the upper mediastinum
- Virchow's node—an enlarged left-side supraclavicular lymph node, which is usually firm and irregular and may be fixed. This finding was initially described in the context of advanced gastric cancer, but other intra-abdominal malignancies can also spread to this node
- Sister Mary Joseph's node—a subcutaneous lymph node in the region of the umbilicus, usually seen in intra-abdominal malignancy, classically ovarian cancer
- increasing fluid accumulating in body cavities—e.g. ascites, pleural effusion, pericardial effusion
- painless jaundice—may be an indication of a malignant biliary obstruction
- changing nevus or new hyperpigmented cutaneous lesion—melanoma should be considered.

Diagnostic tests

Despite the most convincing clinical evidence, a histological confirmation of the diagnosis is always required. This will involve one of the following biopsy procedures:

- fine-needle aspiration (FNA) cytology
- core biopsy
- excision biopsy.

The tissue obtained is examined with standard tissue staining (hematoxylin and eosin, H&E) enabling assessment of:

- the cancer cell appearance, and
- the architecture of the tissue.

Subsequent immunohistochemistry (IHC) will enable a more detailed analysis and support a specific diagnosis, although results are not themselves diagnostic.

Immunohistochemistry (IHC)

The following markers are useful in clinical practice:

- cytokeratins—cancer of epithelial origin, i.e. adeno-carcinoma or squamous-cell carcinoma
  - » CK7—lung
  - » CK20—gastrointestinal tract
- thyroid transcription factor (TTF)—lung cancer, thyroid cancer
- prostate-specific antigen (PSA)—prostate (specific)
- synaptophysin/chromogranin—neuroendocrine tumor, small-cell carcinoma
- CD117 (= c-kit)—gastrointestinal stromal tumor (GIST)
- lymphocyte common antigen (LCA)—lymphoma
- CD20—lymphoma.

PROGNOSIS

Each cancer has a unique biological behavior. The following are factors associated with worsening prognosis.

Cancer factors

- Stage—the more advanced the stage, the poorer the prognosis.
- Differentiation—the poorer the differentiation (equates to higher grade), then the poorer the prognosis. The caveat is that for some cancers, notably lymphoma, a higher grade represents a poor prognostic factor without treatment but a more responsive and potentially curable lymphoma when treated.
- Critical organ involvement.
- Certain gene mutations, e.g. *BRAF* mutation in stage 4 colon cancer.

Patient factors

- Performance status—this is a measure of the overall fitness of patients. It takes into account mobility and the capacity to engage in activities of daily living, including self-care. The poorer the performance status, the worse the prognosis. Commonly used scores include the Eastern Cooperative Oncology Group (ECOG) performance status (0–5) or the Karnofsky Performance Score (0–100).
- Lactase dehydrogenase (LDH)—high LDH is a marker of increased tumor bulk, faster cell turnover, and tumor hypoxia. A high level often indicates a poorer prognosis.
- Albumin—a low level can be a negative acute-phase reactant, a marker of malnutrition, and is a negative prognostic factor.
- Weight loss—increased catabolism is a poor prognostic factor.

- High or low white cell count (WCC), including the neutrophil to lymphocyte ratio, is a validated poor prognostic factor, and may be related to cancer-induced cytokine production.

Prognostic vs predictive factors

- A **prognostic factor** is related to the overall outcome of patient survival, and has an association that is independent of any treatment effects. The effect on survival outcome is independent of intervention (therapy).
- A **predictive factor** predicts the benefit, or lack of benefit, related to an intervention (therapy). The predictive factor has relevance only in relation to the therapy. In the absence of intervention, the predictive factor has no influence in the outcome.

Examples of prognostic factors:

- *BRAF* mutation in advanced colorectal cancer
- microsatellite instability (MSI) status in early-stage bowel cancer (stages II and III)
- LDH level in lymphoma.

Examples of predictive factors:

- Epidermal growth factor receptor (EGFR) gene mutation and tyrosine kinase inhibitor (TKI) therapy in advanced non-small-cell lung cancer
- *K-ras* mutation in pre-treated advanced colon cancer.
- PD-L1 IHC expression and response to immunotherapy in non-small-cell lung cancer
- Microsatelite instability (MSI) and response to immunotherapy in stage 4 colorectal cancer.

Some biomarkers can be both—e.g. human epidermal growth factor receptor 2 (HER2) in breast cancer.

TREATMENT PRINCIPLES

Defining treatment goals

1 *Cure*—accept the potential for more toxicity, consider long-term consequences of therapies.
2 *Extend survival time but not cure*—weigh up the benefits of therapy against toxicity, and aim to prolong life while maintaining or improving quality of life.
3 *Palliate*—aim to optimize symptom control and quality of life above all else.

The six principal treatment modalities in cancer are:

1 surgery
2 radiotherapy
3 chemotherapy
4 hormonal therapy
5 molecular targeted therapy, including monoclonal antibodies and TKIs
6 immunomodulatory therapy, including programmed cell death protein 1 (PD-1) and programmed cell death ligand 1 (PD-L1) inhibitors; cytotoxic T lymphocyte antigen 4 (CTLA-4) modulators; interferon; and vaccines.

Adjuvant therapy

Adjuvant therapy is given after a treatment (usually surgery) has apparently eliminated or removed the cancer. There is therefore no detectable cancer, and the aim of the adjuvant therapy is to prevent a recurrence of cancer. It is thought that the therapy can eliminate disease that may still be present but is too small to be detected. The concept of the cancer stem cell is also potentially important here. Such stem cells may be cleared by the adjuvant therapy.

Postoperative adjuvant therapy has been proven to be of benefit in increasing survival for a proportion of patients, as outlined below.

- **Postoperative adjuvant chemotherapy**
  - » Stage III colon cancer—5-fluorouracil (5FU), capecitabine, oxaliplatin + 5FU
  - » Stage II colon cancer—survival benefit of <5%, but should be considered in patients with high-risk features (e.g. T4, bowel perforation)
  - » Early-stage breast cancer
  - » Stage II and III non–small-cell lung cancer
  - » Pancreatic cancer
  - » Gastric cancer
  - » Ovarian cancer
- **Postoperative adjuvant radiotherapy**
  - » Breast cancer
  - » Head and neck cancer
  - » Endometrial cancer
  - » Brain tumors
- **Postoperative adjuvant monoclonal antibody therapy**
  - » Breast cancer—HER2-positive; trastuzumab
  - » The other monoclonal antibodies have not been associated with survival benefit as adjuvant therapies; studies investigating bevacizumab and cetuximab have been performed in early-stage colorectal cancer, but the studies failed to demonstrate a survival advantage
- **Postoperative tyrosine kinase inhibitors**
  - » Imatinib in gastrointestinal stromal tumor (GIST)—use of imatinib after the complete removal of a GIST tumor that has intermediate or high-risk features for recurrence (these features are based on the size of the tumor and the number of mitoses per high-power field)
  - » No benefit has been observed through the use of epidermal growth factor receptor (EGFR) tyrosine kinase inhibitors after surgery as an adjuvant therapy in lung cancer.

Neoadjuvant therapy

For neoadjuvant treatment, the additional therapies are administered before the definitive treatment (usually surgery). This usually comprises of chemotherapy with or without radiotherapy. The advantages of giving the treatment before surgery include:

- making the primary tumor smaller ('down-staging'), which may increase the chance of complete surgical clearance

- giving the systemic treatment earlier may allow a greater effect against micro-metastatic disease, as such disease would be of smaller volume before as compared with after surgery
- patients may be physically fitter before the surgery and may tolerate the chemotherapy and radiotherapy better.

Some examples of where neoadjuvant therapy is in routine use include:

- locally advanced rectal cancer
- esophageal cancer
- breast cancer (for locally advanced disease).

Supportive management

It is important to consider the additional management that patients will require to manage either the symptoms of the cancer or the adverse effects associated with the therapies for treating cancer.

- These supportive therapies may include antiemetics, analgesics, laxatives or antidiarrheal agents, antibiotics, parenteral nutrition or feeding through a percutaneous endoscopic gastrostomy (PEG) tube, and mouth rinses.
- The additional contribution of allied health services can provide a significant benefit for patients and their families. These services may include specialised cancer nurses or cancer care coordinators, social work, dietitian input, dental care, physiotherapy, psychology and counseling services.

Maintenance therapy

Attempts to prolong the period of cancer control through longer administration of treatment such as chemotherapy or monoclonal antibodies have proven to improve outcomes in certain situations.

- The use of rituximab after completion of an initial chemotherapy + rituximab course has been proven to prolong the time of lymphoma control (i.e. prolong progression-free survival) for patients with low-grade non-Hodgkin lymphoma.
- Use of the cytotoxic drug pemetrexed after an initial course of chemotherapy for non–small-cell lung cancer has been associated with prolongation of survival.

Aside from these situations, the use of maintenance chemotherapy has not been shown to improve overall survival, but may prolong the time to disease progression. This benefit has to be balanced against the cumulative side-effects of therapy.

PRINCIPLES OF CHEMOTHERAPY

In common medical parlance, chemotherapy has come to mean treatment with agents that are classified as *cytotoxic*. These drugs exert their impact principally on cells that are actively dividing, hence their impact on cells within the bone marrow (causing cytopenias) or lining the gastrointestinal tract (causing mouth ulceration or diarrhea).

- With each dose of chemotherapy, a fixed percentage of cells is killed (log kill) rather than an absolute number of cells (see Figure 14-2).
- The optimal dose of chemotherapy and the frequency of administration is determined through phase I clinical trials, and is determined by the degree and duration of myelosuppression and non-hematological toxicity.
- The *maximal tolerated dose* is that dose which is tolerated by a predefined proportion of patients without the need for dose attenuation.

Toxicity is graded by applying international scales, such as the National Cancer Institute Common Toxicity Criteria. Chemotherapy is delayed if toxicity persists or significant cytopenia is present on the day that chemotherapy is due. Dose attenuation is also usually considered if significant toxicity develops.

Attitudes to chemotherapy

When asked for their preferences, patients who already have advanced cancer, including medical and nursing professionals, are much more likely to opt for radical treatment with minimal chance of benefit than people who do not have cancer.

In a study of non-small-cell lung cancer patients, 22% stated that they would choose chemotherapy for a survival benefit of 3 months. For a substantial reduction in symptoms without prolonging life, 68% would choose chemotherapy.

Toxicity of cytotoxic chemotherapy

Cytotoxic drugs often cause:

- nausea and vomiting
- bone marrow suppression
- alopecia.

Etoposide, taxanes and anthracyclines usually cause alopecia. When used as single agents, 5FU, vinorelbine, gemcitabine, pemetrexed and carboplatin cause little hair loss.

Cytotoxics that are relatively non-myelosuppressive

1 Vincristine
2 Bleomycin
3 Cisplatin
4 Streptozotocin

CLINICAL PEARL

Most cytotoxics that are myelosuppressive cause a nadir at 10–14 days after treatment, but some alkylating agents (e.g. busulfan, melphalan, procarbazine) can have stem-cell toxic effects which cause severe myelosuppression with a delayed nadir 6–8 weeks after therapy.

Cytotoxics that require dose reduction or avoidance in renal disease

1 Increased toxicity systemically occurs with methotrexate, cyclophosphamide, oral capecitabine, bleomycin and bis-chloroethylnitrosourea (BCNU).
2 Increased renal damage occurs with cisplatin, mithramycin, BCNU, streptozotocin and high-dose methotrexate.

Cytotoxics that cause prolonged azoospermia

1 Chlorambucil
2 Cyclophosphamide
3 Cisplatin

Cytotoxics that cause ovarian failure

Most combinations of cytotoxic chemotherapy will induce ovarian failure. Women in their 40s generally do not regain ovarian function. Younger women are more likely to retain ovarian function and fertility. Chemotherapy particularly associated with reduced ovarian function includes:

1 Cyclophosphamide
2 Chlorambucil
3 Nitrogen-mustard
4 Mitomycin C
5 Procarbazine

Drugs which tend to increase the rate of second cancers

Since part of the mechanism of action of cytotoxic chemotherapy is to damage DNA, there is a small risk of second cancers with most cytotoxic drugs. Most of these are hematological malignancies due to previous exposure to alkylating agents. The drugs most often associated with secondary leukemia are etoposide and alkylating agents.

PRINCIPLES OF RADIOTHERAPY

Radiotherapy provides localized treatment for cancer.

- The main mechanism for cell death as a result of radiotherapy is damage to DNA. Malignant cells are far less able to repair damage, so there is a differential effect sparing normal cells.
- There may also be a contribution from apoptosis (programmed cell death), release of cytokines, and the switching on of signal transduction pathways.
- Although at times cells are not killed with radiotherapy, they may be rendered unable to replicate.

Chemotherapy is sometimes used concurrently with radiotherapy to potentiate the effects of radiotherapy. Examples of this include 5–fluorouracil chemotherapy in rectal cancer, and platinum-based chemotherapy in non-small-cell lung, cervical and head and neck cancers.

Various sources of radiotherapy are available. These include:

- gamma rays from cobalt-60 decay
- photons generated as X-rays or electrons in a linear accelerator
- neutrons and protons in a cyclotron.

The dose of therapy is measured in Grays (Gy). One Gy equals one joule of energy per kilogram of tissue.

Fractionation

Cells are most sensitive to ionizing radiation immediately before mitosis. Multiple exposures to radiotherapy increase the likelihood of finding the cell in this particular part of the cycle. Fractionation also serves to limit the damage to normal tissues.

Radiation effects

All normal tissues have a dose beyond which recovery will not occur after exposure to radiation, due predominantly to irreversible damage to the microvasculature. This defines the maximum dose of radiotherapy.

Short-term toxicity

1 Dry and moist desquamation
2 Epilation
3 Mucosal damage—gastrointestinal tract, respiratory tract and bladder
4 Acute organ damage/failure with high-dose radiotherapy involving the lung, brain, kidney and large volumes of bone marrow

Long-term toxicity

1 Skin fragility
2 Second malignancies
3 Direct damage to mucosal surfaces (late proctitis or cystitis, dry mouth)
4 Scarring (small-volume bladder)

TREATMENT RESPONSIVENESS

Endocrine responsive

1 Breast cancer (anti-estrogen)
2 Endometrial cancer (progesterone)
3 Prostate cancer (androgen blockade)
4 Thyroid cancer (thyroxine, which suppresses thyroid-stimulating hormone [TSH])
5 Carcinoid (somatostatin)

Potentially curable following chemotherapy alone

1 Germ-cell tumors (mainly testicular cancer)
2 Hodgkin lymphoma
3 Non-Hodgkin lymphoma (certain subtypes)
4 Acute leukemia
5 Wilms' tumor
6 Ewing sarcoma and rhabdomyosarcoma (embryonal)

Tumors very sensitive to chemotherapy

(≥80% response rate)
1 Small-cell lung cancer
2 Non-Hodgkin lymphoma
3 Ovarian cancer

Potentially curable following radiotherapy

1 Seminoma (early stage)
2 Hodgkin lymphoma (early stage)
3 Head and neck, or laryngeal cancers (early stage)
4 Cervical carcinoma (early stage)
5 Prostate cancer (early stage)
6 Bladder cancer (early stage)

CLINICAL PEARL

Renal cell carcinoma and melanoma are relatively resistant to cytotoxics and radiation. Recent advances in immunotherapy, however, have shown these cancers to be very responsive to immunotherapy.

PERSONALIZED MEDICINE

Recent advances in cancer therapy have focused on an individualized approach to management, focusing novel treatment on specific targets and utilizing predictive biomarkers for optimal patient selection.

- Biomarkers include immunohistochemical staining patterns, fluorescent or chromogenic *in-situ* hybridization (FISH) staining patterns, or gene mutation analysis.
- Pharmacogenetic biomarkers may help to predict tumor sensitivity, but as yet have not become routine or accepted practice nor shown improved outcomes at a population level.

Gene expression profiling using sequence technology may help to rapidly identify a molecular profile of a tumor that will identify risk of recurrence and allow treatment selection.

- Multiple gene panels are in commercial development, and are currently available for risk stratification and decision-making regarding adjuvant chemotherapy for early-stage breast and bowel cancer. Such an approach is not universally accepted.

MOLECULAR TARGETED THERAPY

(The 'ABs' and the 'IBs'.)

Relatively recent advances in the medical therapy of cancer have focused on treatments that target recently discovered or previously known molecular signals or pathways that are critical for the survival and propagation of particular cancers.

The new drugs have mainly comprised either monoclonal antibodies or tyrosine kinase inhibitors.

Monoclonal antibodies (the 'ABs')

- These are large protein-based structures that inhibit either extracellular receptors that initiate growth signals (e.g. trastuzumab, cetuximab, panitumumab, rituximab), or the ligands of the receptors (bevacizumab).

- They are usually given intravenously.
- Side-effects can include hypersensitivity infusion reactions. Each antibody has its own side-effects:
  - » cetuximab—rash
  - » trastuzumab—cardiotoxicity
  - » bevacizumab—hypertension, arterial thrombotic events, small risk of bowel perforation.

Tyrosine kinase inhibitors (the 'IBs')

- TKIs are small molecules that inhibit either specific or multiple tyrosine kinases (e.g. imatinib, gefitinib, erlotinib, sorafenib, sunitinib, lapatinib, osimertinib).
- They are given orally in tablet or capsule form.
- Side-effects are peculiar to each TKI, although skin toxicity is common.
  - » erlotinib and gefitinib—rash
  - » sunitinib—fatigue, thyroid function disturbance.
- Despite promising activity in tumors that often are resistant to chemotherapy (e.g. renal cell cancer, gastrointestinal stromal tumors), with prolonged responses and good tolerability, these treatments are not considered curative. In general, treatments are usually continued indefinitely in cancers of advanced stage as discontinuation has led to earlier cancer progression.
- Aside from imatinib in GIST, these targeted therapies do not have proven roles as adjuvant therapies following surgical excision of cancer of early stages.

Other

Other potential molecular pathways targeted as part of novel cancer therapy approaches include mTOR (in which the inhibitor is everolimus), the hedgehog pathway (in which the inhibitor is GDC-0449), integrins, PI3K, PARP, CDK4/6 and proteasomes. Only some of these approaches are part of standard treatment to date and will be discussed in subsequent sections.

FAMILIAL CANCERS AND CANCER GENETICS

Cancers can develop in the context of a familial syndrome. These cancers may be associated with specific gene mutations and predispose to particular cancers, sometimes occurring at a young age. Patients with such syndromes may be at risk of multiple cancers and so should be subject to more intensive cancer surveillance. Sometimes preventative measures should be considered, including prophylactic surgery or pharmacotherapy.

- **Lynch syndrome, also known as hereditary non-polyposis colon cancer (HNPCC)**, is an autosomal dominant disorder with a high penetrance of cancer in mutation carriers (approximately 80%). Lynch syndrome accounts for 3% of all colonic adenocarcinomas and endometrial carcinoma develops in up to 60% of women. Other cancers that develop as part of the syndrome include those of the ovary, stomach, small bowel, hepatobiliary system, and renal pelvis or ureter.
  - » In this context, consideration should be given to increased frequency of cancer surveillance (Chapter 11)
  - » This should include annual colonoscopy commencing at an age that is at least 10 years younger than the youngest affected family member, annual urinalysis, upper gastrointestinal endoscopy, screening for endometrial cancer with endometrial biopsy and ovarian cancer with CA-125, and transvaginal ultrasound.
  - » There should also be discussion about the possibility of prophylactic hysterectomy and salpingo-oophorectomy at the end of the childbearing years.
- **BRCA1 and BRCA2 gene mutations** can lead to hereditary breast and ovarian cancer (HBOC) syndrome. The lifetime risk of developing breast cancer is 30–60% for carriers of the mutation. Men have increased risk for breast and prostate cancer, while both men and women have other cancer risks, such as increased risk of pancreatic cancer and colon cancer. Effective strategies for breast and ovarian cancer risk-reduction include cancer surveillance, risk-reducing surgery and/or chemoprevention such as tamoxifen. The likelihood of this being the underlying cause of breast cancer is higher in women who are diagnosed under the age of 40 years, those with so-called 'triple negative' breast cancers (negative for estrogen, progesterone and Her-2 receptors) as well as women with multiple family members diagnosed with breast or ovarian cancer.
- **Li–Fraumeni syndrome** is a cancer predisposition syndrome associated with germ-line abnormalities of the TP53 gene. The syndrome is associated with several cancers usually occurring at an early age, including breast cancer, sarcomas, brain tumors and adrenocortical carcinomas. The management of malignancies is the same as for other individuals. However, in women with breast cancer, mastectomy rather than lumpectomy plus radiation therapy is generally indicated because of the risk of second malignancies due to radiation-induced tumors.

The familial aspects of these syndromes need to be carefully considered. Counseling through specialized cancer genetics services is recommended. Particular issues to contemplate include risk quantification, cancer surveillance strategies and preventative measures such as prophylactic surgery or preventative chemotherapy. These matters need to be handled sensitively and professionally, as there are potential implications to family planning, insurance, body image, guilt and family relationships.

ONCOLOGICAL EMERGENCIES

Spinal cord compression

- Spinal cord compression should be suspected if the patient complains of back pain, difficulties in walking, altered bowel habit (usually constipation, but sometimes diarrhea with loss of anal tone), or urinary retention.
- It is essential to check anal tone and check for a sensory level.
- The best way to investigate is with magnetic resonance imaging (MRI) of the spine (Figure 14-3).

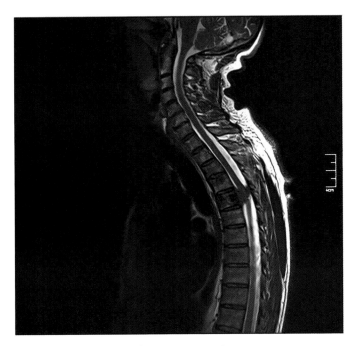

Figure 14-3 Magnetic resonance image demonstrating spinal cord compression

- Clinical judgment will be required to determine the location of the lesion causing the symptoms, as some patients have multiple lesions.
- Treatment is with analgesia, corticosteroids and radiotherapy.
- Surgery may be needed depending on the nature of the lesion as well as the overall condition of the patient.

Febrile neutropenia

Patients undergoing cytotoxic chemotherapy are expected to have a fall in their white cell count with most cytotoxic drugs 10–14 days after their administration.

- If patients are unwell or febrile with this, it should be assumed they are neutropenic until proven otherwise. This is a medical emergency as, if untreated, overwhelming sepsis can lead to death within a very short time.
- Patients should receive broad-spectrum antibiotics immediately after appropriate blood cultures are taken even if the neutrophil count is not yet known.

Patients may have:
- fevers (>38.0°C), chills, rigors
- a flu–like illness
- malaise without fever or signs of sepsis.

The likelihood of sepsis increases with the length of time the absolute neutrophil count is <1.0×10^9/L. The risk increases further if the neutrophil count is <0.5×10^9/L.

- Patients are at higher risk of bacteremia or septicemia if they have evidence of mucosal damage (mouth ulcers or diarrhea), advancing age, or other comorbidities.
- Blood cultures are often negative even in the presence of overwhelming sepsis.

CLINICAL PEARL

In the febrile neutropenic cancer patient, an empirical antibacterial regimen should be started immediately.
- The regimen should have a broad spectrum of activity (including activity against *Pseudomonas aeruginosa*), the ability to achieve high serum bactericidal levels, and be effective in the absence of neutrophils (e.g. aminoglycoside plus an anti-pseudomonal beta-lactam such as ticarcillin-clavulanate, piperacillin, or ceftazidime).
- If no infection is documented yet fever and neutropenia are still present on day 7, consideration should be given to adding an antifungal drug.
- In a patient with a central venous catheter, there should be a low threshold for considering the addition of an antibiotic that has methicillin-resistant Gram-positive bactericidal activity, for example vancomycin.

Cardiac tamponade

Clinical symptoms and signs

- In the setting of malignant pericardial effusion, dyspnea and reduced level of consciousness are symptoms suggesting an emergency due to cardiac tamponade.
- Elevated jugular venous pressure, dyspnoea, tachycardia, hypotension and pulsus paradoxus demonstrate hemodynamic compromise. The heart sounds may be muffled by the fluid in the pericardial sac.

Diagnosis

- An urgent echocardiogram should be obtained. This will confirm the diagnosis and help guide pericardiocentesis, if needed.
- Other imaging techniques may also reveal the diagnosis, for example CT scanning (Figure 14-4).

Management

- Supplemental oxygen should be administered as required.
- Other comorbidities should be excluded (e.g. coagulopathy).

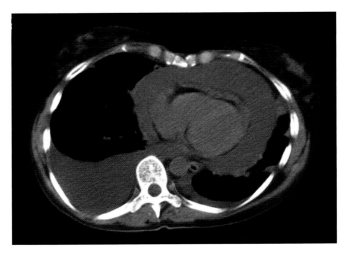

Figure 14-4 Pericardial effusion with large right pleural effusion

- Pericardiocentesis may be needed urgently, or a pericardial window may need to be inserted for longer-term management.

Addisonian crisis

(See Chapter 9.)

- This can occur due to tumor involvement of the adrenals, drugs that block the adrenal function, or withdrawal of corticosteroids that occurs too quickly.
- It presents with weakness, orthostatic hypotension, and pigmentation (if chronic).
- Serum chemistry will reveal hyponatremia and hyperkalemia.
- Treatment is with replacement of corticosteroid.

Disseminated intravascular coagulation (DIC)

(See Chapter 12.)

This can occur in any malignancy, but most commonly in carcinoma of the prostate and acute promyelocytic leukemia.

Hypercalcemia

- Hypercalcemia (see Chapter 9) can be due to lytic bone metastases, parathyroid hormone (PTH)-related peptide production or ectopic PTH production.
- It is most commonly seen in myeloma and breast, head and neck, and lung cancers.
- In the patient with cancer it can also be due to non-malignant causes, including endocrine causes, medications (thiazides, vitamin D, lithium) and other conditions (sarcoidosis).
- Immobilization can precipitate or aggravate hypercalcemia.
- Signs and symptoms include lethargy, nausea, weakness, dehydration and decreased reflexes.

Treatment of hypercalcemia is discussed in Chapter 9. In some patients, hypercalcemia may be a manifestation of advanced disease and treating it may be inappropriate.

Hyponatremia

Hyponatremia can be due to the syndrome of inappropriate antidiuretic hormone (ADH) secretion, of which small-cell lung cancer is the most common oncological cause, but sometimes it is due to liver failure, cardiac failure, overuse of diuretics, spurious causes (e.g. drawing blood from the intravenous line) or medications (tricyclic antidepressants).

Investigation and treatment of hyponatremia is discussed in Chapter 8.

Superior vena cava (SVC) obstruction

- SVC obstruction leads to edema of the face and orbits, facial plethora, dyspnea and orthopnea.
- Examination of the neck will reveal distended veins, with raised jugular venous pressure and loss of normal wave forms.

- Both MRI and computed tomography (CT) are effective in providing the diagnosis.
- Corticosteroids and radiation therapy may relieve obstruction and allow for specific chemotherapy to be used if appropriate.

CLINICAL PEARL

Superior vena cava obstruction may result from central venous cannulation. In this circumstance, anticoagulation will be required.

Raised intracranial pressure (ICP)

- Both primary and secondary intracranial malignancies can result in raised ICP. This should be suspected if nausea, vomiting and headache are present.
- Physical examination may reveal reduced level of consciousness, cerebellar and brain stem neurological signs, and papilledema.
- MRI is a sensitive test for detecting raised ICP.
- Lumbar puncture must be avoided until raised ICP pressure is excluded.
- High-dose corticosteroids will often reduce ICP while definitive therapy is awaited.
- Treatment may include intravenous mannitol, corticosteroids and urgent neurosurgical intervention.

TUMOR MARKERS IN SERUM

Tumor markers predominantly have a role for following the course of disease rather than for establishing the diagnosis. Almost all of these markers can also be raised in non-malignant conditions.

1 **Carcinoembryonic antigen (CEA).** Causes of an elevated level include:
   a colonic cancer (higher levels if the tumor is more differentiated or the cancer is at an advanced stage)
   b other cancers, including lung and breast cancer
   c seminoma
   d cigarette smoking
   e GI tract conditions: cirrhosis, inflammatory bowel disease, rectal polyps, pancreatitis
   f advanced age.

   CEA is of no value in the preoperative diagnosis of colonic cancer or as a prognostic indicator, except for operable liver metastases where a very high level does predict a higher risk of cancer relapse after liver resection. CEA *is* of value in the follow-up of resected colonic cancer; a consistently rising titer suggests metastatic disease and further diagnostic evaluation is indicated.

2 **Alpha fetoprotein (AFP).** Causes of an elevated level include:
   a hepatocellular cancer—very high titers (>500 ng/mL) or a rising titer are strongly suggestive, but >10% of patients do not have an elevated level

b hepatic regeneration, including cirrhosis, and alcoholic or viral hepatitis

c cancer of the stomach, colon, pancreas or lung

d teratocarcinoma or embryonal cell carcinoma (testis, ovary, extra-gonadal)

e pregnancy

f ataxia-telangiectasia

g normal variant.

3 **CA-19-9.** Causes of an elevated level include:

a pancreatic carcinoma (80% with advanced, well-differentiated cancer have an elevated level)

b other gastrointestinal cancers: colon, stomach, bile duct

c other solid tumors, e.g. breast cancer, ovarian cancer, peritoneal carcinoma

d acute or chronic pancreatitis

e chronic liver disease

f cholestasis (any benign or malignant cause)

g cholangitis.

Patients who cannot synthesize Lewis blood group antigens (about 5% of the population) do not produce CA-19-9 antigen.

4 **hCG (human chorionic gonadotropin)**

a non-seminomatous germ-cell tumors (50%), pure seminoma (10%)

b choriocarcinoma (nearly 100%)

c solid tumors, e.g. lung, colon, stomach, pancreas.

5 **Prostate-specific antigen (PSA)**—prostatic carcinoma or any inflammatory condition of the prostate such as prostatitis.

6 **CA-125**—raised in ovarian cancer, peritoneal carcinoma or peritoneal inflammation. CA-125 is not a screening test, but useful for following disease and response to treatment.

7 **CA-15-3**—raised in a range of solid tumors including breast cancer, and can be used to follow disease and response to treatment.

PARANEOPLASTIC SYNDROME

Paraneoplastic syndromes represent a group of clinical scenarios or a constellation of signs and symptoms that occur in association with particular cancers. The cancer is the underlying driver of the syndrome, although the specific pathophysiology that underlies the syndrome may not be fully understood.

The common paraneoplastic syndromes are:

- The 'B' symptoms—anorexia, weight loss, fever.
- Endocrine:
  » hypercalcemia secondary to parathyroid hormone-related peptide (PTHrP), especially squamous-cell carcinomas
  » hyponatremia due to the syndrome of inappropriate secretion of antidiuretic hormone (SIADH)
  » ectopic adrenocorticotropic hormone (ACTH) production, most often seen in small-cell carcinoma
  » carcinoid syndrome from neuroendocrine tumors
  » gynecomastia due to gonadotropin production
  » hypoglycemia due to secretion of insulin–like peptide from squamous-cell carcinoma or mesothelioma
  » hypercalcitoninemia which is usually asymptomatic.

- Neuromuscular:
  » Eaton–Lambert syndrome
  » peripheral neuropathy
  » subacute cerebellar degeneration
  » polymyositis
  » cortical degeneration.
- Connective tissue and bone, including:
  » acanthosis nigricans
  » clubbing
  » hypertrophic osteoarthropathy (due to small-cell lung carcinoma)
  » scleroderma (alveolar cell cancer, adenocarcinoma).
- Hematological:
  » anemia
  » leukoerythroblastosis
  » disseminated intravascular coagulation
  » migrating venous thrombophlebitis.
- Nephrotic syndrome due to membranous glomerulonephritis.

CANCER WITH UNKNOWN PRIMARY (CUP)

The primary site of a cancer is not always known, and up to 5% of cancers are considered to be of 'unknown primary'.

The most common reasons for an undefined primary site are because the primary lesion is too small for detection, there has been removal or elimination of the primary site with surviving metastases, or multiple sites of involvement are present making determination of the primary site imprecise.

Diagnosis

Exhaustive diagnostic investigations, including whole-body imaging with PET scans, are often unrewarding. Careful evaluation of the tumor tissue is important and may provide evidence to support a possible primary location.

Potentially treatable subgroups of CUP

It is important that potentially curable cancers or those responsive to specific therapies are considered in formulating a treatment plan. Potentially treatable subgroups are:

1 Females with isolated axillary lymphadenopathy should be treated as breast cancer, even with a normal mammogram and negative estrogen/progesterone receptor status on biopsy.

2 Females with peritoneal carcinomatosis, which often behaves like ovarian cancer, should be offered treatment with platinum-based chemotherapy.

3 Males with an elevated PSA and blastic bone lesions should be treated as though they have metastatic prostate cancer.

4 Squamous-cell carcinoma in lymph nodes of the upper two-thirds of the head and neck without an obvious primary should be treated aggressively, as 5-year survival rates may then be as high as 30% in this subgroup.

5 Males who fit the classification of midline germ-cell tumor—age <50 years, mediastinal or retroperitoneal tumors (which may not stain for AFP or beta-hCG) may respond to platinum-based chemotherapy like that for germ-cell tumors, with the possibility of long-term survival.

6 Patients with neuroendocrine histology may also respond well to platinum-based chemotherapy.

> ### CLINICAL PEARLS
> - Consider 'treatable' subsets of cancer with unknown primary (CUP) which have better prognosis.
> - Most CUPs are diagnosed at an extensive stage and have a poor outlook.
> - There is no standard chemotherapy regimen.

Recent research and future directions

- PET scan—detects primary cancers in only 40% of cases, usually lung or pancreas.
- Molecular profiling may provide a 'signature' for diagnosis of primary cancer, but currently there is no validated approach to guide therapy.

LUNG CANCER

Clinical presentation

- Cough
- Hemoptysis
- Chest pain
- Dyspnea
- Constitutional symptoms
- Incidental finding on a chest X-ray

Risk factors

- Smoking (90–95% of all cases)
- Increasing age
- Asbestos exposure (both carcinoma and mesothelioma); smoking is synergistic
- Radiation exposure—especially in uranium workers; smoking is synergistic
- Other occupational exposure (aromatic hydrocarbons, arsenic, vinyl chloride, chromium, nickel, hematite, chromate, methyl ether)
- Previous lung cancer resected—5% per year risk of a second primary
- Interstitial lung disease

Epidemiology and pathology

- Fifth most common cancer in men and women
- Most common cause of cancer death (18.9%)
- Median age at diagnosis is 72 years of age.

The two main histological subtypes are non-small cell and small cell lung cancer.

Non-small-cell lung cancer (NSCLC)

- Represents 85% of lung cancers
- Includes the following histologies:
    » adenocarcinoma (40% of all NSCLCs)—this type of cancer represents a greater percentage of NSCLCs in non-smokers and in cancer affecting people from East Asia
    » squamous cell carcinoma (30% of all NSCLCs). These tumors are frequently central lesions with areas of cavitation.
    » large cell carcinoma (10% of all NSCLCs)—usually a poorly differentiated cancer that cannot be characterized as adenocarcinoma or squamous cell carcinoma
    » other rarer subtypes (<5% of all NSCLCs) e.g. mixed histology, sarcomatoid. Staging of NSCLC is outlined in Table 14-1.

Molecular profiling

Molecular profiling is indicated in select patients with advanced lung cancer to identify those individuals with targeted driver mutations for which oral targeted therapies are available in the clinical setting.

All patients with non-squamous cell histology should have molecular profiling of their tumor tissue. This should include EGFR, ALK and ROS-1 testing as a minimum requirement. Any patient with squamous cell histology with unusual clinical characteristics (e.g. non-smoker) should also be considered for molecular testing.

All patients with advanced disease should have PD-L1 immunohistochemistry analysis performed to select those patients who may derive benefit from immune therapy.

Table 14-1 Staging of non-small-cell lung cancer

STAGE	DESCRIPTION
1	Lung cancer <3 cm in diameter and without lymph node involvement
2	Lung cancer >4 cm in diameter with ipsilateral peribronchial or hilar lymph node involvement
3	Lung cancer >5 cm in diameter; or cancer directly invading local structures including pleura, chest wall, heart, great vessels, carina; or cancer with mediastinal lymph node involvement
4	Cancer with malignant pleural effusion, separate tumor nodules in contralateral lobe, or distant metastases

Prognosis

Figure 14-5 (overleaf) shows cumulative survival rates following treatment.

Management

Treatment of different stages is outlined in Table 14-2, overleaf.

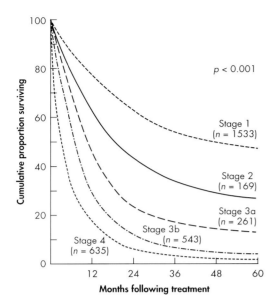

Figure 14-5 Cumulative survival of non-small-cell lung cancer after treatment, according to clinical stage

Redrawn from Mountain CF. A new international staging system for lung cancer. Chest 1966;89(4 Suppl):S225–S233.

Table 14-2 Treatment of non-small-cell lung cancer

STAGE	TREATMENT
I	Surgery*
II	Surgery* + consider adjuvant chemotherapy
IIIA	Possible surgery ± chemotherapy If inoperable, for definitive chemoradiotherapy followed by maintenance immune therapy
IIIB	Definitive chemoradiotherapy followed by maintenance immune therapy
IV	Chemotherapy, immune therapy, targeted therapies, palliative radiotherapy
* Radical radiotherapy if patient is not a surgical candidate.	

Treatment of stage IV NSCLC

The results of molecular profiling and PD-L1 analysis guide the choice of first-line systemic therapy. For those patients with no actionable mutation and PD-L1 levels <50%, chemotherapy or a combination of chemotherapy and immune therapy are the standard treatment options. Chemotherapy can provide a benefit for patients with advanced lung cancer:

- it improves median overall survival
- it delays cancer progression
- it sustains or improves the quality of life
- it results in symptom improvement.

First-line chemotherapy

Key information:

- Platinum doublet chemotherapy regimens confer a survival advantage.
- Combination therapy with two drugs is better than single agent chemotherapy alone.
- Patients with a poor performance status do not derive benefit from combination treatment.

Monoclonal antibodies

- Monoclonal antibodies have shown benefits in NSCLC:
  » Bevacizumab when combined with chemotherapy (carboplatin and paclitaxel) prolongs survival in advanced-stage NSCLC.
  » Cetuximab when combined with chemotherapy (vinorelbine and cisplatin) also prolongs survival in advanced-stage NSCLC.
  » The decision to incorporate these monoclonal antibodies into first-line chemotherapy must take into account additional toxicity, patient preference, and cost-effectiveness.

'Maintenance' therapy

Maintenance therapy after first-line chemotherapy can prolong survival or delay the time to cancer progression. These treatments are given after an initial course of chemotherapy, so called first-line chemotherapy, as a means of 'maintaining' or sustaining the response against the cancer. In effect, that time to cancer progression is prolonged. Pemetrexed has demonstrated benefit as maintenance therapy in patients with non-squamous histology.

First-line immune therapy

In patients with NSCLC with high PD-L1 expression (equal to or greater than 50%), first-line immune therapy (pembrolizumab) has been shown to be superior to platinum-based chemotherapy in terms of response rates, progression-free survival and overall survival.

Epidermal growth factor receptor as a treatment target

- Epidermal growth factor receptor (EGFR) activation initiates signal transduction that promotes tumor-cell proliferation and survival.
- Activating EGFR gene mutations are found in 15–20% of NSCLC cases.
- These mutations are more common in females, non-smokers and people from East Asia.
- EGFR TKI (e.g. gefitinib, erlotinib, afatinib) have been shown to be superior to platinum-based chemotherapy in the first-line setting for patients with an underlying EGFR sensitizing mutation.
- Patients will develop resistance to EGFR TKI at a median time of 9–12 months and repeat biopsy should be considered to evaluate the resistance mechanisms to guide further therapy.
- The most common resistance mechanism is the T790M mutation and there are third-generation EGFR TKIs

(e.g. osimertinib) in clinical practice that have activity against this mutation.

Anaplastic lymphoma kinase gene rearrangement as a treatment target

Anaplastic lymphoma kinase (ALK) gene rearrangements are seen in 2–5% of all NSCLCs.

They are typically seen in younger patients with a light smoking history and an adenocarcinoma histology. Signet ring cells are often seen.

ALK inhibitors (e.g. crizotinib and alectinib) have been found to be superior to platinum-based chemotherapy and good central nervous system penetration is seen with this class of drugs.

ROS-1 and other targets

ROS-1 rearrangements are seen in 1–2% of all NSCLC and ROS-1 inhibitors are starting to be used in clinical practice (e.g. crizotinib).

There are other rare genotypes with targeted therapies moving into clinical practice or clinical trials. These include BRAF mutations, NTRK fusions, HER2 mutations, MET abnormalities and RET rearrangements.

Recent developments are focusing on the use of 'liquid biopsies' or blood-based tests.

Small cell lung cancer (SCLC)

- Represents 15% of lung cancers.
- This is one of the most aggressive cancers, with a rapid doubling time.
- It has a tendency to spread early, frequently involving the liver, bones, adrenals and brain.
- It is broadly split into two stages—limited stage and extensive stage.
- A platinum agent and etoposide is the most commonly employed chemotherapy regimen.

Limited stage (Stage I–IIIB)

- Disease is limited to the thorax and encompassed within a radiotherapy field.
- Treatment is with concurrent chemotherapy and radiotherapy.
- Prophylactic cranial irradiation reduces the risk of CNS involvement and may improve overall survival.
- The aim of treatment is cure; this may be achieved in only 15–20% of patients who present with limited disease.

Extensive stage (Stage IIIB–IV)

- The disease has started to spread to other organs and is incurable.
- Without chemotherapy the prognosis is very poor, with an expected survival of less than 3 months.
- While more than 80% of patients will have tumors that respond to chemotherapy, the majority will progress within a short time of completing chemotherapy.

- The expected survival in those who receive chemotherapy is <12 months.
- The addition of immune therapy (atezolizumab, durvalumab) to chemotherapy with continuation of maintenance immune therapy has shown modest improvement in overall survival of 2 months, with no improvement in response rates or progression-free survival.

RENAL CANCER

Background

- The typical presentation of renal cancer is with flank pain, hematuria and abdominal mass.
- Increasingly, renal cancers are found incidentally on radiological scans such as CT imaging and account for 25–30% of presentations.
- The most frequent histological subtypes include clear cell, papillary and chromophobe renal cell carcinoma.
- The *VHL* gene mutation is associated with clear-cell carcinoma.

The risk factors for renal cell carcinoma include:

- smoking
- environmental toxins such as trichloroethylene
- chronic use of certain analgesic agents
- genetic conditions such as von Hippel–Lindau disease
- hereditary papillary renal cell carcinoma

A genetic predisposition may also be a factor.

Diagnosis and staging

- CT imaging of the kidneys will often reveal characteristic features of carcinoma and help with differentiation from simple cysts. Magnetic resonance imaging (MRI) of the kidneys is also being increasingly utilized in both characterization of renal cancer for diagnosis, and surgical work-up.

CLINICAL PEARL

Renal cysts that represent concern for the possibility of renal cell carcinoma have features beyond simple cysts, such as hairline or thick septa, irregular outlines, thickened walls, fine or coarse calcifications in the wall, and solid elements.

- A tissue diagnosis is usually required and involves either a biopsy of the renal mass or a metastatic lesion. However, improved diagnostic imaging tools have negated the need for tissue diagnosis prior to nephrectomy in some circumstances.
- There is no reliable serum tumor marker.
- CT imaging of the chest, abdomen and pelvis will assist with staging.
- A bone scan should be performed if symptoms suggest possible bone involvement.

Much less common forms of kidney cancer include Wilms' tumor (childhood embryonic nephroblastoma) and renal sarcoma.

Treatment

Localized disease

- The aim of treatment for localized renal cancers is curative with surgery, usually with a radical or partial nephrectomy.
  - » Non-surgical treatment options e.g. stereotactic body radiotherapy (SBRT) are being evaluated for patients who are medically unfit for surgery.
  - » Currently, there are no studies of adjuvant treatment which have shown an overall survival benefit in patients with high-risk renal cancer.

Advanced disease

- Chemotherapy has not been shown to be effective in treatment of renal cell carcinoma.
  - » There have been significant advances in the treatment of renal cell carcinoma over the last decade with the use of immunotherapy and VEGF-directed therapy and tyrosine kinase inhibitors.
  - » The role of cytoreductive nephrectomy in the setting of metastatic disease has been controversial; however, recent studies suggest surgery should be reserved for those with symptomatic primary disease such as significant hematuria and flank pain or those with limited or solitary metastases.
  - » There is also a role for metastatectomy in some patients with renal cell cancer.

Immunotherapy

- » The combination of ipilimumab (anti-CTLA-4 monoclonal antibody) and nivolumab (anti-PD-1 antibody) has been shown to improve overall survival, partial response (42% versus 27%) and complete response (9% versus 1%) compared to sunitinib in the first-line setting in patients with intermediate or poor prognostic features.
- » Nivolumab has been shown to improve overall survival and response rates compared to everolimus after the use of first-line tyrosine kinase inhibitors.
- » There are ongoing trials investigating the use of combination immunotherapy or immunotherapy plus tyrosine kinase inhibitors in renal cancers.

VEGF-directed therapy and multi-targeted TKIs

- This is associated with 50–80% tumor shrinkage and a 10–20% partial response rate, but no or few complete responses.
  - » Cabozantinib, sunitinib and pazopanib are used in the first-line setting for renal cancer with cabozantinib shown to have improved progression-free survival and partial or complete response rates over sunitinib.
- Cabozantinib and axitinib are also used in the second-line setting.

mTOR-directed approach

Mammalian target of rapamycin (mTOR) inhibitors such as temsirolimus and everolimus have been studied with modest improvements in progression-free survival.

Prognosis

- The 5-year survival for patients with regional or localized cancer is 70–90%.
- In patients with stage 4 renal cancer, the 5-year survival is approximately 8–12%.

TUMORS OF THE PELVIS, URETER AND BLADDER

Epidemiology

Bladder and ureteric cancer has roughly the same incidence rate as renal cancer, at 21 per 100,000 per year. There are increased rates in men compared with women, and it is more common in individuals of Caucasian genetic origin. In parts of Africa and the Middle East, bladder cancer associated with schistosomiasis is very common and is usually associated with squamous bladder cancers. The median age at presentation is 73 and the 5-year overall survival for all stages is 70–80%, although patients with stage 4 bladder cancer have a 5-year overall survival of ~ 5%.

Risk factors

Incidence rates and overall survival are improving with time. However, in women, 50% of bladder cancer is now known to be smoking-related, due to increased rates of smoking in women. Smoking remains an important risk factor in men. Other risk factors include the following:

- Occupational exposures including to dyes (e.g. aniline dye and aromatic amines; hairdressers, machinists, painters and truck drivers).
- Schistosomiasis.
- Arsenic exposure.
- Chronic bladder problems, such as stones and bladder infections, including in those with paraparesis-related chronic urinary sepsis.
- Exposure to cytotoxic drugs, especially cyclophosphamide (which is of special interest to physicians).
  - » Cyclophosphamide is known to cause acute hemorrhagic cystitis, and lead to a significant increase in the risk of bladder and other renal tract cancers. Protocols related to chemotherapy use for other cancer states include significant prophylaxis against bladder cancer. This is achieved by administration early in the day (not leaving a concentrated amount of chemotherapy drug or its metabolites in the bladder overnight), with adequate hydration, even forced diuresis, and with the bladder protectant Mesna (2-mercaptoethan sulfonate sodium). Mesna detoxifies by reaction with its sulfhydryl group, and by increasing cysteine excretion in the urine is protective against hemorrhagic cystitis.

- Long-term use of compound analgesics. These gain access to the totality of the urinary drainage system by way of their concentration through active excretion in the urinary tract, leading to multiple points of carcinogenesis and thereby multi-focal urethelial tumors.

Bladder cancer can take the form of:

- transitional cell carcinoma (urothelial carcinoma) (90%)
- squamous-cell carcinoma (3–4%)
- adenocarcinoma (1–2%).

These can all occur anywhere in the urinary tract.

Clinical presentation

Bladder cancer should be suspected in those with painless hematuria, and known risk factors. There can be dysuria, and stranguria in the absence of proven urinary tract infection. Other nonspecific symptoms can include frequency and nocturia.

Investigation and diagnosis

- Early diagnosis and screening in those susceptible is best achieved by cystoscopic examination, with retrograde examination of the ureters.
- Urinary cytology may be useful also in a sufficiently concentrated sample.
- Imaging modalities including intravesical ultrasound, and abdominopelvic CT or MRI may be necessary to determine extension beyond the bladder wall, and pelvic or retroperitoneal extension or spread.

Treatment

- The mainstay of bladder cancer treatment is resection of the tumors by endoscopic procedures in those with non-muscle invasive bladder cancer. This may be followed by treatment with intravesical Bacillus Calmette-Guérin (BCG) therapy to prevent disease recurrence.
  - » In patients with muscle-invasive bladder cancer, treatment usually involves radical cystectomy and extended pelvic lymphadenectomy with either neo-adjuvant or adjuvant chemotherapy or combination chemoradiotherapy for patients who are medically unfit for surgery.
- Treatment of early or low-grade tumors is with laser-induced interstitial thermotherapy or hyperthermia, or photodynamic therapy after using a photosensitizing agent.
  - » In patients with metastatic disease or those with muscle-invasive bladder cancers who are unfit for surgery, chemotherapy options include platinum-based therapy with cisplatin or carboplatin.
  - » Recently, trials with immunotherapy have been very promising with pembrolizumab and nivolumab used in the non-first-line setting. There are ongoing trials investigating the use of immunotherapy with or without chemotherapy in the first-line and the neoadjuvant settings.

PROSTATE CANCER

Epidemiology

- The most common malignancy diagnosed in males.
- Although most men do not die of prostate cancer, it still represents the second most common cause of cancer-related death in men.
- BRCA1/2 mutations should be considered in patients with younger onset prostate cancer or those with aggressive disease. Genetic testing should also be considered for those with a strong family history of breast and prostate cancer due to the 3–8-fold increase in prostate cancer risk for those with BRCA1 or 2 mutations.

Screening

- At a population level, serum PSA testing will detect pre-clinical cases of cancer but the overall survival benefit has not been verified. There are no national population-based screening programs and the adoption of PSA screening as a population-based tool is controversial.
- Individual management of prostate cancer risk relies on a strong history and presentation at age <60 years.

Staging

A Incidental finding at transurethral resection.

B Palpable nodule involving one lobe of the prostate.

C Peri-prostatic tissue involved (C2 involves the seminal vesicles).

D Metastatic disease including regional lymph nodes.

The Gleason score, a pathological grading system based on the microscopic appearance of the cancer, informs prognosis and may guide therapy. It is used as a pathological measure of the biology of the cancer. A higher score usually indicates a more aggressive (faster growing, poorer prognosis) cancer.

- » Diagnostic staging scans include CT chest/abdomen and pelvis and bone scan as the most common sites of metastases are bone (90%), lymph nodes (70%) and lung.
- » Recently, the use of prostate-specific membrane antigen (PSMA)/positron emission tomography (PET) scans have been widely utilized to increase the diagnostic and staging accuracy of patients with prostate cancer.

Management

Stages A–C

Surgery and/or radical radiotherapy is the treatment of choice.

- The decision between surgery or radical radiotherapy relies on a careful weighing of the risks of each strategy. Usually, locally advanced disease or localized cancers with a high PSA and a high Gleason score are managed with radiotherapy. Those with a relatively low PSA and Gleason score may be managed with either approach.

- » Risks of surgery can include erectile dysfunction and incontinence.
- » Risks of radiation include radiation proctitis and cystitis.
- In men without symptoms and a low PSA/low Gleason score, a reasonable policy may be to monitor only, as clinically significant disease may take more than 10 years to develop.
- In younger men with PSA <15 ng/dL, surgery is often recommended.

Stage D

- Stage D may be treated by hormonal manipulation when patients are symptomatic.
  - » LHRH agonists (e.g. goserelin or leuprorelin, degarelix) or LHRH antagonists such as degarelix administered by regular subcutaneous depot injection downregulate the LHRH receptor to cause a chemical castration. Depending on the formulation used, these injections can be administered monthly to 3- or 4-monthly.
  - » Anti-androgens (flutamide, bicalutamide, cyproterone acetate) block androgen receptors on tumor cells and are used ideally in combination with medical or surgical castration ('total androgen blockade'). The timing of total androgen blockade (at the time of diagnosis or when symptoms manifest) remains controversial.
  - » Castrate-resistant prostate cancer refers to a rise in PSA despite the use of androgen deprivation therapy and when serum testosterone is in the castrate range. This may occur in either the absence or the presence of metastases.
  - » In the setting of metastatic castrate-resistant prostate cancer, chemotherapy including docetaxel and cabazitaxel have been shown to improve overall survival in the first- and second-line settings. Abiraterone, a novel hormone therapy targeting inhibition of CYP17 and enzalutamide, an androgen receptor inhibitor has also been shown to improve survival used either prior to or following chemotherapy.
  - » Recently, the use of docetaxel chemotherapy or abiraterone at the time of diagnosis with metastatic disease in the addition of androgen deprivation therapy (castrate-sensitive prostate cancer) has also been shown to significantly improve overall survival.
  - » Radium-223 has also been shown to improve overall survival in patients with bone metastases, although this treatment is not widely available.
- A prostate cancer autologous vaccine, Sipuleucel-T, is an immune-stimulant that has been associated with a prolongation of survival of 4.1 months in a large randomized controlled trial. This became the first FDA-approved cancer vaccine, but the expense has precluded widespread uptake.
- New radioisotope therapeutic strategies are in development. Denosumab and zoledronic acid are used in patients with castrate-resistant prostate cancer and bone metastases for prevention of skeletal-related events. These treatments have not been shown to improve survival in prostate cancer. Significant adverse events include hypocalcemia and osteonecrosis of the jaw.

TESTIS CANCER

Epidemiology and risk

- The incidence of testis cancer has risen, having doubled in the past 40 years.
- Testis cancer represents 1% of male cancers.
- It is the most common cancer in men aged 20–34 years.
- The lifetime risk in Caucasians is 0.2%; it is less common in people of Asian or African origin.

Risk factors

- Cryptorchidism
- Contralateral testicular tumor: 2–5% risk
- Orchitis
- Testicular injury
- Estrogen exposure
- Low sperm count
- Elevated follicle-stimulating hormone (FSH)

Pathology

- 95% are germ cell tumors (GCTs): seminoma and non-seminomatous germ cell tumor (NSGCT).
- Carcinoma *in situ* (CIS) is a precursor, and if present there is a 50% risk of developing cancer at 5 years.
- NSGCT is classified into:
  - » malignant teratoma undifferentiated (MTU) (embryonal)
  - » teratoma differentiated (TD) (mature teratoma)
  - » choriocarcinoma
  - » yolk sac tumor.

Testicular cancer is a highly curable cancer. The 5-year overall survival is 98%. It is considered highly sensitive to chemotherapy.

Diagnosis

Clinical features

- Scrotal or testicular mass; 75% are painless
- Scrotal or testicular pain
- Hydrocele
- Lymphadenopathy
- Symptoms due to metastases

Investigations and staging

- Testicular ultrasound is the appropriate initial investigation to assess a suspicious testicular mass.

- Confirmation of the diagnosis will require orchidectomy.
- CT scanning is used for staging—25% of cancers are, however, under-staged by CT.
- Tumor markers (AFP, hCG, LDH) are an important determinant of the presence of occult metastatic disease after orchidectomy.
- PET scanning is increasingly used; note that it requires specialist interpretation and has not yet been established as improving outcomes.

Staging according to the Union for International Cancer Control is given in Table 14-3.

Table 14-3 UICC staging system

Clinical stage I	Pathology confined to the testis Tumor markers normal (or falling at expected rate) Radiological investigations normal
Pathological stage I	As per clinical stage I, but no evidence of lymph-node involvement in retroperitoneal lymph nodes following resection
Stage II	Regional lymph-node involvement, including retroperitoneal nodes
Stage III	Distant nodes or visceral/bone metastases

UICC, Union for International Cancer Control.

Adapted from Sobin LH, Gospodariwicz M and Wittekind C (eds). TNM classification of malignant tumors. UICC International Union Against Cancer, 7th ed. Wiley-Blackwell, 2009.

Prognostic factors in stage I NSGCT

Studies show that there is one consistent histological prognostic factor in this condition, which is vascular invasion (VI).

- VI is an important predictor of retroperitoneal lymph-node involvement in clinical stage 1 disease.
- VI predicts the risk of relapse (usually visceral) in pathological stage I disease after retroperitoneal lymph-node dissection.

Treatment

Sperm storage should be offered to all patients before chemotherapy.

Radical orchidectomy

The procedure describes orchidectomy plus retroperitoneal lymph-node dissection (RPLND).

- It is part of primary 'treatment' in the USA and Germany, but not a routine staging or therapeutic procedure in the rest of Europe or in Australia.
- As imaging techniques improve, the need for RPLND should lessen.
- It carries a risk of causing ejaculatory dysfunction.
- Routine RPLND detects metastases in 25–30% of patients, therefore 70–75% are having an unnecessary procedure.

- The incidence of visceral metastases following RPLND is 10% when lymph node is negative for tumor.

Seminoma

Stage I

- Adjuvant para-aortic radiotherapy.
- Single-agent chemotherapy: 1 cycle of carboplatin.
  » Active surveillance.

Stage II

- If the disease is bulky (>5 cm), treatment is with chemotherapy: bleomycin, etoposide and cisplatin (BEP), or etoposide and cisplatin (EP).
- If the disease is not bulky, radiotherapy is another option.

Stage III

Treatment is with chemotherapy, either with BEP or with EP in better prognosis disease.

NSGCT

Stage I

- The choice of treatment in stage I disease is between surveillance alone and adjuvant chemotherapy with 2 cycles of BEP.
- The decision should take into account relapse risk, prognostic histological factors, and compliance with surveillance.

The arguments *against* adjuvant therapy are:

- There are outstanding results in stage II/III disease, with >90% long-term disease-free survival. So, with close surveillance a cancer recurrence can be detected and successful therapy implemented.
- Many patients who are cured by surgery will receive chemotherapy when they do not need it.

The arguments *for* adjuvant chemotherapy are:

- The risk of recurrence is very low after adjuvant therapy—only 1% will develop cancer recurrence.
- The total dose (i.e. number of cycles) will be less when giving adjuvant therapy, with less cumulative toxicity, than the chemotherapy needed to treat a cancer recurrence.

Stages II and III

Treatment is with chemotherapy, either with BEP or with EP in better-prognosis disease.

Intermediate- or poor-prognosis metastatic disease

Treat with chemotherapy (3 cycles of BEP, then 1 cycle of EP).

Post-chemotherapy residual masses

Residual masses are commonly seen after primary chemotherapy, particularly in seminoma and differentiated teratoma, and less commonly with embryonal carcinoma.

- 45–50% of masses are found to be lymph nodes which contain necrotic tissue and fibrosis.
- 35% of teratomas are differentiated (mature teratoma).
- 15–20% contain viable carcinoma (vital malignant tumor).

After salvage chemotherapy for residual masses, approximately 50% of lesions will still contain carcinoma, so resection should be considered.

Relapsed disease

Salvage chemotherapy for relapsed GCT

- Overall, 10–30% of patients with GCT will relapse.
- It can be difficult to differentiate relapsed disease versus residual mass or mature teratoma.
- Patients can be cured with second-line chemotherapy, with the long-term survival of 20–30%.
- Seminoma and NSGCT are treated in essentially the same manner upon relapse following primary chemotherapy.
- Consideration should be given to surgical resection for late relapses, as such cancers are more likely to be resistant to chemotherapy.
- Most relapses occur in the first 2 years and are still curable even in those who have had prior chemotherapy.

High-dose chemotherapy (HDCT)

This is usually given following conventional-dose salvage chemotherapy or in high-risk/poor-prognosis situations, such as:

- an extragonadal primary site
- progressive disease after an incomplete response to primary therapy
- poor response or progression after treatment with cisplatin plus ifosfamide-containing conventional salvage therapy.

HEAD AND NECK CANCER

A multidisciplinary approach, involving surgeons, medical oncologists and radiation oncologists as well as dentists, dietitians, speech pathologists and rehabilitation therapists, is generally required for treatment planning and management of patients with head and neck cancer.

- Optimal therapy will depend upon tumor site and stage, the risks of therapy, and patient performance status, comorbidities and preference.
- Patients often have a history of excessive alcohol intake and smoking.
- Human papillomavirus (HPV) is becoming increasingly associated with oropharyngeal cancers (see below).

Early-stage disease

Small primary tumors with no nodal or distal metastases are generally managed with single-modality treatments (either surgery or radiation therapy).

Advanced-stage disease

Advanced head and neck cancer—large primary tumor and/or nodal involvement—is usually managed with multimodality treatments.

- Options include:
  » primary surgery followed by either postoperative radiotherapy or concurrent chemotherapy and radiation
  » induction chemotherapy (the addition of chemotherapy prior to surgery and/or radiotherapy)
  » concurrent chemoradiotherapy
  » sequential therapy (induction chemotherapy followed by concurrent chemoradiotherapy).
- Palliative chemotherapy and/or supportive care is recommended for recurrent or metastatic disease. Immune therapy may have a role in patients who have developed progression post platinum-based chemotherapy.
- Select patients with disease confined to the head and neck may benefit from surgical salvage and/or re-irradiation.
- Cetuximab also provides a benefit in patients with inoperable localized disease when used in combination with radiotherapy, particularly in patients not considered suitable for chemotherapy.

Human papillomavirus (HPV) infection

- Human papillomavirus is associated with over one-half of all head and neck squamous-cell cancers, primarily in the tonsils and the base of the tongue.
- Younger patients without a history of excessive exposure to alcohol and tobacco are often affected.

ESOPHAGEAL CANCER

Pathology and epidemiology

- The majority of cases of esophageal cancer are either adenocarcinoma, for which the incidence is rising, or squamous-cell carcinoma, for which the incidence is falling.
- The male:female ratio is 4:1.
- Risk factors include smoking, alcohol consumption, obesity, dry salted foods and, most importantly, Barrett's esophagus for adenocarcinoma.
- *Helicobacter pylori* is a protective factor for adenocarcinoma (lowers gastric acid).
- Barrett's esophagus is the major risk factor for adenocarcinoma.

Clinical presentation

The three major symptoms of esophageal cancer are:

- dysphagia
- nausea
- weight loss.

Less commonly, patients may experience chest pain or GI tract bleeding.

Diagnosis and screening

- Endoscopy allows for visualization of lesions and biopsy to confirm the diagnosis.
- Endoscopic ultrasound allows assessment of loco-regional extent of disease.
- FDG-PET scanning and/or diagnostic laparoscopy may be used to determine if there is metastatic disease.
- CT imaging of the thorax and abdomen allows assessment for local spread and metastatic disease.
- No survival advantage has yet been demonstrated for population-based screening for Barrett's esophagus.

Management

Early-stage disease

Multiple treatment strategies are available:

- surgery alone
- radiotherapy alone
- chemoradiotherapy alone
- surgery followed by chemoradiotherapy
- chemotherapy followed by surgery
- perioperative chemotherapy.

There is no evidence of the curative potential for chemotherapy alone without surgery or radiotherapy.

- Radiotherapy is usually given concurrently with a platinum-based chemotherapy regimen.
- For cancers of the lower esophagus, perioperative chemotherapy (before and after surgery) has been shown to improve outcomes.

Metastatic disease

- Metastatic disease is not curable.
- Chemotherapy delivers modest survival benefit over best supportive care, and may also help to alleviate symptoms.
- Overall, the 5-year survival rate for esophageal cancer is 20%.

GASTRIC CANCER

Epidemiology

- There is a decline in incidence in Western countries of gastric cancer, although it remains high in Southeast Asia.
- It is the second most common cause of cancer death worldwide. Tumors of the cardia and gastroesophageal junction are increasing.
- *Helicobacter pylori* is the major cause; autoimmune atrophic gastritis (pernicious anemia) is less common.
- Hereditary diffuse gastric cancer is autosomal dominant, leading to early gastric cancer.

Clinical presentation

- Gastric cancer often presents with locally advanced disease.
- Dyspepsia and nausea are common symptoms.
- Weight loss, anorexia, early satiety, and pain are common in the advanced stages of disease.
- Rarer presentations include gastrointestinal bleeding, and prominent vomiting may be a clue to linitis plastica or gastric outlet obstruction, where diffuse infiltration of tumor reduces gastric distensibility.

CLINICAL PEARLS

- Remember, all gastric ulcers need repeat endoscopy to ensure healing.
- Early cancers are impossible to reliably distinguish from benign ulcers on appearance alone.

Diagnosis

- Endoscopy should be performed on symptomatic patients to determine location and allow for biopsies. Endoscopic ultrasound allows assessment of the depth of lesions.
- Staging investigations should include abdomino-pelvic CT.
- Although PET is useful for distant metastases it may not define peritoneal disease, for which a preoperative laparoscopy may be of benefit.

Treatment

Surgery

- Surgical resection has the greatest chance of cure.
- While there is increased operative mortality for total gastrectomy, it is recommended if there is diffuse involvement of the stomach or involvement of the cardia.

Adjuvant therapy

Adjuvant chemotherapy

Meta-analyses reveal a survival benefit with the use of adjuvant chemotherapy.

- Peri-operative chemotherapy (epirubicin, cisplatin and 5FU given before and after surgery) prolongs survival in the management of operable gastric cancer compared with surgery alone.
- Following initial gastrectomy, the application of both chemotherapy and radiotherapy may prolong survival and lower the risk of cancer recurrence.

Chemotherapy for metastatic disease

- A survival benefit has been demonstrated through the use of chemotherapy compared with best supportive care (BSC).

- Response rates generally range from 25% to 50%.
- Overall survival usually ranges from 6–9 months, but is usually less than 12 months in large, randomized trials.
- Trastuzumab combined with chemotherapy should be used for patients with advanced gastroesophageal cancer that is HER2-positive on immunohistochemistry. HER2-positive disease accounts for 20% of advanced gastric cancers.
- Combination chemotherapy is associated with palliative benefit with acceptable toxicity.
- There has been little recent change in case fatality in Western countries, with a 5-year survival rate of 20%. This contrasts with a 50% 5-year survival rate in Japan.

Gastric MALT lymphoma

- Gastric mucosa-associated lymphoid tissue (MALT) lymphoma is a form of extranodal marginal-zone B-cell lymphoma.
- Chronic immune stimulation, most commonly from *Helicobacter pylori* infection, is causative. Early lesions often respond to *H. pylori* eradication, and more than 90% of patients with MALT lymphoma are infected with *H. pylori*.
- More advanced disease requires systemic chemotherapy.

COLORECTAL CANCER

Pathology and epidemiology

- The transformation from normal colonic epithelium to an invasive cancer is a multi-step gene mutation process.
  » Adenomatous polyposis coli (APC) and hereditary non-polyposis colon cancer (HNPCC) are driven by single germ-line mutations.
  » Sporadic cancers result from the stepwise accumulation of multiple somatic mutations.
  » Microsatellite instability high (MSI-H) expression is associated with HNPCC and is also observed in approximately 10–15% of sporadic colorectal cancers.
  » Most cancers develop from polyps via the adenoma-to-carcinoma sequence.
- The incidence and mortality from colorectal cancer can be reduced through population screening for colorectal cancer, using fecal occult blood testing or colonoscopy.

CLINICAL PEARL

20–30% of cases of colorectal cancer will present with stage IV (metastatic) disease, with the liver, lungs and lymph nodes being the most common sites of cancer spread.

Colorectal cancer (CRC) risk factors

- Age >50
- Inflammatory bowel disease
- Smoking
- History of adenomatous polyps
- First-degree relatives with colon cancer or adenomatous polyps
- Familial polyposis (FAP) syndromes
- HNPCC
- Obesity, fatty and high-calorie diet and type 2 diabetes
- *BRCA1* mutation
- Female genital or breast cancer
- Acromegaly

Diagnosis and staging

- Common presenting symptoms include change in bowel habit, bleeding per rectum, abdominal bloating or pain.
- Fatigue can be a presenting feature related to iron-deficiency anemia.
- Colonoscopy can localize and biopsy lesions throughout the large bowel, and polyps can be removed.
- Preoperative clinical staging involves physical examination, CT scan of the abdomen and pelvis, and chest imaging (CT or chest X-ray).
- Digital rectal examination, rigid sigmoidoscopy, trans-rectal endoscopic ultrasound, and/or MRI are indicated for loco-regional staging of patients with rectal cancer, to select the surgical approach and identify those patients who are candidates for initial radiotherapy or chemoradiotherapy rather than up-front surgery.
- PET scanning is not required prior to resection of localized bowel cancer, but are performed prior to hepatic resection for liver metastases.
- Serum carcinoembryonic antigen (CEA) is not useful in the primary diagnosis of colorectal cancer, but can be a useful biomarker to monitor patients after initial treatment of bowel cancer. A rising CEA level usually indicates cancer progression or recurrence.
- The optimal follow-up schedule for patients with early-stage CRC after completion of surgery and adjuvant therapies has not been defined. The approach usually includes periodic physical examination, CEA, colonoscopy and liver imaging (ultrasound or CT scan).

Staging of bowel cancer is outlined in Table 14-4.

CLINICAL PEARL

Important red flags for colorectal cancer when taking the history:
- hematochezia, melena, altered bowel habits, weight loss, iron-deficiency anemia and onset of symptoms after the age of 45 years
- endocarditis or sepsis caused by either *Streptococcus gallolyticus* or *Clostridium septicum*.

Table 14-4 Staging of bowel cancer

STAGE	DESCRIPTION
I	Cancer restricted to the bowel wall, extending from mucosa to submucosa and involvement of muscularis layer but not through to serosal surface
II	Cancer extending through the bowel wall to the serosal surface and may even extend beyond the serosa but not to regional lymph nodes
III	Cancer spread to local lymph nodes
IV	Cancer spread to distant sites (metastases)

Management

Early-stage bowel cancer

- Complete surgical excision remains the curative option.
- Following potentially curative resection of colon cancer, the goal of adjuvant chemotherapy is to eradicate micro-metastases, thereby reducing the likelihood of disease recurrence and increasing the cure rate.
- The benefits of adjuvant chemotherapy have been most clearly demonstrated in stage III (node-positive) disease.
- The benefit remains contentious for stage II disease.

Stage I

No further therapy after surgery.

Stage II

- The survival benefit associated with adjuvant chemotherapy is very small or absent.
  - » Without high-risk features, observation (without adjuvant therapy) is an acceptable approach.
  - » If high-risk features are present, such as bowel obstruction, bowel perforation, T4, high-grade tumor or lymphovascular invasion, adjuvant chemotherapy may provide a survival benefit across the population.
  - » A low number of lymph nodes examined (<12) is also considered a potential feature associated with a higher risk of cancer recurrence, and such patients should be considered for adjuvant chemotherapy.
- Adjuvant chemotherapy may comprise of single-agent fluoropyrimidine (e.g. 5FU/leucovorin or capecitabine) or FOLFOX (5FU/leucovorin and oxaliplatin) or CAPOX (capecitabine and oxaliplatin), although combination chemotherapy has not been demonstrated to provide a survival benefit over single-agent fluoropyrimidine chemotherapy in stage II disease.
- Patients without high-risk features who have MSI-H–deficient mismatch-repair tumors have a favorable prognosis and are not likely to benefit from adjuvant fluoropyrimidine-based therapy.

Stage III

- Adjuvant chemotherapy provides a survival benefit, with a relative reduction in the risk of disease recurrence of 30% and a mortality reduction of 25%.
- The most commonly used regimen is FOLFOX or CAPOX. The duration of treatment is usually 6 months; however, recent studies have shown that 3 months of adjuvant chemotherapy for patients with low-risk stage III CRC is non-inferior to 6 months of treatment.
- Peripheral neuropathy can be a long-term complication of oxaliplatin.
- Single-agent capecitabine can also provide a survival benefit.
- There is no evidence of benefit with the addition of bevacizumab.
- No evidence has been found for improved outcomes when cetuximab is added to chemotherapy in *K-ras* wild-type stage III colon cancer.
- Older patients may not benefit from oxaliplatin doublet chemotherapy, but they do benefit from 5FU-based adjuvant chemotherapy as much as younger patients do.

Metastatic bowel cancer—stage IV

- The intent of therapy is palliative in almost all people.
- A subset of patients with liver, and in select cases lung-limited, disease can undergo resection of metastases with curative intent.
- Although long-term prognosis is poor for patients with unresectable metastatic CRC, palliative chemotherapy can relieve symptoms, improve quality of life and prolong survival.
  - » Active drugs include the fluoropyrimidines, oxaliplatin, irinotecan, and the therapeutic monoclonal antibodies bevacizumab, cetuximab, and panitumumab.
  - » The optimal way to combine and sequence these agents is not yet established. In general, exposure to all active drugs is more important than the specific sequence of administration.
- Commonly used chemotherapy regimens include a chemotherapy doublet:
  - » FOLFOX = folinic acid, 5FU, oxaliplatin
  - » XELOX = Xeloda (capecitabine) and oxaliplatin
  - » FOLFIRI = folinic acid, 5FU, irinotecan.
- Long-term survival can be achieved in as many as 50% of cases. Down-staging with neoadjuvant chemotherapy may permit successful resection in a small number of people.

VEGF targeted therapies (bevacizumab and aflibercept)

- Addition of bevacizumab to chemotherapy can prolong survival and progression-free survival.
- The benefit needs to be weighed against the acute risks, including bowel perforation (1%), arterial thrombotic events, hypertension and headache, wound-healing complications and fistula formation.

» Because of the risk of impaired wound healing, bowel perforation and fistula formation, at least 1 month should elapse between major surgery and administration of bevacizumab.

- Aflibercept, another VEGF inhibitor, has also been associated with prolongation of survival when combined with chemotherapy as part of second-line treatment of metastatic colorectal cancer.
  » Pembrolizumab immunotherapy is associated with clinically significant response rates in chemotherapy-pretreated patients with MSI-H colorectal cancer; however, only approximately 5% of patients with stage IV CRC have MSI-H disease.
  » Regorafenib and tifuldine-tipiracil have also been shown to have modest response rates (10–15%) in patients with heavily pre-treated colorectal cancer.

EGFR monoclonal antibodies (cetuximab or panitumumab)

These antibodies have been proven to prolong survival for patients with advanced *K-ras* wild-type colorectal cancer. They have no proven role as part of adjuvant therapy in early-stage *K-ras* wild-type CRC.

Rectal cancer

- Neoadjuvant chemoradiotherapy (i.e. concurrent chemotherapy, in the form of 5FU infusion or capecitabine, and radiotherapy given for 5–6 weeks as an initial treatment measure before surgery) is an increasingly used strategy for patients with rectal cancer, particularly if the tumor is locally advanced.
- Preoperative chemoradiotherapy might allow some patients to undergo sphincter-preserving low anterior resection (LAR) rather than an abdominoperineal resection (APR).
- A short course (5 days) of high dose per fraction neoadjuvant radiotherapy is another option that is recommended by some practitioners.
- Postoperative chemotherapy may also be advised after initial neoadjuvant therapy, although the benefit has not been quantified in randomized controlled trials.
- Combining oxaliplatin with fluoropyrimidine and radiotherapy in early-stage rectal cancer is being evaluated, but early results have revealed more toxicity without improved outcomes.

Future directions

The rationale for use of multiple biomarkers such as circulating tumor DNA to select the most appropriate therapy, particularly new molecular targeted therapies, remains a topic of intense investigation.

PANCREATIC CANCER

The pancreas can harbor malignancies arising from several cell types. These can be grouped into:
- exocrine pancreatic cancers
- neuroendocrine pancreatic cancers (e.g. glucagonoma, insulinoma).

Neuroendocrine pancreatic cancers are discussed in Chapter 10.

Key points

- Pancreatic cancer has a poor prognosis.
- When detected early, it may be cured by complete surgical resection (Whipple's procedure) or by resection of the tail of the pancreas if this is where disease is located.
- Following complete surgical resection, adjuvant chemotherapy can lower the risk of cancer recurrence and provide a survival benefit.
- Current treatments of advanced disease provide only modest improvement in median survival.

Epidemiology

- Pancreatic cancer occurs more commonly as age increases.
- It represents the fifth most common cause of cancer-related death.
- Prognosis is very poor, with 5-year survival in the order of 5%.
- Risk factors include smoking, chronic pancreatitis, diabetes mellitus and those with a genetic (familial) predisposition.
- At the time of diagnosis, 20% of patients will present with localized and operable disease, 40% will have locally advanced inoperable disease, and 40% will have metastatic disease.

Diagnosis

- Tumors in the pancreatic body or tail usually present with pain and weight loss.
- Tumors in the head of the pancreas typically present with jaundice, pain, weight loss, and steatorrhea.
- The most common sites of distant metastases are the liver, peritoneum and lungs.
- Contrast-enhanced multi-slice helical CT scan is the preferred method to diagnose and stage.
- Endoscopic ultrasound is another method to assess vascular invasion, and an endoscopic ultrasonography (EUS)-guided FNA can establish histological confirmation of the diagnosis.

CLINICAL PEARLS

New-onset diabetes mellitus in persons aged 50 years and above with normal weight should raise suspicion of pancreatic cancer. Also, unexplained episodes of pancreatitis or thrombophlebitis can be manifestations of pancreatic cancer.

Management

- Complete resection will achieve the best chance of cure, but only a minority of patients present with resectable disease.

» Even when a complete resection is achieved, the majority of patients eventually develop recurrence.

» Systemic chemotherapy (5FU in combination with other agents) applied after R0 or R1 surgical excision can improve outcomes.

- Pancreatic cancer is often deemed unresectable due to vascular involvement or nodal disease (locally advanced inoperable disease), or due to the finding of metastases at the time of diagnosis.

- For recurrent or metastatic disease, treatment goals are palliative.

- Adjuvant radiotherapy, either alone or in combination with chemotherapy, has not demonstrated improved cure rates.

- For locally advanced, inoperable cancer, chemotherapy can prolong survival to a modest degree, with median survival increments of weeks to a few months possible. Current standard chemotherapy regimens include single-agent gemcitabine, oxaliplatin + 5FU (FOLFOX), oxaliplatin + 5FU + irinotecan (FOLFIRINOX).

- The above regimens, as well as nab-paclitaxel in combination with gemcitabine, have been associated with prolongation of survival for patients with advanced inoperable pancreatic cancer.

HEPATOCELLULAR CARCINOMA (HCC)

Key points

- Hepatocellular carcinoma is the third leading cause of cancer death worldwide.

- The number of deaths matches the incidence, indicating a high case fatality rate.

- Eighty percent of cases develop in association with chronic hepatitis B or C infection.

- There is high geographical variation, with the highest incidence reported in eastern Asia and parts of Africa. Forty percent of HCC cases worldwide originate from China.

- Men are between two and five times more likely to be affected than women.

- Underlying chronic liver disease or cirrhosis is common.

Risk factors

- The most common etiological factor is chronic hepatitis B or C infection.

- Other causes include excessive alcohol intake, Wilson's disease, and hemochromatosis.

- Cases may be idiopathic.

Prognosis

There are a number of methods of predicting prognosis in patients with HCC. The Tumor Node Metastasis (TNM) system is recommended for patients that undergo surgical resection. The Barcelona Clinic Liver Cancer (BCLC) system is thought to be more appropriate for patients with advanced HCC who are not candidates for surgery.

Treatment

- 20% of tumors are resectable at presentation.

- 70% develop recurrence post-resection (90% within 3 years).

Liver transplant

Liver transplant can be considered for patients with unresectable disease. Patients are usually considered unresectable due to their underlying liver function rather than the extent of the tumor.

Liver-directed strategies

This is the preferred approach where possible. Options include:

- partial hepatectomy
- alcohol injection
- transarterial chemotherapy embolization (TACE)
- radiofrequency ablation (RFA)
- cryoablation
- radiotherapeutic microspheres.

Chemotherapy

Systemic chemotherapy has no proven survival benefit or palliative role.

Molecular targeted therapy

- Sorafenib, a vascular endothelial growth factor (VEGF)-targeted TKI, may delay cancer progression and prolong survival in a small number of cases.

Regional chemotherapy

(e.g. TACE)

- Hepatocellular tumors are preferentially supplied by the hepatic artery. Delivery of chemotherapy directly to the tumor provides increased local drug concentration and decreased systemic effects.
  » Angiography is performed with injection of a chemotherapy/lipiodol conjugate and an embolic agent into the tumor via the hepatic artery.
  » Ischemia due to the embolization increases tumor kill.
  » Patients may require repeated treatments.

- Contraindications are:
  » portal vein occlusion
  » impairment of hepatic function
  » large tumor >50% of liver volume.

- Toxicities from regional chemotherapy include fever (>95%), abdominal pain (>60%), anorexia (>60%), and deterioration in liver function.

- The response rate is 50–80%.

- There is no consensus on appropriate drugs or technique. Usually anthracyclines or cisplatin are used.

BRAIN TUMORS

Low-grade glioma (astrocytoma and oligodendroglioma)

Key points

- Almost all patients have progressive disease and will require some form of therapy.
- Surgery is usually not curative in intent.
- Radiotherapy can be effective, but there are late toxicity concerns.
- The role of chemotherapy is not clearly defined.
- There is little randomized evidence to guide management.

Diagnosis

Brain tumors are diagnosed on MRI scan appearance and biopsy.

Treatment

Surgery

- Complete resection is rarely possible. Most surgeons will biopsy if radiological appearances are consistent with low-grade glioma.
- The role of subtotal resection is debatable.
- Surgery has an important role in the management of intracranial hypertension, hydrocephalus, control of epilepsy, and symptom palliation.
- Surgery is estimated from historical series to improve or control symptoms in about 80% of patients.

Radiotherapy

- The true benefit of radiotherapy is difficult to determine because of the heterogeneity of patient groups and many treatment-related variables.
- Retrospective reviews reveal a long-term survival advantage for radiotherapy after surgery.
  - » Postoperative radiotherapy for oligodendroglioma will provide a survival benefit for a subtotally resected tumor, but this benefit is only observed after 5 years of follow-up.
  - » There is no clear survival benefit from radiotherapy if there is a true complete surgical resection.
  - » Improvement in 5-year progression-free survival is observed if radiotherapy is given early after surgical biopsy rather than waiting for progression, but no difference in 5-year overall survival.
- Radiotherapy does not induce malignant transformation of low-grade glioma.
- A 'wait and see' policy can be justified in younger patients with seizures only.
  - » Treatment should not be delayed in patients with focal signs, raised intracranial pressure, symptoms or cognitive deficits.
- The effect of radiotherapy on quality of life is still uncertain.

- » There is no justification for radiotherapy doses above 50 Gy using the current conformal techniques, as higher-dose radiotherapy is no more effective and potentially more toxic, with late toxicity a particular problem.
- Most progression after radiotherapy still occurs in the radiotherapy field, suggesting that the currently used radiation doses are inadequate for cure.
- The role for intensity-modulation radiotherapy (IMRT) and targeted dose escalation remains unclear.

Adjuvant treatment

Up-front chemotherapy may be indicated, especially for patients with large tumors.

Glioblastoma multiforme (GBM)

Epidemiology

The most common and most aggressive malignant primary brain tumor, it represents 2% of all cancer-related deaths.

Diagnosis

- Patients may present with neurological symptoms and signs. Sometimes, a seizure may be the first manifestation.
- MRI imaging is superior to CT imaging in the diagnosis of GBM.
- A tissue sample should be obtained by neurosurgical resection or stereotactic biopsy.
- Molecular characterization for isocitrate dehydrogenase (IDH) mutation testing and testing for O6-methyl-guanine-DNA methyltransferase (MGMT) promotor methylation status are important for prognostication and treatment.

Treatment

- Following the brain biopsy, treatment is usually commenced with combined chemotherapy (particularly temozolomide) and radiotherapy. This treatment runs for approximately 6 weeks, with the oral chemotherapy given daily.
- One month following completion of the chemoradiotherapy, patients then begin regular courses of temozolomide, given for 5 consecutive days every 4 weeks; 6 cycles are usually given.
- Treatment may induce imaging changes that are difficult to distinguish from progressive disease.
- Bevacizumab has reduced requirements for corticosteroid therapy and has been associated with imaging evidence of tumor response.
- Despite the use of a combined modality approach, most patients eventually relapse.

LYMPHOMA

See Chapter 12, Hematology.

MELANOMA

Pathology and epidemiology

There are four principal histological types of melanoma, each including an *in situ* form:

1 **Superficial spreading melanoma**—plaque-type lesions with irregular borders and variegated color. Malignant melanocytes spread through the layers of the epidermis, and in the vertical growth phase move to the dermis.

2 **Lentigo maligna melanoma**—discolored, usually brown, macular lesions that enlarge gradually and eventually become palpable when they invade into the dermis. Malignant melanocytes involve the dermal–epidermal junction in a lentiginous pattern.

3 **Acral lentiginous melanoma**—usually arises on palmar, plantar, subungual and mucosal surfaces. Histology usually reveals large junctional nests of atypical melanocytes with scant cytoplasm.

4 **Nodular melanoma**—vertical growth phase melanomas. They present as darkly pigmented nodules, sometimes ulcerated. Neoplastic cells form a nodular structure in the dermis, with no recognizable adjacent radial growth phase. The neoplastic melanocytes are epithelioid or spindle cells and the mitotic index is usually high.

Diagnosis and staging

- Discolored nodule or plaque-like lesions are the hallmark feature, but they are not always dark (e.g. amelanotic melanoma).
- Melanomas are diagnosed on histology; immunohistochemistry (markers S-100 and HMB-45) can be helpful in confirming the diagnosis.
- An excisional biopsy with a 1–2 mm rim of normal-appearing tissue should be used for lesions suspected to be a melanoma.
- When an excisional biopsy is not technically feasible, an incisional or punch biopsy can provide a definitive diagnosis.

Staging of melanoma is described in Table 14-5.

Table 14-5 Staging of melanoma

STAGE	DESCRIPTION
I	Melanoma <1 mm thick (ulcerated or unulcerated) ulcerated, or 1–2 mm thick and not ulcerated
IIA/B	Melanoma 1–2 mm thick and ulcerated, or 2–4 mm thick and not ulcerated
IIC	Melanoma >4 mm thick and ulcerated
III	Melanoma has spread to involve lymph nodes
IV	Melanoma has spread to distant organs

Management

Resectable disease

- Once a diagnosis of melanoma has been established, surgical excision with an adequate margin of normal tissue is required.
- Lymphatic mapping and sentinel lymph-node biopsy are indicated in the initial management of melanomas with a thickness ≥1 mm, or high-risk features such as ulceration or mitoses >1/mm² in otherwise healthy patients.
- Adjuvant immune therapy with nivolumab or pembrolizumab is recommended for patients with resected stage III (lymph node positive) melanoma.
- Radiation therapy may also decrease the incidence of local recurrences in carefully selected patients, although no impact on survival has been demonstrated.

Advanced disease

Targeted therapy

- Mutations in the *BRAF* gene, which are present in approximately 40–60% of advanced cutaneous melanomas, may be an important driver of melanoma cell growth.
  » The presence of a V600E in the *BRAF* gene predicts for responsiveness to targeted therapies that induce *BRAF* inhibition, such as vemurafenib or dabrafenib.
- Combining BRAF inhibitors with inhibitors of downstream MEK (e.g. trametinib) result in improved survival compared to BRAF inhibitors alone.
  » Ipilimumab, an anti-CTLA-4 monoclonal antibody, significantly prolongs overall survival in patients with metastatic melanoma compared with dacarbazine, independent of the mutation status of *BRAF*.

Immune therapy

- Checkpoint blockade with anti-programmed cell death (PD-1) antibody is an integral component of treatment for metastatic melanoma.
- The addition of an anti-cytotoxic T lymphocyte associated protein 4 (CTLA-4) antibody results in higher response rates and improved progression-free survival.

NON-MELANOMA SKIN CANCER

Non-melanoma skin cancer consists of basal cell carcinoma (BCC; ~70%) and squamous cell carcinoma (SCC; ~30%).

Risk factors

- sun exposure
- multiple dysplastic nevi

- tendency to sunburn
- prior skin cancer
- immunosuppression, in particular solid organ transplant recipients.

Management

- Most can be treated with local treatment by a variety of methods—excision, cryotherapy, curettage.
- Topical treatments including immune modifiers e.g. imiquimod, or chemotherapy e.g. topical 5-fluorouracil are sometimes used.
- Non-melanoma skin cancers rarely metastasize. For those that do, treatment options include radiotherapy, targeted therapy, chemotherapy or immune therapy, although strong clinical trial evidence is scarce for any approach owing to the rarity of the disease.

SARCOMA

Clinical presentation

- Soft-tissue sarcomas are a heterogeneous group of tumors of mesenchymal origin. There are more than 50 different histological subtypes and each has a different biology and clinical course.
- They usually present as an enlarging, painless mass, often well circumscribed and localized, involving the trunk or extremities.
- The presence of distant metastatic disease at the time of initial diagnosis is more likely in large and high-grade sarcomas. About 80% of metastases are located in the lungs.

Diagnosis

- Pathological diagnosis is based on histological morphology, immunohistochemistry, and sometimes molecular testing.
- Referral of a patient with a suspect soft-tissue mass to a specialized center with a multidisciplinary sarcoma team is recommended.
- An excision or a core needle biopsy is required. Ideally, all pathology specimens of suspected soft-tissue sarcomas should be reviewed by a pathologist who specializes in this tumor.
- CT or MRI is used to determine the stage of the sarcoma.
- Imaging of the brain with CT scanning is suggested for patients with high-grade sarcoma or angiosarcoma, due to the high propensity of these tumors for CNS metastases.
- In addition to tumor stage, other prognostic variables include histological grade and subtype, tumor size, anatomical site and patient age.

Treatment

Patients should be managed in a center with multidisciplinary expertise in the management of soft-tissue sarcomas.

Surgery

- Surgical resection is the principal curative treatment modality.
- Consideration must be given to the functional consequences of intervention, as surgery may require limb amputation.
- Surgical resection of limited metastatic disease can provide long-term relapse-free survival and perhaps cure in selected patients, the majority of whom have isolated pulmonary metastatic disease.

Preoperative (neoadjuvant) therapy

- The combination of surgery and radiotherapy achieves better outcomes than either treatment alone for nearly all intermediate- and high-grade soft-tissue sarcomas >5 cm in the greatest dimension.
- Neoadjuvant therapy can provide a benefit when used to treat large (>10 cm), potentially resectable soft-tissue sarcomas or if there is concern for adverse functional outcomes from initial surgery, e.g. limb surgery.
- Neoadjuvant therapy could consist of chemotherapy alone, radiotherapy alone, or the combination either sequentially or concurrently. There is no proven 'gold standard' approach.

Postoperative (adjuvant) therapy

Adjuvant chemotherapy may improve survival, but the evidence remains contentious.

Chemotherapy

- Systemic chemotherapy is a routine component of treatment for several soft-tissue sarcomas that occur predominantly in children (e.g. rhabdomyosarcoma, Ewing sarcoma).
- For asymptomatic patients with unresectable disease and low-grade histologies, surveillance may be the preferred initial management approach.
- Chemotherapy-sensitive histologies include synovial sarcoma, liposarcoma, leiomyosarcoma, and high-grade pleomorphic unclassified sarcoma.
- Anthracycline or anthracycline + ifosfamide remain the recommended first-line treatments for these patients.

Ewing sarcoma

- Ewing sarcoma and peripheral primitive neuroectodermal tumors (PNETs) comprise a spectrum of neoplastic diseases known as the Ewing sarcoma family of tumors (EFT).
- These tumors are thought to share the same cell of origin and chromosome translocations, in particular the 11;22 translocation involving the *EWSR1* gene on chromosome 22q12.
- Although rare, these tumors represent the second most common bone tumor in children and adolescents.
- Patients with EFT require referral to centers that have multidisciplinary teams of sarcoma specialists.
- Combination chemotherapy and definitive local therapy is usually required.

- Up to 40% of patients with limited pulmonary metastatic disease who undergo intensive chemotherapy and pulmonary resection with or without radiation therapy may be long-term survivors.
- The prognosis for other subsets of patients with advanced disease is less favorable, but patients are treated aggressively with the aim of long-term survival or cure.

BREAST CANCER

Epidemiology

- Lifetime risk—1 in 12 women (some series quote as high as 1 in 8).
- 1 in 33 lifetime risk of dying from breast cancer.
- Incidence increases with age.

Risk factors

- Long, unopposed estrogen stimulation of breast tissue (early menarche, late menopause).
- Late first pregnancy, nulliparity.
- Hormone replacement therapy/oral contraceptive pill use is associated with a small increased risk counterbalanced by benefits.
- Previous radiation exposure to breast tissue, particularly during the breast development period through puberty or early adulthood.
- Family history of breast cancer.

Pathology

- Ductal carcinoma *in situ*—a pre-cancerous change, often a 'field' change (the *in situ* changes are seen in multiple areas or can be diffuse).
- Invasive ductal carcinoma—usually localized, palpable, and accounts for more than 80% of breast cancers.
- Lobular carcinoma—may be multicentric, sometimes bilateral with impalpable disease, and accounts for 10% of breast cancer histology.
- More than 50% of breast cancers are hormone-receptor positive (estrogen and/or progesterone), and the majority of these will respond to endocrine manipulation.
- HER2 receptor status is also examined, as receptor positivity predicts benefits from treatment utilizing the monoclonal antibody trastuzumab. Twenty percent of breast cancers are HER2-positive. HER2 status is determined by the evaluation of breast cancer tissue by immunohistochemistry or by *in situ* hybridization techniques.

Screening

- The principle is based on improved prognosis when treating breast cancer of an earlier stage (smaller tumor, less or no lymph node involvement).
- Randomized trials demonstrate a reduction in breast-cancer-related death of 20–30% with the use of screening mammography every 2–3 years.
- The effect is greatest in women aged 50–69 years.

Diagnosis and staging

For early-stage breast cancer, the following investigations are usually performed:

- clinical examination of the breast
- mammography
- ultrasound examination of breast ± guided biopsy
- chest X-ray
- whole-body bone scan.

The following are not performed routinely, but may be considered depending on other clinical findings and symptoms:

- CT scan
- PET scan.

For patients with metastatic disease, CT imaging of the chest, abdomen and pelvis should be performed. CT of the head may also be performed if other clinical parameters raise concern that the brain is involved. If disease is involving the spine and neurological symptoms are present, then an MRI scan may be recommended.

Staging of breast cancer is given in Table 14-6.

Table 14-6 Staging of breast cancer

Stage I	Localized to breast
Stage II	Breast and lymph-node involvement
Stage III	Locally advanced or inflammatory tumor
Stage IV	Metastases to distant sites

Management

- For early-stage breast cancer (disease limited to the breast and adjacent lymph nodes), the treatment goal is to achieve a cure.
- For metastatic disease, the treatment goals are to prolong survival time, alleviate symptoms, and maintain or improve the quality of life. The treatment will not be curative.

Surgical options—stages I and II

1. a Breast-conserving surgery—offered to women except in the setting of multi-focal breast disease or where the tumor is large (especially in relation to the total volume of breast tissue).
   b Total mastectomy.
2. Sentinel lymph-node (SLN) biopsy—if negative, axillary node clearance can be avoided. SLN positivity can be used to predict the need for adjuvant therapy, but subsequent axillary clearance does not improve survival and may be avoided.

Endocrine therapy—hormone-receptor-positive cancers

Ovarian ablation

This reduces the risk of cancer relapse after surgery and improves overall survival in pre-menopausal women with hormone-receptor-positive cancers.

- It can be achieved surgically, with radiation, or with the use of luteinizing hormone releasing hormone (LHRH) analogues.
- It is effective in both early and advanced disease.

Tamoxifen

Tamoxifen reduces the risk of breast cancer recurrence when used after breast surgery for patients with cancer that is hormone-receptor-positive.

- The optimal duration of adjuvant therapy is 5 years.
- Tamoxifen can also help reduce the size of tumors or delay the progression of disease in patients with metastatic disease.
- The benefit of tamoxifen is seen in both pre-menopausal and post-menopausal patients.
- It has an anti-estrogenic effect in breast cancer tissue but some pro-estrogenic effects in other tissues, reducing age-related bone loss and the risk of heart disease.
- Tamoxifen is associated with an increased risk of endometrial cancer and thromboembolism.

Aromatase inhibitors (AIs)

These inhibit the conversion of androstenedione to estrone in adipose tissue, a process that requires aromatases (enzymes produced by the adrenal glands).

- They are effective only in post-menopausal women where estrogen production is predominantly reliant on aromatases, and ineffective in pre-menopausal patients.
- They reduce the risk of cancer recurrence after surgery in post-menopausal women.
- The optimal duration of therapy is 5 years.
- Tamoxifen and AIs should not be given concurrently. Tamoxifen and AIs can be used *sequentially*, for example using tamoxifen for 2–3 years and then an AI for 2–3 years.
- AIs can also be used in the management of metastatic disease.
- A principal concern with long-term AI usage is the development of osteoporosis.
- The most common reason for stopping therapy is arthralgia.

Chemotherapy

Chemotherapy reduces the risk of cancer recurrence after surgery and improves overall survival, but the magnitude of benefit varies according to the stage of the cancer and the biological characteristics of the tumor. A careful balance of risk against benefit needs to be considered. Even patients with small tumors (<1.0 cm) without lymph node involvement may benefit from chemotherapy, but the absolute magnitude of benefit is less than 5%.

CLINICAL PEARL

A 2% absolute benefit for overall survival means that for every 100 women treated there will be a survival difference in 2 of them. The magnitude may be small, but the outcome variable—survival—is major. This 'small' benefit may still be considered worthwhile by patients.

Active drugs include:
- taxanes, e.g. docetaxel (Taxotere [T]), paclitaxel (Taxol)
- anthracyclines, e.g. doxorubicin (Adriamycin [A]), epirubicin (E)
- alkylating agents, e.g. cyclophosphamide (C)
- antimetabolites, e.g. 5-fluorouracil (F), methotrexate (M).

Combinations of chemotherapy are more active than single agents. Commonly used combinations include:
- CMF—cyclophosphamide, methotrexate, 5-fluorouracil
- AC—Adriamycin (doxorubicin), cyclophosphamide
- FEC—5FU, epirubicin, cyclophosphamide
- DC—docetaxel, cyclophosphamide
- TAC—Taxotere (docetaxel), Adriamycin (doxorubicin), cyclophosphamide.

There are several acceptable chemotherapy regimens but no universally accepted 'gold standard'. Clinical trials evaluating adjuvant chemotherapy have shown that:
- 6 cycles of CMF improves overall survival
- 4 cycles of AC is equivalent to 6 cycles of CMF
- 6 cycles of FEC may be better than CMF
- AC followed by paclitaxel is better than AC alone
- 4 cycles of AC is equivalent to 4 cycles of DC
- TAC is better than FAC
- accelerating the chemotherapy to a shorter schedule (shorter intervals between doses) may provide a small benefit, but this requires granulocyte growth factor support.

HER2-targeted therapy

Trastuzumab

- Trastuzumab, a monoclonal antibody that targets the HER2 receptor, reduces the risk of cancer recurrence and improves overall survival in early-stage HER2-positive breast cancer.
- The current recommended duration of adjuvant therapy is 12 months.
- Trastuzumab also improves survival in the management of metastatic breast cancer, whether used as a single agent or in combination with chemotherapy.
- The principal risk associated with trastuzumab is cardiac failure, which occurs in up to 5% of patients.

Lapatinib

- Lapatinib, a HER2 tyrosine kinase inhibitor, has been demonstrated to prolong the time to cancer progression in patients with HER2-positive metastatic breast cancer when used alone or in combination with capecitabine.

- Preliminary results from a randomized controlled trial indicate that lapatinib is inferior to trastuzumab when used as adjuvant therapy in early-stage breast cancer.
- Skin toxicity and diarrhea are the principal toxicities.

New HER2-directed therapies

- **Pertuzumab**—this monoclonal antibody exhibits an anti-tumor effect through inhibition of HER-dimerization. Dimerization of HER receptors is required to activate HER2 and initiate downstream signaling in the cancer cell, which is required for cancer cell growth. The addition of pertuzumab to the combination of trastuzumab and docetaxel has been shown to prolong progression-free survival. Pertuzumab did not increase the risk of cardiotoxicity.
- **Trastuzumab emtansine** (T-DM1)—this is an antibody–drug conjugate that consists of the monoclonal antibody trastuzumab with the cytotoxic agent mertansine (DM1). Trastuzumab acts as a transporter, enabling DM1 to enter cancer cells and inhibit tubulin. T-DM1 has been shown to prolong the survival of patients with advanced breast cancer that is resistant to trastuzumab alone, compared with the combination of lapatinib and capecitabine.

Metastatic breast cancer

The most frequent sites of metastatic disease include bone, liver, lung and brain. HER2-positive disease is particularly prone to the development of central nervous system (CNS) involvement. When metastatic, breast cancer is not considered curable. Measures that can improve quality of life and prolong survival include endocrine therapies and systemic chemotherapy. Radiotherapy is useful for local disease, in particular to manage bone pain.

The median time to development of breast cancer recurrence in patients with hormone-receptor-negative disease is 2 years, and for hormone-receptor-positive disease 6 years. Later recurrences do occur.

Bisphosphonates

- Bisphosphonates reduce skeletal complications associated with metastatic breast cancer involving bones, including bone pain, malignancy-associated hypercalcemia, and skeletal fractures.
- They include intravenous bisphosphonates such as zoledronic acid and pamidronate, and oral bisphosphonates such as ibandronate and clodronate.
- A particular adverse event associated with bisphosphonate use is osteonecrosis of the jaw (ONJ), with an incidence of 1% or less in most recent series, although there are reports of ONJ rates as high as 5%. The risk of ONJ is related to the duration of therapy and underlying dental health.
- Receptor activator of nuclear factor kappa-B (RANK)-ligand inhibitors (e.g. denosumab) may be better at preventing skeletal complications in metastatic breast cancer than bisphosphonates.

Recent research and future directions

- SLN positivity can be used to predict the need for adjuvant therapy, but subsequent axillary clearance does not improve survival and may be avoided.
- Molecular markers or signatures may be used to predict benefit from adjuvant hormonal therapy, not just hormone receptor status.
- Tamoxifen and aromatase inhibitors have been shown to reduce the risk of breast cancer in individuals considered to be at greater risk. A careful balance of risk vs benefit is needed when considering using such hormonal therapy as a preventive measure.
- New HER2-targeted therapies may improve or prolong response.
- Bevacizumab prolongs time to cancer progression but not overall survival.

OVARIAN CANCER

Key points

- While most tumors are adenocarcinomas, the ovaries can be affected by a wide variety of cancer pathologies.
- Treatment depends on the stage, but optimal surgical clearance remains the cornerstone of successful intervention.
- For advanced-stage disease, chemotherapy after surgery improves survival.

Pathology and epidemiology

- Most ovarian cancers derive from epithelial cells on the surface of the ovary, and are effectively adenocarcinomas.
- Germ-line mutations in *BRCA1*, *BRCA2* and other genes have been implicated in some cases, but in the majority no mutation is found.
- Papillary serous histology accounts for as many as 75% of ovarian cancers. Mucinous and endometrioid tumors account for 10% each. Less than 10% of ovarian cancers of epithelial origin are represented by clear-cell tumors, Brenner (transitional-cell) tumors, or undifferentiated carcinomas. Rarer cancers such as germ-cell tumors or sex cord-stromal tumors arise from other cell types.
- Tumors of low malignant potential are called *borderline tumors* and represent approximately 10% of malignant ovarian neoplasms defined histologically by atypical epithelial proliferation without stromal invasion.
- Ovarian cancer is the second most common gynecological malignancy in the developed world, but the most common cause of death among women with gynecological cancer and the fifth leading cause of cancer death in all women.
- The lifetime risk of ovarian cancer in the general population of women is 1.4%.
  - » Risk factors for ovarian cancer include nulligravidity, infertility, endometriosis, and hereditary

ovarian cancer syndromes (*BRCA* mutations, Lynch syndrome).

» Protective factors include oral contraceptives, tubal ligation, hysterectomy, and breastfeeding.

Diagnosis

- Symptoms of early-stage ovarian cancer are often ill-defined.
- The majority of cases are at an advanced stage at the time of diagnosis.
- A typical presentation of ovarian cancer is a woman with a fixed, irregular pelvic mass and an upper abdominal mass and/or ascites.
- Ultrasound examination is the most useful noninvasive diagnostic test in women with an adnexal mass and will reveal sonographic features suggestive of malignancy.
- The serum CA-125 is elevated in 80% of women with epithelial ovarian cancer, as well as in some women with benign and other malignant lesions.
- Routine imaging following therapy has not been shown to improve outcome, and is usually reserved to investigate symptoms or suspected recurrence rather than for routine surveillance.
- Primary peritoneal carcinoma (also known as papillary serous carcinoma of the peritoneum) is closely associated with, but distinct from, epithelial ovarian cancer and histologically is indistinguishable from papillary serous ovarian carcinoma.

Management

- For early-stage disease, surgery alone is usually optimal therapy.
- For all other disease, chemotherapy is recommended after surgery.
- Approximately 75% of women have disease involving the peritoneal cavity or lymph nodes, or spread to more distant sites. A standard approach for these women is maximal surgical cytoreduction followed by chemotherapy. However, initial chemotherapy may be appropriate for patients whose performance status makes them unsuitable for a prolonged surgical effort, or with extensive disease that precludes optimal cytoreduction.
  » Optimal cytoreduction, if technically feasible, involves removing all visible tumor and is the goal of primary surgery.
- For optimally debulked disease not extending beyond the peritoneal cavity, chemotherapy after surgery provides a survival benefit, with up to 20% of patients becoming long-term cancer-free survivors. Single-agent carboplatin or a combination of paclitaxel and carboplatin are the regimens of choice, usually applied in 6 cycles.
- For disease that cannot be optimally cytoreduced (i.e. residual tumor ≥1 cm), there is a survival benefit associated with using a paclitaxel-platinum regimen after surgery. Usually surgery is followed by 6 cycles

of intravenous carboplatin + paclitaxel. Dose-dense (weekly paclitaxel plus 3-weekly carboplatin) chemotherapy is also an option.

- Further chemotherapy is usually given after cancer recurrence or progression, but the goals of second-line therapy and beyond are palliative and survival benefit is modest. Chemotherapy agents that have activity include topotecan, liposomal doxorubicin, etoposide and gemcitabine.
- If disease progression occurs at least 6 months after previous platinum-based chemotherapy, then the cancer may still be platinum-sensitive and further platinum-based chemotherapy may induce a response and provide a benefit.

CLINICAL PEARL

The role of monitoring CA-125 after surgery is controversial, as this has not been demonstrated to improve outcomes despite allowing for earlier detection of recurrence.

Future directions

- Bevacizumab-containing chemotherapy—either first-line or following recurrence—may prolong progression-free survival.
- There is a possible role for maintenance chemotherapy, in particular paclitaxel. The potential progression-free survival benefit must be weighed against cumulative toxicity.

ENDOMETRIAL CANCER

Pathology and epidemiology

- Endometrioid tumors account for 80% of cases and are related to stimulation by estrogen.
- Papillary serous or clear-cell tumors account for 20% of cases and are hormone-independent.
- Risk factors include estrogen exposure in the absence of adequate exposure to progestins. High-risk situations include tamoxifen use, obesity, type 2 diabetes, and anovulation.
- Use of oral contraceptives decreases risk.

Diagnosis

- Abnormal uterine bleeding is the most common presenting symptom and occurs in 90% of cases.
- Post-menopausal bleeding in a woman not on hormone replacement therapy should always be investigated to exclude endometrial cancer.
- Endometrial biopsy, dilatation and curettage, or hysteroscopy with directed biopsy and curettage are the principal diagnostic strategies.

Management

- Surgery is the principal treatment modality.
- Adjuvant radiotherapy will reduce the risk of recurrence for disease that has invaded down to the muscle level and beyond.
- Adjuvant chemotherapy is also recommended in higher-stage cancer.
- Chemotherapy may improve symptoms and provide a modest survival prolongation in metastatic endometrial cancer.

CANCER SURVIVORSHIP

With recent advances in screening, diagnostics and personalized treatment, increasing numbers of patients are being cured of their cancer or are living their lives with cancer.

A cancer survivor is any individual who has been diagnosed with cancer. Cancer survivors may be on any part of this continuum from the time of diagnosis through to end of life care. Their care needs are complex and may vary depending upon the particular stage in their cancer trajectory.

Cancer survivorship care is multidisciplinary and includes the following components:

- Cancer surveillance and assessment of recurrence
- Screening for second primary cancers
- Assessment and treatment of medical and psychosocial late effects of cancer and/or its treatment
- Education and implementation of preventative health measures
- Coordinated and integrated care between the primary health provider, community and specialist teams.

SELF-ASSESSMENT QUESTIONS

1 Which of the following population-based screening programs has been proven to reduce cancer-specific mortality?

A Computed tomography (CT) scans of lungs in men aged 50 and over
B Prostate-specific antigen (PSA) screening in men aged 70 and over
C Cancer-associated antigen 125 (CA-125) measurement in all women aged 50 years
D Fecal occult blood test (FOBT) for all adults aged 50 and over
E Bronchoscopy every 5 years in smokers aged 50 and over

2 Which of the following statements is correct?

A A prognostic factor allows you to select the best therapy for a particular subgroup of patients.
B A predictive factor exerts an influence on outcome that is independent of therapy.
C It is not possible for a biomarker to exert both predictive and prognostic properties.
D Predictive factors do not have any effect of the potential cost-effectiveness of a new therapy.
E A prognostic factor is related to the outcome of patient survival and has an association that is independent of any treatment effect.

3 Which of the following serum tumor markers is *not* helpful in the clinical monitoring of patients after therapy?

A Lactase dehydrogenase (LDH) level in non-Hodgkin lymphoma
B Carcinoembryonic antigen (CEA) level in colon cancer
C Prostate-specific antigen (PSA) in prostate cancer
D Human chorionic gonadotropin (hCG) level in non-seminomatous germ-cell tumor
E Cancer-associated antigen 125 (CA-125) in the monitoring of squamous-cell carcinoma of the lung

4 In which of the following situations is treatment administered with the expectation that the majority of patients will not be cured?

A Radical radiotherapy with concurrent chemotherapy for inoperable stage III non-small-cell lung cancer (NSCLC)
B Surgery followed by adjuvant chemotherapy for stage I breast cancer
C Chemotherapy for metastatic seminoma involving the lungs and multiple lymph nodes above and below the diaphragm
D Nodular sclerosing Hodgkin lymphoma involving the mediastinum in a 22-year-old patient
E Surgery followed by chemotherapy in a patient with stage III colon cancer that involves 2 out of 12 lymph nodes

5 When a patient who received chemotherapy 10 days previously presents with a fever of 39°C, the optimal treatment approach is:

A Take blood cultures and check the blood count. If neutropenia is found, admit the patient for observation and commence appropriate antibiotics based on the blood culture results and the observed antibiotic sensitivities.
B Commence Gram-positive antibiotic cover immediately, then wait for blood cultures in case further antibiotics are needed.
C Take blood cultures and check the blood count. If neutropenia is found, then start antibiotics immediately to cover possible Gram-negative bacteremia including *Pseudomonas* sepsis.
D No action is needed unless the fever persists for more than 24 hours.
E Start antibiotics only if the patient is either hypoxic or hypotensive, otherwise observe and apply supportive measures until the fever settles.

6 Which of the following scenarios of cancer of unknown primary (CUP) may still be cured with chemotherapy?

A Well-differentiated adenocarcinoma found in the lung, bone and inguinal lymph nodes of a 42-year-old female
B Malignant ascites with carcinoma proven on cytological examination in a 77-year-old man
C Carcinoma involving multiple sites of the liver and considered inoperable
D Poorly differentiated carcinoma found in a retro-peritoneal mass in a 24-year-old male
E Squamous-cell carcinoma in the supraclavicular lymph node and also involving the 5th lumbar vertebral body

7 Which of the following statements associating gene mutation with clinical implication is *not* correct?

A Advanced colon cancer with *K-ras* mutations are more likely to respond to cetuximab.
B Epidermal growth factor gene mutations have been associated with responsiveness to first-line therapy for advanced non-small-cell lung cancer using EGFR tyrosine kinase inhibitors.
C *BRAF* mutations predict a poorer prognosis in advanced colon cancer.
D The presence of V600E *BRAF* mutations predict responsiveness to vemurafenib in melanoma.
E *ALK* mutations predict responsiveness to crizotinib in non-small-cell lung cancer.

8 Chemotherapy has not been demonstrated to prolong survival for which of the following scenarios?

A First-line therapy with carboplatin and paclitaxel in advanced ovarian cancer
B Second-line chemotherapy for advanced pancreatic cancer
C Second-line chemotherapy for advanced colon cancer
D Inoperable non-small-cell lung cancer
E Combined with radiotherapy in glioblastoma multiforme

9   Which of the following targeted therapies does not provide a benefit for the associated clinical scenario?
   A   Third-line therapy with cetuximab in *K-ras* wild-type advanced colon cancer
   B   Bevacizumab in the first-line therapy of advanced colon cancer
   C   Adjuvant therapy with cetuximab in high-risk stage III *K-ras* wild-type colon cancer
   D   Trastuzumab in HER2-positive advanced gastric cancer
   E   Lapatinib in metastatic HER2-positive breast cancer

ANSWERS

1   D.

Only FOBT has been associated with improved survival. The other screening tests may enable earlier detection, but this has not been associated with prolongation of overall survival.

2   E.

It is important to understand the difference between a *prognostic* factor (a factor associated with prognosis, independent of a treatment effect) and a *predictive* factor (a factor that helps select a patient who is most likely to benefit from an intervention or therapy).

3   E.

CA-125 is a nonspecific tumor marker and is not a reliable indicator of disease response or prognosis in the context of lung cancer. The other markers listed all have a role in assessing disease response and in monitoring patient status after therapy during surveillance.

4   A.

While patients with inoperable NSCLC treated with chemoradiotherapy can achieve long-term survival, in randomized controlled trials of selected patients only 15–20% of patients become long-term survivors. The other cancers all have expected long-term survival rates of above 50%.

5   C.

This answer relates to the optimal treatment strategy, and sequence, when patients present with presumed febrile neutropenia. Taking blood cultures before antibiotics are commenced is important to allow the best chance of identifying a pathogen. Antibiotics that cover Gram-negative organisms, especially *Pseudomonas*, are important as such an infection can cause rapid and overwhelming sepsis.

6   D.

Consider the possibility of a retro-peritoneal germ cell tumor in such a clinical situation. Such tumors are curable with chemotherapy.

7   A.

The predictive value of *K-ras* is well established in metastatic colorectal cancer. Those with *K-ras* mutations are less likely to respond or benefit from cetuximab. In fact, the benefit is restricted to the wild-type cetuximab subgroup, and no benefit is seen in patients with tumors that harbor *K-ras* mutations.

8   B.

Pancreatic cancer remains a cancer associated with a poor prognosis, particularly when inoperable or metastatic. Second-line chemotherapy trials have yielded uniformly disappointing results so far.

9   C.

Monoclonal antibodies such as cetuximab have been studied in the adjuvant context, and so far the trials have been negative. The other scenarios are all associated with a clinical benefit for the molecular targeted therapies.

CHAPTER 15

PALLIATIVE MEDICINE

Meera Agar, Katherine Clark and David Currow

CHAPTER OUTLINE

- PAIN
  - Definition
  - Impact of the problem
  - Pathophysiological basis
  - Interventions to palliate the problem

- MUCOSITIS
  - Definition
  - Impact of the problem
  - Pathophysiological basis
  - Interventions

- FATIGUE
  - Impact of the problem
  - Pathophysiological basis
  - Interventions to palliate the problem

- NAUSEA AND VOMITING
  - Definition
  - Impact of the problem
  - Pathophysiological basis
  - Interventions to palliate the problem

- CACHEXIA AND ANOREXIA
  - Definition
  - Impact of the problems

  - Underlying pathophysiological basis
  - Interventions

- BREATHLESSNESS
  - Definition
  - Impact of the problem
  - Pathophysiological basis
  - Interventions to palliate the problem

- CONSTIPATION
  - Definition
  - Impact of the problem
  - Pathophysiological basis
  - Interventions to palliate the problem

- DELIRIUM
  - Definition
  - Impact of the problem
  - Pathophysiological basis
  - Interventions to palliate the problem

- INSOMNIA
  - Definition
  - Impact of the problem
  - Pathophysiological basis
  - Interventions to palliate the problem

PAIN

Definition

According to the International Association of Pain, pain is 'an unpleasant sensory and emotional experience associated with actual or potential tissue damage, or described in terms of such damage'. Pain is a complex experience, and there are usually multiple contributing factors in any individual. It is also important to recognize the prevalence of chronic pain, including the more complex neuropathic pain.

Impact of the problem

Pain at cancer diagnosis occurs in 20–50% of patients, and in 75–90% of people with advanced cancer. Pain can be experienced at multiple anatomical sites, with varying intensity, frequency and clinical characteristics, and is often driven by different mechanisms.

If pain is poorly managed it can restrict function, the ability to participate in work or other meaningful activities, the ability to care for oneself and one's quality of life. These adverse effects also negatively affect caregivers' quality of life. Pain is a subjective and individual experience that may result in fear, anxiety, depression, a sense of lack of control and/or hopelessness if not adequately addressed.

Pathophysiological basis

The neurophysiology of cancer pain is complex.

- Primary afferent sensory neurons transmit *noxious* (C and A-delta fibers) and *non-noxious* (A-alpha and A-beta fibers) stimuli (Figure 15-1). C and A-delta fibers end within the dorsal horn of the spinal cord at superficial levels, whereas A-alpha and A-beta fibers

end in the deep aspect of the dorsal horn and in the dorsal column nuclei.

- Sensory neurons synapse onto second-order neurons in the spinal cord or dorsal column nuclei. These second-order neurons then ascend to higher centers of the brain, including the thalamus, from which projections go to the somatosensory cortex, the anterior cingulate and the insular cortices, all of which modulate the experience of pain.
- Peripheral sensitization (through sensitizing peripheral afferent fibers) and central sensitization occur after prolonged exposure to C-fiber nociceptive drive, and this is thought to be mediated through glutamate and substance P, which alters the N-methyl-D-aspartate (NMDA) receptor.
- Long-term potentiation, possibly mediated in the hippocampus, also leads to sustained excitability of dorsal horn pain transmission neurons.

Interventions to palliate the problem

A multidisciplinary and multidimensional assessment and management approach is required. Thorough history and examination, and regular reassessment are needed to adequately manage pain. A written pain management plan and patient/caregiver education about cancer pain and its management are useful, including discussion of opioid myths and concerns.

Non-pharmacological approaches

Psychological strategies that promote self-efficacy and manage coexisting anxiety and depression may be helpful. Therapeutic exercise, graded and purposeful activity, massage and soft-tissue mobilization, transcutaneous electrical nerve

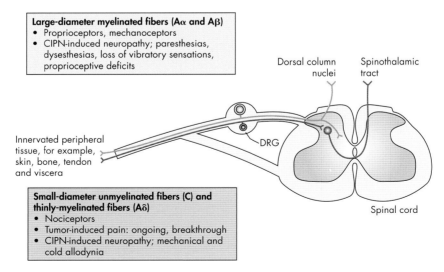

Figure 15-1 Primary afferent sensory nerve fibers involved in generating the pain and/or neuropathy induced by tumors and anti-tumor therapies. CIPN, chemotherapy-induced peripheral neuropathy; DRG, dorsal root ganglion

From Mantyh PW. Cancer pain and its impact on diagnosis, survival and quality of life. Nature Rev Neurosci 2006; 7:797–809. doi:10.1038/nrn1914

stimulation (TENS), postural re-education and heat/cold therapy can be helpful in some patients. Adapted activities and lifestyle adjustments may be required. Physical and occupational therapy assessments are crucial to optimize function.

Pharmacological approaches

Cancer pain management may require the use of opioids and co-analgesics. Selection of the appropriate agent depends on the severity of pain, the safety and efficacy of the agents in the particular pain syndrome, comorbidities, patient preference, convenience, and cost.

Opioid receptors

Opioid receptors are coupled to inhibitory G-proteins. Endogenous opioids are dynorphins, endorphins, endomorphins, nociceptin and enkephalins. The mu-opioid receptor is the primary receptor mediating the action of opioid analgesics, including morphine, fentanyl and methadone.

- Genetic variations have been identified in the human mu-opioid receptor (MOP) gene (*OPRM1*) which reduce the response to opioid analgesia.
- COMT (catechol-O-methyltransferase) variants cause up-regulation of the mu-opioid receptor, resulting in the need for lower dosages of exogenous opioids.
- P-glycoprotein efflux transporter gene (*ABCB1*) variants have an increased response to some opioids while those with poor metabolizer variants in the *CYP2D6* gene have reduced response to some opioids that produce metabolites with mu-opioid receptor activity (codeine, tramadol, oxycodone).

Table 15-1 lists opioid receptors and their respective endogenous and exogenous ligands.

> ## CLINICAL PEARLS
>
> - Opioids remain the mainstay of cancer pain treatment.
> - For continuous pain, it is appropriate to give opioids on a regular schedule and ensure that the patient has 'as needed' doses prescribed for breakthrough pain.

When commencing an opioid, a short-acting formulation (usually oral) or a low-dose long-acting formulation is given and titrated to effect. A short-acting formulation (of the same opioid where possible) should be provided on an 'as needed' basis for breakthrough pain.

- The appropriate dose is the dose that relieves the patient's pain throughout the dosing interval, with recurrence of pain prior to the next dose being a sign that a further dose increase may be needed in people with opioid-responsive pain.
- Renal and hepatic function changes may increase a patient's propensity to adverse effects and may require selection of an alternative opioid.
- When converting between different opioids and also between different routes of administration, it is important to be aware of the relative potency and dose equivalents to ensure that pain control is maximized. It is

Table 15-1 Opioid receptors and their ligands

OPIOID RECEPTOR	EXOGENOUS LIGAND (OPIOID MEDICATION)	ENDO-GENOUS LIGAND
Mu	Methadone Morphine Fentanyl, alfentanil, sufentanil, ramifentanil Codeine Tramadol (also modulates serotonin/noradrenaline) Hydromorphone Oxycodone	Many Beta-endorphin Endomorphins
Kappa	Morphine Codeine Meperidine (pethidine) Oxycodone	Dynorphin A
Delta	Morphine Codeine Meperidine (pethidine) Fentanyl	Enkephalins

recommended that a dose conversion chart or calculator is used to avoid errors.

Pharmacokinetic considerations

- Accumulation of morphine metabolites can occur in renal impairment, over a wide range of creatinine clearances, with some patients with severe renal impairment not being affected and others with minor impairment showing reduced clearance.
- There is delayed elimination of oxycodone and its metabolite oxymorphone (the active metabolite) in renal failure.
- Hydromorphone has several metabolites, with no evidence that they accumulate in renal failure; however, toxicity has been reported in renal failure.
- Fentanyl and alfentanil do not have active metabolites, and have been successfully used in renal failure.
- Codeine is bioactivated to morphine by cytochrome P450 2D6, and there is evidence that codeine-6- glucuronide, a major bioactive metabolite of codeine, also contributes to central nervous system side-effects, in addition to the morphine metabolites byproducts.

Opioid rotation

Opioid rotation is defined as substituting one strong opioid with another when a satisfactory balance between pain relief and adverse effects is not achieved with the first opioid.

The biological mechanisms underpinning why better pain relief and reduced adverse effects have been seen in some clinical observations when switching from one mu-opioid receptor agonist to another is not fully understood, but could relate to inter-individual variations in pharmacokinetics and pharmacodynamics, such as speed of crossing biological barriers (e.g. P-glycoprotein variants), changes in tolerance of the mu-receptor system, or changes in metabolism and clearance.

Co-analgesics, interventional and antineoplastic therapies

Co-analgesics can be useful for pain associated with inflammation, nerve compression, or pain which is neuropathic in its pathophysiology.

- For pain related to inflammation, non-steroidal anti-inflammatory drugs (NSAIDs) or glucocorticosteroids can be used: the choice is related to the relative risk of adverse effects (based on the physiological characteristics of the patient, e.g. renal function, and other comorbidities).

- Bisphosphonates can be helpful to manage bone pain, in particular in multiple myeloma and breast cancer.

- For neuropathic pain, a trial of an antidepressant such as amitriptyline or an anticonvulsant such as pregabalin can be helpful. The choice of antineuropathic agent should be guided by the efficacy of the agent and its toxicity profile.

Intrathecal infusions, celiac plexus blocks and nerve blockade can be extremely effective in carefully selected patients.

MUCOSITIS

Definition

Oral mucositis is inflammation and ulceration of the oral mucosa with pseudomembrane formation. The initial presentation is erythema, followed by painful, white desquamating plaques.

Pseudomembrane formation and ulceration results from epithelial crusting and a fibrin exudate. Similar processes may occur anywhere along the gastrointestinal tract. With the advent of new targeted therapies, other patterns are seen. For example, mammalian target of rapamycin (mTOR) inhibitors cause oral aphthous-like ulcers (mTOR-inhibitor–associated stomatitis).

Impact of the problem

Oral mucositis secondary to chemotherapy or radiotherapy affects more than 40% of cancer patients, resulting in pain, and difficulty in swallowing and eating. It is a potential source of infection, which, in extreme cases, may result in death, particularly if accompanied by neutropenia.

Pathophysiological basis

The pathophysiology of mucositis involves a complex interaction of local tissue damage, oral environment, myelosuppression, and intrinsic genetic predisposition (e.g. single-nucleotide polymorphisms). The current working biological model for oral mucositis has five phases:

1 Initiation phase, due to the generation of free radicals and DNA damage from anticancer therapies.

2 Message generation phase, in which transcription factors (e.g. nuclear factor kappa-B [NFkB]) are activated, leading to up-regulation of pro-inflammatory cytokines (interleukin [IL]-1-beta and tumor necrosis factor-alpha [TNF-alpha]). These cytokines mediate inflammation and vasodilatation, and increase the local concentration of anticancer agents, which all lead to tissue damage.

3 Signaling and amplification phase—microtrauma from speech, swallowing and mastication leads to further ulceration. Inflammation is accelerated due to increased signal feedback.

4 Ulcerative/bacteriological phase (during which neutropenia is common)—bacterial colonization of ulcers occurs, and the endotoxins lead to release of more IL-1 and TNF-alpha. This is likely to be the phase most responsible for the clinical pain and morbidity associated with oral mucositis.

5 Healing phase, in which cell proliferation occurs with re-epithelialization of ulcers, with epithelial cells migrating and proliferating underneath the pseudomembrane (fibrin clot) of the ulcer. The direct relationship between resolution of neutropenia and oral mucositis is uncertain.

Interventions

- Benzydamine can assist in the prevention of radiation-induced mucositis.

- Keratinocyte growth factor 1 (palifermin) is helpful in stem cell transplantation recipients with mucositis.

- Low-level He–Ne laser therapy accelerates the healing of tissue; however, it is expensive and not readily available.

- Loperamide can be used to control diarrhea.

- Oral sulfasalazine helps reduce radiation enteropathy when a patient is receiving pelvic external beam radiotherapy.

- Sucralfate enemas, specifically formulated in hospital, can reduce rectal bleeding from proctitis.

- Proton pump inhibitors or 5-HT_3 antagonists can assist with epigastric pain.

- Amifostine can be used as a cytoprotective agent in some settings.

- Topical antiseptic and antimicrobial agents are not helpful.

FATIGUE

CLINICAL PEARL

Fatigue is often poorly assessed, with little consideration given as to how other symptoms may contribute, including anemia, mood disorders and pain.

Definition

Although fatigue is common, no universally agreed definition exists. Fatigue is highly subjective, with the diagnosis based on self-report of tiredness *unrelieved by rest*.

Impact of the problem

Approximately 70% of people with advanced cancers or end-stage organ failure experience fatigue which is acknowledged as distressing, debilitating and negatively affecting people's quality of life. There are few evidence-based therapeutic options.

Pathophysiological basis

Fatigue in cancer patients is usually a result of multiple contributing factors, as outlined in Box 15-1.

Interventions to palliate the problem

Limited data support pharmacological interventions including corticosteroids, with other agents under investigation including modafinil, amantadine and methylphenidate.

Non-pharmacological interventions include resistive load training and supportive counseling, with the best outcomes expected for people who have better functional status at the time that supportive measures are instituted.

NAUSEA AND VOMITING

Definition

Nausea is defined as the unpleasant sensation of needing to vomit. While often accompanied by vomiting, nausea and vomiting are separate clinical entities.

Box 15-1
Contributing issues in cancer-related fatigue

Symptom burden
- Pain
- Anxiety
- Depression
- Sleep dysfunction
  » Obstructive sleep apnea
  » Restless leg syndrome
  » Narcolepsy
  » Insomnia

Nutritional imbalances
- Weight changes
- Changes in caloric intake
- Fluid and electrolyte imbalances
- Motility disorders

Physical function changes
- Decreased physical activity
- Decreased physical conditioning

Medical issues
- Anemia (from various etiologies)
- Other comorbidities
  » Infection

» Cardiac dysfunction
» Connective tissue diseases
» Pulmonary dysfunction
» Renal dysfunction
» Hepatic dysfunction
» Neurological dysfunction
» Endocrine dysfunction
  – hypothyroidism
  – hypogonadism
  – diabetes mellitus
  – adrenal insufficiency

Medications
- Sedating agents (hypnotics, opioids, neuropathic agents)
- Beta-blockers
- Other (drug interactions and other medication side-effects)

Cancer treatment effects
- Chemotherapy
- Radiation therapy
- Surgery
- Bone marrow transplantation
- Biological response modifiers
- Hormonal treatment

From Escalante CP and Manzullo EF. Cancer-related fatigue: the approach and treatment. J Gen Int Med 2009;24(2):S412–S416.

Impact of the problem

Nausea and vomiting secondary to tumor-modifying treatments

Up to 80% of people treated with chemotherapy and radiotherapy are likely to experience nausea and vomiting, with more severe problems resulting from chemotherapy. Failure to manage chemotherapy-induced nausea and vomiting (CINV) has implications for the patient's ongoing capacity to tolerate treatment.

CINV is complex, with people at risk of immediate and delayed presentations. Risk factors include both the chemotherapy regimen and individual factors that include female gender, younger people and a past history of nausea and vomiting with chemotherapy. Nausea is less likely to occur when people have a past history of heavy alcohol use.

Nausea and vomiting secondary to progressive disease

Quite separate to CINV is the problem of nausea and vomiting which is likely to affect 70% of patients with advanced cancer, especially late in the course of the disease.

Pathophysiological basis

- **Nausea and vomiting secondary to tumor-modifying treatments**—CINV occurs as the result of activation of peripheral afferent nerve fibers, predominantly in the gastrointestinal tract and cerebral cortex, as summarized in Figure 15-2.

- **Nausea and vomiting secondary to progressive disease**—while the same afferent pathways summarized in Figure 15-2 are presumed to underlie the problem of nausea and vomiting in advanced disease, there is little objective evidence to support this.

Interventions to palliate the problem

- **Nausea and vomiting secondary to tumor-modifying treatments**—evidence-based recommendations support the prescription of combination antiemetics. The emetogenic potential of the tumor-modifying treatment underlies the choice of antiemetics. For the acute phase of highly emetogenic platinum-based chemotherapy, 5-HT$_3$ antagonists in combination with corticosteroids and a neurokinin-1 (NK$_1$) antagonist are the treatment of choice.

- **Nausea and vomiting secondary to progressive disease**—although there are numerous published clinical guidelines to advise clinicians on the palliation of nausea and vomiting, the evidence that supports the majority of guidelines remains poor. As people approach death, there is even less information to identify which antiemetic is likely to be the most effective. In this situation, the choice is guided by which agent is least likely to cause adverse effects and by ready availability. The antiemetic that has the most robust evidence base is metoclopramide.

Table 15-2 lists antiemetic agents and their recommended uses.

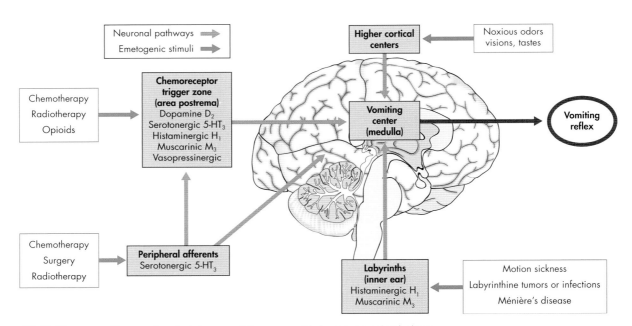

Figure 15-2 The vomiting reflex is triggered from multiple anatomical sites

Based on Nedivjon B and Chaudhary R. Controlling emesis: evolving challenges, novel strategies. J Supportive Oncol 2010;8(4 Suppl 2):1–10.

Table 15-2 Antiemetic drugs

ANTIEMETIC CLASS	MECHANISM OF ACTION	RECOMMENDED USES	LEVEL OF EVIDENCE TO SUPPORT USE IN CANCER-RELATED NAUSEA AND VOMITING
Corticosteroid: Dexamethasone	Unknown, possibly reduced prostaglandin activity in the brain	Treatment-related nausea and vomiting Nausea and vomiting secondary to raised intracranial pressure	High
		Vomiting secondary to bowel obstruction	Low
5-HT$_3$ antagonist: Granisetron Ondansetron Palonasetron Dolasetron	Inhibit visceral afferents by blocking binding of peripheral 5-HT to serotonin (type 3) receptors along the vagus nerve in the GI tract	Treatment-related nausea and vomiting Opioid-induced nausea and vomiting Nausea of advanced cancer	High
NK$_1$ antagonist: Aprepitant Fosaprepitant	Blockade of the binding of substance P to NK$_1$ receptors in the chemotrigger zone of the *area postrema*	Treatment-related nausea and vomiting	High
Benzodiazepine: Lorazepam Alprazolam	Presumably due to anxiolytic, sedative and anterograde amnesic effects of these medications centrally Especially useful in delayed or anticipatory nausea as adjuvant agents	Adjuvant support for the management of treatment-related nausea and vomiting, particularly when nausea associated with anxiety	High
Atypical antipsychotic: Olanzapine	Antipsychotic in the thienobenzodiazepine drug class that blocks multiple neurotransmitters, including: —dopamine at D$_1$, D$_2$, D$_3$ and D$_4$ brain receptors —serotonin at 5-HT$_{2a}$, 5-HT$_{2c}$, 5-HT$_3$ and 5-HT$_6$ receptors —catecholamines at alpha-1 adrenergic receptors —acetylcholine at muscarinic receptors —histamine at H$_1$ receptors	Adjuvant agent to manage treatment-related nausea and vomiting	Moderate
Antihistamine: Diphenhydramine Promethazine	Predominantly histamine antagonist in vestibular nucleus and chemotrigger zone Central dopamine and acetylcholine antagonist	Adjuvant, especially when the extra-pyramidal effects of dopamine antagonists are considered problematic	Moderate
Butyrophenone: Haloperidol Droperidol	Dopaminergic (D$_2$ subtype) receptor antagonists	Adjuvant	Moderate

continues

Table 15-2 Antiemetic drugs *continued*

ANTIEMETIC CLASS	MECHANISM OF ACTION	RECOMMENDED USES	LEVEL OF EVIDENCE TO SUPPORT USE IN CANCER-RELATED NAUSEA AND VOMITING
Phenothiazine: Prochlorperazine	Dopamine antagonist Histamine antagonist Acetylcholine antagonist	Adjuvant	High
Dopamine$_2$-antagonist: Metoclopramide	Competitive antagonist at central dopaminergic (D$_2$) receptors Weak competitive antagonist peripherally at GI 5-HT$_3$ receptors (at high dose) 5-HT$_4$ agonist Increased lower esophageal sphincter pressure Enhanced rate of gastric emptying	Adjuvant Gastric stasis Opioid-induced nausea and vomiting Nausea of advanced disease	High

5-HT, 5-hydroxytryptamine; GI, gastrointestinal; NK$_1$, neurokinin-1.

CLINICAL PEARL

Chemotherapy-induced nausea and vomiting is best managed pre-emptively with antiemetic medications commenced before the initiation of treatment and routinely prescribed for 1–3 days post-treatment.
- For highly emetogenic chemotherapy, a combination of a 5-HT$_3$ antagonist, an NK$_1$ antagonist and dexamethasone minimizes the risks of nausea and vomiting.
- Moderately emetic treatments require a 5-HT$_3$ antagonist and dexamethasone.
- Low-emetic treatments require dexamethasone.

CACHEXIA AND ANOREXIA

Definition

Although often considered in tandem, anorexia and cachexia are separate entities that often coexist.

- Cancer-associated cachexia occurs as the result of an inflammatory state leading to profound muscle wasting.
- This is typically accompanied by anorexia, loss of subcutaneous fat, increasing insulin resistance and inflammation.
- The core of the problem is that, by definition cachexia cannot be reversed with nutritional support, and leads to progressive weakness, weight loss and functional decline.

Although cancer-associated anorexia may be worsened by other poorly controlled symptoms such as pain or nausea, like cachexia, increasing evidence indicates that anorexia is secondary to a profound state of cancer-induced inflammation driven by cytokines.

Impact of the problems

Cachexia accompanies up to 20% of cancer patients at the time of diagnosis, especially those with upper gastrointestinal and lung cancers. It is identified as a poor prognostic sign, increasing the likelihood that people will be unable to tolerate chemotherapy and other tumor-modifying treatments.

The only possible treatment of cachexia requires treatment of the underlying cause. There are no clinical or biological factors that systematically differentiate between cachexia, age-related sarcopenia and malnutrition. For many people with advanced disease, weight loss is a result of all three factors. Emerging data suggest that ghrelin agonists and selective androgen receptor modulators can increase lean body (muscle) mass and appetite for sustained benefit without virilizing side-effects.

CLINICAL PEARL

Aside from physical problems, cachexia may cause significant existential suffering for both the patient and the family. Contributing factors include worsening body image, anxiety and distress.

Underlying pathophysiological basis

- At present there are no reliable biological markers of cachexia, although it is increasingly recognized as a complex inflammatory state with the key drivers being cytokines.
- As with cachexia, there is no biological marker for anorexia.
- Anorexia is also presumed to be cytokine-driven.

Interventions

- If the etiology of cachexia is unclear, enteral or parenteral feeding should not be excluded, particularly in the early stages of illness where cure is the therapeutic goal.
  - » The reason that nutritional supplements should be considered early in the disease is that the best outcomes are achieved for people who respond to tumor-modifying treatments, and nutritional support may help in tolerating anticancer therapies.
  - » This situation changes with progressive disease, especially when disease-modifying treatments are exhausted and the risks are unlikely to outweigh the benefits.

BREATHLESSNESS

Definition

Breathlessness is a subjective experience of breathing discomfort that may be frightening and distressing, often worsening as life shortens.

Impact of the problem

Up to 70% of people are likely to experience breathlessness near the end of life. A debilitating condition, breathlessness is a poor prognostic sign in life-limiting illnesses and is directly correlated with poor physical and mental quality of life.

Pathophysiological basis

The pathophysiology of breathlessness is complex, with multiple afferent receptors implicated (Table 15-3).

Most recently, 3D neuroimaging studies have shown that breathlessness causes separate areas of the cerebral cortex to be activated (anterior right insula, the cerebellar vermis, the amygdala, the anterior cingulate cortex, and the posterior cingulate cortex). These areas of the brain are also activated by pain. Both endogenous and exogenous opioids may improve breathlessness by altering the central processing of unpleasant sensations associated with breathlessness. The role of opioids in mediating the sensation of breathlessness through peripheral opioid receptors is not clear.

Table 15-3 Possible afferent sources for respiratory sensation

SOURCE OF SENSATION	ADEQUATE STIMULUS
Medullary respiratory corollary discharge	Drives to automatic breathing (hypercapnia, hypoxia, exercise)
Primary motor cortex corollary discharge	Voluntary respiratory drive
Limbic motor corollary discharge	Emotions
Carotid and aortic bodies	Hypercapnia, hypoxemia, acidosis
Medullary chemoreceptors	Hypercapnia
Slowly adapting pulmonary stretch receptors	Lung inflation
Rapidly adapting pulmonary stretch receptors	Airway collapse, irritant substances, large fast (sudden) lung inflations/deflations
Pulmonary C-fibers (J-receptors)	Pulmonary vascular congestion
Airway C-fibers	Irritant substances
Upper airway 'flow' receptors	Cooling of airway mucosa
Muscle spindles in respiratory pump muscles	Muscle length change with breathing motion
Tendon organs in respiratory pump muscles	Muscle active force with breathing motion
Metaboreceptors in respiratory pump muscles	Metabolic activity of respiratory pump
Vascular receptors (heart and lung)	Distension of vascular structures
Trigeminal skin receptors	Facial skin cooling
Chest wall joint and skin receptors	Tidal breathing motion

From Parshall MB, Schwartzstein RM, Adams L et al., ATS Committee on Dyspnea. An official American Thoracic Society statement: update on the mechanisms, assessment, and management of dyspnea. Am J Respir Crit Care Med 2012;185(4):435–52.

Interventions to palliate the problem

The degree of reversibility of the problem needs to be assessed. Palliative approaches include both pharmacological and non–pharmacological interventions.

- Non-pharmacological interventions include advice regarding positioning, including the use of walking frames, breathing exercises, cognitive therapy and exercise programs, and moving air over the face with hand-held fans.
- With regard to the pharmacological palliation of chronic breathlessness, administration of regular, low-dose, sustained-release morphine has been shown to reduce the severity of the chronic breathlessness experienced without respiratory compromise. Immediate release opioids should not be co-prescribed for episodic breathlessness.

CLINICAL PEARL

The administration of oxygen has not been shown to produce significant benefits in the palliation of chronic breathlessness when people are not hypoxic, and thus should not be routinely prescribed in this population. Supplemental oxygen is unlikely to improve chronic breathlessness when oxygen saturations are greater than 90%.

CONSTIPATION

Definition

While there is no currently agreed definition for constipation in palliative care, it is generally accepted that changes in usual bowel habits frequently complicate the lives of people with advanced illness. Unlike functional constipation, no single cause can be identified as many factors contribute to constipation in palliative and supportive care.

Impact of the problem

The current lack of agreed diagnostic criteria make it difficult to assess the true prevalence of the problem of constipation in the hospice/palliative care population. Recent observations support the notion that constipation, like some other physical symptoms, may worsen as life expectancy shortens. It is associated with an increased likelihood of hospitalization.

Pathophysiological basis

Constipation is defined as a disorder of neuromuscular function of either the colon or the pelvic floor. Opioids slow gastric emptying, and slow small bowel and colon transit times. Other factors likely to contribute include the use of medications with anticholinergic effects, reduced performance status and reduced oral intake.

Interventions to palliate the problem

- Reversible causes should be addressed.
- Assessment should include a rectal examination, which is important to diagnose fecal impaction. A plain abdominal radiograph is only useful to exclude a bowel obstruction and should not be used as the basis of a diagnosis of constipation.

- There are few data to define the optimal laxatives to use; clinical guidelines mostly recommend either a senna-based treatment or a macrogol initially.

CLINICAL PEARL

Opioids remain the most cited risk factor for constipation; despite this, the use of peripheral opioid-antagonists still requires concurrent administration of other laxatives. If the predominant cause of the constipation is opioids, then methylnaltrexone may be added to other agents.

DELIRIUM

Definition

Delirium is a common clinical syndrome, characterized by disturbed consciousness and changed cognitive function that develops over a short period of time (usually hours to days), due to the direct physiological consequences of a medical condition.

- The features of delirium can vary between individual patients. They include: impairment in memory and attention; disorientation to person, place and/or time; perceptual disturbances (hallucinations, delusions); and disturbance of the sleep–wake cycle.
- A diagnosis of delirium rests solely on clinical skills, aided by the use of questionnaires that can guide clinical assessment, as no diagnostic test exists.

There are three clinical subtypes of delirium: *hyperactive* (characterized by perceptual disturbances, agitation, restlessness, psychomotor overactivity, and disorientation); *hypoactive* (characterized by drowsiness, lack of interest in the activities of living, slowed cognition, and poor initiation of movement); or *mixed* (where the features oscillate between the two other subtypes).

Impact of the problem

The prevalence of delirium in oncology settings has been cited as 16–18%; however, in palliative settings it ranges from 25% to 90% in the more advanced or terminal stages of illness.

Delirium is associated with increased mortality, increased length of hospital stay, worse physical and cognitive recovery, and increased need for institutional care.

CLINICAL PEARLS

- Delirium is associated with high morbidity and mortality, especially if detected late or missed. In people with advanced disease, delirium is an independent predictor of mortality.
- Witnessing delirium symptoms is associated with a markedly increased risk of generalized anxiety in bereaved caregivers.
- Delirium is a distressing experience, with more than 50% of cancer patients with resolution of delirium recalling the experience.

Pathophysiological basis

In a person who was previously well, a major insult would be required to cause delirium (e.g. serious infection), whereas someone with multiple risk factors can develop delirium with a minor perturbation (change in medication, mild hypercalcemia).

There is an average of 3 precipitants per episode of delirium. Risk factors in cancer include: advanced age; severity of illness; prior delirium; the use of benzodiazepines, opioids or corticosteroids; low albumin levels; bone, liver, brain or leptomeningeal metastases; and hematological malignancies.

There are multiple neurotransmitter abnormalities in delirium (Figure 15-3). The neurotransmitter and neurobiological pathways implicated include acetylcholine and dopamine, serotonin, gamma-aminobutyric acid (GABA), cortisol, cytokines, and oxygen free-radicals. There are also emerging data supporting evidence for involvement in limbic hypothalamic–pituitary–adrenal axis dysfunction, priming of microglia such that they respond more vigorously to systemic inflammatory events in at-risk individuals, and exaggerated inflammation-induced illness.

Interventions to palliate the problem

Effective strategies for delirium prevention include regular re-orientation, therapeutic activity, early mobilization, management of sleep or anxiety with non-pharmacological strategies, maintaining nutrition and hydration, and correcting vision and hearing with relevant aids (if possible).

Management of delirium relies on early identification, and immediate assessment and treatment of precipitants.

Even in advanced cancer, delirium is reversible in at least 50% of cases. During an episode of delirium, supportive care includes management of hypoxia, maintaining hydration and nutrition, minimizing the time spent lying in bed, regular mobilization, and avoidance of restraints.

The role of psychotropic medications in delirium is still to be established, with systematic reviews not demonstrating more rapid resolution of delirium. Low-dose benzodiazepines in order to sedate in the short term while reversible causes are sought only if a patient poses a risk to themselves or others.

INSOMNIA

Definition

Insomnia is a subjective complaint by the patient of sleep disturbance despite adequate opportunity to sleep. This includes difficulty initiating or maintaining sleep, interrupted sleep and poor quality ('non-restorative') sleep.

Impact of the problem

Sleep disturbance can lead to daytime fatigue and somnolence, and also psychological distress if time spent awake at night is associated with negative thoughts. Often there is also an impact on caregivers.

Pathophysiological basis

The restorative function of sleep depends on well-organized and uninterrupted 'sleep architecture' with the order and

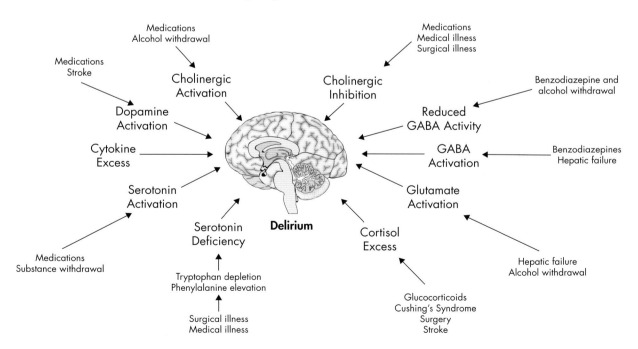

Figure 15-3 Pathophysiology of delirium. The evidence supports multiple mechanisms of delirium, which may pertain in different clinical situations

Reproduced from Flacker JM and Lipsitz LA. Neural mechanisms of delirium: current hypotheses and evolving concepts. J Gerontol 1999:54A(6):B239–B246.

duration of non-rapid eye movement (NREM) and rapid-eye movement (REM) sleep maintained. Sleep is also a mediating factor in pain regulation and immune function (cytokine and natural killer cell activity). The major categories of sleep disorders are:

- primary insomnia
- sleep-related breathing disorders (e.g. obstructive and central sleep apnea)
- hypersomnolence (e.g. narcolepsy)
- circadian rhythm disorders (e.g. shift work, jetlag)
- movement disorders (e.g. restless leg syndrome)
- parasomnias (e.g. night terrors, sleepwalking).

Common contributing factors to insomnia at the end of life include anxiety and depression, delirium, direct involvement of the brain with primary or secondary cancer, fever and sweats (especially if nocturnal), unrelieved symptoms (in particular pain, breathlessness, nausea and vomiting), medications (stimulants, corticosteroids, bronchodilators, activating antidepressants, and withdrawal syndromes), restless leg syndrome (peripheral neuropathies, uremia), and psychological factors (poor sleep habits, negative expectations).

Interventions to palliate the problem

Sleep hygiene strategies can be helpful; these include:

- maintaining a regular sleep–wake schedule
- avoiding unnecessary time in bed during the day
- providing cognitive and physical stimulation during daytime hours, in particular for bedridden patients
- avoiding stimulating medication and other substances (caffeine, nicotine) at night
- minimizing noise at night
- maintaining adequate pain relief through the night.

Cognitive behavioral therapy and muscle relaxation techniques may be helpful in some individuals.

Short-term use of a benzodiazepine hypnotic may be indicated in some patients, with careful consideration of the potential for complications, side-effects and rapid tolerance.

CLINICAL PEARL

Sleep hygiene strategies need to be tailored to individual etiologies, and sedative hypnotics considered in highly selected situations for short-term use.

SELF-ASSESSMENT QUESTIONS

1   A 56-year-old woman with metastatic breast cancer presents with a new painful lytic lesion in her distal right humerus. Plain-film radiography suggests that the lesion is occupying less than one-third of the bony cortex, and therefore surgical consultation is not sought. Discussions with her radiation oncologist are initiated. In the short term, what other strategies may be useful to improve her pain control?

    A   Bisphosphonate infusion
    B   Regular opioid analgesia
    C   A non-steroidal anti-inflammatory drug
    D   A neuropathic agent
    E   All of the above

2   A 71-year-old man is receiving combination cisplatin-based chemotherapy plus conventional radiotherapy for a head and neck cancer. Despite good mouth care and regular reviews, he develops painful oropharyngeal mucositis. Which of the following is *not* true?

    A   Mucositis is associated with increased mortality.
    B   Poor oral health is a risk factor for mucositis.
    C   Mucositis is always due to infections.
    D   5-fluorouracil is no longer recommended as concurrent treatment.
    E   Pain management is the most important aspect of treatment.

3   A 52-year-old man with adenocarcinoma of the pancreas has recently been diagnosed with liver metastases. In the outpatient clinic he advises his oncologist that the main and most distressing problem he is experiencing is fatigue. Which of the following statements is the most correct?

    A   There is a clearly defined association between tumor necrosis factor alpha and fatigue.
    B   Burst dexamethasone is strongly recommended to improve fatigue.
    C   Exercise programs are likely to worsen fatigue.
    D   Regardless of life expectancy, depression may contribute to fatigue.
    E   The best advice is to rest as, like tiredness, fatigue improves with rest.

4   An 80-year-old man presents with an inoperable cecal cancer which, at diagnosis, has already spread to the liver and lungs. He is symptomatic with right upper quadrant pain, increasing shortness of breath, and constant nausea for which he is unable to articulate factors that exacerbate or relieve this problem. He feels that if he could just improve his nausea enough to eat, he would be much better. Which of the following statements is the most correct in situations like this?

    A   The mechanisms that underlie nausea of progressive disease are well defined.
    B   Aprepitant is a useful antiemetic in this situation.
    C   Poorly controlled nausea is a poor prognostic sign.
    D   Expect that <20% of people with advanced cancer will have nausea at the end of life.
    E   Dexamethasone is a useful agent to try for this man.

5   A 58-year-old woman is diagnosed with stage IIIB adenocarcinoma of the lung. At presentation, her main symptoms are cough and weight loss. Her husband is distressed by the weight loss, constantly berating her to try harder to eat more. He is concerned that she has just given up and is frustrated with her because of this. With regard to the cancer cachexia, which of the following is the most correct?

    A   Parenteral feeding should not be considered.
    B   The benefits of parenteral feeding usually outweigh the risks.
    C   Cancer cachexia is easily differentiated from other causes of weight loss in cancer.
    D   Cachexia may be a source of conflict between patients and families.
    E   Dexamethasone is the most useful agent to help people gain weight.

6   A 62-year-old man with extensive small-cell cancer of the lung is referred to the palliative care consult team of the cancer center. His main symptom is breathlessness, which he and his family are finding frightening and distressing. He tells you he is too scared to sleep at night in case he suffocates. He is requesting home oxygen. However, you note that his oxygen saturations are 94% on room air. What other interventions may be useful to improve palliation of his breathlessness?

    A   Prescribe oxygen, as this is always useful regardless of oxygen saturations.
    B   Advise him to avoid morphine, as this will suppress his respiratory drive.
    C   Refer him to physiotherapy for advice about breathing exercises and positioning techniques.
    D   Advise him to rest as much as possible to avoid exacerbating his breathlessness.
    E   Prescribe regular nebulized 0.9% sodium chloride (NaCl) every 4 hours.

7   A patient with stage IV colon cancer presents complaining of increased abdominal distension, nausea without vomiting, and increasingly infrequent bowel actions. At presentation, he describes a situation where he has not experienced a bowel action for 4 days. His regular medications include sustained-release morphine 40 mg daily and

regular sennoside 2 tablets twice daily. He notes that prior to his cancer diagnosis he had very regular bowel actions. What is the next most appropriate step to address the fact that his bowels have not moved for 4 days?

    A   Organize a plain-film radiograph to assess the degree of fecal loading.

    B   Organize a plain-film radiograph to exclude a bowel obstruction.

    C   Undertake a rectal examination to exclude fecal impaction.

    D   Administer subcutaneous methylnatrexone for opioid-induced constipation.

8 A 62-year-old man with pancreatic cancer and biliary obstruction presents with increasing jaundice and disorientation. His wife says that he has been awake all night, has displayed evidence of hallucinations and will not take his medication as he thinks it is poison. Which of the following statements is true?

    A   Delirium does not affect mortality in advanced cancer.

    B   The cause of the presentation is most likely due to brain metastases.

    C   Most patients with delirium have one identified precipitant.

    D   Delirium is not a distressing experience as patients cannot recall it when it resolves.

    E   Delirium pathophysiology involves multiple neurotransmitters.

ANSWERS

1 E.

The management of bone pain requires multiple modalities to achieve analgesia. All of the suggested interventions have been identified as useful in the management of this often distressing problem.

2 C.

Mucositis involves a complex interaction of local tissue damage, the oral environment, myelosuppression and intrinsic genetic predisposition.

3 D.

Although a common problem in advanced cancer, the underlying etiology of fatigue remains unclear. Furthermore, the optimal management is also unclear. However, in a void of knowledge, the best clinical practice in palliative care recommendations are that as far as possible underlying factors are identified and reversed.

4 C.

Nausea is a common problem in advanced cancer. As life shortens, there are likely to be numerous contributing factors occurring simultaneously. Aside from metoclopramide, the evidence base to support other antiemetics in this palliative situation is currently limited.

5 D.

The underlying etiology of cancer cachexia is not yet clearly defined. As a result, intervention options are still being explored. In the absence of well-defined pharmacological approaches, other work has identified this to be a source of significant conflict between patients and families.

6 C.

Evidence suggests that non-hypoxic patients may not derive symptomatic benefit from the prescription of oxygen. More robust evidence supports the use of non-pharmacological approaches to breathlessness and the concurrent prescription of low-dose sustained-release morphine.

7 C.

Disturbed bowel function is very common in palliative care, with numerous contributing factors including opioids and other factors such as poor performance status, proximity to death and other medications. Fecal impaction is likely to complicate the lives of palliative care patients, and this is most easily diagnosed with a rectal examination. Prior to the administration of methylnaltrexone in constipation believed to be opioid-induced, a bowel obstruction must be excluded.

8 E.

Delirium in advanced cancer is an independent predictor of mortality, and multiple neurotransmitters are implicated in the pathophysiology. Although brain metastases may be a cause, several other precipitants are also possible, and on average patients with delirium have three or more precipitating causes for any episode of delirium. There is good evidence that patients recall delirium after resolution and find the experience highly distressing.

CHAPTER 16

IMMUNOLOGY

Brad Frankum, Monique Wei Meng Lee and Jessie A Lee

CHAPTER OUTLINE

KEY CONCEPTS IN IMMUNOBIOLOGY

- Innate and adaptive immunity are unique but heavily interdependent entities.
- Specificity and diversity are the foundation for successful adaptive immunity.
- Immunological memory is the basis for immunity and immunization.
- Hypersensitivity, autoimmunity and immunodeficiency are the key drivers of immunopathology.
- Immunity, inflammation and tissue repair are essential and interdependent components of a complex system to maintain health.
- Understanding immunobiology is the key to logical diagnosis and treatment of infection.
- Manipulation of the immune system is central to the current, and future, treatment of a vast range of human diseases: allergy, autoimmunity, malignancy, infection and transplantation.

Innate and adaptive immunity

Innate and adaptive immunity are unique but heavily interdependent entities. Their key features are described in Table 16-1.

Innate immune response

Innate immunity refers to that section of the immune system that does not require specific antigen recognition to eliminate a pathogen. It includes barrier functions such as integrity of the skin and mucous membranes, and physiological mechanisms such as coughing, sneezing, urination, and mucus production.

- The innate immune response is rapid, first-line, and prevents tissue invasion in most instances.
- Epithelial surfaces also provide chemical barriers to infection in the form of secreted antimicrobial peptides, antibacterial enzymes and fatty acids, as well as microbiological barriers in the form of commensal microbiota that compete with pathogens.
- Phagocytic cells can recognize a restricted number of cell-surface molecules on microbial pathogens, and be directly activated. These molecules are known as pathogen-associated molecular patterns (PAMPs). Examples of receptors that can recognize PAMPs include Toll-like receptors, and mannose-binding lectin (MBL).
- There are also receptors in the cytoplasm of cells that can recognize microbial products. This is obviously important for dealing with pathogens that have evaded defense mechanisms in the extracellular environment. Examples include NOD-like and RIG-1-like receptors and MDA-5.
- The innate immune system also recognizes molecules released from damaged or infected cells. These molecules are known as DAMPs, or damage-associated molecular patterns.
  » DAMPs help to activate both the innate immune response and the inflammatory response.
- Complement is a set of plasma proteins that form a cascade to ensure amplification of both innate and adaptive immune responses.
  » Complement can be activated by the presence of microbial cell surfaces, by the presence of immune complexes, or by the binding of MBL.

Table 16-1 Innate versus adaptive immunity

KEY FEATURES	INNATE IMMUNE SYSTEM	ADAPTIVE IMMUNE SYSTEM
Cells	Neutrophils, monocyte-macrophages, eosinophils, basophils, mast cells, dendritic cells, natural killer cells	B and T lymphocytes, plasma cells
Receptors	PRRs, Toll-like receptors	B-cell receptors (immunoglobulins), T-cell receptors
Effectors	Molecular—complement, acute phase reactants, cytokines Cellular—phagocytes (neutrophils, monocyte-macrophages), cells that produce inflammatory mediators (eosinophils, basophils, mast cells), natural killer cells	Humoral—B cells, antibody Cell-mediated—cytotoxic T cells
Specificity	Absent	Antigen-specific
Memory	Absent (does not require prior contact)	Antigen-specific (requires prior contact)
Response time	Immediate	Delayed
Response magnitude	Not enhanced by prior contact	Enhanced by prior contact
PRR, pattern-recognition receptor.		

» Activated complement proteins have chemotactic actions to trigger phagocytosis, as well as effector function, resulting in cell killing through the membrane attack complex.

Activation of the innate immune response results in recruitment of the adaptive response. This is achieved predominantly via antigen presentation by dendritic cells and macrophages to lymphocytes, but is augmented by changes in cytokine milieu.

In turn, the adaptive immune response utilizes effector cells of the innate system.

Adaptive immune response

The three key components of the adaptive immune response are diversity, specificity and memory.

- **Diversity** is manifested by the deliberate generation of many lymphocyte clones, but selecting only those that recognize foreign but not self-antigen for survival.
- **Specificity** refers to each lymphocyte clone having receptors of one specificity, and responding to that specific antigen only.
- **Memory** is maintained by retention of antigen-specific clones of both B and T lymphocytes, and the ongoing production of specific antibody, in perpetuity.

A number of different cells are involved (Figure 16-1):

- B cells differentiate into plasma cells to secrete antibody.
- CD4+ T-helper cells direct other cells to perform effector functions.
- CD8+ cytotoxic T cells, when activated, kill cells infected by intracellular organisms, e.g. viruses.
- T-regulatory cells:
  » are a subset of CD4+ T cells which express high levels of CD25, and a transcription factor called FoxP3
  » are generated centrally in the thymus, or peripherally in secondary lymphoid tissue

Box 16-1

The five stages of the adaptive immune response

1 Antigen capture
2 Recognition of antigen
3 Activation of lymphocytes
4 Antigen elimination
5 Decline of immune response

» are the cells which recognize self-antigen, so are antigen-specific, but develop in such a way as to suppress response toward self-antigen rather than initiate it
» function to maintain self-tolerance and suppress inflammatory responses.

The adaptive immune response proceeds through the five stages listed in Box 16-1.

The major histocompatibility complex (MHC) is a set of genes which encode for cell-surface proteins that represent a critical step in presenting foreign antigen to the effector cells of the immune system.

- Cells which are able to stimulate CD8+ cytotoxic T cells must be able to process cytosolic antigen, and present the antigen to the cell surface in conjunction with **MHC class I antigens**. These are *all* nucleated cells.
- Cells which are able to present antigen to CD4+ T-helper cells, and stimulate them, must be able to process endocytosed antigen, and express **MHC class II antigens** in conjunction with the foreign antigen on the cell surface. These are dendritic cells, monocyte-macrophages and B lymphocytes, and are collectively referred to as *antigen-presenting cells*.

Specificity and diversity

Specificity and diversity are the foundation for successful adaptive immunity.

- During development in the bone marrow (B cells) and the thymus (T cells), millions of different genetic recombinations occur in the genes that encode for lymphocyte receptors.
- **Immunological specificity** refers to the ability of the immune system to possess cells that are capable of recognizing one specific antigen only. This is the function of the lymphocyte.
  » B lymphocytes express cell-surface receptor (immunoglobulin) which is specific for one antigen. When secreted, this immunoglobulin can be arranged as a pentamer (IgM), dimer (IgA) or monomer (IgG, IgE, IgD), but still remains specific for one antigen only.
  » T lymphocytes express the T-cell receptor which is also specific for one antigen only.
- **Immunological diversity** refers to the capacity of the immune system to have lymphocytes capable of

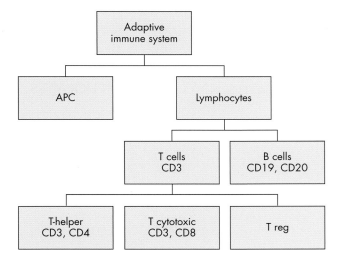

Figure 16-1 Cells of the adaptive immune system. APC, antigen-presenting cell; T reg = T-regulatory cell

recognizing every conceivable antigen. The vastness of this repertoire is staggering.

» In generating sufficient diversity amongst the lymphocyte population, the immune system needs a system in place during the requisite genetic rearrangements that allows production of clones responsive to foreign antigen, but disallows clones that are self-reactive.

» Failure to delete these autoreactive clones from being generated, or failure to recognize and deal with those that escape, is the basis for autoimmunity.

Immunological memory

Immunological memory is the basis for immunity and immunization.

- Lymphocytes exist in three states: naïve, effector and memory (Table 16–2).
  - » **Naïve lymphocytes**
    - Naïve lymphocytes have not encountered specific antigen, and survive for several months only if not exposed to antigen. There is a steady-state replacement process for these naïve cells. This may wane in older people when immunosenescence occurs.
    - Naïve T lymphocytes can be recognized by the cell-surface marker CD45RA.
    - Naïve B lymphocytes express IgM or IgD on their surface and have low expression of the cell-surface marker CD 27.
    - Naïve lymphocytes circulate predominantly to lymph nodes, and have low expression of surface molecules such as adhesion molecules that would draw them to sites of inflammation.
  - » **Effector lymphocytes**
    - Effector lymphocytes arise after specific antigen exposure.
    - They have a short half-life.

- Effector T lymphocytes are either cytotoxic T lymphocytes or T-helper cells.
- Effector B lymphocytes are plasma cells, which secrete antibody.

- Upon exposure to antigen, naïve lymphocytes transform into lymphoblasts, which are larger, more metabolically active cells. Some of these lymphoblasts then differentiate into effector cells.

- Cytotoxic T cells can be recognized by the cell-surface markers CD45, CD3 and CD8.
  - » T-helper cells express CD45, CD3 and CD4. They produce cytokines that stimulate B lymphocytes and macrophages.
  - » Both cytotoxic and T-helper cells express molecules that draw them to sites of inflammation, such as adhesion molecules.

- Activated (effector) B cells express IgG, IgA and IgE on their surface predominantly. They have high expression of CD27.

- After resolution of the effector response to specific antigen, a population of **memory lymphocytes** persists in the circulation.
  - » These cells may survive for months or years.
  - » Like plasma cells, memory B cells express IgG, IgA or IgE, but can be distinguished by being small with less cytoplasm. Memory B lymphocytes can be distinguished from naïve B cells by high expression of CD27.
  - » Like effector T cells, memory T lymphocytes express surface molecules that draw them to sites of inflammation, such as adhesion molecules. They also predominantly express CD45RO. Memory T lymphocytes differ from effector T cells, however, by expressing high amounts of CD127.

The unique qualities of memory cells make them far more efficient at responding to antigen challenge than naïve cells.

Table 16-2 Features of naïve, effector and memory lymphocytes

FEATURE	NAÏVE LYMPHOCYTES	EFFECTOR LYMPHOCYTES (B CELLS = PLASMA CELLS; T CELLS = T-HELPER CELLS, CYTOTOXIC T CELLS)	MEMORY LYMPHOCYTES
Survival	Several months	Days	Months to years
B cell surface markers	IgM, IgD Low CD27	IgG, IgA, IgE, high CD27	IgG, IgA, IgE, high CD27
T cell surface markers	CD45RA	T-helper cells: CD4+, CD25, CD40 ligand, CD45RO, low CD127 Cytotoxic T cells: CD8+, CD25, CD45RO, low CD127	CD45RO High CD127
T cell adhesion molecule expression	Low	High	High
Cytoplasm size	Small	Large	Small

This forms the basis of adaptive immunity. It also explains the efficacy of vaccination:

- For a given antigen, there are larger numbers of memory than naïve lymphocytes. This proportion increases with age.
- Memory T lymphocytes are more readily drawn to sites of infection and inflammation.
- Memory B lymphocytes have already class-switched to express the higher-affinity cell-surface immunoglobulins —IgG, IgA and IgE.
- Memory lymphocytes respond to antigen stimulation several days faster than do naïve lymphocytes.

Hypersensitivity, autoimmunity and immunodeficiency

Hypersensitivity, autoimmunity and immunodeficiency are the key drivers of immunopathology.

- Immunological reactions that are inappropriate in intensity, inappropriately targeted or inadequately regulated are labeled *hypersensitivity disorders*.
- There are four classic types of hypersensitivity (see Table 16-3).

Autoimmunity is the basis for a large amount of human disease.

- Autoimmune disease may be organ-specific, as in Hashimoto's thyroiditis and pernicious anemia; or systemic, as in systemic lupus erythematosus (SLE).
- Autoimmunity results from a combination of genetic and environmental factors. For example, patients with certain human leukocyte antigen (HLA) subtypes, and with certain inherited complement component

deficiencies, are more prone to SLE. When they incur tissue damage, e.g. with exposure to ultraviolet (UV) radiation or through infection, they are then more likely to suffer a disease flare. The cell breakdown that occurs from the environmental factor releases more autoantigen (in the case of SLE this is cellular nuclear material), and the autoreactive cells then produce more antibody, which combines with the autoantigen. The resultant immune complexes then elicit an inflammatory response through combination with Fc receptors on phagocytes, and via complement activation.

Immunodeficiency can be congenital or acquired.

- Most congenital (primary) immunodeficiency is genetically based. All components of the immune system can be thus affected, although severe forms of primary immunodeficiency are rare.
- Acquired immunodeficiency can result from environmental factors such as infection (e.g. human immunodeficiency virus [HIV] infection), or malnutrition, or from aging, or malignancy. Iatrogenic factors such as cancer chemotherapy or immunosuppressive drugs are also important.

Immunity, inflammation and tissue repair

Immunity, inflammation and tissue repair are essential and interdependent components of a complex system to maintain health.

- Infection or tissue damage incites an inflammatory response.
- Immune system activation results in the release of a variety of cytokines (chemokines) that function to attract effector cells.

Table 16-3 Classification of hypersensitivity

	TYPE			
	I	II	III	IV
Mechanism	Immediate	Antibody-mediated	Immune-complex-mediated	T-cell-mediated
Immunopathology	IgE-mediated Mast-cell degranulation Production of prostaglandins and leukotrienes	Antibody directed at tissue antigens Complement activation Fc-receptor-mediated inflammation	Deposition of immune complexes in vascular beds Fixation of complement Fc-receptor-mediated inflammation	Mediated by CD4+ T-helper cells of the TH1 or TH17 subsets, or by cytotoxic T lymphocytes May be inappropriately directed against self-antigens, or foreign antigens (e.g. nickel in jewelry causing contact dermatitis) There may be collateral damage in responses against intracellular infection (e.g. viral hepatitis)
Disease examples	Allergic rhinitis Asthma Food allergy Anaphylaxis	Pernicious anemia Hashimoto's thyroiditis Myasthenia gravis	Serum sickness Lupus nephritis Post-streptococcal GN	Contact dermatitis Multiple sclerosis Type I diabetes mellitus

GN, glomerulonephritis.

- Other cytokines are inflammatory, resulting in effects such as vasodilatation, increased vascular permeability, fever and pain, all of which enhance the effectiveness of the immune response in limiting damage caused by the injury or infection.
- Clotting mechanisms are enhanced by inflammatory cytokines. This both results in limitation of blood loss from damaged tissue, and hinders travel of infection to distant sites.
- Yet other cytokines trigger tissue repair in order to restore tissues once the insult has been dealt with.

For the most part, these systems function smoothly to maintain homeostasis, and control mechanisms are in place to curtail responses when function is restored. When components of the systems are deficient, or control mechanisms fail to limit an excessive inflammatory response, disease results.

Understanding immunobiology

Understanding immunobiology is the key to logical diagnosis and treatment of infection.

- The response of the immune system to dealing with a variety of different pathogens forms the basis of effective treatment.
- Deficiencies in components of the innate immune system, for example neutropenia, will make the individual especially susceptible to bacterial and fungal infection, and thus antibiotic or antifungal therapy should be considered promptly in the setting of early signs of infection.
- Antibody deficiencies will similarly predispose to extracellular infection.
- Cellular immune deficiency predisposes to infection with intracellular organisms such as viruses and mycobacteria. The approach to an ill patient in this setting will therefore differ both diagnostically and therapeutically.
- At present the capacity to iatrogenically 'boost' the immune system is limited. Replacing immunoglobulin in those who are deficient is of proven benefit, but the use of pooled donor immunoglobulin for infection otherwise is not. T-cell deficiencies are even more problematic, with a very small number of congenital, severe immunodeficiencies being managed with bone marrow transplantation though with variable results.
- Rarely, the administration of cytokines for therapy is used. An example is the success of interferon-gamma for chronic granulomatous disease.

Manipulation of the immune system

Manipulation of the immune system is central to the current, and future, treatment of a vast range of human disease: allergy, autoimmunity, malignancy, infection, and transplantation.

- While immunosuppression remains the mainstay of treatment for a large number of immunologically mediated diseases, newer and more sophisticated approaches, especially the growing use of biological agents, offer increasing hope for more targeted and less toxic therapy.
- Strategies for dealing with allergic disease include:
  - » treatments that block the release of mediators (mast-cell stabilizers) or the effect of mediators (antihistamines, leukotriene antagonists, corticosteroids)
  - » treatments that suppress the immune system to counteract the activity of B lymphocytes producing IgE, or effector T lymphocytes (corticosteroids, other immunosuppressives)
  - » treatments that manipulate and ameliorate the allergic response (immunotherapy)
  - » specific anti-IgE therapy (omalizumab).
- Autoimmune disease will predominantly require immunosuppression to counteract the effect of pathological antibody production or autoreactive T cells.
- Agents such as corticosteroids and methotrexate have both anti-inflammatory and immunosuppressive actions, depending on dose.
- Targeted biological therapy, using monoclonal antibodies against cellular receptors or cytokines, is increasingly being used to treat both malignancies and autoimmune disease (Table 16-4).
- Although largely unhelpful for treating infection in immune-competent hosts, pooled human immunoglobulin can be very effective to modify immune responses in the setting of autoimmunity (Box 16-2).
- Manipulation of the immune system has enabled the use of tissue transplantation to treat a variety of life-threatening diseases.
  - » Organs can now be transplanted from donors who are less immunologically matched to the recipient than ever before.

Table 16-4 Biological agents with a role in autoimmune disease

BIOLOGICAL AGENT	ANTIBODY TARGET
Infliximab Etanercept Adalimumab Golimumab Certolizumab	TNF-alpha
Anakinra	IL-1R
Tocilizumab	IL-6
Rituximab Ocreluzimab Ofatumumab	CD20 (anti-B cell)
Abatacept	CD80 and CD86
Belimumab	BAFF
Natalizumab	alpha-4 integrin
Efalizumab	CD11a

BAFF, B-cell activating factor; IL, interleukin; IL-1R, interleukin-1 receptor; TNF, tumor necrosis factor.

Box 16-2

Evidence-based uses for high-dose immunoglobulin therapy in autoimmune disease

Neurological disease
- Myasthenia gravis
- CIDP (chronic inflammatory demyelinating polyneuropathy)
- Guillain–Barré syndrome
- Dermatomyositis
- Multifocal motor neuropathy
- Lambert–Eaton syndrome
- Stiff person syndrome

Hematological disease
- Immune thrombocytopenic purpura
- Immune neutropenia
- Immune hemolytic anemia
- Parvovirus B19-associated aplasia in immunocompromised patients

Other autoimmune disease
- Kawasaki disease
- Vasculitis (some forms, limited evidence)

» So successful has been immunosuppression to suppress tissue rejection, that the major risks to the transplanted patient lie in the susceptibility to infection and the long-term threats of metabolic disease and malignancy, rather than from organ rejection *per se*.

- Similarly, the role of immunotherapy is likely to increase in the treatment of malignancy in the future, both by activating immune mechanisms directed toward cancer cells and by supporting the immune system in those who have been immunosuppressed by the effects of chemotherapy, radiotherapy or targeted biological therapy.

- Highly tissue-damaging consequences can result from the inflammatory response induced by a variety of infections. This is largely through the systemic effects of pro-inflammatory cytokines.
  - » A limited role has been defined for the use of immunotherapy that counteracts this excessive inflammatory response, but it is likely that agents will be discovered in the future.
  - » It is also possible that more specific and safer therapies will be developed in the future that can augment components of the immune response to infection, enhancing eradication of pathogens while preserving tissue integrity and function simultaneously.

ALLERGIC DISEASE

Anaphylaxis

Epidemiology

Anaphylaxis is a life-threatening disorder, with a lifetime prevalence that is unknown but may be as high as 2%. The incidence is increasing. Children and young adults are affected more frequently. The diagnosis is often missed. Fatalities due to anaphylaxis are rare, but, again, may be under-reported. Common causes are shown in Box 16-3.

Pathophysiology

- Anaphylaxis results from widespread mast-cell and/or basophil degranulation, resulting in the immediate release of pre-formed vasoactive and smooth-muscle-reactive

---

Box 16-3

Causes of anaphylaxis

IgE-dependent
- Foods—peanuts and tree nuts, eggs, crustaceans, seeds, cow's milk
- Drugs—beta-lactam antibiotics, neuromuscular blocking drugs, local anesthetic agents, insulin, chemotherapy agents, monoclonal antibodies, immunotherapy allergens
- Insect stings— *Hymenoptera* venom (bee, yellowjacket/wasp, hornet)
- Latex, chlorhexidine
- Inhalants rarely—horse hair, cat hair

Non-IgE-dependent
- Radiocontrast media
- Drugs—non-steroidal anti-inflammatories, opioids
- Physical causes— exercise, cold, heat
- Idiopathic anaphylaxis
- Systemic mastocytosis

---

chemicals such as histamine, and rapid production of others such as leukotrienes and prostaglandins.

- This can be triggered by IgE-dependent or non-IgE dependent mechanisms.

- Non-IgE-dependent mechanisms may be IgG- or complement-driven, or a result of direct mast-cell activation.

Clinical features

- The majority of patients with anaphylaxis have cutaneous involvement of the skin and mucous membranes, in the form of urticaria and angioedema.

- Generalized flushing can also occur.

- Pruritus is usual.

- Respiratory involvement in the form of stridor, secondary to laryngeal and upper airway edema, or wheezing, secondary to bronchospasm, is necessary for diagnosis, unless there is hypotension plus skin involvement.

- Hypotension may result in syncope, confusion or incontinence.
- Gastrointestinal involvement in the form of nausea, abdominal cramps, vomiting and/or diarrhea is common.

Differential diagnosis

- The diagnosis of anaphylaxis is clinical, but elevated serum tryptase in a sample taken within 3 hours of the event, or serum histamine taken within 1 hour, is usually confirmatory.
- Other causes of shock need to be considered, especially if there is no evident mucocutaneous involvement.
- When anaphylaxis is suspected, it is important to attempt to ascertain the trigger through careful history taking, and confirmatory tests where relevant such as allergen skin-prick tests or serum-specific IgE for foods, drugs or venoms.

Management

The key to the management of anaphylaxis is the early administration of epinephrine (adrenaline), and fluid resuscitation. Fluid volume expansion may need to be aggressive to restore adequate circulation.

> **CLINICAL PEARL**
>
> The dose of epinephrine (adrenaline) to be used in anaphylaxis should be 0.01 mg/kg, up to a maximum dose of 0.5 mg. This should be given intramuscularly (1:1000 dilution) or intravenously (1:10,000 dilution). Intravenous epinephrine administration should only occur in the setting of cardiac monitoring. Doses can be repeated as needed if response is poor.

- H₁ antihistamines and corticosteroids are useful adjuncts in treatment, but should never be used as an alternative to epinephrine (adrenaline).
- Any patient with anaphylaxis should be observed in hospital for at least 4 hours, and up to 24 hours in severe cases.
- Long term, patients must be instructed to strictly avoid identified triggers, and subsequent challenge to assess for ongoing clinical risk should only ever be undertaken in a hospital setting under the supervision of appropriate specialists.
- Allergen immunotherapy is only used in the setting of anaphylaxis for *Hymenoptera* venom allergy, and more recently for single food allergy with the use of oral immunotherapy for peanut allergy.

Prognosis

- Death is unusual in anaphylaxis, but is probably under-recognized.
- Prognosis is worse in patients with coexisting asthma, other respiratory disorders, and underlying cardiovascular disease.

- Patients on beta-adrenoceptor blockers are at increased risk, due to antagonism of the effect of epinephrine.
- Lack of preparedness for community self-management in those at risk, through the availability of and ability to appropriately use an adrenaline self-injecting device, also confers a worse prognosis.

> **CLINICAL PEARL**
>
> Anaphylaxis is a clinical syndrome, with no distinction made between IgE-mediated and non-IgE-mediated causes. The term 'anaphylactoid' is no longer used.

Allergic rhinitis (AR) and allergic conjunctivitis (AC)

Epidemiology

- Allergic rhinitis and allergic conjunctivitis affect up to 30% of the population.
- They are more common in developed countries and temperate climates.
- They frequently coexist in the same individual, but AR is more common than AC. It is uncommon to see AC in an individual without AR, but this can occur.
- Both genders are affected equally.
- AR and AC form part of the atopic phenotype, with affected individuals more likely to suffer from asthma, food allergy and/or atopic dermatitis.
- In particular, asthma is found in 15–38% of patients with AR, and nasal symptoms are present in up to 85% of patients with asthma. AR is a risk factor for asthma, and uncontrolled moderate-to-severe AR affects asthma control.
- Onset is typically in childhood after the age of about 5 years until young adulthood, but can come on later in life, especially with a change in geographical location.

Pathophysiology

Both AR and AC result from allergic sensitization to inhalant allergens.

- Nasal mucosal and/or conjunctival mast cells have surface IgE that is specific for allergen in affected individuals.
- Combination of allergen with IgE bound to the mast-cell surface after inhalation into the nose, or settling on the conjunctival surface, results in cross-linking of IgE and triggering of the allergic reaction locally.
- Common allergens implicated in AR are the house dust mite, grass and tree pollen, and animal danders (see Box 16-4). Sufferers may be mono-sensitized, but more commonly react to multiple allergens.

Box 16-4
Common airborne allergens

Perennial allergens

- House dust mite—*Dermatophagoides pteronyssinus, D. farinae*
- Animal danders—dog, cat (Fel d 1), horse hair
- Cockroach—German and American species
- Molds—e.g. *Alternaria tenuis, Cladosporium herbarum*

Seasonal allergens

- Grass pollen—e.g. perennial ryegrass, Bermuda grass, ragweed
- Tree pollen—e.g. birch, pine

CLINICAL PEARLS

- The demonstration of a specific IgE to an allergen in an individual confirms **sensitization** to that allergen rather than clinical **allergy**.
- Many individuals are sensitized to allergens that cause no clinical symptoms.
- Both *in vivo* (skin-prick tests) and *in vitro* (serum-specific IgE testing) testing are highly sensitive for the detection of allergic sensitization. Skin-prick testing, in expert hands, is more sensitive and specific, and allows clearer identification of individual allergens, whereas specific IgE tests can be used when patients have skin disease that renders skin testing difficult, or when the patient is taking antihistamines, which will give false-negative skin-prick testing.

Clinical features

- AR is characterized by nasal congestion and blockage, rhinorrhea (usually watery), excessive sneezing, and nasal itch, in varying combinations. The local allergic reaction can also result in palatal itch, or itch within the ear.
- AC results in redness, excessive tearing, and itching of the eyes.
- Sufferers of AR and AC frequently complain of fatigue and irritability.
- In AR, physical examination reveals pale, swollen inferior nasal turbinates. There may be partial to complete nasal occlusion.
- In AC, conjunctivae may be injected, with variable chemosis.
- In general, symptoms will be perennial when due to dust mite or animal danders, or seasonal with grass and tree pollen. This, however, may vary with climatic conditions and geography.
- 'Hayfever' is a historical term that refers to the intense rhinoconjunctivitis that occurs in the springtime in individuals with pollen sensitization.

Differential diagnosis

Diagnosis is usually not difficult, and can be confirmed by the demonstration of specific IgE to an appropriate allergen, either by skin-prick testing (Figure 16-2) or by the detection of specific IgE in serum by various techniques.

- Non-allergic rhinitis can cause similar symptoms to AR, in the absence of demonstrable allergic sensitization. The etiology is unknown.
  - » Vasomotor rhinitis is a subset of non-allergic rhinitis, and is characterized by nasal congestion and rhinorrhea that is provoked by non-specific environmental stimuli such as rapid temperature change and strong odors.
  - » NARES is non-allergic rhinitis with eosinophilia, where excess eosinophils are found on a nasal smear. This is presumed to be due to local mucosal allergic sensitization where the culprit allergen/s is not demonstrable systemically.
- Chronic rhinosinusitis is more likely if the individual has thick or purulent nasal discharge, sinus and/or dental pain, post-nasal drip and/or hyposmia or anosmia.
- Nasal congestion can occur in the latter stages of pregnancy, and is known as pregnancy rhinitis.
- Inappropriate long-term use of nasal decongestant sprays can cause rebound nasal mucosal congestion, and is known as rhinitis medicamentosa.

Management

Management of AR and AC is outlined in Box 16-5, overleaf.

Prognosis

- AR and AC have been shown to adversely affect quality of life when not treated, or treated sub-optimally.
- Symptoms generally persist for decades in the absence of allergen-specific immunotherapy, only abating in most cases in middle age.

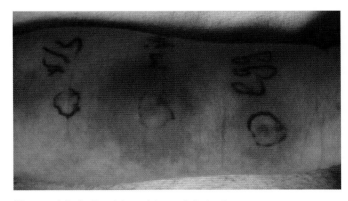

Figure 16-2 Positive skin-prick tests

From Yu M-C et al. Allergic colitis in infants related to cow's milk: clinical characteristics, pathologic changes and immunologic findings. Pediatr Neonatol 2013;54(1):49–55.

Box 16-5
Management of allergic rhinitis and allergic conjunctivitis

Allergen avoidance
- May be useful for house dust mite and animal danders, although it is difficult to achieve
- Not possible for grass and tree pollens
- Of limited overall efficacy

Intranasal corticosteroids
- Mometasone
- Fluticasone propionate
- Fluticasone furoate
- Budesonide
- Ciclesonide
- Triamcinolone
- Beclomethasone
- Once daily; safe for long-term use
- Adherence often limits efficacy

Intranasal antihistamines
- Azelastine
- Levocabastine
- Equally effective alternative to oral antihistamines but faster onset of action

Intranasal anti-muscarinic
- Ipratropium
- Rapid onset and prolonged action
- Useful adjunct if there is marked rhinorrhea

Systemic H_1 antihistamines
- Cetirizine
- Fexofenadine

- Loratadine
- Desloratadine
- Safe. More effective for itching and rhinorrhea; less effect on nasal blockage
- Useful adjunct when used with other modalities

Topical ocular therapy
- Lubricants
- Antihistamines
- Mast-cell stabilizers
- Multiple-action drugs
- Corticosteroids
- Need to be used multiple times per day. Corticosteroids are not safe for long-term use (cataracts, infection)
- Adherence is often poor
- Costly

Allergen-specific immunotherapy
- Subcutaneous or sublingual: single or multiple allergens, with less evidence for efficacy for multiple allergens
- Oral tablet immunotherapy is now also available for house dust mite and grass pollen
- Risk of anaphylaxis with subcutaneous immunotherapy, therefore requires expert administration and specialist supervision
- Offers potential for long-term disease modification
- Costly, but cost-effective in the long term

Chronic rhinosinusitis

Epidemiology

- Chronic rhinosinusitis (CRS) is classified as CRS without nasal polyps or CRS with nasal polyps.
- The condition causes considerable morbidity.
- Prevalence data suggest that CRS is common, perhaps affecting up to 5% of the population. The type without nasal polyps is more common.

Pathophysiology

The etiology of CRS is unknown. It occurs more frequently in atopic than non-atopic individuals, suggesting a role for allergic sensitization in some cases.

Humoral immunodeficiency is a risk factor for CRS, which raises suspicion for the role of infection, as both bacteria and fungi can be isolated in many cases. Treatment with antibiotics and antifungal agents is, however, disappointing.

This contrasts with acute bacterial sinusitis, for which antibiotics are generally efficacious.

Other risk factors for CRS include:
- ciliary dyskinesia
- cystic fibrosis
- aspirin sensitivity
- asthma.

Clinical features

Chronic rhinosinusitis is generally subacute in onset, presenting with:
- persistent nasal blockage (often with nocturnal snoring)
- facial pain and frontal headache
- post-nasal drip.

Other symptoms may include:
- dental pain
- hyposmia or anosmia

- ear pain, fullness, or blockage
- persistent cough, with or without expectoration.

Physical examination may be unremarkable, or reveal:

- tenderness over the sinuses
- mucopurulent secretions in the nasal passages or pharynx
- nasal obstruction.

Differential diagnosis

- The diagnosis of CRS can be confirmed with computed tomography (CT) or magnetic resonance imaging (MRI) of the paranasal sinuses, and/or direct visualization with nasendoscopy.
- Both persistent allergic rhinitis and non-allergic rhinitis are less likely to cause facial pain, headache, post-nasal drip, and alteration in the sense of smell than CRS.
- ANCA-positive vasculitis should always be considered in a patient with chronic sinus–related symptomatology, especially if there is associated epistaxis, lower respiratory tract symptoms, or the patient is systemically unwell.
- Paranasal sinus tumors are very rare, but should be obvious on imaging.
- Some patients are prone to recurrent bouts of acute infective sinusitis. The patient should be symptom-free between episodes. The majority of cases of acute infective sinusitis are, in fact, viral in origin, and resolve without specific treatment.
- If nasal ulceration or a saddle-nose deformity is found, the following conditions should be considered:
  » granulomatosis with polyangiitis (Wegener's granulomatosis)
  » midline granuloma (non-caseating granuloma without vasculitis)
  » tumor—carcinoma, lymphoma
  » relapsing polychondritis
  » infection—tuberculosis, leprosy, syphilis, histoplasmosis
  » cocaine sniffing.

Causes of nasal blockage are listed in Box 16-6.

CLINICAL PEARL

Samter's triad (aspirin-exacerbated respiratory disease, AERD) consists of sinonasal polyposis, aspirin hypersensitivity and asthma. It should be remembered that approximately 10% of all asthmatics will have aspirin-exacerbated asthma, but a much smaller number have Samter's triad. It is extremely important to inquire about aspirin or non-steroidal anti-inflammatory drug (NSAID)-related symptoms in asthmatics, because anaphylaxis may occur with inadvertent use.

Aspirin 'desensitization' (the graduated introduction of increasing doses of aspirin, commencing with minute quantities) can be an effective treatment in Samter's triad, but is dangerous due to the risk of severe asthma or anaphylaxis and should only be performed under strict specialist guidance. Those patients who do tolerate the regimen often then have gastrointestinal side-effects from the high daily doses of aspirin that are required for maintenance of effective desensitization.

Box 16-6

Causes of nasal blockage

- Nasal mucosal conditions
  » Allergic rhinitis
  » Non-allergic rhinitis
  » Infective rhinitis
  » Chronic rhinosinusitis (with or without nasal polyps)
- Adenoidal hypertrophy
- Vasculitic conditions
  » ANCA-positive vasculitis
- Granulomatous disorders
  » Sarcoidosis
- Mass lesions
  » Tumors of the nasal cavity, paranasal sinuses, or nasopharynx
- Anatomical obstruction
  » Nasal septal deviation
  » Trauma
  » Foreign bodies

Management

- CRS tends to be very corticosteroid-responsive, and often a short course of moderate-dose prednisolone will relieve symptoms and result in significant shrinkage of polyp size. Effects are, however, temporary and patients can become inappropriately reliant upon ongoing steroid medication.
- Intranasal steroids may benefit a minority of patients, if used continuously.
- Daily nasal lavage with saline solutions can help alleviate symptoms.
- Patients with severe and ongoing disease will often require surgical intervention. While often effective in the short term, disease will often recur after surgery.
- Patients with concurrent allergic rhinitis should be treated for that problem.
- Leukotriene antagonists reduce symptoms in a minority of patients.
- Antibiotic therapy should be used for acute flares of the condition. Intranasal antibiotics used long-term are of limited benefit.
- The monoclonal antibodies omalizumab, mepolizumab and dupilumab have all been shown to improve chronic rhinosinusitis with nasal polyps, although availability is variable for this indication, largely due to high cost.

Prognosis

CRS is a chronic disease that requires ongoing management.

- Few patients are symptom-free at 5 years.
- Patients should be monitored for the development of obstructive sleep apnea.
- Frequent or long-term corticosteroid use will require monitoring for the usual complications.

Atopic dermatitis (AD)

Atopic dermatitis is a common, chronic, pruritic skin condition which has significant adverse effects on quality of life. The term 'eczema' is often used synonymously, but is less precise and is best avoided.

Epidemiology

- Atopic dermatitis is estimated to affect more than 10% of young children. The prevalence decreases with age.
- AD is more common in Western industrialized nations.
- The majority of patients have the atopic phenotype, with significant risk of concurrent or future food allergy, asthma and allergic rhinoconjunctivitis.

Pathophysiology

The development of AD results from a complex interplay of immune dysregulation, skin barrier dysfunction and microbiome imbalance, together with environmental insults. While it is clear that an abnormal Th2 response in the skin in AD leads to the overproduction of Th2 cytokines (see Table 16-5), which then drive excessive IgE production in response to a variety of food and environmental allergens, it is often incorrectly assumed that AD results solely from exposure to these allergens. Patients and parents of affected children often despair when the strict avoidance of allergens to which they or their children are sensitized fails to adequately control the disease.

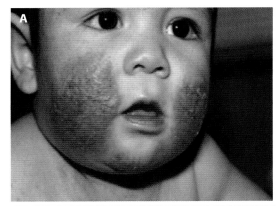
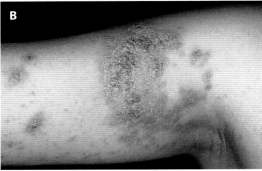

Figure 16-3 Typical patterns of atopic dermatitis in (**A**) an infant and (**B**) an adult

From: (A) Weston WL, Lane AT and Morelli JG. Color textbook of pediatric dermatology, 4th ed. Elsevier, 2007. (B) Dr Harout Tanielian/Science Photo Library.

Table 16-5 TH2 cytokines in AD

CYTOKINE	ACTION IN AD
IL4/IL13	- Epidermal barrier dysfunction - Inflammatory cell migration into AD lesions - Innate immune suppression - Pruritus
IL5	- Maturation, activation and migration of eosinophils
IL31	- Binds to receptors on sensory neurons and may directly induce pruritus

Other components of this complex, multifactorial disease include:

- Skin dryness contributes toward poor barrier function. Filaggrin is a structural skin protein important for physical integrity and prevention of water loss. Patients with loss of function mutations in the Filaggrin gene suffer from a particularly severe form of AD.
- Chronic cutaneous bacterial colonization with Staphylococcus and fungal colonization with Malassezia are known to contribute to skin flares and severe AD.
- Pruritus, resulting in persistent scratching and further damage to barrier function, and risk of infection.

CLINICAL PEARL

Detection of allergic sensitization by demonstration of specific IgE by skin-prick or serum-specific IgE testing remains important in atopic dermatitis (AD), but results must be interpreted in the context of the individual patient.
- A child whose AD is under good control with topical treatment, and is tolerating foods such as wheat or milk with no flare in their disease after consuming these foods—even if they have demonstrable specific IgE to these foods—should not be advised to remove wheat and milk from their diet.
- A child who has demonstrable specific IgE to the house dust mite may gain some benefit from dust mite reduction methods in the home, but the AD is very unlikely to be driven by this alone, so common sense should prevail as to the extent to which allergen avoidance measures are pursued.

Studies have shown that the presence of AD in children predisposes to subsequent food allergen sensitization and aeroallergen sensitization and is the first step in the atopic march toward the development of food allergy, allergic rhinitis and asthma.

Clinical features

The rash of AD:

- is characterized by scaly, erythematous patches
- is very pruritic
- may be discoid
- occurs on very dry skin.

The pattern of rash in AD (Figure 16-3) typically evolves with increasing age, although at any point it may be generalized:

- Infants—cheeks, torso, nappy area
- Toddlers—cheeks, perioral, flexures, nappy area
- Children—eyelids, behind ears, flexures, torso
- Adults—flexures, limbs, hands, face, back.

Secondary infection is common, and may be manifested by pustules, weeping, or worsening erythema.

Differential diagnosis

Pruritic, erythematous skin rashes are common. AD is best distinguished by the age of onset and the pattern of rash, but may be mistaken for the following:

- Allergic contact dermatitis, common causes of which are:
  - » nickel sulfate (jewelry)
  - » potassium dichromate (cement, leathers, paint)
  - » paraphenylenediamine (hair dyes, cosmetics)
  - » para-aminobenzoic acid (sunscreen)
  - » formaldehyde (cosmetics, shampoos)
- Irritant contact dermatitis
- Psoriasis
- Scabies
- Drug eruptions.

Biopsy of the rash is rarely necessary, with the majority of patients displaying other atopic conditions.

> **CLINICAL PEARL**
>
> In a patient with a generalized erythrodermic dermatosis, a markedly elevated total serum IgE is highly suggestive of atopic dermatitis.

Treatment

Topical treatment is the mainstay of successful management of AD.

- Minimum twice-daily application of moisturizers and/or emollients.
- Adequate cleansing of the skin, while avoiding drying soaps.
- Sterilization of the skin with dilute bleach baths 2–3 times per week can be useful.
- Liberal application of topical corticosteroids.
  - » AD that is worse than mild should be treated with moderate- to high-potency steroid creams or ointments (e.g. mometasone, methylprednisolone) for as long as it takes to get the disease under control.

- » Mild disease, and facial AD, can be safely treated with topical 1% hydrocortisone.
- 1% pimecrolimus cream can be safely used for facial dermatitis, including eyelid dermatitis. Tacrolimus cream may be effective in severe cases.
- Wet dressings or bandages used for several hours per day can be highly effective for moisturization.

Patients who fail to improve despite adequate topical therapy should be considered for **systemic therapy**. The following agents have been shown to be effective:

- cyclosporine (ciclosporin)
- azathioprine
- methotrexate.

Several biologic agents have been proven effective in the treatment of AD, while a number of others are under investigation. See Table 16-6. Where possible, oral corticosteroids should be avoided in the long-term management of AD. Rebound flaring is usual when oral steroids are withdrawn, and it is difficult to justify the long-term side-effects of steroids in all but the most disabling cases of AD.

Treatment of **superimposed infection** is important.

- Short courses of anti-staphylococcal antibiotics should be used for obvious infection, or with disease flares.
- Long-term low-dose antibiotics, e.g. once-daily co-trimoxazole, may be of benefit in some patients.
- Intermittent application of intranasal mupirocin may reduce staphylococcal carriage.

Prognosis

- Many affected children improve with age.
- Adult AD can be severe, and relatively resistant to therapy.
- An explanation for the exacerbations and remissions seen in the disease over time is not always obvious, and these may not be only on the basis of varying allergen exposure.

Food allergy

Adverse reactions to foods can be IgE- or non-IgE-mediated, due to immune or non-immune mechanisms. The term 'allergy' should be reserved for immune-mediated reactions.

Epidemiology

- An epidemic of food allergy is being observed in the developed world. The incidence of food allergy is increasing sharply, and levels of up to 10% are being observed in preschool-aged children in the developed world.
- Prevalence is much higher in children; not all children 'grow out of' their food allergies, so prevalence in adults will increase over the next decades.
- Adults can develop food allergy de novo.

Pathophysiology

- Non-IgE-mediated food reactions tend to mainly cause gastrointestinal symptoms, such as bloating, cramping, and diarrhea.
- This may be chemically or immunologically mediated through non-IgE mechanisms, e.g. celiac disease.

Table 16-6 Biological agents in AD

BIOLOGICAL AGENT	MECHANISM OF ACTION	EFFECTIVENESS IN AD
Dupilumab	Anti-IL4 receptor alpha.	Approved for AD treatment. Significantly improved AD severity, pruritus, quality of life, sleep.
Lebrikizumab Tralokinumab	Anti-IL13.	Significantly improved AD severity, improved skin clearance, quality of life, pruritus. Phase IIb.
Nemolizumab	Anti-IL-31 receptor alpha.	Significant reduction in pruritus and AD severity. Phase II.
Baricitinib Upadacitinib	JAK 1/2 inhibitor. JAK 1 inhibitor.	Significantly improved AD severity, pruritus and sleep. Phase II.
Crisaborole	Inhibitor of phosphodiesterase-4.	Approved for mild to moderate AD for adults and children 2 years and older.
Ustekinumab	Anti-IL-12/IL23 p40.	May provide some benefit for AD; more investigation needed.

Box 16-7

Common causes of food allergy

Infants	Toddlers	Children	Adults
Cow's milk	Hen's eggs	Hen's eggs	Peanuts
Soya bean	Cow's milk	Peanuts	Tree nuts
Hen's eggs	Peanuts	Tree nuts	Seeds, e.g. sesame
	Tree nuts	Seeds, e.g. sesame	Crustaceans
		Fish	Fruits and some vegetables
		Crustaceans	
		Fruits and some vegetables	

- Systemic reactions resembling anaphylaxis, or components of anaphylaxis such as generalized urticaria, can occur through non–IgE mechanisms and can be dangerous. These can be due to a wide variety of food components. Examples may include preservatives such as sulfites, or food-coloring agents. In these cases, it is presumed that release of histamine and other vasoactive molecules through non–IgE-mediated mechanisms is responsible.
- It is increasingly recognized that food components exacerbate symptoms of irritable bowel syndrome in significant numbers of sufferers.
- Atopic dermatitis can be exacerbated by both IgE and non–IgE food reactions.
- Allergy to a very wide variety of foods has been demonstrated in individuals, but allergy to meats, cereals and vegetables are rare. Common causes of food allergy are listed in Box 16-7.

Clinical features

Oral allergy syndrome (OAS)

- Oral allergy syndrome results in oral and pharyngeal tingling, itching, and sometimes swelling.
- OAS uncommonly results in systemic symptoms or airway obstruction.

- It is often caused by ingestion of fruits and some raw vegetables, and is more common in those who are sensitized to tree and grass pollen and suffer from seasonal allergic rhinitis.
- Reactions may be more common, and more severe, in the pollen season.
- Cooking will often denature the allergenic components of fruits and vegetables in OAS, and may allow consumption.

Systemic food reactions

- Angioedema of the lips, face and upper airway can result from ingestion of culprit foods within minutes.
- Gastrointestinal reactions of nausea, vomiting and diarrhea are common.
- Urticaria can be generalized.
- Anaphylaxis with circulatory collapse and/or airway obstruction can result in death.

Differential diagnosis

- When symptoms occur immediately after food ingestion, it is usually obvious that the reaction is due to a specific food, but young children may ingest culprit foods when their carers are not watching them.

- Food allergy almost always occurs rapidly.
- Non-IgE-mediated adverse food reactions may occur some hours after ingestion, and may result from components of several foods rather than an individual one.
- Patients frequently attribute a wide range of symptoms to food. The physician needs to take a careful history to see if this is likely.
- Testing for specific IgE with skin-prick tests or serum-specific IgE is generally sensitive for detecting food-allergen sensitization. For skin-prick testing, fresh fruits, vegetables, seafoods and meats are more reliable than commercially available extracts.

CLINICAL PEARL

The size of the positive skin-prick reaction to a food, or the absolute level of serum-specific IgE to that food, is a guide to that person's risk of an allergic reaction occurring with ingestion but not the severity of the reaction. The result must be used in conjunction with the history and in comparison with the size of previous reactions, or levels, to assess an individual's risk.

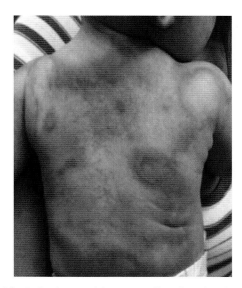

Figure 16-4 Patient with generalized urticaria

From Callen JP and Jorrizo JL, eds. Dermatological signs of internal disease, 4th ed. Elsevier, 2009.

Treatment

- Strict avoidance of culprit foods is essential.
- Emergency action plans should be in place for all food-allergy sufferers.
- Epinephrine self-injecting devices must be carried at all times by patients with food allergy who are assessed to be at risk of anaphylaxis.
- Determining the level of risk is often difficult, and requires specialist assessment.
- Food challenge testing is appropriate in individuals when there is evidence of developing tolerance, usually evidenced by reduction in skin-prick reactivity or a lower specific IgE value, but must be conducted in specialist clinics under strict protocols.
- Introduction of common allergenic foods to infants should not be delayed, and all infants should be given allergenic solid foods in the first year of life, including those at high risk of allergy. These foods include cow's milk products, peanut butter, cooked egg and wheat products.
- In particular, early introduction of peanut in the first year of life considerably reduces the risk of peanut allergy in many children.
- Immunotherapy (oral, sublingual and epicutaneous) for the treatment of food allergy is under clinical trial and remains experimental.

Urticaria and angioedema

Urticaria (Figure 16-4) refers to raised, erythematous, typically pruritic lesions that last for less than 24 hours. *Angioedema* (Figure 16-5) is non-pitting swelling that typically involves mucous membranes but can also affect the skin, with a predilection for face, hands and feet, and genitalia. Angioedema can affect the gut.

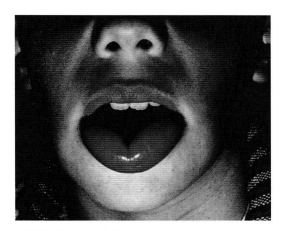

Figure 16-5 Patient with lip angioedema

From James WD, Berger T and Elston D. Andrew's Diseases of the skin: clinical dermatology, 11th ed. Elsevier, 2011.

- Acute urticaria or angioedema refers to short-lived and self-limited episodes of disease. Causes are listed in Box 16-8.
- Chronic urticaria or angioedema refers to episodes occurring daily, or almost daily, for a minimum period of 6 weeks.
- At times the definition of the condition as either acute or chronic can be problematic when frequent or recurrent acute episodes are occurring, but it is important to make this judgment, given the differing pathophysiology and management approaches of the two conditions.
- Around 50% of patients will have both urticaria and angioedema simultaneously or successively, whereas 40% will have urticaria alone, and 10% exclusively angioedema.

> **Box 16-8**
>
> **Causes of acute urticaria and angioedema**
>
> | **IgE-mediated** | **Non-IgE-mediated** |
> |---|---|
> | Food allergy | Adverse food reactions |
> | Insect sting allergy | Drug reactions, e.g. aspirin sensitivity |
> | Drug allergy | Radiocontrast media |
> | Aeroallergen allergy, e.g. horse hair | Physical factors—cold, heat, exercise, sun |
> | | Inherited angioedema |
> | | Idiopathic |
> | | Infection, especially in children |

CLINICAL PEARLS

- The patient who suffers episodes of angioedema without any history of urticaria should be assessed for hereditary or acquired angioedema due to complement component deficiency or dysfunction. It is inappropriate to do this if urticaria is present.
- Angioedema without urticaria can also be the result of treatment with angiotensin-converting enzyme inhibitors and gliptins (dipeptidyl peptidase-4 inhibitors).

Epidemiology

- It is estimated that approximately 20% of individuals will have an episode of acute urticaria during their life.
- Chronic urticaria is less common, with an estimated prevalence of 0.5–5%.

Pathophysiology

- Various environmental and food allergens can also cause *contact urticaria*. This usually remains confined to the area of skin or mucous membrane that the allergen directly contacts, but can occasionally generalize. An example might be a cutaneous reaction to a plant experienced by a gardener.
- Approximately 50% of cases of chronic urticaria and angioedema are autoimmune.
- Autoimmune cases of chronic urticaria and angioedema are characterized by IgG antibodies directed against autologous IgE, demonstrable by a positive wheal and flare to autologous serum on skin-prick testing.
- *Physical urticaria* refers to urticaria and angioedema provoked by physical factors (Table 16-7, overleaf).

Regardless of the cause, the manifestations of the disease are the result of the release of histamine and other vasoactive factors from mast cells, resulting in vasodilatation and increased vessel permeability.

Differential diagnosis

- Other pruritic skin conditions can occasionally urticate, especially after extensive scratching, e.g. atopic dermatitis.
- Cellulitis is sometimes mistaken for angioedema, but is generally painful and associated with systemic symptoms such as fever.
- Serum IgE is often moderately elevated in the setting of chronic urticaria. This should not be interpreted as indicating an 'allergic' cause.
- Approximately 10% of those with chronic urticaria will have demonstrable thyroid autoantibodies. Actual thyroid dysfunction is much less common, but these patients should remain under surveillance prospectively for the development of hypothyroidism.

CLINICAL PEARL

Urticarial lesions that are painful or burn, last longer than 24 hours, or leave a bruise or stain, could be due to urticarial vasculitis. A skin biopsy is indicated in this circumstance.

Hereditary angioedema (HAE)

Hereditary angioedema is a rare but important cause of recurrent bouts of angioedema occurring in approximately 1 in 50,000 individuals. Urticaria is absent in this condition.

- It is an autosomal dominant disorder that generally manifests in early childhood.
- Episodes frequently affect the airway, and can be life-threatening. Intestinal involvement is also frequent, causing severe abdominal pain and frequent misdiagnosis.
- Episodes are often precipitated by events such as minor trauma, surgery or dental work.
- It is due to a genetic defect in the complement system, specifically in the absolute quantity of C1-esterase inhibitor (type 1 HAE) or in its function (type II HAE).
- The primary mediator of swelling is bradykinin, which predominantly acts on the bradykinin B2 receptor to induce increased vascular permeability. Bradykinin is rapidly metabolised by endogenous metalloproteases including angiotensin converting enzyme
- Diagnosis is made by demonstrating low C4 levels, and low C1 inhibitor levels or function.
- On-demand treatment of all attacks as early as possible is recommended and all patients should carry on-demand medications at all times sufficient to treat two attacks.
- Attacks should be treated with C1 inhibitor concentrate, icatibant, which is a selective bradykinin B2 receptor antagonist or ecallantide, a kallikrein inhibitor.
- Pre-procedural or short-term prophylaxis should be administered prior to surgery, childbirth or dental surgery in the form of C1 inhibitor concentrate, as close as possible to the start of the procedure.
- All patients should be assessed for long-term prophylaxis with C1 inhibitor or androgens.

Table 16-7 Physical urticaria

PHYSICAL FACTOR	CLINICAL FEATURES
Dermographism	Common condition Wheals only appear after scratching Benign, usually self-limited condition
Heat = cholinergic urticaria	Small, transient hives directly after skin becomes hot, e.g. showering Not associated with angioedema
Cold = cold-induced urticaria	Generally affects exposed skin Can produce angioedema Anaphylaxis is a risk, e.g. with immersion in cold water
Exercise = exercise-induced urticaria	Often only occurs after moderate to strenuous exercising Anaphylaxis can result
Water = aquagenic urticaria	Occurs with any water contact on skin, regardless of temperature Generally does not affect mucous membranes, e.g. with drinking.
Sun exposure = solar urticaria	Presumed to be due to UV radiation
Vibration = vibratory urticaria	Occurs particularly with repetitive stimuli, e.g. using a jackhammer Angioedema is frequent
Delayed-pressure = delayed-pressure urticaria	Frequently produces angioedema Occurs on skin subject to prolonged pressure, e.g. under tight clothes Often antihistamine-resistant, and can be difficult to control
Food-dependent, exercise-induced	Occurs after exercise, but only if specific food is consumed immediately beforehand Especially occurs with wheat and seafood Can cause anaphylaxis

- C1-esterase inhibitor deficiency can be acquired, in about 15% of cases. This is generally in the setting of hematological malignancy and patients often have depressed C1q levels.

Treatment of urticaria and angioedema

Acute episodes of urticaria and angioedema with an identified cause should, as much as possible, be managed long-term with avoidance of identified culprits.

Antihistamine therapy

- Adequate doses of second-generation, non-sedating H_1 antihistamines are the mainstay of treatment for both acute and chronic urticaria, and angioedema.
- The superiority of newer, non-sedating agents such as fexofenadine, cetirizine, loratadine, and desloratadine over the older, sedating agents is well established. A standard dose of one of these second-generation H_1 antihistamines is the initial treatment. Patients who do not achieve adequate symptom control at 2–4 weeks should increase to up to 4 times the usual recommended dose of antihistamines.
- Patients with CSU who have not responded to a 2–4 week trial of 4 times the standard dose of a second-generation antihistamine should be considered for omalizumab, a monoclonal antibody against IgE, as add-on therapy.

- Cyclosporine may be used as fourth-line therapy if there has been no response to 6 months of treatment with omalizumab.
- Daily prophylactic antihistamine therapy should be used for extended periods in the setting of chronic urticaria and angioedema. Many patients make the mistake of relying upon p.r.n. (as required) treatment in this setting, with disappointing results.
- Prophylactic H_1 antihistamines may alleviate or reduce the severity of physical urticaria (e.g. taken prior to exercise or cold exposure).
- Addition of H_2 antihistamines such as ranitidine or famotidine may have a synergistic effect with H_1 antihistamines, but are ineffective by themselves.

Alternative treatments

- Acute severe urticaria or angioedema may occasionally require a dose of subcutaneous epinephrine.
- Leukotriene antagonists such as montelukast can be tried for cases unresponsive to antihistamine.
- Short courses of corticosteroids can alleviate acute severe episodes.
- Long-term corticosteroids should be avoided for chronic cases, unless all other pharmacotherapy has failed.

- Azathioprine, mycophenolate, cyclosporine and methotrexate should be used only under specialist supervision and monitoring.

Prognosis

Approximately 20% of chronic urticaria patients will have ongoing symptoms after 5 years.

Drug allergy

Adverse reactions to drugs are extremely common, and may be predictably dose-related or idiosyncratic. The term 'drug allergy' should be reserved for reactions that are likely to be immunologically mediated.

- IgE-mediated drug reactions can result in anaphylaxis, and can be fatal.
- Non-IgE-mediated reactions can also be extremely dangerous, and indeed fatal, e.g. Stevens–Johnson syndrome and toxic epidermal necrolysis.

Epidemiology

- Allergic drug reactions are clearly under-reported, making estimation of the incidence of drug allergy very difficult. Anaphylaxis is, however, rare.
- Patient self-reporting of drug allergy is unreliable. This is particularly the case for antibiotics. Many patients (and practitioners) mistake the viral exanthem that is exacerbated by the administration of antibiotics in childhood for a drug allergy.
- Antibiotics remain the most common cause of drug allergy, especially those of the beta-lactam class.

Pathophysiology

Drugs can cause hypersensitivity via type I, II, III and IV reactions, although there is likely to be overlap between mechanisms in some instances.

- Type I reactions are characterized by rapidity of onset, due to the presence of specific IgE to that drug on the surface of mast cells and basophils.
- Type III (serum-sickness) reactions will often occur 10–14 days after commencement of a drug. These reactions may last for up to 3 weeks, due to persistence of immune complexes.
- Most drug allergic reactions are likely to be T-cell mediated, and therefore fall within the type IV hypersensitivity category. This explains the likelihood of onset of symptoms after approximately 48 hours of drug use.
- Type II reactions are less common. An example is hemolysis resulting from treatment with penicillin. In this instance, penicillin binds to erythrocyte membrane proteins, resulting in antibody-directed attack against the cell and clearance by macrophages.

Clinical features

The clinical history, with very specific noting of all drugs taken and the timing of onset of symptoms and/or signs, is the key to making an accurate diagnosis of drug allergy. Supplementary testing is unavailable, or inadequate, for all but a few drugs.

- Type I reactions may result in urticaria, angioedema, upper airway obstruction, bronchoconstriction, vomiting and diarrhea, or circulatory collapse.
- Type III reactions often manifest with fever, malaise, arthritis, maculopapular or vasculitic rash. Urinalysis may be abnormal due to glomerulonephritis.
- Cutaneous abnormalities due to drug reactions are numerous, and include maculopapular rash, vasculitis, urticaria, photosensitivity, erythema, erythema multiforme, cutaneous lupus, and fixed eruptions. These may result from all types of hypersensitivity.

Table 16-8 outlines specific serious drug reaction syndromes.

Differential diagnosis

- Any new symptoms which occur after commencing a new drug should be considered as possibly drug-related.
- Given the array of different cutaneous manifestations that may represent drug allergy or adverse drug reactions, skin biopsy is of limited value. However, biopsy may be useful to confirm vasculitis or exclude other pathologies.
- Peripheral eosinophilia, eosinophiluria, and acutely abnormal liver function tests are suggestive of drug allergic reactions.
- Skin-prick and intradermal allergy testing is a validated tool for suspected allergy to penicillin and to local and general anesthetic agents. Cephalosporin testing is also increasingly being performed. Positive tests have a high positive predictive value for IgE-mediated drug allergy.
- Negative testing for penicillin should be followed up with a carefully supervised oral challenge with one of the penicillin drugs. It is very unusual in this instance for anaphylaxis to occur, although delayed-onset rash may occur, confirming a non-IgE-mediated immunological reaction.

CLINICAL PEARL

Cross-reactivity between IgE-mediated penicillin and cephalosporin allergy is relatively uncommon, with estimated rates <5%. If anaphylaxis has occurred to one of the agents, however, it is prudent to seek specialty consultation and allergy skin testing prior to prescription of the other class. Reactions less severe than anaphylaxis do not require testing, but observation of the patient upon administration of the first dose is advisable.

Treatment

- Suspected or proven drug allergy necessitates strict avoidance of the offending drug.
- Patients should be advised to wear emergency identification jewelry if anaphylaxis or other life-threatening drug reactions have occurred.
- Emergency rapid desensitization is possible to some antibiotics, e.g. penicillin, platinum and taxane chemotherapy agents, aspirin and some biologic agents, if there is no possible alternative for an inpatient with a life-threatening problem. This procedure is high risk, and should only

Table 16-8 Specific serious drug reaction syndromes

SYNDROME	CLINICAL FEATURES	COMMON CULPRIT DRUGS	TREATMENT
Stevens–Johnson syndrome	Maculopapular rash, which may blister, ulcerate and necrose Mucosal ulceration (Figure 16-6) Fever Usually a drug reaction, but may follow infection or malignancy, or be idiopathic	Allopurinol Carbamazepine Phenytoin Antibiotics, esp. sulfonamides	**Medical emergency** Cease suspected culprit medications Hemodynamic support Burns-style dressings and nursing care Corticosteroids unproven but generally used in moderate to high doses
Toxic epidermal necrolysis (TEN)	Fever Maculopapular rash Skin ulceration and necrosis affecting >30% of body surface area Mucosal ulceration Usually a drug reaction, but may follow infection or malignancy, or be idiopathic	Allopurinol Carbamazepine Phenytoin Antibiotics, esp. sulfonamides	**Medical emergency** Cease suspected culprit medications Hemodynamic support Burns-style dressings and nursing care Corticosteroids unproven but generally used in moderate to high doses, in conjunction with high-dose IV immunoglobulin
DRESS (drug reaction with eosinophilia and systemic symptoms)	Fever Onset >10 days after commencement of drug Maculopapular or vasculitic rash Eosinophilia Abnormal LFTs Interstitial nephritis Pericarditis	Anticonvulsants Allopurinol NSAIDs Sulfonamides Abacavir	Withdraw offending drug Oral corticosteroids
Erythema multiforme	Urticaria Target lesions Bullae Mucosal lesions may occur Usually associated with infection, esp. herpesviruses, but may be a drug reaction	Beta-lactam antibiotics Allopurinol Carbamazepine Phenytoin Sulfonamide antibiotics	Cease suspected offending drug Antihistamines if itch prominent

IV, intravenous; LFT, liver function test; NSAID, non-steroidal anti-inflammatory drug.

be performed by allergy specialists. It is also important to note that once the drug is discontinued or doses are missed, the patient's sensitivity to the medication returns over days to weeks.

Insect venom allergy

Anaphylaxis to stinging insects is a life-threatening and unpredictable form of allergic disease.

- Insects of the *Hymenoptera* order are the usual culprits. These are bees, yellowjackets/wasps, hornets and ants. Systemic allergic sting reactions have been reported in up to 7.5% of adults and 3.5% of children.
- Anaphylaxis also can result from bites from a number of species of fly.

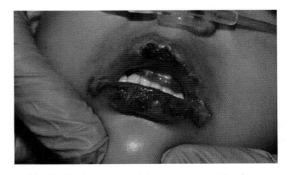

Figure 16-6 Oral mucosal involvement in Stevens–Johnson syndrome

From Eichenfield LF et al. (eds). Neonatal and infant dermatology. 3rd ed. Philadelphia: Elsevier, 2015.

- Neither atopy nor family history is a risk factor for *Hymenoptera* anaphylaxis, but repeated stings, e.g. in beekeepers, does confer increased risk.

Clinical features

Clinical reactions to *Hymenoptera* stings take three general forms:

1 Typical local reactions are localized pain, erythema, and edema. Pruritus may be prominent.
2 Large local reactions consist of extensive swelling and erythema, contiguous with the sting site. Even if an entire limb swells, it is classified as a local reaction if contiguous with the sting site.
3 Systemic reactions—can range from generalized urticaria through to full-blown anaphylaxis.

Differential diagnosis

- It is usual for a patient to clearly have experienced the sting, due to pain, and a stinger will often remain *in situ* following a bee or wasp sting.
- The patient may have trouble distinguishing the insect, and may not recognize the species of wasp particularly.
- Insect sting should be considered in any patient with 'idiopathic' anaphylaxis.
- Skin-prick and intradermal testing to different *Hymenoptera* species is very sensitive to diagnose sensitization.

Treatment

The clinical history determines the appropriate course of treatment.

- H_1 antihistamines, NSAIDs and oral corticosteroids can be used for large local reactions.
- All patients with systemic reactions should have an anaphylaxis action plan and carry an epinephrine self-injection device.

CLINICAL PEARL

Subcutaneous immunotherapy to the specific insect venom is essential for any adult or child patient following a systemic-allergic reaction exceeding generalized skin symptoms with documented sensitization to the culprit insect venom with either specific serum IgE tests and/or skin-prick tests. Immunotherapy reduces the risk of anaphylaxis with subsequent stings from >50% to <5%, so is highly effective. Immunotherapy is neither effective nor appropriate for local reactions, however large.

EOSINOPHILIA

Eosinophilia is classified according to the absolute level of eosinophils in the peripheral blood:

- mild eosinophilia: 0.5–1.5×10^9/L
- moderate eosinophilia: 1.5–5.0×10^9/L
- severe eosinophilia: $>5.0 \times 10^9$/L.

Hypereosinophilia is defined as a peripheral blood eosinophil count of $>1.5 \times 10^9$/L.

Eosinophils have multiple functions in innate immunity, and inflammation:

- their production is stimulated by interleukins 5 and 3, and GM-CSF (granulocyte–monocyte colony stimulating factor)
- they release a variety of cytotoxic, chemotactic and vasoactive molecules
- they are involved in tissue repair.

Causes of eosinophilia are listed in Box 16-9.

Box 16-9
Causes of eosinophilia

Common causes of eosinophilia
- Allergic disease
- Helminthic parasitic infection
- Drug reactions

Primary eosinophilic disorders
- Eosinophilic pneumonia
- Organ-specific eosinophilic syndromes, e.g. eosinophilic esophagitis
- Eosinophilic fasciitis

Disorders with secondary eosinophilia
- Allergic bronchopulmonary aspergillosis
- Eosinophilic granulomatosis with polyangiitis (Churg–Strauss vasculitis)
- Dermatitis herpetiformis
- Systemic mastocytosis
- Malignancy, e.g. lymphoma, adenocarcinoma
- Hyper-IgE syndrome
- Omenn syndrome

Eosinophilic clonal disorders
- Myeloproliferative hypereosinophilic syndrome (M-HES)
- Lymphoproliferative hypereosinophilic syndrome (L-HES)
- Eosinophilic leukemia (extremely rare)
- Otherwise unclassified HES

Hypereosinophilic syndrome (HES)

- HES is defined as hypereosinophilia ($>1.5 \times 10^9$/L eosinophils in peripheral blood) or excessive tissue eosinophilia in the setting of clinical manifestations attributable to the eosinophilia, in the absence of an identifiable secondary cause.
- Patients present with a range of clinical problems including thromboembolism, pulmonary infiltrates, endomyocardial fibrosis, lymphadenopathy, splenomegaly, and myelofibrosis.
- Specific cytogenetic abnormalities are detectable in bone marrow in some subsets, including myeloproliferative HES (M-HES) in which a tyrosine kinase mutation is present.

- Corticosteroids are the mainstay of treatment for most variants of HES.
- M-HES is responsive to tyrosine kinase inhibitors, e.g. imatinib.
- Anti-IL5 monoclonal antibody therapy is increasingly being used for all variants of HES and remains under active clinical investigation.

MAST CELL DISORDERS

Cutaneous and systemic mastocytosis represent a spectrum of malignant mast cell disorders. They are predominantly due to mutations in the *KIT*-oncogene, which results in abnormal activation of the gene with uncontrolled proliferation of mast cells.

Cutaneous mastocytosis (CM)

- Cutaneous mastocytosis is the most common presentation of mast cell disease, representing 90% of cases. Urticaria pigmentosa produces a raised red, brown or purple papular rash (Figure 16-7) which can occur anywhere other than the face. The rash urticates on scratching (Darier's sign).
- It is due to the accumulation of mast cells in the skin.
- Approximately 25% of those with CM will have systemic symptoms, but without demonstrable mast cell accumulation in tissues other than the skin, most notably the bone marrow.
- CM affects both children and adults. The childhood form may regress spontaneously.
- Diagnosis is made by skin biopsy.

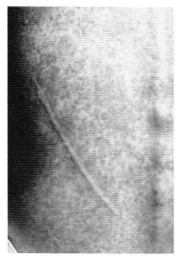

Figure 16-7 Typical appearance of pigmented rash in urticaria pigmentosa, and demonstrating Darier's sign

From Skarin AT (ed). Atlas of diagnostic oncology, 4th ed. Philadelphia: Elsevier, 2010.

Systemic mastocytosis (SM)

- Skin involvement is seen in >50% of cases of SM.
- Systemic features typically manifest with pruritus, urticaria, flushing, diarrhea, abdominal pain, bronchospasm, and recurrent anaphylaxis.
- Organ involvement can result in weight loss, lymphadenopathy, and hepatosplenomegaly. Bone marrow involvement is most common outside of skin involvement.
- Cardiac and neurological involvement is rare, but has been described.
- Bone involvement with either osteopenia or osteosclerosis is frequent.
- Serum tryptase is elevated.
- Cytopenias may result from bone marrow infiltration.
- Diagnosis is confirmed with excess mast cells seen on bone marrow biopsy. The majority of patients will have somatic mutations in the KIT gene (CD117 receptor) as well as CD25 expression on clonal mast cells.

Treatment

- High-dose H_1 and H_2 antihistamine therapy is the mainstay of treatment.
- UV therapy may offer some relief for urticaria pigmentosa.
- Oral sodium cromolyn should be used for gastrointestinal symptoms, and may relieve some systemic symptoms by preventing mast cell degranulation. Leukotriene antagonists may be useful as second line for pruritus.
- The oral multiple tyrosine kinase inhibitor midostaurin has been shown to be highly effective in patients with advanced SM. Other tyrosine kinase inhibitors such as imatinib are only effective in patients without a KIT mutation and thus are not appropriate for a majority of patients.
- Corticosteroids may relieve symptoms in some cases of SM.
- Aggressive cases of SM are usually treated with cytotoxic chemotherapy.
- Anaphylactic reactions are common, occurring in approximately half of all adult SM patients. Patients with SM should carry an epinephrine self-injecting device if there is a history of anaphylaxis.
- All patients should be aware of potential triggers of mast cell degranulation in particular *Hymenoptera* stings, infection, trauma, emotional stress and drugs such as alcohol, aspirin, NSAIDs, opioids and general anesthetic agents.
- SM patients can suffer severe anaphylaxis in response to insect stings. All patients with anaphylaxis to *Hymenoptera* sting should be offered venom immunotherapy if found to be sensitized.
- Pre-medication with antihistamines and corticosteroids is usually administered prior to surgical procedures.

- Omalizumab should be considered in patients with severe symptoms such as recurrent anaphylaxis unresponsive to the aforementioned treatment measures.
- Allogeneic hematopoeitic stem cell transplant is the only potential for cure in patients with advanced SM.
- SM patients should wear emergency identification jewelry.

SYSTEMIC AUTOIMMUNE DISEASE

- The diagnosis of one of the forms of systemic autoimmune disease is frequently devastating for a patient. This group of diseases is chronic and incurable. Treatment is often associated with significant short- and long-term morbidity.
- Diagnostic uncertainty is an issue in many cases, with patients potentially displaying clinical features which overlap between conditions, and laboratory investigations with imperfect sensitivity and specificity (see Table 16-9 later in the chapter).
- The relatively low prevalence of most systemic autoimmune diseases, combined with the heterogeneity of clinical patterns, makes development of precise treatment protocols difficult. Clinicians will need to individualize their approach in all cases.

The following systemic autoimmune conditions will be considered in this section:
- systemic lupus erythematosus
- Sjögren's syndrome
- polymyositis
- dermatomyositis
- scleroderma
- CREST syndrome
- mixed connective tissue disease
- primary antiphospholipid syndrome
- IgG4-related disease.

Rheumatoid arthritis is covered in Chapter 17.

Systemic lupus erythematosus (SLE)

Systemic lupus erythematosus is a multisystem disorder of unknown etiology, thought to affect approximately 1 in 1000 people. Females outnumber males in a ratio of 8–10:1. Rare in childhood but not unheard of, onset is frequently in the young adult years. Manifestations of the disease are protean, and can be mild through to lethal (Box 16-10).

Pathophysiology

Systemic lupus erythematosus results from the formation of pathogenic autoantibodies targeting nucleic acid-bound antigens. Much of the tissue damage is thought to result from:
- the formation of immune complexes, subsequent immune complex deposition, and initiation of inflammation via complement and Fc-receptor activation

- direct antibody-directed cellular cytotoxicity
- thrombus formation with resultant tissue ischemia.

Immunological abnormalities which have been demonstrated in SLE include:
- abnormalities in T cell number and function
- an excess of autoreactive B cells but with overall B cell lymphopenia, and hyperactivation of the BAFF pathway, a T cell independent B cell survival pathway
- reduced number and function of natural killer cells
- high levels of circulating immune complexes, and decreased clearance by the reticuloendothelial system
- abnormal cytokine profiles, including strong type 1 interferon signature
- excess and impaired degradation of neutrophil extracellular traps, resulting in increased nucleic acid antigen production

Known risk factors aside from gender include:
- Inherited complement component deficiencies (C1q, C2, C4). Complement deficiency results in reduced ability to clear apoptotic cells, with consequent increased exposure of cellular material on cell-surface blebs to immunologically active cells, and the formation of autoantibodies.
- Family history. Monozygotic twins have an approximate 1 in 4 chance of disease concordance, with only 3% of dizygotic twins affected.
- Certain HLA alleles. HLA subtypes A1, B8, DR2, and DR3 show an increased frequency in SLE patients.
- Certain drugs. Drug-induced lupus is associated with multiple medications, including procainamide, carbamazepine and isoniazid, and newer biological agents such as infliximab and etanercept.
- Race. SLE is more common in Southeast Asians and African-Americans.

Flares in disease may be associated with situations in which there is higher than normal cell damage or turnover, such as after exposure to UV radiation, or infection, or during pregnancy. The disease may manifest with exacerbations and remissions, or pursue a relentless course.

Diagnosis

Diagnosis is based on:
- the totality of clinical manifestations
- autoimmune serology
- tissue diagnosis where possible and appropriate; histopathology is particularly important in the setting of renal disease (see Chapter 9), and with skin disease where the diagnosis is not clear.

Criteria have been developed in an attempt to increase the precision of diagnosis, and are important when attempting to standardize patient populations for research and treatment protocols. Those given in Box 16-11 are from the Systemic Lupus International Collaborating Clinics (2012), which has high sensitivity (94.6%) and specificity (95.5%) for the diagnosis of adult SLE.

Box 16-10
Clinical features of systemic lupus erythematosus (SLE)

Incidence of clinical manifestations in SLE (in approximate descending order)

- Arthralgia (or arthritis)
- Fatigue
- Cutaneous—malar rash (Figure 16-8), photosensitivity, discoid lupus (Figure 16-9), alopecia, cutaneous vasculitis, subacute sclerosing lesions
- Myalgia (or uncommonly myositis)
- Renal—recurrent urinary tract infection, glomerulonephritis

- Hematological—normocytic anemia, hemolysis, lymphopenia, thrombocytopenia
- Serositis—pericarditis, pleuritis
- Raynaud's phenomenon
- Oral ulceration
- Neuropsychiatric—cerebritis, cerebral vasculitis, peripheral neuropathy, psychosis, seizures
- Gastrointestinal—hepatitis, intestinal vasculitis
- Anti-phospholipid-related—recurrent miscarriage, thrombosis
- Pulmonary—pneumonitis, pleuritis
- Cardiac—pericarditis, non-infective endocarditis
- Generalized lymphadenopathy

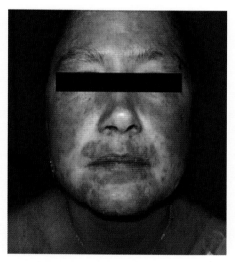

Figure 16-8 This picture displays the malar (or butterfly) rash typical of SLE. Note the sparing of the nasolabial folds, which distinguishes it from seborrheic dermatitis

From Wallace D and Hahn BH (eds). Dubois' Lupus erythematosus and related syndromes, 8th ed. Philadelphia: Elsevier, 2013.

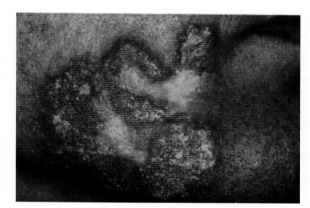

Figure 16-9 A discoid lupus lesion on the face. Note the predilection for the face, scaly appearance, and lighter color in the center of the lesion, as is typical in discoid lupus

From Tsokos C, Gordon C and Smolen JS (eds). Systemic lupus erythematosus. St Louis: Elsevier, 2007.

CLINICAL PEARL

Patients with nonspecific symptoms such as fatigue and arthralgia are often labeled as having 'a mild case of lupus'. They may be an adult female with a detectable low-titer antinuclear antibody in the absence of any objective clinical signs or specific laboratory abnormalities. Such spurious diagnostic labeling can have a profoundly negative long-term effect on an individual, with resultant unnecessary investigation and excessive specialist consultation. Potentially, iatrogenic harm will result from inappropriate use of toxic therapies. Always consider non-immunological physical or psychological causes when faced with this type of scenario.

Autoantibodies in SLE

Demonstration of the presence of autoantibodies helps significantly with diagnosis and classification of systemic autoimmune disease. However, clinical features remain the 'gold standard' for diagnosis, as:

- a significant minority of the population will have detectable autoantibodies in the absence of any autoimmune disease
- up to 20% of asymptomatic relatives of SLE patients will have detectable antinuclear antibodies (ANA)
- the presence of low-titer ANA increases with age, especially in women.

Conversely, SLE is very rare in the absence of ANA, so caution must be exercised when diagnosing 'ANA-negative lupus'.

Box 16-11

SLICC classification criteria for systemic lupus erythematosus (SLE)

Requirements: ≥4 criteria (at least 1 clinical and 1 laboratory criterion) *or* biopsy-proven lupus nephritis with positive ANA or anti-DNA. *See notes for criteria details.

Clinical criteria

1. Acute cutaneous lupus*
2. Chronic cutaneous lupus*
3. Oral or nasal ulcers*
4. Non-scarring alopecia
5. Arthritis*
6. Serositis*
7. Renal*
8. Neurological*
9. Hemolytic anemia
10. Leukopenia*
11. Thrombocytopenia (<100,000/mm^3)

Immunological criteria

1. ANA
2. Anti-DNA
3. Anti-Smith antibodies
4. Antiphospholid antibodies
5. Low complement (C3, C4, CH50)
6. Direct Coombs' test (do not count in the presence of hemolytic anemia)

Notes

CLINICAL CRITERIA

1. Acute cutaneous lupus OR subacute cutaneous lupus

- Acute cutaneous lupus: lupus malar rash (do not count if malar discoid), bullous lupus, toxic epidermal necrolysis variant of SLE, maculopapular lupus rash, photosensitive lupus rash (in the absence of dermatomyositis)
- Subacute cutaneous lupus: nonindurated psoriaform and/or annular polycyclic lesions that resolve without scarring, although occasionally with postinflammatory dyspigmentation or telangiectasias)

2. Chronic cutaneous lupus

- Classic discoid rash localized (above the neck) or generalized (above and below the neck), hypertrophic (verrucous) lupus, lupus panniculitis (profundus), mucosal lupus, lupus erythematosus tumidus, chillblains lupus, discoid lupus/lichen planus overlap

3. Oral ulcers OR nasal ulcers

- Oral: palate, buccal, tongue
- Nasal ulcers
- In the absence of other causes, such as vasculitis, Behçet's disease, infection (herpesvirus), inflammatory bowel disease, reactive arthritis, and acidic foods

4. Non-scarring alopecia

- Diffuse thinning or hair fragility with visible broken hairs, in the absence of other causes such as alopecia areata, drugs, iron deficiency, and androgenic alopecia

5. Synovitis involving 2 or more joints

- Characterized by swelling or effusion
- OR tenderness in 2 or more joints and at least 30 minutes of morning stiffness

6. Serositis

- Typical pleurisy for more than 1 day OR pleural effusions OR pleural rub
- Typical pericardial pain (pain with recumbency improved by sitting forward) for more than 1 day OR pericardial effusion OR pericardial rub OR pericarditis by electrocardiography
- In the absence of other causes, such as infection, uremia and Dressler's pericarditis

7. Renal

- Urine protein-to-creatinine ratio (or 24-hour urine protein) representing 500 mg protein/24 hours OR red blood cell casts

8. Neurological

- Seizures, psychosis, mononeuritis multiplex (in the absence of other known causes such as primary vasculitis), myelitis, peripheral or cranial neuropathy (in the absence of other known causes such as primary vasculitis, infection and diabetes mellitus), acute confusional state (in the absence of other causes, including toxic/metabolic, uremia, drugs)

9. Hemolytic anemia

10. Leukopenia (<4000/mm^3) OR lymphopenia (<1000/mm^3)

- Leukopenia at least once in the absence of other known causes such as Felty's syndrome, drugs, and portal hypertension
- Lymphopenia at least once in the absence of other known causes such as corticosteroids, drugs, and infection

11. Thrombocytopenia (<100,000/mm^3)

- At least once in the absence of other known causes such as drugs, portal hypertension, and thrombotic thrombocytopenic purpura

IMMUNOLOGICAL CRITERIA

1. ANA level above laboratory reference range

2. Anti-dsDNA antibody level above laboratory reference range (or 2-fold the reference range if tested by ELISA)

3. Anti-Sm: presence of antibody to Sm nuclear antigen

4. Antiphospholipid antibody positivity, as determined by
- Positive test for lupus anticoagulant

- False-positive test result for rapid plasma reagin
- Medium- or high-titer anti-cardiolipin antibody level (IgA, IgG or IgM)
- Positive test result for anti-beta-2 glycoprotein 1 (IgA, IgG or IgM)

5. Low complement (C3, C4 or CH50)

6. Direct Coombs' test (in the absence of hemolytic anemia)

ANA, antinuclear antibodies; anti-dsDNA, anti-double stranded DNA; anti-Sm, anti-Smith antibody; DNA, deoxyribonucleic acid; dsDNA, double-stranded DNA; Ig, immunoglobulin; SLICC, Systemic Lupus International Collaborating Clinics Collaboration.

From Petri M et al. Derivation and validation of Systemic Lupus International Collaborating Clinics classification criteria for systemic lupus erythematosus. Arthritis Rheum 2012;64(8):2677–86.

Table 16-9 Autoantibodies found in systemic lupus erythematosus (SLE)

AUTOANTIBODY	SENSITIVITY	COMMENT
Antinuclear antibodies (ANA)	>95%	More specific with increasing titer Titers <1:320 not considered significant in most laboratories Homogeneous pattern more specific for SLE No relationship with disease activity
Double-stranded DNA (dsDNA)	~50%	Good specificity for SLE, which increases with higher titer Titer may reflect disease activity Risk factor for renal disease
SS-A (Ro)	30–50%	Also found in Sjögren's syndrome Associated with subacute cutaneous disease 2% of babies born to SS-A-positive mothers develop congenital heart block
SS-B (La)	10%	More sensitive and specific for SS
Anti-Sm (Smith)	20–30%	Highly specific for SLE
Anti-histone	High for drug-induced lupus	Not found in association with anti-TNF-therapy-associated drug-induced lupus (infliximab, etanercept)
Anti-cardiolipin antibodies (including lupus inhibitor)	25%	May be associated with anti-phospholipid syndrome, or asymptomatic

TNF, tumor necrosis factor.

Table 16-9 describes autoantibodies found in SLE.

Neonatal lupus

- Neonatal lupus results from the passage of IgG anti-SSA (Ro) antibodies from mothers with SLE or Sjögren's syndrome to the fetus via the placenta.

- Clinical features in the newborn include complete heart block, which is frequently irreversible and may be associated with congestive heart failure if the heart block develops sufficiently early before delivery; skin rash; and hematological abnormalities including hemolytic anemia and thrombocytopenia.

- Severity of maternal illness does not correlate with the risk of development of neonatal lupus, but the risk is significant if previous pregnancies were affected.

- All but the cardiac lesions resolve by 3 months of age (commensurate with the half-life of maternal IgG).

Monitoring of disease activity

Clinical history and physical examination will provide the most accurate gauge of disease activity, but laboratory investigations are a useful supplement. A patient with active inflammatory disease will characteristically demonstrate evidence of an acute-phase response and active consumption of complement.

A disease flare may be accompanied by:
- a rising titer of anti-ds-DNA antibodies
- an elevated erythrocyte sedimentation rate (ESR)
- normochromic, normocytic anemia
- active urinary sediment

- reduced levels of complement components C3 and C4, and total hemolytic complement.

CLINICAL PEARL

C-reactive protein (CRP) is often not elevated in the setting of systemic lupus erythematosus. A rise in CRP in a lupus patient with a previously normal CRP should raise the prospect of concurrent infection.

Treatment and prognosis

In general terms, treatment for SLE is symptomatic for manifestations that are non-organ- or non-life-threatening, but immunosuppressive for the more serious complications.

- Non-steroidal anti-inflammatory drugs (NSAIDs) may be helpful for arthralgia and myalgia, and sometimes for pericarditis.
- Hydroxychloroquine has important immune modulation and disease-modifying actions and is the only drug shown to improve survival in SLE patients, as well as reduce lupus flares and prevent organ damage. It should be used for every SLE patient unless there is a clear contraindication, at a dose of 200–400 mg daily. Hydroxychloroquine also improves cutaneous manifestations and arthritis.
- Vitamin D should be supplemented in all patients with insufficiency, and has anti-fibrotic and immunomodulatory effects associated with improved global disease activity.
- Corticosteroids have been widely used for their anti-inflammatory and immunosuppressive actions, with higher doses used as initial, urgent therapy particularly for nephritis, neuropsychiatric disease or severe cytopenias. However, emerging studies suggest corticosteroids might not be necessary to control lupus manifestations and there is an increasing move to avoid oral corticosteroids as much as possible due to the significantly increased risk of cardiovascular events and later organ damage.
- Intravenous (IV) high-dose methylprednisolone is the most rapidly-acting immunosuppressive agent available, but does carry the risk of causing avascular osteonecrosis, particularly of the femoral head.
- Cyclophosphamide is a highly toxic alkylating agent that was widely used in the past for the induction and maintenance treatment of severe forms of lupus such as lupus nephritis and neuropsychiatric disease. It has, however, now been largely replaced by less toxic immunosuppressive medications.

There are now several less toxic, effective immunosuppressive agents, as well as biological agents.

- Mycophenolate is effective for the induction and maintenance of lupus nephritis, with similar efficacy compared to cyclophosphamide. It has also been shown to be superior to azathioprine for controlling disease activity and preventing both renal and non-renal flares.
- Azathioprine has been used for the treatment of renal and extra-renal SLE for many decades, and remains an excellent option to control disease activity in pregnancy.

- Calcineurin inhibitors including tacrolimus and cyclosporine have been shown to be effective for lupus nephritis.

Several biological agents show great promise in the treatment of lupus.

- Belimumab is a monoclonal antibody against BAFF (B cell activating factor of the TNF family), an important T cell independent B cell survival factor. It is effective in the treatment of non-renal lupus and also significantly reduces flares.
- Rituximab is an anti-CD20 monoclonal antibody that has shown clinical efficacy in lupus nephritis patients refractory to conventional therapy; however, data remains controversial.

All patients should be advised to avoid known disease triggers including UV, through adequate sun protection and use of at least SPF50 sunscreen. Infections are common and patients should receive influenza and pneumococcal vaccinations in addition to the local immunization schedule. Osteoporosis is more frequent in SLE patients, and bone health should be optimized in all patients. Table 16-10 summarizes the mechanism of action and major toxicities of drugs used to treat SLE. Given the chronic nature of SLE, much of the long-term morbidity is due to the effects of treatment, particularly corticosteroids. Table 16-11 provides a guide that may be useful in systematic monitoring of patients on long-term steroids and/or immunosuppressants.

Patients with SLE have a 5-year survival rate of >90%. Given the heterogeneity of the condition, prognostication is difficult, and clearly is worse in those with significant renal, neurological or pulmonary disease. The major long-term risk to health is likely to be due to medication toxicity, through increased risk of:

- malignancy
- infection
- metabolic disease.

There is some evidence that SLE is an independent risk factor for atherosclerotic vascular disease, presumably due to the atherogenic consequences of chronic inflammation. The risk of cardiovascular events is increased by 2.66-fold and aggressive management of modifiable cardiovascular risk factors is essential.

Sjögren's syndrome (SS)

Primary Sjögren's syndrome is a chronic, relentless, systemic autoimmune disease characterized by autoimmune destruction of exocrine glands, and sometimes accompanied by vasculitis. The classic clinical features of SS are:

- dry eyes due to keratoconjunctivitis sicca, secondary to destruction of the lacrimal glands
- dry mouth (xerostomia), due to destruction of the salivary glands.

The disease is generally not life-threatening, but serious complications such as nephritis and pneumonitis can occur (Table 16-12).

- It should be kept in mind that patients have a significantly increased risk of lymphoma.

Table 16-10 Mechanism of action and major toxicities of drugs commonly used to treat SLE

DRUG	MECHANISM OF ACTION	MAJOR TOXICITIES
Hydroxychloroquine	Inhibits B cell receptor and toll-like receptor signaling, interferes with MHC-antigen binding by increasing lysosomal pH, which affects autoantigen processing and cytokine secretion Has anti-type 1 interferon activity	Retinal toxicity
Prednisolone	Inhibits leukocyte migration Reduces cytokine production Suppresses antibody production	Weight gain, osteoporosis, glucose intolerance/diabetes mellitus, hypertension, Cushing's syndrome, poor wound healing, avascular osteonecrosis, immunosuppression
Azathioprine	Inhibits DNA synthesis in dividing cells, therefore is cytotoxic to lymphocytes Blocks CD28 co-stimulation, so prevents activation of naïve lymphocytes	Hepatitis, GI intolerance, myelosuppression, skin malignancy, immunosuppression
Methotrexate	Inhibits enzyme dihydrofolate reductase, which leads to impairment of thymidylate synthesis, and impairment of DNA synthesis The anti-inflammatory effect results from the impairment of leukocyte function	GI tract disturbance, mucositis, myelosuppression, hepatic fibrosis, pulmonary fibrosis, immunosuppression
Cyclosporine (ciclosporin)	Inhibits production of IL-2 by T lymphocytes, thus reducing induction of cytotoxic T cells and T-cell-dependent B cell responses	Renal impairment, hypertension, glucose intolerance, gum hypertrophy, hirsutism, immunosuppression, skin malignancy
Cyclophosphamide	Alkylating agent which cross-links DNA Has a pronounced effect on reducing the function of lymphocytes	Myelosuppression, especially neutropenia, hemorrhagic cystitis, nausea and vomiting, bladder cancer, skin malignancy, immunosuppression, pulmonary fibrosis
Mycophenolate	Inhibits purine synthesis, resulting in reduced guanine nucleotides especially in lymphocytes, resulting in reduced function	GI tract disturbance, anemia, immunosuppression

GI, gastrointestinal; IL, interleukin; SLE, systemic lupus erythematosus.

- When xerophthalmia or xerostomia occurs in association with other systemic autoimmune disease, such as rheumatoid arthritis or SLE, this is known as *secondary Sjögren's syndrome*, which is generally less severe than primary Sjogren's syndrome.

Pathophysiology

- The etiology of SS is unknown.
- It is predominantly a disease of middle-aged women.
- It is likely that by the time of diagnosis, most of the damage to the exocrine glands has been done. This explains the lack of efficacy of immunosuppressive medication in this condition, which is generally contraindicated except when vasculitis occurs.
- Histopathology reveals intense lymphocytic infiltration of involved structures in SS.
- The tissue damage is likely a result of type IV (cell-mediated) immune hypersensitivity.
- The autoantigen is unknown.

Diagnosis

Diagnosis is generally based on the American-European consensus group (AECG) classification, with SS diagnosed when 4 of the following 6 items are present:

1. Subjective presence of ocular dryness
2. Subjective presence of oral dryness
3. Objective measures of ocular dryness by Schirmer's test or corneal staining
4. Focus score >2 in salivary gland biopsy
5. Salivary scintigraphy showing reduced salivary flow and/or diffuse sialectasis
6. Positive autoantibodies against SS-A and/or SS-B.

Either salivary gland biopsy or presence of autoantibodies is mandatory.

The classic autoimmune serology found in SS consists of:

- high-titer antinuclear antibody (ANA) in speckled pattern.
- positive SS-A and SS-B (Ro and La) antibodies
- positive rheumatoid factor.

Table 16-11 Monitoring of patients on long-term immunosuppressants

DRUG	EVERY 3 MONTHS	EVERY 6 MONTHS	ANNUALLY
Corticosteroids	Blood sugar levels Blood pressure monitoring	Lipid monitoring	Bone densitometry
Cyclophosphamide	Full blood count (more frequently depending on protocol being used)	Urinalysis, for hematuria; cystoscopy if positive	Skin examination (for pre-malignant and malignant change) Papanicolaou (Pap) tests (females)
Azathioprine	Liver function tests Full blood count		Skin examination (for pre-malignant and malignant change) Pap tests (females)
Methotrexate	Liver function tests Full blood count (more frequently in initiation of treatment phase) Clinical screening for cough or dyspnea (risk of pulmonary fibrosis)		Skin examination (for pre-malignant and malignant change) Pap tests (females)
Cyclosporine (ciclosporin)	Blood sugar levels Blood pressure monitoring Renal function and electrolytes Oral examination (for gum hypertrophy)	Lipid monitoring	Skin examination (for pre-malignant and malignant change) Pap tests (females) Biannual renal DTPA scans
Mycophenolate	Full blood count		Skin examination (for pre-malignant and malignant change) Pap tests (females)

DTPA, diethylene triamine pentaacetic acid.

Table 16-12 Major clinical manifestations of Sjögren's syndrome

MANIFESTATION	CAUSE
Keratoconjunctivitis sicca	Destruction of lacrimal glands
Xerostomia	Destruction of salivary glands
Dry skin	Destruction of sebaceous glands
Dry cough	Due to lack of respiratory tract mucus
Dental caries/gingivitis/periodontitis	Due to lack of saliva
Parotitis	May have recurrent painful episodes, or chronic inflammation with gradual parotidomegaly Be aware of possibility of malignant transformation
Pancreatitis	Rare
Pneumonitis	May lead to 'shrinking lung syndrome'
Cerebral vasculitis	Likely to result in focal neurological signs, or organic brain syndrome
Interstitial nephritis	Renal tubular acidosis a likely outcome. Can progress to renal failure
Glomerulonephritis	May progress to end-stage renal disease
Cutaneous vasculitis	Often affects lower limbs, and tends to be recurrent
Fatigue	
Lymphoma	Most often in parotid glands

It is typical to find:

- significant polyclonal hypergammaglobulinemia
- markedly elevated erythrocyte sedimentation rate (ESR).

It is advisable for the physician to involve an ophthalmologist in the long-term care of the SS patient.

Treatment

Treatment is largely symptomatic.

- Preservative-free lubricant eyedrops such as methylcellulose are important both for comfort and to prevent scarring of the eye surface. They should be applied every couple of hours during the day.
- Lubricant ocular gel can be applied prior to bed.

CLINICAL PEARL

Cyclosporine (ciclosporin) eyedrops can be quite successful at restoring some tear production and reducing the severity of keratoconjunctivitis sicca, which is interesting given the lack of efficacy of systemic immunosuppression in SS.

- Dry mouth is difficult to treat.
  - » Patients may benefit from using an atomizer to spray water into the mouth if frequent water-sipping causes polyuria.
  - » Pilocarpine mouth washes may help stimulate residual salivary gland function.
  - » Regular dental care is essential to attempt to avoid progressive tooth damage.
- Methotrexate and hydroxychloroquine are used for the treatment of arthritis in pSS patients.
- There is some evidence that rituximab shows beneficial effects on B cell activity, glandular morphology, fatigue, dryness and several extraglandular manifestations, and may be considered for systemic disease manifestations.

Patients should be regularly monitored for development of complications such as interstitial nephritis or glomerulonephritis, although unfortunately immunosuppression is frequently ineffective at altering disease course. Lymphoma needs to be kept in mind as a long-term risk.

Inflammatory myopathies

The classification of idiopathic inflammatory myopathies (IIM) is evolving and now includes the following subgroups: sporadic inclusion-body myositis; polymyositis; dermatomyositis; non-specific (or overlap) myositis, and immune-mediated necrotizing myopathy. A comparison of the different subgroups is summarized in Table 16-13.

Patients typically present with:

- progressive symmetrical, usually proximal, weakness of skeletal muscle
- muscle aching or pain, although this is variable
- cutaneous changes in the case of dermatomyositis
- clinical features and autoantibodies that overlap with other connective tissue disorders in overlap myositis

- elevated creatine kinase in the vast majority of cases
- characteristic electromyographic changes of fibrillations and positive sharp waves.

These diseases are rare and approximately twice as common in women as men. The etiology is unknown, although there are associations with certain HLA alleles. Onset is more common in middle age, but can occur in childhood.

Anti-synthetase syndrome

- This is a separate subgroup of IIM that is associated with the presence of anti-synthetase antibodies.
- 75% of patients will have Jo-1 antibodies.
- Other antibodies include PL-7; PL-12; EJ; OJ; KS; Zo.
- The syndrome includes interstitial lung disease, non-erosive arthritis, and a characteristic hyperkeratotic dermatosis known as mechanic's hands (Figure 16-10).
- Raynaud's phenomenon may be prominent, and fever may occur.

Diagnosis

The diagnosis can be established to a satisfactory degree of certainty with the combination of:

- clinical features
- elevated creatine kinase levels
- characteristic electromyographic features
- positive autoimmune serology is helpful in defining the clinical phenotype
- rheumatoid factor positivity in approximately 50% of patients
- muscle biopsy remains the gold standard for diagnosis and differentiation of the subgroups of IIM
- MRI has become increasing useful for diagnosis, guiding muscle biopsies and monitoring response to treatment.

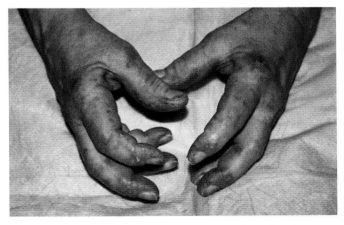

Figure 16-10 The hyperkeratosis and fissuring known as mechanic's hands

From James WD, Berger T and Elston D. Andrews' Diseases of the skin: clinical dermatology, 11th ed. Elsevier, 2011.

Table 16-13 Inflammatory myopathies

INCLUSION BODY MYOSITIS (IBM)	POLYMYOSITIS (PM)	DERMATOMYOSITIS (DM)	IMMUNE-MEDIATED NECROTIZING MYOPATHY (IMNM)
No skin involvement	No skin involvement	Pathognomonic cutaneous signs: — Violaceous (heliotrope) rash on and around top eyelids (Figure 16-11) — Gottron's nodules/papules over extensor surfaces of hands (Figure 16-12) Non-pathognomonic cutaneous signs: — Facial erythema — Poikiloderma (Figure 16-13)	No skin involvement
May start asymmetrically. Hip flexors, quadriceps and finger flexors preferentially affected. More common in men	Progressive symmetrical muscle pain and weakness	Progressive symmetrical muscle pain and weakness	Significant proximal symmetric weakness
Muscle biopsy shows internalization of nuclei in muscle fibers, CD8+ T cells; congophilic amyloid deposits; scant inflammation	Muscle biopsy shows perifascicular muscle atrophy and regeneration; infiltration with CD4+ T cells	Muscle biopsy shows muscle fiber infiltration by cytotoxic (CD8+) T cells, and macrophages	Muscle biopsy shows necrotic fibers with macrophages. Absence of CD8+ T cells.
Antibodies against Mup44; Anti-cytosolic 5'-Nucleotidase 1A (cN1A) (not routinely assessed)	Not currently associated with any myositis-specific antibodies	Antibodies against Mi-2; SAE; MDA5; TIF1-gamma; TIF1-beta; NXP2	Antibodies against SRP; HMG-Co A reductase
Malignancy is rarely associated	Increased risk of malignancy, but less so than in DM	Significantly increased risk of malignancy compared with general population	Increased risk of malignancy, but less so than in DM

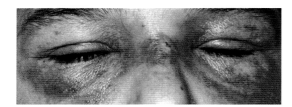

Figure 16-11 Heliotrope rash around the eyes in a patient with dermatomyositis

From Paller AS and Mancini AJ. Hurwitz Clinical paediatric dermatology, 4th ed. Philadelphia: Elsevier, 2011.

Treatment

- Corticosteroids are the mainstay of treatment and are generally effective, but often at unacceptably high doses with excessive toxicity.
- A steroid-sparing agent such as methotrexate, azathioprine, mycophenolate or rituximab is frequently required.
- High-dose IV immunoglobulin is a treatment for which there is an evidence base. It does not result in immunosuppression, so is useful if effective.
- IBM is typically resistant to immunosuppression.

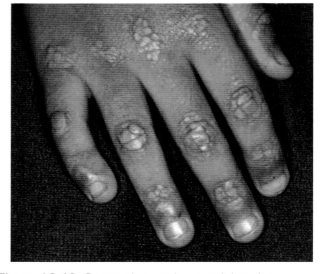

Figure 16-12 Gottron's papules overlying the metacarpophalangeal, proximal interphalangeal, and distal interphalangeal joints

From Paller AS and Mancini AJ. Hurwitz Clinical paediatric dermatology, 4th ed. Philadelphia: Elsevier, 2011.

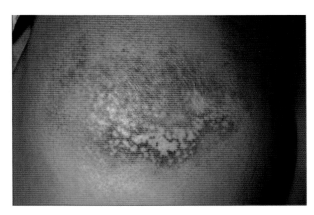

Figure 16-13 Poikiloderma, as may be found in dermatomyositis. Note the combination of hyper- and hypo-pigmentation, and erythema

From Bolognia JL et al. Dermatology, 2nd ed. St Louis: Elsevier, 2008.

CLINICAL PEARL

Steroid-sparing immunosuppressive agents will frequently be required in the setting of systemic autoimmune disease, given that these diseases are chronic and often life-threatening. The rarity, and heterogeneity, of systemic autoimmune disease limits the availability of evidence-based treatment guidelines for many clinical scenarios, unlike in common diseases such as hypertension or ischemic heart disease. The skill in managing systemic autoimmune disease lies therefore in striking a balance between efficacy, short- and long-term toxicity, patient adherence to treatment, drug cost and availability, and individual patient factors. For example, a young female with dermatomyositis who has become Cushingoid with high doses of prednisolone may be best started on azathioprine rather than cyclosporine (ciclosporin) or mycophenolate, because:

- there is concern that she may not be fully adherent with contraception (mycophenolate is highly teratogenic, azathioprine is better established as safer in pregnancy than cyclosporine)
- her blood pressure is 125/85 mmHg (cyclosporine is likely to make this worse)
- there is a strong family history of type 2 diabetes mellitus (cyclosporine predisposes to glucose intolerance).

Scleroderma and CREST syndrome

Also known as diffuse and limited systemic sclerosis, this is a disease spectrum involving autoimmune inflammation with vascular involvement and connective tissue scarring in the skin and multiple other organs. It is thought to have an incidence of around 1 in 10,000.

Clinical manifestations

- Diffuse scleroderma nearly always involves the skin both below and above the elbows and knees, including the face and trunk (Box 16-12). Patients are at increased risk of pulmonary, gastrointestinal, renal and cardiac involvement (Box 16-13).

Box 16-12

Skin changes in scleroderma

- Thickening and edema of digits (sclerodactyly) (Figure 16-14)
- Prominent telangiectasiae, especially on digits and face
- Skin tightening on face, resulting in reduction in oral aperture, and 'beaking' of nose
- Calcinotic nodules and/or ulcers, especially on digits
- Pulp atrophy of digits
- Thickening and edema of skin on trunk

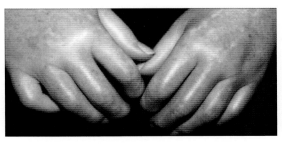

Figure 16-14 The typical swollen and shiny appearance of hands due to sclerodactyly. Note also the fixed flexion position of the fingers

From Marks JG and Miller JJ. Lookingbill & Marks' Principles of dermatology, 4th ed. Philadelphia: Elsevier, 2006.

Box 16-13

Organ involvement in scleroderma

Pulmonary
- Interstitial fibrosis
- Pulmonary arterial hypertension
- Pleural effusion

Gastrointestinal
- Reflux esophagitis
- Dysphagia due to strictures
- Intestinal fibrosis leading to dysmotility and absorptive abnormalities
- Vascular ectasia in the stomach (watermelon stomach)

Renal
- Accelerated hypertension
- Rapidly progressive renal failure due to renal vasculopathy

Cardiac
- Pericarditis
- Myocarditis
- Cardiac failure

- In limited scleroderma, skin involvement is usually confined to the distal limbs, although facial changes can occur. The label CREST syndrome is often given, due to the prominence of **C**alcinosis, **R**aynaud's phenomenon, **E**sophageal dysfunction, **S**clerodactyly and **T**elangiectases.

- CREST patients will often have digital ulcers, and are at risk of pulmonary arterial hypertension.
- Nail-fold capillaroscopy will reveal abnormalities in most patients with both limited and diffuse disease. Changes include reduction in numbers of capillaries, with those remaining forming giant loops.
- Raynaud's phenomenon is often an early manifestation, occurs almost invariably, and reflects the vascular abnormality with propensity to vasospasm. This contributes to digital ulceration in around half of cases, and can be further complicated by digital gangrene, infection with osteomyelitis, and autoamputation.
- Digital ulceration is extremely painful, and disabling.

The etiology of scleroderma is not known and the pathogenesis is complex, with abnormalities demonstrable in the function of endothelium, epithelium, fibroblasts and lymphocytes. The end result is accumulation of abnormal and excessive extracellular matrix, which gradually fibroses and causes tissue dysfunction. A variety of autoantibodies are detectable in this condition, the pattern of which can be helpful in distinguishing subtypes.

Diagnosis

- The diagnosis of scleroderma is made on clinical grounds, with the appearance of the hands being of greatest utility.
- Tissue biopsy is rarely indicated.
- Autoantibodies are detectable in the majority of cases, with a nucleolar-pattern ANA present in 70–90%.
- Anti-centromere antibodies have sensitivity of >50% for limited scleroderma, with a small percentage of patients with diffuse disease also positive. Anti-centromere is highly specific for scleroderma.
- Anti-Scl-70 antibody, whose target is DNA topoisomerase 1, is more common in patients with diffuse disease.
- Pulmonary fibrosis can be detected on high-resolution CT scanning and with pulmonary function tests (PFTs).
  » PFTs are the most useful tool for monitoring the progression of lung disease, along with the 6-minute walk test.
- Echocardiography is generally used for screening for pulmonary arterial hypertension.
- Endoscopy will detect the presence of esophagitis.

Differential diagnosis of skin findings is outlined in Box 16-14.

Treatment

- Lung disease, and particularly pulmonary fibrosis, is the major cause of mortality in scleroderma.
  » Interstitial lung disease is the only indication for immunosuppression in the form of high-dose corticosteroids and other agents such as cyclophosphamide, but results are disappointing.
- Early detection of pulmonary arterial hypertension in scleroderma patients is critical, with evidence that commencement of endothelin-receptor antagonists such as bosentan, and possibly phosphodiesterase-5 inhibitors such as sildenafil, can delay progression and improve prognosis.

> ### Box 16-14
> ### Differential diagnosis of thickened and tethered skin
>
> - CREST syndrome, scleroderma, or mixed connective tissue disease
> - Eosinophilic fasciitis
> - Localized morphea—small areas of sclerosis
> - Chemicals—vinyl chloride, pentazocine, bleomycin, toxic oil syndrome
> - Pseudoscleroderma—secondary to porphyria cutanea tarda, acromegaly, carcinoid syndrome
> - Scleredema—diabetics develop thick skin over the shoulders and upper back
> - Graft-versus-host disease
> - Silicosis

- Autologous human stem-cell transplantation should be considered in a patient with progressive skin and/or lung disease in the presence of normal cardiac function.
- Scleroderma renal crisis is uncommon, at around 5% of cases. It is characterized by marked hyper-reninemia, so early detection of hypertension and institution of angiotensin-converting enzyme inhibitor (ACEI) therapy is vital.
- Raynaud's phenomenon and digital ulceration may be improved with the use of calcium-channel antagonists such as felodipine or nifedipine, via vasodilatation.
- Acute digit- or limb-threatening ischemia can be treated with IV prostacyclin.

Patients with scleroderma frequently face great challenges with activities of daily living, chronic pain, and depression. Treatment aimed at providing physical and psychological support, and palliative care when appropriate, needs to be part of the overall approach to management.

Mixed connective tissue disease (MCTD)

This rare condition is characterized by features of SLE, polymyositis, scleroderma and rheumatoid arthritis, in the presence of autoantibodies against U1 ribonucleoprotein (RNP). The U1 RNP antigen is actually a complex of polypeptides, a number of which can act as the epitope. The ANA is usually markedly elevated in a speckled pattern.

Patients present with a variety of symptoms that can develop and occur sequentially over time. Common symptoms are:

- Raynaud's phenomenon
- sclerodactyly
- hand swelling
- esophageal reflux
- myositis.

Less common symptoms are:

- pulmonary arterial hypertension
- glomerulonephritis
- Sjögren's syndrome
- skin changes
- hematological abnormalities.

MCTD is more common in women. It can occur, rarely, in childhood.

Treatment is dictated by the nature of the organ involvement in the individual patient, along the lines that would be used for the separate disease entities.

Antiphospholipid syndrome (APS)

- Antiphospholipid syndrome is characterized by:
  - » recurrent fetal loss, and/or
  - » recurrent venous or arterial thrombosis (Box 16-15).
- Diagnosis is based on the presence of clinical features and, for diagnosis, persistent antibodies (>12 weeks) against phospholipid in the form of:
  - » anti-cardiolipin antibodies
  - » anti β_2 Glycoprotein1 antibodies, or
  - » lupus inhibitor.
- APS occurs frequently in patients with SLE, with 25–50% demonstrating autoantibodies, but an estimated 10–15% developing the clinical syndrome. Conversely, only 5–10% of individuals with APS also have lupus.
- The etiology of the condition is unknown, but APS is more common in females.
- A rapidly progressive form of the disease in which multiple organs can be affected by infarction, including the liver and kidneys, resulting in multi-organ failure, is known as catastrophic APS.
- Antiphospholipid antibodies bind to phospholipids or phospholipid-binding proteins on cell surfaces. This triggers thrombus formation within vessels, via a number of mechanisms, including:
  - » Binding of phospholipid on platelet surfaces leads to expresssion of thrombogenic glycoprotein 2b-3a and increased production of thromboxane A2.
  - » Binding on endothelial cell and monocyte surfaces stimulates expression of adhesion molecules as well as inflammatory and prothrombotic cytokines.
  - » Phospholipid-binding proteins are anticoagulants, so binding of these by antibody results in inhibition of their function, and favors thrombosis.

Box 16-15

Clinical manifestations of APS

- Venous thrombosis
- Arterial thrombosis
  - » Pre-term birth due to eclampsia or preeclampsia (prior to 34 weeks of gestation, fetus normal); or
  - » Fetal death beyond 10 weeks of gestation; or
  - » 3 or more consecutive spontaneous abortions at <10 weeks of gestation
- Thrombocytopenia
- Livedo reticularis
- Hemolysis
- Stroke
- Neurological disease—chorea; migraine
- Cardiac valvular disease
- Renal thrombotic microangiopathy

Laboratory considerations

- The presence of antiphospholipid antibodies in a serum sample interferes with the activated partial thromboplastin time (APTT) in the laboratory, leading to prolongation. This, paradoxically, gives an *in vitro* elevated APTT in the setting of an *in vivo* propensity to thrombosis. It also renders the APTT essentially invalid for use to monitor therapy with unfractionated heparin. The prolonged APTT is only partially correctable with mixing with normal serum in the laboratory, demonstrating the presence of an inhibitor.
- Demonstration of lupus inhibitor confers an adverse prognosis to the patient, with increased likelihood of both fetal loss and thrombosis.
- Most laboratories measure both IgG and IgM anti-cardiolipin antibodies, but the IgG form is more predictive of development of the clinical syndrome.
- Thrombocytopenia is found in up to 25% of cases.

Treatment

- Lifelong anticoagulation is usually required for patients with thrombotic complications of APS, with warfarin the first choice of drug.
- Direct oral anticoagulants are less effective than warfarin in preventing thrombosis, particularly in high-risk patients.
- There are no clear evidence-based guidelines for the patient who has antiphospholipid antibodies but is asymptomatic. Use of long-term anti-platelet therapy needs to be balanced against the increased risk of intracerebral hemorrhage in this situation.
- Treatment of pregnant patients with APS is dealt with in Chapter 25.

IgG4-related disease

This is an increasingly recognized cluster of rare conditions, characterized pathologically by swelling, fibroinflammatory changes, and IgG4 plasma cell infiltration of the affected organs, and elevated serum IgG4 in most cases.

- Conditions now recognized to form part of this spectrum include:
  - » autoimmune pancreatitis
  - » Mikulicz's syndrome
  - » retroperitoneal fibrosis
  - » Riedel's thyroiditis
  - » Kuttner's tumor
  - » periaortitis and periarteritis
  - » mediastinal fibrosis
  - » inflammatory pseudotumor
  - » eosinophilic angiocentric fibrosis
  - » multifocal fibrosclerosis
  - » inflammatory aortic aneurysm
  - » idiopathic hypocomplementemic tubulointerstitial nephritis with extensive tubulointerstitial deposits.
- Organs known to be potentially involved in this process include the pancreas, periorbits, biliary tract, thyroid, salivary glands, retroperitoneum, lung, breast, skin, meninges, pericardium, prostate, aorta, lymph nodes, kidneys, and mediastinum.

- The pathogenesis of this condition is unknown, but there is evidence of autoimmune and allergic dysregulation. The IgG4 antibodies are not thought to be pathogenic. It is more common in elderly males.
- Tissue biopsy is required to make the diagnosis. At times, tissue can be replaced by tumefactive masses, making IgG4-related disease a differential diagnosis for malignancy.
- When recognized, the patient should be screened for potential disease in other target organs.
- Treatment requires immunosuppression.
  - » Corticosteroids are the mainstay of initial treatment.
  - » Second-line agents such as azathioprine, mycophenolate or rituximab, are often required for steroid-sparing effect.

PRIMARY VASCULITIS

- Vasculitis can be a localized problem, or part of a systemic process.
- Vasculitic disease may be primary, or occur as part of a systemic disorder such as SLE or rheumatoid arthritis.
- Systemic vasculitic illnesses are generally autoimmune in basis and life-threatening, requiring aggressive immunosuppressive therapy.

The following section will focus on the primary systemic vasculitides.

Classification of the vasculitides is confusing. Some authors classify according to the size of the vessels involved, while others recommend groupings based on association with anti-neutrophil cytoplasmic antibodies (ANCAs). Box 16-16 groups the illnesses taking both features into account.

More recently, a revised, more comprehensive classification system has been recommended (Box 16-17). This system will be used to discuss the diseases addressed below.

Box 16-16

Classification of vasculitides

Large-vessel, non-ANCA-associated
- Giant-cell arteritis/Polymyalgia rheumatica
- Takayasu arteritis

Medium-vessel, non-ANCA-associated
- Polyarteritis nodosa
- Kawasaki disease

Small-vessel, ANCA-associated
- Granulomatosis with polyangiitis (GPA, previously Wegener's granulomatosis)
- Eosinophilic granulomatosis with polyangiitis (EGPA, previously Churg-Strauss vasculitis)
- Microscopic polyarteritis

Small-vessel, non-ANCA-associated
- Leukocytoclastic vasculitis
- Essential cryoglobulinemia (see Chapter 9)
- Henoch–Schönlein purpura

Large-vessel vasculitis

Polymyalgia rheumatica (PMR)

Clinical characteristics
- Polymyalgia rheumatica is a disease of unknown etiology, characterized by stiffness and aching in the limb girdle, particularly in the mornings.
- Incidence increases progressively in people over the age of 50 years, and is more than twice as common in females as males.
- The pain centers around the shoulders in up to 95% of patients, the neck and hips in the majority, and the lower back in some.
- PMR causes systemic symptoms in approximately half of those affected, in the form of malaise and fatigue, and can cause fevers and night sweats.
- Peripheral arthritis can occur.

Pathophysiology
- There is some evidence that the pathological lesion is a low-grade synovitis, rich in CD4-positive T lymphocytes, and macrophages.
- Vasculitis is not a feature, but PMR forms part of a disease spectrum with giant-cell arteritis (GCA), with approximately 20% of PMR patients developing GCA and around 50% of GCA patients also suffering PMR.

Diagnosis
- PMR is invariably accompanied by an acute phase response, resulting in elevated ESR, CRP, and at times abnormal liver function tests and a normocytic anemia, although there are cases described with a normal ESR.
- MRI or bone scanning may demonstrate synovitis in proximal joints.
- The diagnosis is clinical.

Treatment
- Failure of symptoms to resolve with low-dose corticosteroids, usually with a starting dose of 15 mg/day, should prompt reconsideration of the diagnosis.
- Patients may need long-term treatment, or the disease may eventually spontaneously remit.
- Patients should be counseled to seek urgent review if they develop symptoms suggestive of GCA, such as headache or visual disturbance.

Giant-cell arteritis (GCA)

- GCA is a life-threatening vasculitis involving large and medium-sized muscular arteries, especially those of the external carotid system. GCA typically involves the temporal arteries—hence its alternative, but less accurate, name 'temporal arteritis'.

Clinical characteristics
- Patients are usually elderly.
- Atherosclerosis, heavy smoking, and the HLA-DRB1 haplotype are risk factors.

Box 16-17

Names for vasculitides adopted by the 2012 International Chapel Hill Consensus Conference on the Nomenclature of Vasculitides

Large-vessel vasculitis (LVV)
- Takayasu arteritis (TAK)
- Giant-cell arteritis (GCA)

Medium-vessel vasculitis (MVV)
- Polyarteritis nodosa (PAN)
- Kawasaki disease (KD)

Small-vessel vasculitis (SVV)
- Anti-neutrophil cytoplasmic antibody (ANCA)–associated vasculitis (AAV)
- Microscopic polyangiitis (MPA)
- Granulomatosis with polyangiitis (Wegener's) (GPA)
- Eosinophilic granulomatosis with polyangiitis (Churg–Strauss syndrome) (EGPA)
- Immune complex SVV
- Anti–glomerular basement membrane (anti-GBM) disease
- Cryoglobulinemic vasculitis (CV)
- IgA vasculitis (Henoch–Schönlein) (IgAV)
- Hypocomplementemic urticarial vasculitis (HUV) (anti-C1q vasculitis)

Variable-vessel vasculitis (VVV)
- Behçet's disease (BD)
- Cogan's syndrome (CS)

Single-organ vasculitis (SOV)
- Cutaneous leukocytoclastic angiitis
- Cutaneous arteritis
- Primary central nervous system vasculitis
- Isolated aortitis
- Others

Vasculitis associated with systemic disease
- Lupus vasculitis
- Rheumatoid vasculitis
- Sarcoid vasculitis
- Others

Vasculitis associated with probable etiology
- Hepatitis C virus–associated cryoglobulinemic vasculitis
- Hepatitis B virus–associated vasculitis
- Syphilis-associated aortitis
- Drug-associated immune complex vasculitis
- Drug-associated ANCA-associated vasculitis
- Cancer-associated vasculitis
- Others

Jennette JC et al. 2012 Revised International Chapel Hill Consensus Conference Nomenclature of Vasculitides. Arthritis Rheumatism 2013;65(1):1–11.

- Patients present with severe headache, scalp tenderness, malaise, fevers, and weight loss.
- Focal neurological symptoms can occur, depending on pattern of vessel involvement.
- Jaw claudication with chewing, and tongue claudication are not pathognomonic, but have a high positive predictive value for this condition.
- Aortic arch syndrome and neuropathy occur in a minority.
- Physical examination will usually reveal fever, and marked tenderness over the scalp with thickened, tender temporal arteries which may have lost their pulse.
- **Visual symptoms are a medical emergency**, as they indicate embolization or vasculitis of the ophthalmic artery, which is a branch of the external carotid. Sudden blindness may result.

Investigations
- Laboratory investigations reveal markedly elevated ESR and CRP, and often a normocytic anemia, thrombocytosis, and abnormalities on liver function tests.

- Diagnosis is supported by temporal artery biopsy revealing granulomatous inflammation of the full thickness of the arterial wall, with infiltration by multinucleated giant cells, lymphocytes and fibroblasts. The intima is often markedly hyperplastic, with stenosis and occlusion of the vessel. False negatives can occur due to 'skip' lesions, and biopsies should be taken within 1 week of the commencement of corticosteroids. A negative result does not exclude the diagnosis, and treatment should not be delayed for a biopsy to be performed.
- Imaging techniques of the temporal arteries such as with ultrasound or MRI do not yet have a defined role.

Treatment
- High-dose corticosteroids need to be administered immediately upon suspicion of the diagnosis of GCA, either orally (≥1 mg/kg/day of prednisolone) or intravenously (methylprednisolone 500 mg daily for 3 days followed by high-dose oral prednisolone).
- Once clinical and serological parameters return to normal, gradual dosage tapering can occur with careful monitoring.

- If unacceptably high doses of steroids are required for disease control, a second immunosuppressive agent such as cyclophosphamide or methotrexate may be required.
- There is growing evidence for the use of IL-6 receptor antagonist tocilizumab in this condition.

Many patients will go into apparent long-term remission after a period of immunosuppression, but approximately 50% of patients suffer a flare with steroid reduction.

Takayasu arteritis

Takayasu arteritis is a disease that mainly affects young females, with greatest prevalence in Asia.

- It is a granulomatous vasculitis of the proximal aorta and its major branches.
- Fibroproliferative changes are found in the intima of the affected vessels, resulting in variable stenosis, thrombosis, and aneurysmal dilatation.

Clinical presentation is invariably with ischemia of the affected region. It is often referred to as 'pulseless disease'. Patients may present with:

- transient ischemic attacks
- strokes
- limb claudication
- visceral ischemia
- hypertension that can result from renal artery stenosis
- constitutional symptoms of fever, malaise, and weight loss (frequent)
- serological evidence of an acute-phase response
- absent peripheral pulses
- vascular bruits
- aortic regurgitation due to dilatation of the aortic root.

Imaging with MRI and CT angiography is a mainstay in the diagnosis of the disease. PET scan is increasingly used, but its role in diagnosis remains unclear.

Treatment consists of:

- Immunosuppression for the vasculitis.
- Corticosteroids in high doses are used for initial remission induction.
- Second agents such as methotrexate, cyclophosphamide or mycophenolate may be needed for remission maintenance. Biological agents such as anti-TNF antibodies are showing promise in this condition.
- Surgical methods to restore blood flow in occluded vessels where possible.
  - » Surgical approaches depend on the location and severity of lesions, and range from percutaneous angioplasty through to stenting and bypass.

Medium-vessel vasculitis

Polyarteritis nodosa (PAN)

- Polyarteritis nodosa is a rare vasculitis of unknown etiology affecting medium to small arteries. The disease has a propensity for mesenteric, renal and coronary arteries.

- Approximately 30% of patients will be hepatitis B surface-antigen positive; it is important to identify patients with active hepatitis B infection, as the treatment will differ despite the disease being identical.
- PAN has also been associated with other infections such as HIV, hepatitis C and cytomegalovirus (CMV), with autoimmune disease such as rheumatoid arthritis, and with malignancy e.g. Hodgkin's lymphoma and hairy-cell leukemia.
- PAN is more common in men.

Most patients have marked constitutional symptoms of fever, night sweats, weight loss, fatigue, and malaise. More specific symptoms and signs (Box 16-18) will generally be due to organ ischemia.

Diagnosis and treatment

- There is no specific diagnostic test for PAN, other than demonstration of necrotizing vasculitis on tissue biopsy. Testicular biopsy is relatively safe, and can be diagnostic in patients with testicular symptoms.
- Imaging may demonstrate irregularities of vessels such as stenosis or aneurysm formation.
- Treatment is with immunosuppression, generally commencing with high-dose corticosteroids and then with a second agent such as cyclophosphamide.
- Patients with hepatitis B should be treated with antiviral medication.

Kawasaki disease

- Kawasaki disease is a disease almost exclusively of childhood that commences with high fever and causes systemic vasculitis of medium-sized arteries.
- The acute phase of the illness is characterized by high fever which lasts for upward of a week. The more prolonged the fever, the greater the risk of cardiac complications.
- Kawasaki disease is common in East Asia. Up to 90% of cases occur before age 5. The etiology is unknown.

Box 16-18

Clinical features in patients with polyarteritis nodosa

- Angina pectoris
- Myocardial infarction
- Mesenteric angina
- Intestinal infarction
- Peripheral neuropathy
- Mononeuritis multiplex
- Stroke
- Cutaneous vasculitis
- Asymmetric polyarthritis
- Testicular pain
- Splenic infarction
- Hypertension
- Renal infarction

Box 16-19

Clinical manifestations of Kawasaki disease

Common
- Prolonged fever
- Cervical lymphadenopathy
- Mucocutaneous lesions: conjunctivitis, diffuse maculopapular rash, strawberry tongue, inflamed lips, pharyngitis, edema of the palms and soles, desquamation of the fingers

Less common
- Arthralgia
- Arthritis
- Diarrhea
- Myocarditis/pericarditis
- Aseptic meningitis
- Pneumonia
- Hepatitis

- The clinical abnormalities (Box 16-19) are due to vasculitis, and this is also responsible for the feared complication of aneurysmal dilatation of arteries, especially the coronary arteries. This in turn can lead to rupture or thrombosis of the vessel, leading to myocardial ischemia or infarction. Aneurysm formation generally occurs between 2 and 12 weeks of disease onset.

Diagnosis and treatment
- There is no specific diagnostic test for Kawasaki disease, so clinical features are key.
- A high index of suspicion is necessary, given the importance of instituting treatment promptly to lessen the risk of aneurysm formation.
- Most patients display an acute phase response.
- High-dose IV immunoglobulin should be administered as soon as the diagnosis is made. If fever does not resolve promptly, a second dose should be given.
- Aspirin also improves prognosis and is used in low doses to reduce the risk of thrombosis.

CLINICAL PEARL

Aspirin is generally contraindicated in children because of the risk of Reye's syndrome. Kawasaki disease is one of the rare exceptions to this rule, as benefit outweighs risk in this case.

Small-vessel vasculitis

Granulomatosis with polyangiitis (GPA)/ Wegener's granulomatosis (WG)

- Granulomatosis with polyangiitis is a systemic vasculitis with a propensity to involve the respiratory system and the kidneys.
- It is one of the ANCA-associated vasculitides, with up to 90% of sufferers ANCA-positive, especially those with systemic rather than localized disease.

- GPA can be a fulminant, life-threatening disease, and lung involvement is frequently misdiagnosed as infection in the first instance, resulting in considerable peril for the patient.

CLINICAL PEARL

Granulomatosis with polyangiitis should be a differential diagnosis in any patient with a pulmonary–renal syndrome, hemoptysis, or respiratory tract symptoms that fail to respond to antibiotics. Delays in diagnosis significantly worsen both the pulmonary and the renal prognosis.

Box 16-20 lists the clinical manifestations of GPA.
- The majority of patients present with upper respiratory tract symptoms of variable duration and severity, prior to the development of systemic constitutional features and those related to involvement of various organs.
- Cavitating lung lesions are typical, with or without interstitial changes.
- The renal lesion is a pauci-immune, focal necrotizing glomerulonephritis.
- Development of renal failure can be rapid.

Diagnosis
- The detection of a c-ANCA (cytoplasmic pattern ANCA) with anti-PR3 (proteinase 3) antibodies in a patient with consistent clinical features is diagnostic of GPA.
  » Rarely, p-ANCA (perinuclear pattern ANCA) is found in patients with the more typical clinical phenotype of GPA than microscopic polyangiitis (which is described below).
  » In ANCA-negative patients, tissue diagnosis will be required. This will usually be in the setting of sinonasal disease, so biopsy of the nasal mucosa may reveal vasculitis.

Box 16-20

Clinical manifestations of GPA

Rhinosinusitis

Epistaxis

Cough

Dyspnea

Dysphonia

Hemoptysis

Respiratory failure

Fever

Renal failure

Hypertension

Arthralgia

Headache

Focal neurological symptoms

- While tissue biopsy will reveal granulomatous necrotizing vasculitis, this may not always be possible in the setting of an acutely unwell patient. Treatment needs to be instituted immediately when respiratory, renal or neurological involvement is present.
- There is usually serological evidence of an acute phase reaction.
- Microscopic urine examination, determination of renal function, and lung imaging is essential in all patients. It is worthwhile to obtain CT imaging of the paranasal sinuses.
- Baseline testing of pulmonary function should be performed.

Treatment

- Without aggressive immunosuppression, the prognosis of GPA is dismal.
- The use of cyclophosphamide has resulted in a 5-year survival rate of >90%, although progression to end-stage kidney disease remains a risk.
- High-dose IV corticosteroids should be instituted immediately for any patient with lung or kidney disease, concurrently with cyclophosphamide or rituximab.
  » Some patients may be able to be maintained on methotrexate or mycophenolate, given the significant long-term toxicity associated with cumulative doses of cyclophosphamide.
  » It is recommended that patients on long-term immunosuppression be treated with prophylaxis for *Pneumocystis jirovecii* in the form of low-dose oral trimethoprim-sulfamethoxazole.
- The aim of treatment is to achieve remission. This can be assessed by clearing of respiratory tract lesions, and normalization or stabilization of renal function.
- The titer of c-ANCA and PR3 antibodies may be a guide to disease activity, and can be used for long-term monitoring of patients.
- Occasionally, fulminant disease requires plasma exchange.

Microscopic polyangiitis (MPA)

Similar to GPA, MPA is a small-vessel vasculitis associated with ANCA.

Clinical characteristics

- Patients with MPA generally present with constitutional symptoms, and renal impairment with active urinary sediment.
- Lung disease will often cause hemoptysis secondary to pulmonary vasculitis.
- Upper airway involvement is not usual, in contrast to GPA.
- Skin, joint, and neurological complications affect a minority.
- The ratio of lung:renal involvement is reversed compared with GPA, whereby renal involvement in MPA is present in 90% of patients.

Diagnosis and treatment

- MPA is characterized by p-ANCA (perinuclear ANCA) and the presence of antibodies to MPO (myeloperoxidase) in about 80% of cases.
  » Occasionally, c-ANCA is detected in patients who behave clinically more like MPA than GPA.
- The presence of a positive p-ANCA and MPO antibodies has high positive predictive value for the diagnosis of MPA. Renal biopsy is desirable, however, for both definitive diagnosis and prognostic reasons.
- Determination of renal and pulmonary function at baseline is essential, as is lung imaging.

The treatment approach is similar to that described for GPA.

Eosinophilic granulomatosis with polyangiitis (EGPA)/Churg–Strauss syndrome (CSS)

Clinical characteristics

- Eosinophilic granulomatosis with polyangiitis is a rare eosinophilic vasculitis of small vessels that arises in patients with a history of atopic disease. Most patients will have a history, often for many years, of allergic rhinosinusitis and asthma.
- When vasculitis develops, patients present with a combination of blood eosinophilia and pulmonary infiltrates, sometimes with hemoptysis, vasculitic skin rash, and neurological features in the form of either symmetrical peripheral neuropathy or mononeuritis multiplex.

Diagnosis

- Around half of patients are p-ANCA-positive.
- Tissue biopsy of skin or sural nerve may be helpful for diagnosis if cutaneous or neurological disease is present. An eosinophilic vasculitis is diagnostic.
- Lung biopsy is generally not needed when characteristic radiological abnormalities are present in an atopic patient.
- Bronchoalveolar lavage will reveal eosinophil-rich fluid if performed.

Treatment

As is typical for most eosinophilic disorders, corticosteroids are effective, however, some patients require ongoing therapy with unacceptably high doses. For those with severe, multi-organ disease, cyclophosphamide can be used to induce remission. A second agent such as azathioprine or mycophenolate may be required to maintain remission or to allow reduction of the corticosteroid dose. Anti-IL-5 monoclonal antibodies, such as mepolizumab also appear to be effective in this condition.

IgA vasculitis (IgAV)/Henoch-Schönlein purpura (HSP)

IgA vasculitis is a systemic vasculitis which is much more common in children than adults. The disease results from deposition of IgA-containing immune complexes in vessel walls, stimulating an inflammatory response.

Clinical characteristics

- Palpable purpura of the lower extremities is invariable, very often extending up to the buttocks (Figure 16-15).
- Joint involvement and abdominal pain occur in the majority of cases.
  - » The arthritis mainly affects the joints of the lower limbs.
  - » The abdominal pain may be accompanied by bloody diarrhea.
- Around 40% of sufferers will have microscopic hematuria.
- Renal impairment is rare, but a small number of patients, usually adults, will progress to end-stage renal disease.
- IgAV usually follows on from infection, mostly of the upper respiratory tract. Both *Streptococcus* and *Staphylococcus* have been implicated in some case series.

Diagnosis

- Diagnosis is generally obvious when faced with the combination of the lower extremity purpura, and joint, GI tract or renal disease.
- Renal biopsy changes are identical to IgA nephropathy when the kidneys are involved.

Treatment

- Most episodes resolve without treatment within 3 weeks.

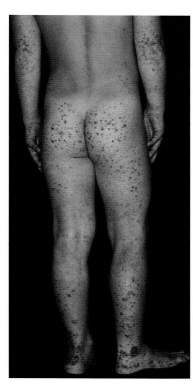

Figure 16-15 The typical palpable purpura seen in Henoch-Schönlein purpura (IgA vasculitis)

From Habif TB. Clinical dermatology, 5th ed. St Louis: Elsevier, 2009.

- Severe episodes, and those with renal impairment or evidence of organ failure, require treatment with systemic corticosteroids and possibly second-line agents such as cyclophosphamide or mycophenolate.

Single-organ vasculitis

Cutaneous leukocytoclastic angiitis

This may occur in isolation, or in association with a systemic vasculitis or autoimmune disease (Box 16-21).

- Drug reactions are a common cause when there is no associated systemic illness.
- Reactions to vaccines or foods are also a possibility.
- Sometimes the disease appears to be idiopathic.
- Systemic diseases include SLE, SS, IgAV, rheumatoid arthritis (RA), and cryoglobulinemia, with the pathogenetic mechanism being immune-complex deposition.

Clinically, patients have tender, non-blanching purpuric or petechial lesions which nearly always start on the distal lower limbs, but may spread proximally. Biopsy reveals perivascular neutrophils with fibrinoid necrosis (leukocytoclasis; Figure 16-16, overleaf).

- The rash is self-limited once the inciting antigen (e.g. antibiotic) is withdrawn.
- When associated with systemic disease, treatment is according to the usual protocols for that disease.

Variable-vessel vasculitis

Behçet's disease

- Behçet's disease is a rare disorder characterized by painful oral (Figure 16-17, overleaf) and genital aphthous ulceration, uveitis, and vasculitis that can affect multiple organs, including the central nervous system, retina and skin.

Box 16-21

Differential diagnosis of palpable purpura

Leukocytoclastic vasculitis (angiitis)

- Idiopathic
- Cryoglobulinemia
- Malignancy
- IgA vasculitis (Henoch-Schönlein purpura)
- Malignancy
- Systemic autoimmune disease—systemic lupus erythematosus, Sjögren's syndrome, rheumatoid arthritis

Cutaneous emboli

Infection

- *Meningococcus*
- *Gonococcus*
- *Rickettsia* (e.g. Rocky Mountain spotted fever)

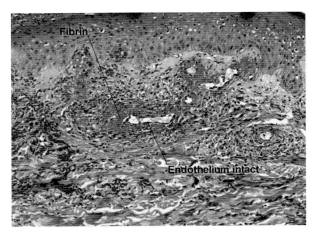

Figure 16-16 This photomicrograph shows leukocytoclasis, with evidence of fibrinoid necrosis and polymorphonuclear cells surrounding the blood vessel

From Elston D et al. Dermatopathology. Philadelphia: Elsevier, 2008.

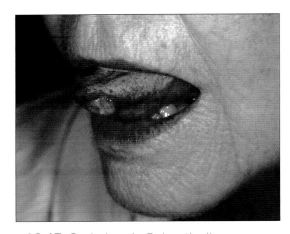

Figure 16-17 Oral ulcer in Behçet's disease

From Krachmer JH, Mannis MJ and Holland EH. Cornea, 3rd ed. St Louis: Elsevier, 2010.

- An oligoarthritis, recurrent abdominal pain, and pulmonary vasculitis rarely may occur.
- More common in women, there is a striking racial disposition with Behçet's mainly affecting those from Iran, Turkey and East Asia.
- Behçet's does not result in autoantibody formation, but will usually be accompanied by an acute phase response.
- The skin of most patients with Behçet's displays pathergy—puncturing the skin with a needle results in the formation of a pustule after 24–48 hours.

Treatment

- Recurrent ulceration may be ameliorated by treatment with colchicine.
- Both dapsone and thalidomide have been reported to display efficacy.

- Vasculitic complications require immunosuppression with corticosteroids and often second-line agents.
- Ocular disease especially needs an aggressive approach, with anti-TNF monoclonal therapy gaining favor in this situation.

AUTOINFLAMMATORY DISORDERS

These are a group of monogenic syndromes that result in inflammasome dysregulation and overproduction of pro-inflammatory cytokines, especially IL-1-beta. Characteristic features include fever, rash, and serositis. Mostly very rare, there are now a large number of identified syndromes, but Familial Mediterranean fever and TNF-receptor-associated periodic syndrome are the most prevalent of these.

Familial Mediterranean fever (FMF)

Clinical characteristics

This most common of the autoinflammatory syndromes affects predominantly those of ethnicity from the populations located around the Mediterranean Sea. FMF results from a mutation in the *MEFV* gene, and is autosomal recessive.

- Most patients present in childhood or adolescence.
- The disease is characterized by recurrent acute attacks of peritonitis, high fever, and a typically large-joint monoarthritis.
- Pleuritis, pericarditis, and testicular pain can also occur, as can an intensely erythematous rash that mainly affects the lower limbs.
- Attacks occur at variable frequency. In severe cases they may be weekly.
- Many patients undergo abdominal surgery due to uncertainty regarding the cause of peritonitis.
- Those with frequent attacks over a prolonged period are at risk of the development of secondary amyloidosis as a result of prolonged elevation in levels of the acute phase reactant serum amyloid A protein. Renal amyloidosis is the most common site.

Diagnosis

- Inflammatory markers are raised during an attack. ESR, CRP, white cell count, and platelets are usually markedly elevated.
- These parameters usually normalize between attacks.
- The definitive test is demonstration of the abnormal *MEFV* gene.

Treatment

- Long-term administration of colchicine at a dose of 0.5–1.5 mg daily reduces the number and severity of attacks, and the risk of amyloidosis, in the majority of patients.

- Interleukin-1 (IL-1) inhibition with monoclonal antibody therapy (anakinra, rilonacept, canakinumab) is safe and effective in those unresponsive to or intolerant of colchicine.

TNF-receptor-associated periodic syndrome (TRAPS)

Less common than FMF, TRAPS is an autosomal dominant condition resulting from a mutation in the *TNFRFS 1A* gene which encodes the TNF (tumor necrosis factor) receptor.

Clinical characteristics

- Onset is generally in early childhood (<10 years) but can be delayed until adulthood.
- Fever often lasts for 10–14 days.
- Abdominal pain is typical, and often severe.
- Myalgia and arthralgia occur frequently, along with headache, pleuritis, a variety of skin rashes, and ocular inflammation in the form of conjunctivitis or uveitis.
- Secondary amyloidosis can be a chronic complication.

Diagnosis

- Inflammatory markers are raised during an attack. ESR, CRP, white cell count, and platelets are usually elevated, often markedly so. These do not always return to normal between attacks.
- Definitive diagnosis depends on detection of the abnormal *TNFRFS 1A* gene.

Treatment

- IL-1 inhibition is the mainstay of treatment in this disorder.
- TNF blockade with etanercept is effective or partially effective in some patients.

IMMUNODEFICIENCY

Deficiencies of the immune system are common, and can be divided into *primary* (congenital) and *secondary* (acquired).

- Primary immunodeficiency refers to a defective component, or components, of the immune system due to a genetic mutation.
- Secondary immunodeficiency occurs as a result of a wide array of diseases, and their treatments.

Table 16-14 gives examples of deficiencies of each type.

For the clinician, the challenge will often be:

- to recognize when a patient with infection is immunodeficient, and thus be in a position to adapt treatment appropriately
- to look at ways to protect the patient from future risk, for example through prophylaxis, replacement therapy, or immunization.

Table 16-14 Primary and secondary immunodeficiency

TYPE	EXAMPLE(S)
Primary immunodeficiency	
Predominant antibody deficiencies	Common variable immunodeficiency
Phagocyte defects	Chronic granulomatous disease
Combined T and B cell deficiencies	Severe combined immunodeficiency
Combined T and B cell deficiencies with syndromic features	DiGeorge syndrome
Secondary immunodeficiency	
Environmental	Malnutrition
Infection	Human immunodeficiency virus
Disease-related	Malignancy; protein-losing enteropathy; burns; widespread skin disease
Iatrogenic	Cancer chemotherapy; Immunosuppressive drugs

CLINICAL PEARL

Immunodeficiency should be suspected in the setting of:
- recurrent or chronic infection
- infection with low-virulence organisms
- evidence of end-organ damage, e.g. bronchiectasis
- poor response to standard antimicrobial therapy
- recurrent infection with the same organism.

Primary immunodeficiency

The true incidence of primary immunodeficiency is unknown, but is relatively common if selective IgA deficiency is taken into account. Approximately 65% of cases are antibody deficiencies. Unfortunately, many cases are missed worldwide; however, neonatal screening for some conditions has been implemented in certain countries.

- Diagnosis is frequently delayed for an average of over 5 years.
- Given that earlier diagnosis improves prognosis, many patients will have developed complications by the time their underlying immunodeficiency is recognized.
- Consanguinity is the major risk factor for primary immunodeficiency.

Box 16-22 (overleaf) outlines clinical clues to diagnosis at different ages.

CLINICAL PEARL

Infection is the major complication of immunodeficiency, but it is important to remember that immunodeficiency is also associated with immune dysregulation. Some patients will develop autoimmunity, allergy and malignancy as a result of their immunodeficiency.

Box 16-22

When to consider a diagnosis of primary immunodeficiency

Infancy
- Failure to thrive
- Family history of primary immunodeficiency
- Omphalitis
- Congenital defects
- Consanguinous parents

Childhood
- 8 or more infections in 1 year, especially ear infections
- Persistent candidiasis
- Recurrent skin infection
- Recurrent abscesses

Any age
- Opportunistic infection, e.g. with *Pneumocystis jirovecii*
- Recurrent pneumonia or sinusitis
- Evidence of end-organ damage, e.g. bronchiectasis
- Failure of response to standard antibiotics
- Autoimmune disease

Primary antibody defects

Antibody defects generally manifest with recurrent sinopulmonary infection in the form of otitis media, sinusitis and pneumonia (Table 16-15). Frequent, recurrent, and chronic infection should raise suspicion.

Investigating antibody deficiency

The initial investigation of a patient with suspected primary antibody deficiency should be with:

- full blood count
- serum immunoglobulins
- specific antibody responses following vaccination with protein antigens (tetanus, pertussis), and polysaccharide antigens (*Pneumococcus*).

If these are normal:

- investigate for complement deficiency: CH50, AH50, C2, C4, C3.

If there is evidence of lymphopenia and/or hypogammaglobulinemia, follow-up testing should be sought with:

- lymphocyte subsets
- specific gene testing.

CLINICAL PEARL

Differential diagnosis in recurrent sinopulmonary infection:
- primary or secondary immunodeficiency
- allergic rhinosinusitis
- chronic rhinosinusitis with or without polyposis
- cystic fibrosis
- ciliary dyskinesia
- anatomical sinonasal obstruction.

Long-term management of antibody deficiency

Patients who are on long-term immunoglobulin replacement therapy should be kept in regular review:

- IgG levels should be monitored to ensure adequate replacement
- lung function testing and imaging should be performed at regular intervals to screen for bronchiectasis

- paranasal sinus imaging should be performed if patients are symptomatic
- patients are unlikely to have an adequate response to most immunization
- hyperimmune globulin should be used where available if exposure to a relevant infection is reasonably suspected.

Phagocyte deficiency

Phagocyte deficiency accounts for approximately 10% of primary immunodeficiency. Most deficiency in phagocyte number or function is acquired, secondary to infection, medication, nutrition or malignancy, with the primary forms being due to rare genetic defects.

Primary neutropenia

Cyclic neutropenia and severe congenital neutropenia are rare conditions with defined genetic mutations.

Combined antibody and cellular immunodeficiencies

Congenital T-cell deficiency has a profound effect on the development and function of B cells also, and hence patients present with problems related to both cell-mediated and humoral immunodeficiency.

Patients generally present as infants, and without treatment do not survive.

Severe combined immunodeficiency

- Rare; approximately 1:65,000.
- Consanguinity is a major risk factor.
- Infants present with sepsis, failure to thrive, and opportunistic infections.
- Multiple gene defects have been identified, e.g. adenosine deaminase deficiency, *JAK3* deficiency.
- Treatment involves stem–cell transplantation or gene therapy.

Chronic granulomatous disease (CGD)

- This is a rare condition with an incidence of approximately 1:250,000.

Table 16-15 Primary antibody deficiencies

PRIMARY IM-MUNODEFI-CIENCY	INCIDENCE	GENETIC DEFECT	CLINICAL FEATURES	DIAGNOSIS	TREATMENT
Selective IgA deficiency	Common; 1:500 to 1:700	Unknown	80% asymptomatic Recurrent sinopulmonary infection Celiac disease Autoimmune disease	No measurable IgA	Antibiotic therapy as required
Common variable immunodeficiency (CVID)	1:25,000 to 1:50,000	Mutations defined in about 15%; includes *TACI, ICOS* genes	Onset may be delayed until teenage years or young adulthood Recurrent bacterial infection, especially sinopulmonary; septicemia, abscesses Bronchiectasis Autoimmune disease	Low IgG Low IgM and IgA is usual Poor or absent specific antibody response to vaccination	Regular replacement therapy with pooled donor immunoglobulin
Specific antibody deficiency	Unknown	Unknown	Recurrent bacterial infection, especially sinopulmonary; otitis media	Absent or sub-normal response to vaccination (e.g. pneumo-coccal, tetanus)	Regular replacement therapy with pooled donor immunoglobulin
IgG sub-class deficiency	Unknown	Unknown	Clinical significance unclear No longer recommended in screening for immunodeficiency	Low levels of one or more IgG sub-classes in presence of normal total IgG	Nil
X-linked agamma-globulinemia	1:70,000 to 1:400,000	*BTK* gene	Almost exclusively seen in boys; presents in childhood with recurrent bacterial infection	Absent B cells Low or absent IgG, IgM, IgA *BTK* gene abnormality	Regular replacement with pooled donor immunoglobulin

BTK, Bruton's tyrosine kinase; *ICOS*, inducible co-stimulator; *TACI*, transmembrane activator and calcium-modulator and cyclophilin-ligand interactor.

- Patients with CGD tend to present with recurrent deep-seated infections due to *Staphylococcus aureus*, *Burkholderia cepacia*, *Serratia marcescens*, *Nocardia* spp. and *Aspergillus* spp. Hepatic and pulmonary infections are frequent.
- CGD is caused by mutation in one of the five genes that encode the nicotinamide adenine dinucleotide phosphate (NADPH) phagocyte oxidase complex (Phox) which is responsible for the respiratory burst that kills phagocytosed bacteria in neutrophils.
- Diagnosis is by demonstration of reduced phagocyte oxidase activity, either by a negative NBT (nitroblue tetrazolium) test by or a reduction in the dihydro-rhodamine 123 assay.
- Treatment is with long-term administration of gamma-interferon, prophylactic antibiotics (trimethoprim-sulfamethoxazole) and antifungals (itraconazole).

Combined antibody and cellular immunodeficiencies with syndromic features

These are outlined in Table 16-16 (overleaf).

CLINICAL PEARL

Relatively few pathology tests need to be employed in the initial screening of a patient with suspected primary immunodeficiency:
- full blood count and film
- serum immunoglobulins
- complement levels
- specific antibody responses.

If all of these are normal, primary immunodeficiency is unlikely. If the lymphocyte count is low, specific B- and T-cell subsets should be measured. If Howell−Jolly bodies are present on blood film, asplenia is likely.

Table 16-16 Examples of primary combined immunodeficiencies with syndromic features

T-CELL IMMUNO-DEFICIENCY	INCIDENCE	GENE DEFECT	CLINICAL FEATURES	DIAGNOSIS
DiGeorge syndrome	1:4,000	Deletion of chromosome 22q11.2	Typical facies (Figure 16-18) Recurrent infections Hypocalcemia due to parathyroid hypoplasia Schizophrenia Developmental delay Thymic hypoplasia Cardiac anomalies	Reduction in T-cell numbers Decreased antibody responses to protein antigens
Ataxia-telangiectasia	1:100,000	*ATM*	Progressive ataxia Ocular and cutaneous telangiectasia from age 3–5 years Recurrent bacterial infections	Low Ig levels B and T cell lymphopenia Poor antibody responses Elevated alpha-fetoprotein
Wiskott–Aldrich syndrome	1:100,000 to 1:1,000,000	*WASP* X-linked recessive	Severe eczema; recurrent bacterial infection, frequently staphylococcal	Thrombocytopenia with small platelets Decreased T cells Low Ig levels
Hyper-IgE	1:100,000	*STAT3*	Eczema; skin abscesses (Figure 16-19) Recurrent staphylococcal infection Pneumatoceles Candidiasis Typical facies Retention of primary teeth (Figure 16-19)	Very high total serum IgE Eosinophilia

Ig, immunoglobulin.

Vaccination in PID

- Live viral and bacterial vaccines should not be given.
  - » Specifically, oral polio vaccine, bacille Calmette-Guérin (BCG), measles-mumps-rubella (MMR) vaccine, yellow fever, live typhoid, varicella vaccine, live influenza vaccine, and live oral rotavirus vaccine should be avoided.
- Inactivated and sub-unit vaccines are safe, but may be ineffective; antibody response should be measured to check efficacy.
- Passive immunization should be considered where appropriate, e.g. VZV (varicella zoster virus) immunoglobulin.

Secondary (acquired) immunodeficiency

The majority of cases of secondary immunodeficiency globally result from poor nutrition and chronic infection secondary to poor living conditions, or communicable disease. In the developed world, aging of the population with the accompanying immunosenescence accounts for a substantial proportion of the increased susceptibility to infection, along with immunosuppressive treatments used in the treatment of a variety of malignant and autoimmune conditions, and in the management of transplanted organs.

HIV/AIDS

The human immunodeficiency virus (HIV) pandemic has presented unique global challenges both clinically and ethically. The acquired immune deficiency syndrome (AIDS) has affected all nations and all sections of society. There have been deep insights into the understanding of both the intact and the disordered immune system as a result of this disease. A previously nearly universally fatal condition has turned into a chronic, treatable condition due to the advent of effective antiretroviral therapy.

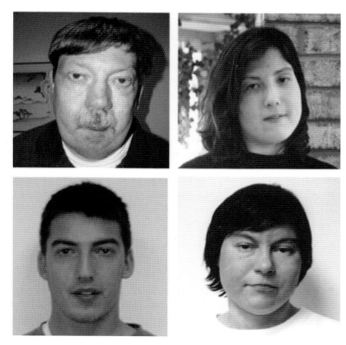

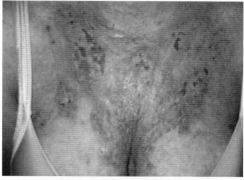

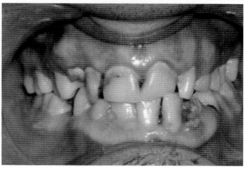

Figure 16-18 Patients with typical facies for DiGeorge syndrome

From Fung WLA et al. Extracardiac features predicting 22q11.2 deletion syndrome in adult congenital heart disease. Int J Cardiol 2007;131(1):51–58.

Figure 16-19 Patient with hyper-IgE syndrome, demonstrating severe atopic dermatitis (above) and retention of primary teeth (below)

From Esposito L et al. Hyper-IgE syndrome: dental implications. Oral Surg Oral Med Oral Pathol Oral Radiol 2012;114(2):147–53.

Epidemiology

UNAIDS, the Joint United Nations Programme on HIV/AIDS, estimates that in 2019:

- 36.9 million people are infected with HIV globally
- 21.7 million people were accessing antiretroviral therapy
- 940,000 people died of the disease
- 1.8 million people were newly infected, but new infections were reduced by 47% since the peak in 1996
- sub-Saharan Africa accounts for the majority of people living with the infection
  - » 79% of new infections in 10- to 19-year-olds were in females
- high rates of infection are found in South America, Asia and Eastern Europe.

Risk factors for HIV infection

- Heterosexual transmission remains the predominant mode of acquisition of the virus globally.
- Male-to-male sex carries the highest risk in developed Western countries and is an important risk factor elsewhere.

Other key risk groups include:

- children, through perinatal transmission
- people who inject drugs
- sex workers.

Other risk factors include:

- concurrent genital infection
- uncircumcised males
- transfusion of infected blood products
- exposure from medical or dental procedures.

Pathophysiology

- HIV is transmitted through blood, genital fluids or breast milk.
- HIV gains entry to cells through the CD4 molecule found on the surface of CD4+ cells, T-helper lymphocytes, monocyte–macrophages, and dendritic cells.
  - » The CD4 molecule acts as the receptor for an HIV envelope protein known as gp120.
  - » For successful entry into the cell, HIV gp120 must also bind a co-receptor, which is usually a protein in a class known as chemokine receptors.
  - » The two major chemokine receptors used by HIV for cell entry are CCR5 and/or CXCR4. Differences in gp120 protein structure determine tropism for either of these co-receptors. **CCR5 blockade** is one therapeutic target in HIV treatment.
- To enter the cell, the virus undergoes fusion with the membrane, a step that can be blocked by **fusion inhibitors**.
- HIV is a single-stranded RNA retrovirus that requires reverse transcription in the cell cytoplasm, through the

action of the enzyme reverse transcriptase, to form single-stranded and then double-stranded DNA. This step can be blocked by **reverse transcriptase inhibitors**.

- For the newly formed HIV DNA to be copied, it must next be integrated into the host cell genome via the action of the enzyme integrase. This is the next target for therapeutic blocking of the process, with the use of **integrase inhibitors**.

- Following successful transcription, the newly formed viral polypeptides are spliced by the enzyme protease into their functional forms, a step susceptible to the action of **protease inhibitors**.

- The viral particles and structural proteins are then assembled in the cytoplasm into mature virus which is ready for release.

Most individuals mount a prompt and vigorous immune response to acute HIV infection, via formation of antibody and the action of cytotoxic T cells and natural killer cells.

- A high viral load and a sudden drop in CD4+ T-cell numbers during the acute infection phase is typically seen, followed by restoration as the immune response kicks in.

- The virus is directly cytopathic to CD4+ T cells. In addition, infected cells are targeted by cytotoxic T lymphocytes, and by antibody. It is less cytopathic toward macrophages and dendritic cells.

- Viral replication continues in lymphoid tissue at varying rates, and a steady decline is seen in CD4+ lymphocyte numbers and immune function over years, with consequent increase in plasma viral load unless effective treatment is instigated.

- As immune function declines, patients become susceptible to a range of infective, autoimmune and neoplastic complications.

Clinical features and diagnosis

Acute HIV infection

- More than 50%, and possibly up to 90%, of patients will suffer an acute (seroconversion) illness from 3 to 6 weeks after being infected with the virus. Clinical features are outlined in Box 16-23.

Box 16-23

Clinical features of acute HIV infection

Common
- Fever
- Generalized lymphadenopathy
- Maculopapular rash
- Headache
- Pharyngitis
- Myalgia
- Constitutional symptoms

Less common
- Oral candidiasis
- Splenomegaly
- Diarrhea
- Arthralgia
- Night sweats
- Productive cough
- Meningitis

- Severe acute illness with high levels of viremia is poorly prognostic.

- Highly-sensitive enzyme immunoassays are used as screening tests, but confirmation of HIV infection requires a positive Western blot test. Recommended baseline investigations are outlined in Box 16-24.

- The formation of HIV antibodies signals the end of the seroconversion phase, but antibodies—although detectable at 3 months in the vast majority—may occasionally take up to 6 months or even longer to be detectable in serum. For this reason, earlier diagnosis can require detection of viral antigen in the serum, with p24 antigen testing or nucleic acid amplification testing.

Chronic HIV infection

- Untreated, the majority of patients decline physically and immunologically after a variable-length clinically latent period.

- Autoimmune phenomena may be seen prior to the development of significant immunodeficiency (Box 16-25). This is often associated with a CD8+ lymphocytosis, and affected organs may also demonstrate infiltration with cytotoxic T cells. Generalized lymphadenopathy may persist during this phase.

As immunodeficiency progresses, opportunistic infection begins to appear. Early such infections include:
- recurrent or persistent herpes simplex
- herpes zoster

Box 16-24

Recommended baseline investigations for the newly diagnosed HIV patient

- CD4+ T cell count
- HIV viral load
- HIV resistance assay (genotypic/phenotypic, depending on local availability)
- Full blood count
- Electrolytes, urea, creatinine
- Liver function tests
- Fasting lipids and glucose
- Urinalysis
- Hepatitis B and C serology
- Toxoplasma serology
- Serum cryptococcal antigen
- CMV serology
- Screening for other STIs (syphilis, chlamydia, gonorrhea)
- HLAB*5701 (to detect risk of abacavir hypersensitivity)

CMV, cytomegalovirus; HIV, human immunodeficiency virus; STI, sexually transmitted infection.

Adapted from: http://aidsinfo.nih.gov/contentfiles/AdultARV_GL_Table3.jpg

---

Box 16-25
Autoimmune diseases seen in HIV infection

Immune thrombocytopenic purpura
Polymyositis
Lymphoid interstitial pneumonitis
Bell's palsy
Sjögren's syndrome
Autoimmune thyroid disease
Antiphospholipid syndrome
Guillain–Barré syndrome

- oral hairy leukoplakia
- oropharyngeal candidiasis.

When immunodeficiency becomes profound, generally coinciding with a CD4+ T lymphocyte count of <200/m^3, life-threatening infections such as pneumocystis pneumonia (Figure 16-20) and malignancies such as Kaposi's sarcoma (Figure 16-21) become frequent.

Management

Comprehensive management of the HIV-infected patient requires attention to the psychological, environmental, socioeconomic, sexual and physical factors affecting each individual. Access to medical treatment, specifically antiretroviral therapy, is obviously a key consideration.

The complexities of such management are beyond the scope of this text. The principles of pharmacotherapy, however, are key to the successful treatment of the disease, as outlined in Table 16-17 (overleaf).

Combined antiretroviral therapy (cART)

Aims of therapy

- Control viral replication.
- Maintain or restore immune function (specifically CD4+ T cells) and reduce HIV-associated morbidity.
- Prevent emergence of resistance (at least three antiviral agents aimed at two molecular targets).
- cART is also used for pre-exposure prophylaxis (PrEP) and post-exposure prophylaxis (PEP).

When to initiate therapy

Current guidelines are:

- cART is recommended for all infected individuals, regardless of CD4+ T cell count.
- Commence with three effective drugs
  » A 'backbone' of two nucleos(t)ide reverse transcriptase inhibitors
  » An 'anchor' of a non-nucleotide reverse transcriptase inhibitor, a boosted protease inhibitor or an integrase inhibitor.
- The earlier cART is initiated after infection, the better the prognosis. However, this needs to be weighed

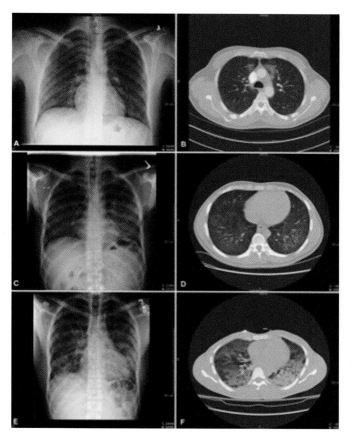

Figure 16-20 Chest X-rays and corresponding CT scans of pneumocystis pneumonia in chronic HIV infection; note the interstitial changes progressing to ground-glass appearance

From Goldman L and Schafer AI. Goldman's Cecil medicine, 24th ed. Philadelphia: Elsevier, 2012.

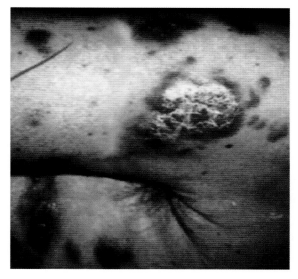

Figure 16-21 Cutaneous Kaposi's sarcoma in an AIDS patient

From Hoffman R et al. Hematology, basic principles and practice, 5th ed. Philadelphia: Elsevier, 2009.

Table 16-17 AIDS-defining conditions and their treatment

CONDITION	TREATMENT PRINCIPLES
Infections	
Esophageal, bronchial, tracheal or pulmonary candidiasis	Azole antifungals
Pneumocystis jirovecii pneumonia	High-dose oral or IV co-trimoxazole, or IV pentamidine, plus prednisolone 1 mg/kg/day for 21 days if $PaO_2 < 70$ mmHg on room air
Cerebral toxoplasmosis	Pyrimethamine, plus sulfadiazine or clindamycin
Cytomegalovirus	IV ganciclovir or foscarnet, or oral valganciclovir Longer duration of treatment required for CMV retinitis
Cryptosporidiosis	Restoration of immune function essential; paromomycin, azithromycin not proven to be effective
Coccidioidomycosis, disseminated or extrapulmonary	Amphotericin-B or azole antifungals
Cryptococcosis, extrapulmonary	IV amphotericin-B with flucytosine, followed by oral fluconazole
Herpes simplex bronchitis, pneumonitis, esophagitis, or ulcer lasting >1 month	Acyclovir (aciclovir), valacyclovir or famciclovir
Histoplasmosis, disseminated or extrapulmonary	Amphotericin-B or azole antifungals
Chronic intestinal isosporiasis	Co-trimoxazole
Mycobacterium tuberculosis infection	Standard four-drug therapy as first-line: rifamycin, isoniazid, pyrazinamide, ethambutol Multi-drug resistance is found in many parts of the world, necessitating local protocols Interactions with ARVs are complex and must be considered
Mycobacterium avium complex or *M. kansasii*	Clarithromycin, ethambutol, rifabutin
Recurrent salmonella septicemia	As per standard treatment guidelines
Recurrent bacterial pneumonia	As per standard treatment guidelines
Progressive multifocal leukoencephalopathy	Combination ART
Malignancy	
Kaposi's sarcoma	Control of HIV infection with ART; radiotherapy or combination chemotherapy in rare instances
Cerebral lymphoma	As per standard treatment guidelines
Burkitt's lymphoma	As per standard treatment guidelines
Immunoblastic lymphoma	As per standard treatment guidelines
Invasive cervical cancer	As per standard treatment guidelines
Other	
HIV-associated wasting (>10% body weight plus diarrhea, weakness and fever)	Control of HIV infection with ART
HIV-associated dementia	Control of HIV infection with ART
ART, antiretroviral therapy; ARV, antiretroviral drug; HIV, human immunodeficiency virus.	

against the patient's preferences and psychosocial context, and the cost-effectiveness of early treatment.

- Effective treatment with cART can reduce the risk of HIV infection by any mode of transmission.

> **CLINICAL PEARL**
>
> The institution of antiretroviral therapy (ART) carries the risk of triggering immune reconstitution disease (IRD). The risk is higher in patients who are more immunosuppressed at initiation of ART (lower CD4 count), and those who have existing opportunistic infection, even if treated. In IRD, the recovering immune system triggers a dysregulated, often exuberant, inflammatory response to the existing opportunistic infection. This can result in clinical flares of disease that carry a high risk of mortality, especially with cryptococcal and mycobacterial infections. A range of autoimmune phenomena can also occur. Patients with IRD may require corticosteroid therapy.

Factors impairing efficacy of therapy

- Non-adherence.
- Poor tolerability.
- Drug interactions between antivirals, or other medications, that reduce effective drug levels.

Toxicities of antitretroviral drugs (ARVs) are outlined in Table 16-18.

Drug resistance

Drug resistance has been documented in:

- therapy-näive patients who have been infected with resistant virus

- patients who have experienced treatment failure; non-adherence is a major risk factor for this
- all classes of ARV.

It should be tested for in:

- therapy-näive patients
- patients who have experienced treatment failure, to guide treatment changes.

In the virally-suppressed patient on long-term HIV treatment, it is important to screen for and manage potential comorbidities:

- hyperlipidemia
- hypertension
- glucose intolerance and diabetes mellitus
- proteinuria
- osteoporosis.
- depression and other psychosocial issues.

Prognosis

- Prognosis has improved dramatically in all areas of the world where treatment with ARVs is available.
- Prognosis is adversely affected by socioeconomic factors, and concurrent morbidities, especially pulmonary tuberculosis in the developing world.
- Non-AIDS events are now the major cause of death in patients receiving treatment, and the management of HIV in an aging population is a new concern.
- While modern ARVs have improved safety profiles, the challenge now is to further minimise drug toxicity and to manage each patient's comorbid risk factors.

Table 16-18 Antiretroviral drugs

DRUG TARGET	DRUG EXAMPLES	IMPORTANT SPECIFIC DRUG TOXICITIES
Preventing viral entry—chemokine receptor antagonists	Maraviroc	Hepatotoxicity Rash Pyrexia Upper respiratory tract infection Cough GI intolerance
Preventing viral entry—fusion inhibitors; prevent gp41 from achieving fusion-active conformation	Enfuvirtide (T20)	Injection site reactions GI intolerance Fatigue
Preventing reverse transcription—nucleoside reverse transcriptase inhibitors; analogues of native nucleoside substrates	Abacavir Emtricitabine Lamivudine Zalcitabine	Abacavir—hypersensitivity reaction in those with HLA-B*5701; rash; increased cardiovascular risk Zidovudine—bone-marrow suppression

continues

Table 16-18 Antiretroviral drugs *continued*

DRUG TARGET	DRUG EXAMPLES	IMPORTANT SPECIFIC DRUG TOXICITIES
Preventing reverse transcription—nucleotide reverse transcriptase inhibitors	Tenofovir disoproxil fumarate (TDF) Tenofovir alafenamide (TAF)	TDF—renal impairment, reduced bone mineral density
Preventing reverse transcription—non-nucleoside reverse transcriptase inhibitors binding to reverse transcriptase, preventing its action	Etravirine Delavirdine Efavirenz Nevirapine Rilpivirine	Efavirenz—neuropsychiatric changes; nightmares; teratogenic Nevirapine—rash; hepatotoxicity
Preventing integration of HIV into host cell genome—integrase inhibitors	Elvitegravir Raltegravir Dolutegravir Bictegravir	Raltegravir—rhabdomyolysis Dolutegravir—neuropsychiatric changes
Preventing viral polypeptide splicing—protease inhibitors	Atazanavir Fosamprenavir Darunavir Indinavir Saquinavir Ritonavir (used to inhibit metabolism and enhance blood levels of other protease inhibitors)	Class toxicities—hyperlipidemia; hepatotoxicity Atazanavir—hyperbilirubinemia; prolonged PR interval; nephrolithiasis Lopinavir—diabetes
GI, gastrointestinal.		

SELF-ASSESSMENT QUESTIONS

1 A 16-year-old male has perennial symptoms of nasal blockage, excessive sneezing and ocular itch. Which of the following statements is most likely to be TRUE for this patient?

A Skin-prick allergy tests will be strongly positive for birch and ryegrass.
B Allergen avoidance has no role in the management of his condition.
C A cow's-milk-free diet may improve his symptoms.
D Positive serum-specific IgE for *Dermatophagoides pteronyssinus* probably explains the cause of his problem.
E Effective treatment of this problem is unlikely to improve the management of his coexistent bronchial asthma.

2 A 44-year-old female presents with daily episodes of urticaria for approximately 6 months. The urticarial lesions are occurring in a generalized distribution. There have also been four episodes of moderately severe angioedema, affecting the lips and periorbital tissues. The patient has not noted any physical factors that provoke the problem. Which of the following actions would be most appropriate in this circumstance?

A Organize for skin-prick allergy tests to a broad range of foods and aeroallergens.
B Prescribe fexofenadine 180 mg twice daily for a minimum period of 2 months.
C Prescribe a short course of prednisolone 50 mg daily to achieve control of the problem.
D Place the patient on a modified diet that excludes common allergenic foods.
E Order testing for complement components C4 and C1q to exclude hereditary or acquired angioedema.

3 A 50-year-old man suffers acute hypotension during an operation to remove his gallbladder under general anesthesia. The anesthetist notes some urticarial lesions on the torso and increased airway pressures, and treats the patient with epinephrine and fluid volume expansion with good effect. Which *two* of the following actions would constitute appropriate follow-up?

A Take blood immediately for serum tryptase measurement.
B Organize for skin-prick and intradermal testing to the anesthetic drugs used during the procedure as an outpatient.
C Strictly avoid all drugs used during the procedure in future.
D Prescribe the patient an epinephrine self-injecting device.
E Perform a skin test with the agents being used for future anesthesia in the anesthetic bay prior to any further anesthesia, to ensure no new allergies have developed.

4 A 25-year-old male presents with central chest pain of subacute onset, made worse by inspiration and somewhat relieved by leaning forward. He has noticed a rash over his cheeks in recent weeks, and has been feeling fatigued. His wrists and fingers have been aching, especially in the mornings. Physical examination reveals a malar rash with sparing of the nasolabial folds. There are no abnormal cardiac signs, and no obvious joint swelling. Dipstick urinalysis is negative for blood and protein. Laboratory investigations reveal erythrocyte sedimentation rate 45 mm/h (reference range [RR] 1–35 mm/h), C-reactive protein 4.8 mg/L (RR 0.0–5.0 mg/L), antinuclear antibodies 1:640 (homogeneous pattern), double-stranded DNA antibody negative, and microscopic urine examination normal. Which of the following statements is correct in this case?

A The patient should be commenced on prednisolone at a dose of 1 mg/kg/day.
B The chest pain is unlikely to be related to the other symptoms.
C Hydroxychloroquine at a dose of 200 mg twice daily should relieve the symptoms within 48 hours.
D Lack of a pericardial rub makes pericarditis unlikely.
E An electrocardiogram, full blood count and extractable nuclear antigen (ENA) test would be appropriate in this situation.

5 A 75-year-old female with a 50-year history of smoking 30 cigarettes per day presents with severe headaches for 2 weeks. She has been taking prednisolone 5 mg daily for 4 months for the diagnosis of polymyalgia rheumatica (PMR). She denies ocular symptoms or night sweats. She has recently lost several kilograms in weight. She has a longstanding cough with morning sputum production, which has worsened over the past few months. Physical examination reveals a thin woman with a temperature of 37.8°C. There is mild bilateral scalp tenderness but no obvious thickening of the temporal arteries. Which of the following approaches would be appropriate in this situation?

A Arrange for chest radiograph and head computed tomography (CT) for the presumptive diagnosis of lung cancer with cerebral metastases.
B Organize an urgent temporal artery biopsy to exclude giant-cell arteritis (GCA).
C Increase the prednisolone dose to 50 mg daily and organize an urgent temporal artery biopsy.
D Arrange urgent ophthalmological review to exclude ophthalmic artery vasculitis.
E Arrange for urgent erythrocyte sedimentation rate (ESR) and full blood count, and only increase the steroid dose if these have shown substantial change from previous levels.

Questions continue overleaf.

6 A 60-year-old female patient develops pallor and pain of the right hand while camping in cold weather, which last for about an hour. She subsequently develops a persistent dry cough, mild dyspnea on exertion, and feels 'weak'. Physical examination reveals bilateral basal inspiratory lung crackles, no signs of pulmonary hypertension, and marked symmetrical weakness of proximal muscle groups. Which combination of abnormal laboratory results is most likely to correspond to this clinical situation?

A Antinuclear antibodies positive 1:1280, anti-Jo-1 antibodies positive, CK (creatine kinase) 853 U/L (reference range [RR] 26−140 U/L)

B Antinuclear antibodies positive 1:320, anti-RNP antibodies positive, CK 299 U/L (RR 26−140 U/L)

C Antinuclear antibodies positive 1:2560, anti-SS-A antibodies positive, anti-SS-B antibodies positive, rheumatoid factor 42 IU/mL (RR 0−14 IU/mL), CK 130 U/L (RR 26−140 U/L)

D Antinuclear antibodies negative, rheumatoid factor 102 (RR 0−14 IU/mL), CK 53 U/L (RR 26−140 U/L)

E Antinuclear antibodies positive 1:2560, anti-ds-DNA 27 IU/mL (RR 0−6 IU/mL), anti-Sm antibodies positive, CK 330 U/L (RR 26−140 U/L)

7 A 52-year-old non-smoking male presents with a left-hemisphere ischemic stroke. Subsequent investigations reveal:

Activated partial thromboplastin time (APTT)	37 seconds	Reference range (RR) 25−39 seconds
Dilute Russell viper venom time (DRVVT) and phospholipid neutralization:		
Patient DRVVT	40 seconds	RR 32−42 seconds
DRVVT + phospholipid	36 seconds	
DRVVT (normalized) ratio	1.0 seconds	<1.2 = negative 1.2−1.5 = weak positive 1.6−2.0 = moderate positive >2.0 = strong positive
Kaolin ratio	1.1	(RR <1.2)
Cardiolipin IgG antibodies	75 GPL	(RR <5 GPL)
Cardiolipin IgM Abs	45 MPL	(RR <5 MPL)
Beta-2-glycoprotein 1 Abs	33 SGU	(RR <20 SGU)

GPL, unit equivalent to 1 microg of immunoglobulin G; MPL, unit equivalent to 1 microg of immunoglobulin M; SGU, standard IgG anti-beta glycoprotein 2 international units.

Which of the following management approaches would be most appropriate in this situation?

A Aspirin 100 mg daily long-term.

B Subcutaneous therapeutic-dose enoxaparin for 3 months, then recheck cardiolipin antibody levels. If levels remain positive, institute lifelong warfarin therapy.

C Therapeutic-dose intravenous unfractionated heparin until warfarin therapy has been instituted to therapeutic levels. Continue warfarin therapy lifelong.

D Standard therapy for stroke. Recheck cardiolipin antibodies in 3 months. If the IgG cardiolipin antibody level remains positive, institute lifelong warfarin therapy.

E Immediately commence aspirin, intravenous heparin, and warfarin. Once therapeutically warfarinized, discontinue heparin but continue aspirin and warfarin

8 A 21-year-old woman has had five significant episodes of sinusitis and three of pneumonia in the previous 12 months. Which of the following pathology results would be consistent with the most likely diagnosis in this case?

A Normal total IgG levels, but reduced IgG2 and IgG4

B Reduced total hemolytic complement level

C Persistent reduction in the absolute neutrophil count

D Reduced levels of blood CD4+ lymphocytes on flow cytometry

E *TACI* mutation

9 A 35-year-old man with stable human immunodeficiency (HIV) infection for 5 years on treatment with two nucleoside reverse transcriptase inhibitors and efavirenz is found to have detectable HIV viremia (at a low level) for the first time since commencing antiretroviral therapy. Which of the following would be the most appropriate course of action?

A Perform antiretroviral resistance testing, and add a protease inhibitor.

B Suspend antiretroviral therapy while waiting for antiretroviral resistance testing and CD4+ T-cell numbers.

C Perform antiretroviral resistance testing and change to a different three-drug regimen.

D Perform antiretroviral resistance testing, CD4+ T-cell numbers, and maintain the current regimen pending the results.

E Review and reinforce medication adherence, and arrange to re-examine HIV viral load at the next clinical review.

ANSWERS

1 D.

This is a typical case of persistent allergic rhinoconjunctivitis, which is usually caused by exposure to perennial allergens such as house dust mite or animal danders. The demonstration of specific IgE to *Dermatophagoides pteronyssinus* strongly suggests that the house dust mite is the cause. Specific house dust mite reduction measures, particularly in the bedroom, may help alleviate symptoms, and should be employed in addition to other therapy. Cow's milk does not cause persistent allergic rhinoconjunctivitis. Birch or ryegrass allergy causes seasonal (spring and summer) symptoms rather than perennial ones. There is evidence that improved control of allergic rhinitis symptoms results in improved asthma control.

2 B.

Of the options given, prescription of a prolonged course of adequate-dose non-sedating H_1 antihistamines is the appropriate course of action in chronic idiopathic urticaria and angioedema (CIU/A). CIU/A is not an allergic or diet-related condition, so allergy testing and elimination diets are not appropriate. Corticosteroids should be avoided in CIU/A if at all possible, as this is a chronic problem, and reliance on steroids is likely to cause significant morbidity. The exception would be if a severe bout of angioedema was present. Angioedema secondary to a complement deficiency is not associated with urticaria. Failure of high-dose antihistamine therapy to control the symptoms should prompt consideration of the use of omalizumab.

3 A and B.

This is a typical history of anaphylaxis to general anesthesia. Measuring serum tryptase promptly will help confirm the diagnosis of anaphylaxis. Formal skin testing in a specialized clinic for allergy to the agents used—and generally to a standard panel of anesthetic drugs—is essential to identify the culprit. This will also allow the patient to have access to the drugs which were not the cause of the reaction in the future. It may be very difficult to avoid all of the drugs which were administered on this occasion in the future if the patient requires further surgery. The patient does not need an epinephrine self-injecting device if his only anaphylaxis risk is general anesthesia! Non-standardized skin testing is not a safe way to diagnose drug allergy.

4 E.

This patient most likely has acute pericarditis in the setting of systemic lupus erythematosus (SLE). A combination of malar rash, arthralgia and positive antinuclear antibody in a young male has a high positive predictive value for the disease. Elevated erythocyte sediment rate (ESR) with normal C-reactive protein is typical of SLE. Pericardial rub is an insensitive sign for pericarditis, so an electrocardiogram and echocardiogram should be performed. The presence of anti-Sm, anti-SS-A, or anti-SS-B on ENA testing would be strong evidence of SLE, although sensitivity is low. Evidence of a lymphopenia or normochromic, normocytic anemia would also be consistent with SLE. Treatment in this situation would be appropriate with non-steroidal anti-inflammatories, and possibly low-dose corticosteroids. There is no apparent indication for high-dose steroids. Hydroxychloroquine is a good choice for ongoing therapy, but its effect is not rapid so other treatment is needed in the short term.

5 C.

Approximately 20% of patients with PMR will go on to develop GCA. Being on low-dose corticosteroids may disguise some of the symptoms and signs of GCA, so the lack of visual symptoms or palpable temporal arteries should not reassure the clinician that GCA has not developed. Similarly, the lack of serological evidence of an acute phase response, while being unusual, does not exclude GCA altogether. Headache is the most common symptom of GCA. To miss the diagnosis of GCA and not treat it, only to have a patient go blind or have a stroke, is a disaster. The approach should always be to treat the patient for GCA while organizing diagnostic tests. While involvement of an ophthalmologist in the case may be important, they will not usually be able to diagnose changes due to GCA in the absence of ocular symptoms.

6 A.

The combination of Raynaud's phenomenon, myopathy and probable interstitial lung disease is a classic presentation of the anti-synthetase variant of polymyositis. The presence of antinuclear antibodies and anti-Jo-1 antibodies would be consistent with this, and the markedly elevated CK level would indicate significant myositis. Answer B would be more consistent with mixed connective tissue disease, where pulmonary fibrosis would be unlikely. Answer C is likely to be Sjögren's syndrome. The findings in answer D could be present in rheumatoid arthritis, where one would not expect a myopathy. Answer E is consistent with systemic lupus erythematosus, where myopathy to this degree and rapidly developing pulmonary fibrosis would be unusual.

Table 16-19 summarizes disease associations with autoantibodies.

Table 16-19 Autoantibodies and disease associations

DISEASE	AUTOANTIBODY	PREVALENCE/COMMENT
Systemic lupus erythematosus (SLE)	ANA	>95%; homogeneous pattern more specific
	ds-DNA	~50%; high specificity; risk factor for renal disease
	SS-A	30–50%; also found in Sjögren's syndrome
	SS-B	10%; also found in Sjögren's syndrome
	Sm	20–30%; high specificity
Drug-induced lupus	Histone	>70% specificity; not associated with drug-induced lupus due to anti-TNF (tumor necrosis factor) therapy (infliximab, etanercept)
Sjögren's syndrome	ANA	Up to 80%; speckled pattern associated with SS-A and SS-B
	SS-A (Ro)	60–95%; responsible for neonatal lupus (only about 2% of SS-A-positive women will have babies with neonatal lupus)
	SS-B (La)	40–90%
Polymyositis (PM)/ dermatomyositis (DM)	ANA	60–90%; variable pattern
	Myositis-specific antibodies: Anti-synthetase including Jo-1	20%; associated with anti-synthetase syndrome; more common in PM than DM
	Anti-signal recognition	Not routinely measured
	Anti-Mi-2	Not routinely measured
	Myositis-associated antibodies: includes anti-PM-Scl, anti-U1RNP, anti-Ku	Not routinely measured
Scleroderma	ANA	Up to 90%; nucleolar pattern reasonably specific
	Scl-70	~50%
	Centromere	~10%
CREST syndrome	ANA	Up to 90%; nucleolar pattern reasonably specific
	Centromere	~80%
	Scl-70	<10%
Mixed connective tissue disease	ANA	>90%
	RNP	Approaches 100% sensitivity; also found in SLE and scleroderma
Antiphospholipid syndrome (APS)	Cardiolipin Lupus inhibitor Beta$_2$-GP-1	Demonstration of one of these antiphospholipid antibodies necessary for diagnosis of APS; 25% of SLE patients are antibody-positive
Granulomatosis with polyangiitis (Wegener's granulomatosis)	c-ANCA (proteinase 3)	>90%
	p-ANCA (myeloperoxidase)	Occasional
Microscopic polyangiitis	p-ANCA (myeloperoxidase)	80%
	c-ANCA (proteinase 3)	Occasional
Eosinophilic granulomatosis with polyangiitis (Churg–Strauss syndrome)	p-ANCA (myeloperoxidase)	50%
	c-ANCA (proteinase 3)	Occasional

7 C.

The results show strongly positive anti-cardiolipin and beta-2-glycoprotein 1 antibodies, consistent with the anti-phospholipid syndrome (APS), and very likely to have caused a thromboembolic stroke. The lupus inhibitor is not present, as evidenced by the normal DRVVT and phospholipid neutralization, and normal APTT.

Russell viper venom (RVV) contains a coagulant that activates factor X, which in turn converts prothrombin into thrombin in the presence of phospholipid and factor V. The DRVVT will therefore be prolonged in the case of either the presence of an inhibitor of phospholipid or a deficiency of factor V or prothrombin. In the laboratory, a standard sample of RVV and phospholipid is used that will give a clotting time within a range when combined with normal serum. Abnormal serum that contains some types of antiphospholipid antibody will result in a prolonged time. The lupus inhibitor prolongs the DRVVT, whereas most other anti-cardiolipin and beta-2-glycoprotein 1 antibodies do not.

Without anti-coagulation, this patient is at high risk of further thrombosis. Antiplatelet therapy is not adequate therapy, and there is no evidence that both anticoagulation and antiplatelet therapy need to be used concurrently in APS. Technically, the presence of the anti-cardiolipin antibodies needs to be documented on two occasions 12 weeks apart for the diagnosis of APS, but there is no reason to use enoxaparin for 3 months rather than warfarin.

In the unlikely event that the anti-cardiolipin antibody levels are no longer elevated when checked at 3 months, and if no other predisposing factors to stroke have been identified in this patient, it would still be advisable to continue lifelong anticoagulation.

8 E.

A mutation in *TACI* is found in a small number of patients with common variable immunodeficiency (CVID). This case history is typical of CVID, which tends to come on in teenagers or young adults, and classically results in recurrent respiratory tract infection. IgG subclass deficiency has not been shown to significantly increase the risk of recurrent infection. Complement deficiencies usually present with invasive infection due to encapsulated organisms, such as *Neisseria meningitides* or *Streptococcus pneumoniae*. Neutropenic disorders are more likely to present with abscesses, septicemia, and oral mucosal infections. Reduced levels of T cells are associated with opportunistic viral and fungal infections.

9 D.

In this situation, the most likely explanation for the loss of viremic control is non-adherence to therapy. There are multiple possible explanations for this: adverse drug reactions, concern over long-term medication use, psychosocial factors, or simple difficulty with remembering to take daily medication. It is important to explore these issues with the patient and use this opportunity to reinforce the importance of adherence. Drug resistance is very possible if adherence has been patchy; however, testing may not be able to be performed if there is low level viraemia only. Any change in treatment, however, is best made with knowledge of the resistance pattern.

CHAPTER 17

MUSCULOSKELETAL MEDICINE

Carlos El Haddad and Kevin Pile

CHAPTER OUTLINE

Musculoskeletal disease and/or injury is an almost universal human experience. Multiple branches of medicine deal with varying aspects of the musculoskeletal system, but it is the internist who will often be required to make the more difficult diagnoses, and institute and supervise an increasingly sophisticated array of available treatments, particularly for chronic conditions.

AN APPROACH TO A PATIENT WITH PAINFUL JOINTS

History

You should assess the following:

- Are the symptoms related to a musculoskeletal problem, and which part?
- Was there an identified trigger or precipitant?
- Why has the patient presented at this time?
- What has been the pattern or progression of symptoms?
- Are there features of a systemic illness or inflammatory symptoms?
- Has anything helped the problem?

Pain and loss of function are primary presenting symptoms, and while usually coexistent this is not always the case.

- Is the pain in a joint; in a related joint structure such as tendon, ligament or bursa; or in a bone?
- What is the nature of the pain; when does it occur; and what is the effect of movement? The red flag for malignant pain is a dull, deep ache within a bone that occurs at night or when resting. Similar symptoms may occur with Paget's disease or with a fracture.

The cardinal features of the joint pain will often help distinguish inflammatory from mechanical etiologies (Box 17-1).

- Onset of symptoms following specific trauma self-evidently supports mechanical disruption of a joint, its surrounding capsule and ligaments, or a bone fracture.

Box 17-1

Differentiators of joint pain

Inflammatory musculoskeletal pain	Non-inflammatory/ mechanical pain
• Pain and stiffness predominant in the morning and at the end of the day • Stiffness for >30 minutes • Symptoms lessen with activity • Pain does not improve with rest • Localized erythema, swelling, tenderness • Systemic features— fatigue, weight loss	• Short-lived joint stiffness • Pain worsens with activity • Pain improves with rest

---

- Less obvious triggers to explore are infectious exposures (Box 17-2), which should include vaccinations (rubella) and recent travel (Lyme disease after tick bites).
  - » The *Togaviridae* family of viruses, which include the arthropod-borne alphavirus, and rubella virus are a significant cause of arthritis worldwide.
  - » Viruses such as Ross River, chikungunya, o'nyong-nyong, Barmah Forest, Mayaro and Sindbis are associated with outbreaks of viral arthritis in South America, Europe, Africa, Asia and Australia.
- Several infections may not be overtly symptomatic (e.g. a rash may not be seen or may be quite mild in Ross River or Barmah Forest virus infection), or the site of infection may produce no symptoms (e.g. chlamydial urethritis/cervicitis with resultant reactive arthritis). The connection between genitourinary symptoms and arthritis will not be self-evident to patients.
- The majority of viral arthropathies resolve within 6–8 weeks, and can be excluded from the differential diagnosis of chronic arthropathies.

Box 17-2

Common infections associated with arthritis

Viral*	Gastrointestinal	Genitourinary
Hepatitis B, hepatitis C	*Salmonella typhimurium*	*Chlamydia trachomatis*
Rubella	*Shigella flexneri*	*Gonococcus* spp.
Parvovirus	*Yersinia enterocolitica*	
Arbovirus	*Campylobacter jejuni*	
Coxsackievirus		
Cytomegalovirus		
Varicella		
Human immunodeficiency virus		

*Serology should be tested according to exposure.

A comprehensive family history is a key part of each and every history.

- A familial pattern of a specific diagnosis such as rheumatoid arthritis, ankylosing spondylitis or systemic lupus erythematosus (SLE) highlights that particular diagnosis and may also raise related diagnoses that are particularly relevant for seronegative spondyloarthritides, such as psoriasis or inflammatory bowel disease in first-degree relatives.
- A family history of other, non-musculoskeletal autoimmunity such as thyroid disease or type 1 diabetes mellitus is also a risk factor for autoimmune arthritis.

Examination

The examination of a patient with arthritis identifies the pattern and number of joints involved and whether extra-articular features are present, as detailed in Table 17-1. The cardinal features of inflammation are sought:

- *systemic features*—temperature, pulse and blood pressure
- *joint features*—localized erythema and warmth, tenderness to touch, soft boggy inflammation obscuring the joint margins, and reduced function.

Due to its prevalence, coexisting osteoarthritis is common, and hence the patient may well have the hard bony swelling of osteophytes in the distal interphalangeal (DIP) and proximal interphalangeal (PIP) joints of the hands, in addition to the inflammatory findings.

Examination will reveal:

- how many joints are involved, separating monoarthritis from oligoarthritis (≤4 joints) and polyarthritis (>4 joints)
- whether these joints are large or small
- whether there is spinal (particularly sacroiliac) involvement.

Distal to the wrist and ankle there are at least 56 joints, so that as the number of joints increases in the hands and feet, the pattern becomes increasingly 'symmetrical'.

As well as a joint focus, the fingernails are assessed for pitting or onycholysis suggestive of psoriasis, and the scalp, umbilicus, natal cleft and extensor surfaces of the knee and elbow should be inspected. The presence of a malar rash or photosensitive rash in a young woman who has additional constitutional features would elevate SLE in the differential diagnosis.

CLINICAL PEARL

Parvovirus B-19 may cause an acute symmetric polyarthritis and aplastic anemia with a positive rheumatoid factor.

Table 17-1 Patterns of arthritis

	PATTERN				
	MONO-ARTHRITIS	INFLAMMATORY SPINAL DISEASE SACROILIITIS	ASYMMETRICAL LARGE JOINT ARTHRITIS	SYMMETRICAL SMALL JOINT ARTHRITIS (MCP, PIP, MTP)	DIP HANDS
Differential diagnosis	Trauma Hemophilia Septic Gout Pseudogout	Ankylosing spondylitis Psoriatic arthritis IBD	Psoriatic arthritis Reactive arthritis IBD	RA SLE Psoriatic arthritis	Inflammatory OA (if involves PIP and 1st CMC) Psoriatic arthritis
Further investigations	X-ray Aspirate for crystals and culture	Review personal and family history HLA-B27 X-ray lumbar spine and SI joints MRI sacroiliac joints	Review personal and family history Examine scalp and buttocks for psoriasis Examine for conjunctivitis and urethritis Infection screen	Examine for rheumatoid nodules, skin rashes, serositis or mucositis Urinalysis RF, CCP antibodies, ANA X-ray hands and feet	X-ray hands

ANA, anti-nuclear antibodies; CCP, cyclic citrullinated peptides; CMC, carpometacarpophalangeal; DIP, distal interphalangeal; HLA, human leukocyte antigen; IBD, inflammatory bowel disease; MCP, metacarpophalangeal; MTP, metatarsophalangeal; OA, osteoarthritis; PIP, proximal interphalangeal; RA, rheumatoid arthritis; RF, rheumatoid factor; SI, sacroiliac; SLE, systemic lupus erythematosus.

Investigations

Investigations serve four purposes:

1. to confirm or refute a diagnosis
2. to monitor for known complications of the disease or the treatment
3. to identify a parameter that changes with disease activity or treatment
4. to contextualize the presenting problem, e.g. are there coexisting medical conditions in the patient which may have an impact on the diagnostic or therapeutic process?

The last includes the non-specific inflammatory markers ESR (erythrocyte sedimentation rate) and CRP (C-reactive protein). If a person's joints are hot and swollen upon examination, the ESR or CRP result is not diagnostic but it is a parameter to monitor.

CLINICAL PEARLS

- Whenever the possibility of a septic joint is considered, aspiration of the joint is mandatory. Aspirated fluid should be sent to the laboratory for crystal microscopy, cell count and differential, Gram staining, culture and sensitivities. Specific tests for tuberculosis and fungal infection may be indicated.
- On a joint aspiration, $\leq 5000/mm^3$ white cells suggests rheumatoid arthritis, spondyloarthopathies, gout or pseudogout; ≥ 5000 white cells/mm^3 is likely to be septic arthritis.

RHEUMATOID ARTHRITIS (RA)

Rheumatoid arthritis is a chronic inflammatory disease affecting the synovium, and leading to joint damage and absorption of adjacent bone.

- The overall incidence of RA is 20–50 per 100,000 per year, and the prevalence ranges from 0.3–1.1%.
- Age of onset peaks in the 5th decade, and females are 2–3 times more likely to be affected than males, although the sex distribution becomes less apparent with increasing age.
- Apart from the suffering and disability caused by the disease, it also has a significant impact on life expectancy, with RA patients living on average 3–10 years less than unaffected patients in the background population.

Genetics and environmental contribution to RA

The etiology of RA is complex, involving interplay between genetic and environmental factors (see Figure 17-1).

- The prevalence of RA in first-degree relatives of RA sufferers is approximately 10 times that of the background population.
- The major susceptibility gene for RA (*HLA-DRB1*) is located in the class II histocompatibility region on chromosome 6p.

- Risk of RA is associated with human leukocyte antigen (HLA) DR4 and DR1 alleles, which have similar beta-chain sequences, potentially affecting the selection and presentation of arthritogenic peptides to CD4+ T cells.
- The HLA component accounts for only 30% of the genetic risk of RA, and other genes associated with RA include tumor necrosis factor alpha (TNF-alpha); peptidyl arginine deaminases (PADIs) that catalyze the citrullination of arginine residues and, therefore, determine the level of citrullinated peptides; and PTNP22 (tyrosine phosphate non-receptor type 22) that has also been linked with type 1 diabetes and autoimmune thyroid disease, due to reduced deletion of autoreactive T cells.

Smoking is the most potent environmental trigger, with smokers at two- to fourfold increased risk of RA and heavy smokers being at higher risk than light smokers.

- Smoking is associated with citrullination of alveolar proteins throughout the body, with citrullinated antigens binding with more affinity to HLA-DR4.
- More severe rheumatoid disease is seen in smokers with erosive arthropathy, rheumatoid nodules, and vasculitis.
- The increased risk of RA persists for up to 20 years after cessation of smoking.

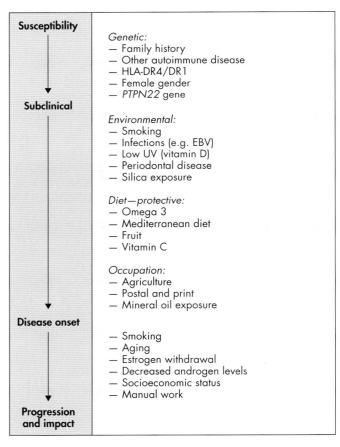

Figure 17-1 Development of rheumatoid arthritis. EBV, Epstein–Barr virus; HLA, human leukocyte antigen; PTPN22, protein tyrosine phosphatase non-receptor type 22

Workers exposed to silica dust (drilling or crushing rock) are at up to a threefold risk of RA.

It is not clear why the prevalence of RA is so much higher in women compared with men. Estrogen exposure in women has a protective effect, with a decreased incidence of RA noted among users of oral contraceptive pills. This is consistent with increased risk of the disease after the menopause, and the slight protective effect of using hormone replacement therapy.

The strongest evidence of an infectious trigger for RA is with Epstein–Barr virus (EBV), the glycoprotein of which has cross-reactivity with the HLA-DRB1 shared epitope. Increased incidence and levels of EBV DNA have been reported in peripheral blood mononuclear cells and synovial fluid of RA patients, and the virus is well described to have immunomodulatory properties.

One of the more interesting infectious links brings together the long-described association of periodontitis with RA, and the more recent anti-cyclic citrullinated peptide antibodies (anti-CCP antibody; sensitivity 76%; specificity 96%).

Pathology

The underlying pathology of RA transforms the synovium into a chronically inflamed tissue.

- The normally thin synovial layer thickens dramatically due to accumulation of macrophage-like and fibroblast-like synoviocytes.
- The sub-synovial layer becomes edematous, hypervascular, and hypercellular with the accumulation of macrophages, mast cells, CD4+ T cells, CD8+ T cells, natural killer (NK) cells, B cells and plasma cells.
- The increased number of cells in the synovium in RA is believed to result from recruitment of blood-derived leukocytes, as well as increased proliferation and reduced apoptosis.
- Neutrophils are abundant in rheumatoid synovial fluid but are sparse within the synovium.

In concert with this inflammatory process, the inflamed synovium invades adjacent cartilage and bone.

- Cartilage injury is caused by the generation of degradative enzymes including matrix metalloproteinases, and aggrecanases.
- Cytokines released from synovial tissue affect distant chondrocyte production in the extracellular matrix.
- Bone injury is separately mediated by a process of osteoclast activation. Osteoclast activation occurs via a receptor known as RANK (receptor activator of nuclear factor kappa-B). The ligand system for this receptor, RANKL, is a member of the TNF superfamily. It is produced in the inflammatory setting by osteoclasts after stimulation by cytokines released from macrophages and/or fibroblasts.

CLINICAL PEARL

Rheumatoid arthritis involves the metacarpophalangeal (MCP) and proximal interphalangeal (PIP) joints, but not the distal interphalangeal (DIP) joints.

Box 17-3
1987 ACR criteria for RA

1 Morning stiffness of greater than 1 hour's duration.
2 Objective evidence of joint inflammation such as soft-tissue swelling or fluid in 3 of 14 defined joint areas (being right or left PIP, MCP, wrist, elbow, knee, ankle, and MTP joints).
3 At least one of the joint areas demonstrating inflammation must be in the hands.
4 Simultaneous involvement of the same joint area bilaterally in at least one pair.
5 Rheumatoid nodules.
6 A positive rheumatoid factor using a method that is positive in <5% of normal subjects.
7 Typical changes of RA in hand and wrist X-rays, which must include erosions or unequivocal periarticular osteopenia.

ACR, American College of Rheumatology; MCP, metacarpophalangeal; MTP, metatarsophalangeal; PIP, proximal interphalangeal; RA, rheumatoid arthritis.

Diagnosis

The American College of Rheumatology (ACR) has developed criteria for the epidemiological classification of RA (requires a patient to meet four of seven criteria; Box 17-3). Clinical features should have been present for at least 6 weeks.

The newer 2010 ACR criteria (Table 17-2, overleaf) allow the diagnosis of RA to be made earlier, but include a greater percentage of persons who subsequently go into remission and may not have had classical RA. Definite RA requires a score of 6 or greater.

CLINICAL PEARL

The American College of Rheumatology scoring system reinforces the mental picture of rheumatoid arthritis (RA) as one of peripheral small joint polyarthritis of greater than 6 weeks' duration, with laboratory evidence of acute inflammation and serology suggestive of RA.

Clinical features and complications

Rheumatoid arthritis is a systemic disease with predominant articular manifestations, but also includes myriad extra-articular disease encompassing most systems.

- Synovitis manifests as tender, hot and functionally restricted joints, and in RA has a predilection for the PIP, MCP, wrist and MTP joints.
  - » More proximal joints such as ankle, knee, shoulder, cervical spine and temperomandibular joint can also be involved.
  - » Synovial tissue also surrounds many tendons, with resultant swelling and pain.
- As disease progresses, the synovial inflammation secondarily destabilizes the supporting joint ligaments and tendon pulleys, allowing subluxation.

Table 17-2 2010 ACR criteria for RA

	SCORE
A. Joint involvement	
1 large joint (shoulder, elbow, hip, knee, ankle)	0
2–10 large joints	1
1–3 small joints (MCP, MTP, PIP, wrist)	2
4–10 small joints	3
>10 joints (at least 1 small joint)	5
B. Serology (at least one result needed)	
Negative RF and negative CCP antibodies	0
Low positive RF or low positive CCP (1–3 × upper limit of normal [ULN])	2
High positive RF or high positive CCP	3
C. Acute-phase reactants (at least one needed)	
Normal CRP and normal ESR	0
Abnormal CRP or abnormal ESR	1
D. Duration	
<6 weeks	0
≥6 weeks	1

ACR, American College of Rheumatology; CCP, cyclic citrullinated peptides; CRP, C-reactive protein; ESR, erythrocyte sedimentation rate; MCP, metacarpophalangeal; MTP, metatarsophalangeal; PIP, proximal interphalangeal; RA, rheumatoid arthritis, RF, rheumatoid factor.

» The classical deformities of RA are volar subluxation of the hand at the wrist with ulnar deviation, and subluxation of the fingers at the MCP joints with ulnar deviation.

» The fingers themselves may develop either 'swan-neck' deformity (hyperextension of the PIP joint, with flexion of the DIP joint) or 'boutonniere' deformity (flexion of PIP joint, with hyperextension of the DIP joint)—and both may occur within the same person. See Figure 17-2.

CLINICAL PEARL

While the presenting complaint may relate to the hands, an examination and palpation of the metatarsophalangeal joints is essential and will often reveal unrecognized synovitis, which often begins in the 4th joint. Later dorsal subluxation at this joint leads to severe pain due to weightbearing on the metatarsal heads, callous formation on the soles of the feet, and abrasions on the subluxed toes from rubbing on footwear.

Extra-articular manifestations should be considered. They include:

- scleritis and corneal thinning leading to rupture
- pleural effusions
- pulmonary fibrosis
- pericarditis
- vasculitic ulcers—particularly nailfold infarcts, leg ulcers
- rheumatoid nodules—skin and lungs
- mononeuritis multiplex
- atlanto–axial subluxation with spinal cord compression (C1–C8 dermatomes and any paresthesiae or hyper-reflexia should be checked for)
- Felty's syndrome (splenomegaly, neutropenia)

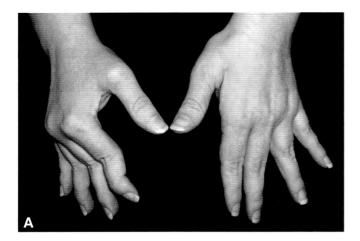
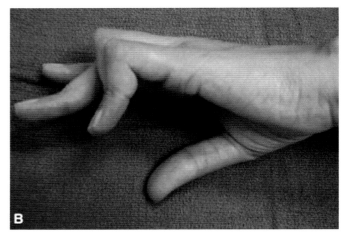

Figure 17-2 (**A**) Hyperextension of the proximal interphalangeal (PIP) joints and hyperflexion of the distal interphalangeal (DIP) joints in the right hand, demonstrating the swan neck deformity. (**B**) Hyperflexion of the PIP and hyperextension of the DIP joints, which is the boutonnière deformity

From: (A) Sebastin SD and Chung KC. Reconstruction of digital deformities in rheumatoid arthritis. Hand Clinics 2011;27(1):87–104. (B) Canale ST and Beaty JH (eds). Campbell's Operative orthopaedics, 12th ed. Philadelphia: Elsevier, 2013.

- large granular lymphocyte (LGL) syndrome (splenomegaly, neutropenia, infections, risk of leukemia)
- Raynaud's phenomenon
- cricoarytenoiditis (if an RA patient has neck pain, sore throat or hoarseness, cricoarytenoiditis must be ruled out before intubating because of the risk of airway collapse)
- pyoderma
- secondary Sjögren's syndrome
- anemia
- thrombocytosis
- peripheral neuropathy.

Investigations

There are no specific tests to confirm the diagnosis of RA. Investigations are undertaken to:

- support the differential diagnosis
- clarify the impact and severity of the diagnosis at that time
- detect physiological changes that will affect management.

Rheumatoid factor (RF) is a polyclonal antibody predominantly of the IgM and IgG (immunoglobulin) classes, which targets the Fc region of IgG.

- While commonly thought to have diagnostic significance by both doctors and patients, it has a very poor predictive value, being present in only 70% of RA cohorts and also present in at least 5% of the normal population. The resulting lack of specificity for RA can lead to confusion, and unnecessary treatment.
- RF positivity increases with age, and is positive in any circumstance with prolonged antigen stimulation such as malaria, bronchiectasis, and tuberculosis.

Anti-cyclic citrullinated peptide (anti-CCP) antibody is a useful diagnostic test for RA. The sensitivity is of the same order as RF. The specificity improves when anti-CCP antibodies and RF are present concurrently.

> ### CLINICAL PEARLS
> - Rheumatoid nodules and rheumatoid factor (RF) positivity are linked pathologies, with the presence of nodules almost guaranteeing the presence of RF, but not vice versa. RF positivity is associated with increased joint erosions, and vasculitis.
> - The patient with a swollen calf and RA or osteoarthritis (OA) may have ruptured a Baker's cyst—examine the posterior knee for a cyst.

X-ray changes in RA mirror the joints clinically involved, primarily affecting the hands, the PIP and MCP joints, and the wrists. Soft tissue swelling occurs early, with periarticular osteopenia noted, and subsequently symmetrical joint space narrowing. Erosions, when they occur, begin at the site of synovial lining of the joint capsule, reflecting onto the cartilage/periosteum junctions so that they occur slightly distant from the joint surface.

The inflammatory process affects other investigations nonspecifically, with no findings unique to RA.

- Erythrocyte sedimentation rate (ESR) and C-reactive protein (CRP) will both be raised in accordance with the inflammatory process, and will act as a monitor of therapy with the goal being their normalization.
- CRP is the first to rise and fall after an inflammatory stimulus, and is the preferred measurement for monitoring success in suppressing joint inflammation, particularly in RA.

> ### CLINICAL PEARL
> Despite lack of specificity, C-reactive protein will be the first inflammatory marker to rise and fall, and is the preferred way to monitor joint inflammation.

The blood film commonly will show:

- inflammatory thrombocytosis
- normochromic normocytic anemia
- hypochromic microcytic anemia due to iron deficiency, which can occur after prolonged inflammation due to the inflammatory process blocking the utilization of the body's iron stores; concomitant therapies such as non-steroidal anti-inflammatory drugs (NSAIDs) may cause genuine iron deficiency via gastrointestinal blood loss
- often, a neutrophil leukocytosis induced by corticosteroids.

The standard clinical examination should include urinalysis, with the presence of proteinuria or leukocytes warranting further microscopy and evaluation.

Investigations should also include:

- electrolytes, urea and creatinine
- liver function tests (potential hepatotoxicity with some treatments).

Treatment

To minimize the morbidity of RA, long-term management of patients is required, based on drug treatment, non-pharmacological approaches including physiotherapy, and psychosocial support. As yet there are no reliably curative or disease-remitting therapies, although considerable gains have been made recently with the advent of biological therapies for this condition.

Traditional disease-modifying anti-rheumatic drugs (DMARDs)

There is no way of predicting who will respond to a particular therapy, either a conventional DMARD or a biological DMARD, and therefore a decision pathway must be used. A pathway for treating RA is shown in Figure 17-3 (overleaf), with adjunct therapy of oral steroids, joint injections, and hydroxychloroquine used as required.

- Intra-articular and/or low-dose oral corticosteroids are frequently administered as bridging therapy until the effect of DMARDs is fully established.

- In some patients they are used long-term with DMARDs, in order to satisfactorily suppress the disease.
- Corticosteroids may also be used alone in the elderly for disease control, if this can be achieved with a daily dose equivalent to 7.5 mg prednisolone or less.

Methotrexate underpins current treatment regimens, and may be commenced alone or in combination with leflunomide or sulfasalazine. If disease remission cannot be achieved using these agents within 6–9 months, then consideration of biological agents should be made.

- Methotrexate is currently the 'gold standard' DMARD, with doses accelerated to achieve 20–25 mg/week within 6–8 weeks of commencement, with folic acid supplementation of 5 mg/week.

Objective outcomes need to be recorded, including:

- swollen and tender joint counts
- inflammatory markers (ESR, CRP)
- a quality of life/functional index.

The principal side-effects of methotrexate include:

- bone marrow suppression (note that trimethoprim is an anti-folate and must be avoided because this can induce cytopenia)
- pneumonitis (not dose-related)
- liver fibrosis
- hepatitis
- nausea
- mouth ulcers.

Failure to achieve remission of disease activity after a maximum of 3–4 months of methotrexate therapy should result in an escalation to combination therapy, or switching of therapy.

- Leflunomide is administered at 20 mg daily, and sulfasalazine is commenced at 500 mg daily and increased at 500 mg/week to 2 g daily, and occasionally to 3 g daily.

- Biological agents targeting specific cytokines such as TNF (adalimumab, golimumab, infliximab, etanercept, certolizumab), and interleukin-6 (tocilizumab), or that block cell-to-cell signaling such as that through CTLA$_4$-Ig (abatacept) are becoming increasingly used in those who do not respond quickly to 'standard' therapy, and may become standard or first-line therapy as cost reduction alters their cost–benefit profile. Janus kinase (JAK) inhibitors (e.g. tofacitinib, baricitinib) are now also available to treat rheumatoid arthritis, with similar efficacy to biological agents.

CLINICAL PEARLS

- Despite the development of biological agents, methotrexate remains the anchor drug (alone or in combination) for the majority of patients with rheumatoid arthritis.
- Anti-tumor necrosis factor therapy should not be utilized in patients with any demyelinating disorder, or severe congestive heart failure.

Omega-3 oil supplementation

Inflammation is characterized by the production of arachidonic-acid-derived eicosanoids (prostaglandins, thromboxanes, leukotrienes). Long-chain omega-3 fatty acids, eicosapentaenoic acid (EPA) and docosahexaenoic acid (DHA) have anti-inflammatory properties when taken in doses greater than 2.7 g daily, and are of proven benefit in RA—including reduced morning stiffness, decreased tender joint count, and a lessened need for treatment with NSAIDs.

Monitoring of DMARD and biological therapies

All RA patients requiring immunosuppressive therapy should be screened for hepatitis B and C and for tuberculosis, according to local guidelines.

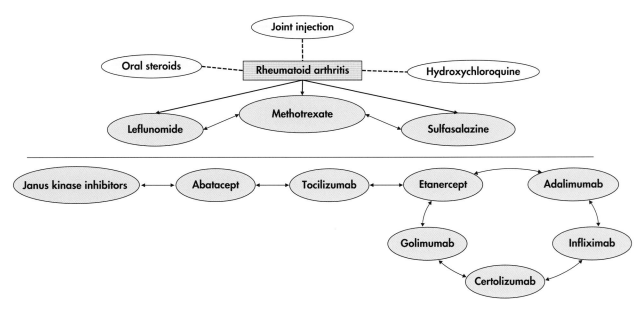

Figure 17-3 Schema of rheumatoid arthritis therapy

Table 17-3 Monitoring of anti-rheumatic therapy

THERAPY	BASELINE MONITORING	PERIODIC MONITORING
NSAIDs	BP, edema, K$^+$, creatinine	K$^+$ and creatinine at 1 week BP and edema at each clinical visit Annual FBC
Methotrexate	Chest X-ray, hepatitis B and C serology, FBC, LFT	FBC, LFT at 4–6 weekly intervals Chest auscultation at each clinical visit
Sulfasalazine	FBC, LFT	FBC, LFT monthly × 3, then 3-monthly
Leflunomide	Chest X-ray, hepatitis B and C serology, FBC, LFT	FBC, LFT at 4–6 weekly intervals; extend to 12-weekly when stable Chest auscultation at each clinical visit
Biological therapy	Chest X-ray, hepatitis B and C serology Screen for latent TB, as per local guidelines	As clinically indicated

BP, blood pressure; K$^+$, serum potassium; FBC, full blood count/screen; LFT liver function tests; NSAIDs, non-steroidal anti-inflammatory drugs; TB, tuberculosis; TNF, tumor necrosis factor.

Table 17-3 describes a guide for monitoring anti-rheumatic therapy.

Conclusions

Early recognition of RA and undifferentiated poor-prognosis arthritis, and prompt disease suppression with DMARDs and prednisolone, are key to the initial improvement of the patient's quality of life and to minimizing subsequent progressive joint damage.

Methotrexate retains its key role in the treatment of RA and, while there remains controversy over unequivocal demonstration of the superiority of combination therapy, several studies do support the concept. Some of the best evidence in support of combination therapy is that of TNF blockers when combined with methotrexate, in which the combination is significantly superior to monotherapy with either agent with respect to clinical, functional and radiographical outcome.

SPONDYLOARTHROPATHIES

The spondyloarthropathies are a group of disorders characterized by inflammation of the spine and sacroiliac joints, and may include an oligoarthritis with a preference for hip and shoulder joints. Ankylosing spondylitis (AS) is the prototypic disease, and as a group they share several common factors, as depicted in Figure 17-4.

The principal diagnoses are AS, psoriatic arthritis (PsA), reactive arthritis (ReA), and inflammatory bowel disease (IBD)-associated arthritis. Common to many classifications is an undifferentiated spondyloarthropathy and a juvenile-onset chronic arthritis. Despite the separate diagnoses and mucocutaneous manifestations, there is significant overlap, with:

- subtle colitis and terminal ileitis in AS
- the palmar lesions of reactive arthritis being histologically indistinguishable from pustular psoriasis

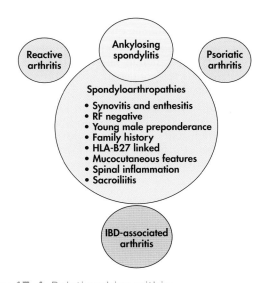

Figure 17-4 Relationships within spondyloarthropathies. HLA, human leukocyte antigen; IBD, inflammatory bowel disease; RF, rheumatoid factor

- the presence of high bacterial populations in psoriatic plaques possibly inciting a reactive component.

The key and unique pathology of spondyloarthropathies is enthesitis/enthesial inflammation (inflammation of tendon and ligament insertions into bone), which occurs at sites of physical stress.

- Easily identified sites of enthesitis are plantar fasciitis, or Achilles tendinitis.
- The same pathology occurs within the axial skeleton, where inflammation of the spinal longitudinal ligament and intervertebral disc insertions causes pain on movement and ultimately calcification and fusion.

- This fibrotic response at sites of inflammation also links the spondyloarthropathies with:
  - » ascending aortitis
  - » anterior uveitis
  - » apical lung fibrosis.
- Synovitis varies between different group members, but is usually an asymmetric small- and large-joint lower-limb arthritis that may represent an extension of enthesitis from the surrounding joint capsule into the synovium.

The spondyloarthropathies present a clinical spectrum, with AS as a strongly HLA-B27 related spinal/sacroiliac disorder, ReA as a predominantly lower-limb asymmetric arthropathy only moderately associated with HLA-B27, and PsA in between (see Figure 17-5).

Ankylosing spondylitis (AS)

Ankylosing spondylitis is a chronic progressive inflammatory disorder predominantly affecting the sacroiliac joints and spine (spondylitis), leading to fusion of vertebrae (ankylosis).

- Affecting 0.1–1.4% of the population, its prevalence is underestimated due to misdiagnosis of degenerative back disease.
- The typical age of onset is between 17 and 35 years, with a male predominance of 3:1.
- With an over 90% genetic contribution there is a strong family history to be elicited, and the HLA-B27 association explains 20–50% of genetics, possibly via dysregulated immunity to gut bacteria.

Sacroiliac (SI) inflammation causes pain localized over the SI joints, with pain extending into the buttocks that may radiate to the thighs but not below the knee. The presenting symptoms are of insidious low-back pain persistent for at least 3 months, worsened by inactivity and improved by exercise.

> ### CLINICAL PEARL
> Features strongly indicative of an inflammatory basis of back pain are insidious onset at age <40 years, improvement with exercise and no improvement with rest, with pain at night (particularly the early morning).

The consequence of enthesial inflammation of the spine is progressive spinal pain, and restriction of movement in all directions that is clinically evident first in the lumbar region and progresses to involve the whole spine.

Over time the classical AS posture (Figure 17-6) develops:
- forward thrust and flexed neck
- increased abdominal girth
- loss of lumbar lordosis
- flexed hips and knees.

Objective documentation of spinal disease includes:
- occiput to wall distance
- degree of cervical rotation and lateral flexion
- reduced chest expansion (supplemented by pulmonary function testing)
- lumbar flexion measured as Schober's index—the Schober's test is a clinical measurement of lumbar spine mobility, and a reduction of the index is likely in AS
- lumbar lateral flexion measured as fingertip to floor distance.

The ability to 'touch your toes' is a composite of lumbar flexion, hip movement and hamstring stretch, and is unreliable in AS.

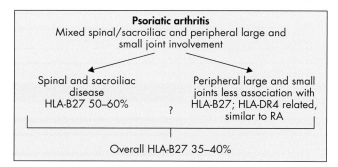

Figure 17-5 Relationship of the spondyloarthropathies to HLA-B27

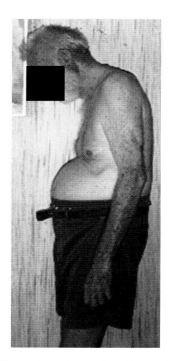

Figure 17-6 Typical posture of patient with ankylosing spondylitis; note the flexed neck, protruberant abdomen, and loss of lumbar lordosis

CLINICAL PEARLS

- Ankylosing spondylitis restricts spinal movement in all directions. Degenerative spinal disease is predominantly in one plane.
- Dactylitis (or a sausage-shaped digit) is caused by both synovitis and enthesitis in more than one digit, and is a key sign of a spondyloarthropathy.

Nonspecific constitutional features of inflammation, such as fatigue, anorexia and weight loss, are present proportional to disease activity, although profound weight loss warrants investigation for IBD.

Ankylosis of the spine, in addition to restricting a range of daily activities, increases the risk of spinal fracture from minor trauma, with potential spinal cord injury or cauda equina syndrome.

Additional extra-articular complications are:

- uveitis
- aortitis with aortic insufficiency
- cardiac conduction defects
- restrictive lung disease secondary to pulmonary fibrosis
- restricted thoracic wall movement; this may lead to reliance on diaphragmatic breathing, with marked abdominal wall excursion
- Achilles tendinitis.

Diagnosis

The ASAS (Assessment of SpondyloArthritis International Society) classification criteria for ankylosing spondylitis in a person aged <45 years, with back pain for >3 months, are:

- sacroiliitis on X-ray or magnetic resonance imaging (which will detect earlier features) plus one or more additional feature

or

- the presence of HLA-B27 and two features from:
  - » inflammatory back pain
  - » arthritis
  - » enthesitis
  - » uveitis
  - » dactylitis
  - » family history of spondyloarthritis
  - » psoriasis
  - » raised CRP
  - » inflammatory bowel disease
  - » NSAID-responsive.

CLINICAL PEARL

Sacroiliitis is not always present on plain X-rays. Reliance on the presence of unequivocal sacroiliitis on plain X-rays delays both the diagnosis and the management, and in 5–10% of cases will prevent the diagnosis being made at all.

Laboratory testing

Before testing HLA-B27, you need to consider the family history and your clinical confidence.

- AS has a 95% association with HLA-B27, so if AS is present in a first-degree relative then there is 50% random chance of finding a positive result.
- 8–10% of the normal population carry HLA-B27, so a positive result with an uncertain clinical presentation is unlikely to help, although the absence of HLA-B27 would make you rethink the diagnosis.

Treatment

- A key platform of therapy is exercise to maintain the spine in an erect and normal position, with maintenance of a normal range of spinal movements, and spinal muscle strength.
- NSAIDs assist in reducing symptoms to allow exercise to be undertaken, with participation in group activities aiding adherence.
- Regular NSAID use may slow X-ray progression, but has to be balanced against gastrointestinal and renal toxicity.
- Sulfasalazine, and methotrexate and other DMARDs, have no proven benefit in axial arthritis but may be useful in peripheral joint disease.
- Anti-TNF agents have made a large difference to the management of AS. They significantly improve patient-reported outcomes of disease activity, pain and fatigue, along with reduced acute phase reactants and spinal movement scores. Retardation of radiological progression is yet to be demonstrated. Anti-IL17 antibodies (e.g. secukinumab) are also effective in the management of ankylosing spondylitis.

Psoriatic arthritis (PsA)

Skin disease

- Psoriasis is characterized by red, scaly, raised silvery plaques within a well-demarcated patch, typically occurring on the scalp, elbows and knees.
- Pitting of the nails is a strong clue that a rash may be psoriatic. Psoriasis is common in Caucasians, with a prevalence of around 2%. It is much less common in Asians.
- There is a family history of psoriasis in one-third of patients.

Joint disease

- Arthritis occurs in 10–40% of cases. A clinical clue is sausage-shaped digits.
- Compared with AS there is a more equal sex distribution.
- 85% of patients have developed skin lesions in the 5–10 years before the onset of joint disease.
- Around 10% develop psoriasis and PsA contemporaneously.
- 5% have a pattern of PsA with psoriasis developing later.

As illustrated in Figure 17-5 above, the spectrum of PsA is broad and may mimic any form of inflammatory arthritis. Table 17-4 (overleaf) compares PsA with RA.

Table 17-4 Comparison of psoriatic arthritis and rheumatoid arthritis

	PSORIATIC ARTHRITIS	RHEUMATOID ARTHRITIS
Small-joint involvement	++	+++
DIP involvement	+++	+
Spine, sacroiliac involvement	++	C-spine late
Enthesitis	+++	−
Synovitis	++	+++
Subcutaneous nodules	−	++
Skin lesions	+++	+
RF-positive	+	+++
Anti-CCP antibodies	−	+++
Inflammatory markers	++	+++
Family history	+++	+

CCP, cyclic citrullinated peptide; C-spine, cervical spine; DIP, distal interphalangeal. RF, rheumatoid factor.

CLINICAL PEARL

40% of patients with psoriatic arthritis will have only spinal and sacroiliac disease resembling ankylosing spondylitis, with the most common pattern an oligo-arthritis of large and small joints.

- Less common in PsA is the small joint peripheral poly-arthritis which resembles RA; the DIP-only pattern; and the <5% pattern of arthritis mutilans in which destruction of the PIP and DIP joints leads to opera-glass fingers.
- When assessing a patient for PsA, in addition to a confirmed personal or family history of psoriasis, examination of the scalp, natal cleft, umbilicus and extensor surfaces for unrecognized psoriasis is required.
- Psoriatic nail changes of pitting, transverse ridging and onycholysis should be carefully sought.

There is no relationship between the extent of psoriatic skin disease and the prevalence or severity of PsA.

CLINICAL PEARLS

- Useful clues to psoriatic arthritis are distal interphalangeal inflammatory disease, synovitis of interphalangeal (IP) joints in the toes, and sausage digits—representing synovitis of proximal and distal IP joints with tenosynovitis and periostitis.
- Sausage-shaped digits occur commonly in psoriatic arthritis and reactive arthritis.

Treatment

As with all inflammatory joint disease, a program that maintains joint mobility and the strength of the supporting muscles is required. PsA can have an insidious pattern of joint involvement so that at any one time the disease burden is low, but it progressively damages and restrict joints and function, particularly in the hands.

- Physiotherapy and splintage assist with joint protection, and single or small numbers of inflamed joints can be injected with corticosteroids.
- Care is required with the use of oral corticosteroids as they may cause rebound skin lesions if rapidly reduced.
- In patients with predominant synovitis the management is similar to RA, with methotrexate used to treat both skin and joint lesions. Sulfasalazine and leflunomide may also be used.
- Numerous biological and novel agents are being increasingly used in PsA. These include anti-TNF agents, anti-IL12/23 antibodies, anti-IL17 antibodies, and JAK inhibitors.

Reactive arthritis (ReA)

Reactive arthritis is an aseptic joint inflammation that occurs distant in both time and place from an inciting infection that is usually of gastrointestinal or genitourinary origin.

- Typically it affects young adults, with a very slight overall male predominance.
- Onset is usually 7–21 days after the trigger.
- HLA-B27 positivity is present in 65–95% of cases.
- Less than 5% of exposed persons will develop ReA.
- The most common genitourinary trigger is *Chlamydia trachomatis*, which can be detected by polymerase chain reaction (PCR) analysis of a morning urine sample. Chlamydial infection is commonly asymptomatic in women, and should be tested in a woman presenting with knee monoarthritis.
- Gastrointestinal triggers are common 'food poisoning' organisms, which will be evident on personal and household contact history. PCR is replacing stool culture, and will allow detection of *Salmonella typhimurium*, *Shigella flexneri*, *Yersinia enterocolitica* and *Campylobacter jejuni*.
- Rarer triggers include post-streptococcal ReA, and *Neisseria* spp.
- There is a high prevalence of human immunodeficiency virus (HIV) infection in people with reactive arthritis, and it may occur in the setting of acute infection.

The joint disease in ReA is an asymmetrical oligoarthritis, or monoarthritis, usually of the lower limb. Most commonly there is involvement of the knee, ankle and hip, and less often the shoulder and wrist. Enthesitis of the plantar fascia and Achilles' tendon are common.

The mucocutaneous manifestations of ReA are a sterile urethritis, balanitis, cervicitis, and conjunctivitis/uveitis. An infrequent skin involvement is keratoderma blennorrhagica on the palms and soles, which is a pustular variant of psoriasis.

Treatment

If the inciting trigger is identified, then this should be treated and if possible avoided in the future. Most cases resolve within 3 months, and require only simple management involving analgesia, NSAIDs and intra-articular steroids. However, a significant minority have disease severe enough to require DMARDs. The morbidity from eye disease can be severe, and necessitates specialist intervention.

CLINICAL PEARL

A small percentage of patients with reactive arthritis develop a chronic destructive arthropathy requiring the full range of disease-modifying agents (DMARDs), initially with sulfasalazine, and at times progressing to biological therapies.

IBD-associated spondyloarthropathy

- An AS-type spondyloarthropathy is found in 2–20% of patients with ulcerative colitis or Crohn's disease, and up to 60% of patients with AS are found to have subclinical inflammatory bowel disease (IBD) if the colon and terminal ileum is examined and biopsied.
- The HLA-B27 allele associates with the presence of sacroiliitis, which may be asymmetrical compared with the symmetry of AS.
- Peripheral arthritis is not HLA-B27-associated and is an asymmetrical oligoarthritis, often monoarthritis, involving knees, ankles and MTP joints.
- Treatment of the IBD generally also reduces the joint disease.

Adult-onset Still's disease (AOSD)

This is an inflammatory disorder typically presenting with polyarthritis, fevers, and an 'evanescent' salmon-pink rash. The underlying etiology remains unclear. Fevers often occur daily ('quotidian') and can be accompanied by the rash, which may resolve as the fever settles. Abnormal liver function tests and markedly elevated serum ferritin levels are characteristic. No specific antibodies are diagnostic for AOSD, and the diagnosis is often made after more common conditions are excluded (e.g. viral infections).

Treatment depends on the severity of the disease, but usually involves immunosuppression. Various medications have been used in conjunction with prednisolone, including biological agents.

CRYSTAL ARTHROPATHIES

Gout

Gout is an intensely painful acute inflammatory response to monosodium urate crystals within the joint.

- More than 1% of adult men in Western countries have gout, with significant increases in prevalence occurring secondary to obesity, insulin resistance, low-dose aspirin, diuretics for hypertension, and longevity.
- Gout affects men four times more than women, and most often develops after the age of 45 years, although earlier gout occurs particularly in men with a family history of gout or a history of heavy alcohol consumption.
- In women estrogen has a uricosuric effect, so gout is most often of post-menopausal onset.

Hyperuricemia is the primary risk factor for gout, with a risk that increases exponentially with the serum uric acid (UA) level.

- The prevalence of hyperuricemia is 10–20% in some populations, although the majority of patients with hyperuricemia do not develop gout.
- Currently, asymptomatic hyperuricemia does not warrant treatment, but this is likely to require review with increasing evidence of a relationship between hyperuricemia and hypertension, renal disease, metabolic syndrome, diabetes, and cardiovascular disease.
- Serum UA levels are determined principally by genetic polymorphisms of renal urate transporters and glucokinase regulatory proteins.
- Genetically predisposed people may subsequently develop gout if they are exposed to other risk factors such as a high purine diet, obesity, increased alcohol consumption, or diuretic use.

Etiology

- Uric acid is the end-product of purine metabolism in humans (Figure 17-7), due to the absence of uricase activity.
- This lack of uricase activity, combined with kidneys that efficiently reabsorb 90% of filtered UA, and eating habits that create high amounts of purine, result in a UA normal range of 0.36–0.42 mmol/L, which is very close to or above the 0.41 mmol/L saturation concentration of many tissues and exceeds that of cooler peripheries. This contributes to UA crystallization within the joints and to the creation of tophi (Figure 17-8, overleaf).

Box 17-4 (overleaf) lists secondary factors to be considered.

CLINICAL PEARL

An elevated uric acid level does not indicate that the diagnosis is gout—it only indicates an increased risk of gout.

Diet and alcohol

- The relative risk of gout is higher in people who eat a diet high in red meat.
- Diets high in purine-rich vegetables (peas, beans, lentils, mushrooms and asparagus) do not increase the risk.
- Diets high in low-fat dairy products are associated with reduced risk.
- Fructose-rich fruits (apples, oranges) are associated with a modestly increased risk of gout.
- Coffee consumption reduces the risk of gout.
- In prospective studies, beer has the greatest effect on gout risk, then spirits, whereas wine has no increased risk.

Stages of gout

- The first stage is asymptomatic hyperuricemia, a common physiological abnormality which in most people is not associated with the development of gout. Asymptomatic hyperuricemia does not need to be treated.
- The second stage is characterized by periodic attacks of acute gout with asymptomatic interludes. The frequency, duration and severity of the acute gout tends to increase over time. Patients develop a marked systemic illness with fevers, chills and intense pain that escalates over 6–12 hours.
- Finally, chronic gout may develop with the development of tophaceous deposits and a chronic arthropathy overlaid with intermittent flares.

Acute gout

Acute gout attacks can be triggered by direct trauma to the joint, dehydration, acidosis, alcohol intake, administration of chemotherapy, or rapid weight loss. A common trigger is intercurrent illness, or surgery, that causes an acute phase response, causing an increased urinary excretion of UA, subsequent lowering of serum UA levels with partial crystal dissolution, and encouragement of crystal shedding into the joint fluid.

- The vast majority of first attacks affect only a single joint, typically the great toe MTP joint (podagra), but oligoarticular and polyarticular gout can occur, especially in the elderly.
- Distal and cooler joints are characteristically targeted, possibly due to the reduced solubility of UA in these joints: midfoot, ankle, finger joints, wrists, and knees.
- Attacks commonly start in the early morning, awakening the patient from sleep with rapid development of severe pain and tenderness over 6–24 hours.
- One of the characteristic features of acute gout attacks is that they are self-limiting, and resolve spontaneously regardless of treatment within several to 14 days.

Diagnosing gout

- The purist approach is to establish the presence of negatively birefringent intracellular UA crystals in the joint

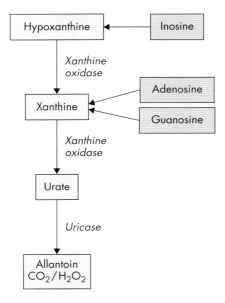

Figure 17-7 Purine pathway producing urate

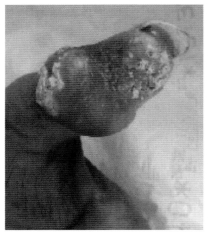
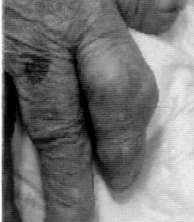
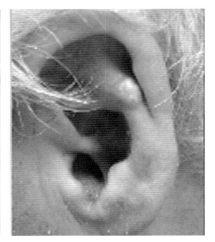

Figure 17-8 Tophaceous gout

Box 17-4
Causes of hyperuricemia

A. Increased uric acid production (10%)

- Obesity
- Myeloproliferative disease
- Paget's disease
- Alcohol
- Polycythemia rubra vera
- Psoriasis
- Hemolysis
- Rhabdomyolysis
- Glycogen storage diseases (types III, V, and VII)
- Inborn errors of metabolism (including hypoxanthine–guanine phosphoribosyltransferase [HPRT] deficiency)

B. Decreased uric acid excretion (90%)

- Renal impairment
- Starvation
- Polycystic kidney disease
- Acidosis (ketoacidosis, lactic acidosis)
- Toxemia of pregnancy
- Hypothyroidism
- Hyperparathyroidism
- Bartter syndrome
- Diabetes insipidus
- Down syndrome
- Sarcoidosis
- Lead poisoning
- Drugs:
  - » aspirin
  - » diuretics
  - » cyclosporine (ciclosporin)
  - » ethambutol
  - » L-dopa (levodopa)
  - » pyrazinamide

---

fluid of an inflamed joint (Figure 17-9). In reality, the classically inflamed podagra/1st MTP joint is a difficult joint to aspirate.

- A practical diagnosis can be made using a typical presentation such as podagra with a current or recent history of hyperuricemia.
- Strong supporting evidence is the presence of tophi, or documented joint crystals during an inter-critical (clinically quiescent) period.

CLINICAL PEARL

If septic arthritis is suspected, or if a larger joint is involved, then joint aspiration for Gram staining and culture in addition to crystal identification is required.

- Gout and septic arthritis can coexist, and joint aspiration can also identify the calcium pyrophosphate dihydrate (CPPD) crystals of pseudogout.

CLINICAL PEARL

Remember the joint aspiration changes in gout and pseudogout:
- Gout—negative birefringence, yellow needles
- Pseudogout—weakly positive birefringence, blue rhomboids

Figure 17-9 Needle-shaped urate crystals (yellow and blue) under polarizing microscopy (crystal color depends on orientation relative to the polarizer; the blue crystals are at 90° to the yellow)

Acute gout management

Acute gout will spontaneously get better, so the goal of therapy is provision of pain relief and reduction in the duration of acute inflammation. NSAIDs and colchicine are the most widely prescribed agents, with corticosteroids (oral, intramuscular, intra-articular) also of value.

- NSAIDs are effective in reducing pain if used in full doses; options include indomethacin 50 mg three times daily, diclofenac 50 mg three times daily, celecoxib 100 mg twice daily, and etoricoxib 120 mg daily. All of these agents work quickly but should be limited to 7 days' duration.
- Colchicine use for the management of acute gout should be restricted to when NSAIDs and corticosteroids are contraindicated, ineffective or cause unacceptable side-effects. Start with two 0.5 mg tablets followed by 0.5 mg one hour later, and then 0.5 mg twice daily for 2–4 days maximum.
  » Colchicine adverse effects of nausea, vomiting and diarrhea occur in 25–75% of patients prescribed 1.5–4.5 mg daily, and occur in all patients on higher doses. Severe adverse effects include bone marrow suppression, neuromyopathy and rhabdomyolysis.

CLINICAL PEARL

Colchicine should not be prescribed 'to be taken until diarrhea develops'.

- Oral corticosteroids are useful in patients in whom NSAIDs or colchicine are contraindicated due to comorbid factors.
  » Prednisolone or prednisone 25–50 mg daily is often needed to ensure adequate control of acute gout.
  » Comparative studies equate prednisolone 30–35 mg/day to indomethacin 50 mg three times daily and naproxen 500 mg twice daily respectively, with equal efficacy in reduction of pain, and similar adverse events.
- In those in whom you wish to avoid oral steroids, intra-articular steroid injection can be undertaken.

Chronic gout management/urate-lowering options

- In a patient with recurring attacks of acute gout, the goal is to reduce the frequency and severity of acute attacks over the next 12–18 months, so that they eventually disappear.
- The initiation of therapy may induce 'mobilization' flares of gout, and a plan of managing these acute attacks needs to be in place.
- In addition to medical therapy, a dietary review should take place, and patients should be advised to maintain a high water intake to assist with urate excretion.

CLINICAL PEARL

Urate-lowering agents need to be used long-term, and currently lifelong therapies should be commenced when gout is severe, as indicated by:
- recurrent flares (particularly polyarticular)
- deforming and destructive tophaceous deposits
- the presence of renal calculi.

The goal of therapy is to achieve a serum urate level of 0.30–0.36 mmol/L, and therapy is stepwise escalated until this target is reached. Treatment is initiated slowly and at low levels during a quiescent phase of gout, although in some patients with frequent attacks it can be initiated when the acute attack is controlled and while the NSAID or corticosteroid is being continued.

Allopurinol

Allopurinol blocks the metabolic conversion of hypoxanthine to uric acid (Figure 17-7), and can cause a rapid reduction in serum UA, resulting in mobilization flares.

- Allopurinol should be commenced at 50 mg/day for 2 weeks, prior to increasing to 100 mg/day.
- Subsequently, serum UA should be measured 3–4 weeks after the dose increase, and stepwise increases of 100 mg continued until the target serum UA of 0.30 mmol/L is achieved.
- Minor self-limiting drug reactions are relatively common, affecting 2–10% of patients, and include itching, rash and gastrointestinal problems.
- The more serious and potentially fatal allopurinol hypersensitivity is far less common, estimated at 0.002–0.4% of patients. It occurs 2–6 weeks after treatment is started, with features of toxic epidermal necrolysis, exfoliative dermatitis, fever, eosinophilia, liver and renal dysfunction, vasculitis, and bone-marrow suppression. Allopurinol should never be re-tried in such situations. Extreme caution is required with the co-administration of allopurinol, azathioprine, or mercaptopurine.
- The co-prescription of ampicillin/amoxicillin with allopurinol should also be avoided due to an increased frequency of skin rash.

CLINICAL PEARL

Urate-lowering agents such as allopurinol or probenecid should not be initiated, ceased or adjusted during an acute attack of gout. The unstable serum uric acid level will cause additional crystal shedding and worsen the attack.

Probenecid

Probenecid blocks the proximal tubular reabsorption of uric acid.

- Its starting dose is 250 mg daily for 1 week, increasing to 250 mg twice daily, and then very gradually the dose is titrated against serum UA up to a maximum of 1000 mg twice daily.
- The net effect of probenecid is increased urinary excretion of UA, and it is contraindicated in patients with coexisting renal stones.
- Probenecid may potentiate the toxicity of methotrexate, and aspirin should be avoided as at any dose it antagonizes the action of probenecid.

Febuxostat

Febuxostat is a non-purine selective inhibitor of xanthine oxidase which decreases the serum uric acid levels by preventing the formation of uric acid from xanthine. The severe allopurinol hypersensitivity reaction (see above) has also been reported with febuxostat.

The dose ranges typically from 40–80 mg daily.

There is uncertainty regarding the long-term cardiovascular safety of febuxostat, so caution is advised in patients with significant cardiovascular risk factors.

Pseudogout

The most frequent manifestation of CPPD-deposition disease is chondrocalcinosis, the asymptomatic radiographical finding of calcification of articular or fibro-cartilage.

- Up to 5% of the world's population show radiographical evidence of chondrocalcinosis, with the incidence rising with age to 15–40% of those >60 years of age, and 30–60% of those >85 years old.

- The acute symptomatic presentation of chondrocalcinosis is termed *pseudogout*, on the basis of its similarity to gout in terms of acute and painful joint inflammation.

- A less common chronic arthropathy is most common in elderly women; while usually mild, it can lead to quite severe and rapidly destructive arthritis. The 2nd and 3rd MCP joints are most commonly those severely affected.

The presentation of pseudogout is of an inflammatory arthropathy with loss of function, early-morning stiffness and improvement with activity. Other manifestations include: atypical forms of OA; severe destruction mimicking neuropathic arthropathy; a symmetrical synovitis similar to RA; and calcification of the intervertebral discs and longitudinal spinal ligaments leading to restricted spinal mobility, and hence resembling ankylosing spondylitis but without sacroiliitis.

CPPD deposition is associated with acute attacks of pseudogout, characterized by joint effusions with marked neutrophilia.

- The release of CPPD crystals into a joint space is followed by neutrophilic phagocytosis, with subsequent release of potent chemoattractant and inflammatory mediators.

- Pseudogout most commonly involves the knees, followed by the wrists, metacarpophalangeal joints, hips, shoulders, elbows, and ankles.

- The joint distribution may provide a clue to CPPD disease, as primary OA rarely involves the MCP joint, wrist, elbow, shoulder or ankle. CPPD crystals, however, may also be found in the synovial fluids of primary OA, either alone or in association with basic calcium phosphate crystals.

- Tenosynovitis is also reported, and is associated with tendon rupture.

- Soft tissue CPPD deposits may present as tumor-like masses.

Acute attacks of pseudogout may be precipitated by local events that induce crystal shedding from cartilage into the synovial fluid, such as trauma, arthroscopy or intra-articular injection of high-molecular-weight hyaluronic acid as a viscosupplement. Systemic changes affecting calcium concentration, such as rapid changes in fluid balance, medical illness, commencement of thyroxine replacement, or parathyroid surgery, can also induce an acute attack.

CLINICAL PEARL

A systemic response to pseudogout is noted in half of patients with fever, neutrophil leukocytosis, and raised inflammatory markers.

A definitive diagnosis of CPPD-deposition disease requires unequivocal identification of weakly positively birefringent rhomboid or rod-shaped CPPD crystals in joint fluid or articular cartilage.

- Aspirated fluid is often turbid or bloodstained, with reduced viscosity and a marked neutrophil leukocytosis.

- Articular cartilage at any site may demonstrate chondrocalcinosis, with the classical sites being the triangular ligament of the wrist, the pubic symphysis, and the menisci of the knee.

- It has been proposed that the presence of CPPD crystals in synovial fluid combined with radiographically observed calcification of the cartilage would make a definitive diagnosis and either one would make a probable diagnosis. The absence of chondrocalcinosis does not exclude the diagnosis of CPPD.

- Although many metabolic and endocrine diseases are reported to predispose to CPPD deposition, the better evidence for an association lies with hyperparathyroidism, hemochromatosis, hypophosphatasia, and hypomagnesemia (see Box 17-5 and Figure 17-10). The presence of a CPPD arthropathy in a patient younger than 50 years, or in those with florid polyarticular chondrocalcinosis, should lead to a complete investigation for an underlying metabolic disorder.

Box 17-5

Conditions associated with calcium pyrophosphate dihydrate (CPPD)-deposition disease

Secondary to underlying medical conditions

- Hyperparathyroidism
- Hypophosphatasia
- Hemochromatosis
- Hypomagnesemia
- Familial hypocalciuric hypercalcemia
- Possibly hypothyroidism
- Chronic gout

Secondary to underlying cartilage alterations

- Aging and possibly osteoarthritis
- Postmeniscectomy
- Epiphyseal dysplasia

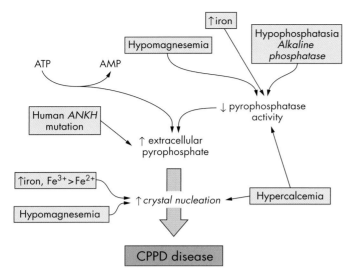

Figure 17-10 Metabolic factors predisposing to calcium pyrophosphate dihydrate (CPPD)-deposition disease. AMP, adenosine monophosphate; ANKH, inorganic pyrophosphate transport regulator; ATP, adenosine triphosphate

Treatment

The therapeutic options for pseudogout are more limited than for gout. Symptomatic therapy with NSAIDs, colchicine, joint aspirations, intra-articular steroids, and non-pharmacological support are the main approaches to acute management of the acutely inflamed joint. There is currently no specific treatment to slow or prevent the gradual joint deterioration due to chondrocalcinosis, or the progression of the crystal deposition itself, other than treatment of any underlying biochemical or metabolic disorders.

RELAPSING POLYCHONDRITIS (RP)

Relapsing polychondritis is a rare condition of unknown etiology characterized by repeated inflammation of cartilaginous structures. An autoimmune, cell-mediated response to type II collagen leads to inflammation of the elastic cartilage of ears and nose, the hyaline cartilage of peripheral joints, vertebral fibro-cartilage, and tracheo-bronchial cartilage.

- The classical presentation is of acute painful inflammation of the cartilaginous pinna of the ear, with sparing of the ear lobule. Often misdiagnosed as infection, the sparing of the non-cartilaginous lobe is a clue, and often the attacks become bilateral.
- Nasal chondritis and inflammation of eyelids occurs, with saddle-nose deformity (Figure 17-11) a complication of distal septal inflammation.
- Arthritis is the second most common presentation, with involvement of the small joints of the hands, knees and ankles.

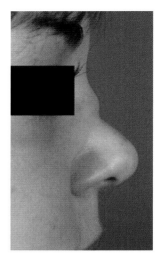

Figure 17-11 Saddle-nose deformity

From Bennett HS and Reilly PG. Restylane—a temporary alternative for saddle nose deformity in nasal Wegener's granulomatosis: how we do it. Br J Oral Maxillofacial Surg 2011;49(4):e3–e5.

- Recurrent involvement of the trachea can lead to tracheomalacia and obstruction.
- During the course of the illness, nearly half the patients will experience deafness due to involvement of Eustachian tube inflammation, and vestibulo-cochlear nerve inflammation.
- Less commonly, aortitis and aortic regurgitation can develop, along with large vessel and leukocytoclastic vasculitis.

RP has been described in association with major vasculitides, and connective tissue disorders such as RA and systemic lupus erythematosus. There are no specific investigations, with diagnosis being made on clinical grounds.

RP is a relapsing disorder, and the treatment depends on the severity of disease and the end organs involved.

- Mild symptoms may only require analgesics and NSAIDs, with colchicine and dapsone used for more persistent symptoms.
- Severe manifestations require pulse and oral prednisolone, with additional therapy as per vasculitis and renal involvement utilizing methotrexate, cyclophosphamide and mycophenolate.

CLINICAL PEARL

Saddle-nose deformity (nasal septal collapse) occurs in granulomatosis with polyangiitis and relapsing polychondritis.

OSTEOARTHRITIS (OA)

The global impact of osteoarthritis on the health system is enormous, particularly in an aging population with its associated obesity and metabolic disorders. It is crucial to identify and promptly provide effective treatment to these patients to reduce pain, improve quality of life, and avoid potentially painful and crippling sequelae of the disease. Individual therapeutic strategies continue to provide sub-optimal management, and future research directions will include new therapies and combine multiple therapies.

Types of osteoarthritis

Osteoarthritis can be subdivided into *primary* or *secondary* types, as described below.

1 Primary or idiopathic osteoarthritis can be subclassified into *localized* or *generalized*, with commonly affected sites including the hands, feet, knees, hips and spine. Generalized osteoarthritis usually affects three or more joints.

2 Conditions that alter the balance of cartilage wear or damage, and repair processes, may contribute to the development of secondary osteoarthritis. These conditions or diseases include:

   a joint inflammation, e.g. RA, that induces enzymatic destruction of the collagen matrix and aggrecan molecules which are integral to cartilage

   b direct trauma to cartilage or its vascular supply, and secondary biomechanical derangement, increasing local wear

   c congenital and acquired disorders of joint morphometry, which leads to local wear

   d obesity with increased mechanical load, and concomitant decreased mobility

   e obesity-associated metabolic syndrome with insulin resistance, which causes elevated inflammatory cytokines secondary to the accumulation, and activation of proinflammatory cells within the adipose tissue, particularly the abdomen

   f certain occupations (e.g. farmers), and repetitive high-impact sports

   g other diseases such as diabetes mellitus, acromegaly, hypothyroidism

   h neuropathic (Charcot) arthropathy.

Clinical features

> ### CLINICAL PEARL
>
> Pain is the predominant symptom in patients with osteoarthritis, which is typically worse with activity and relieved by rest. Pain occurring at rest and at night signifies more advanced disease. Evening stiffness is the hallmark of osteoarthritis, while morning stiffness lasting longer than 30 minutes is more suggestive of an inflammatory arthropathy.

Signs of osteoarthritis include the following:

- Altered gait from hip, knee, ankle or foot involvement.
- Joint tenderness on palpation, which is easily elicited on superficial peripheral joints such as the hands, knees and feet, and is not necessarily accompanied by joint swelling.
- Crepitus or creaking from the joints, which may be both felt and heard by the patient, and can be elicited by placing a palm on the joint and objectively feeling for disrupted joint movements.

- Osteophytes, which may be palpable as bony protrusions along the edge of the joint, and are easily seen and felt at the DIP joints of the hand.
- Joint effusions which, if present, are usually cool to the touch.
- Analysis of synovial fluid shows mild inflammation (white cell count of less than 2000 cells/mm^3), and slightly elevated protein levels. It should be negative for culture and crystals.

CPPD-deposition disease may mimic the clinical course of osteoarthritis or cause secondary osteoarthritis, which may be evident radiographically.

Psoriatic arthritis is the great mimic, and can present in many forms, including only DIP joint disease. Marked inflammation of the DIP joints, without palpable osteophytes, and with concomitant evidence of psoriasis in the nails or skin, is suggestive of PsA. Synovitis of the interphalangeal joints of the toes is also a helpful clue which points to psoriatic arthritis rather than osteoarthritis.

Specific joint involvement

Hands

- The hands are commonly involved in OA, with bony osteophytic changes known as Heberden's nodes (Figure 17-12) and Bouchard's nodes affecting the distal and proximal interphalangeal joints, respectively.
- The first carpometacarpal joint can also be affected, giving the physical appearance of a squared hand due to subluxation of the thumb under the palm.

Feet

Varying degrees of foot involvement can occur.

- The first metatarsophalangeal joint can cause a 'bunion' (hallux valgus) deformity (Figure 17-13) or hallux rigidus.
- Ankle disease of the talonavicular and subtalar joints is often secondary to trauma and ligamentous instability.

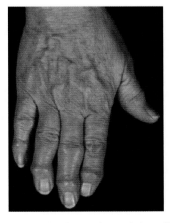

Figure 17-12 Heberden's nodes of the distal interphalangeal joints

From Abishek A and Doherty M. Diagnosis and clinical presentation of osteoarthritis. Rheum Dis Clin North Am 2013;39(1):45–66.

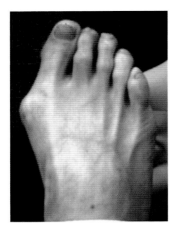

Figure 17-13 Hallux valgus

From Coughlin MJ, Saltzman CL and Anderson RB (eds). Mann's Surgery of the foot and ankle, 9th ed. Philadelphia: Elsevier, 2014.

Knees

- Physical findings on examination of the knees may underestimate the degree of knee involvement.
- Malalignment of the knees may occur in advanced disease, giving the physical appearance of genu varum (bowed legs) or genu valgum (knocked knees), and is associated with more rapid progression of OA of the knees.
- Baker's cyst, a fluctuant swelling in the posterior aspect of the knees, may also be elicited.

Hips

- OA of the hip is typically associated with pain and limited range of motion, and the development of a limp aimed at reducing pain.
- It is important to distinguish referred pain to the hip (from the lumbosacral spine or knee) from greater trochanteric bursitis, which is felt laterally with a normal range of passive motion.
- Pain worsens with weightbearing and is usually localized to the groin or medial thigh.

Spine

- OA of the spine typically occurs in the areas of greatest spinal flexibility, at levels C5 to C7 and L3 to L5, with relative sparing of the thoracic spine.
- It is important to recognize that cervical and lumbar spondylosis may occur due to osteophytes originating from the diarthrodial facet joints, combined with intervertebral disc narrowing and hypertrophic vertebral spur formation, which impinges on the spinal canal or exiting nerve root, potentially causing neurological deficits. Paraspinal muscle spasm is a common clinical finding.
- In severe OA, spondylolisthesis (forward slipping of a vertebral body) can be seen. It is usually demonstrated at levels L4 to L5.

Shoulders

- Glenohumeral joint involvement typically causes chronic anterior shoulder pain, made worse on movement, particularly abduction.
- Acromioclavicular joint involvement may cause diffuse shoulder pain, or pain in the anterior shoulder, and may not be immediately evident as OA of the shoulder.

Investigations

Uncomplicated OA with typical clinical characteristics rarely warrants further investigation. However, further laboratory testing and imaging may be carried out in patients with:

- isolated knee or hip symptoms, without other evidence of OA
- atypical joint involvement (e.g. shoulder, elbow, wrist and ankle)
- sudden onset of severe joint pain.

This is to ensure that important inflammatory and infective causes are not missed.

- Septic arthritis should always be considered in a systemically unwell patient, and requires joint aspiration and culture even in joints classically affected by OA.
- Radiographical severity may not correlate with clinical severity, and early findings are often nonspecific. X-ray distinctions between OA and RA are shown in Table 17-5.

Treatment

In general, therapeutic options are non–pharmacological, pharmacological and surgical (Figure 17-14). Factors to consider when managing a patient with OA include:

- prior perception and knowledge of OA, including its treatment
- treatment efficacy and adverse effects
- cost, availability and logistics of treatment modality
- the presence of comorbid disease
- functional activity, including work and recreational aspirations.

Non-pharmacological options

Non-pharmacological therapy should always be part of a patient's management strategy, because it may significantly reduce pain and disability and may reduce or negate the need for pharmacological treatment.

- Exercise and activity should be prescribed to all patients with large joint involvement, regardless of their age. It provides a distraction as part of a cognitive–behavioral approach to pain management, utilizes endorphin release, and provides psychological benefit from improved overall wellbeing and control of pain.
- Some patients may benefit from physiotherapy sessions.
- Aerobic exercise improves wellbeing, and benefits patients with obesity and hypertension.
- Local neuromuscular training increases muscle strength, and range of joint motion.

Table 17-5 Comparison of radiographical features of osteoarthritis and rheumatoid arthritis

RADIOGRAPHICAL FEATURE	OSTEOARTHRITIS	RHEUMATOID ARTHRITIS
Clinical pattern	Distal interphalangeal and 1st carpometacarpal joints, and less often proximal interphalangeal joints	Proximal interphalangeal and metacarpophalangeal joints, and wrist, plus deformities
Joint-space narrowing	Localized to one side, or compartment of joint	Diffusely throughout joint
Periarticular erosions	Absent	Present
Subchondral bony change	Sclerosis	Osteopenia
Subchondral cysts	Present	Absent
Osteophytes	Present	Absent

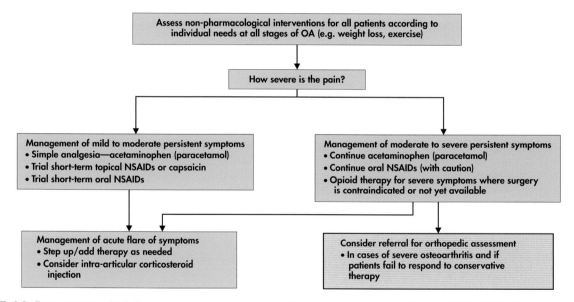

Figure 17-14 Recommended therapeutic approach to hip and knee osteoarthritis (OA). NSAIDs, non-steroidal anti-inflammatory drugs

- There is clear evidence that even modest weight loss improves function and reduces pain in overweight patients with OA, especially of the hip and knee.
- Appropriate footwear (e.g. thick, soft soles; insoles), walking aids, braces and slings are available, and may improve symptoms of osteoarthritis significantly.
- Transcutaneous electrical nerve stimulation (TENS) and thermotherapy are safe and effective adjunct therapies in most patients with OA.
- T'ai chi and acupuncture may be of benefit by improving muscle tone and balance, especially if patients are at risk or have a fear of falling.

Pharmacological options

- Acetaminophen (paracetamol) is recommended as a first-line option for patients with OA. It is inexpensive, effective and well tolerated.

  » Doses of up to 1 g four times daily may be used; however, under-dosing is common mainly due to patients' perceptions of its safety and the number of tablets involved. Slow-release formulations allow dosing three times daily.

  » Acetaminophen is thought to work via inhibition of COX-3, and has little prostaglandin inhibition and therefore no gastrointestinal, cardiovascular or renal toxicity.

- Topical NSAIDs are a popular option with patients and are safer than oral NSAIDs (achieving systemic levels 15% that of orally taken NSAIDs).
- Topical capsaicin is also a viable alternative.
- Oral NSAIDs may be an option in patients unresponsive to acetaminophen or topical NSAIDs.

  » They may be used in combination with other agents; however, potential side-effects include gastrointestinal, liver, renal and cardiovascular toxicity, especially in the elderly. NSAIDs should be used at the lowest effective dose for the shortest time possible.

» If a patient has a history of peptic ulcer disease, the use of antiulcer prophylaxis or a selective COX-2 inhibitor should be considered. NSAIDs should also be used with caution in patients taking concomitant warfarin, because of the increased risk of bleeding via NSAID-induced platelet dysfunction.

» There has been increasing global withdrawal of COX-2 inhibitors from the market because of increased adverse cardiovascular events in users. COX-2 inhibitors may be an option for patients at low cardiovascular risk, who have a history of intolerance to COX-1 NSAIDs, or peptic ulcer disease.

- Opioids should be avoided if possible, and their need should alert the physician to the need for specialist referral and consideration for surgery, or the use of a regional nerve block.

- Low-dose amitriptyline (25–50 mg daily taken 2 hours before bedtime) should be considered in patients with refractory pain and poor sleep.

- Depression is a common comorbidity, and should not be overlooked.

- Intra-articular glucocorticoids may be useful in patients with mono- or oligo-articular involvement, and with persistent symptoms despite the use of regular acetaminophen and/or NSAIDs. They may be utilized every 3 months.

Surgery

- Arthroplasty should be considered in patients with severe and disabling hip or knee OA because it provides the potential for pain control, restoration of function, and improvement in quality of life.

- Referral should be made before severe protracted pain and functional limitation set in, because this may affect the outcome negatively.

- An aging yet active obese population affects the timing of joint replacement surgery. The early and immediate gain in quality of life needs to be balanced against the increasing number of patients requiring revision of their joint replacements later in life, with its currently poorer outcome and increased perioperative morbidity and mortality.

GENETIC CONNECTIVE TISSUE DISORDERS

A number of inherited disorders of connective tissue, specifically mutations in genes encoding for collagen and elastin, result in significant musculoskeletal abnormalities in addition to other organ defects. Three of the important diseases are outlined in Table 17-6.

PAINFUL SHOULDERS

Shoulder pain is an almost unavoidable life experience, with 7% of an adult population reporting at least 1 month of shoulder pain in the previous year, and a quarter of 85-year-olds suffering from chronic shoulder pain and restriction.

- The peak annual incidence of shoulder disorders is in the 4th and 5th decades, at a rate of 0.25%, with roughly an equal sex incidence.

- Up to 20% of patients with chronic shoulder pain, and 65% of all diagnoses, relate to lesions of the rotator cuff.

Table 17-6 Genetic connective tissue disorders

	EHLERS–DANLOS SYNDROME	OSTEOGENESIS IMPERFECTA	MARFAN SYNDROME
Genetics	1:5000 births Abnormality in structure of collagen due to 1 of 3 types of mutation in the collagen gene, affecting types I, III, and V collagen	1:10,000 births Abnormality in type I collagen gene	1:4000 births Abnormality in elastin due to fibrillin gene mutation
Clinical features	Joint hypermobility Hyperextensible skin Easy bruising Delayed wound healing Blood vessel abnormalities	Brittle bones with multiple pathological fractures Blue sclerae Abnormal dentition	Overgrowth of long bones High arched palate Dislocated ocular lenses Mitral valve disease Aortic root aneurysms with aortic incompetence
Diagnosis	Clinical; genetic testing may be available	Skin biopsy—abnormal collagen production by fibroblasts	Clinical grounds
Treatment	Supportive	Bisphosphonates	Individual complications are treated as they arise

CLINICAL PEARLS

The localization of pain may be diagnostically helpful.
- The pain-sensitive structures of the shoulder are mainly innervated by the 5th cervical segment (C5), so that pain from these structures is referred to the C5 dermatome, creating the sensation of pain over the anterior arm, especially the deltoid insertion.
- The acromioclavicular joint is innervated by the C4 segment, so that pain arising here is felt at the joint itself, and radiates over the top of the shoulder into the trapezius muscle and up to the side of the neck.

Clinical assessment

In the elderly a history of trauma, marked night pain, and weakness on resisted abduction strongly suggests a rotator cuff tear. The sleeping position that induces night pain is an important clue in the history.

- Shoulder pain that results in awakening when *not* lying on the affected shoulder is found in frozen shoulder (adhesive capsulitis) and inflammatory arthritis.
- Pain when lying on the affected shoulder is seen in acromioclavicular joint disease and rotator cuff disease.

Prior shoulder problems suggest rotator cuff disease with chronic impingement or calcific tendinitis.

- A history of marked shoulder joint swelling suggests an inflammatory arthropathy, with the presence of an anterior bulge in the shoulder usually secondary to a subacromial bursa effusion.

- Glenohumeral OA is characterized by morning stiffness, pain with use, and chronicity of symptoms. OA is, however, significantly less common than rotator cuff dysfunction.

Causes and characteristics of shoulder pain are outlined in Table 17-7.

Examination

- The contours of the shoulder are examined for wasting, asymmetry and muscle fasciculations.
- Palpation should proceed from the sternoclavicular joint along the clavicle to the acromioclavicular joint, to the tip of the acromion, and the humeral head beneath the acromion.
- The shoulder range of movement should be examined both actively and passively, with muscle strength and pain on resistance assessed. There are essentially three movements to test in the shoulder:
  » abduction due to supraspinatus contraction
  » external rotation as a result of infraspinatus and teres minor movement
  » internal rotation due to subscapularis movement.

Rotator cuff disease

- The glenohumeral joint is, by virtue of its anatomical shape, reliant for its stability on the tendons and ligaments of the rotator cuff as well as the rotator cuff muscles (supraspinatus, infraspinatus, subscapularis, teres minor) for additional stability.

Table 17-7 Causes and clinical characteristics of shoulder pain

CATEGORY	CAUSE	CLINICAL FEATURES
Extracapsular lesions	Rotator cuff, and subacromial bursa—e.g. impingement syndromes, calcific tendinitis, cuff tears, bursitis	Painful arc of abduction (Figure 17-15) Pain on resisted cuff muscle movements, with intact passive movement (allowing for pain and guarding) Pain on impingement maneuvers as the inflamed rotator cuff tendons impinge on the inferior surface of the acromion, and coracoacromial arch
Intracapsular lesions	Glenohumeral joint—inflammatory arthritis, i.e. rheumatoid arthritis, spondyloarthritis, pseudogout Joint capsule—adhesive capsulitis Bone disease—Paget's disease, metastases	Loss of both active and passive movement Reduced glenohumeral range Night pain Muscle strength, allowing for pain, is intact
Referred pain	Cervical spine—facet joint root impingement, discitis Brachial plexus—brachial amyotrophy Thorax—Pancoast's tumor Thoracic outlet syndrome Suprascapular nerve entrapment Subdiaphragmatic—abscess, blood, hepatic lesions	Arm and hand pain with paresthesia Marked muscle weakness and wasting Neck pain and stiffness Herpes zoster rash Systemic features with weight loss

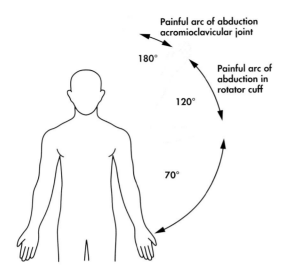

Painful arc of abduction acromioclavicular joint

180°

Painful arc of abduction in rotator cuff

120°

70°

Figure 17-15 Painful arc. The patient slowly abducts the arm as high as possible, describing symptoms as the arm rises

- The rotator cuff becomes compressed in the subacromial space as the arm is elevated, with impingement of the cuff between the proximal humerus and the acromioclavicular arch occurring from anomalies of the coracoacromial arch (structural impingement), and from instability due to joint hyperlaxity or weak rotator cuff muscles (functional impingement).
- Acquired impingement occurs secondary to osteophytes growing from the acromioclavicular joint, or calcification of the acromioclavicular ligament.
- Complications of impingement include a frozen shoulder, rupture of the rotator cuff tendons, or rupture of the long head of biceps.

CLINICAL PEARL

Three positive clinical tests (supraspinatus weakness, weakness of external rotation, and impingement), or two positive results for a patient older than 60 years, are highly predictive of a rotator cuff tear.

Treatment

Treatment depends on the mechanism of impingement.

- Patients with functional impingement are treated with a resting sling for 24–36 hours, pendular exercises, and full-dose NSAIDs.
- Structural impingement is treated similarly, but the surgical options of arthroscopic surgery to remove osteophytes or trim the acromion are available, after an adequate trial of conservative therapy.
- Corticosteroid injection to the subacromial space can be combined with an initial 4–7 days of pendulum exercises and avoidance of abduction, prior to a program of shoulder-strengthening exercises.

Frozen shoulder/adhesive capsulitis

This common disorder (2% cumulative risk in an at-risk population annually) is frequently misdiagnosed, and is characterized by painful restriction of all shoulder movements, both active and passive, with characteristic restriction in the glenohumeral range.

- There is marked reduction, or absence, of shoulder external rotation at 0° abduction, reduction of both internal and external rotation at 90° abduction, as well as prominent restriction of placing the hand behind the back on internal rotation.
- Frozen shoulder is characterized pathologically by fibrosis and retraction affecting predominantly the anterior and inferior structures of the glenohumeral joint capsule.
- Patients usually present in the 6th decade of life, and onset before the age of 40 is very uncommon.

Box 17-6 lists the diseases associated with frozen shoulder, diabetes being the most significant. Diabetes, particularly longstanding type 1 diabetes mellitus, is associated with glycosylation of subcutaneous collagen and the development of soft-tissue contraction—so-called diabetic cheiroarthropathy.

CLINICAL PEARL

When a diabetic patient presents with adhesive capsulitis, other diabetic complications, especially retinopathy and nephropathy, are seen more frequently and should be searched for.

Box 17-6

Common disorders associated with frozen shoulder

- Acute shoulder trauma, and shoulder immobilization
- Diabetes mellitus
- Thyroid disease (both hyper- and hypothyroidism)
- Cardiac disease, particularly after cardiac surgery
- Neurological disease with loss of consciousness, or hemiplegia
- Pulmonary disease—tuberculosis, carcinoma
- Rotator cuff disease, especially cuff tear
- Acute glenohumeral joint inflammation

Three phases of frozen shoulder are recognized.

1. **Painful inflammatory phase:** beginning insidiously with often only a minor injury being recalled, nocturnal awakening pain develops. The pain may be constant, and prevents the patient lying on the shoulder. Studies suggest that this phase lasts 2–9 months.
2. **Frozen shoulder:** with time, the night and rest pain eases but the shoulder remains 'frozen'. Mean duration is 4–12 months.
3. **Recovery phase:** after a mean delay of 5–26 months, in the majority of patients shoulder limitation slowly

recovers toward normal range (usually a 10–30% loss of motion which is often undetected by the patient). The total duration of symptoms lasts 12–42 months, with mean disease duration of 30 months.

Interestingly, 10–20% of patients develop a contralateral frozen shoulder, usually milder than the first, while the original shoulder is 'thawing'.

Management

- It is important to educate patients that the condition will spontaneously resolve and the stiffness will greatly reduce.
- NSAIDs and analgesics can be used.
- Exercise within the limits of pain achieves a better long-term outcome than intensive physiotherapy.
- Patients who receive an intra-articular injection earlier in the course of the disease recover more quickly compared with placebo.
- For those unable to tolerate the pain and disability of a frozen shoulder, manipulation under anesthesia (MUA) is a reliable way to improve the range of movement. It is particularly indicated when disability persists after 6 months of non-operative therapy. Other surgical approaches include arthroscopic release of adhesions, and hydrodilatation.
- Oral corticosteroid initially improves a frozen shoulder with a modest benefit on pain and disability, and ability to move the shoulder, but the effect does not last beyond 6 weeks.

TENNIS ELBOW AND GOLFER'S ELBOW

Tennis elbow (lateral epicondylitis)

Tennis elbow, or lateral epicondylitis, is considered to be an overload injury, which occurs after minor or unrecognized microtrauma to the proximal insertion of the extensor muscles of the forearm—particularly extensor carpi radialis brevis.

- It is the most frequently diagnosed elbow condition, occurring most commonly in middle life (35–55 years of age), and has an incidence in general practice of 4–7 cases per 1000 patients.
- Despite its common name, most cases occur in non-tennis players, and it is frequently a work-related enthesopathy affecting up to 15% of workers in at-risk industries which are characterized by highly repetitive activities.
- Both traction injury and ischemia appear to play a role in the development of this lesion.

The clue to the diagnosis is exquisite tenderness distal to, or anterior to, the lateral epicondyle. Resisted movement that tightens the fascial origin of the extensor carpi radialis brevis, i.e. resisted wrist dorsiflexion and resisted finger extension, worsens the pain.

> **CLINICAL PEARL**
>
> Diagnosis of tennis elbow:
> - Lateral elbow pain with tenderness on palpation just distal to the lateral epicondyle
> - Worsening pain localizing to the lateral epicondyle on resisted wrist dorsiflexion

Treatment

- It is usually a self-limiting condition, with the average duration of a typical episode being 6 months to 2 years, with 90% recovering within 1 year.
- Various conservative interventions exist for the treatment of this condition, including pain-relieving medications, corticosteroid injections, physiotherapy, elbow supports, acupuncture, surgery, and shockwave therapy.
- Most important in treatment is activity modification; both the frequency and the method of performance. In the work setting a review by an occupational therapist is recommended, focusing particularly on pronation/supination movements and grip size.
- A physiotherapy program that includes strengthening exercises for the entire upper limb, and a graded resistive program for wrist dorsiflexors, is recommended.
- Injection of corticosteroid with local anesthetic into the inflamed tendon may give short-term relief, but may be offset by a poorer long-term outcome.
- There may be a role for injection of platelet-rich plasma into the tendon.

A small number of patients have recalcitrant lateral epicondylitis, and are considered for operative intervention—open, arthroscopic, and percutaneous.

Golfer's elbow (medial epicondylitis)

Golfer's elbow, or medial epicondylitis, is the mirror image of tennis elbow and is thought also to relate to repetitive traction stress, and to microtears at the insertion of the forearm flexors (flexor carpi radialis) and pronator teres into the medial epicondyle.

- It occurs in both professional and amateur sports players, as well as manual workers such as bricklayers.
- It is much less common than tennis elbow, being approximately one-twentieth as common.
- Similarly to tennis elbow the diagnosis is clinical, with localized tenderness which worsens on resisted wrist flexion and forearm pronation.

> **CLINICAL PEARL**
>
> Golfer's elbow:
> - Elbow pain at the medial epicondyle
> - Increasing symptoms on resisted wrist flexion, and resisted forearm pronation
> - Treatment includes modification of activities, upper limb exercises, and analgesics

Box 17-7

Diagnosis of plantar fasciitis

- Chronic inferior heel pain on weightbearing: throbbing, searing, piercing in character
- Pain worst with the first steps in the morning, or after rest
- Pain reduces after mobilization, to recur with continued activity
- Walking barefoot, on toes, or upstairs exacerbates pain
- Tenderness around medial calcaneal tuberosity at the plantar aponeurosis
- Bilateral plantar fasciitis is highly suggestive of a spondyloarthropathy

Box 17-8

Therapeutic recommendations for treating plantar fasciitis

- Off-the-shelf (non-magnetic) insoles
- Plantar fascia stretching is more effective than calf stretching, and should be recommended to all patients
- Corticosteroid iontophoresis should be considered for short-term relief if initial therapy fails
- Custom-made night splints
- Walking casts in those who have failed conservative therapy
- Open or endoscopic surgery for those who have failed all conservative measures

PLANTAR FASCIITIS

Plantar fasciitis commonly causes inferior heel pain, and has been reported to occur in up to 10% of the US population.

- It affects both active and sedentary adults of all ages, but is more likely to occur in those who are obese, who spend most of the day on their feet, or who have limited ankle dorsiflexion.
- Plantar fasciitis is a musculoskeletal disorder primarily affecting the fascial enthesis. Although poorly understood, the development of plantar fasciitis is thought to have a mechanical origin.
- The diagnosis is based on the history and physical examination (Box 17-7).
- Unaccustomed walking in the sedentary, or prolonged running in the athlete, may induce fatigue tears of the plantar fascia, and avulsion fracture may cause pain at the medial calcaneal tuberosity. The same area is involved in spondyloarthropathy (ankylosing spondylitis, psoriatic arthritis and reactive arthritis) as plantar fascia enthesitis.
- 50% of patients with plantar fasciitis and 20% of persons without plantar fasciitis have heel spurs. The presence or absence of heel spurs is not helpful in diagnosing plantar fasciitis.

Most patients with plantar fasciitis eventually improve, although slowly, with 80% of patients treated conservatively in complete remission at 4 years. A variety of therapies are utilized in the treatment of plantar fasciitis, including exercise, and the key recommendations are summarized in Box 17-8.

Limited evidence supports the use of corticosteroid injections to manage plantar fasciitis; the benefit is short-lived, and may be associated with serious adverse effects such as fascial rupture.

FIBROMYALGIA

Fibromyalgia syndrome (FMS) is a soft-tissue musculoskeletal condition with many features in common with chronic fatigue syndrome (CFS), the major difference being the predominance of musculoskeletal features in FMS. Clinical features of FMS are:

- pain on both sides of the body
- pain above and below the waist
- pain in an axial distribution
- increased tenderness on palpation, although a specific number of trigger points is no longer required for diagnosis.

FMS diagnosis is based on a composite Widespread Pain Index (0–19) and Symptom Severity Score (0–12), with a score ≥13 consistent with fibromyalgia (Figure 17-16). The pain is often defined as 'aching' or 'burning', and may vary in intensity and location from day to day. Almost all people with FMS will describe muscular pain, fatigue, insomnia, joint pain and headache, half having memory impairment, poor concentration and paresthesiae, and one-third to one-fifth experiencing anxiety and depression.

- Musculoskeletal pain is, by definition, the most consistent feature of FMS.
- Fatigue, for some patients, can be almost as debilitating.
- Disordered sleep is also a very frequent feature, and clearly contributes to the general feeling of fatigue and to the mood disturbances. Sleep abnormalities are strongly correlated with the alpha-EEG abnormality on an electroencephalogram, and with movement disorders including the periodic jerking of arms and legs, teeth grinding (bruxism), and restless legs.
- Gastroesophageal reflux disease (GERD) occurs with high frequency, as does irritable bowel syndrome.
- Headaches are a major feature in at least 60%, and may be of the migraine or tension type.
- Facial pain is also relatively common, including discomfort related to temperomandibular joint dysfunction.
- Psychological and psychiatric morbidity is also increased in patients with FMS. This may range from minor mood disturbance to major depression. There is also a very high prevalence of anxiety disorders, including obsessive compulsive disorder and post-traumatic stress disorder.

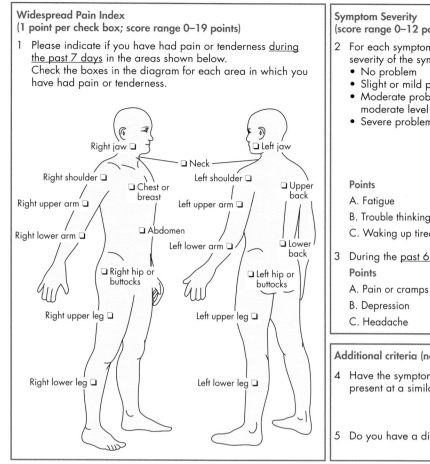

Widespread Pain Index
(1 point per check box; score range 0–19 points)

1 Please indicate if you have had pain or tenderness <u>during the past 7 days</u> in the areas shown below.
Check the boxes in the diagram for each area in which you have had pain or tenderness.

Right jaw ❏
❏ Left jaw
❏ Neck
Right shoulder ❏
Left shoulder ❏
❏ Upper back
❏ Chest or breast
Right upper arm ❏
Left upper arm ❏
Right lower arm ❏
❏ Abdomen
Left lower arm ❏
❏ Lower back
❏ Right hip or buttocks
❏ Left hip or buttocks
Right upper leg ❏
Left upper leg ❏
Right lower leg ❏
Left lower leg ❏

Symptom Severity
(score range 0–12 points)

2 For each symptom listed below, use the following scale to indicate the severity of the symptom <u>during the past 7 days</u>.
• No problem
• Slight or mild problem: generally mild or intermittent
• Moderate problem: considerable problems; often present and/or at a moderate level
• Severe problem: continuous, life-disturbing problems.

	No problem	Slight or mild problem	Moderate problem	Severe problem
Points	0	1	2	3
A. Fatigue	❏	❏	❏	❏
B. Trouble thinking or remembering	❏	❏	❏	❏
C. Waking up tired (unrefreshed)	❏	❏	❏	❏

3 During the <u>past 6 months</u> have you had any of the following symptoms?

Points	0	1
A. Pain or cramps in lower abdomen	❏ No	❏ Yes
B. Depression	❏ No	❏ Yes
C. Headache	❏ No	❏ Yes

Additional criteria (no score)

4 Have the symptoms in questions 2 and 3 and widespread pain been present at a similar level for at <u>least 3 months</u>?
❏ No   ❏ Yes

5 Do you have a disorder that would otherwise explain the pain?
❏ No   ❏ Yes

Figure 17-16 Criteria worksheet for fibromyalgia

From Wolfe FI et al. The American College of Rheumatology preliminary diagnostic criteria for fibromyalgia and measurement of symptom severity. Arthritis Care Res 2010;62(5):600–10.

Epidemiology and etiology

An estimated prevalence of FMS is 1–4%, and it is 2–6 times more likely to occur in women than men. The incidence in the female population has been estimated at 11.3 per 1000 person years. Although it can occur at any age, the condition becomes more common with advancing years.

It is highly unlikely a single underlying cause for FMS will be found, with a strong interplay between physical and psychological factors.

• The onset of illness may be triggered by physical illness, including intercurrent infection; or by trauma, including surgery.

• There is some suggestion that heredity may play a part, with components of the serotonergic and dopaminergic systems being candidate genes.

• Some of the symptomatology around the trigger points may be due to increased acetylcholine at the motor end-plate, causing contraction and shortening of the sarcomere. This may lead to increased energy consumption and increased local blood supply, with resulting local tenderness.

• A number of local and systemic mediators have been implicated in the pathogenesis. These include bradykinin, calcitonin gene-related peptide (CGRP), substance P, TNF-alpha, interleukin-1 (IL-1), noradrenaline, and serotonin.

Investigations

• Routine investigations including full blood count, biochemistry, ESR, CRP and other inflammatory markers are all within the normal range.

• X-rays, CT and MRI are likewise generally normal, and there are no specific abnormalities on muscle biopsy, electromyography (EMG) or nerve conduction studies (NCS).

• Electroencephalography (EEG) for more formal sleep studies may be requested in patients who have marked sleep disturbance. This may reveal abnormalities including periodic limb movement disorder, rapid eye movement (REM) sleep disorder, or sleep apnea.

The diagnosis of FMS is basically one of exclusion, and is made clinically.

Prognosis, differential diagnosis and treatment

- The outlook for a patient with classic FMS is very variable, and the condition tends to become chronic.
- More widespread understanding and a clearer definition of the syndrome, along with a more highly developed treatment flow, is beginning to streamline management and improve the outlook for a proportion of patients.
- There is no specific treatment. Therapeutic measures depend upon the precise complaints of the patient, and should take into account other aspects of the patient's health.

Treatment measures include the following.

- **Appropriate investigation and making a clear diagnosis.** Educating the patient as to the nature of the diagnosis, and reassuring them about the prognosis and treatment. Liaison with support organizations for education, and self-help groups.
- **Attention to psychological and social factors**, and encouraging the patient to have a normal sleep pattern and to engage in physical activity consistent with the state of health and preferences.
- **Pain relief.** This may range from simple analgesics such as acetaminophen (paracetamol), to more powerful agents. Inappropriate use of powerful opioid analgesics should be avoided, as this may lead to dependence and seldom alleviates the symptoms in the long term. NSAIDs have marginal benefits over simple analgesics. Tramadol is a weak opioid, with some action to inhibit the uptake of serotonin; this agent sometimes proves to be of great benefit.
- **Antidepressants.** Either tricyclic antidepressants or selective serotonin reuptake inhibitors (SSRIs) are of benefit in many cases. Some patients benefit from these agents even when there is no major evidence of depression. Dual inhibitors of both noradrenaline and serotonin uptake, such as duloxetine, may be of particular benefit. Duloxetine is FDA-approved for the treatment of fibromyalgia.
- **Alpha$_2$–adrenergic agonists** such as clonidine or tizanidine are of benefit to some patients, and may act by inhibiting the action of neurotransmitters such as glutamate or substance P within the central nervous system.
- **Anticonvulsants** may contribute to pain relief. There is increasing experience with agents such as pregabalin and gabapentin, which reduce the release of the central pain transmitters glutamate and substance P, resulting in improvement in pain and quality of sleep.
- **Trigger point injection.** This may be undertaken with local anesthetic, steroid or botulinum toxin. Botulinum may be more effective than steroid injection, and may act by diminishing acetylcholine release, thus decreasing muscle activity and local ischemia.
- **Postural training, exercise, and ergonomic adjustments** (particularly in the workplace) may all help patients to adapt to disability associated with FMS.
- **Stress reduction** may be achieved with a variety of techniques, including cognitive–behavioral therapy, relaxation techniques and biofeedback methods.
- **Physical therapies** such as acupuncture, massage, transcutaneous electrical nerve stimulation (TENS), and ultrasound may all be helpful. Hydrotherapy is strongly recommended for all fibromyalgia patients.

SEPTIC ARTHRITIS

An acutely swollen knee is one of the most common presentations of a monoarthritis; and fortunately, due to the ease of aspirating this joint, it is also a monoarthritis with a good chance of a diagnosis being made. Although redness may occur in any acute arthritis regardless of the etiology, its presence evokes a more limited diagnosis. The differential diagnosis of monoarthritis is listed in Box 17-9.

- Elevated temperature suggests infection, and questioning should cover the systemic aspects of infection as well as questioning and examination for local and more distal sites of infection.
- Septic arthritis is usually exquisitely tender to examination, with resistance to joint movement.
- *Staphylococcus* is the most common cause of musculoskeletal sepsis, accounting for 80% of infections, with the prevalence of both streptococcal and mycobacterial infection increasing.
- With staphylococci, streptococci, Gram-negative bacteria and anerobes, only one joint is usually involved.
- Polyarticular involvement is more likely in the elderly or the immunosuppressed, with infection by *Haemophilus influenzae*, meningococcus, and *Neisseria gonorrhoeae* tending to be polyarticular.
- Lyme disease can present with knee involvement, although the diagnosis can be quickly excluded if there has been no exposure to the tick vector of *Borrelia burgdorferi*.
- *H. influenzae* is the most common organism in children under 5 years who have not been immunized.
- A particular clinical situation is suspected septic arthritis in a postoperative shoulder, in which *Propionibacterium acnes* should be considered.

Box 17-9

Differential diagnosis of monoarthritis

- Trauma—meniscal or ligamentous tears with or without hemarthrosis
- Sepsis—gonococcal arthritis, *Staphylococcus aureus*, penetrating injury, or foreign body
- Reactive arthritis—post gastrointestinal or genitourinary infection
- Hemophilia
- Crystal arthritis—gout or pseudogout
- Inflammatory—a single joint presentation of an ultimately polyarthritic process, e.g. rheumatoid, psoriatic or reactive arthritis

---

If septic arthritis is clinically suspected, prompt evaluation of the synovial fluid is mandatory prior to the administration of antibiotics. Accompanying clinical features may include fever and acute onset of symptoms. The presence of risk factors should be looked for, and these include:

- age >80 years
- diabetes mellitus
- rheumatoid arthritis and other joint disease
- prosthetic joint
- recent joint surgery
- skin infection, cutaneous ulcers
- intravenous drug use, alcoholism
- previous intra-articular corticosteroid injection.

Gonococcal septic arthritis will not have systemic or cutaneous manifestations in 50% of cases. This diagnosis should be considered in all sexually active patients. In young adults, gonococcal arthritis is a common cause of non-traumatic acute monoarthritis, and questioning regarding either a change in sexual partners or genitourinary symptoms needs to be undertaken.

- In addition to the often polyarticular arthritis, tenosynovitis and a pustular rash of the extremities should be examined for.
- Gonococcal arthritis is 3–4 times more common in women, who often develop the arthritis in the perimenstrual period.
- Men will often experience a urethritis as dysuria and may notice a morning discharge, whereas women may be asymptomatic.

Investigations

The key investigation of a suspected septic joint is aspiration of the joint. A relatively small volume of only 1–2 mL of fluid is sufficient to complete all investigations; however, the joint should be aspirated of as much fluid as can be obtained without increasing the trauma of the procedure.

- Substantial pain relief is achieved by aspirating a tense effusion, and while re-accumulation will occur, it buys some time while the preliminary results are received from the laboratory.

- Note should be taken of the color, viscosity and turbidity of the aspirate. Normal synovial fluid is similar to egg white, and is both viscous and acellular.
- As the degree of inflammation increases, from the negligible amount found in OA to the mid-range of RA and the extreme of septic arthritis, the viscosity decreases and the cellularity and turbidity increase.

CLINICAL PEARL

Blood-colored effusions are suggestive of either trauma or calcium pyrophosphate arthropathy.

Comparisons of synovial fluid analysis are shown in Table 17-8.

Tests requested should include an urgent Gram stain, cell count and differential, crystal examination using polarized light microscopy, and culture.

Treatment

- The presence of bacteria on Gram staining, or subsequent bacterial growth, requires specialist medical and orthopedic review, to combine antibiotic therapy with joint lavage.
- Empirical therapy for septic arthritis using intravenous antibiotics covering *S. aureus* and *N. gonorrhoeae* should be commenced after the synovial fluid aspirate has been obtained.
- Adequate analgesics, antipyretics and rest should be employed, with the joint aspiration or lavage itself often affording considerable pain relief.

ACUTE LOW BACK PAIN

Low back pain (LBP) is a common human experience with an annual incidence of 2–5%, and 70–90% of the general population experiencing an episode of LBP at some point in their lives, with a peak prevalence at 65 years. Fortunately, 90% of individuals with acute LBP improve within 4–8 weeks, and only 5% of patients develop persistent or chronic LBP lasting >3 months. Risk factors for low back pain are shown in Table 17-9.

Table 17-8 Synovial fluid characteristics in health and disease

	NORMAL	NON-INFLAMMATORY	INFLAMMATORY	SEPTIC
Color	Clear	Straw yellow	Yellow	Variable
Clarity	Transparent	Transparent	Hazy opaque	Opaque
Viscosity	High	High	Low	Low–thick
WBC count (per mm³)	0–200	200–2000	2000–75,000	>75,000
Neutrophils	<25%	<25%	25–50%	>75%
WBC, white blood cell.				

Table 17-9 Risk factors for low back pain

Strongest risk factor	Previous history of back pain
Strong risk factors	Poor job satisfaction
	Emotional distress
	Manual laborer, involving heavy lifting
	Prolonged sitting or standing
Moderate risk factors	Vibration-tool use
	Smoking
	Obesity
	Poor physical fitness

Box 17-10

Causes of acute low back pain (LBP)

97% mechanical LBP
- 80%: idiopathic
- 20%:
  » prolapsed intervertebral disc
  » lumbar spondylosis
  » spondylolisthesis
  » spinal stenosis
  » fracture
  » Scheuermann's disease

1% non-mechanical spinal pain
- Inflammatory spondyloarthritis

1–2% visceral disease
- Infection
- Neoplasia

The cause of the vast majority of LBP is unknown, with no pathological cause for the pain found in at least 80% of cases (Box 17-10). Based on the history and physical examination, LBP is classified as:

- nonspecific LBP or simple backache
- nerve-root or spinal–nerve compromise
- potentially serious spinal pathology (including infection, cancer, fracture, inflammatory back pain, and cauda equina syndrome).

Serious pathology as a cause of back pain is uncommon, <5% having compression fractures, and <1% cancer, infection, inflammatory disorders, or cauda equina syndrome. Red flags of suspicion are listed in Box 17-11.

CLINICAL PEARL

Indicators of nerve root problems:
- Unilateral leg pain > low back pain
- Radiates to foot or toes
- Numbness and paresthesia in same distribution
- Straight leg raising induces more leg pain
- Neurological deficit confined to one nerve root distribution

- Simple backache does not benefit from extensive investigation, which may even be harmful if leading to the management of benign abnormalities such as disc bulge on imaging, despite these being rarely related to LBP.
- In those few cases where further diagnostic investigation is required, it should be aimed at confirming a specific pathological lesion that would explain the patient's symptoms or findings.
- Cauda equina syndrome should be suspected when leg pain that includes several spinal nerve levels is accompanied by widespread motor and/or sensory weakness, and importantly when there is associated bladder or bowel dysfunction.

Box 17-11

'Red flags' of low back pain

Weight loss, fever, night sweats
Nocturnal pain
History of malignancy
Recent or current infection
Acute onset <20 or >55 years
Constant or progressive pain
Bilateral or alternating symptoms
Neurological or sphincter disturbance
Morning stiffness
Claudication or peripheral ischemia

Specific pathology leading to acute low back pain

The spine is commonly described as a three-joint complex, consisting of the intervertebral disc anteriorly and the two facet joints posterolaterally. These border the triangular-shaped spinal canal, as depicted diagrammatically in Figure 17-17.

- Deformity of the three-joint complex, anterior or posterior subluxation (spondylolisthesis) of a vertebral body, as well as deformity of the posterior longitudinal ligament and ligamentum flavum, can lead to nerve-root impingement in the lower spine or to spinal cord compression at higher levels.
- The spinal cord ends at approximately the level of L1–L2, so that neurological manifestations in LBP syndromes are lower motor neuron lesions affecting the peripheral nerve roots.
- The most common site of disc prolapse is the L4 or L5 disc, and at that level a posterolateral protrusion

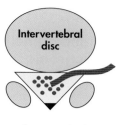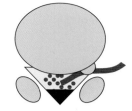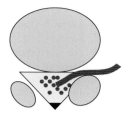

| Normal intervertebral disc, facet joints and exiting nerve root | Central disc bulge and posterolateral bulge with ligamentum flavum hypertrophy | Facet joint hypertrophy |

Figure 17-17 Nerve root pain

impinges on the L5 nerve root. A centrally placed bulge may affect multiple lower nerve roots in a bilateral fashion, causing a cauda equina syndrome.

- The combined pathologies of facet joint hypertrophy/osteophyte formation, disc bulges, and deformity of the long ligaments effectively stenoses the spinal canal and is a common spinal disorder in the elderly, presenting with pseudoclaudication, sciatica, and dysfunction of the cauda equina.

Abnormalities in X-ray and MRI are poorly associated with the occurrence of nonspecific LBP.

- Abnormalities found when imaging people without back pain are just as prevalent as those found in patients with LBP, and it needs to be remembered that radiological abnormalities of degeneration and spondylosis have been reported in 40–50% in people without LBP.
- Many people with LBP show no abnormalities, which has led to the recommendations to be restrictive in imaging unless 'red flags' are present.
- CT and MRI are equally effective in diagnosing lumbar disc herniation and stenosis, but are only meaningful if compatible with the clinical findings.
- MRI is the modality of choice for suspected infection or malignancy, although these are relatively rare causes of LBP.

Prolapsed intervertebral disc

The intervertebral disc is composed of the inner nucleus pulposus and the outer annulus fibrosus. The outer third of the annulus is innervated such that mechanoreceptors respond to distortion. Prolapsed disc is a result of the nucleus pulposus protruding through a defect in the annulus fibrosus, usually a tear in the posterolateral portion. While this is generally due to degeneration in the annulus fibrosus, it can result from mechanical forces, e.g. heavy lifting. The tear results in a local inflammatory response.

Spinal fracture

The older patient, particularly female, who presents with sudden-onset localized back pain after minor or inconsequential trauma should be suspected to have an osteoporotic compression fracture, particularly in the presence of additional underlying risk factors for osteoporosis.

Cancer

Features predictive of malignancy as a cause of LBP are:

1. previous history of cancer
2. age 50 years or older
3. failure of conservative therapy
4. weight loss >4.5 kg.

Using these indicators, patients with a past history of cancer should undergo MRI investigation; with any other indicator, a CT scan or plain-film radiograph is ordered.

Infection

A history of immunosuppression, or risk factors for breaches in the normal barriers to bacteremia, should be elicited from the patient and coupled with an examination looking for septic foci. In 40% of cases of spinal osteomyelitis there is hematogenous spread from an identifiable extraosseous source, most commonly genitourinary, skin or respiratory. The most commonly identified organism is *Staphylococcus aureus*, with Gram-negative organisms in the elderly or intravenous drug users.

Management

Treatment guidelines are summarized in Box 17-12.

Outcome

Most guidelines for the management of acute LBP identify the following as poor prognostic factors: fear avoidance

---

Box 17-12

Summary of treatment guidelines for acute low back pain

- Reassure patient of favorable prognosis
- Advise patient to remain active, and discourage bed rest
- Do not prescribe specific back exercises
- Prescribe regular medication consisting of
  » acetaminophen (paracetamol)
  » non-steroidal anti-inflammatory drugs
- Consider net benefit of muscle relaxants

---

behavior, leg pain, and low job satisfaction. Overall, however, it is consistently reported that more than 90% of patients improve by 6–12 weeks.

Recurrences of LBP are common, with an estimated three-quarters having a recurrence within a 1-year period. The severity, however, is usually less, and does not always lead to a new visit to the physician.

CHRONIC LOW BACK PAIN

In patients with chronic LBP the terms 'nonspecific' or 'mechanical' low back pain are used with an implication that an anatomical or pathological basis is understood as the cause of the patient's symptoms. In reality, the etiology remains unknown for the majority of such patients.

Clinical assessment

- Observation is used to determine alteration in posture, muscle wasting, changes in the physiological lordoses, and the effects of movement on the alignment of the spine.
- Palpation can be undertaken to assist in evaluating movement at a segmental level, and also to identify local tenderness.

Conservative treatment

- Strong evidence supports the use of exercise and intensive multidisciplinary pain-treatment programs for chronic LBP.
- Cognitive–behavioral therapy, analgesics, antidepressants, NSAIDs, back schools, and spinal manipulation are supported only by weak evidence.
- Regrettably, however, for most effective treatments the effects are usually only small and short-term.

Box 17-13

Recommended guidelines for the treatment of chronic low back pain

- Recommend cognitive–behavioral therapy, supervised exercise, brief educational interventions, multidisciplinary (biopsychosocial) treatments
- Advise patient to remain active
- Short-term use of non-steroidal anti-inflammatory drugs and weak opioids
- Consider the net benefit of muscle relaxants, back schools, anti-depressants, and manipulation
- Avoid passive treatment such as ultrasound and shortwave
- Invasive treatments such as facet joint injections are generally not recommended

---

- No evidence supports using interventions such as steroid injections, lumbar supports, and traction.

Treatment guidelines are outlined in Box 17-13.

Invasive treatment

The efficacy of invasive interventions in the form of facet joint, epidural, trigger point and sclerosant injections have clearly been shown to be ineffective for the treatment of LBP and sciatica.

No sound evidence is available for the efficacy of spinal stenosis surgery, although surgical discectomy may be considered in those with sciatica due to lumbar disc prolapse, who have failed to respond to conservative management.

SELF-ASSESSMENT QUESTIONS

1 A 28-year-old woman presents with an 8-week history of pain and swelling in her left knee. She is afebrile, has moderate effusion of the left knee, mild left quadriceps wasting, and a 'sausage digit' of the right 3rd toe. Her erythrocyte sedimentation rate (ESR) is 58 mm/h (normal <18) and C-reactive protein (CRP) 45 mg/dL (normal <5). Which of the following statements is correct in this case?

A The absence of psoriasis on examination excludes psoriatic arthritis as a likely diagnosis.

B Quadriceps wasting and an 8-week history indicate a chronic arthritis that is not part of the post-infectious arthritis spectrum.

C Investigation should include an early morning urine for *Chlamydia trachomatis* polymerase chain reaction (PCR) testing.

D Her anti-nuclear antibodies (ANA) will be positive with a homogeneous pattern and titer >1:1280, with anti-double-stranded DNA antibodies elevated above the reference level.

E The prominent inflammatory marker elevation indicates sepsis, and intravenous flucloxacillin should be administered pending further investigation.

2 A 54-year-old bricklayer has had progressive pain and swelling in his hands over the past 4–6 months. He finds it hard to dress himself in the morning, with pain under his feet when first standing. He can only begin carrying bricks when he has warmed up in the sun, around 10 a.m. A local family physician commenced him on prednisolone 7.5 mg daily for the past 2 weeks, and he feels much better. When examined, he winces when shaking hands, and has palpable synovial swelling of his metacarpophalangeal (MCP) and proximal interphalangeal (PIP) joints. His erythrocyte sedimentation rate (ESR) and C-reactive protein (CRP) are normal, rheumatoid factor (RF) testing is negative, and anti-cyclic citrullinated peptide (CCP) antibody strongly positive. Which of the following approaches is most appropriate?

A No additional therapy is needed, as his normal inflammatory markers will soon be matched by resolution of his clinical findings, and the prednisolone will then be able to be withdrawn.

B The absence of RF indicates a seronegative disease, such as psoriatic arthritis. Initiation of anti-interleukin 12/23 therapy will treat both the arthritis and his psoriasis.

C A chest X-ray is not required.

D Information and prescriptions for hydroxychloroquine, methotrexate, folic acid and omega-3 oil supplementation should be provided.

E Bricklaying will accelerate his joint destruction and he should cease employment and seek an occupation that does not require manual labor.

3 You have been managing an overweight patient with gout for some time. He presents after a week of pain and swelling in the right knee and more recently his left midfoot. Both joints are warm, pink and tender. Which of the following is correct regarding this presentation?

A His acute gout should be managed with non-steroidal anti-inflammatory drugs (NSAIDs) or corticosteroids before prescribing colchicine.

B He should cease his allopurinol during the acute attack and recommence when his joints have been quiet for at least 2 weeks.

C Today's serum urate, 0.38 mmol/L, is within the normal range (0.36–0.42 mmol/L), making acute gout very unlikely.

D He has continued to have attacks of gout despite reliably taking his allopurinol 300 mg tablet daily, and has 'failed' this therapy. It should be ceased and an alternative agent trialed.

E He has been losing weight rapidly, using a diet which includes peas, beans, mushrooms and asparagus. These are rich in purines, and will have brought on this attack of gout.

4 Vera is a 64-year-old book-keeper who now finds it hard to operate her computer and to pick up objects. The pain in her hands has worsened over the past few years, and she has had to stop her hobby of needlework. She has had psoriasis of the scalp for most of her life. Examination is of square hands, with swelling of all distal interphalangeal (DIP) joints and most of her proximal interphalangeal (PIP) joints. Blood tests showed a rheumatoid factor (RF) of 16 IU (normal <14) and C-reactive protein (CRP) of 7 (normal <5). Which of the following is correct?

A Symmetrical interphalangeal swelling combined with a positive RF indicates a diagnosis of rheumatoid arthritis.

B Careful examination of the joints is needed to differentiate hard bony swelling from soft boggy swelling.

C An X-ray of the hands is needed to confirm the diagnosis.

D Topical non-steroidal anti-inflammatory drugs (NSAIDs) are less efficacious than oral agents.

E The presence of elevated inflammatory markers warrants the addition of an anti-rheumatic agent such as methotrexate.

ANSWERS

1 C.

An oligoarthritis with dactylitis (synovitis of both interphalangeal joints and tenosynovitis) is highly suggestive of a seronegative spondyloarthritis, the differential diagnosis for which includes psoriatic arthritis. Diagnostic criteria for psoriatic arthritis are weighted toward current psoriasis on examination, but previous psoriasis or a family history of psoriasis can be considered. In up to 10% of cases the psoriatic skin rash will develop after the arthritis.

Gastrointestinal and genitourinary infections can be associated with a longer-lasting reactive arthritis, and symptoms of infection should be sought. *Chlamydia trachomatis* infection is often asymptomatic and a missed infection may adversely affect future fertility, hence the importance of PCR testing in this case. If there has been travel through areas prone to arthropod-borne viruses, this can cause an arthritis that is often of short duration, but there are exceptions with some patients having chronic symptoms.

Systemic lupus erythematosus is often associated with arthralgia or a symmetrical small-joint arthritis, and in the absence of other systemic features is lower on the differential diagnosis. A screening ANA test may be undertaken, with subsequent testing dependent on the result; extractable nuclear antigen testing if a speckled ANA pattern is found, and anti-dsDNA antibodies if a rim or homogeneous pattern is found.

Septic arthritis is a diagnosis 'not to be missed'; however, in an afebrile, immunocompetent patient with a long history, bacterial infection is unlikely. Positive culture results from synovial fluid aspiration are well below 100%, but synovial aspirate for Gram stain, cell count and differential, and culture should be undertaken prior to antibiotic commencement.

2 D.

Prednisolone may have ameliorated the cytokine-driven ESR and CRP response, but the presence of synovitis in the MCP and PIP joints indicates a joint count of at least 20, which is severe disease. The treatment target will be undetectable clinical synovitis, in addition to normalization of his inflammatory markers.

Psoriatic arthritis is the great mimic and can present with any pattern of joint inflammation; a symmetrical rheumatoid arthritis (RA)-like picture occurring in 10% of psoriatic arthritis. While approximately 70% of RA patients are RF-positive, the absence does not exclude RA (nor does the presence prove RA). Absence of RF would not dissuade you from a diagnosis of RA, particularly in the presence of anti-CCP antibodies, which are most specific for RA and are present in some of the RF-negative RA patients. Anti-CCP antibodies are a poor prognostic factor, correlating with increased joint damage and extra-articular manifestations.

The available information fulfills points 2, 3 and 4 of the 1987 American College of Rheumatology criteria for RA which did not include anti-citrullinated peptide status. Using the newer 2010 criteria, this man has definite RA on the basis of joint count (5 points), high positive anti-CCP antibodies (3 points), and duration >6 weeks (1 point). Low-dose prednisolone can quickly ameliorate disease, and should be combined with methotrexate and folic acid. Methotrexate is slow-acting over 6–8 weeks, after which the prednisolone can be withdrawn. Hydroxychloroquine is synergistic with methotrexate therapy. As most patients are interested in diet and natural therapies, constructive guidance on the use of 2.7 g daily of EPA/DHA long-chain omega-3 fatty acids to reduce symptoms and lessen the need for therapy with non-steroidal anti-inflammatory agents with associated side-effects will be well received.

A chest X-ray is indicated due to smoking being one of the strongest environmental triggers for RA, and pulmonary fibrosis can occur as part of the disease process and as a reaction to medications such as methotrexate and leflunomide. A baseline for comparison is a handy reference, and it is also part of the screen for tuberculosis, which is recommended, along with hepatitis serology, in patients likely to receive long-term immunosuppression.

RA reduces life expectancy; up to 50% of RA patients will no longer be in employment at 10 years, and this is more likely in a manual worker. However, this is not inevitable, and the array of treatment options has meant remission is an achievable target. Each clinic visit should amend therapy to minimize objective measures of disease impact on joint count, inflammatory markers, and patient quality of life.

3 A.

Untreated gout will progress from intermittent acute monoarthritis to increasingly frequent and severe attacks that will involve more proximal joints, and become polyarticular. Once commenced, allopurinol should only be ceased for an allergic reaction or adverse event. Ceasing or commencing a urate-lowering therapy during an acute attack creates friable uric acid crystals within the joint, and will worsen and prolong the attack, and patients are likely to abandon the therapy as it makes their gout worse.

Up to 30% of patients will have a normal urate level during an acute attack, particularly if measured a few days into the attack. This is falsely low due to the acute phase response and does not exclude the diagnosis of gout. Once urate-lowering therapy is commenced, treatment is adjusted until a urate level of 0.30–0.36 mmol/L is reached. In this example, his normal urate is still above target and his allopurinol should be increased to 400 mg after the acute attack has settled. One 300 mg tablet is insufficient therapy in the majority of patients, and allopurinol should not be abandoned but instead slowly titrated to achieve the target at lowest possible dose, with doses up to 900 mg daily approved.

Vegetable-derived purines have no negative effect on gout and can be safely incorporated into diets aimed at reducing meat and seafood intake, while increasing low-fat dairy intake. His rapid weight-loss diet may have induced a ketotic/starvation state leading to reduced renal excretion of urate, and may have precipitated his gout.

Increasing awareness of the toxicity of colchicine has meant that it should only be used in acute attacks if NSAIDs and corticosteroids are ineffective or contraindicated, which is a rare event. If used, the dose needs to be strictly monitored and used for no longer than 4 days, with a 2- to 3-day gap between courses.

4 B.

Osteoarthritis is the most common form of arthritis, and typically involves the DIP joints, leading to osteophytic expansion of the joint line, known as Heberden's nodes. The 1st carpometacarpal joint is involved similarly, leading to subluxation of the joint which moves the thumb toward the palm of the hand to give a square appearance to the hand in the prone position. Osteophytes of the PIP joint (Bouchard's nodes) are less common than Heberden's nodes. A low-level RF occurs in at least 5% of the healthy population, and needs to be interpreted in the clinical context. Osteoarthritis is relatively non-inflammatory compared, for example, with gout or rheumatoid arthritis, but can cause mild elevation of markers as seen in this case. Methotrexate is not indicated in osteoarthritis.

Psoriatic arthritis occurs in 25–33% of patients with psoriasis. Clinical examination to differentiate hard bony swelling from soft boggy swelling distinguishes osteoarthritis from psoriatic arthritis. Clinical examination provides the pattern of joint involvement, and will differentiate inflammatory synovitis from degenerative osteophytes; an X-ray will not provide more information in these circumstances.

Effective therapy for osteoarthritis remains problematic, with many studies showing large placebo effects. In comparative studies, topical NSAIDs have a larger effect size than oral agents.

CHAPTER 18

NEUROLOGY

Christopher Levi and Thomas Wellings

CHAPTER OUTLINE

- **DISORDERS OF CONSCIOUSNESS**
  - Definitions
  - Levels of consciousness
  - Causes of coma
  - Assessment of the patient with impaired consciousness

- **HEADACHE**
  - Primary headache syndromes
  - Secondary headache

- **STROKE**
  - Acute assessment and management
  - Thrombolysis
  - Neurosurgical intervention
  - General care measures
  - Early secondary prevention

- **INTRACEREBRAL HEMORRHAGE**
  - Medical treatment
  - Surgical management

- **SUBARACHNOID HEMORRHAGE (SAH)**
  - Natural history and outcome of an aneurysmal SAH
  - Surgical versus endovascular management of SAH

- **TRANSIENT ISCHEMIC ATTACK (TIA)**
  - Definition
  - Differential diagnosis of transient neurological disturbances

  - Pathophysiology
  - Investigation
  - Recurrent event risk
  - Prevention of recurrent events

- **DEMENTIA**
  - Diagnosis
  - Major dementia syndromes
  - Diagnostic work-up of the dementia patient
  - Other dementia syndromes

- **SEIZURES AND THE EPILEPSIES**
  - Seizure types
  - Assessing a patient after a seizure
  - Investigation of a first seizure
  - The epilepsies
  - Important epilepsy syndromes
  - Choice of anticonvulsant therapy
  - Status epilepticus
  - Non-epileptic seizures

- **BALANCE, DIZZINESS AND VERTIGO**
  - Hemodynamic dizziness or 'lightheadedness'
  - Vertigo
  - Central pathologies
  - Treatment of vertiginous patients
  - Other balance disorders

- **MOVEMENT DISORDERS**
  - Tremor
  - Parkinson's disease (PD)
  - Dementia with Lewy bodies (DLB)
  - Multisystem atrophy (MSA)
  - Progressive supranuclear palsy (PSP)

- Corticobasal syndrome
- Dystonia
- Hyperkinetic movement disorders
- NMDA encephalitis

• MULTIPLE SCLEROSIS AND CNS INFLAMMATION
  - Multiple sclerosis (MS)
  - Neuromyelitis optica (NMO; 'Devic's disease')
  - Acute disseminated encephalomyelitis (ADEM) and transverse myelitis (TM)
  - Neurological manifestations of sarcoidosis and Behçet's disease

• NEUROMUSCULAR DISEASE
  - Myopathy
  - Genetic muscle disorders
  - Disorders of the neuromuscular junction
  - Disorders of peripheral nerves
  - Motor neuron disease (MND)/amyotrophic lateral sclerosis
  - Demyelinating neuropathy and Guillain–Barré syndrome (GBS)
  - Peripheral neuropathy

DISORDERS OF CONSCIOUSNESS

Definitions

- Consciousness is the state of responsiveness of an individual to the environment.
- The most severe form of impairment of consciousness is coma, a state of unresponsiveness where the person is unable to be aroused.
- The ascending reticular formation (reticular activating system, RAS) is the central neuroanatomical structure responsible for maintaining consciousness. It comprises a network of neurons extending from the medulla to the thalamus, receiving projections from all major sensory pathways and sending projections diffusely to the cerebral cortex.

Levels of consciousness

- *Normal consciousness*—alert wakefulness with orientation, and prompt and appropriate response to stimuli.
- *Confusion and delirium*—clouding of consciousness with impaired attention, concentration and capacity for clear thought and understanding. There is often slowed or inappropriate response to stimuli, progressing to disorientation, distractability, agitation, and restlessness. In severe forms, anxiety, behavioral disturbance and hallucinations are seen.
- *Stupor and obtundation*—drowsiness, progressing to absence of spontaneous motor activity, and responsiveness only evident to vigorous stimulation or pain.
- *Coma*—unrousability, where no appropriate response can be elicited by external stimuli.

Causes of coma

Coma is the result of either dysfunction of the RAS or diffuse processes affecting both cerebral hemispheres.

- It is important to note that structural lesions in the brainstem and the cerebral hemisphere will not necessarily cause impairment of consciousness.

  » Focal brainstem lesions need to be strategic, with the location directly damaging the RAS in the ventral medulla and peri-aqueductal region of the ventral pons and midbrain.
  » Hemispheric lesions need to be causing significant mass effect with lateral and/or downward displacement, and secondary mass effect on the diencephalic structures containing the upper extent of the RAS.

- The most common cause of coma is diffuse (Box 18-1) and widespread disturbance of brain function secondary to factors such as neurotropic drugs, and toxic, metabolic and electrical disturbances of brain function.

Box 18-1

Causes of coma

Structural or focal brain pathology (approx. 30%)

(Supratentorial 15%, infratentorial 15%)

- Stroke
- Meningitis
- Encephalitis
- Cerebral abscess
- Brain tumor
- Head injury

Diffuse disturbances of brain function (approx. 70%)

- Metabolic:
  » Hypoxia
  » Hyponatremia
  » Hypercalcemia
  » Uremia
  » Hypoglycemia
  » Hepatic encephalopathy
- Toxic substances:
  » Hypnosedative drugs
  » Narcotics
- Seizure-related:
  » Post-ictal coma
  » Persistent subclinical seizure activity
- Psychogenic (rare)

Table 18-1 Glasgow Coma Scale

	SCORE					
	1	2	3	4	5	6
Eyes	Does not open eyes	Eyes open to pain	Eyes open to command	Eyes open spontaneously		
Verbal	Makes no sound	Incomprehensible sounds, groans	Inappropriate words	Confused, disorientated	Alert and converses normally	
Motor	No movement	Extension to pain (*decerebrate* response)	Abnormal flexion to pain (*decorticate* response)	Flexion or withdrawal to painful stimuli	Localizes to pain	Obeys commands

Note that the scale goes from a total of 3 to 15. A score less than 3 is not possible.

CLINICAL PEARL

Relatively common and serious but potentially reversible causes of sudden-onset coma include:
- acute basilar artery occlusion with brainstem stroke
- subarachnoid hemorrhage
- fulminating meningitis
- generalized seizure with ongoing non-convulsive seizure activity
- hypnosedative drug overdose.

Assessment of the patient with impaired consciousness

- A detailed immediate, recent and past history is essential in formulating the differential diagnosis in a patient with stupor or coma.
  - » It is particularly important to interview family members and reliable witnesses to gain insight into antecedent events, recent health status, past medical problems, evidence of recent behavioral change, seizures, and alcohol or drug abuse.
  - » It is also essential to obtain a detailed medication history, and to consider the possibility of a drug overdose.
- Thorough physical examination is essential (see below).
- Structural brain imaging with computed tomography (CT) or magnetic resonance imaging (MRI) will reveal structural pathology in approximately 30% of patients.
- Cerebrospinal fluid (CSF) analysis will assist to identify meningitis and encephalitis.
- Electroencephalography (EEG) will identify patients with ongoing seizure activity.

Physical examination can often provide important diagnostic clues. General examination should include:
- assessment of temperature
- careful inspection of the skin for rashes, and for needle marks which would provide evidence of intravenous drug use or insulin-requiring diabetes

Table 18-2 Key pupillary abnormalities in the patient with impaired consciousness

PUPILLARY ABNORMALITY	LIKELY PATHOLOGY
Dilatation of one pupil with poor or no response to light	Ipsilateral 3rd nerve palsy
Non-reactive, sometimes irregular mid-position pupils	Midbrain pathology
Pinpoint pupils	Pontine pathology or narcotic excess
Small, reactive pupils	Toxic/metabolic encephalopathy
Fixed, dilated pupils	Major brainstem damage

- observation of respiratory patterns—abnormal patterns can be seen in brainstem pathology and with metabolic disturbances
- cardiorespiratory examination, particularly looking for evidence of heart valve or lung infection, or circulatory failure.

Neurological examination should include an initial assessment of the level of consciousness using the Glasgow Coma Scale (Table 18-1).

A structured neurological examination should then be conducted to examine a hierarchy of brainstem function. Examination should include the following components:
- Pupil size and reactivity (Table 18-2).
- Eye position and movements (Table 18-3, overleaf).
- Corneal reflexes—these may be absent in light coma due to toxic or metabolic causes, but are usually retained until severe levels of coma develop. Their absence generally suggests a poor prognosis.
- Oculocephalic reflexes—the so-called 'doll's-eye maneuver' examines the vestibulo-ocular reflexes (VORs) and is induced by lateral rotation of the head:

Table 18-3 Eye movement abnormalities in the patient with impaired consciousness

EYE MOVEMENT ABNORMALITY	LIKELY PATHOLOGY
Lateral conjugate gaze deviation away from side of lesion	Lateral pontine structural pathology
Lateral conjugate gaze deviation toward side of lesion	Frontal hemispheric structural pathology
Forced lateral gaze deviation	Active fronto-temporal seizure foci
Skew deviation and ocular bobbing (a rhythmic downward jerking of both eyes)	Low pontine or ponto-medullary pathology
Major dysconjugate eye positioning	Generally suggests either 3rd nerve palsy, 6th nerve palsy (nuclear or infranuclear for either) or an internuclear ophthalmoplegia. Pathology could be either pontine or midbrain
Conjugate depression of both eyes or eyes jerking back into the orbits (refractory nystagmus)	Suggests midbrain pathology
Roving eye movements or minor dysconjugate movements	Commonly seen in coma and are of no adverse prognostic significance
Ping-pong gaze (rhythmic lateral conjugate eye movements)	These are poorly localized brainstem phenomena

  » lateral rotation with intact brainstem vestibular nuclei results in conjugate movements of the eyes in the opposite direction to head movement
  » the loss of brainstem VOR results in the eyes remaining fixed, looking in the direction of movement, and with no conjugate shift.
- Caloric reflexes—this test also examines the VORs, and is performed by irrigating the external auditory canal with ice-cold water:
  » an intact VOR results in the eyes deviating tonically toward the irrigated side and suggests the possibility that the cause of the coma is pathology above the pons
  » an absent or dysconjugate caloric response suggests brainstem pathology.

A general neurological examination should then be completed, with assessment of character and symmetry of tone, reflexes, plantar responses and fundoscopy.

HEADACHE

Headache is thought to arise from a number of pathophysiological mechanisms:

- irritation of pain-sensitive structures within the cranium, such as the blood vessels and meninges
- release of chemical mediators activating central pain pathways, such as in migraine
- stimulation of extracranial nociceptive pathways by muscle contraction, such as in tension headache.

Less commonly, extracranial pathologies may lead to headache:

- damage to or inflammation of extracranial blood vessels
- structural/inflammatory pathology in paranasal sinuses
- referred pain from cervical spine pathology.

A systematic approach to assessment and management of headache is illustrated in Figure 18-1.

Primary headache syndromes

Migraine

Migraine is one of the commonest neurological disorders, affecting 1 in 5 people.

- The condition causes considerable burden in terms of quality of life and societal economic impact.
- It is a complex multifactorial illness with pathophysiology that is incompletely understood.
- There are defined links to the phenomenon of cortical spreading depression, and also to activation of the trigeminovascular system, inducing inflammatory changes in intracranial vessels and the dura.

Figures 18-2 and 18-3 (overleaf) describe the cortical, subcortical and upper cervical cord pathways linking to the dura, and blood vessel innervation via the trigeminovascular system.

Presentation

- Migraines typically present with recurrent severe headache associated with autonomic symptoms.
- 10–15% of migraine sufferers experience migraines with aura.
- The severity of the pain, duration of the headache, and frequency of attacks is variable, and migraine lasting longer than 72 hours is often termed 'status migrainosus'.

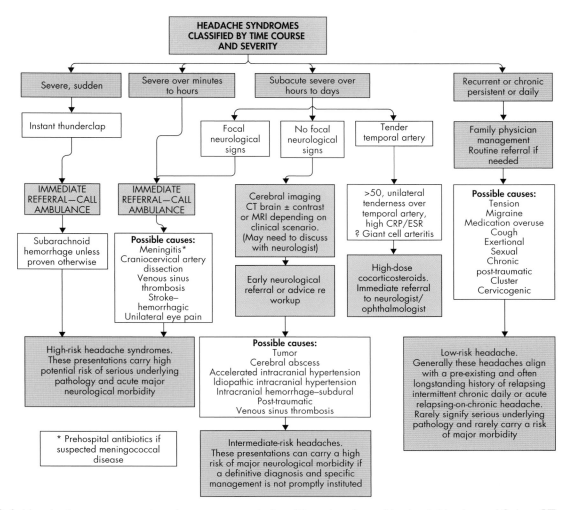

Figure 18-1 Headache assessment and management algorithm developed by Levi, Magin and Sales. CT, computed tomography; CRP, C-reactive protein; ESR, erythrocyte sedimentation rate; MRI, magnetic resonance imaging

The described phases of a migraine attack are:

1 prodrome—which occurs hours or days before the headache

2 aura—generally immediately precedes the headache but can occur in association with it

3 headache phase

4 postdromal period.

Prodromal symptoms occur in approximately 50% of migraine sufferers.

- This phase may consist of altered mood, fatigue, sleepiness, and a variety of nonspecific symptoms.

- These symptoms usually precede the headache phase of the migraine attack by several hours or days.

Aura (most commonly visual, but also somatosensory, dysphasic or vertiginous) comprises focal neurological phenomena that precede or accompany the attack.

- Aura appear gradually over 5–20 minutes and generally last less than 60 minutes, and mirror the cortical spreading depression phenomenon.

- Visual aura is the most common of the neurological accompaniments, and most often consists of unformed flashes of white and/or black, or rarely of multicolored lights (photopsia) or formations of dazzling zigzag lines.

- Some patients complain of blurred or shimmering or cloudy vision, as though they are looking at an area above a heated surface, or looking through stained glass.

- The visual aura is commonly associated with an area of visual loss—either scotomatous or at times hemianopic.

The **headache** phase of the migraine attack usually begins within 60 minutes of the end of the aura phase.

- The typical migraine headache is unilateral, throbbing, and moderate to severe, and can be aggravated by physical activity.

- The pain may be bilateral at the onset, or start on one side and become generalized, and may occur primarily on one side or alternate sides from one attack to the next.

- The onset is usually gradual. The pain peaks and then subsides and usually lasts 2–72 hours in adults and 1–48 hours in children.

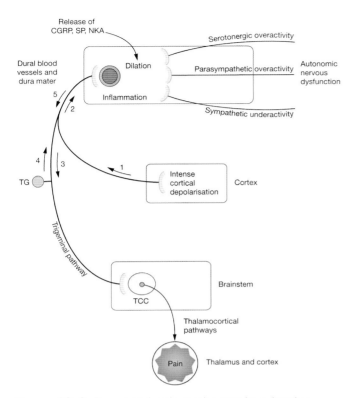

Figure 18-2 Proposed pain pathways in migraine. In this scenario, the trigger is a wave of cortical depression (1) which sensitizes and stimulates the trigeminal pathway in either direction (2, 3). This results in stimulation of the trigeminocervical complex (TCC) (3) in the brainstem; onward stimulation of the thalamus and other areas can cause pain and nausea. Other reflex pathways from the brainstem via the superior salivatory nucleus to the dural blood vessels, which result in vasodilatation, can also be activated at this stage. The stimulation of trigeminal nerves innervating the dural blood vessels (2, 4) results in the release of mediators such as calcitonin gene-related peptide (CGRP), substance P (SP) and neurokinin A (NKA), which cause vasodilatation and participate in inflammation. CGRP and possibly other mediators are able to stimulate nociceptors in the trigeminal nerve endings, resulting in further activation of the pathways to the TCC and thalamus (5) and consequently further pain. The control of vascular tone in the dural blood vessels is complex, with sympathetic, parasympathetic and serotonergic systems contributing to the migraine process. Vasoconstrictor innervation of these vessels is by sympathetic nerves and vasodilatation occurs by parasympathetic innervation. Serotonergic pathways produce vasoconstriction by stimulation of 5-HT_{1B} receptors and vasodilation via 5-HT_2 receptors. TG, trigeminal ganglion

From Waller DG et al. Medical pharmacology and therapeutics, 4th ed. Saunders, 2014.

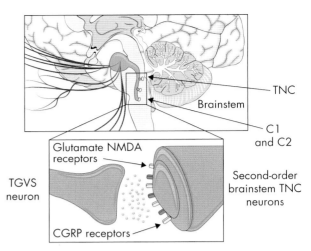

Figure 18-3 Pain pathways in headache. CGRP, calcitonin gene-related peptide; NMDA, *N*-methyl-D-aspartate; TGVS, trigeminovascular system; TNC, trigeminal nucleus caudalis

Based on Goadsby PJ and Bartsch T. On the functional neuroanatomy of neck pain. Cephalalgia 2008;28(Suppl 1):1–7.

- The frequency of attacks is extremely variable, from a few in a lifetime to several per week; the average sufferer experiences 1–3 headaches a month.
- The head pain varies greatly in intensity, and can be very severe.
- The pain of migraine is invariably accompanied by autonomic features, particularly nausea, which occurs in almost 90% of patients, with vomiting occurring in about one-third. There may be localized edema of the scalp or face, scalp tenderness (migranous hygroma), prominence of a vein or artery in the temple, or stiffness and tenderness of the neck.

The effects of migraine may persist for some days after the main headache has ended (**postdrome** period). Many sufferers report feeling tired or 'washed out' with impaired concentration for a few days after the headache has passed.

The International Classification of Headache Disorders published by the Headache Classification Subcommittee of the International Headache Society in 2004 classifies migraine as follows:

- *Migraine without aura*, or 'common migraine', involves migraine headaches that are not accompanied by an aura.
- *Migraine with aura*, or 'classic migraine', usually involves migraine headaches accompanied by an aura. Less commonly, an aura can occur without a headache, or with a non-migraine headache.
- Two other varieties are *familial hemiplegic migraine* and *sporadic hemiplegic migraine*, in which a patient has migraines with aura, and with accompanying motor weakness. If a close relative has had the same condition, it is called 'familial'; otherwise it is called 'sporadic'.
- Another variety is *basilar-type migraine*, where a headache and aura are accompanied by difficulty speaking, vertigo, ringing in the ears or a number of other brainstem-related symptoms, but not motor weakness.

- *Childhood periodic syndromes that are commonly precursors of migraine* include cyclical vomiting (occasional intense periods of vomiting), abdominal migraine (abdominal pain, usually accompanied by nausea), and benign paroxysmal vertigo of childhood (occasional attacks of vertigo).
- *Retinal migraine* involves migraine headaches accompanied by visual disturbances, or even temporary blindness in one eye.
- *Complicated migraine* includes migraine headaches and/or auras that are unusually long or unusually frequent, or are associated with a seizure or brain lesion.
- *Probable migraine* describes conditions that have some characteristics of migraine, but where there is not enough evidence to diagnose it as a migraine with certainty (in the presence of concurrent medication overuse).
- Vestibular migraine describes the symptom complex of vertigo that occurs spontaneously in migraine sufferers. It should coexist with headache >50% of the time, but is thought to have a different mechanism to that seen with migraine aura. Vertigo attacks last from seconds to days, and may be brought on by complex and contrasting visual patterns.

Migraine management

The general approach to management depends on the characteristics, frequency and severity of attacks.

- Infrequent, relatively mild attacks may need little more therapy than prompt simple analgesics or non-steroidal anti-inflammatory medication.
- More severe and refractory migraine may require the use of tryptan medication.
- If attacks occur frequently, generally twice or more per month, then it is reasonable to use prophylactic agents.

Acute-phase treatment

- Non-steroidal anti-inflammatory drugs (NSAIDs)
  » NSAIDs with evidence from randomized, placebo-controlled trials include single-dose aspirin (650–1000 mg), ibuprofen (400–1200 mg), naproxen (750–1250 mg) and diclofenac (50–100 mg). Some of these studies are limited by varying outcome measures and definitions of migraine, but all NSAIDs may be beneficial in patients who have migraine, with or without aura.
  » Indomethacin as acute-phase treatment for migraine, including the suppository form for nauseated patients, can also be effective.
  » There are no studies comparing the relative efficacy of different NSAIDs; in general, if one NSAID is ineffective then a different drug may be tried.
- Triptans
  » The serotonin 1B/1D agonists (triptans) are 'specific' therapies for acute migraine, working to dampen activity in the trigeminovascular system by inhibiting release of vasoactive neurotransmitted peptides such as calcitonin gene-related peptide (CGRP). Oral triptans include sumatriptan, zolmitriptan, naratriptan, rizatriptan and eletriptan. Sumatriptan can also be given as a subcutaneous injection and as a nasal spray for patients with vomiting. Randomized, controlled trials and systematic reviews have found all of the triptans to be effective for the treatment of acute migraine.

Prophylactic treatment

- Beta-blockers
  » Numerous placebo-controlled trials show evidence that propranolol (in doses of 40–160 mg daily) is significantly more effective than placebo for reducing migraine frequency. Other beta-blockers may also be used for migraine prophylaxis but have less evidence.
  » Beta-blockers should be avoided in patients with erectile dysfunction, peripheral vascular disease, baseline bradycardia or low blood pressure, and used cautiously in elderly patients, asthmatics, diabetics, and patients with cardiac conduction disturbances.
- Pizotifen
  » Placebo-controlled trials demonstrate that pizotifen (in three divided doses starting at 1.5 mg daily, dosage range 1.5–3 mg daily) is superior to placebo for migraine prophylaxis.
  » Weight gain and sedation are the most common adverse events.
- Calcium-channel blockers are widely used for migraine prophylaxis. However, the data supporting the efficacy of calcium-channel blockers are relatively weak.
- Antidepressants
  » Amitriptyline (starting dose 10 mg nocte, dosage range 20–50 mg) was effective in randomized trials for migraine prophylaxis in four trials. Anecdotal evidence suggests that amitriptyline is most effective in migraine associated with sleep disturbance and mild affective symptoms. Other tricyclic antidepressants have no proven benefit.
  » Side-effects of tricyclic antidepressants include sedation, dry mouth, constipation, tachycardia, palpitations, orthostatic hypotension, weight gain, blurred vision, and urinary retention. Confusion can occur, particularly in the elderly.
- The serotonin/norepinephrine reuptake inhibitor venlafaxine (starting at 37.5 mg once a day, dosage range 75–150 mg once a day) can also be effective as prophylaxis for migraine.
- Anticonvulsants—sodium valproate, gabapentin and topiramate are all more effective than placebo for reducing the frequency of migraine attacks.
- Other prophylactic agents:
  » Botulinum toxin—several randomized placebo-controlled trials have found no consistent, statistically significant benefits for botulinum toxin injection in the treatment of episodic migraine headache; however, there is evidence to support its use in 'chronic migraine/tension headache'.
  » Methysergide—an ergot derivative and a specific serotonin receptor antagonist (primarily $5HT_2$), has been demonstrated in open-label and controlled studies to be effective in migraine prophylaxis. Long-term use is associated with a low risk of retroperitoneal, pleural and heart valve fibrosis, and therapy duration of >4 months is not recommended. The use of triptans in combination for acute attacks is also not recommended, due to risk of vasospasm.

» Monoclonal antibodies to CGRP (galcanezumab and fremanezumab) and CGRP-receptors (erenumab) have also now entered usage in the management of chronic migraine, and may play a larger role in management in the future.

Non-pharmacological therapies

Cognitive–behavioral therapy is as effective as drug therapy in preventing migraine, and is useful in all age groups including children and adolescents. Relaxation exercises, stress-management training, acupuncture and reduction in caffeine intake are also beneficial. They may be more effective when combined with preventive drug therapy.

Menstrual migraine

Migraine can be sensitive to changes in estrogen concentrations. When estrogen levels are stable (e.g. during pregnancy or after menopause), women are often relatively free of migraine attacks. Estrogen concentrations fall immediately before menstruation and can trigger a migraine attack.

Cluster headache

Cluster headache is rare, and is mainly seen in males with attacks of severe, generally periorbital headache typically accompanied by unilateral rhinorrhea, lacrimation, or conjunctival congestion. Attacks typically last from 15 minutes to 3 hours, recurring in separate bouts, often nocturnally, with 1–8 attacks per day for several weeks or months. Prevention of further attacks is the main focus of cluster headache treatment.

Preventive treatment options

- Verapamil sustained-release 160 or 180 mg orally, once daily, up to 360 mg daily.
- Lithium 250 mg orally, twice daily, titrated according to clinical response and tolerance, and guided by serum concentration levels.

Preventive treatment is continued until attacks have ceased for 1 week or more. The same preventive drug is usually effective if attacks recur. In some cases, multiple preventive drugs may need to be used in combination.

Bridging treatment with corticosteroids can be used while prophylaxis is taking effect:

- prednisolone 50 mg orally, daily in the morning for 7–10 days, then tapered off over 3 weeks.
- Greater occipital nerve blocks with local anesthetic and steroid can manage the acute cluster in some patients, and may allow time to introduce preventative therapy in other individuals.

Acute treatment

- High-flow oxygen—100% by inhalation, for up to 15 minutes at 10 L/min using a tight-fitting, non-rebreathing mask is effective in relieving cluster headache in a large proportion of patients.
- Sumatriptan 6 mg subcutaneously, sumatriptan 20 mg intranasally, dihydroergotamine 1 mg intramuscularly, or lignocaine 4% solution instilled into the nose on the side of the pain can all be effective for acute attacks.

Tension headache

Tension headache is the most common form of headache.

- It is usually characterized by bilateral, dull ache, described as a feeling of tightness or pressure that may extend like a band around the head and down the neck.
- Affective symptoms are more common in this group, as are environmental stressors.
- Stress is a common trigger for exacerbations.
- The term 'chronic daily headache' is sometimes used to describe frequent attacks or constant (chronic unremitting) tension headache, which usually evolves from infrequent tension headache over many years.

Non-pharmacological management

- Massage, stretching, heat and postural correction can relieve pain.
- Cognitive–behavioral therapy is as effective as drug therapy in episodic and constant tension headache.
- Relaxation exercises, stress-management training, and reduction in caffeine intake are also beneficial.

Pharmacological management

- Simple analgesics are effective for short-lived attacks of tension headache; however, medication-overuse (rebound) headache may develop if analgesics are used regularly for more than 2–3 days in a week.
- Frequent attacks or chronic tension headaches are best treated with a combination of non-pharmacological approaches and preventive medication in the form of amitriptyline 50–75 mg daily. If amitriptyline produces unacceptable adverse effects, nortriptyline or dothiepin can be used.

Preventive medications may take several weeks to act, and their effect may be blocked by frequent analgesic consumption and then development of medication-rebound headache. Preventive medication should be continued for a minimum of 3–6 months, and then tapered off and ceased.

Secondary headache

Headache is present in a wide range of pathologies, from intracerebral hemorrhage and stroke to malignant hypertension and even intracranial infection. Most of these conditions are discussed in their relevant chapters. There are, however, a few disorders presenting primarily with headache that should be specifically discussed.

Headaches with increased intracranial pressure

Venous sinus thrombosis (VST)

A disorder requiring a high threshold of suspicion, VST may present at any age, but often occurs in young patients with a history of venous thrombosis.

- It presents with a headache often described as a pressure inside the head, sometimes with pulsation. Due to raised intracranial pressure, it is usually worse when lying flat or with coughing or straining.
- With time papilledema develops, though in very acute VST this may be absent.

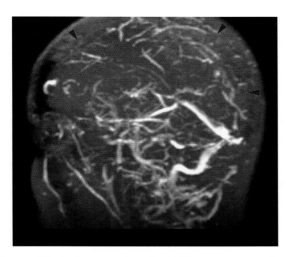

Figure 18-4 A reconstructed MR venogram of a patient with extensive venous sinus thrombosis. Note obliteration of the superior sagittal sinus

- It can be associated with venous stasis, and venous infarction of superficial cerebral cortex.
- Seizures often occur.
- Small-convexity subarachnoid bleeds may be seen, distant to any typical sites of aneurysms.

Diagnosis

Diagnosis is with dedicated cerebral imaging with CT venography or MRI venography (Figure 18-4).

Treatment

Even in patients with subarachnoid bleeds, urgent anticoagulation is the mainstay of treatment. Investigation for thrombophilia should be routine in these patients.

Idiopathic intracranial hypertension (IIH)

Previously termed 'benign intracranial hypertension', IIH is most certainly not benign.

- It commonly affects overweight young women, and is a disease on the rise.
- It presents with insidious onset of headache, with similar features to VST although less acute in onset. It is worse with lying and better upright. It is worse with coughing or straining.
- Risk factors apart from weight, age and gender include the use of tetracyclic antibiotics (tetracycline, doxycycline), and retinoids for acne.
- IIH is frequently associated with visual symptoms, including transient visual obscurations with bending, coughing or straining (when a brief rise in intracranial pressure impairs retinal perfusion), and at times blurring of vision.
- A scotoma consistent with an increased blind spot may be noted.
- Diplopia may occur, commonly due to abducens palsy (or bilateral palsies) due to compression from intracranial pressure.
- Patients usually present with florid papilledema and are referred for urgent investigation and management.

Diagnosis

- Urgent imaging of the brain should be performed to exclude venous sinus thrombosis or mass lesion.
- IIH is typically diagnosed on the basis of appropriate history, examination, and absence of thrombosis on imaging.
- It can be confirmed and treated by performing a lumbar puncture in a left lateral position. Normal opening pressure in this position is less than 20 cmH$_2$O, while in patients with IIH the pressure is usually well over 25 cmH$_2$O. A minimum of 30 mL of CSF should be removed as a therapeutic procedure, and sent for assessment including biochemistry, cell count and cytology to exclude other abnormality within the meninges resulting in raised intracranial pressures.

Management

- Weight loss is the cornerstone of IIH management, and 10% weight loss can result in substantial improvements in symptoms.
  - » In patients with morbid obesity, early intervention should be considered if weight loss does not occur while undergoing supportive management.
- When present, retinoids and tetracyclic antibiotics must be ceased.
- Medical management involves the use of acetazolamide at doses of 250–750 mg twice daily to reduce CSF production. A carbonic anhydrase inhibitor, acetazolamide induces a mild metabolic acidosis and may cause acral paresthesiae, and increases the risk of kidney stones. It causes carbonated beverages to taste unpleasant.
  - » Topiramate may be used to augment this effect, with the additional benefits of appetite suppression and headache reduction. Topiramate is of similar efficacy to acetazolamide as a single agent in IIH in trials.
- Serial lumbar punctures may be used to treat recurrent headache.

In patients poorly responsive to medication or with vision-threatening ocular symptoms, more invasive procedures may be required.

- Optic nerve sheath fenestration may be performed to reduce pressure on the optic nerve head if vision is threatened. Other symptoms of IIH are not treated.
- Shunting is occasionally performed, though placement of shunts is often difficult and shunts commonly fail.
- In patients with significant stenosis of venous outflow, venous stenting is also considered when medical intervention has failed.

Headaches with low pressure

Spontaneous low-pressure headache is rare. It is seen far more commonly following lumbar puncture (LP), especially when a large-gauge 'cutting' needle is used.

- The headache occurs due to low CSF pressure, and occurs with an upright posture. It improves dramatically with a return to a supine position.
- Low-pressure headache following LP is typically treated by pushing oral fluids, giving caffeine (which increases

CSF production) and restricting the patient to strict bed rest in a supine position for 24–48 hours.

- If this fails to work, blood patch may be performed.

The rare presentation of spontaneous low-pressure headache can be diagnosed through the combination of a typical clinical presentation and MRI imaging demonstrating an increased CSF space, often with gadolinium enhancement. Specialized imaging (MRI or nuclear scintigraphy) can isolate the source of the leak, and treatment is with large-volume or targeted blood patch.

STROKE

Stroke is a heterogeneous collection of pathological entities, but may be divided into broad pathogenic subgroups: 85% ischemic, 10% intracerebral hemorrhage, 5% subarachnoid hemorrhage.

- An understanding of stroke pathophysiology is important in determining the most appropriate acute therapy and preventive treatment.
- Brain imaging with CT or MRI is required to accurately differentiate ischemic from hemorrhagic stroke.
- Clinical features and brain imaging findings should be used to determine the affected brain topography (e.g. anterior or posterior circulation, cortical or subcortical). This can give some clues to the underlying etiology and help guide further investigation. For example, subcortical syndromes such as lacunar stroke are often due to small vessel disease, while cortical syndromes should prompt a search for cardiac emboli or carotid stenosis.

Although traditionally included as a type of stroke, *subarachnoid hemorrhage* is a distinct clinical entity with acute onset of severe headache or sudden loss of consciousness, and is diagnosed by acute CT scan. All cases of suspected subarachnoid hemorrhage require immediate evaluation in hospital.

Stroke may be classified as described in Box 18-2. The incidence of different causes of ischemic stroke are given in Table 18-4.

CLINICAL PEARL

Atrial fibrillation accounts for 85% of thromboembolic stroke and 36% of ischemic stroke.

Acute assessment and management

- Any patient with sudden onset of focal neurological symptoms or signs should be considered to have an acute stroke, and should be urgently evaluated in hospital with transport to hospital by ambulance.
- Ideally, health systems should have pre-hospital stroke assessment and triage protocols to facilitate rapid access for stroke sufferers to hospital, and thereby maximize potential eligibility for time-limited acute therapy.

Clinical assessment remains the cornerstone of diagnosis of acute stroke.

- The clinician must rule out a stroke mimic, determine the severity of the neurological deficit (ideally using

---

Box 18-2

The TOAST stroke classification system

The TOAST (Trial of Org 10172 in Acute Stroke Treatment) classification is based on clinical symptoms as well as the results of further investigations. Based on this, a stroke is classified as being due to:

1 Thrombosis or embolism due to atherosclerosis of a large artery
2 Embolism of cardiac origin
3 Occlusion of a small blood vessel
4 Other determined cause
5 Undetermined cause:
   a two possible causes
   b no cause identified
   c incomplete investigation.

Determination of the subtype is important for:

- classifying patients for therapeutic decision-making in daily practice
- describing patients' characteristics in a clinical trial
- grouping patients in an epidemiological study
- careful phenotyping of patients in a genetic study.

From Adams HP Jr, et al. Classification of subtype of acute ischemic stroke. Definitions for use in a multicenter clinical trial. TOAST. Trial of Org 10172 in Acute Stroke Treatment. Stroke 1993;24:35–41.

Table 18-4 Causes of ischemic stroke

CAUSE	% OF CASES
Cardioembolic	42
Large artery atherosclerosis	16
Small vessel disease	11
Undetermined	25
Other causes	6

a validated stroke scale such as the National Institutes of Health Stroke Scale score), and arrange immediate investigations.

- In a patient presenting acutely, immediate brain imaging is required to determine the pathology and exclude a stroke mimic. CT scanning (Figure 18-5) is used acutely to exclude hemorrhage and may show evidence of infarction, but MRI—particularly diffusion-weighted imaging—is much more sensitive for detection of ischemia.
- Advanced CT and MRI techniques may help guide immediate therapy decisions, and can potentially define brain tissue that may be salvaged by reperfusion therapies, possibly beyond the conventional time window for treatment (Figures 18-6 and 18-7). This is currently being studied in trials, and is not recommended in routine clinical practice.

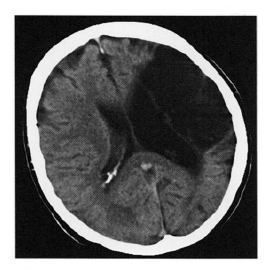

Figure 18-5 CT scan of infarction in the distribution of the frontoparietal branch of the middle cerebral artery

From Perkin DG et al. Atlas of Clinical Neurology, 3rd ed. Philadelphia: Elsevier, 2011.

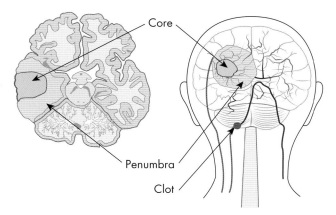

Figure 18-6 The ischemic penumbra. The ischemic penumbra is the region of critically under-perfused tissue at risk of progressing to infarction if reperfusion does not occur promptly. The penumbra is maintained by collateral flow and varies in extent and duration across individual patients with similar vessel occlusions at similar points in time from stroke onset. The ischemic penumbra can now be imaged with advanced magnetic resonance and computed tomography perfusion methods

- Perfusion CTs and MRI techniques now allow selection of patients for extended thrombolysis well beyond the 4.5 hour standard time window. The EXTEND trial demonstrated efficacy for thrombolysis to 9 hours in patients with appropriately selected perfusion imaging. Endovascular clot retrieval may be indicated to 24 hours in patients with appropriate imaging.

- Despite these extensions of the window for intervention, there is still progressive loss of brain tissue with time in stroke, and urgent treatment remains critical in achieving best clinical outcomes for patients.

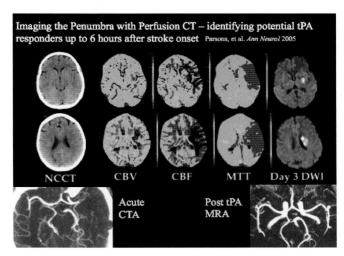

Figure 18-7 Imaging the ischemic penumbra. The ischemic penumbra can be imaged with magnetic resonance imaging and advanced perfusion computed tomography (CT). Penumbral imaging with advanced CT is now a validated technique and can be used to identify those patients most likely to respond to reperfusion therapies. The penumbral 'signature' is tissue that has marker delay in contrast transit (see MTT [mean transit time] map above) in the setting of relatively preserved cerebral blood flow and volume. CBF, cerebral blood flow; CBV, cerebral blood volume; CTA, CT angiogram; DWI, diffusion weighted image; MRA, magnetic resonance angiogram; MTT, mean transit time; NCCT, non-contrast CT; tPA = tissue plasminogen activator

From Parsons MW et al. Perfusion computed tomography: prediction of final infarct extent and stroke outcome. Ann Neurol 2006;59:726.

- Clinical and radiological assessment can also suggest the subtype of ischemic stroke (e.g. lacunar stroke), but this is not always accurate.

- In almost all patients, the clinician should search for a cardiac or carotid (where appropriate, as in an anterior circulation territory stroke) source of embolus.

The best stroke care involves admission to a dedicated stroke unit; the evidence in support of stroke unit care is overwhelming. Organized care in a stroke unit reduces mortality and dependency by approximately 20%, increases the likelihood of discharge to home, and does not increase the length of hospital stay. The benefits are seen regardless of age, gender or severity of stroke. Key components of a stroke unit include specialized staff, a coordinated multidisciplinary team, location in a geographically discrete unit, and early mobilization.

Thrombolysis

CLINICAL PEARL

The time between onset of brain ischemia and commencement of reperfusion is one of the critical factors determining the outcome of thrombolysis. Every minute saved can make a difference to clinical outcome.

Intravenous alteplase (a recombinant tissue-plasminogen activator) is an effective treatment for selected patients with nonhemorrhagic stroke.

- When administered within 4.5 hours of symptom onset, alteplase (0.9 mg/kg up to 90 mg intravenously [IV] over 1 hour, with 10% of the dose given as an initial bolus) increases the likelihood of independence (discharge to home) by 30%.

- Delivery of treatment within 90 minutes from stroke onset is associated with a number needed to treat for rapid complete recovery of 3. The absolute benefit reduces with time between onset and alteplase delivery.

- The major complication of alteplase is symptomatic intracranial hemorrhage, which occurs in around 6% of patients.

- At present, use of alteplase beyond 4.5 hours is not guideline-recommended in some countries, and clinical trials are exploring the efficacy and safety of different types of thrombolytic drug up to 9 hours after stroke onset, some using advanced brain-imaging techniques.

- In the traditional setting of decision-making based on non-contrast CT brain, treatment with thrombolysis is only of benefit to 4.5 hours from symptom onset, with a greater benefit with shorter time windows. However, thrombolysis may now be considered with advanced imaging under the instruction of experienced clinicians to 9 hours from symptom onset.

CLINICAL PEARL

If pre-hospital and hospital systems of care are well organized, stroke units should be aiming to treat approximately 20% of their ischemic stroke patients with alteplase.

- Thrombolysis must be given in a setting with expert staff, and close monitoring of blood pressure and neurological status is required for 24 hours following alteplase infusion.
  » Hypertension should be treated promptly if blood pressure exceeds 185/110 mmHg, aiming to maintain blood pressure below this level.

- Neurointerventional therapy, with intra-arterial thrombolysis or clot retrieval, is possible in a few highly specialized stroke centers.
  » Intra-arterial approaches may be considered for patients with proximal middle cerebral artery, distal internal carotid artery, and basilar occlusions, as these respond poorly to intravenous thrombolysis.
  » Evidence supports intra-arterial thrombolysis within 9 hours, but data for clot retrieval suggests benefit for as long as 24 hours in appropriately selected patients, lifting the importance of this therapy. The number needed to treat (NNT) to restore independence in a patient with large vessel stroke is between 2 and 3.

Neurosurgical intervention

In the setting of extensive hemispheric infarction (typically complete distal carotid or middle cerebral artery occlusion), cerebral edema results in mortality rates of above 80%.

- In such patients, neurosurgical hemicraniectomy can be performed to reduce intracranial pressure and improve

---

Box 18-3

Exclusion criteria and relative exclusion criteria for thrombolytic therapy in stroke

Exclusion criteria

- Head trauma or prior stroke in previous 3 months
- Symptoms suggest subarachnoid hemorrhage
- Arterial puncture at non-compressible site in previous 7 days
- History of previous intracranial hemorrhage
- Elevated blood pressure (systolic >185 mmHg or diastolic >110 mmHg)
- Acute bleeding diathesis, including but not limited to:
  » Platelet count <100,000/mm^3
  » Heparin received within 48 hours, resulting in APTT > upper limit of normal
  » Current use of anticoagulant with INR >1.7 or PT >15 seconds
- Blood glucose concentration <50 mg/dL (2.7 mmol/L)
- CT demonstrates multilobar infarction (hypodensity > $^1/_3$ cerebral hemisphere)

Relative exclusion criteria

Recent experience suggests that under some circumstances—with careful consideration and weighing of risk to benefit—some patients may receive fibrinolytic therapy despite 1 or more relative contraindications. Consider risk to benefit of recombinant tissue plasminogen activator (rtPA/alteplase) administration carefully if any of these relative contraindications is present:

- Only minor or rapidly improving stroke symptoms (clearing spontaneously)
- Seizure at onset with post-ictal residual neurological impairments
- Major surgery or serious trauma within previous 14 days
- Recent gastrointestinal or urinary tract hemorrhage (within previous 21 days)
- Recent acute myocardial infarction (within previous 3 months)

APTT, activated partial thromboplastin time; CT, computed tomography; INR, international normalized ratio; PT, prothrombin time.

From Levi CR et al. The implementation of intravenous tissue plasminogen activator in acute ischaemic stroke–a scientific position statement from the National Stroke Foundation and the Stroke Society of Australasia. Int Med J 2009;39:317–24.

---

cerebral perfusion. Randomized controlled trials show that this treatment reduces the mortality rate by 50%. However, most survivors are left with some degree of disability.

- Hemicraniectomy should be considered within 48 hours of stroke onset for patients aged between 18 and 60 years. The younger the patient, the greater the benefit, and beyond the age of 60 the benefits are doubtful. The decision-making process should involve experienced stroke specialists and neurosurgeons working in highly specialized stroke units.

Cerebellar hemorrhages and large cerebellar infarcts are associated with a mortality of >80%. Ventricular drainage, to relieve acute hydrocephalus, and posterior fossa decompression are the treatments of choice for space-occupying cerebellar hemorrhages and infarcts.

General care measures

Multidisciplinary stroke care involves screening and assessment of swallowing ability, management of fluid balance and nutrition, guideline-based management of physiological variables such as blood sugar, temperature and blood pressure, and early mobilization and physical therapies for weak limbs including adequate management of shoulder positioning.

- Blood pressure is often elevated after an acute ischemic stroke; in most instances this settles spontaneously. In general, blood pressure lowering should be avoided in the acute phase of stroke (first 48 hours); exceptions may include patients with malignant hypertension, hypertensive encephalopathy or those receiving alteplase.
- Patients who are hypoxic should be given supplemental oxygen, but routine use is not supported.
- Fever should be lowered with acetaminophen (paracetamol).
- Hyperglycemia is associated with worse outcomes after stroke, and IV fluids containing glucose should be avoided. Around 20% of patients admitted with acute stroke are found to have unrecognized diabetes. Blood glucose levels should be monitored, with action taken to maintain euglycemia, but intense and aggressive management of blood glucose is not recommended.
- Early mobilization, adequate hydration and antiplatelet therapy can help to prevent deep vein thrombosis in all patients with ischemic stroke. Patients immobilized by the ischemic stroke should receive low-molecular-weight heparin. The use of graduated compression stockings is not recommended.

Early secondary prevention

Most recurrent ischemic events occur within the initial few weeks of the primary event. Prompt introduction of pathophysiologically tailored secondary prevention is critical.

Antiplatelet therapy

- Aspirin reduces the risk of subsequent stroke by approximately 13% and all vascular events by 20%. There is no discernible difference in efficacy between the different doses of aspirin down to 30 mg daily. Low doses are associated with less risk of hemorrhagic complications. Both men and women benefit from aspirin.
- Several studies and meta-analyses found that the combination of dipyridamole plus aspirin was marginally more effective than aspirin alone. Dipyridamole plus aspirin is preferred in patients with moderate or greater absolute risk of recurrent stroke events. It should also be considered in patients with recurrent stroke events despite aspirin therapy, but has more adverse effects. Headache is the most frequent adverse effect and may be overcome by initiating treatment with smaller doses.
- Clopidogrel is modestly more effective than aspirin in the prevention of serious high-risk vascular outcomes (stroke, myocardial infarction, vascular death). Clopidogrel is mainly used as second-line therapy in patients who are either intolerant of aspirin or have developed recurrent cerebral ischemic events while on aspirin.
- The combination of clopidogrel plus aspirin has been the subject of several randomized controlled trials. There is no benefit to this combination because a reduction in ischemic events is offset by an increase in serious bleeding. The combination is not recommended for long-term stroke prevention; however, it is often used as short-term therapy for around 30 days. It may be continued, with care, if there are clear cardiac indications.

Warfarin

- The recurrent stroke risk in patients with atrial fibrillation can be as high as 15–20% per year on no antithrombotic therapy. There is strong evidence that anticoagulation is better than antiplatelet therapy for long-term secondary prevention of ischemic stroke in patients with atrial fibrillation, reducing the incidence of further events by approximately 66% per year.
- In patients without atrial fibrillation or another clear source of cardiogenic embolism (e.g. mural thrombus), there is no benefit of warfarin over antiplatelet therapy.
- With careful control of the international normalized ratio (INR), the risk of serious intracranial bleeding is 0.5% and extracranial bleeding is 2.5% per year.
- The best time to commence warfarin after stroke is not known. Guidelines generally suggest delaying treatment for a week or two after acute stroke and using an antiplatelet agent in the interim.
- In patients with atrial fibrillation who are unable to take warfarin, the combination of aspirin and clopidogrel reduces the rate of stroke compared with aspirin alone, but with a higher risk of major bleeding complications.

Direct/Novel Oral Anticoagulants (DOACs/NOACs)

These medications now have broad usage in anticoagulation in atrial fibrillation, as well as venous thromboembolism. They are used with caution in renal failure, and are not used in place of warfarin in prosthetic heart valves and the antiphospholipid syndrome.

Dabigratran, a direct thrombin inhibitor, shows superior ischaemic stroke protection against warfarin. It can be rapidly reversed with idarucizumab in case of haemorrhage.

Factor Xa inhibitors (rivaroxaban, apixaban spelled incorrectly in text at present) have non-inferiority to Warfarin in protecting against stroke. Apixaban has particular utility given an extremely low bleeding risk. These agents can be reversed with andexanet alfa, though the effect is slower and this agent is not widely available outside of the United States at the time of publication.

Blood pressure lowering

Hypertension is the major reversible risk factor for first and recurrent stroke.

For secondary prevention of stroke, the importance of blood pressure lowering has been shown in a meta-analysis of 10 randomized controlled trials of antihypertensive therapy. Both recurrent strokes and cardiovascular events were reduced by around 30% per year. The reduction of blood pressure was often modest and the initial blood pressure of many patients was in the normal range, yet all experienced benefit. The data are primarily from studies that used angiotensin-converting enzyme inhibitors (ACEIs) alone or in combination with a diuretic, but almost all antihypertensive agents are effective.

Cholesterol lowering

- Studies consistently show that cholesterol lowering with an HMG-CoA reductase inhibitor (statin) reduces the risk of further strokes.
- Overall, statins reduce the risk of stroke by 12% (a 20% reduction in ischemic stroke was offset by an increase in risk of hemorrhagic stroke), and all serious vascular events by 25%.
- Cholesterol lowering with a statin should be considered in most patients following ischemic stroke, regardless of their initial cholesterol levels.

Management of carotid stenosis

- Carotid endarterectomy (CEA) is effective in secondary prevention after minor stroke or TIA (transient ischemic attack). The benefit is greatest when the stenosis is severe (more than 70%), the stroke event was recent, and the patient is male or over 75 years of age. The benefit is marginal for patients with 50–69% symptomatic stenosis, or if the surgery is delayed beyond 3 months. The success of the procedure is critically dependent on the skill of the surgeon, who must have a perioperative complication rate of less than 3%.
- Percutaneous transluminal cerebrovascular angioplasty and stenting (PTCAS) is less effective than CEA, largely because of significant greater early periprocedural hazard. PTCAS is not routinely recommended for management of carotid stenosis. It may be considered in circumstances where CEA is not feasible, or risk of surgery excessive.

INTRACEREBRAL HEMORRHAGE

Medical treatment

Blood pressure lowering in acute intracerebral hemorrhage may reduce hematoma expansion, and a recent large randomized trial (INTERACT2) suggested that aiming for a blood pressure target of 140/90 mmHg showed a strong trend to better long-term functional outcome.

- Current consensus guidelines recommend urgent blood pressure lowering if above 180/110 mmHg, aiming for a target systolic blood pressure of 160 mmHg or possibly now 140 mmHg.
- Warfarin-related intracerebral hemorrhage can be treated by urgent reversal with a combination of pro-thrombin complex concentrate, fresh frozen plasma (FFP) and vitamin K; however, this therapy is generally not effective and prognosis is generally very poor.

- In patients immobilized by their intracerebral hemorrhage and requiring prophylaxis for deep vein thrombosis, it is common practice to commence low-molecular-weight heparin 48 hours after the hemorrhage.

Surgical management

In patients with intracerebral hemorrhage, neurosurgical intervention may be undertaken to evacuate supratentorial hematomas. Evidence to support this practice, however, is very limited, with one large randomized trial suggesting no significant benefit above medical management.

- Decompression of cerebellar hematomas larger than 3 cm in diameter can be life-saving and result in favorable outcomes in many patients.
- CSF drainage devices (to reduce the risk of secondary deterioration due to hydrocephalus caused by obstruction of the fourth ventricle) can be an effective adjunctive therapy to decompression.

SUBARACHNOID HEMORRHAGE (SAH)

- Subarachnoid hemorrhage is a common and devastating condition, with mortality rates as high as 45% and significant morbidity among survivors.
- The incidence increases with age, occurring most commonly between 40 and 60 years of age (mean age ≥50 years). SAH is about 1.6 times higher in women than men.
- Risk factors for SAH include hypertension, smoking, female gender and heavy alcohol use.
- Cocaine-related SAH occurs in younger patients.
- Familial intracranial aneurysm (FIA) syndrome occurs when two first- through third-degree relatives have intracranial aneurysms.

Natural history and outcome of an aneurysmal SAH

- 30-day mortality rate after SAH ranges from 33% to 50%.
- Severity of initial hemorrhage, age, sex, time to treatment, and medical comorbidities affect SAH outcome.
- Aneurysm size, location in the posterior circulation, and morphology also influence outcome.
- Up to 14% of SAH patients may experience re-bleeding within 2 hours of the initial hemorrhage.

Surgical versus endovascular management of SAH

Endovascular coil insertion and surgical aneurysm clipping both dramatically reduce early re-bleeding rates in SAH. The choice of therapy will depend on local facilities and expertise.

TRANSIENT ISCHEMIC ATTACK (TIA)

CLINICAL PEARL

As for ischemic stroke, prompt determination of the mechanism or underlying pathophysiology of an ischemic event is the key to appropriate and most effective secondary prevention. The earlier appropriate prevention can be commenced, the better the chance of preventing the next event.

Definition

Transient ischemic attack is defined as a transient neurological event of presumed vascular etiology with symptoms and/or signs that last for <24 hours. The majority of TIAs have clinical features lasting <1 hour.

There has been a recent recommendation to define TIA using MRI as a transient neurological event of presumed vascular cause without associated changes of infarction on diffusion-weighted MRI (DWI). This new imaging-based definition is gaining favor and illustrates the fact that approximately 50% of TIAs that have a symptom duration exceeding 4 hours will be accompanied by evidence of infarction on DWI.

Differential diagnosis of transient neurological disturbances

There are a number of common causes of transient neurological disturbances (transient neurological attacks, TNAs) that mimic the TIA syndromes. These are generally distinguishable by using detailed symptom analysis and neuroimaging.

- The most common TIA mimic is migraine with aura; however, other less common mimic syndromes are partial seizures, hypoglycemia, transient global amnesia, and functional or non-organic attacks including hyperventilation syndrome.
- Pre-syncope and syncope are often referred to the neurologist for assessment of possible TIA; however, TIA and stroke are extremely rare causes of transient loss of consciousness alone.
- Neuroimaging is important to rule out certain TIA mimic syndromes such as small deep hemorrhages that can cause transient symptoms, subdural hemorrhages, cerebral neoplasms, and other structural pathologies that could predispose to partial seizures.
- Amyloid angiopathy is a syndrome of micro- (and macro-) hemorrhages associated with small vessel disease. It occurs due to deposition of an Alzheimer's-like amyloid protein within vessel walls. Patients may present with ischaemic or hemorrhagic stroke, but also frequently experience 'amyloid spells' with some features of TIA and others suggestive of seizure. Optimal treatment of these recurrent symptoms remains unclear at present.

Pathophysiology

TIA and ischemic stroke share the same vascular risk factors and the same pathophysiology.

There is no reliable way to clinically determine whether the abrupt onset of a neurological deficit will be reversible; hence, if a patient is seen with clinical signs of significant neurological impairment they should be regarded as being in the process of having a stroke.

CLINICAL PEARL

Overall only approximately 10–15% of all ischemic cerebrovascular events will spontaneously resolve. In general, therefore, all patients presenting with sudden neurological symptoms and signs should be managed with urgency.

Investigation

- A clinical and radiological (non-contrast CT as a minimum standard) diagnosis of TIA should be followed, as done in ischemic stroke, by investigation to determine the pathophysiology of ischemia.
- The two very high recurrent stroke risk pathophysiologies to identify and manage within the initial 24 hours of presentation are:
  » severe large vessel occlusive disease
  » atrial fibrillation (either persistent or transient).
- The key investigations required, therefore, are imaging of the extracranial and intracranial large vessels (ultrasound, CT angiogram or MRI angiogram), electrocardiography (EKG) and, if the EKG is negative, Holter monitoring and/or echocardiography.

Recurrent event risk

- The risk of recurrent stroke after a TIA or a minor stroke averages approximately 10% in the first month following the index event.
- There are, however, some patients with much higher risk—up to 20% in the initial week. This subgroup at very high risk generally has underlying severe large vessel disease or unrecognized/untreated atrial fibrillation (AF).
- It is important to recognize that patients with high-risk pathophysiologies, and all clinico-radiologically proven TIA cases, should undergo screening for high-grade large vessel disease and AF.
- An additional high-risk scenario is crescendo TIA (≥2 TIAs in a week) where, again, the risk of early recurrent stroke is high.

Prevention of recurrent events

The specific therapies for stroke prevention following TIA are identical to those described above for ischemic stroke.

- As in ischemic stroke, the selection of therapies for the prevention of recurrent events is based around determination of the underlying pathophysiology.
- Recurrent stroke risk following TIA is 'front loaded', meaning that the majority of the recurrent events occur within the first days to weeks after the index event.
- Early commencement of appropriate antithrombotic therapy, blood pressure lowering and lipid lowering therapies, along with carotid intervention for high-grade carotid stenosis, is of paramount importance.

DEMENTIA

Dementia is characterized by impairment of memory and at least one additional cognitive domain where there is impairment (e.g. aphasia, apraxia, agnosia, executive function), with decline from previous level of function severe enough to interfere with daily function and independence.

Diagnosis

Dementia is a clinical diagnosis and does lack precision when the neurodegenerative process is in the early stages.

- Presentation is often via a spouse or other informant who brings a problem with memory and/or personality and behavioral change to attention.
- The normal cognitive decline associated with aging consists primarily of mild changes in memory and the rate of information processing, which are not progressive and do not affect daily function.
- Patients with dementia often have difficulty with functions such as learning and retaining new information, handling complex tasks, reasoning, spatial ability, orientation and navigation, speech and language function, and social interaction and behavior.

The diagnosis of *dementia* must be distinguished from *delirium* and *depression*.

- Delirium is usually acute in onset and is associated with a clouding or fluctuation of consciousness, difficulty with attention and concentration.
- Patients with depression are more likely to complain about memory loss than those with dementia.
- Patients with dementia are frequently brought to physicians by their families, while depressed patients often present by themselves.
- Patients with depression may have signs of psychomotor slowing and produce a poor effort on testing.

Mild cognitive impairment (MCI) is generally defined by the presence of memory difficulty and objective memory impairment but preserved ability to function in daily life. Patients with MCI appear to be at increased risk of dementia.

Major dementia syndromes

Alzheimer disease (AD)

Alzheimer disease, the most common cause of dementia, is a neurodegenerative disorder of uncertain cause and pathogenesis that primarily affects older adults.

- The main clinical manifestations of AD are selective memory impairment and dementia.
- While treatments are available that can modulate the course of the disease and/or ameliorate some symptoms, there is no cure, and the disease inevitably progresses in all patients.
- It is not rare for Alzheimer pathology to coexist with other processes, including vascular lesions and vascular dementia, cortical Lewy bodies and Parkinson's disease.

- While the diagnosis is clinical, high-resolution MRI scanning can quantify hippocampal volumes and may aid diagnosis.

Genetic testing is not recommended in the routine evaluation.

- However, genotyping for apolipoprotein E ε4 adds marginally to the predictive value of clinical criteria for AD and may stratify risk of conversion of amnesic MCI to AD.
- Genetic testing for presenilin 1 mutations is commercially available, but should be reserved for cases of onset at <60 years of age in the setting of a positive family history.

Patients with AD have reduced cerebral production of choline acetyltransferase, which leads to a decrease in acetylcholine synthesis and impaired cortical cholinergic function.

- Cholinesterase inhibitors increase cholinergic transmission by inhibiting cholinesterase at the synaptic cleft, and have been proved to mitigate symptoms and the rate of symptom progression.
- A treatment trial with a cholinesterase inhibitor is generally recommended for patients with mild to moderate dementia (Mini-Mental State Examination score 10–26).

Dementia with Lewy bodies (DLB)

Dementia with Lewy bodies is increasingly recognized clinically as the second commonest type of degenerative dementia after Alzheimer disease.

- In addition to dementia, distinctive clinical features include visual hallucinations, parkinsonism, cognitive fluctuations, dysautonomia, sleep disorders, and neuroleptic sensitivity.
- Cholinesterase inhibitors may represent a first-line pharmacological treatment in DLB. Research suggests that cholinesterase inhibitors are effective in symptomatic treatment of DLB, with reported benefit not only in cognition but also for fluctuations, psychotic symptoms, and parkinsonian symptoms.

Frontotemporal dementia (FTD)

- Frontotemporal dementia typically presents as either a progressive change in personality and social behavior or as a progressive form of aphasia. In both cases there is progression ultimately to a dementia.
- The most common presentation of FTD is that of a progressive change of personality and behavior, with personality change, lack of insight, loss of social awareness, emotional blunting and mental rigidity.
- Cognitive functioning may be relatively intact early in the course, with minimal memory loss and normal Mini-Mental State Examination (MMSE) scores; however, over time, impairment of executive functions, problem-solving, judgment, attention, organization and planning develop. For this reason the Montreal Cognitive Assessment (MoCA) is preferred, as it specifically assesses some of these domains.
- Rarer forms of FTD are a predominant aphasia, either progressive expressive and/or receptive, FTD associated

with motor neuron disease, and FTD associated with corticobasal degeneration—a syndrome of asymmetric rigidity and apraxia.

- Patients with progressive supranuclear palsy (PSP), a clinical syndrome of supranuclear vertical-gaze palsy, axial dystonia, bradykinesia, rigidity and falls, often also develop a dementia syndrome with features that overlap with FTD.

Pharmacological treatment in FTD is symptomatic and aimed at alleviating neurobehavioral symptoms. However, there is limited evidence of the efficacy of pharmacological treatments modifying FTD.

Vascular (multi-infarct) dementia (VaD)

Vascular dementia is a heterogeneous syndrome in which the underlying cause is cerebrovascular disease in some form, and its ultimate manifestation is dementia.

There is considerable overlap between AD and VaD with regard to comorbidity as well as shared risk factors and even pathogenesis. The combination of pathologies may be more common than either in isolation, and it is not generally easy to identify the primary etiological entity.

Preventative agents and treatments for VaD are essentially those for prevention of small vessel and large vessel cerebrovascular disease—antiplatelet therapy, blood pressure lowering and lipid lowering therapies.

Parkinson's disease (PD) with dementia

While PD can coexist with other common causes of dementia, such as Alzheimer disease and vascular dementia, dementia is increasingly recognized as a common feature of PD itself.

- The clinical characteristics and course of dementia, its pathological features, and the most appropriate treatment are areas of current investigation.
- Clinical features can generally distinguish between PD and other movement disorders associated with dementia. However, whether PD dementia (PDD) and dementia with Lewy bodies (DLB) are distinct disorders or represent different presentations of the same disease is an area of debate and investigation.

Diagnostic work-up of the dementia patient

- History relayed by the patient but most importantly also that relayed by family members will provide much of the diagnostic information.
- Physical examination and initial objective cognitive screening with the MMSE or MoCA is then generally followed by laboratory and imaging studies (Table 18-5, overleaf).
- Investigations are largely performed to rule out reversible or partially reversible pathologies such as hydrocephalus, central nervous system (CNS) infection, occult structural pathology such as subdural hematomas and low-grade tumors, and low-grade inflammatory processes such as cerebral vasculitis. A diagnosis of depression

should be pursued with formal psychiatric assessment in situations where there is any clinical suspicion.

There are many examination schemata for bedside testing of memory and cognition. The MMSE (Figure 18-8, overleaf) is commonly used, though it is now under copyright. Other testing schemes such as the Montreal Cognitive Assessment are available, and may be more sensitive. It is critical to be aware of the limitations of any simple questionnaire, and that they are performed within the limits of attention, language, the environment and education.

- An MMSE score of less than 24 points is suggestive of either dementia or delirium.
- Using a cut-off of 24 points, the MMSE has a sensitivity of 87% and a specificity of 82%; however, the test is not sensitive for mild dementia, and scores may be influenced by age and education as well as language, motor and visual impairments.
- Studies suggest that high scores ($\geq$23) and low scores (<19) can be highly predictive in discriminating broad mental competency from incompetency.
- The MMSE has limitations for assessing progressive cognitive decline in individual patients over time. Changes of 2 points or less are of uncertain clinical significance.

Other dementia syndromes

Normal pressure hydrocephalus (NPH)

Normal pressure hydrocephalus refers to a condition of pathologically enlarged ventricular size with normal opening pressures on lumbar puncture.

CLINICAL PEARL

Normal pressure hydrocephalus is associated with a classic triad of dementia, gait disturbance and urinary incontinence.

Because NPH is potentially reversible by the placement of a ventriculoperitoneal shunt, it is important to recognize and accurately diagnose. However, there is little consensus regarding the diagnosis of NPH and the selection of patients for shunt placement.

- MRI scanning can give some diagnostic guidance, with reports that increased aqueduct of Sylvius flow is associated with the condition.
- A generally used 'confirmatory' test is the CSF 'tap' test where 30–50 mL of CSF is removed with documentation of the patient's gait and cognitive function before and 30–60 minutes after the procedure. Common parameters measured before and after CSF removal include measures of gait speed, stride length, and tests of verbal memory and attention. Documented improvement in one or more parameters following the tap test has a high positive predictive value.
- It is generally considered that gait impairment is most responsive to shunting.

Cognitive impairment is more resistant to shunt therapy but can improve, especially if not severe at the time of intervention.

Table 18-5 Pathology work-up for dementia

TEST	INDICATION	INTERPRETATION
Blood tests, includes FBC, biochemical profile, TSH, vitamin B_{12}	Routine	Useful for detection of systemic illness which may present with cognitive slowing such as hypothyroidism Also may reveal changes of chronic alcohol abuse and chronic illness
Syphilis screening, HIV serology	Anyone at risk	Assesses for the possibility of HIV dementia and syphilis-related dementia
Copper studies	Young patient with psychiatric presentation	Screen for Wilson's disease; also check LFTs and for Kayser–Fleischer rings
Brain imaging	Routine	Assesses for treatable forms of dementia, e.g. normal pressure hydrocephalus, unrecognized vascular disease May help stratify diagnosis AD—frequently shows atrophy, with hippocampal atrophy prominent DLB—frequently normal FTD—may show asymmetrical frontal (FTD) or temporal (progressive non-fluent aphasia, semantic dementia) atrophy VaD—diffuse evidence of small- and/or large-vessel infarction with volume loss* CJD—may show cortical DWI restriction and changes in basal ganglia
Lumbar puncture	Young or rapidly progressive *or* Clinical picture of NPH	May reveal subtle inflammation (chronic meningitis, limbic encephalitis), infiltrative processes (meningeal metastases) and allow protein 14-3-3 testing May allow CSF tap test in patients with imaging and clinical presentation of normal pressure hydrocephalus (take 20–30 mL)
Protein 14-3-3	Rapidly progressive dementia with clinical picture of CJD	A marker of rapid neuronal death, this is sensitive and specific for CJD in an *appropriately selected population*. It should not be used as a screening tool in general
Genetic testing	Strong family history or very young onset	Testing of presenilin 1 can be considered in patients with very-young-onset AD Familial FTD-MND may also be tested for an expanding number of genes
PET/SPECT scanning	Complex cases only	Used only in complex cases, where the diagnosis is not clinically apparent
Brain biopsy	Last resort	In rapidly progressive cases where the diagnosis remains unclear despite comprehensive investigation (e.g. atypical presentation of CJD with autoantibodies *or* progressive imaging changes consistent with intravascular lymphoma)

* Some microvascular change is common in older patients presenting with dementia. For a diagnosis of vascular dementia, the imaging findings need to be congruent to the clinical history.

AD, Alzheimer disease; CJD, Creutzfeldt–Jakob disease; CSF, cerebrospinal fluid; DLB, dementia with Lewy bodies; DWI, diffusion-weighted imaging; FBC, full blood count; FTD, frontotemporal dementia; LFT, liver function test; MND, motor neuron disease; NPH, normal pressure hydrocephalus; PET, positron emission tomography; SPECT, single-photon-emission computed tomography; TSH, thyroid-stimulating hormone; VaD, vascular dementia.

Creutzfeldt–Jakob disease (CJD)

Creutzfeldt–Jakob disease is the most common human prion disease, although it is still rare with an approximate incidence of 1 case of sporadic CJD per 1,000,000 population per year.

- Prion diseases share the common neuropathological features of neuronal loss, proliferation of glial cells, absence of an inflammatory response, and the presence of small vacuoles within the neuropil, producing a spongiform appearance.

- *Sporadic, familial, iatrogenic* and *variant* forms of CJD are the recognized forms.

- The vast majority of CJD cases are sporadic (85–95%), while 5–15% are familial and iatrogenic cases account for less than 1%.

MMSE SAMPLE QUESTIONS

Orientation to time

What is the date?   Score _____ out of 5

Registration

Listen carefully. I am going to say three words. You say them back after I stop.

Ready? Here they are...

APPLE (*pause*), PENNY (*pause*), TABLE (*pause*). Now repeat those words back
to me.   Score _____ out of 3

Naming

What is this? [Point to a pencil or pen.]   Score _____ out of 1

Reading

Please read this and do what it says. [Show examinee the words on the
stimulus form.]   Score _____ out of 1

CLOSE YOUR EYES

Figure 18-8 Sample questions from the Mini Mental State Examination

Questions reproduced by special permission of the Publisher, Psychological Assessment Resources, Inc., 16204 North Florida Avenue, Lutz, Florida 33549, from the Mini Mental State Examination, by Marshal Folstein and Susan Folstein, Copyright 1975, 1998, 2001 by Mini Mental LLC, Inc. Published 2001 by Psychological Assessment Resources, Inc. Further reproduction is prohibited without permission of PAR, Inc. The MMSE can be purchased from PAR, Inc. by calling (1 813) 968-3003.

- Variant CJD has developed as a result of bovine-to-human transmission of the prion disease of cattle bovine spongiform encephalopathy (BSE). Variant CJD can be distinguished from cases of typical sporadic disease by patients being of considerably younger age at the onset of symptoms, showing less rapid progression of illness, and also by distinctive differences in neuropathological features including the presence of prominent amyloid plaques which stain intensely for prion protein.

Brain biopsy remains the 'gold standard' diagnostic test; however, MRI scanning can show relatively specific features with increased T2 and FLAIR signal intensity in the putamen and head of the caudate and, less commonly, areas of T2 and FLAIR signal hyperintensity being seen in the globus pallidus, thalamus, cerebral and cerebellar cortex, and white matter.

SEIZURES AND THE EPILEPSIES

Seizures can be defined as a transient occurrence with signs and symptoms due to abnormal, excessive or synchronous neuronal electrical activity within the brain.

They are a common symptom of a multitude of pathologies, some transient and some long-lasting, with ongoing susceptibility to seizures (epilepsy). Due to issues in the social domain of personal safety, in particular driving, there is morbidity associated with seizures well outside the scope of the seizure itself.

Seizure types

Seizures may be described as *focal* (formerly *partial*; affecting part of the brain), or *generalized* (affecting both hemispheres). Focal seizures may spread from their initial site of activity to involve both hemispheres, and the seizure is then referred to as *secondarily generalized*.

- When the brain is diffusely involved as in a generalized seizure, consciousness is lost; but in focal seizures, consciousness may remain intact throughout the seizure, termed 'simple partial', or focal with preserved awareness, or may be lost after an aura or focal motor onset, termed 'simple partial with secondary generalization'.

- When awareness is lost rapidly but there are clear focal signs at onset, the seizure is usually referred to as 'focal with impaired awareness'.

- When describing seizure phenomena, an emphasis is placed on the motor appearance of the seizure (Table 18-6, overleaf), especially when generalized. The motor phenomena frequently help with the underlying diagnosis of a patient with recurrent seizures.

Table 18-6 Appearance of seizures

TYPE	NOTES
Tonic	Sustained contraction of muscles with stiffening of the limb(s) or trunk
Clonic	Brief jerking movements, typically waxing then waning in rate
Tonic–clonic	Tonic phase followed by clonic phase
Myoclonic	Brief shock-like jerks of the body or limbs. May cause dropping of objects in the patient's hands
Atonic	Sudden loss of tone in the body, resulting in a fall to the ground. These seizures are the hallmark of Lennox–Gastaut syndrome and are usually only present in severe epilepsy syndromes with developmental delay. Injury frequently results if unprotected
Absence*	One of the few seizure types not defined by motor features, these episodes are generalized events with loss of awareness but maintained tone

* It is important not to equate absence seizures with episodes of loss of awareness without tonic–clonic activity. Many such episodes do demonstrate focal motor signs such as head turning or eye deviation.

- In a patient with recurrent seizures, it is also important to ask about other seizure types, as patients may have several types of seizures in some syndromes and may not have recognized the significance of them (e.g. juvenile myoclonic epilepsy with generalized tonic–clonic, myoclonic and absence seizures).

Assessing a patient after a seizure

In assessing a patient with a seizure, it is critical to first assess whether indeed it *is* a seizure. The main differential for a seizure is a syncopal episode, and with an adequate history it is often possible to reliably distinguish these episodes. In considering the differential, it is important to consider the following aspects.

The situation

- Events occurring in emotional situations or with prolonged standing in a stationary position are often syncopal events. Syncope may also occur with micturition or in the shower with peripheral vasodilatation.
- Events occurring during sleep while supine are much more likely to be seizures than syncope.

The prodrome

- Syncope frequently, though not always, has a prodrome with lightheadedness, sweating, pallor, vision and aural symptoms and collapse.
- Seizures may have an 'aura', which is in fact a focal seizure within the brain, of which the patient is aware. It is varied from patient to patient, but should be the same (allowing scope for severity) within one patient for each seizure focus.
- It is important to note that seizures arising from the temporal lobe may trigger a rising feeling, anxiety and at times déjà vu. This can be difficult to distinguish from panic attacks, especially with anxiety and depression frequently comorbid with epilepsy.

- In patients with generalized epilepsy (e.g. juvenile myoclonic epilepsy), there may be a longer prodrome, inconsistent with an aura, in which patients are aware that they are more likely to have a seizure.

The event

- Frequently the least useful piece of history, 'twitching' and 'eyes rolling back in the head' are often commented upon but have no specific diagnostic value.
- It should be noted that syncope frequently results in brief seizure activity due to cerebral hypoxia, termed 'convulsive syncope'.
- The presence or absence of tongue-biting and incontinence is neither sensitive nor specific and cannot be relied upon.
- A clear tonic then clonic phase may help suggest a generalized seizure.
- Focal arm raising or hand posturing with specific head turning and spread of jerking ('Jacksonian march') is helpful in identifying focal-onset seizures.

The post-ictal stage

- A prolonged drowsy state, especially if focal neurology is present, is suggestive of a seizure.
- Briefer post-ictal phases may be syncope, seizure or non-epileptic in origin.

CLINICAL PEARL

In the modern day of cell (mobile) phones with video recorders, ask if anyone has a video of the event(s). This may allow better assessment of the nature of the event. Remember, the most useful piece of equipment in the neurologist's office is often a telephone!

Table 18-7 Causes of seizures

ETIOLOGY	EXAMPLES
Infection and inflammation	Infective (meningo)encephalitis
	Chronic CNS infection (e.g. neurocysticercosis)
	Autoimmune limbic encephalitis (may present bizarrely)
	Cerebral lupus
Neoplasia	Gliomas and other primary CNS neoplasms
	Metastases
	Lymphoma
Vascular	Stroke*
	Subarachnoid hemorrhage*
	Subdural hematoma
	Eclampsia
	Hypertensive encephalopathy
Metabolic	Hyponatremia
	Hypoglycemia
	Hypocalcemia
	Uremia
	Porphyria
Trauma	Head injury*
	Neurosurgery*
Drugs and withdrawal	Alcohol
	Amphetamines, MDMA
	Pethidine
	Benzodiazepine or barbiturate withdrawal
	Many others
Neurodegeneration	Alzheimer disease
	Creutzfeldt–Jakob disease
Epilepsy	Multiple causes
Psychiatric	Psychogenic non-epileptic seizures

* May occur at the time of the insult, or may occur up to years later.

CNS, central nervous system; MDMA, 3,4-methylenedioxy-*N*-methylamphetamine (Ecstasy).

Causes

Seizures are a *symptom*, and in an acute first seizure it is imperative to consider the possible causes (Table 18-7).

Investigation of a first seizure

All patients with a first seizure warrant a thorough history, and screening for an obvious cause (e.g. a first seizure in a young type I diabetic at night with a blood glucose of 1.5 g/L). Family history is important given the frequent genetic basis of epileptic disorders.

Examination is frequently normal, but clinical findings of ongoing Todd's paresis, previous sequelae of strokes, or clinical features of alcohol abuse are examples of physical signs suggesting possible underlying etiologies.

Investigations are outlined in Table 18-8, overleaf.

> **CLINICAL PEARL**
>
> Generalized epilepsy can only be *excluded* by an electroencephalogram if performed during an attack.

The epilepsies

Often considered by the greater public to be a single disease, the epilepsies are disorders grouped together by the predisposition to seizures, although there are many disparate causes, treatments and prognoses. They can be focal or generalized, consist of one or more seizure types, and have a specific age range of onset and, in some cases, of resolution.

Recognition of the correct seizure type(s) is critical to appropriate treatment, and incorrect treatment may make seizures worse. Indeed, anticonvulsants have a spectrum of activity in a manner similar to antibiotics, and identification of the correct seizure disorder is as important as recognition of a bacterial pathogen causing infection.

In the past, epilepsies were defined as 'idiopathic' where genetics may have played a role, or 'symptomatic' when seizures accompanied structural features. However, with modern genetics, many epilepsy types have been identified as having genetic causes from formerly 'idiopathic generalized epilepsies' to the more severe syndromes with encephalopathy and refractory seizures.

For this reason, the nomenclature of epilepsy syndromes has changed, though the old names are still frequently used, making an understanding of both important.

With modern genetics, many syndromes with cognitive impairment (e.g. Dravet syndrome) have been identified as having distinct genetic causes. As such, there has been a move toward classifying epilepsies as 'genetic', 'structural' or 'unknown'.

The importance of making a correct diagnosis for a patient with epilepsy is manifold.

1. It allows selection of the most appropriate therapy to maximize effectiveness and minimize dose and side-effects.
2. It can provide prognosis as well as explanation for seizures.
3. It can have genetic implications for parents and siblings in the case of children with epilepsy.
4. Some epilepsies are surgically amenable if refractory.

Important epilepsy syndromes

Genetic generalized epilepsies

These epilepsies are notable for seizures that are electrographically generalized at onset on EEG. There is a significant contribution from genetic factors. Sodium valproate is typically the first-line treatment in males, though the potential teratogenic effects leads to it being avoided in young women of childbearing age.

Table 18-8 Investigations for seizures

TEST	NOTES
Full blood count	Infection, chronic disease, alcohol abuse
Electrolytes, urea, creatinine	Hyponatremia, uremia, hypocalcemia or severe hypomagnesemia
Blood glucose levels	Hypoglycemia
Liver function tests	Alcohol abuse
Prolactin	Not for routine use. Can be elevated after syncope or with the use of psychotropic drugs, as well as after a seizure. May occasionally help distinguish a psychogenic cause from generalized seizure
Electrocardiograph	To exclude arrhythmogenic abnormalities that may lead to syncope, e.g. prolonged QT syndrome, heart block
Brain imaging	Computed tomography—acutely, to exclude hemorrhage or mass Magnetic resonance imaging—to define etiology, e.g. mesial temporal sclerosis, cortical dysplasia, old hemorrhages, subtle inflammation
CSF examination	If suspected acute or chronic infection, meningeal malignancy, or autoimmune encephalitis (NMDA antibodies)
Electroencephalogram (EEG)	Depending on the history and the seizure type, EEG has a variable sensitivity in detecting epilepsy. Techniques such as hyperventilation and photic stimulation (flashing lights) may further increase sensitivity. An EEG is almost always abnormal during a seizure (though some focal seizures may be difficult to detect, and interictal abnormality may be present in many patients. However, a normal interictal EEG *cannot* exclude epilepsy When a clinical history is compelling for epilepsy, further provocation is usually undertaken in the form of a sleep-deprived EEG, improving the likelihood of an intermittent abnormality being found

CSF, cerebrospinal fluid; NMDA, *N*-methyl-ᴅ-aspartate.

Childhood absence epilepsy

- Coming on in the childhood years (ages 4–9), children have typical absence episodes in which they stop suddenly mid-activity for usually between 5 and 20 seconds, from one or two to hundreds of times per day.
- They are unresponsive during this period, and maintain body tone.
- They often return to their activity afterwards as if they had never stopped.
- It is readily controlled by sodium valproate or ethosuximide.
- Prognosis is usually good, with most children growing out of it by adolescence.
- EEG tends to be sensitive, with 3 Hz spike–wave discharges the hallmark, often brought on by hyperventilation.

Juvenile myoclonic epilepsy (JME)

Usually presenting in the 2nd decade of life, this epilepsy is notable for:

1. myoclonus—often in the morning and when tired
2. generalized tonic–clonic seizures (often with sleep deprivation or alcohol)
3. absence episodes.

Not all patients will have all three seizure types.

- EEG is once again reasonably sensitive, with a >3 Hz polyspike-wave pattern.
- Sodium valproate is usually first-line treatment, although it may be problematic in young women of childbearing age when pregnancy is likely.
- Lamotrigine is second-line treatment, with levetiracetam and other broad-spectrum anticonvulsants used in cases of ongoing seizures.
- Most patients will have JME lifelong, and withdrawal of medication even after 5 or more years of good control is usually unsuccessful.

Epileptic encephalopathies

These epilepsy syndromes are also notable for generalized activity on EEG (but in different patterns), but have a much worse prognosis. Most are associated with at least mild and often more significant developmental delay.

West syndrome

- Coming on usually before the age of 1 year, infants with West syndrome suffer intermittent flexor spasms ('salaam spasms').
- EEG reveals hypsarrhythmia, and treatment is frequently with corticosteroids or vigabatrin.
- With development, most children develop Lennox–Gastaut syndrome.

Lennox–Gastaut syndrome (LGS)

- The most common form of intractable epilepsy, children who develop this syndrome often have seizures throughout their lives and into adulthood. Many have significant developmental delay, making them reliant on the care and support of others.
- The hallmark of LGS is atonic seizures or 'drop attacks', in which the patient loses all tone and drops to the ground, often injuring themselves.
- They may also have absence episodes, tonic seizures, tonic–clonic seizures, and may develop non-convulsive status epilepticus, appearing 'not themselves' and being less interactive.
- Medication with a clear role includes sodium valproate, lamotrigine, topiramate, phenytoin, clonazepam, clobazam, and phenobarbitone. Many other anticonvulsants may, paradoxically, worsen the situation, and should be monitored carefully when used.

Dravet syndrome

(Generalized epilepsy with febrile seizures plus.)

- Coming on at around 1 year of life, this syndrome is fortunately rare.
- It initially presents as febrile convulsions in an otherwise normally developing child.
- Over the next year, seizures become more common and may be brought on by heat.
- Seizures frequently appear focal, although generalized and focal abnormalities may be present on EEG.
- Patients with Dravet syndrome are often resistant to medication, and treatment is best through specialized units.

Common focal epilepsies

Temporal lobe epilepsy (TLE)

- Temporal lobe epilepsy is the most common form of epilepsy and may arise from any part of the temporal lobe, although it usually arises as a consequence of scarring of the hippocampus, termed 'mesial temporal sclerosis'.
- The pathology underlying this change is not well understood, although patients often have a history of febrile convulsion.
- Unlike the rest of the brain, seizures arising in the mesial temporal lobe need not spread rapidly to cause loss of consciousness. This results in frequent reports of sensory 'aura' at onset, which are in fact simple partial seizures.
- Frequent descriptions include a particular smell or taste, a rising feeling in the chest, anxiety or fear, a feeling of déjà vu (having done something before) or jamais vu (everything feeling unfamiliar), as well as music or a stereotyped sound.
- At times patients may have secondary generalized seizures, while others may have frequent 'aura' in isolation.

Diagnosis

- MRI is of particular utility in identifying mesial temporal sclerosis (Figure 18-9, overleaf).
- EEG can confirm unilateral temporal dysfunction or seizure.

Treatment

- Treatment is usually with carbamazepine or lamotrigine, although a wide variety of anticonvulsants may be used. Unfortunately, in some patients, seizures may be resistant to medication and require high doses of medication or multiple anticonvulsants.
- In intractable seizures, epilepsy surgery may be considered in patients with TLE, by removing the anterior temporal lobe on the symptomatic side. However, patient selection is critical due to the potential for resection of brain involved in language and memory and that which is also important for mood. This assessment should be performed through a specialist epilepsy unit.

Epilepsy associated with neuronal migration disorder (e.g. cortical dysplasia)

- In some patients, epilepsy arises as a consequence of disordered migration of gray matter within the brain during development. This can sometimes be attributed to a fetal or neonatal trauma, although sometimes no cause is identified.
- Most neuronal migration disorders can be identified with dedicated, careful MRI sequences and even more careful review of films. More extreme abnormalities such as megalencephaly (overgrowth of one or both hemispheres), polymicrogyria (multiple small disordered gyri) and, in the extreme, schizencephaly (a fissure in the brain connecting the surface with the ventricle) should all be more readily identified.
- Treatment is carbamazepine or lamotrigine as first-line therapy, with multiple second-line options.
- Surgery is not usually possible due to microscopic dysplasia, often extending outside the radiologically apparent region.

Epilepsy as a symptom of acquired cortical injury (e.g. stroke, tumor)

- This is a common cause for seizures in the elderly.
- Patients developing symptomatic epilepsy late in life will typically require lifelong therapy.

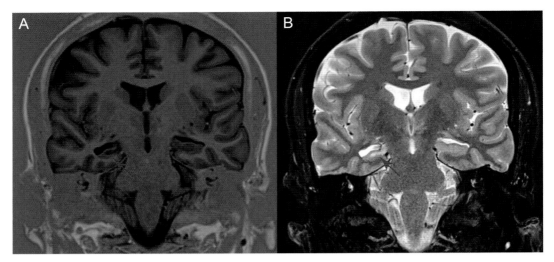

Figure 18-9 (**A**) T1 coronal image through the hippocampi demonstrating reduced volume of the right hippocampus relative to the left. (**B**) T2 image with increased signal within the right hippocampus, consistent with sclerosis

Choice of anticonvulsant therapy

All anticonvulsants have specific uses, as well as potential side-effects. It is important when starting patients on anticonvulsants to do so with an understanding of:

1 the certainty of diagnosis
2 the type of epilepsy
3 side-effects
4 the implications for pregnancy.

Table 18-9 outlines important anticonvulsant medications and indications for their use.

Status epilepticus

CLINICAL PEARL

Status epilepticus refers to a seizure that does not remit for a period of 5–10 minutes or more, or multiple seizures without a return to normal consciousness between them. It is a medical emergency.

Status epilepticus may occur in patients with epilepsy who have been poorly adherent, or when other precipitants have led to a deterioration in control. It may be seen *de novo* in patients when symptomatic of intracranial pathology or drug withdrawal, or in infective or inflammatory pathology.

Treatment

In the community, status epilepticus is usually managed by paramedics with IV midazolam or other short-acting benzodiazepines. This allows termination of a seizure without the risk of longer respiratory depression.

- In brittle epileptic patients, rectal diazepam or buccal midazolam may be used under direction of an epilepsy plan.

In the hospital, a more measured approach is required.

- Parenteral midazolam or diazepam is often useful initially, but in refractory status epilepticus the effect is rapidly lost with resumption of seizures due to rapid metabolism (midazolam) or redistribution (diazepam) of these medications.
- Clonazepam 0.25–0.5 mg is often given intravenously to allow longer effect.

CLINICAL PEARL

Status epilepticus should *not* be managed in-hospital with repeated boluses of diazepam intravenously. Diazepam is rapidly redistributed and the effect is rapidly lost, minimizing effect and maximizing toxicity. The use of a long-acting benzodiazepine such as clonazepam 0.25–0.5 mg is recommended.

- In known epileptic patients with likely non-adherence, where possible it is best to give medication known to be effective. For example, in a patient normally prescribed sodium valproate or levetiracetam, their dose can be given IV.
- When the background of the patient is not known, a loading dose of phenytoin is recommended (15 mg/kg). This should be given slowly through a large vein to avoid venotoxicity and 'purple glove syndrome' (see Figure 18-10).
- In cases refractory to this, patients are often loaded with a further anticonvulsant, for example levetiracetam 1000 mg.

Table 18-9 Anticonvulsant medications

DRUG	MECHANISM OF ACTION	USES	SIDE-EFFECTS
Carbamazepine	Sodium-channel blocking agent	Focal seizures	May worsen generalized seizures Nausea, ataxia, elevated hepatic enzymes, drowsiness, rash Potential for Stevens–Johnson syndrome in Han Chinese ethnicity, so must be avoided Agranulocytosis, which is usually reversible
Sodium valproate	Multiple, including sodium-channel blockade, and increasing cerebral GABA	Multiple actions Broad-spectrum anticonvulsant First-line therapy in generalized epilepsies	Weight gain, tremor, thrombocytopenia, LFT dysfunction Rarely but importantly, hyperammonemic encephalopathy Teratogenic, in particular neural tube defects Interacts with lamotrigine
Lamotrigine	Sodium-channel blocker	Broad-spectrum anticonvulsant Focal epilepsies Useful in generalized epilepsies Second-line therapy in JME	CNS side-effects Stevens–Johnson syndrome
Topiramate	Enhances central GABA activity, and antagonizes AMPA and kainate glutamate receptors	Broad-spectrum anticonvulsant Migraine prophylaxis	Cognitive blunting and speech disturbance Acral paresthesiae Kidney stones Mood disturbance
Levetiracetam and brivaracetam (less neuropsychiatric events)	Not fully known	Broad-spectrum anticonvulsant Renally excreted with minimal interactions	Lethargy Possible neuropsychiatric disturbance with mood change and irritability
Clonazepam + clobazam	Benzodiazepines	Broad-spectrum effect on seizures Predominantly used in the short-term control of epilepsy while titrating other medication	Longer-term use should be limited to intractable epilepsies due to tolerance, difficulty with withdrawal, and the potential for abuse
Phenobarbitone + primidone	Barbiturates	Less commonly used now, but some patients have been on these drugs for many years	Sedation Narrow therapeutic index Withdrawal seizures
Lacosamide	Slow inactivation of sodium channels	Narrow spectrum, usually as add-on therapy Few interactions	Dizziness, diplopia and visual disturbance Nausea and headache
Perampanel	Inhibition of AMPA glutamate excitatory channels	Broad spectrum with uses in generalized and focal epilepsy. Less helpful in absences.	Somnolence, dizziness and behavioural disturbance may occur
Phenytoin	Sodium-channel blocking agent	Status epilepticus (due to availability for IV infusion)	Ataxia, drowsiness, nausea, encephalopathy Multiple drug interactions Gum hypertrophy or cerebellar degeneration possible with long-term use

AMPA, alpha-amino-3-hydroxy-5-methyl-4-isoxazolepropionic acid; CNS, central nervous system; GABA, gamma-aminobutyric acid; IV, intravenous; LFT, liver function test.

- When this is ineffective, infusions of midazolam or thiopentone may be required with respiratory support through intensive care.

Non-epileptic seizures

Clinicians are frequently faced by patients with episodes superficially similar to seizures.

- It is important to mention that some of these events may have an organic basis, and that paroxysmal movement disorders, parasomnias and syncope need to be considered.
- Psychogenic episodes may also present with attacks similar to seizures. They are currently referred to as psychogenic non-epileptic seizures (PNES).
  » 'Hysteria' and 'pseudoseizures' carry negative connotations and are frequently pejorative in their use, negating the distress and discomfort of the patient.
  » Recognizing these attacks as such is critical, as they do not respond to anticonvulsants (although in suggestible patients they may seem to do so initially) and require psychological therapy.
  » More challenging is that PNES may complicate the clinical picture in patients with documented epilepsy.

Some features are very suggestive of PNES, although it is important to remember that frontal lobe seizures or limbic encephalitis may present bizarrely.

- Forced eye closure during a seizure is a common feature of PNES.
- Typical epileptic seizures are usually rhythmic, coordinated and may follow a typical speed up–slow down pattern. PNES are often uncoordinated, arrhythmic, or wax and wane multiple times in a single episode.

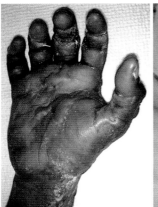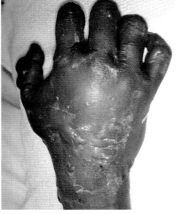

Figure 18-10 Purple glove syndrome following a phenytoin infusion

From Santoshi JA et al. Purple glove syndrome: a case report. Hand surgeons and physicians be aware. J Plastic Reconstruct Aesthetic Surg 2010; 63:e340ee342.

- Other motor manifestations atypical for epilepsy include pelvic thrusting, back arching (opisthotonus), side-to-side movements of the body or head, alternating in the plane of a movement (nodding then shaking the head), or prolonged unresponsive atonia.
- PNES typically occur in the presence of a witness, often in a waiting room or a busy place.
- Epileptic seizures should follow a similar activation pattern in that patient—if video is available demonstrating different motor activation with each event, it is strongly suggestive of PNES.
- Prolonged episodes >5 minutes are very common in PNES, and some may last well in excess of 30 minutes. In patients with prolonged PNES it is especially important to ascertain the diagnosis to avoid inappropriate management as per refractory status epilepticus. Many patients with PNES have ended up intubated in intensive care, due to a failure of recognition of the true diagnosis.
- Tongue biting and incontinence are less common in PNES, but do occur. This feature cannot be relied upon clinically.

Diagnosis

Diagnosis is frequently made with EEG recording during a typical event.

Treatment

Management of patients with PNES is frequently challenging.

- It is best to present the finding of PNES to the patient as a manifestation of stress, but one not under their direct control. Validating that the episodes are distressing and unpleasant is important.
- Likening PNES to another disorder with a significant relationship to stress, such as migraine, may promote acceptance.
- Ongoing supportive care during the transition to psychological therapy is recommended.

BALANCE, DIZZINESS AND VERTIGO

Balance is critical to a person's ability to interface with the world and move through it. Its importance is most evident when its deficiency affects a person.

It is important to remember that the sense of balance is dependent on several discrete factors, and these must be considered and tested separately. They are:

- vestibular function (sensation of head position and movement in space)
- proprioception (joint position sense)
- visual function (providing an alternative means of judging position in space).

Dizziness is often a problem area for the clinician due to the limited precision with which patients may describe it. The term 'dizzy' is often used to describe a number of pathophysiologically very different processes, and as such a great part of the clinical skill of assessing dizziness requires teasing out historical elements to better understand the patient's own complaint. It is also important to realize that nearly 50% of the time, when asked to repeat a description for dizziness, the nature of this will change. As such, in case of doubt it is critical to properly assess a patient for a multi-factorial cause.

Major differential diagnoses for 'dizziness' include:

- hemodynamic dizziness, including postural hypotension ('lightheadedness')
- vertigo (typically a sense of movement of self or world)
- astasia (loss of balance without vertigo)
- cognitive clouding and other nonspecific 'dizziness'.

Hemodynamic dizziness or 'lightheadedness'

- Syncope, and the dizziness beforehand, termed pre-syncope, are the final common pathways of hypo-perfusion of the brain.
- The duration of pre-syncope prior to fainting depends on the degree and tempo of circulatory collapse, from a prolonged period with prominent autonomic symptoms in vasovagal syncope to brief and sudden in cardiac arrhythmia.
- Those with a period of symptomatic pre-syncope may be aware of lightheadedness, sweating or clamminess, a tunneling of vision and alteration in hearing, and will typically become pale. Symptoms typically occur when upright, and recover with a supine position.

The etiology of hemodynamic dizziness is covered in Table 18-10.

Vertigo

Vertigo refers to a sense of movement, which may be rotational ('spinning') or translational (linear movements).

- It is a result of mismatch between visual and vestibular sensory systems, and is often distressing and accompanied by nausea and vomiting.
- It may be caused by pathology in any location within the vestibular system peripherally or centrally, and can be physiological (as seen in amusement rides with prolonged rotation).
- The clinical accompaniment to vertigo is nystagmus, defined by eye movements with a slow drift in a horizontal, vertical or rotational direction (due to the pathological process) with an opposite compensatory fast phase. It is named after the direction of the fast phase, as this is more evident to the observer.
- When symptoms are severe, nystagmus is usually easily evident; but when symptoms are milder, more specialized techniques for assessing eye movements may be necessary for the less skilled observer. It is worth noting that nystagmus need not be accompanied by vertigo, such as in congenital nystagmus, brief optokinetic nystagmus (seen in fellow passengers as a train pulls into

Table 18-10 Etiology of hemodynamic dizziness

GENERAL CLASS	CAUSE
Autonomic	Vasovagal syncope (neurocardiogenic syncope) Autonomic neuropathy or failure Multisystem atrophy
Cardiac	Arrhythmia Aortic stenosis
Hypovolemia	Dehydration Hemorrhage Addisonian state
Drugs	Antihypertensives Antipsychotics
Cerebrovascular	Basilar insufficiency (rare!)

a station), or in gaze paretic nystagmus with lesions within the oculomotor pathway.

The peripheral vestibular system

Each inner ear houses a vestibular labyrinth, with three semicircular canals orientated perpendicularly in a close approximation to paired eye muscles, and two otolith organs, the utricle and the saccule, for horizontal translational accelerations and vertical (especially gravitational) accelerations respectively (Figure 18-11, overleaf).

- The vestibular organs are tonically active, and are balanced such that activation on one side is balanced by proportional deactivation on the opposite side.
- Vertigo often results when there is disturbance in this balance between sides, with either increased activity or silencing of an organ, or loss of connectivity of their pathways more centrally.
- Due to differences in etiology as well as clinical signs, peripheral and central causes tend to be separated in discussion of causes of vertigo (Table 18-11, overleaf).

Vestibular neuritis and labyrinthitis

An acute peripheral lesion of the vestibular system is a common cause of acute severe vertigo presenting as the 'acute vestibular syndrome' of inability to walk, dizziness and nystagmus with the head at rest. With regard to terminology, if auditory function is also involved the condition is termed 'labyrinthitis', whereas sparing of auditory function is termed 'vestibular neuritis'.

The pathology of this process is poorly understood, with an infectious or post-infectious etiology postulated as the predominant cause in most cases. In older patients with vascular risk factors, it should be remembered that the internal auditory artery is a branch of the anterior inferior cerebellar artery (AICA), and an acute vestibular and auditory lesion may be macrovascular in origin.

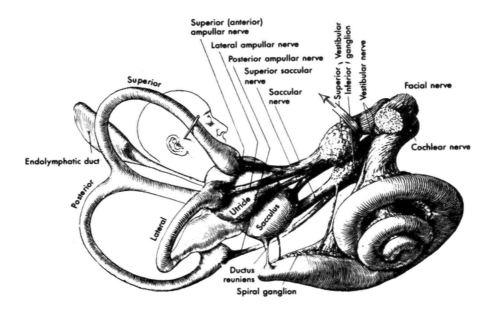

Figure 18-11 The anatomy of the vestibular and cochlear apparatus. Note the three orthogonally orientated semicircular canals and the two otolith organs, the utricle and the saccule

From Minor LB. Physiological principles of vestibular function on earth and in space. Otolaryngology—Head Neck Surgery 1998;118 (3 Suppl):S5–15.

Table 18-11 Important causes of vertigo

CAUSE	CHARACTERISTICS
Peripheral	
Vestibular neuritis	Acute-onset vertigo, usually with severe nausea and vomiting
Ménière's disease	Episodic vertigo with hearing loss and tinnitus
Benign paroxysmal positional vertigo (BPPV)	Paroxysms with movement, usually seconds to a minute or two
Central	
Stroke	Isolated vertigo extremely rare
Migraine	May occur disparate to headache
Demyelination	May have other neurological findings like RAPD (relative afferent pupillary defect)

- In the case of vestibular neuritis, vertigo results from mismatch in vestibular inputs between sides. It presents with acute-onset, usually severe (often to the point of prostrating a patient) vertigo, and usually with severe nausea and vomiting. In the acute phase it is usually associated with persistent nystagmus, which should be evident to the observer. It is always worse with movement, as this stresses an already challenged vestibular system, but does not completely clear when still.
- A hallmark of acute vestibular neuritis is loss of the vestibulo–ocular reflex (VOR), which helps differentiate it from a cerebellar lesion.

Benign paroxysmal positional vertigo (BPPV)

A diagnosis of BPPV implies a very particular pathology that is very distinct from the acute vestibular syndrome, which is usually accompanied by a characteristic history.

- It occurs due to loose crystalline matter within the semicircular canals (otoconia), impacting upon stereocilia and causing vestibular mismatch with movements in a particular direction.
- The commensurate history is one of paroxysms of vertigo, lasting seconds to a minute or two (rarely more), occurring solely with movement and usually in a predictable manner.
- The most common site is the posterior semicircular canal, which results in vertigo on moving from lying to sitting, when bending over and straightening again, when looking up to hang clothing on the line, and particularly on rolling over in bed.

CLINICAL PEARL

Intermittent dizziness which occurs on rolling over in bed or on lying down is very suggestive of benign paroxysmal positional vertigo.

- The diagnosis can be confirmed by normal eye movements with the head still, and usually normal VOR on head impulse testing but an abnormality on performing a Dix–Hallpike test (Figure 18-12).
- In the absence of an abnormality on testing but with a compatible clinical history with recent spontaneous symptom resolution, a diagnosis can still be made with relative confidence.
- Patients may complain of 'dizziness' between movements, and while movement-phobic 'dizziness' can occur in BPPV, it is also important to remember that movements stress an impaired vestibular system and that all vestibular lesions are symptomatically worse with movement.
- Should BPPV be evident on a Dix–Hallpike maneuver, a number of canalith repositioning maneuvers (CRMs) can be performed, including the Epley and Semont maneuvers. These involve a series of head positionings designed to move the canaliths and can be essentially curative, although canalithiasis can recur.

Ménière's disease

- The pathology of Ménière's disease is much discussed and incompletely understood, although it is believed that both fluid and ion homeostasis play roles.
- The pathological correlate is so-called endolymphatic hydrops, although this process may be present in the absence of Ménière's disease.

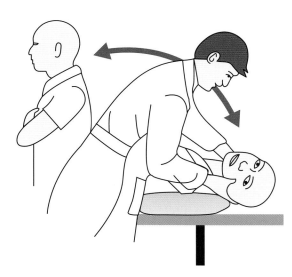

Figure 18-12 The Dix–Hallpike test is performed by lying a patient down from sitting, with the head orientated 30° to the horizontal and turned 45° toward the side being tested. The patient should keep their eyes open (often a problem in the severely dizzy patient), and after a latency, nystagmus will be seen in an 'earth-beating' or geotropic direction. It will then fatigue over seconds to a minute or so

From Hornibrook J. Benign paroxysmal positional vertigo (BPPV): history, pathophysiology, office treatment and future directions. Int J Otolaryngol 2011: 835671.

- The hallmark of this process is concurrent vestibular and audiological symptoms, most often between the ages of 20 and 40, but without any age limit.

The primary symptom complex is that of:

1. Episodic vertigo—usually 20 minutes to 24 hours.
2. Hearing loss:
   a. typically low-frequency, or low- and high-frequency, sparing the middle frequencies
   b. may fluctuate between attacks
   c. progressive with time.
3. Tinnitus—often low-pitch, machinery-like.

Additional symptoms may include nausea and a feeling of aural fullness coinciding with attacks.

There is no definitive diagnostic test for Ménière's disease, although with appropriate vestibular investigation, especially during an attack, a diagnosis should be able to be made with confidence.

- Symptoms can be precipitated by both alcohol and caffeine, and moderation in intake of both of these substances can be of benefit.
- Patients should not receive a diagnosis of Ménière's disease on history alone, but instead need comprehensive audiological and neuro-otological assessment before the diagnosis may be made.
- Salt restriction may also benefit symptoms.

Central pathologies

Migrainous vertigo (vestibular migraine)

Migraine is one of the most common causes of episodic dizziness in the community. Patients have often been mislabeled as suffering Ménière's disease.

- Symptoms are variable, with vertigo and dizziness during and disparate to headaches, although for a definite diagnosis at least some attacks should be concurrent with migrainous headache.
- It typically lasts minutes to hours, but can be brief and paroxysmal or more sustained.
- It may cause a sense of spinning, translational movement, rocking, or some other form of dysequilibrium.

Diagnosis is typically made on clinical history with normal clinical examination, and if assessed, normal vestibular function testing.

- One of the most useful diagnostic aids is the response to migraine prophylaxis.

CLINICAL PEARL

Migrainous vertigo is far more common than previously recognized, with approximately 10% of migraine sufferers experiencing vestibular symptoms, and a population prevalence of nearly 1%.

Stroke

- Stroke is the most critical differential diagnosis in an acutely vertiginous patient.

- Isolated vertigo without any other neurological symptoms or signs is very rare in stroke. However, vertigo may result from a variety of ischemic lesions, and other neurological abnormalities may not be as obvious or distressing as the vertigo so must be properly assessed.

CLINICAL PEARL

Vertigo is very rare as an isolated sign in stroke, but other signs can be missed easily if not properly assessed.

Vertigo may occur in the following strokes:

- cerebellar infarction or hemorrhage
- posterior inferior cerebellar artery (PICA) stroke
- anterior inferior cerebellar artery (AICA) stroke.

Cerebellar stroke

- This often presents with abrupt onset of ataxia with or without vertigo.
- Headache is not specific for ischemia or for hemorrhage, although hemorrhage in particular may also cause severe nausea and vomiting and often leads to drowsiness with mass effect.
- In this setting, nystagmus is usually worst when looking to the side of the lesion, with drift toward the center and fast-correction in the direction of gaze.
- An absence of appendicular ataxia does not preclude a diagnosis of cerebellar stroke, and gait may be solely affected. This results in a difficult assessment in an acutely vertiginous patient.

PICA infarction/lateral medullary syndrome

- An easily recognized syndrome for a clinician looking for it, this diagnosis is also too frequently missed due to inadequate neurological examination.
- This syndrome usually follows infarction in the territory of the posterior inferior cerebellar artery, which is the terminal branch of the vertebral artery before the two sides join in the basilar artery.
- Dissection of a vertebral artery often presents with this syndrome (with or without further posterior infarction), and must be considered.

CLINICAL PEARL

Clinical features of the lateral medullary syndrome:
- Vertigo—nystagmus is usually horizontal in the direction of the lesion
- Ipsilateral ataxia
- Ipsilateral Horner's syndrome
- Contralateral spinothalamic sensory impairment
- Ipsilateral vocal cord paresis ± dysphagia
- Muscle power and fine touch are clinically normal in this syndrome, and limited clinical assessment will be unrevealing. As a minimum, pain and temperature should be assessed in acutely vertiginous patients.

AICA infarction

- The terminal anterior inferior cerebellar artery, a branch of the basilar artery, perfuses the vestibulocochlear end-organ, and so AICA infarction presents with abrupt-onset deafness and peripheral vestibular symptoms analogous to vestibular neuritis.
- If more extensive, other features include:
  » limb ataxia (cerebellar peduncular infarction)
  » facial paresis (lateral pontine infarction).

Demyelination

The presentation of demyelination-induced vertigo will be variable, based on the location of the causative lesion.

Diagnosis in a patient with known multiple sclerosis is not especially challenging, but as a clinically isolated syndrome a high level of suspicion is required, and MRI imaging is the most helpful investigation.

Treatment of vertiginous patients

Acute therapy

Canalith repositioning maneuvers (CRMs)

As discussed above, these can be very effective in BPPV. However, all patients with vertigo get worse with movement, and attempts at CRMs in a severely vertiginous patient at rest can be distressing and unpleasant.

Antiemetics and vestibular sedatives

Phenothiazines, particularly prochlorperazine, are frequently used acutely for antiemesis and have a vestibular-sedative property. They can be helpful in the severely nauseated, prostrated patient, but should not be continued long-term.

Corticosteroids

There have been limited trials of acute corticosteroid therapy in vestibular neuritis, all with different regimens of drug and delivery. There has been some evidence to suggest that brief (5- to 7-day) courses of moderate-dose corticosteroids have benefit in the resolution of symptoms, particularly improving the speed of recovery.

Ongoing therapies

Vestibular rehabilitation

Often overlooked, this technique is one of the most helpful approaches for long-term recovery for an acutely or chronically dizzy patient. It helps provide graded exposure to vestibular stimuli to facilitate central compensation for lesions in the pathway.

Betahistine and diuretic therapy

These medications are thought to be able to reduce vestibular hydrops, and improve both symptoms and progression of Ménière's disease. They are not useful for other causes of vertigo.

Migraine prophylaxis

In vestibular migraine, acute migraine therapies such as analgesics and triptan agents tend to be ineffective. However, a range of prophylactic medications provide a reduction in symptoms, as for migraine.

Other balance disorders

Oscillopsia

Oscillopsia is the result of bilateral vestibular pathology.

- Due to absence of vestibular imbalance, vertigo does not occur but the absence of reflexive control of eye movements with locomotion results in a feeling of the world rapidly 'moving back and forth'.
- Such patients may also have severe balance impairment when visual stimulation is removed, as in Romberg's test.

Similar generalized imbalance and multi-directional nystagmus can be seen with multiple drugs with CNS activities, particularly anticonvulsant (most commonly phenytoin due to its non-linear kinetics), and lithium intoxication.

Chronic dysequilibrium

In addition to hemodynamic and vestibular systems, patients may describe dysequilibrium with a number of other pathologies. These are worth clinically assessing for before trying to make a diagnosis.

- Proprioceptive loss—patients often describe clumsiness, but may also describe sensory symptoms, especially tight band-like feelings in the setting of dorsal column involvement.
- Extrapyramidal postural instability—not to be confused with postural hypotension, early loss of postural righting reflexes is a feature of progressive supranuclear palsy ('Richardson syndrome'), and occurs later in Parkinson's disease. This can be tested with the 'pull test', whereby the examiner instructs the patient to maintain their balance while being sharply but briefly pulled backwards. While helping diagnostically, there is no specific therapy other than risk reduction strategies such as those employed through falls clinics.

The remainder of chronically dizzy patients are a struggle to diagnose and to pigeonhole—something which often distresses them.

In studies of chronically dizzy patients, up to 80% of patients had psychiatric comorbidity at the time of onset of symptoms. This may lead to maladaptive central compensation. Patients may develop symptoms such as 'visual vertigo', a feeling of severe imbalance in busy environments such as shopping centers or traffic, or with flashing lights and strobes. This may represent an inappropriate increase in optokinetic stimulation, but also may have elements of phobic behavior.

A combined vestibular rehabilitation and cognitive–behavioral strategy may be helpful, sometimes requiring additional pharmacological intervention.

MOVEMENT DISORDERS

Patients with movement disorders typically present with clinical symptoms and signs, and a diagnosis can often be made through accurate description of these features. Indeed, there remains no definitive diagnostic test for Parkinson's disease to this day, and a compatible history and examination remains the mainstay of diagnosis for the most part.

However, with the development of imaging tools together with genetic and immunological testing, the field of movement disorders has become clearer on one level (the pathophysiology of the disease process)—but simultaneously more confusing, with the understanding that a single disease may present with either hyperkinetic or hypokinetic features, and sometimes both. Many disease processes can no longer be linked to a single set of signs and symptoms, and a high degree of suspicion needs to be maintained for treatable conditions, such as Wilson's disease, which progress without treatment and may result in death.

The other consideration in reviewing movement disorders is that the majority of these processes involve neural circuitry within the basal ganglia, especially dopaminergic pathways. This circuitry and transmitter is partially shared with the mesolimbic and mesocortical pathways, which are integrally related with psychiatric wellbeing. It is therefore not surprising that a large proportion of patients with movement disorders may have psychiatric symptoms or comorbidities, a finding which challenges the physician seeing a patient with abnormal movements in the absence of other obvious pathology.

Tremor

With an appropriate approach, an accurate description of the phenomenology of a patient with tremor helps greatly to narrow the differential diagnosis. In assessing a patient with tremor, it is important to look carefully at the patient as a whole, even if they have noticed tremor only in a particular region. If their hand is involved, it is important to take note of additional head tremor, jaw tremor or even vocal tremor. Any unusual posturing of the leg or abnormal rotation of the head upon the neck should be noted. Often patients may not be aware of these clinical signs, especially if a friend or relative has prompted their visit.

In then assessing the tremor it is critical to assess it:

- at rest (ideally in a couple of different resting positions)
- held in a static posture (first with arms outstretched, then with fingertips held beneath the nose and elbows up)
- with movement toward a target.

Physiological tremor

Normal individuals have a high-frequency tremor of 10–12 Hz which may be exacerbated by a variety of precipitants to bring them to clinical attention. These can include:

- drugs—caffeine and stimulants, beta-agonists, theophylline or other stimulants of the adrenergic response
- anxiety and stress
- muscle fatigue and sleep deprivation.

Enhanced physiological tremor may be seen in drug or alcohol withdrawal, with thyrotoxicosis, or with fever. A tremor resembling physiological tremor may be seen with drugs such as sodium valproate or lithium.

Essential tremor (ET)

Essential tremor is estimated to have a prevalence of up to 5%. The name 'essential' implies that the tremor is the solitary symptom of the diagnosis, and abnormal posturing or features of other movement disorders all but preclude this diagnosis. It is considered the most common cause of a *postural* tremor, with no tremor typically present at rest.

- It is typically familial, often with a dominant history.
- The tremor is often exacerbated by the same features which increase physiological tremor listed above.
- The term 'benign' should be avoided, as it can be a distressing and disabling problem for the affected individual.

A typical history is one of tremor that worsens with efforts to perform a fine motor task, particularly under stress or in public (e.g. drinking from a glass in public, trying to get money out of a wallet at the cash register).

- It may suppress with alcohol consumption.
- The arms are typically involved (95%), and head (34%), lower limbs (30%) and voice (12%) much less frequently so, usually with the arms still predominant.

Treatment

Treatment is usually with a non-selective beta-blocker such as propranolol, or if not able to be tolerated then a barbiturate such as phenobarbitone or primidone may be used, although this is frequently limited by tolerability.

Differential diagnosis

It is emerging that dystonic tremor may be frequently mistaken as both essential tremor or Parkinson's disease, with a variable pattern of involvement, either resting or postural.

- Unlike with ET, a patient with a dystonic tremor may have abnormal posturing of the affected limb when outstretched, in addition to the tremor.
- As with ET, the tremor will typically worsen with stress or efforts to control it, but typically will not respond to beta-blockers. It may, however, respond to anticholinergics such as benzhexol/trihexyphenidyl or benzodiazepines.

Parkinson's disease (PD)

Since Parkinson's 1817 description, a great deal more has developed in both clinical assessment and treatment of PD. However, the clinical hallmarks remain the same; they can be summarized as in Figure 18-13.

- The **tremor** in Parkinson's disease is a 4–6 Hz resting tremor, and may be noticed by observers before patients themselves.

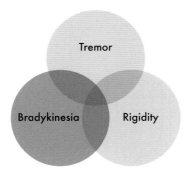

Figure 18-13 Tremor, bradykinesia and rigidity—the parkinsonian triad

» It is usually seen in the hand at presentation, and may be 'pill rolling' although this is not always the case.

» Idiopathic PD (iPD), i.e. drug-responsive Parkinson's disease without additional features of early dementia, falls, gaze paresis or autonomic failure (characteristics of 'Parkinson's plus' disorders) or without a clearly genetic basis, will almost always be asymmetrical in presentation. Symmetry of tremor should prompt further consideration.

- **Bradykinesia** usually begins asymmetrically together with the tremor, although the severity of these symptoms need not be linked. Patients may have tremor-predominant or bradykinetic-rigid presentations of iPD. Its symptoms include not just slowing of movements but also a decrease in amplitude of regular movements. This may be evident through decreased arm swing, reduced facial expression (hypomimia) or decreased volume in the voice (hypophonia).
- **Rigidity** is noted. It is the combination of rigidity and tremor which leads to the 'cog-wheel' movements classically described.
- **Gait disorder** is a common feature of PD, with a decreased stride length (shuffling), and difficulty initiating gait.
  » A person with PD may demonstrate 'festination'—an appearance of hurrying, as their upper body moves ahead of their center of gravity. Difficulty turning is common, and 'turning by numbers' may be noted. Freezing may occur, where a patient is unable to voluntarily initiate gait; cognitive tricks may sometimes help in overcoming this.

Non-motor features

More recently, features of iPD have been described outside of the typical motor symptoms.

- Sleep disorder is very common, taking the form of rapid eye movement (REM) sleep behavior disorder. While dreaming, a person with PD may lash out or enact dreams, while non-affected individuals are paralyzed in REM sleep. This often precedes a diagnosis of iPD by years.
- Hyposmia has been described in PD, and is a research tool in early diagnosis. It does require formal testing if being relied on, as a person's reported sense of smell often fails to correspond with what can be assessed with bedside testing.

Psychiatric disturbances are recognized increasingly frequently in patients treated for PD. They can broadly be separated into *dopa-dysregulation* and *impulse-control* disorders (ICDs).

- Dopa-dysregulation describes the phenomenon seen in some patients where the dose of levodopa may be incrementally increased in the absence of clinical need. Given fluctuation in the degree of symptoms, it may be hard to recognize when a person is requesting more medication inappropriately, and collaborative history and a high index of suspicion are essential.
- ICDs include pathological gambling, shopping, eating, hypersexuality, or repetitive performance of a task to

distraction (from drawing to internet chess), termed 'punding' (Figure 18-14). They most commonly occur with dopamine agonist therapy, especially in high doses.

CLINICAL PEARL

When initiating a person on medication for Parkinson's disease, especially dopamine agonists, it is absolutely essential to disclose the risk of impulse-control disorders to them, as these may have socially and financially devastating consequences.

Dementia has been recognized as a component of PD, but should not be present at diagnosis or within 1 year of diagnosis, as this suggests dementia with Lewy bodies.

- All patients with PD may demonstrate some form of executive dysfunction on complex testing early in their course, but the mean time to diagnosis of dementia in PD is 10 years.

- The pattern differs from Alzheimer disease, with less-prominent memory disturbance and more attentional problems, apathy, language and visuospatial dysfunction.

Diagnosis

The diagnosis is a clinical one, but is supported by a clinically effective trial of treatment. However, as the condition worsens with time, the predictability of medication response becomes less, and often response to a 'dopa trial' becomes more difficult to interpret due to altered oral absorption and a narrower therapeutic window. At such a time, the efficacy of medication may be more evident when medication is inadvertently omitted in a patient on long-term treatment.

- There are tools available for supporting a diagnosis of PD. DaT scanning is available in many countries to assess pre-synaptic dopamine transport via means of a nuclear ligand (Figure 18-15).
  - » This typically shows a decrease in striatal dopamine, with an asymmetry in keeping with the clinical state.
  - » It does not, however, differentiate from other disorders of dopamine activity, from multisystem atrophy to types of spinocerebellar ataxia.
  - » A normal pattern should be seen in drug-induced parkinsonism.

- Due to the availability of this technology, the term SWEDDs (symptoms without evidence of dopamine deficiency) has been coined, with controversy about the pathophysiological nature of patients in this group.

Treatment

Levodopa

- Levodopa is absorbed from the proximal jejunum via amino acid transporters, and is therefore competed against by other dietary proteins.

- It is rapidly degraded by monoamine oxidase (MAO), and thus is always combined in formulation with a peripheral MAO inhibitor.

- After crossing the blood–brain barrier it is metabolized to dopamine, and can then be degraded by cerebral MAO or catechol-O-methyl transferase (COMT).

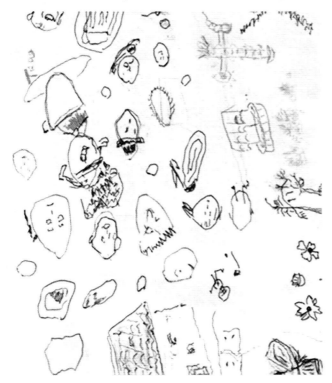

Figure 18-14 An example of doodling punding

From O'Sullivan SS, Evans AH and Lees AJ. Punding in Parkinson's disease. Pract Neurol 2007;7:397–9.

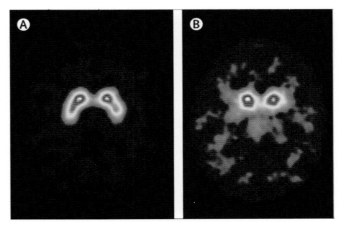

Figure 18-15 (A) Normal DaT scan demonstrating diffuse basal ganglia pre-synaptic activity of dopamine transporter, with a 'comma' shape. **(B)** Abnormal result with asymmetrical activity localized to the heads of the caudate nucleus, indicating disordered dopamine transport consistent with Parkinson's disease, multisystem atrophy or progressive supranuclear palsy

From Kurian MA et al. Clinical and molecular characterisation of hereditary dopamine transporter deficiency syndrome: an observational cohort and experimental study. Lancet Neurol 2011;10(1):54–62.

CLINICAL PEARL

Levodopa competes with other dietary amino acids for absorption, and should be taken at a time away from protein-rich meals.

- With a centrally dopaminergically deplete state, in early stages of Parkinson's disease the benefit of a small dose of levodopa may be marked, with a long, clinically good response.
- With further neurodegeneration of the substantia nigra, doses may be required more frequently, and on average motor fluctuations and dyskinesias occur in 50% of treated individuals by 5 years.
- Patients may begin suffering from peak dose dyskinesias with accompanying choreoathetoid or dystonic movements, which typically trouble them less than 'off' times when they are rigid. It is not infrequent for a clinically dyskinetic patient to ask for an increase in treatment, and this should prompt gathering of more collaborative history and consideration of dopa-dysregulation.
- Levodopa is available in multiple formulations, with 'regular', fast-release and controlled-release forms.
- Treatment side-effects include nausea, and fluctuations in hemodynamic indices, frequently hypotension.

Hallucinations or other psychiatric disturbance early in the treatment should prompt consideration of dementia with Lewy bodies.

Dopamine agonists

Dopamine agonists are used in monotherapy or in combination with other medications, and have a longer half-life than levodopa. As such, they may provide smoother and more predictable pharmacokinetics, particularly in patients with motor fluctuations. Unfortunately, their use is associated with a higher risk of ICDs, and these must be monitored for closely.

Entacapone

A COMT inhibitor, this drug increases the duration of action of levodopa by reducing central metabolism. It is especially helpful in patients requiring frequent dopa administration.

Rasagiline/selegiline/safinamide

- These are centrally active MAO-B inhibitors.
- There is limited evidence to suggest a neuroprotective effect of rasagiline in terms of progression of PD with time.
- These drugs have a very modest effect in monotherapy, and are advocated for early therapy of PD, delaying the time to levodopa and reducing the incidence of motor fluctuations.

Amantadine

- Amantadine has weak dopaminergic action.
- It was previously used in early PD to delay commencing levodopa, due to fear that an earlier start on dopaminergic medication caused faster progression. This assertion has subsequently been proven false, and amantadine has since found its place in the treatment of dyskinesias and peak–dose motor fluctuations.

Anticholinergics

- This group of medications is reserved for younger patients with tremor-predominant PD, and is used uncommonly.
- Side-effects include constipation, dry mouth and confusion.

Apomorphine

- Apomorphine is a highly emetogenic drug and can only be given parenterally, usually via subcutaneous injection.
- It is used in advanced PD and may be given as a 'rescue' medication in a person with severe 'offs' or freezing, usually by a partner, or in some cases as an infusion.
- It is dependent on injection technique, pumps and usually a partner willing to take on the responsibility of its provision.
- It is also very expensive on a yearly basis once costs are considered, and should only be commenced by dedicated units with experience in its use.

Duodopa

- A form of levodopa gel, this medication requires a percutaneous endoscopic gastrostomy tube with jejunal extension (PEG-J tube) to allow continuous delivery into the jejunum.
- While this eliminates variability of absorption with progressive PD, and more direct titration of dose, it has limitations in terms of cost, the willingness of a person to have a PEG-J tube, the mechanics of delivery, and availability.

Deep brain stimulation (DBS)

Prior surgical ablation of sites within the basal ganglia (e.g. thalamotomies) has given way to stimulation by stereotactically inserted pacemaker leads.

- A variety of sites have been described (subthalamic nucleus, globus pallidus interna, zona incerta and pedunculopontine reticular formation), each with its own particular benefits and risks.
- Initially reserved for advanced PD, there is now increasing evidence for a positive cost–benefit balance when used in patients earlier in their course. There are a number of problems that can follow insertion, aside from the surgical complications of infection and hemorrhage.
  - » Patients may develop acute cognitive deterioration, hypophonia, facial paresthesiae, and mood disorder.
  - » DBS is not in general effective for patients with 'on' freezing, nor does it have benefit in loss of postural reflexes and falls.
  - » Patients with cognitive decline or frank dementia should not be considered for DBS.

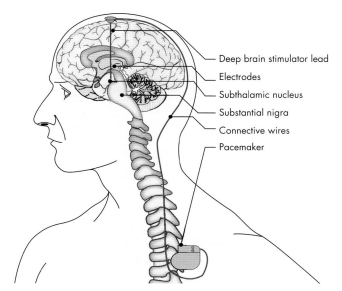

Deep brain stimulator lead
Electrodes
Subthalamic nucleus
Substantial nigra
Connective wires
Pacemaker

Figure 18-16 A schematic for deep brain stimulation

Dementia with Lewy bodies (DLB)

- A 'Parkinson's plus' disorder, DLB is notable for early dementia (at diagnosis or within a year of diagnosis of PD) with marked fluctuations, and sensitivity to both dopaminergic therapy (levodopa agonists) with hallucinations and sometimes confusion, and to dopamine antagonists (haloperidol, risperidone) with severe worsening of mobility when given for hallucinations or confusion.
- Hallucinations are often visual and are frequently fully formed, being of animals or people. They are almost always silent, and insight may be present into the fact they are indeed not real. A patient may be embarrassed about these, and it is important to query about these symptoms in all patients with newly recognized parkinsonism, as they are very specific for the diagnosis of DLB.
- Treatment is probably best with cholinesterase inhibitors.

Multisystem atrophy (MSA)

A more rapidly progressive disorder than idiopathic PD, MSA has no greatly effective therapies. It presents with:

- parkinsonism, often symmetrical with minimal tremor
- autonomic features, including:
  » erectile dysfunction (an early sign in men)
  » bowel and bladder dysfunction (constipation or incontinence)
  » postural hypotension (often severe, and exacerbated by dopaminergic medications)
- hypophonia of speech
- in some, disordered breathing and stridor
- cerebellar degeneration (less common).

Attempts to treat parkinsonism with dopaminergic medications are often met with exacerbations of hypotension. Symptomatic treatment may be beneficial with:

- fludrocortisone (a mineralocorticoid)
- midodrine (an alpha-adrenergic agonist)
- droxidopa (an adrenaline/noradrenaline precursor in late-stage trials).

Progressive supranuclear palsy (PSP)

A syndrome of relentless midbrain degeneration, PSP is marked by:

- symmetrical parkinsonism, often with an extended, upright posture (rather than the flexed, hunched PD posture)
- early falls with loss of postural reflexes
- early dementia
- degeneration of speech and swallow
- eye movement abnormalities, including:
  » vertical-gaze palsy or slowing of saccades (more than horizontal, which may also be affected)
  » loss of convergence.

Dopaminergic therapy is rarely beneficial, and the combination of dementia, impulsivity, and loss of postural reflexes often results in personal injury. Therapy is usually secondary prevention, with hip protectors for frequent falls, early speech therapy and, if necessary, alternative feeding strategies.

Corticobasal syndrome

Once termed 'corticobasal degeneration', only 50% of patients with this clinical syndrome will have the pathological diagnosis on autopsy, and the name has therefore been modified.

It presents with a starkly asymmetrical parkinsonism, usually in the arm with minimal tremor. Features include:

- marked asymmetry
- bradykinesia and rigidity
- loss of cortical sensation in the affected limb (astereognosis, agraphesthesia)
- apraxia
- in some, an 'alien limb' phenomenon
- aphasia.

With progression, a profoundly akinetic rigid limb usually results. Treatment is supportive only.

Dystonia

Dystonia is the phenomenon of sustained or tremulous abnormal posture of part of the body in response to inappropriate contraction of muscle groups, often opposing.

- It may affect any voluntary skeletal muscle group, including the face, limbs, vocal cords, or head and neck.
- It may occur in a localized distribution (*focal*), may affect two or more adjacent body regions in isolation (*segmental*), or may be more diffuse (*generalized*).

- It may occur solely in response to particular activity (writer's cramp, musician's dystonia, golfer's yips), and may be able to be stopped with a seemingly incongruous movement (e.g. a single finger on the chin in cervical dystonia), termed a 'geste antagonistique'.
- It may be associated with considerable pain if muscle spasm is severe.
- Together with a tendency for normal imaging and other investigation, this makes dystonia a challenging clinical diagnosis.

Dystonia may be *primary* (occurring spontaneously for no reason, or in the case of a genetic process), or *secondary* (as a symptom from another process). Causes of secondary dystonia include:

- traumatic brain injury/neonatal cerebral hypoxia
- drugs—especially neuroleptics and dopaminergic antiemetics
- neurodegenerative causes
- Wilson's disease and other metabolic processes.

Treatment

Anticholinergics

- Anticholinergics such as benztropine are used as an antidote to acute dystonia associated with neuroleptic or antiemetic use.
- They may also be useful in long-term dystonia, although are limited by tolerability.
- They may also be useful in a range of other neuroleptic-induced movement disorders, with the exception of tardive dyskinesias which are typically resistant.

Benzodiazepines

These may be useful as muscle relaxants and for sedation in painful dystonia at night; however, increasing requirements and dependency limit use.

Baclofen

- A GABA (gamma-aminobutyric acid) sub-unit agonist, baclofen is less sedating than benzodiazepines, and is often helpful in decreasing muscle spasm.
- In severe cases it may be given intrathecally via a pump under the supervision of a specialized unit.

Tizanidine

- A centrally active alpha$_2$-agonist, tizanidine has better tolerability than baclofen or benzodiazepines, and may be used in their place or in combination with them.
- Liver function abnormality, or rarely hepatocellular necrosis, limits its use in some countries.

Botulinum toxin

- In limited dystonia, injection of botulinum toxin into involved muscle groups may decrease the level of spasm and provide substantial relief. This can be repeated with recurrent need, often on a 3-monthly basis.
- Unfortunately, in more widespread dystonia or when large muscles are involved, toxicity limits dose and botulinum toxin may not be useful.

Levodopa

- In the rare genetic condition dopa-responsive dystonia (DRD or Segawa's disease), a profound response can be seen to levodopa.
- Given the potential for improvement in this subset of patients, a levodopa trial is advocated, especially for children presenting with dystonia.

Hyperkinetic movement disorders

Tics

Tics consist of repetitive, usually brief, irregular movements of distinct muscle groups or vocalizations, which may be preceded by a premonitory sensation of urge.

- Tics may be *simple* (e.g. a jerk, gaze deviation or grunt) or *complex* (mimicry of motor or speech—echopraxia and echolalia, coprolalia, or other mannerisms). They may be incorporated into pseudomeaningful actions (parakinesias).
- Popular culture would have one believe that 'involuntary' shouting of expletives is a common phenomenon, but coprolalia is a rare feature of tic disorders.
- Tics are the hallmark of the genetic process of Tourette syndrome, which demands both motor and vocal tics, but may be seen in other neuropsychiatric processes such as tuberous sclerosis or neuroacanthocytosis (Figure 18-17).
- Tourette syndrome begins in childhood, and is usually accompanied by features of obsessive–compulsive disorder (OCD). It is worsened by stimulant and levodopa administration, and may be suppressed with neuroleptic medications, or monoamine depletors such as tetrabenazine. It is typically combined with an antidepressant for OCD and attentional deficits.

Chorea

Chorea is a phenomenon characterized by involuntary, random, dance-like movements that may involve any part of the body, as well as the inability to sustain motor postures ('motor impersistence'). Chorea is uncommon, and varied in its cause (Box 18-4).

Treatment

Treatment (after managing the underlying cause or removing any potentially causative drugs) is with agents such as tetrabenazine, or with neuroleptics.

Myoclonus

- While grouped with movement disorders, myoclonus and its 'negative' counterpart asterixis may be a feature of a large number of neurological and systemic processes (Box 18-5).
- It is characterized by brief, shock-like movements or loss of muscle tone.

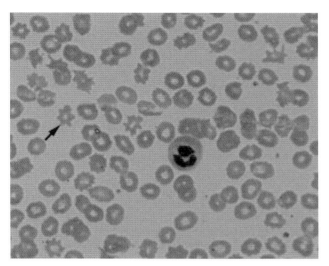

Figure 18-17 A blood film demonstrating plentiful acanthocytes (arrow) from a patient with neuroacanthocytosis

From Bertram KL and Williams DR. Diagnosis of dystonic syndromes: a new eight-question approach. Nature Rev Neurol 2012;8:275–83.

Box 18-4
Causes of chorea

Genetic causes
- Huntington disease
- Huntington-disease-like syndromes

Immunological causes
- Antiphospholipid syndrome
- Rheumatic fever (Sydenham's chorea)
- Systemic lupus erythematosus
- NMDA encephalitis

Infection
- Human immunodeficiency virus
- Syphilis

Metabolic disease
- Wilson's disease
- Porphyria
- Manganese toxicity

Pharmacological causes
- Levodopa
- Amphetamines
- Cocaine
- Phenothiazines

NMDA, N-methyl-D-aspartate.

Box 18-5
Causes of myoclonus

Physiological
- Hypnic jerks

Metabolic causes
- Hepatic encephalopathy
- Uremic encephalopathy
- Electrolyte abnormalities

Drugs
- Opioids
- Lithium
- Antidepressants
- Alcohol withdrawal

Epilepsy syndromes
- Juvenile myoclonic epilepsy
- Myoclonic epilepsy syndromes

Immunological
- Systemic lupus erythematosus
- Post-infective
- Paraneoplastic

Neurodegeneration
- Creutzfeldt–Jakob disease
- Genetic neurodegeneration

Ischemic
- Post-hypoxia

Treatment

Sodium valproate and clonazepam are agents that may be helpful in suppressing myoclonus in the appropriate settings. However, myoclonus should be regarded as a symptom and not a diagnosis.

NMDA encephalitis

Originally described in the setting of ovarian teratoma, this autoimmune process may also occur in the absence of a malignancy. It results from the formation of antibodies against the NMDA (N-methyl-D-aspartate) receptor.

- A typical presentation is one of initial neuropsychiatric disturbance with memory loss, psychotic features and sleep disturbance, which then proceeds to impaired level of consciousness and seizures, sometimes requiring intubation and respiratory support.
- A common feature is the development of a stereotyped movement disorder, often faciobrachial, not accompanied by electrographic seizure.
- Treatment is by urgent excision of any offending tumor (typically an ovarian teratoma) and immunotherapy. This may involve immunomodulation, usually by IVIg (intravenous immunoglobulin) or plasma exchange in

the initial phase, and often requiring ongoing steroid or cyclophosphamide therapy.

MULTIPLE SCLEROSIS AND CNS INFLAMMATION

Central nervous system inflammatory processes are some of the most unusual and capricious pathologies in the field of neuroscience. Their presentation is wide and varied depending on the site of inflammation, from optic involvement through to sphincter dysfunction, which can be contrasted with peripheral nerve demyelination. They may be monophasic, or may relapse and remit over days, weeks or years, or they may be progressive. There is a geographical gradient for prevalence, and racial factors may play a role in the typical nature of a presentation.

Multiple sclerosis (MS)

CLINICAL PEARL

The hallmark of multiple sclerosis is central nervous system demyelinating lesions disseminated in space and time.

Multiple sclerosis is a disorder of patchy inflammation through the brain and/or spinal cord.

- Pathologically, inflammation results in localized demyelination, giving rise to what was originally described macroscopically as 'sclerosis'—a hardening of these regions, which came to be known as 'plaques'.
- Perivascular T-lymphocyte and macrophage infiltration is seen acutely with relative sparing of axons; although more chronically, scarring with glial changes and axonal loss occurs.
- Inflammation is typically seen in areas of rich vascular supply, including the corpus callosum—an area unlikely to be involved in vascular processes.

Classification

Multiple sclerosis can be divided into four main groups, with attendant therapeutic implications.

Relapsing-remitting (RRMS)

- The most common form of MS, some 65% of patients fall into this group.
- An individual has multiple discrete attacks (termed 'relapses'), with improvement between episodes being variable.
- It may appear clinically complete or leave impairment.
- Residual neurological symptoms may compound over time, with resultant disability.

Secondary progressive (SPMS)

- After following a relapsing-remitting pattern for years, a patient may cease having defined relapses, although deficits may slowly worsen.
- The pathology of this process is much debated, but may

relate to secondary neurodegeneration following initial insults.

Primary progressive (PPMS)

- The most feared form of MS, this type is associated with an inexorable deterioration in function over time without any of the typical relapses.
- Epidemiologically, it often affects older individuals, and there is a more equal gender ratio.
- Therapeutic options remain supportive only at this time.

Progressive-relapsing (PRMS)

- While often separated due to little recovery between attacks, this type tends to be treated as per RRMS, due to distinct relapse episodes with or without resolution of acute symptoms between attacks.
- This subtype is notable for ongoing additional clinical progression between acute relapses.

Presentation

The presentation of MS is highly variable, with atypical symptoms and signs common. However, there are some typical presentations and clinical symptoms, which raise the pre-test likelihood of MS.

Optic neuritis

- Optic neuritis is a common initial presentation for MS.
- It presents with acute to subacute unilateral ocular pain on eye movement, which improves, giving way to visual impairment—often in the form of a central scotoma, with impaired acuity and early loss of color discrimination. A relative afferent pupillary defect (RAPD) is seen clinically.

CLINICAL PEARL

Color vision is impaired early in optic neuritis, and normal color sensitivity suggests a different diagnosis in the presence of impaired acuity.

- Bilateral or rapidly sequential optic neuritis is very uncommon in MS, and should raise the possibility of neuromyelitis optica, Leber's hereditary optic neuropathy (a mitochondrial disorder, affecting young men more than women, with painless loss of vision) or neurosarcoidosis. However, asymmetric bilateral symptoms may be seen if the optic chiasm is involved.

Internuclear ophthalmoplegia (INO)

Occurring due to lesions within the medial longitudinal fasciculus, INO results from decoupling of the abducens nucleus (the lateral gaze center) and the contralateral oculomotor nucleus.

- On lateral gaze, the abducting eye rapidly moves to target, while the adducting eye moves either incompletely or more slowly (depending on severity).
- The abducting eye has nystagmus evident until fixation is achieved (Figure 18–18).

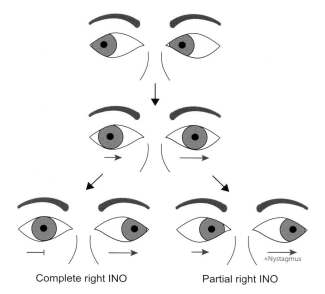

Complete right INO   Partial right INO

Figure 18-18 Internuclear ophthalmoplegia (INO). The top image shows normal gaze to the right. With gaze to the left, the right eye lags behind the left (middle image) and may fail to adduct completely (bottom image). However, in milder INO it may only be a lag in the adducting eye which is evident

This may also be seen in other lesions of the brainstem, such as vascular disease and infiltrative processes, but abrupt-onset INO in a young patient is very suggestive of MS.

Sensory symptoms

- These are common in MS, and almost ubiquitously present in a patient with significant disability.
- The nature and distribution of these may be varied and are multimodal, involving proprioceptive and/or spino-thalamic (pain and temperature) tracts.
- At times a heightened sensitivity or dysesthesia is reported, and pain may be reported.
- Trigeminal neuralgia is sometimes described, and otherwise radicular-sounding symptoms may occur in the limbs or trunk.
- It is frequently seen that sensory involvement seems patchy and does not conform to known dermatomal maps.

Lhermitte's phenomenon

A clinical symptom seen with lesions of the high cervical spine (including non-demyelinating causes), Lhermitte's phenomenon is a brief shock-like sensation radiating from the neck, down into the back or limbs on flexing the neck.

Uhthoff's phenomenon

- This describes the phenomenon by which neurological symptoms worsen with an increased body temperature. It can be seen with exercise, a hot shower or with fevers.
- Patients with MS often remark that their symptoms are worse in summer for this reason.

- This is not seen purely in MS. In myasthenia gravis an identical pattern is seen, and this is used diagnostically with the 'ice-pack' or 'ice-on-eyes' test (see clinical pearl in the section on myasthenia), as neuromuscular transmission improves with cooling.
- This phenomenon also explains why an increased body temperature with infection (such as a urinary tract infection) may make symptoms and signs more prominent, causing what is widely referred to as a 'pseudo-exacerbation'.

Other symptoms

Motor symptoms, vertigo and nystagmus, ataxia, and sphincter dysfunction are all seen with regularity in multiple sclerosis. While these are less suggestive of MS in the acute phase in a *de novo* patient, a high degree of suspicion needs to be maintained.

Other symptoms which become more prevalent with chronicity include:

- fatigue—almost ubiquitous in MS, this can be managed with energy conservation techniques, a rehabilitation approach and at times, medication
- mood disturbance—depression is a common bedfellow of MS, and when unmanaged can lead to further treatable morbidity for an already difficult condition
- cognitive dysfunction—frequently not considered, this may further complicate MS and its management, especially with disease progression.

Diagnosis of multiple sclerosis

The diagnosis of MS is a clinical one, requiring dissemination of CNS-demyelinating lesions in both space and time.

- **Dissemination in space** is demonstrated by:
  - » one or more MRI T2 lesions in at least two of four typical CNS sites—periventricular (Figure 18-19), juxtacortical, infratentorial and spinal

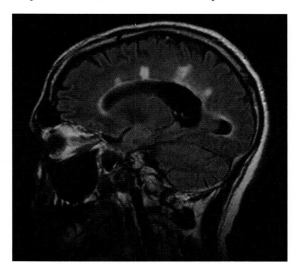

Figure 18-19 Sagittal T2-FLAIR showing typical 'Dawson's fingers', which are an MRI appearance resulting from periventricular plaques. This finding is reasonably specific for multiple sclerosis

or

» additional symptoms not attributable to one of these sites (e.g. optic neuritis with multiple periventricular lesions).

- **Dissemination in time** is demonstrated by:
  » two separate and distinct clinical attacks

or

  » concurrent presence of gadolinium contrast-enhancing and non-enhancing MRI lesions

or

  » development of new lesions, especially if contrast-enhancing, on follow-up MRI (with or without clinical symptoms).

It is also important to note that for a diagnosis of MS, there should be no other more likely diagnosis available.

Clinically isolated syndrome (CIS)

This is a term for a presentation with a single episode of demyelination, with or without other lesions. Approximately 80% of such patients will go on to have a diagnosis of MS given time, although this figure varies depending on the syndrome and the duration of follow-up.

In addition, with MRI more widely available, the concept of *radiologically isolated syndrome* (RIS) has also been described—radiological evidence of demyelination in the absence of clinical symptoms. There is clear evidence of a substantial conversion to clinical MS, but current management for this syndrome is controversial.

Further investigations

Cerebrospinal fluid examination

- Once a routine part of MS diagnostics, CSF examination is now often bypassed in clear cases, although with investigational markers of prognosis and disease activity it may return to use in all patients.
- The pathological hallmark in MS is the presence of unmatched oligoclonal globulin bands (OCBs) in CSF, when compared with plasma.
- OCBs are more sensitive for MS in temperate geographical areas than in equatorial areas.
- There is evidence that those with positive OCBs early in disease face a more rapid progression in disability.
- OCBs, when present in the situation of CIS, are also indicative of increased risk for progression to definite MS.

Electrophysiology

Evoked studies may also be used to assess the integrity of visual and proprioceptive–sensory pathways, with delays seen in previous demyelination.

- Visual evoked responses (VERs) may be tested with flash or a checkerboard pattern. They are sensitive for optic neuritis, even after vision returns to normal. However, adequate vision for fixation is necessary, and in the absence of patient cooperation, absent results cannot be interpreted.
- Somatosensory evoked potentials (SSEPs) are also performed at times, and have their place when spinal

symptoms are present, although they may be positive in around three-quarters of patients with MS even when symptoms are not present. They are most often used in atypical or contradictory cases.

Management of multiple sclerosis

Management of a patient with MS falls into three separate components:

1. Management of acute episodes of neurological symptoms.
2. Management of the underlying disease, with view to disease modification.
3. Symptomatic management of symptoms and disability, from mobility to mood to cognitive disturbance, fatigue and urological function.

The options for long-term management of MS have exploded in recent years. There is a strong case for optimal control of MS early in a patient's course, with a view to preventing long-term disability. Long-term drug management is best provided through a specialist unit, with consideration of safety, efficacy, likelihood of pregnancy and side-effect profile being paramount. (Long-term management of relapsing-remitting MS is outlined in Table 18-12.)

Management of acute exacerbations

> **CLINICAL PEARL**
>
> Prior to initiating treatment for an acute exacerbation of multiple sclerosis, it is important to exclude pseudo-exacerbation due to such complications as urinary tract infection or constipation. This will avoid the risk of unnecessary corticosteroid therapy.

Corticosteroids

- Used both intravenously and orally, as a general rule corticosteroids have a role in MS **only** in the setting of an acute attack.
- The most common form of management is with a 3- to 5-day course of intravenous corticosteroid, commonly methylprednisolone, at a dose of 500–1000 mg/day.
- This is associated with an increased likelihood of improvement or stability of symptoms when compared with placebo at 5 weeks.
- Some clinicians follow with an oral corticosteroid taper, though this has no evidence base.
- It should be noted that gadolinium enhancement on MRI improves with corticosteroids regardless of clinical state, and using this as a surrogate for clinical status is not advised.

> **CLINICAL PEARL**
>
> Oral corticosteroids should be avoided in optic neuritis, as they may be less effective than when used intravenously.

Table 18-12 Long-term drug management of relapsing-remitting multiple sclerosis

DRUG	MECHANISM OF ACTION	SIDE-EFFECTS
Beta-interferons	Immune modulation	Flu-like illness Depression Abnormal LFTs Neutralizing antibodies can reduce efficacy
Glatiramer acetate	Random mixture of peptides made from four amino acids, with antigenic similarity to myelin basic protein, against which it is thought to immunologically compete	Local injection-site complications—pain and redness Syndrome of flushing, sweating, shortness of breath and palpitations
Natalizumab	Alpha-4 integrin inhibitor (monoclonal antibody) Prevents lymphocyte migration across the blood–brain barrier	PML in a small number of patients Herpesvirus reactivations
Fingolimod	Sphingosine analog interfering with lymphocyte migration Lowers lymphocyte count by 20–30% by sequestering them in lymph nodes	Bradycardia at onset—requiring supervised administration on the first dose in a hospital setting Increased risk of both herpesvirus infections and possibly malignancy, including skin cancer PML
Teriflunomide	The active metabolite of leflunomide, teriflunomide interferes with pyrimidine synthesis. This pathway is required by activated lymphocytes to expand	Liver dysfunction, sometimes severe Cytopenias Opportunistic infection Stevens–Johnson syndrome Teratogenic
Dimethyl fumarate	Unknown	Flushing Gastrointestinal symptoms such as nausea, abdominal pain and diarrhea Abnormal LFTs Cytopenias
Cladribine	Lymphocyte-specific chemotherapeutic agent	Teratogenic Myelosuppression Alopecia
Ocrelizumab	CD20 monoclonal antibody with resultant B-cell depletion	Increased respiratory infection Unable to respond to vaccines

LFTs, liver function tests; PML, progressive multifocal leukoencephalopathy.

Symptomatic treatments

Spasticity

- Baclofen, a GABA$_B$ agonist, improves spasticity through activation of inhibitory spinal and other central neurons.
- Use is limited by sedation, frequently occurring above 75 mg/day, in addition to the frequent reduction in tone resulting in significant pyramidal weakness.
- Tizanidine is an alternative when sedation is problematic.
- Baclofen can be given intrathecally in appropriately selected patients.

Lethargy

Multiple factors affect energy levels, and the importance of adequately assessing mood and treating depression if present cannot be understated. Amantadine has been used for fatigue in MS, and has relatively few side-effects at a dose of 100 mg daily or twice a day.

Urinary symptoms

- Urinary urgency is a common symptom in patients with MS, and anticholinergic medication may be of use in such a patient.
- Oxybutinin, solifenacin or newer generations of anti-muscarinic drugs are available, and may be tried after ensuring that voiding is complete.
- In patients with incomplete voiding, anticholinergic use may precipitate urinary retention, and post-void bladder scanning is recommended prior to commencing one of these drugs.

- When significant residuals are present, it is usually necessary to commence intermittent self-catheterization.

CLINICAL PEARL

Check post-void residual bladder volumes before starting anticholinergics for urinary urgency, as they may worsen retention.

Pain

- Pain is common in MS, and therapy should be directed toward the cause of this.
- Pain resulting from spasticity may improve with baclofen or botulinum toxin in extreme cases.
- Neuropathic pain may be improved with adjuvant analgesics, and neuralgia may benefit from the addition of carbamazepine.

Neuromyelitis optica (NMO; 'Devic's disease')

Long thought of as a variant of MS, evidence has mounted over recent years that this is a pathophysiologically distinct disorder, with a more significant humoral etiology.

- NMO is a disorder characterized by severe optic neuritis and transverse myelitis with longitudinally extensive lesions (three or more vertebral segments).
- It has a female preponderance greater than MS, and is not associated with the presence of CSF oligoclonal bands.
- The clinical disorder of NMO is typically relapsing, often with discrete, devastating attacks of demyelination with variable recovery.
- It is associated with the presence of antibodies to aquaporin-4, which are pathogenic.
- Diagnosis is made on the basis of imaging (Figure 18-20), and aquaporin-4 antibodies.

Treatment

- Early treatment is critical, as disability often accrues rapidly.
- Initial treatment is usually with pulse methylprednisolone, 1 g/day for 3–5 days.
- Given the humoral nature of NMO antibodies, plasma exchange is advocated early in those patients not responding to corticosteroids.

Acute disseminated encephalomyelitis (ADEM) and transverse myelitis (TM)

Demyelination is not limited to chronic, relapsing disorders such as MS and NMO. It may also be seen as a monophasic illness, typically post-infectious in etiology. Multiple viral and bacterial infections, including HIV, may precede a presentation with multifocal neurological symptoms and encephalopathy (ADEM) or spinal-cord syndrome (TM).

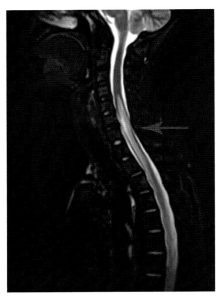

Figure 18-20 Longitudinally extensive transverse myelitis (LETM), typical of neuromyelitis optica

Acute disseminated encephalomyelitis

- ADEM is a disorder predominantly affecting children.
- It follows infection by days to a month or so, although in approximately one-third of cases an antecedent event cannot be identified (more in adults).
- Fever, headache, malaise and meningism may accompany initial symptoms, which typically worsen to nadir over 4–7 days with multifocal demyelination of cerebral, brainstem and spinal-cord white matter.
- Symptoms include unilateral or bilateral pyramidal signs, acute hemiparesis, ataxia, optic neuritis and encephalopathy.
- In adults, peripheral nerve demyelination may also occur.

Diagnosis

- Laboratory investigation may demonstrate CSF pleocytosis or transient oligoclonal bands, although it may also be normal.
- MRI typically shows multifocal white matter lesions without any significant temporal dispersion (Figure 18-21).

Treatment

- Treatment is with pulse steroid therapy with or without a taper, and in unresponsive cases plasma exchange can be considered.
- Prognosis is usually good, although when ADEM follows measles infection recovery may be less optimal.

Transverse myelitis

- TM may also follow infection, although it may also be idiopathic in cause.

- In some cases it may be a symptom of a more systemic process such as sarcoidosis or systemic lupus erythematosus (SLE).
- A majority of the time it is a monophasic illness, although in 5% of cases it may be the first episode of MS.
- Neurological involvement includes motor, sensory and autonomic symptoms, although pain frequently precedes all of these other features.

CLINICAL PEARL

At the clinical nadir of transverse myelitis, approximately half of patients will be paraplegic.

Recovery follows a rule of thirds for complete recovery, partial recovery and significant ongoing disability.

CLINICAL PEARL

Only 5% of patients with transverse myelitis go on to develop multiple sclerosis.

Diagnosis

- As with ADEM, CSF pleocytosis may be seen at times, while oligoclonal bands may also be transiently seen.
- Imaging of the spine typically reveals increased T2 and FLAIR signal in the region of demyelination.

Treatment

Pulse corticosteroid is once again the modality of choice for acute management.

NEUROLOGICAL MANIFESTATIONS OF SARCOIDOSIS AND BEHÇET'S DISEASE

Sarcoidosis

- Neurosarcoid may present peripherally or centrally, and may present in the absence of involvement of pulmonary, cutaneous or other typical sites for sarcoidosis.
- The most common presentation relates to leptomeningeal infiltration by non-caseating granulomas, leading to multiple cranial nerve palsies (typically facial or optic nerves), or endocrine dysfunction due to pituitary involvement (Figure 18-22, overleaf).
- It may also present with parenchymal, spinal or peripheral nerve involvement.

Behçet's disease

- Behçet's disease may cause CNS effects, with a brainstem and posterior fossa inflammatory process causing ataxia and/or hemiparesis (Figure 18-23, overleaf).
- It may also lead to thrombosis of cerebral venous drainage with resultant intracranial hypertension.

NEUROMUSCULAR DISEASE

The peripheral nervous system makes up the entire system outside of the brain and spinal cord, and may be affected by a huge range of pathologies, some of which have also central or systemic features.

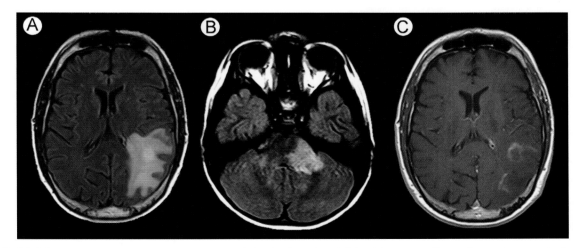

Figure 18-21 T2 magnetic resonance imaging of the brain of a child with acute disseminated encephalomyelitis. (**A**) Tumefactive change in the right temporo-occipital brain, with (**B**) additional T2 signal hyperintensity in the brainstem and cerebellar peduncle. (**C**) Patchy gadolinium enhancement on post-contrast T1

From Bester M, Petracca M and Inglese M. Neuroimaging of multiple sclerosis, acute disseminated encephalomyelitis, and other demyelinating diseases. Semin Roentgenol 2014;49(1):76–85.

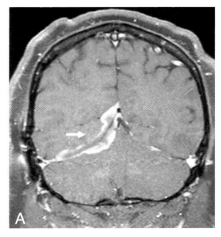

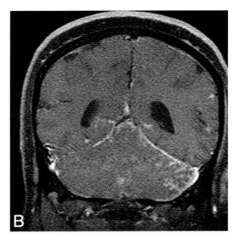

Figure 18-22 Sarcoidosis. (**A**) Gadolinium-enhanced coronal T1 image showing right tentorial durally based mass (arrow). (**B**) Gadolinium-enhanced coronal T1-weighted image showing nodular leptomeningeal enhancement in the basilar cisterns and posterior fossa

From Shah R, Roberson GH and Cur JK. Correlation of MR imaging findings and clinical manifestations in neurosarcoidosis. Am J Neuroradiol 2009;30:953–61 (www.ajnr.org).

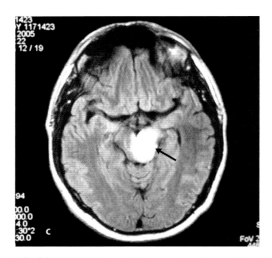

Figure 18-23 FLAIR signal change in the midbrain in a patient with Behçet's disease, extending into the pons and left thalamus on other slices

From Aksel Siva and Sabahattin Saip. The spectrum of nervous system involvement in Behçet's syndrome and its differential diagnosis. J Neurol 2009;256:513–29. DOI 10.1007/s00415-009-0145-6

Myopathy

Disease of muscle presents, not surprisingly, with muscle weakness and, in some disorders, pain. Processes affecting muscle integrity are myriad, and in this area more than any other in the peripheral neuraxis the whole patient must be considered, and indeed myopathy is frequently seen by physicians outside of neurology.

An overview of myopathy is provided in Table 18-13.

Inflammatory myopathy

- Inflammatory myopathy may be seen in isolation, or in the presence of other autoimmune disease.

- It may also be paraneoplastic, and in particular dermatomyositis is associated with an elevated risk of cancer (relative risk 2–7), although this is in a minority of cases.

- Polymyositis and dermatomyositis are often grouped together, separated by the presence of skin rash in the latter. However, while there may appear to be overlap, they are quite different entities pathologically and therefore physiologically.

- They present with proximal myopathy and elevated creatine kinase (CK).

- Diagnosis is made electrophysiologically, with compatible autoantibodies (anti Jo-1 in particular), and biopsy.

- MRI can sometimes show patchy inflammation within muscle.

Treatment

- Treatment is with immunosuppressive therapy, usually with corticosteroids, despite any evidence-based trials.
  - » A dose of 1 mg/kg/day of prednisolone is commonly used. Tapering should be done after a month or so of therapy, based on clinical response.

- Azathioprine and methotrexate are also used as steroid-sparing agents.

Worse weakness, a longer duration of illness, and bulbar features are worse prognostic signs at diagnosis.

Inclusion-body myositis

- Often initially diagnosed as polymyositis, this condition usually presents more insidiously with more notable distal weakness, including wrists and finger flexors.

- Muscle biopsy may display diagnostic features including cytoplasmic inclusions and vacuolar degeneration (Figure 18-24, overleaf).

- Corticosteroids and a variety of immunosuppressive agents have been tried with minimal clinical success,

Table 18-13 An overview of myopathy

PROCESS	CLINICAL FEATURES	CK	NCS/EMG	BIOPSY FINDINGS
Inflammatory				
Polymyositis (PM)	Proximal myopathy, pain in 25% (not prominent)	++	Myopathic (patchy)	Patchy involvement, with inflammation within fascicle
Dermatomyositis	As per PM with skin changes	++	Myopathic	Perivascular inflammation
Inclusion-body myositis* (considered by some to be degenerative)	Proximal, but may have distal involvement (wrists, finger flexors)	Normal or +	Myopathic	Cytoplasmic inclusion bodies
Necrotising Autoimmune Myopathy (NAM)	Rapidly progressive weakness with high CK levels. Often have a history of statin use, but myopathy persists beyond withdrawal.	+++-++++	Myopathic	Muscle necrosis
Mixed connective tissue disease	Should have features of SLE/Sjögren's syndrome/ scleroderma in addition to PM	++	Myopathic	Non-specific necrosis and regeneration
Infective	Often acutely painful	May be +++	not typically done	Depends on etiology
Drugs				
Statins	Myalgias and/or myopathy Can be frank rhabdomyolysis	Normal to +++	May be myopathic	
Corticosteroids	Usually insidious with proximal myopathy	Usually normal	Should be normal	Type II fiber loss
Alcohol	Acute with rhabdomyolysis; chronic with type II atrophy Patients often have neuropathy, cerebral features	+ to +++ Normal in chronic	May be myopathic	Variable depending on clinical picture
Antiretrovirals	Proximal weakness and myalgia/tenderness	+ to ++	Myopathic	Ragged red fibers
Colchicine	Proximal weakness (lower limbs > upper limbs) in long-term use (or overdose)	++	Myopathic with myotonia	May be confused with polymyositis
Endocrine				
Cushing's syndrome	Weight gain, striae	Normal	Usually normal	Type II fiber loss
Hypothyroidism	Weight gain, myxedema	+	Normal or mildly myopathic	Non-specific (TSH much more helpful!)
Thyrotoxicosis	Weight loss, tremor Eye signs in Graves' disease	Normal or +	Normal or mildly myopathic	Variable—may have fiber loss/fibrosis/ necrosis
Metabolic and genetic				
Renal failure	Painless; may have associated neuropathy	May be normal	May be subtle	Type II fibre loss
Mitochondrial disorders	Often progressive; extraocular muscles especially commonly involved	Normal or +	Myopathic changes	Ragged red fibers on biopsy
Disorders of glucose and lipid metabolism	Variable depending on disease; may have exercise-induced rhabdomyolysis	Disease-specific	Disease-specific	Disease-specific
Muscular dystrophies (disorders of muscle structure)	Variable; usually progressive weakness with aging	Disease-specific	Disease-specific	Disease-specific

CK, creatine kinase; SLE, systemic lupus erythematosus; TSH, thyroid-stimulating hormone.

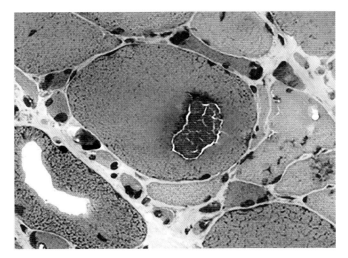

Figure 18-24 A granule-filled cytoplasmic inclusion seen on Gömöri trichrome staining of a muscle biopsy from a patient with inclusion body myositis

From Agamanolis DP. Neuropathology: an illustrated interactive course for medical students and residents. Northeast Ohio Medical University (NEOMED).

which has led some to regard this condition as more of a neurodegenerative process.

Drug-induced myopathy

A variety of drugs can cause acute myopathy with rhabdomyolysis, or chronic myopathy in long-term use.

- Some drugs exert an effect through direct muscle toxicity (alcohol, colchicine), while others affect muscle cellular metabolism leading to secondary toxicity (statins, antiretrovirals).
- Corticosteroids and thyroxine (in supraphysiological doses) cause myopathy through secondary humoral processes.
- A thorough drug history should be taken on any patient presenting with myopathy or myositis, including non-prescribed intake, as recreational drugs such as cocaine and amphetamines may cause muscle toxicity.
- Biopsy is not usually required, but rather treatment is withdrawn and the patient observed for improvement.
- In the case of corticosteroid use for inflammatory or other disorders, often CK levels and electromyography (EMG), together with MRI if necessary, suffice to avoid biopsy.

Endocrine and metabolic processes

- Disordered muscle function may be seen in a Cushingoid state, as well as with both hypothyroidism and thyrotoxicosis.
- Typically, abnormality of electrophysiological or laboratory testing is not found in this case, unless disease is severe. Clinical history and examination is likely to reveal other abnormalities.
- Myopathy may also be seen in renal failure and very

rarely in diabetes mellitus, although they are typically accompanied by features of neuropathy.

Genetic disorders

Making up a small percentage of patients with symptomatic muscle weakness, the number of described muscular disorders continues to expand with improvements in investigative genetic techniques. In many of these disorders cardiac muscle may also be involved, and the involvement of this should always be assessed.

Duchenne muscular dystrophy

Duchenne muscular dystrophy is an X-linked condition, marked by pseudohypertrophy of musculature and progressive weakness during childhood, with a patient (almost always male) typically wheelchair-bound by 12 years of age.

- It is caused by a mutation (typically frameshift) in a myofibrillar protein called dystrophin, and less severe mutations are seen in a less rapidly progressive form referred to as *Becker's muscular dystrophy*.
- Cardiac muscle is involved, and dilated cardiomyopathy often develops in the teenage years.

Other muscular dystrophies

Multiple other genetic causes of muscular dystrophy have now been described (Box 18-6); and with these, variability in the presentation. The core feature is that of proximal muscular weakness, which may progress with time.

Mitochondrial disorders

This includes a large number of distinct disorders, all resulting from defects in the mitochondrial respiratory chain pathway.

- Defects can be in mitochondrial DNA (inherited maternally with variable heteroplasmy), or in autosomal genes coding for mitochondrial proteins.
- Tissues affected include those with a high energy requirement, and therefore muscles and nerves feature highly (Box 18-7).
- The hallmark of mitochondrial disorders where muscle is affected is the presence of ragged red fibers on biopsy, an appearance due to an aggregation of abnormal mitochondria.

Other diagnostic tests that may assist include:

- resting lactate levels
- CSF lactate levels

Box 18-6

Genetic muscular dystrophies

Limb girdle (multiple types)

Facio-scapulo-humeral

Oropharyngeal

Distal

Myotonic

Box 18-7
Features of mitochondrial disorders

Progressive external ophthalmoplegia

Myopathy

Deafness

Diabetes mellitus

Stroke-like episodes

Seizures

Visual failure

Lactic acidosis

Gastrointestinal symptoms

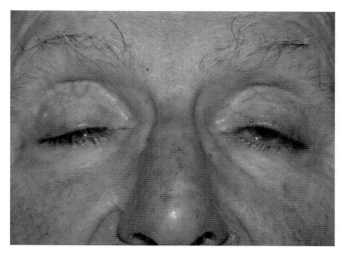

Figure 18-25 Myasthenia gravis patient with bilateral ptosis

From Liu GT, Volpe NJ and Galetta SL. Neuro-ophthalmology: diagnosis and management, 2nd ed. Elsevier, 2010.

- MRI imaging ± magnetic resonance spectroscopy (lactate peaks)
- genetic testing of blood, hair or muscle tissue.

Specialized mitochondrial respiratory chain testing may be performed, but is of very limited availability.

Other disorders of energy production in muscle

A number of disorders have now been described in which muscle may be injured, especially when exerted. This typically occurs in people with episodes of rhabdomyolysis after exertion, and is sometimes life-threatening.

- The two most common disorders are McArdle's disease—a glycogen storage disorder; and CPT (carnitine palmitoyltransferase 1) deficiency—a disorder of fatty-acid metabolism.
- Both can be ascertained by muscle biopsy with appropriate staining by a specialist center.

NEUROMUSCULAR DISORDERS

This group of disorders broadly covers disease states in which symptoms occur due to abnormalities in the transmission of action potentials across the neuromuscular junction, resulting in disordered muscular contraction.

It encompasses myasthenia gravis, Lambert–Eaton myasthenic syndrome (LEMS) and rare congenital myasthenic syndromes.

Myasthenia gravis (MG)

Myasthenia gravis is an autoimmune process that results from production of autoantibodies to proteins involved in the signaling pathways in the postsynaptic neuromuscular junction.

- The predominant feature of MG is fatiguable weakness.
- With often single nerve to single muscle fiber innervation and constant activity, extraocular musculature is most commonly the first site of symptoms, and patients frequently present with fluctuating diplopia or ptosis (Figure 18-25).

  » When more severe, extraocular muscles may have little or no movement, and this can confound the usually fluctuating and fatiguing picture of MG.
  » More than 80% of patients will have ocular symptoms, and myasthenia may be limited to eye movements alone.

- A smaller proportion of patients present with myasthenic involvement of other muscles, notably a dropped neck, bulbar weakness, limb weakness or even respiratory muscle weakness. These features should always warrant a search for fatiguability elsewhere.
- Sensory symptoms should not occur, though are sometimes reported as a 'heavy sensation'.

Pathophysiology

Pathophysiologically, the antibody most commonly implicated is an antibody to inotropic nicotinic receptors to acetylcholine (ACh), hence known as an acetylcholine receptor antibody (AChR Ab), which is present in more than 80% of myasthenic patients but only 50% of myasthenic patients with disease limited to extraocular muscles. An additional antibody to muscle-specific kinase (MuSK), a part of the receptor complex, is seen in more than 50% of the remaining patients.

The antibody leads to inadequate signaling resulting from a single vesicle release pre-synaptically, with reduced receptors or impaired signaling pathways. This results in an increase in the number of vesicles released in response to a single action potential. This may compensate adequately at rest; but with activity, the pre-synaptic store of vesicles may be exhausted and this leads to the development of clinical weakness.

Clinical assessment

- MG is a neurological mimic, and a high degree of suspicion must be maintained in assessing patients with weakness, diplopia or bulbar symptoms, as a routine neurological examination of tone, power and reflexes may not be able to detect the critical feature of fatiguability.

- Fatiguability is tested in ocular musculature by asking a patient to maintain gaze in a position which historically makes the diplopia worse, usually in the midline vertical.
  - » In this position it is critical to observe both pupils for drift of the eye as well as both eyelids for fatiguing ptosis.
- A patient can be asked to count loudly to 20, or if shoulder abduction is strong on testing bilaterally, one arm can be exercised and then shoulders can be tested again.

CLINICAL PEARL

A simple and safe bedside test with good sensitivity and excellent specificity in ocular myasthenia is an ice-pack test (also referred to as an 'ice on eyes' test). In this test, an eye with ptosis or external ophthalmoplegia is covered with a cold pack (wrapped to protect the eye), and after cooling the musculature is re-tested. A clinical improvement should be seen, with deterioration again as cooling wears off. A positive test has excellent specificity. The alternative test, the edrophonium (Tensilon) test, is being used less commonly due to safety concerns and is no more specific.

Diagnostic testing

Edrophonium (Tensilon) test

- Edrophonium is a short-acting acetylcholine esterase inhibitor which facilitates an increase in the amount of acetylcholine at the neuromuscular junction, and therefore improves myasthenic symptoms temporarily.
- It must be given intravenously as a fast push, and has potential cholinergic side-effects including bradycardia, hypotension, sweating and salivation. Bradycardia may be precipitous, and to block this unwanted stimulation of parasympathetic muscarinic receptors, atropine is sometimes given in addition.

- A temporary improvement in clinical signs is seen in a positive test, but when mild or subjective the test is of uncertain value.

Serological tests

- Reliable ACh receptor antibody and MuSK testing is available, and these combined have a >90% sensitivity to the diagnosis of MG.
- In a patient with suspected myasthenic crisis, delays in obtaining results of serological tests may necessitate the use of alternative tests.

Nerve conduction studies

Routine nerve conduction studies and EMG in MG are normal, but pattern of fatigue can be assessed through repetitive stimulation studies, and neuromuscular junction exhaustion is assessed through a technique called single-fiber EMG, both of which have very high sensitivities and specificities (in an appropriate clinical setting) when assessed by an experienced neurophysiologist.

CT scan of the chest

This should be performed in any patient with MG to assess for the presence of a thymoma, which is present in around 15% of patients with another 75% having thymic hyperplasia.

Treatment

The therapy of MG has several components, with treatment aimed at:

- symptoms—pyridostigmine, physostigmine
- disease control—corticosteroids, azathioprine, IVIg, plasma exchange, rituximab, thymectomy (Figure 18-26).

Longer-lasting acetylcholine esterase inhibitors such as pyridostigmine are frequently prescribed to assist symptomatic fatigue of neuromuscular transmission.

- They do not treat the underlying autoimmune biology.

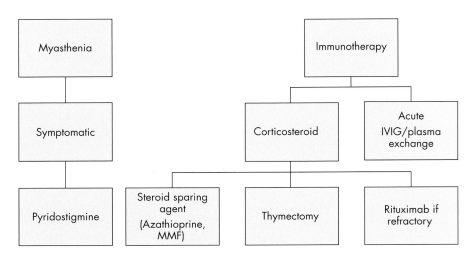

Figure 18-26 Treatment of myasthenia gravis. IVIG, intravenous immunoglobulin; MMF, mycophenolate mofetil

Side-effects include bradycardia and gastrointestinal cramping or diarrhea, which frequently limits dose.

Corticosteroids are first-line agents in the management of the immunological drive of MG, although they can exacerbate weakness if started at too high a dose.

- As such, doses of 10–20 mg/day of prednisolone tend to be a starting dose, with an increase over days or weeks to 1 mg/kg/day. With improvement in symptoms, the dose can then be reduced over time.
- If a faster response is required, either IVIg or plasma exchange may be helpful.
- Azathioprine or mycophenolate can be used in patients with severe or longstanding myasthenia with a view to reducing long-term steroid dose and exposure. There is little evidence for benefit in the first year of therapy, and it is only with prolonged use that patients may be able to reduce their steroid dose.

Thymectomy is indicated in any patient with a thymoma, and is also advocated for patients with chronic disease. Acute thymectomy is dangerous in an uncontrolled patient.

Rituximab is a B-cell-depleting monoclonal antibody which has found a place in patients with chronic intractable myasthenia.

Disorders of peripheral nerves

There are hundreds of causes of peripheral nerve injury, but most present with a fairly restricted group of symptoms: abnormal sensation (numbness, pain or loss of joint position sense) and/or weakness. Because of this, the pattern of involvement is essential to the clinician seeing a person with a peripheral nerve problem, much of which is dependent on the anatomy of the nerve.

Anatomy

Nerve fibers are the axonal processes of the somata of each nerve cell. Disconnection of a distal axon from the soma results in death of the nerve fiber distal to the disconnection, although the nerve proximal to it remains alive.

The somata of nerves are located in different locations for motor neurons (in the anterior horn of the spinal cord),

and in the dorsal root ganglion (outside of the spinal cord) for sensory nerves (Figure 18-27).

Nerves may be *myelinated* (large fibers), facilitating fast speeds of neurotransmission, or *unmyelinated* (small fibers). Different-sized nerve fibers tend to have different functions, which are summarized in Table 18-14, overleaf.

Some pathologies affect one or another type of nerve more than others, with symptoms compatible with the type of fiber affected.

- For example, alcohol abuse (without other vitamin deficiencies) commonly leads to a small-fiber peripheral neuropathy with burning and loss of pain sensation, together with autonomic features.
- In contrast, a lead neuropathy affects large motor fibers, and tends to spare sensory nerves.

The impact on the nerve also depends on where the insult to the nerve is located anatomically, and disorders of peripheral nerves are named for this (Table 18-15, overleaf).

Motor neuron disease (MND)/ amyotrophic lateral sclerosis

- Often grouped with peripheral nerve disorders for ease, it is now understood that MND is a disorder affecting both peripheral motor neurons, with progressive death of cell somata, and central neurons, especially in the frontotemporal regions.
- This causes a picture of frontotemporal cognitive impairment in some patients with frank dementia in others.
- Central features may precede the peripheral findings, and in other patients peripheral features are prominent or present in isolation.

It is this mixed pattern of central and peripheral denervation which gives MND its characteristic clinical features of patchy mixed upper motor neuron involvement (hyper-reflexia, increased tone, jaw jerk) and lower motor neuron involvement (flaccid tone, muscle fasciculations, atrophy). As it is a process involving only motor nerves, sensation should not be affected (although with loss of strength and muscle bulk, occasional compression peripheral neuropathies may also occur).

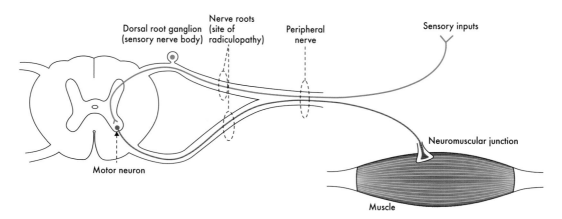

Figure 18-27 The peripheral neuraxis. Disease processes can occur anywhere between the muscle and the spinal cord, and can sometimes be mixed

Table 18-14 Type and function of peripheral nerves

GROUP	MODALITY	SUBGROUP	FUNCTION
A (large myelinated)	Motor	α	Motor neurons
		β and γ	Muscle spindle fibers
	Sensory	α	Muscle spindle and proprioception
		β	Fine touch
		δ	Some pain, temperature, 'electric', crude touch
B (small myelinated)	Autonomic		Presynaptic autonomic nerves
C	Sensory		Pain and temperature, 'burning' and 'itch'
	Autonomic		Post-ganglionic nerves

Table 18-15 Diseases of peripheral nerves

LOCATION OF INSULT	NOMENCLATURE	EXAMPLES
Anterior horn of cord (motor somata)	Motor neuronopathy ('anterior horn cell disease')	Motor neuron disease* Spinomuscular atrophy Poliomyelitis
Nerve roots	Radiculopathy	Meningeal infiltration Foraminal stenosis
Dorsal root ganglion	Sensory neuronopathy	Paraneoplastic Sjögren's syndrome associated Inflammatory
Plexus	Plexitis/plexopathy	Brachial neuritis (inflammatory) Traumatic (e.g. Klumpke's palsy, which affects C8 and T1 nerve roots) Diabetic amyotrophy
Single peripheral nerve	Mononeuropathy	Median neuropathy (carpal tunnel) Radial neuropathy ('Saturday night palsy')
Multiple individual peripheral nerves	Mononeuritis multiplex	Vasculitis Multifocal compressive mononeuropathies
Patchy involvement	Neuropathy	Demyelinating processes (Guillain–Barré, chronic inflammatory demyelinating polyneuropathy)
Diffuse involvement	'Length-dependent' peripheral neuropathy (i.e. longer nerves affected first)	Diabetes mellitus Alcohol Charcot–Marie–Tooth syndrome (some types)

* Disease also affects upper motor neurons, giving characteristic features.

Diagnosis

There is no single investigation capable of diagnosing MND, although neurophysiological studies with a compatible history can come close. A thorough investigation is often performed looking for potential differential diagnoses, given the morbidity associated with this condition.

Neurophysiology

- This can demonstrate evidence of lower motor neuron involvement, with fasciculations as well as other features of denervation a prominent feature. The pattern is typically asymmetric.

- Abnormality is also seen on single-fiber EMG performed in specialized centers.
- More recently, transcranial magnetic stimulation of the cortex has been used to study motor excitability to assess for central involvement in motor pathways, but this is not widely available.

Imaging

MRI of the spinal cord and brain are often done where bulbar or upper motor neuron features predominate, to exclude focal pathology causing bulbar or myelopathic features. Occasionally frontotemporal atrophy may be seen.

Serology

- Investigation is often performed for patchy inflammatory demyelinating processes such as multifocal motor neuropathy, which also presents with asymmetrical lower motor neuron symptoms and is usually strongly responsive to immunomodulation with IVIg or plasma exchange.
- This differential does not cause upper motor neuron signs, and rarely involves cranial nerves (although cranial nerve XII involvement has been reported).

Treatment

- There is very limited pharmacotherapy with any efficacy in MND, although riluzole has been shown to improve survival by approximately 6 months.
- With disordered respiratory musculature, overnight hypoventilation and desaturation are common. In patients with adequate bulbar function to tolerate it, non-invasive ventilatory support may be beneficial for quality of life, and potentially survival.
- Similarly, invasive feeding strategies should be discussed while a patient is fit enough to undergo insertion of gastrostomy tubes, with a view to keeping weight up and preventing additional loss of muscle bulk and fitness.
- Genetic investigations such as testing for mutations in C9ORF72 and SOD1 may become more important in coming years with the development of targeted antisense oligonucleotides.

Demyelinating neuropathy and Guillain–Barré syndrome (GBS)

- With a range of disorders in this group, the clinical history can range from very acute and symmetrical to exceedingly slow and asymmetrical.
- The pathology is one of destruction or functional blockade of myelin on large nerve fibers, through an antibody-mediated process.
- The targets of these antibodies are typically ganglioside molecules; these have structural similarities to a number of bacterial and viral proteins, with antibodies often forming through the process known as 'molecular mimicry'—that is, antibodies formed to pathogens (e.g. *Campylobacter jejuni*) which then cross-react with 'self' molecules.

Acute inflammatory demyelinating polyneuropathies come under the diagnostic umbrella of Guillain–Barré syndrome. They commonly follow an acute gastrointestinal or respiratory tract infection, and typical clinical features include:

1. Ascending bilateral motor weakness (although features start in the hands or face in about 10%).
2. Peripheral sensory impairment:
   a. paresthesiae are common, although often mild
   b. pain is actually very common, present more than 50% of the time, and may be variable in site and extent.
3. Facial and respiratory weakness develop in approximately half and one-third respectively.
4. Dysautonomia is also common, and often not properly considered (constipation, urinary retention, postural hypotension, tachycardia).

It is also worth noting that there are a large number of subtypes of GBS in which sensory or motor features may be present in isolation, or there may be a craniofacial predominance in Miller–Fisher syndrome and Bickerstaff's encephalitis.

GBS typically progresses over 2 weeks, and patients should reach the nadir of neurological deterioration within a month; a slower deterioration suggests an alternative diagnosis such as chronic inflammatory demyelinating polyneuropathy (CIDP).

Diagnosis

Laboratory assessment

- Routine blood examination is typically unremarkable, although on serological studies of ganglioside antibodies a variety of antibodies may be seen. However, the absence of these does not preclude a diagnosis of GBS.
- A lumbar puncture is often performed to assess for evidence of albumino-cytological dissociation—the presence of elevated CSF protein without a pleocytosis. This is present in 80–90% of patients at 1 week.
- GBS is an uncommon seroconversion illness in HIV infection; however, testing for HIV should be considered in an at-risk individual.

Neurophysiological studies

- When performed very early, these may be normal.
- With progression, sensory responses may be absent and slowing of motor conduction as well as conduction may be evident.
- Changes are typically patchy; the nerve should not appear uniformly affected in a typical case of GBS.

Therapy

- After reaching nadir, recovery usually occurs over weeks and months, although this may be incomplete.
- Given that the initial decline may be precipitous, acute therapy is critical.
- The dominant modality of therapy is with IVIg or plasma exchange. Recovery may be much faster than

one may expect in nerve injury, suggestive that part of the symptomatology may relate to functional blockade of molecules with a role in neurotransmission in myelinated fibers, in addition to loss of myelin.

- Corticosteroids are ineffective in GBS.
- Axonal forms of GBS also exist, though these are fortunately rare. Recovery in these variants is exceedingly slow, and often partial. Urgent intervention is therefore indicated in any patient with a clinical phenotype of GBS.
- Supportive care is critical in GBS, especially in patients with facial and bulbar weakness. Close supervision in a facility capable of intubation is indicated in all patients with GBS yet to respond to immunological treatment.

Peripheral neuropathy

- Diffuse peripheral polyneuropathy is a common clinical finding, and typically presents with subacute to chronic sensory disturbance (burning or numbness), starting distally in the feet and slowly progressing proximally.
- Motor weakness may occur as the condition becomes more marked.
- Autonomic nerves are also variably involved, and the degree of involvement may help with differential diagnosis.

Unfortunately for the assessing clinician there are hundreds of causes of peripheral neuropathy, which makes an all-inclusive assessment challenging (Table 18–16).

Table 18-16 Some of the more common causes of peripheral neuropathy

DISEASE	SENSORY	MOTOR	AUTONOMIC	FIBER SIZE	COMMON CLINICAL PRESENTATION
Diabetes	+++	±	++	S > L	Burning starting in feet; 'glove and stocking'
Alcohol	+++	±	++	S > L	Burning in feet Often cerebellar, ocular or cognitive features
Critical illness	++	++	++	Mixed	Weakness, difficulty weaning from ventilator
Vitamin B$_{12}$	+++	−	−	L > S	Sensory ataxia; often dorsal column signs
Uremia	+++	±	+	S > L	Glove and stocking
Malignancy	+++	++	±	Variable	Variable; may have other neurological features; may have cachexia and muscle weakness
Liver failure	+++	+	±	Often S > L	Glove and stocking
Paraprotein Anti-MAG	++	++	−	Both	Slowly progressive glove and stocking
MGUS	++	++	+	S > L	Glove and stocking
POEMS	++	++	+	Both	Progressive sensorimotor involvement with other features of myeloma
Amyloidosis	++	±	+++	S >> L	Painful neuropathy with autonomic dysfunction
Chemotherapy (platinum, taxanes, etc.)	+++	+	±	L>S	Glove and stocking pattern—may be rapidly progressive with repeat exposure
HIV	+++	+	±	Both	Progressive glove and stocking
Hereditary (multiple disorders)	Variable	Variable	Variable	Variable	Typically do not have dysesthesia or pain (may be present late)

HIV, human immunodeficiency virus; L, large; MAG, myelin-associated glycoproteins; MGUS, monoclonal gammopathy of uncertain significance; POEMS = polyneuropathy, organomegaly, endocrinopathy, M-spike, skin changes; S, small. L > S indicates that large fibers are affected more than small fibers.

History is critical, providing information about the tempo of progression, age of onset, pattern of involvement (small fiber/large fiber/motor fiber/autonomic involvement), comorbidities, and other neurological symptoms.

CLINICAL PEARL

If ankle jerks are present clinically, a substantial large-fiber neuropathy is very unlikely.

Investigation

- Neurophysiology may be used to assess for the presence and clinical extent of a neuropathy. However, it only tests large-fiber function, and in a patient with small-fiber symptoms ('burning pain') and a normal examination, a normal nerve conduction study does not rule out small-fiber involvement.
- In some centers psychophysical testing of small fiber-function is possible, but these are dependent on patient attention and motivation and may be difficult to interpret.
- In some centers autonomic function testing is also possible, which is occasionally indicated.

Laboratory investigation

It is near-impossible to perform a screen for all causes of neuropathy; routine investigation should include the investigations shown in Table 18-17.

Treatment

Treatment is aimed at an underlying cause if one can be found, with a view to prevention of progression.

- A low dose of tricyclic antidepressant such as amitriptyline, or gabapentin, may be beneficial for uncomfortable dysesthetic neuropathic symptoms such as burning or sensitivity to pressure.
- Secondary prevention should also be remembered, with regular podiatry review and foot care, well-fitting shoes, and appropriate pressure care.

Table 18-17 Laboratory investigation for neuropathy

INVESTIGATION	RATIONALE
Full blood count	Variety of changes present in vitamin deficiencies, alcohol abuse and malignancies
Urea, electrolytes, creatinine	To assess renal function
Liver function tests	Assesses for evidence of liver failure; albumin as marker of systemic health; review globulin levels
Fasting blood sugar ± glucose tolerance test	Note that symptoms of small-fiber neuropathy may develop with impaired glucose tolerance
Serum and urine protein electrophoresis with immunofixation	Assess for the presence of a paraprotein, including some which are pathogenic in low concentrations
Vitamin B_{12}	Assess for deficiency
Erythrocyte sedimentation rate	Nonspecific—raised in malignancy, paraprotein, (auto)inflammation
Antinuclear antibodies/anti-neutrophil cytoplasmic autoantibody (ANA/ANCA)	Especially if subacute or mononeuritis multiplex—features of vasculitis
Consider HIV/syphilis	If either is possible the patient should be tested

SELF-ASSESSMENT QUESTIONS

1 A 75-year-old man is referred for assessment for possible Parkinson's disease. His family have noticed that he is shuffling in his gait more than previously. Which of the following would make you most concerned about a diagnosis of dementia with Lewy bodies?

A Minimal tremor
B Postural hypotension
C REM (rapid eye movement) sleep behavior disorder
D Early memory loss with frequent falls
E The hallucination of his mother, who visits for tea every day

2 An 18-year-old man is referred to you after two generalized tonic–clonic seizures in 3 months. He reports having had twitches or jerks at times when tired, and in the mornings on and off for a few years. His electroencephalogram demonstrates intermittent generalized polyspike and wave discharges. Which medication is usually considered first-line?

A Carbamazepine
B Phenytoin
C Sodium valproate
D Topiramate
E Clonazepam

3 A 48-year-old woman presents to emergency with acute severe rotatory vertigo present for several hours. She is very nauseated. On examination she has horizontal nystagmus beating toward the right in all positions, worse on gaze to the right, and is deaf in the left ear. There is no tinnitus. She has a positive head impulse test to the left. Clinical examination is unremarkable other than a skew deviation on assessment of eye movements. The most likely diagnosis is:

A Ménière's disease
B Benign positional vertigo
C Vestibular neuritis
D AICA (anterior inferior cerebellar artery) stroke
E Lateral medullary syndrome

4 A 24-year-old man with developmental delay and a history of Lennox–Gastaut syndrome is brought in to the emergency department in status epilepticus from his group home. His medications include sodium valproate 1500 mg twice daily, topiramate 200 mg twice daily and primidone 250 mg three times daily. He has not been unwell and has been taking his medications normally. Despite 4 doses of intravenous diazepam in the ED he continues to seize. The probable reason for this is:

A He takes primidone, which has induced his liver enzymes, clearing diazepam quickly.
B These are behavioral episodes and are unlikely to respond to antiepileptic therapy.
C He has not been loaded with phenytoin.
D Diazepam redistributes rapidly within the various fluid compartments within the body, allowing a return of seizure activity.
E He probably has an intracranial pathology causing new onset of seizures and he requires a computed tomography scan and lumbar puncture.

5 A 73-year-old man with a 5-year history of Parkinson's disease is brought to see you by his wife, as he has been sleeping very poorly. She says that he spends much of the night sitting up playing computer chess, and that he is too tired during the day to be as social as previously. He was diagnosed with tremor-predominant Parkinson's disease, although he had significant REM (rapid eye movement) sleep behavior disorder for the previous 3–4 years. His current medication regimen includes pramipexole extended-release (ER) 3.75 mg/day, levodopa/carbidopa 100/25 mg four times a day and entacapone 200 mg three times daily. He feels that control is pretty good, although he wouldn't mind a little more medication for a period around 2 p.m. when he feels 'slower'. Clinically he looks a little dyskinetic, although his wife says this occurs a minority of the time. What is the most appropriate management step?

A Reduce pramiprexole ER to 3 mg/day
B Increase the pramiprexole ER to 4.5 mg/day
C Add amantadine 100 mg daily
D Check iron studies and arrange a sleep study
E Prescribe some nocturnal zolpidem to help him sleep

6 A 24-year-old woman presents with pain behind the right eye with movement, which resolves as she notices altered vision in that eye. She notices that 'everything looks gray' and her acuity is 6/36. She is given intravenous (IV) methylprednisolone 1 g for 3 days and her symptoms settle. Magnetic resonance imaging (MRI) of the brain at that time is unremarkable. Two months later she has symptoms in her right leg with some difficulty walking, and a band-like sensation around the umbilicus. An MRI shows a small plaque in her thoracic spine. She receives oral prednisolone 100 mg daily for 5 days as she is still mobile and wishes to avoid hospital. She is commenced on beta-interferon as an outpatient, while further assessment is pending. A month later she presents with acute onset paraplegia, coming on over 2 days, and urinary retention. What is the best management strategy?

A IV steroids, continue beta-interferon, re-image the brain and spine, and perform a lumbar puncture
B IV steroids, cease beta-interferon, re-image the brain and spine, and perform a lumbar puncture
C Insert a catheter and treat for a urinary tract infection, hold off on steroids for now
D IV steroids, continue beta-interferon, check for neutralizing antibodies, re-image the spine
E IV steroids, stop beta-interferon and start fingolimod, re-image the brain and spine

7 A 48-year-old man presents with a 1-week history of weakness in the legs and back pain. He has recently been on holiday to Thailand and did have gastroenteritis while there, 2 weeks before. Clinically he is able to walk only with assistance and has grade 2/5 power distally in the legs and 3–4/5 power more proximally. Reflexes are absent throughout. While he has no sensory symptoms, he reports altered cold and vibration sensation distally. He has a history of non-Hodgkin lymphoma for which he received R-CHOP chemotherapy 5 years previously, and is in remission. Which is **not** a possible diagnosis?

A Guillain–Barré syndrome due to campylobacter exposure
B Myasthenia gravis
C Guillain–Barré syndrome secondary to HIV seroconversion illness
D Central nervous system lymphoma recurrence in the cauda equina
E Chemotherapy-induced neuropathy

8 A 55-year-old woman is referred for assessment of progressive proximal muscle weakness causing problems standing from a chair and getting up stairs over 4 months. She has hypothyroidism on thyroxine 100 microg daily, and was on simvastatin for dyslipidemia until 2 months ago when her family physician stopped it due to her symptoms. She has gout, for which she takes allopurinol 300 mg daily. She denies significant muscle pain, although her muscles may become sore with prolonged use. There is no rash. Her creatine kinase is 4000 U/L. Which of the following is most likely?

A Statin myopathy
B Metabolic myopathy due to thyroid disturbance
C Inclusion-body myositis
D Statin-induced autoimmune myositis
E Allopurinol-induced myopathy

9 A 46-year-old women presents with a 4-day history of headache, fever and increasing confusion. She is brought to the emergency department and is noted to be drowsy, disorientated in time and place, and to have difficulty following two-stage commands according to the documented observations on arrival. A non-contrast computed tomography scan of the brain is performed soon after arrival and is reported as normal. You are called to see her as she is found to have become suddenly unresponsive to voice, not opening her eyes, with symmetrical localization to painful stimuli only. Her Glasgow Coma Scale score is measured at 6. The most appropriate advice for the immediate management is:

A Airway support in the ED and lumbar puncture/cerebrospinal fluid examination
B Airway support in the ED and commencement of intravenous anticonvulsant medication
C Urgent magnetic resonance imaging of the brain
D Urgent electroencephalography
E Intensive-care consultation

10 A 55-year-old woman with a past history of depression and migraine with aura presents with a 6-month history of increasing chronic daily generalized throbbing headache, associated with intermittent visual blurring and nausea. She has tried her usual anti-migraine therapy (aspirin 900 mg stat + metoclopramide 10 mg stat orally) on a number of occasions without benefit. On specific questioning she has sleep disturbance and irritability and is concerned about something sinister underlying the headaches. Neurological examination (including good visualization of the optic discs) is normal apart from muscle tenderness in the scalp and over the occiput. Her blood pressure is 145/85 mmHg. The most appropriate initial management recommendation is:

A Urgent brain magnetic resonance imaging (MRI) and a 3-day trial of regular indomethacin
B Addition of a triptan for exacerbations of her headache and physical therapies for neck and scalp discomfort
C Commencement of amitriptyline 25 mg nocte and non-urgent brain computed tomography
D Commencement of a selective serotonin reuptake inhibitor and non-urgent brain MRI
E Trials of bilateral greater occipital nerve local anesthetic/corticosteroid injection

11 A 24-year-old woman with a strong family history of migraine with aura presents with intermittent hemicranial throbbing headache associated with the development of tender swelling over the temple on the side of the headache. The swelling will last up to 1 hour and settles spontaneously. She admits to being very concerned about the possibility of a brain tumor. Neurological examination between events is normal. The most likely initial clinical diagnosis is:

A Anxiety and a non-organic neurological disturbance
B Somatoform disorder
C Migraine with aura
D Migranous hygroma
E Temporo-mandibular joint dysfunction

12 A 64-year-old male is found collapsed in the toilet by his wife at 0330 hours. The wife recalls that he woke her up as he got out of bed to go to the toilet and that she heard him collapse a few moments later. When she attended, he was unable to speak and appeared weak down his right side. He arrives in the emergency department at 0415 hours, and shows clinical features of a major left hemisphere stroke but vital signs are stable. The most important initial aspect of your clinical assessment is:

A Performing a standardized stroke assessment stroke tool to assign a stroke severity score
B Determining the patient's pre-morbid functional status
C Performing a Glasgow Coma Scale
D Performing a checklist for thrombolysis eligibility
E Interviewing the wife to clarify the time of onset

13 A 77-year-old male presents with transient sudden loss of speech and right hand weakness. Symptoms are fully recovered over 45 minutes, and by the time he arrives in hospital and is seen in the emergency department, he is neurologically back to normal. He is a reformed smoker with a past history of coronary artery bypass grafting 5 years previously for triple-vessel disease. His medication includes aspirin 100 mg daily and atorvastatin 40 mg daily. His electrocardiograph (EKG) on arrival captures a brief period of atrial fibrillation. The most appropriate initial management plan for this patient is:

A Add clopidogrel to aspirin after an urgent non-contrast computed tomography (CT) scan is performed, and organize an outpatient Holter monitor and follow-up.
B Arrange magnetic resonance imaging (MRI) scan of the brain and MRI angiography of the extracranial and intracranial vessels for the next day, but make no change in therapy until the results of the scan are known.
C Admit to hospital for EKG telemetry and further investigation of the mechanism of the transient ischemic attack.
D Urgent non-contrast CT scan, and if no hemorrhage commence anticoagulation with low-molecular-weight heparin and arrange outpatient carotid duplex scan.
E Urgent non-contrast CT scan plus CT angiogram of the extracranial and intracranial vessels. If no evidence of intracranial hemorrhage, commence one of the novel oral anticoagulants.

14 A 37-year-old male is found collapsed after being last seen well 6 hours previously. Clinical examination reveals a right hemisphere stroke syndrome. Non-contrast computed tomography (CT) scanning of the brain shows extensive early ischemic change throughout the right hemisphere. CT angiography shows a distal right internal carotid artery occlusion. The most appropriate initial management of this patient is:

A Supportive care in an acute stroke unit
B Stroke-unit care and a repeat CT or magnetic resonance imaging in 12 hours' time if the patient remains clinically stable
C CT perfusion imaging and consideration for endovascular therapy
D Admission to intensive care for induced hypothermia for neuroprotection
E Intravenous thrombolysis with alteplase 0.9 mg/kg

ANSWERS

1 E.

The hallucinations of people, often familiar and typically silent, are a hallmark feature of dementia with Lewy bodies (DLB). Patients, however, are often embarrassed about these and do not describe them unless they are specifically asked about it. It is helpful to know this before treatment, as trials of dopaminergic therapy often worsen hallucinations. Minimal tremor may be present in DLB, but it may also be seen in idiopathic Parkinson's disease (iPD) and other disorders with parkinsonism. Postural hypotension is the hallmark of multisystem atrophy (MSA) when present early, usually with other signs of autonomic failure (erectile dysfunction, bowel and bladder symptoms). REM sleep behavior disorder is often seen in iPD prior to the diagnosis. Early memory loss and frequent falls strongly raise the possibility of progressive supranuclear palsy.

2 C.

The man has presented with a history typical of juvenile myoclonic epilepsy (JME). This diagnosis is significant, as it usually requires lifelong therapy. It is part of the group termed idiopathic generalized epilepsies (IGEs) and sodium valproate is regarded as first-line therapy. More importantly, carbamazepine may *worsen* control.

3 D.

The patient has presented with an acute vestibular syndrome, and the first consideration in the emergency room is to differentiate a peripheral and a central pathology. Clinical assessment has been proven to be more sensitive than *acute* magnetic resonance imaging for this differentiation. It relies upon three elements:

a head impulse testing (*abnormal* in peripheral disease)
b nystagmus description—unidirectional horizontal ± torsional element in peripheral disease; may change direction in central pathology
c assessment for skew deviation (present in central disease).

In this case, the patient presents with some signs consistent with a peripheral process (head impulse test, pattern of nystagmus), but also a skew deviation, which cannot be ignored. This is often seen in AICA infarcts, as the labyrinthine artery (a terminal branch) may be involved, causing infarction of the vestibular organ and cochlear on that side, with other central signs (skew).

4 D.

Lennox–Gastaut syndrome (LGS) is a common cause of medically refractory epilepsy in the community. Even with best medical management, breakthrough seizures are common, sometimes resulting in status epilepticus. This clinical scenario is remarkably common for the neurologist, and demonstrates the importance of using a benzodiazepine with appropriate pharmacokinetics to terminate status epilepticus in a patient such as this. Intravenous clonazepam or a continuous midazolam infusion would be more appropriate strategies. While answer A is correct, it is not the cause for the diazepam failing to work. Behavioral episodes are common in patients with LGS, but should be easily contrasted to status epilepticus. Phenytoin may be necessary, but should not be given without appropriate consideration in patients with a long history of medically refractory epilepsy. Finally, breakthrough seizures are common in patients such as this and, while worthwhile considering, a new pathology causing status epilepticus is uncommon.

5 A.

The patient's disturbance is typical of punding, in which patients develop a compulsive fascination with and performance of a particular task. It is an impulse-control disorder (ICD) and is most commonly seen with dopamine agonists, often at higher dose. Punding warrants reduction in the dose of dopamine agonist, despite patient requests to increase the dose. The disorder does not sound consistent with restless legs syndrome, nor should it warrant regular therapy with a nocturnal sedative. Amantadine is helpful for dyskinesias, but will not treat the presenting complaint.

6 B.

While the patient has a history and presentation which satisfies the criteria for multiple sclerosis (MS), neuromyelitis optica (NMO) requires consideration due to an optico-spinal presentation and increasing severity of attacks over a short duration of time. More importantly, in NMO the treatment required is different and beta-interferon is thought to worsen attacks in NMO. NMO differs from MS in that the number of attacks a patient has is proportional to the disability, so further diagnostic assessment is required. NMO-antibodies should be assessed in cerebrospinal fluid (CSF) and/or serum; CSF oligoclonal bands would be positive in MS but negative in NMO. Repeat imaging of the spine is important, with long segment lesions in the spine another strong indicator of NMO. Cerebral lesions are seen in about 50% of cases of NMO, although usually in a pattern atypical for MS.

While draining the bladder and assessing for urinary tract infection is critical, answer C is incorrect as a pseudoexacerbation due to infection should not be proportionally much worse than an initial presentation. Neutralizing antibodies may form to beta-interferon, causing treatment failure, but this time window would be extremely unusual and unlikely to explain the presentation. Fingolimod should not be commenced without a little more consideration, as NMO would require different treatment.

7 B.

This presentation is not consistent with myasthenia gravis, which usually presents with ocular, bulbar or cervical symptoms and does not have sensory symptoms on clinical examination. The history does suggest an episode of Guillain–Barré syndrome, and in a patient with risk factors for seroconversion illness for HIV (the patient may have also had contact with sex-workers in Thailand), HIV *must* be considered. Options D and E may not explain his signs individually, but in a patient with previous neurotoxic chemotherapy, long-term areflexia due to neuropathy may be present, while his acute symptoms could represent acute cauda equina disease.

8 D.

A newly recognized pathology, anti-HMG-CoA antibody testing may help confirm this diagnosis. Long-term immunosuppression is required, and withdrawal of this may cause disease relapses many years down the track. A typical (toxic) statin myopathy would be expected to settle within 2 months from cessation of treatment. Metabolic myopathy should not cause creatine kinase (CK) up to 4000 U/L. Inclusion-body myositis would not typically be associated with such a high CK, nor acute onset. It commonly affects older individuals. Allopurinol does not cause myopathy, though colchicine, another agent used for gout, can cause a severe myopathy.

9 B.

Meningo-encephalitis is the most likely underlying diagnosis, and urgent airway support plus management for possible non-convulsive seizures is the best initial option.

10 C.

This is a classic clinical scenario of mixed headache syndrome associated with depression of mood—tricyclics are the treatment of choice.

11 D.

This is a rare diagnosis but important to recognize.

12 E.

Defining the time of onset of the acute stroke is the most important initial issue and this will require direct communication with the witness.

13 E.

There is a possibility here of both a cardioembolic and a large-artery embolic mechanism, so there is a need to examine the large vessels but also cover for the atrial fibrillation. NOACs (new oral anticoagulants) are now the best option in terms of efficiency and effectiveness.

14 B.

This patient may be suitable for decompressive hemicraniectomy, and repeat imaging can assist in determining the degree of brain swelling and the timing of this intervention.

CHAPTER 19

PSYCHIATRY FOR THE INTERNIST

Brian Kelly and Lisa Lampe

CHAPTER OUTLINE

- DEPRESSION
- ANXIETY DISORDERS
  - Treatment
- POST-TRAUMATIC STRESS DISORDER (PTSD)
- SOMATIZATION

- EATING DISORDERS
  - Anorexia and bulimia nervosa
- SUICIDE AND DELIBERATE SELF-HARM
- PSYCHOTROPIC AGENTS
  - Lithium carbonate
  - Anticonvulsants
  - Antipsychotic agents
  - Antidepressants

Depression, anxiety and substance-use disorders are the most common psychiatric conditions in the community. Rates of these disorders are significantly elevated among patients with physical illness, e.g. stroke, diabetes mellitus, cancer, chronic renal or respiratory disease, epilepsy, or disorders associated with chronic pain. The relationship between psychiatric disorder and physical illness operates in a number of directions. Psychiatric disorder such as depression may increase the risk of developing a serious physical illness, and physical illness may be a trigger to the development of a depressive or anxiety disorder. These psychiatric conditions also commonly coexist, hence patients with one disorder (e.g. depression) will often have

symptoms of another condition such as anxiety or, in some cases, problematic substance use (e.g. alcohol misuse).

It is important to recognize and treat these disorders early. They contribute to significant suffering and increases in levels of disability. Having a coexisting psychiatric illness increases the functional impairment associated with physical illness, and can have an adverse effect on the outcomes of the physical illness.

DEPRESSION

The core features of depression reflect persistent disturbance in mood that interferes with a person's functioning in areas such as relationships, work and family or social roles. They include:

- low mood
- loss of interest
- loss of capacity for pleasure/enjoyment.

These are typically accompanied by indecision, irritability, feelings of guilt and hopelessness, and/or suicidal ideation. Low self-worth is a key feature that often discriminates

CLINICAL PEARL

Even though a patient's symptoms of depression or anxiety may seem like an 'understandable' response to life stress, especially when coping with significant physical illness, their distress and psychological symptoms may be indicative of a significant psychiatric disorder such as major depression or an anxiety disorder, requiring further assessment and specific treatment.

major depression from other states associated with low mood (e.g. bereavement).

Depression usually causes a range of physical somatic symptoms alongside these psychological features. These *physical symptoms* are often the key presenting complaints for many patients. The most common presenting symptoms are:

- fatigue and malaise
- poor sleep (particularly early morning wakening)
- weight changes
- loss of sexual drive or problems with sexual function
- complaints of physical pain (e.g. muscle aches or pains, or headaches).

It is always important to remember to ask about depressive symptoms, as depression is a common but frequently missed treatable condition. Many patients are initially hesitant to discuss their emotional concerns, and can be more comfortable discussing physical symptoms. This requires the clinician to confidently and sensitively ask about the patient's feelings and emotions.

- Patients may not use the term 'depression' themselves to describe their problem. Asking them to explain what they have been experiencing in their own words is useful.
- Simple questions such as 'How have you been feeling in general lately?' or 'How would you describe your mood?' can be useful ways to begin the discussion.
- It should also be noted that the physical symptoms are less sensitive in detecting depressive disorder than psychological symptoms such as low mood, guilt, hopelessness and worthlessness, especially in people with established physical illness.

In making a diagnosis of *major depression*, a focus on the core mood symptoms outlined above is necessary, alongside attention to the key clinical signs of these mood disorders (e.g. patient being withdrawn, avoiding eye contact, appearing sad, tearful or disinterested, or restless and agitated).

As is the case with other psychiatric syndromes, depression may occur as a *direct physiological effect of an underlying physical illness*. The potential 'organic' causes of depression are extensive, but include:

- malignancy (e.g. lung, pancreatic and other gastrointestinal malignancies, and central nervous system tumors)
- infection (especially chronic infection e.g. with human immunodeficiency virus, Epstein–Barr virus)
- substance misuse, including intoxication and withdrawal (e.g. alcohol, amphetamines)
- prescribed drugs (e.g. antihypertensives, corticosteroids)
- hematological conditions (e.g. anemia)
- neurological conditions (such as Parkinson's disease, multiple sclerosis, dementia especially subcortical dementias)
- endocrine disorders (e.g. Cushing's disease, Addison's disease, hypothyroidism).

CLINICAL PEARL

Slowed thinking, poor concentration and memory impairment may occur in depression, and especially in the elderly may mimic a dementia-like clinical deterioration (so-called 'depressive pseudodementia'), which improves with treatment of the underlying depressive disorder.

ANXIETY DISORDERS

Anxiety is a universal experience. It may cross the threshold to disorder when it is recognized by the individual as excessive in the circumstances, and is persistent, uncontrollable, distressing and impairing. Anxiety problems are best understood and treated by considering key domains of symptoms: cognitive/emotional, physiological and behavioral. The physiological manifestations are frequently what lead the patient to seek medical attention. Symptoms can be severe and frightening and warrant an initial thorough assessment. The most common behavioral response is avoidance of situations that are feared because of their ability to trigger anxiety; avoidance is the main source of impairment and disability. Two main cognitive/emotional categories of symptoms are recognized: fear and anxious apprehension. Fears concern objects or situations, and the content of the fear determines the anxiety diagnosis. Fear-related symptoms tend to be triggered acutely and are associated with often marked autonomic arousal—the classic flight or fight response. When severe, the anxiety may reach the level of a panic attack. Symptoms can occur 'from head to toe', and to the lay person may appear to represent a serious physical illness, such as a heart attack, stroke or even imminent death—this is key to understanding the fear that results. Panic attacks may occur in any anxiety disorder, if symptoms are severe enough. Where panic attacks are recurring or there is ongoing fear of further panic attacks, with associated distress, an individual may have panic disorder.

Anxious apprehension is most typical of generalized anxiety disorder, and the key cognitive feature of this disorder is worry. The worry concerns the likelihood of future loss or adversity, and typically occurs across a number of domains, including work, relationships, health of self and others, and finances. The worry may be constant and is perceived as unwanted but difficult to control. Autonomic arousal is usually less acute and severe than in panic attacks, but can be problematic in leading to insomnia, fatigue and muscle aches and pains.

In panic disorder, the fear is that the panic symptoms represent or may lead to serious and even life-threatening physical ill health. Hence, the most feared symptoms tend to be those most likely to be interpreted as physical illness, such as pounding heart, shortness of breath, and light-headedness. Individuals may also worry about losing control of their mind or behavior. Phobic disorders represent the combination of specific fears that can trigger acute anxiety or panic attacks, and attempts to avoid identified triggers. Agoraphobia represents avoidance of situations in which panic attacks may be triggered, due to fear of the panic attacks themselves (or, more accurately, the feared physical consequences of panic attacks). Social anxiety disorder (formerly referred to as social phobia) represents a fear of negative evaluation from others: the person fears embarrassing themselves or being thought of as odd, weak, or inept, for example. The most distressing physiological symptoms tend to be those that could signal anxiety to others, such as blushing, sweating and shaking. Situations that are feared and avoided are those involving interpersonal interaction, or performance of some activity (writing, using the phone, public speaking) under actual or possible observation by others.

Prior to DSM-5, post-traumatic stress disorder (PTSD) and obsessive compulsive disorder (OCD) were also included as anxiety disorders, but these are now classified under separate categories. Both are typically associated with high levels of anxiety. The individual with PTSD will have a history of exposure to a highly distressing or life-threatening event precipitating a persistent anxiety state, in which intrusive memories and reminders of the event are a significant problem, for example through 'flashbacks' and nightmares. OCD is associated with specific fears, but the diagnostic behavioral response is the 'compulsion': behaviour designed to remove or diminish the feared outcome. For example, a person with an excessive and unreasonable fear of becoming ill through contact with everyday 'dirty' objects, such as handles that other people have used, may wash their hands with excessive frequency and thoroughness, to the point that their hands become dry, and the skin cracked and bleeding.

Of particular relevance in primary care is the inclusion in the DSM-5 of the new category of 'illness anxiety disorder'. This is conceptualised as a fearful preoccupation around having or acquiring a serious physical illness, which can lead to safety-seeking behaviors such as frequent visits to the doctor with requests for investigations or onward referral, on-line searches for health-related information, and excessive self-examination. Individuals with these concerns may find it hard to accept reassurance following appropriate examination and investigation, prompting further visits to the same or other doctors. They may be at risk of repeated or increasingly intrusive investigations carrying a higher risk of adverse effects. The frustration that many doctors feel when repeatedly consulted by patients with these concerns can be challenging, and may present a further risk to the patient that new or different symptoms that may reflect an underlying physical cause are missed or not addressed.

> **CLINICAL PEARL**
>
> An appropriate level of investigation is important. The differential diagnosis of panic disorder or severe anxiety symptoms includes the following medical conditions:
> * serotonin toxicity
> * pheochromocytoma
> * hyperthyroidism
> * hypoglycemia
> * sedative or alcohol withdrawal
> * cardiac arrhythmia.
> Excessive caffeine consumption can also be a contributing factor for some patients.

> **CLINICAL PEARL**
>
> The initial presentation of anxiety is overwhelmingly prior to the fifth decade of life. Depression, medical illness and substance misuse are more likely causes of anxiety presenting for the first time in later life.

Treatment

Both cognitive-behavior therapy (CBT) and antidepressant medication (with a SSRI or SNRI) have level 1 evidence of efficacy, when used alone or together. Every patient should receive advice not to avoid feared situations. Beta-blockers, benzodiazepines and antipsychotic medications should not be used. Most classes of antidepressant apart from SSRIs and SNRIs have limited evidence of efficacy in panic and phobic disorders.

POST-TRAUMATIC STRESS DISORDER (PTSD)

Post-traumatic stress disorder refers to persistent distress following major events. Situations that typically trigger post-traumatic stress symptoms are typically outside the range of usual experience and often entail threat to life, or confrontation with the death or injury of others (e.g. accidents, injuries, assaults, or even the diagnosis of a life-threatening physical illness), or exposure to major disaster events (e.g. cyclones, bushfires) where there is loss of life and/or property.

The symptoms of PTSD are typically intrusive (e.g. unwanted distressing images or memories, as if reliving aspects of the event) or feelings of being emotionally numb, disconnected, or avoiding reminders of the event or similar situations or places. Sleep disturbance, often with nightmares, is very common. PTSD is often associated with symptoms of both anxiety and depression and, especially when chronic, may be complicated by substance misuse, often as a response to unrelieved distress.

SOMATIZATION

Somatization refers to the expression of a person's emotional distress in the form of physical or so-called 'somatic' symptoms (the term 'somatoform disorders' for a set of conditions in which medically unexplained physical symptoms are the chief complaints). 'Abnormal illness behavior' is another term sometimes used to describe maladaptive ways of perceiving and responding to one's health status.

* Somatization may be brief and transient in situations of high stress and resolve as the underlying psychological distress is addressed.

* In other situations it may manifest as severe and persistent medically unexplained symptoms in one or more body systems (e.g. persistent unexplained neurological symptoms such as pain, sensory disturbance or loss of function) that cause significant distress and disruption to

the person's life. These symptoms may or may not exist alongside another medical condition.

- A person may be described as having 'illness anxiety disorder' when there is a persistent and unfounded fear of disease.
- In 'conversion disorder' there is usually a loss of function (e.g. movement of a limb, or loss of sensation mimicking a neurological condition), often triggered by psychological stress and usually with a prior history of similar symptoms.
- Appropriate diagnosis is essential. This is supported by a pattern of persistent and excessive attention to bodily complaints sometimes with unfounded conviction of the presence of disease, failure to be reassured to the contrary, repeated presentations for help, and excessive focus devoted to the health concerns. Concurrent psychosocial stress is often present and contributing.

CLINICAL PEARL

Remember that 'somatoform disorder' is not a diagnosis based solely on the exclusion of physical illnesses. It also requires positive supporting evidence of concurrent psychological or social triggers, and usually a prior history of presentation with medically unexplained symptoms. It tends to have its onset in the adolescent and young adult years, and there should be great caution making the diagnosis for the first time in an elderly person.

Longitudinal studies have indicated a high rate of undiagnosed medical conditions in patients diagnosed with this group of disorders. Adequate investigation of potential organic causes is important, but should be undertaken alongside early assessment of a potential psychological contribution to the patient's symptoms and behavior. Somatoform disorders can also occur in people with existing physical illness, and contribute to otherwise unexplained exacerbations of their symptoms. An example is the patient with established epilepsy who presents with pseudoseizures at a time of family conflict.

- In some cases the physical symptoms may directly reflect the somatic symptoms of anxiety or depression. For example, a person with persistent anxiety may focus on persistent GI disturbance (epigastric discomfort, diarrhea) or cardiorespiratory symptoms of a panic attack. A patient with depression may present with persistent fatigue and malaise, or persistent weight loss.
- A comprehensive history and examination addressing both psychological and physical symptoms and signs, and judicious investigation of potential organic causes of symptoms, is usually necessary. Early recognition of such somatic presentations of distress is beneficial.

By virtue of their persistence and repeated presentation to physicians despite reassurance and investigation, these conditions are very susceptible to sometimes frustrated or judgmental responses from clinicians, over-investigation or over-treatment, and iatrogenic illness. Patients may find it difficult to consider the psychological component of their problems, and be sensitive to feeling that they are not being 'believed' or taken seriously by their physician. Hence it is

not uncommon for conflict to emerge between patients and physicians or between clinicians involved in the patient's care.

- It is important to assess and treat any depressive and anxiety disorders that can give rise to somatic symptom presentations (secondary somatization).
- The condition can be debilitating if unaddressed. It is important to remember that these conditions represent significant and potentially treatable clinical disorders. Treatment requires a clear understanding of the problem and its causes (by all involved), early psychiatric consultation, a nonjudgmental attitude to patients, and efforts to draw the patient's attention to the psychological factors that may be contributing to their distress. Explaining the interaction and link between emotional states and physical health can sometimes do this. It can be important to schedule regular appointments, acknowledge the patient's distress and concern, but also to be judicious in the use of diagnostic investigations or procedures in order to avoid reinforcement of the somatic concerns and avoid iatrogenic complications of medical procedures. Multidisciplinary care can be very beneficial in engaging the patient in strategies to improve function and reduce the focus on physical symptoms (e.g. multidisciplinary behavioral approaches to pain, exercise interventions to promote improved physical functioning). Cognitive-behaviour therapy and other psychological therapies (including addressing family responses or stress) can be effective to address contributing background psychosocial factors. Antidepressant medication (such as SSRIs) can be helpful in addressing coexisting anxiety and depressive symptoms.

The term factitious disorder refers to the falsification of physical (or psychological) symptoms. This can include deliberately inducing injury or disease. While malingering refers to such behaviors being undertaken for clear personal gain (e.g. financial gain), in factitious disorder the gains are generally psychological in nature, such as to maintain the sick role and related medical care.

In rare instances, patients with psychosis may develop delusions concerning physical symptoms (e.g. that they have cancer and are dying, such as in depression with psychosis); psychiatric inpatient treatment is usually required in these cases.

EATING DISORDERS

Eating disorders include anorexia and bulimia nervosa, binge-eating disorder and clinical presentations with subsyndromal or mixed features of both conditions.

- Anorexia and bulimia nervosa occur much more commonly in women than in men. They tend to present to physicians with symptoms relating to abnormal dietary patterns, including the consequences of efforts to reduce weight (e.g. self-induced vomiting, laxative or diuretic abuse) or, in the case of anorexia, the metabolic and endocrine consequences of dietary restriction.
- Binge-eating disorder is more likely to present in the context of weight disorder.

Anorexia and bulimia nervosa

Anorexia nervosa is characterized by:

- significantly low bodyweight (<85% of normal weight for age and height; the disorder is classified as severe when BMI is 15-15.99 kg/m², and extreme when below 15 kg/m²)
- altered body image with relentless pursuit of thinness
- refusal to maintain normal bodyweight
- extreme fear of gaining weight, with marked caloric restriction
- weight-controlling behaviors such as excessive exercise, laxative abuse or purging.

Anorexia nervosa carries a high mortality rate, chiefly due to the chronic metabolic effects of starvation. The condition also carries a markedly elevated risk of suicide.

In **bulimia nervosa**, weight may be within normal or overweight range and is characterized by:

- regular episodes of uncontrolled eating of large amounts of food
- weight-control mechanisms (including self-induced vomiting, diuretic and/or laxative abuse)
- often-excessive guilt and remorse about binge-eating.

In both instances there is a preoccupation with weight and shape, food and diet.

Complications

The chief physical complications of an eating disorder include:

- metabolic disturbances (e.g. hypokalemia), due to repeated vomiting or laxative and/or diuretic abuse (this may also occur in bulimia nervosa)
- endocrine complications—hyopogonadism with amenorrhea and loss of secondary sexual characteristics, osteoporosis with an increased risk of fractures
- fatigue and weakness
- bradycardia and hypothermia
- hair loss and lanugo body hair
- dependent edema
- dehydration
- cognitive changes and potentially reversible cerebral atrophic changes
- eroded dental enamel as a consequence of repeated vomiting (also occurs in bulimia nervosa).

Diagnosis and management

- The differential diagnosis for anorexia nervosa should include any condition that could lead to severe weight loss and the metabolic changes outlined above. This includes primary endocrine and metabolic disorders (e.g. Addison's disease, hypopituitarism), chronic infection leading to weight loss, or primary central nervous system (CNS) disorders.
- Differential diagnosis of bulimia includes disorders such as gastric outlet obstruction, and neurological disorders (such as CNS tumors), especially conditions associated with hyperphagia; including rare disorders such as Kluver–Bucy syndrome.

Common presenting symptoms of an eating disorder include amenorrhea, striking weight loss, fatigue, or unexplained metabolic disturbance (e.g. hypokalemia).

Overall, effective treatment generally entails close links between psychiatric and medical management.

- Behavioral management of disordered eating patterns, and individual psychotherapy (often with family intervention and education), are the mainstay of psychiatric management. Antidepressant medication has been beneficial in the treatment of bulimia.
- Medical management of starvation and re-feeding needs to address potentially life-threatening metabolic disturbance (e.g. hypophosphatemia), necessitating electrolyte and vitamin supplementation.
- Patients with eating disorders often have concurrent anxiety disorders and/or major depressive disorder, and symptoms of disordered eating (e.g. binge-eating and purging) can be exacerbated by a depressive disorder. Treatment of the depression will then improve the abnormal eating behavior.

SUICIDE AND DELIBERATE SELF-HARM

- Suicide and attempted suicide (i.e. deliberate harm with the intention of suicide) are usually associated with an underlying psychiatric disorder.
- Deliberate self-harm (DSH, also called 'parasuicidal behavior') is a term used to refer to self-injury which may be motivated by frustration or distress but not necessarily an intention to die (e.g. cutting).

It can often be difficult to differentiate these in the acute presentation.

- The behaviors in DSH can be very dangerous and life-threatening, and in general it is best to assume that the behavior is with suicidal intent until assessment indicates otherwise.
- It can be difficult to interpret suicidal intent from the behaviors alone (what seems like a trivial overdose may have been undertaken with serious intent to die by the patient who has limited knowledge of drug effects). In general, though, actions that are more violent and potentially irreversible (such as shooting, hanging, jumping from buildings) or those where careful planning is evident (e.g. carbon monoxide poisoning) indicate a stronger intention to die.

It is also important to ask about children who may be in the care of the patient, and consider any child protection issues.

Assessment of suicide risk involves careful review of the following:

- Presence of suicidal thoughts—'Ever thought you did not want to go on with your life?' or 'Ever considered taking your own life?'

- Degree of suicidal intent—'What have you considered doing?' or 'What did you think would happen as a result of … ?'
- Presence of suicidal plans—'Did you ever find yourself taking steps to end your life or thinking through what you would do to end your life?'
- Assessment of hopelessness. Hopelessness is an important indicator of future suicide risk, so it is important to ask about future life plans and expectations (e.g. hope that current problems can be improved, or hope for resolution of current difficulties, or specific positive future plans).
- The presence of alcohol or substance abuse. This can significantly increase the risk of suicide.
- Connection to others can be protective (e.g. children or others dependent on the person). Conversely, social isolation increases the risk of suicide.
- Severity of depression or other psychiatric symptoms. In some cases, severely depressed people may believe that their suicide will relieve others of the burden of the person's problems ('they would be better off'); hence, asking about how others might be affected by the person's self-harm or suicidal behavior is important.
- A prior history of suicide attempt or deliberate self-harm, or a family history of suicide/attempted suicide, are associated with elevated risk of suicide.

Factors that are associated with an increased risk of suicide include:

- the presence of current psychiatric disorder (commonly depression, anxiety and substance-use disorder, especially alcohol abuse)
- psychotic illness (e.g. schizophrenia or current depression with psychosis)
- the presence of a chronic physical illness
- social isolation or lack of social support
- recent loss or interpersonal conflict (including separation or threatened separation)
- recent stress, such as financial strain.

CLINICAL PEARL

Remember: the best clinical approach to suicide prevention is to ask patients about suicidal thoughts or behaviors, respond with appropriate clinical steps to ensure safety, and assess for and instigate appropriate management of the psychiatric disorders that usually accompany these conditions.

It is important to ask about alcohol use. Alcohol intoxication is often associated with suicidal behaviors. Alcohol use can lower mood, and intoxication impairs judgment and can increase the likelihood of a person acting on suicidal feelings. It is important to address problematic alcohol use in the management plan.

In general, people who are suicidal require urgent psychiatric assessment and treatment, usually in an inpatient facility to ensure safety and supervision until improvement occurs.

PSYCHOTROPIC AGENTS

The following section details specific medical considerations in the use of commonly prescribed psychotropic agents.

Lithium carbonate

Lithium carbonate is used in the treatment of bipolar disorder and, in some instances, for recurrent depressive disorder. There are a number of key issues in the care of the patient receiving lithium.

- Lithium is closely monitored using serum levels, with a recommended therapeutic range of 0.6–0.8 mmol/L for maintenance treatment and 0.8–1.2 mmol/L for acute treatment (e.g. of a manic episode).
- Symptoms of lithium toxicity include polyuria, polydipsia, tremor, dysarthria, poor concentration and, as levels increase, sometimes delirium. Lithium toxicity is potentially fatal, and may require saline diuresis and dialysis to reduce serum levels.
- Lithium is excreted via the kidney. Any reduction in renal function (e.g. coexisting renal disease, advancing age) can increase the risk of lithium toxicity. This includes dehydration or fluid restriction. Drugs such as non-steroidal anti-inflammatory drugs (NSAIDs), angiotensin-converting enzyme inhibitors (ACEIs), angiotensin II receptor antagonists (ATRAs) or thiazide diuretics can also cause lithium toxicity through reducing renal excretion.
- Long-term complications of lithium therapy include hypothyroidism, nephrogenic diabetes insipidus and progressive decline in glomerular filtration rate. Hypothyroidism is not usually a reason for stopping lithium, although thyroxine supplementation may be required.
- Lithium therapy requires monitoring of lithium levels, thyroid function and renal function. After achieving a stable serum level of lithium, lithium levels should be checked every 3–6 months, along with serum creatinine and electrolytes. Thyroid function (including thyroid-stimulating hormone, TSH) should be checked regularly also (every 6–12 months).
- Lithium is contraindicated in the 1st trimester of pregnancy due to its association with cardiac abnormalities such as Ebstein's anomaly. Any woman who has been exposed to lithium during pregnancy should have a high-resolution fetal echocardiogram around 18–20 weeks of gestation.

Anticonvulsants

Anticonvulsant medication such as sodium valproate, carbamazepine and lamotrigine have an established role as mood stabilizers in people suffering recurrent major depression or bipolar disorder, including acute mania.

- Common side-effects include weight gain, GI symptoms, sedation, tremor and mild elevation in hepatic enzymes.
- Recommended monitoring varies between agents, but includes regular assessment of weight, full blood count, liver function, glucose and lipid profiles, and serum

drug levels to establish therapeutic dosage (noting that this differs in range from levels recommended for epilepsy management).

- These agents carry a risk of teratogenicity, particularly neural tube defects.

Antipsychotic agents

This class of drugs is generally used in the treatment of acute and chronic psychotic disorders (e.g. schizophrenia, bipolar affective disorders). Their therapeutic effect is chiefly mediated by dopamine receptor (D_2) blockade in the CNS. They are often sub-classified as:

- *'typical'* antipsychotics (e.g. chlorpromazine, haloperidol), which have stronger affinity for the D_2 receptor, including those receptors in the basal ganglia, hence conferring greater potential for extrapyramidal side effects
- *'atypical'* or 2nd-generation antipsychotics, with less affinity for the extrapyramidal D_2 receptor (e.g. clozapine, olanzapine, risperidone).

Most antipsychotic drugs are absorbed rapidly from the gut and are highly lipid-soluble, and there is high interpatient variability in the pharmacokinetics of and responses to these drugs.

Neurological side-effects of these agents include the following.

- Sedation
- Extrapyramidal disorders:
  - » Acute dystonias (including potentially fatal laryngeal dystonia)—these require urgent treatment with rapid-acting antiparkinsonian agents (e.g. intramuscular benztropine).
  - » Drug-induced parkinsonism—if cessation of antipsychotic is not possible, the condition is treated with concurrent use of antiparkinsonian drugs.
  - » Longer-term, potentially irreversible tardive dyskinesia (TD). Treatment includes reduction in the dose of antipsychotic agents if possible, or the use of an alternative antipsychotic agent if necessary (such as clozapine) with less potential to induce

TD. Gamma-aminobutyric acid (GABA) agonists (e.g. baclofen, sodium valproate) have been trialed in treatment of TD, and tetrabenazine has been approved for use in TD.

  - » Akathisia—characterized by persistent motor restlessness, this can occur at low dose and is highly distressing. *Akathisia needs to be differentiated from agitation* due to psychosis or mood disturbance, as the latter may necessitate increased dose whereas akathisia is treated with cessation of the antipsychotic agent if possible. Beta-blockers and benzodiazepines have been used to treat akathisia.

- Neuroleptic malignant syndrome—this can occur at any time during treatment with antipsychotic agents, reflecting dopamine receptor antagonism. This potentially fatal condition is characterized by hyperthermia, diaphoresis, hypertonia and bradyreflexia, delirium and autonomic dysfunction (tachycardia, tachypnea and hypertension). The syndrome is most consistently associated with an elevated creatine kinase and leukocytosis. Risk factors include intercurrent dehydration and recent dose increase. The key differential diagnoses are (see Table 19-1):
  - » malignant hyperthermia
  - » serotonin toxicity
  - » systemic infection and other causes of elevated body temperature.

Metabolic and endocrinological effects include the following:

- Weight gain, hyperglycemia and dyslipidemia can occur.
- Patients receiving antipsychotic medication are at increased risk of developing metabolic syndrome. Monitoring of weight and the development of insulin resistance and dyslipidemia are important aspects of clinical management.
- Hyperprolactinemia can occur due to dopamine blockade, and lead to galactorrhea and amenorrhea.
- Sexual side-effects include reduced libido, impaired sexual arousal, erectile dysfunction and anorgasmia (due to dopamine, acetylcholine and alpha-receptor blockade).

Table 19-1 Differentiating serotonin toxicity from neuroleptic malignant and other syndromes

CONDITION	DRUG	PUPIL SIZE	MUSCLE TONE	TENDON REFLEXES	ONSET
Serotonin toxicity	SSRIs	Mydriasis	↑↑	↑	<12 h
Neuroleptic malignant syndrome (NMS)	Dopamine agonists	Normal	Lead-pipe rigidity	Sluggish	1–3 days
Malignant hyperthermia	Anesthetic agents	Normal	Rigid	↓	30 min–24 h
Anticholinergic syndrome	TCAs or other ACh-blocking agents	Mydriasis	Normal	Normal	1–3 days

ACh, acetylcholine; SSRIs, selective serotonin reuptake inhibitors; TCAs, tricyclic antidepressants.

Clozapine

Clozapine is an atypical antipsychotic agent with a specific role in severe chronic schizophrenia unresponsive to other treatments. Unlike other antipsychotic agents, clozapine treatment is monitored using serum levels.

Important aspects of clozapine treatment include the need to monitor white cell count for the development of potentially fatal neutropenia *and* agranulocytosis, cardiac ultrasound for potential clozapine-induced cardiomyopathy, and monitoring for the development of the metabolic syndrome. Common side-effects are sedation and sialorrhea.

Antidepressants

Selective serotonin reuptake inhibitors (SSRIs)

(e.g. fluoxetine, sertraline, citalopram)

The adverse effects of this class of antidepressants reflect central and peripheral manifestations of serotonin overactivity, e.g. diaphoresis, tremor, hyperthermia, myoclonus, ataxia, hyper-reflexia, diarrhea, agitation and (in toxicity) delirium. Sexual dysfunction is a common side-effect.

- Serotonin toxicity is a serious complication of these drugs, and is characterized by the acute development of symptoms. This is commonly triggered by either deliberate SSRI overdosage or concomitant use of other drugs with serotonergic activity (e.g. other antidepressant agents such as tricyclic antidepressants or monoamine oxidase inhibitors [MAOIs] with serotonergic activity, analgesic agents such as tramadol, or through inhibition of CYP450 enzymes responsible for metabolizing SSRIs by agents such as fluconazole and ciprofloxacin).

- SSRIs have also been associated with the development of inappropriate ADH (antidiuretic hormone) secretion, leading to clinically significant hyponatremia. With prompt recognition and treatment, the prognosis is generally good.

Treatment involves withdrawal of the SSRIs and other contributing or related drugs. In severe cases (with hyperthermia, delirium and autonomic instability), hospitalization is necessary, with supportive care including hydration and antipyretic agents. Benzodiazepines may be useful for tremor and agitation, and cyproheptadine is usually recommended.

Serotonin–noradrenaline reuptake inhibitors (SNRIs)

(e.g. venlafaxine, desvenlafaxine, mirtazapine, duloxetine)

In addition to the potential to cause symptoms of serotonin overactivity and serotonin toxicity (see above), other side-effects of drugs in this class include sedation and weight gain (mirtazapine). Venlafaxine is associated with hypertension at higher doses and with cardiac effects (e.g. QRS widening).

See Table 19-1 for the differential diagnosis of serotonin toxicity and other key conditions.

Tricyclic antidepressants (TCAs)

(e.g. amitriptyline, imipramine, doxepin, nortriptyline)

TCAs have significant side-effects including the following.

- Anticholinergic effects—the basis of most significant side-effects: urinary retention, constipation, precipitation of narrow-angle glaucoma, and propensity to delirium.

- Cardiac toxicity is characterized by increasing sinus tachycardia; increased duration of refractory period; delays in atrioventricular (AV) conduction, including AV block, with prolongation of QRS duration and QT intervals, and T-wave changes; and potential for supraventricular tachycardia and ventricular arrhythmias. These effects are potentially life-threatening in overdose.

- Postural hypotension may occur due to alpha-adrenergic blockade.

- Other common adverse effects include sedation, mild intention tremor, and sexual dysfunction (e.g. erectile dysfunction and anorgasmia).

SELF-ASSESSMENT QUESTIONS

1 An 18-year-old female university student has recently been admitted to hospital for investigation of unexplained hypokalemia. She is an accomplished triathlete. She has been amenorrheic for 6 months and her body mass index is 13 kg/m2. Which of the following is the most likely to indicate the presence of an eating disorder in this patient?

A Excessive fear of gaining weight
B Excessive exercise
C Very low BMI
D Unexplained vomiting

2 A 55-year-old man has been receiving sertraline 250 mg/day for treatment of a major depressive disorder. He was recently prescribed tramadol for acute musculoskeletal pain. He presents feeling generally unwell, with diarrhea, excessive sweating, tremor and mild fever. He has difficulty concentrating and has an unsteady gait. Which of the following would be the most consistent with the likely diagnosis?

A Tachycardia
B QTc prolongation
C Agitation
D Hyperreflexia
E Leg cramps

3 A 58-year-old man with a longstanding history of bipolar affective disorder presents distressed, complaining of feeling generally unwell with unusual neurological symptoms including recent onset of intention tremor and unsteady gait. He also complains of recent loose bowel motions. He has had no previous symptoms of this nature. On examination, he is afebrile and has a marked intention tremor but normal muscle tone. His medications include lithium carbonate 750 mg/day and olanzapine 5 mg/day and he has recently commenced lisinopril 10 mg/day, for hypertension. The most likely diagnosis is:

A Lithium toxicity
B Somatoform disorder
C Neuroleptic malignant syndrome
D Drug-induced parkinsonism
E Hypochondriasis

ANSWERS

1 A

The patient's body mass index is indicative of her being severely underweight. Excessive fear of gaining weight despite weight loss indicates disturbance of body image that is essential for the diagnosis of anorexia nervosa. Excessive exercise, weight loss and vomiting may also occur in this condition, and help in making a diagnosis (but also require the fear of gaining weight), but alone they are less indicative.

2 D

This man has serotonin toxicity clinically. Tramadol, an opioid analgesic, is a serotonin-releasing drug. Hyperreflexia, in the context of selective serotonin reuptake inhibitor (SSRI) use, is the most indicative of serotonin toxicity from this list of options. Tachycardia and agitation may occur but are not specific to this syndrome. Prolongation of QTc interval occurs with other psychotropic agents (e.g. antipsychotic agents or tricyclic antidepressants), but is not a typical feature of this syndrome.

3 A

The symptoms are typical of early lithium toxicity. The addition of lisinopril is likely to have increased his serum lithium levels (by reducing the renal excretion of lithium) and to have precipitated toxicity at doses that were previously well tolerated. While a somatic symptom disorder can present with neurological symptoms, this is most unlikely in a man of this age in the absence of prior unexplained symptoms or any apparent precipitating events. Furthermore, such a premature diagnosis of somatic symptom disorder would place this patient at serious risk of life-threatening undetected lithium toxicity. Neuroleptic malignant syndrome is important to consider in any patient taking a dopamine antagonist (in this instance olanzapine), but would usually be associated with elevated temperature and muscle rigidity. Drug-induced parkinsonism would cause a typical resting tremor and increased muscle tone.

CHAPTER 20

CLINICAL INFECTIOUS DISEASES

Iain Gosbell and D Ashley R Watson

CHAPTER OUTLINE

CLINICAL APPROACH TO INFECTIOUS DISEASES

Overview

Despite vast improvements in public health, sanitation and vaccination, and huge technological advances in medicine, infectious diseases remain a major cause of morbidity and mortality.

Many infectious diseases exhibit a characteristic pattern of symptoms and signs, aiding diagnosis:

- clinically obvious signs and symptoms, e.g. chickenpox
- obvious system involvement without the pathogen being clear, e.g. pneumonia
- obvious infection present, but not localized, e.g. fever.

The extent of initial investigation, and provision of empirical treatment, depends on a number of factors:

- the severity of the manifestations
- the time course of progression of the illness
- the vulnerability of the underlying host; an immunosuppressed host may display more subtle clinical signs of infection
- public health or infection control significance.

CLINICAL PEARL

The time course of most infectious diseases, and their response to treatment, is well known. Deviation from the expected time course should prompt a reappraisal of the initial diagnosis and the treatment, and potentially the collection of further specimens. Monitoring of acute phase reactants such as C-reactive protein or pro-calcitonin may help inform the clinician regarding response to treatment.

History

Key features in the history include the following.

- Onset and time course—for example, sudden onset of fever and chills suggests bacterial infection.
- Systemic symptoms—fever, chills, sweats, malaise, weight loss, fatigue, lethargy, anorexia.
- Localizing symptoms may help pinpoint the site of infection.
- Medication history is pivotal, including previous antibiotics and other drugs.
- Past medical history—immunosuppression, vaccination.
- Exposure history, including:
  - » sexual
  - » family
  - » occupational
  - » travel.
- Recent surgery or injury.

Examination

Physical examination in infectious diseases aims to establish the following.

- Is the patient febrile? Is there tachycardia or relative bradycardia? Is there tachypnea?
- Is septicemia or shock present?
- Is the illness systemic, or organ-based?
- Are there any features highly suggestive of particular infections?

The vital signs answer the first two questions; the rest of the physical examination the other two.

- Ophthalmic examination may reveal conjunctivitis with some systemic infections. There may be hemorrhages in infective endocarditis, and scleral jaundice may be detectable in hepatic infections.
- Central nervous system (CNS) examination involves assessment of mental status. If headache is prominent, evidence of meningitis (photophobia, neck stiffness, difficulty with straight leg raising) should be sought.
- Cardiovascular examination includes inspecting for peripheral stigmata of infective endocarditis and murmurs. Heart failure, pericardial rub and tamponade should be sought.
- Respiratory examination is important to identify lower respiratory infections.
- Abdominal examination specifically seeks evidence of splenomegaly, hepatomegaly, tenderness, and peritonism.
- Genitourinary examination is required if symptoms relating to this system are present, or if there is any evidence in the history and examination of sexually transmitted diseases.
- If the patient reports musculoskeletal symptoms, it is important to ascertain whether there is muscle tenderness or induration, which could indicate pyomyositis or underlying osteomyelitis. Similarly, evidence of arthritis should be sought.
- ENT (ear, nose, throat) examination is particularly important in children. The pharynx should be inspected, cervical lymphadenopathy sought, sinus tenderness examined for, and auroscopic examination performed.
- All medical devices, especially intravenous and other catheters, should be examined for evidence of local inflammation.

It is important to examine areas of the body which are covered by bedclothes or medical apparatus such as casts. It is not infrequent to discover suppurating wounds and bedsores in this way, especially in an obtunded patient.

Important physical signs

Body temperature

- Fever is characteristic of most infections but can be absent, particularly in the old and the immunosuppressed.
- Patients with hypothermia are often septic.
- Sometimes the pattern of temperature over time can suggest particular diagnoses.
  - » If malaria remains untreated for some time, synchronization of parasite release from red cells can cause fevers every 2 or 3 days; this is rarely seen in practice.

» Brucellosis characteristically causes an undulant fever that waxes and wanes over a several-day cycle.
» Hectic fevers with high peaks accompanied by chills and rigors are characteristic of abscesses.
» If the cause of the fever is unclear, examination for goiter and evidence of thyrotoxicosis and features of Graves' disease is required.
» Mostly, however, temperature patterns do not correlate with specific diagnoses.

Rash

The presence of rash can be diagnostic, e.g. chickenpox, herpes zoster, meningococcal disease and measles, so the time course, distribution and morphology need to be carefully noted.

Lymphadenopathy

Viral infections such as human immunodeficiency virus, Epstein–Barr virus or cytomegalovirus can manifest with widespread lymphadenopathy, and splenomegaly. Conversely, localized lymphadenopathy is seen with local suppurative conditions such as cellulitis. In migrants from Africa and Asia, persistent cervical or axillary lymphadenopathy is often due to tuberculosis. Secondary syphilis is classically manifested by lymphadenopathy associated with fever, rash and pale mucosal lesions known as mucous patches.

DIAGNOSTICS IN INFECTIOUS DISEASES

Pre-analytical considerations

One of the pivotal choices in infectious diseases is knowing whom to investigate, and then which investigations to choose.

- Infections that are minor and self-limiting or easily treated, such as mild cellulitis, cystitis, gastroenteritis or mild upper respiratory infections, do not require diagnostic tests.
- However, if the result of the investigation makes a material difference to management, or the patient is seriously ill, or the initial diagnosis of a minor condition appears to be incorrect, or might affect anti-infective choice or direct public health interventions, then such tests should be ordered.

Analytical considerations

Diagnostic microbiology is still labor-intensive in terms of setting up assays, interpretation and reporting of results. It is very helpful if the laboratory is provided with a clinical vignette, especially in special scenarios such as illness in a returned traveler or immunosuppression. It is often helpful to have a discussion with a clinical microbiologist in selecting a suitable range of tests.

Microscopy and culture

Microscopic techniques that are commonly used include Gram stains, but also wet films (e.g. urine and cerebrospinal fluid examinations) and other microscopic techniques such as immunofluorescence. Direct microscopy results are quick but less reliable; culture is much more sensitive at the expense of specificity, particularly for sites that are normally not sterile.

Antigen detection

Antigen tests are used to identify pathogens in bodily fluids and include those performed on nasopharyngeal aspirates to detect respiratory viruses, fecal antigen tests to detect *Clostridium difficile* and *Giardia intestinalis*, and those performed on serum samples to detect the hepatitis B antigen.

Nucleic acid detection

Nucleic acid detection (the polymerase chain reaction [PCR] and similar methods) is particularly useful for those organisms that are hard to culture.

- Nucleic acid detection is useful in diagnosing respiratory pathogens such as influenza, human metapneumovirus, respiratory syncytial virus (RSV) and *Pneumocystis jiroveci*, sexually transmitted pathogens, such as *Neisseria gonorrhoeae*, *Chlamydia* spp., pathogens causing meningitis, such as *Neisseria meningitidis*, *Streptococcus pneumoniae*, enteroviruses and varicella zoster virus (VZV), and in the evaluation of immunosuppressed patients (especially when viruses of the herpes family are suspected).
- For pathogens such as cytomegalovirus (CMV), human immunodeficiency virus (HIV), hepatitis B virus (HBV) and hepatitis C virus (HCV), quantitation (viral load) can be performed, which can be informative to the state of disease and the response to therapy.
- Laboratories now offer panels of nucleic acid tests for particular specimens, such as a gastrointestinal panel for stool specimens, a respiratory virus panel for respiratory specimens, and a central nervous system panel for meningitis pathogens for CSF. Note that if an organism is a commensal as well as a pathogen in a particular site, such as *Streptococcus pneumoniae* in the respiratory tract, adding such organisms to the panel will not be diagnostically useful for that specimen.

Serology

Serological tests which measure the humoral response to infectious agents or an antigen expressed by it are especially useful for difficult-to-cultivate pathogens. Generally the immunoglobulin M (IgM) response occurs in acute infection, followed by the IgG response. A fourfold rise in IgG titer is still considered a gold standard of serological diagnosis.

The preferred format and sensitivity and specificity of serology tests vary pathogen by pathogen. Results in serological testing should generally be interpreted in the light of other information.

Post-analytical considerations

Many considerations come into the interpretation of microbiology results. If a bacteriology specimen came from a site that normally harbors commensal flora, growth of bacteria might not reflect the organisms actually causing the infection. In general, cultures of specimens taken from normally sterile sites such as blood, joint fluid, and cerebrospinal fluid are more reliable. As any demonstration of an organism may be significant, noting that skin commensals may contaminate such specimens in which case demonstration of the same organism from further specimens may be needed.

SELECTED COMMON CLINICALLY IMPORTANT ORGANISMS

Selected bacteria

A working classification of commonly encountered pathogenic bacteria is shown in Table 20-1.

> **CLINICAL PEARL**
>
> Beware the following four bacteria that can cause rapid overwhelming sepsis and death in normal hosts:
>
> 1 *Neisseria meningitidis*
> 2 *Staphylococcus aureus*
> 3 *Streptococcus pneumoniae*
> 4 *Streptococcus pyogenes*.

Staphylococcus aureus

At any given time 20% of people are colonized with *Staphylococcus aureus*, yet it can also cause disease ranging from minor skin and soft tissue infections to overwhelming sepsis and death. It also causes many healthcare-associated infections such as intravenous catheter sepsis and surgical site infections.

- *S. aureus* has the propensity to acquire resistance genes via horizontal gene transfer. Methicillin-resistant *S. aureus* (MRSA) strains caused outbreaks in hospitals in the 1970s and became established in hospitals in many countries (notably, not northern Europe), with strains being characteristically multi-drug-resistant and only susceptible to a few, non-beta lactam, antibiotics.

- Community MRSA strains emerged in Chicago intravenous (IV) drug users in the 1980s and in multiple countries simultaneously in the 1990s. These strains were genetically distinct, frequently caused skin and soft tissue infections, particularly large boils, were more frequent in Indigenous peoples and those from lower socioeconomic groups, and were usually susceptible to most, if not all, non-beta-lactams. Strains causing boils and also pneumonia typically produces Panton-Valentine leukocidin. For this reason, macrolide antibiotics have been recommended here as protein translation is interfered with by this class of antibiotics, and theoretically, the production of this exotoxin should be reduced.

- With respect to invasive disease due to *S. aureus*, it is important to define the extent of disease. In *S. aureus* bacteremia, echocardiography should be performed to identify or rule out endocarditis, and the patient questioned at intervals about bone and joint pain, which, if present, may indicate a need to investigate for septic arthritis or osteomyelitis. If a focus of infection is identified, then control of the sepsis by drainage of pus and/or surgery (commonly known as 'source control') will result in more rapid control of sepsis. If no focus or metastatic complication of bacteremia is identified, a minimum of 2 weeks of IV antibiotics is required; complicated bacteremia requires longer treatment. Invasive disease can be due to methicillin-resistant strains (Figure 20-1).

Streptococcus pneumoniae

Streptococcus pneumoniae may be a commensal of the human upper and lower respiratory tract, but on occasion can cause invasive disease ranging from otitis media to pneumonia, bacteremia, septicemia and meningitis.

Table 20-1 Common pathogenic bacteria encountered in medicine

GRAM STAIN RESULT	GENUS/GENERA	TYPICAL PATHOGENIC SPECIES
Gram-positive cocci	*Staphylococcus*	*Staphylococcus aureus*
	Streptococcus	*Streptococcus pneumoniae* Beta-hemolytic streptococci (including *S. pyogenes, S. agalactiae, S. dysgalactiae*) Alpha- and non-hemolytic streptococci
	Enterococcus	*Enterococcus faecalis* *Enterococcus faecium*
Gram-negative bacilli	*Enterobacteriaceae* ('coliforms')	*Escherichia coli, Klebsiella* spp., *Proteus* spp. ESCAPPM or SPACE organisms
	Respiratory tract GNRs	*Haemophilus influenzae, Moraxella catarrhalis*
	Pseudomonads	*Pseudomonas aeruginosa*
Gram-negative cocci	*Neisseria* spp.	*Neisseria meningitidis, Neisseria gonorrhoeae*
Anaerobes	Multiple	*Bacteroides fragilis*, other Gram-negative and Gram-positive anaerobic species

ESCAPPM, *Enterobacter, Serratia, Citrobacter, Hafnia, Acinetobacter, Proteus (vulgaris), Providencia* and *Morganella* spp.; GNRs, Gram-negative rods; SPACE, *Serratia, Proteus, Acinetobacter, Citrobacter* and *Enterobacter* spp.

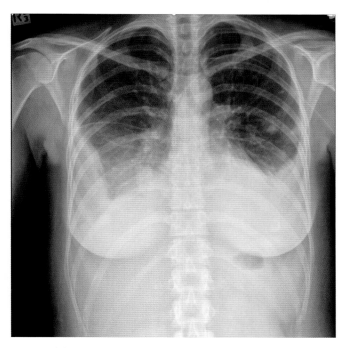

Figure 20-1 Empyema due to community-acquired methicillin-resistant *Staphylococcus aureus*

- Pneumococcal infections are more common at the extremes of life and in immunocompromised individuals. In particular, persons with asplenia and defective humoral immunity are unable to clear opsonized encapsulated bacteria, and are at substantial risk of overwhelming pneumococcal sepsis.
- Vaccines utilizing capsular polysaccharides produce an evanescent immune response; conjugation of the polysaccharide to an immunogenic carrier protein increases the intensity and duration of the humoral response. Technically, only a few serotypes can be included in these conjugated vaccines.
- Diagnosis of pneumococcal disease at times can be difficult.
  » Isolation of bacteria in blood or CSF is diagnostic but many cases have negative cultures, particularly if antibiotics are being given prior to cultures.
  » The organism is part of normal respiratory flora, so isolation of *S. pneumoniae* here is not diagnostic of invasive disease. A sputum or tracheal sample revealing neutrophils with Gram-positive diplococci is more indicative of clinical disease.
  » PCR is quite sensitive in detecting pneumococci in CSF, although is less sensitive in blood. Recently developed urinary antigen tests are more sensitive and specific for invasive disease.

Streptococcus pyogenes

Streptococcus pyogenes may be a commensal of the human nasopharynx and can cause a wide range of diseases by direct invasion, such as pharyngitis, cellulitis and bacteremia, or through immunological phenomena such as rheumatic fever, post-streptococcal glomerulonephritis, and erythema nodosum.

- The organism has never been reported to be resistant to penicillin but is acquiring resistances to other drugs such as macrolides and tetracyclines. This is significant clinically, as drugs such as clindamycin that interfere with ribosomal protein translation, at least *in vitro*, decrease exotoxin production and are recommended in severe invasive disease such as necrotizing fasciitis.
- The isolation of *S. pyogenes* from throat is not specific for pharyngitis. Isolation from wound culture is more suggestive of clinical disease. Blood cultures are usually negative in common syndromes such as pharyngitis and cellulitis, but, if positive, are absolutely specific for invasive disease.
- Patients with invasive or immune disease sometimes have anti-streptolysin O and/or anti-DNase B antibodies.

Neisseria meningitidis

Neisseria meningitidis is a common commensal of the upper respiratory tract that can cause invasive disease including bacteremia and meningitis, and on occasion unusual manifestations such as peritonitis and septic arthritis. Septicemic cases often have the typical petechial rash which can evolve into purpura fulminans.

- Infection is more common in young children and in situations with close crowding, such as in barracks, day-care centers, and where there are aggregations of people. In Western countries, serogroups B and C were the typical pathogens until conjugated serogroup C vaccine was introduced. Serogroups W and Y have recently become more common. Serogroup A is particularly associated with the so-called 'meningitis belt' of west and central Africa.
- People with terminal complement deficiencies are at increased risk of developing invasive meningococcal disease, although typically the case fatality rate is markedly less than in more classic cases.
- Diagnostic tests include rapid tests such as Gram stain of CSF or material from skin lesions; and PCR on CSF and blood, which is the most sensitive test. Traditional tests include culturing the organism from blood and CSF. Serology is occasionally useful in PCR and culture-negative patients.
- *N. meningitidis* remains sensitive to penicillin, and suspected infection should be treated urgently—typically with ceftriaxone. Supportive care, including inotropes and organ support, is often needed. Corticosteroid is typically administered immediately before the antibiotic in suspected cases of meningococcal meningitis.

Alpha- and non-hemolytic streptococci

These are commensal flora in the upper respiratory tract and GI tract. Their main clinical significance is as causes of endocarditis (see Chapter 7).

CLINICAL PEARL

The rash of invasive meningococcal disease may be nonspecific early in the course of infection: carefully examine the chest, back and abdomen for a sparse maculopapular rash when assessing a young patient with an unexplained fever and headache.

Enterococcus species

- The two main species causing human infections are *Enterococcus faecalis* and *E. faecium*.
- All enterococci are resistant to cephalosporins; penicillins are bacteriostatic, but are rendered bactericidal with the addition of aminoglycosides such as gentamicin. For the synergistic and effective treatment of endocarditis, the addition of either gentamicin or, for *E. faecalis*, high-dose ceftriaxone is usually required. Enterococci are resistant to most nonbetalactams, with the exception of vancomycin and newer agents such as daptomycin, pristinamycin (only *E. faecium*), and linezolid.
- Vancomycin-resistant enterococci (VRE) have emerged in recent years and are proving very difficult to control. Most patients with VRE are only colonized, but these patients are an important reservoir of risk to immunocompromised patients and those with intravascular devices, particularly prosthetic heart valves. Bacteremia with VRE has about 40% mortality.
- Control of VRE transmission has proven to be very difficult and involves a multifaceted approach to address environmental reservoirs, optimize hand hygiene practices, impose strict infection-control strategies, and implement robust antibiotic stewardship policies.

Escherichia coli, Klebsiella species and *Proteus* species

- These species are normal flora of the GI tract and are seen in community-onset infections relating to the GI and urinary tracts.
- Various types of *E. coli* can cause toxin-related disease, including gastroenteritis and hemolytic uremic syndrome.
- In general these species are more susceptible to antibiotics than other groups of gram-negative organisms, although antimicrobial resistance is increasing: 50% of *E. coli* in Western countries are now resistant to amoxicillin/ampicillin, and increasingly resistances to quinolones and other drugs including 3rd-generation cephalosporins are being seen.

ESCHAPPM organisms

- ESCHAPPM = *Enterobacter, Serratia, Citrobacter, Hafnia, Acinetobacter, Proteus (vulgaris), Providentia* and *Morganella* spp.
- Infections caused by these organisms are typical of those caused by the *Enterobacteriaceae*, i.e. GI-tract-related infections, urinary tract infections, IV line infections, bacteremia and septicemia, but are more frequently seen in patients with hospital contact and are more resistant to antibiotics. They frequently (especially with *Enterobacter*

species) have inductible cephalosporinases selected out by 3rd-generation cephalosporins.

Pseudomonas aeruginosa

- *Pseudomonas aeruginosa* is an environmental saprophyte which can colonize patients with leg ulcers, chronic respiratory disease (chronic obstructive pulmonary disease [COPD], bronchiectasis, and cystic fibrosis), and biliary tract abnormalities: obstructions, stents, and following ERCP (endoscopic retrograde cholangiopancreatography).
- *P. aeruginosa* is intrinsically resistant to most antibiotics but is covered by anti-pseudomonal penicillins (e.g. piperacillin), anti-pseudomonal cephalosporins (e.g. ceftazidime, cefepime), carbapenems (e.g. meropenem), and aminoglycosides or quinolones, and readily develops resistance to these agents.

Bacteroides fragilis and other anaerobic Gram-negative and Gram-positive species

Anaerobic organisms are usually considered as a group because the infections they cause are usually polymicrobial infections related to mucosal surfaces, secondary to a mucosal breach, and often involve other organisms such as *Enterobacteriaceae*, streptococci and enterococci. Anaerobic (and mixed) infections above the diaphragm are typically caused by organisms normally resident in the oral cavity; those occurring below the diaphragm (i.e. intra-abdominal infections) are typically caused by bowel anaerobes (commonly *Bacteroides* and *Prevotella* species).

Selected viruses

Human immunodeficiency virus, hepatitis B virus and hepatitis C virus are covered in other chapters of this book (HIV in Chapter 16, and hepatitis in Chapter 12).

Herpes simplex virus 1 (HSV-1) and 2 (HSV-2)

- Herpes simplex viruses are acquired by mucosal contact from other people.
- Characteristically there is a primary infection, which can be severe, then a period when the virus lies dormant in cranial nerve or dorsal root ganglia from which it can reactivate to cause recurrent infections.
- HSV-1 usually causes oro-labial manifestations and HSV-2 usually causes genital lesions, although there is substantial overlap between the two syndromes.
- Primary oral herpes infection is typically manifested as unpleasant stomatitis, being more extensive within the oral cavity than recurrent attacks (cold sores).
- There is often a warning tingling and numbness sensation just prior to the onset of an outbreak of lesions, which are often very painful. The characteristic lesions are small vesicles on a red base. Occasionally, particularly with primary episodes and with severe disease, dissemination and/or neurological manifestations may occur.
- Transmission from mother to baby can occur if a woman has an active herpetic lesion in the vagina or vulva during parturition. Neonatal HSV-2 is a severe, generalized infection with septicemia, hepatitis, thrombocytopenia, other organ dysfunctions, and widespread mucocutaneous herpetic lesions. Pregnant women with

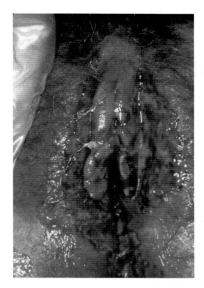

Figure 20-2 Primary genital herpes simplex virus type 2 infection of the vulva

From Mandell GL, Bennett JE and Dolin R. Mandell, Douglas, and Bennett's Principles and practice of infectious diseases, 7th ed. Philadelphia: Elsevier, 2009.

a history of genital herpes require careful genital examination (Figure 20-2), and cesarean section should be performed if there are any lesions detected.

Treatment

- Drugs such as acyclovir (aciclovir, famciclovir and valaciclovir) are highly active against HSV-1 and -2.

- For minor infections in the normal host, antiviral treatment is most effective if given in the first 48 hours after vesicle appearance.

- Severe infections may require IV aciclovir, famciclovir or valaciclovir. Primary infection and recurrences are more severe and slower to respond to treatment if there is T-cell immune deficiency; in this setting, secondary prevention is required.

Vaccines against HSV-1 and -2 are in development and are likely to be clinically available soon.

CLINICAL PEARL

Herpes simplex encephalitis needs to be considered in any patient presenting with unexplained fever and confusion. Diagnosis is with polymerase chain reaction of cerebrospinal fluid. Serology is not helpful here. Characteristically, magnetic resonance imaging shows temporal lobe involvement. Treatment with intravenous acyclovir (aciclovir) is safe and extremely effective.

Varicella zoster virus (VZV)

Varicella zoster virus is a human herpesvirus (HHV-3) that causes chickenpox/varicella (primary infection) and shingles/zoster (reactivation).

- Chickenpox is highly contagious. It is manifested by a systemic infection with a rash consisting of vesicles on a red base, involving most of the body. The vesicles often have tiny central pits, particularly when more than a day or two old. Some patients develop pneumonitis, particularly if the patient is adolescent or adult. Other complications include encephalitis and hepatitis. Chickenpox is more severe in the immunosuppressed.

- On resolution, the virus lies dormant in cranial nerve and dorsal root ganglia and from where, in a substantial proportion of the aging population, the virus may reactivate and erupt in a dermatomal distribution. This occurs most frequently on the trunk, but sometimes in other areas like the divisions of the trigeminal nerve.

- Shingles occurring in those younger than 50 years, or more than once, should raise the suspicion of underlying immunosuppression as shingles (zoster).

Diagnosis and treatment

- Diagnosis of chickenpox and shingles is usually self-evident; appearances can be atypical in the immunosuppressed and testing is more useful here.
  - » The best test is PCR on fluid and cells from the base of vesicles.
  - » Immunofluorescence tests are now rarely requested or readily available.
  - » Culture is usually negative and is not recommended.
  - » Serology is occasionally useful in the diagnosis of atypical cases, but mostly to determine whether a pregnant or immunocompromised patient or healthcare worker is nonimmune and therefore susceptible to primary infection (chickenpox).

- Therapy for primary and recurrent VZV is with antiviral drugs such as acyclovir (aciclovir). These drugs are most efficacious if started within 48–72 hours of the onset of lesions. They may be still effective beyond that, particularly in the immunosuppressed or in severe disease.

- If there is a VZV exposure event, those who are IgG-negative are regarded as susceptible.
  - » Exposed nonimmune healthcare workers are excluded from work from days 0–21 in case they develop chickenpox.
  - » Varicella zoster immune globulin (VZIG) is given to immunosuppressed, nonimmune contacts including pregnant women.
  - » The incubation period of chickenpox may be prolonged if VZIG or antivirals are given.

- An efficacious live vaccine against shingles is now available and is incorporated into immunization schedules. It is contraindicated in people with significant immunocompromise. The vaccine protects against shingles in those aged above 50 years. A recombinant shingles vaccine is also available in some countries and is safe to administer to immuncompromised individuals.

Epstein–Barr virus (EBV)

- Epstein–Barr virus is usually acquired during childhood, adolescence or young adult life by mucosal contact with other people.

- In older individuals it characteristically manifests with pharyngitis and widespread lymphadenopathy, and sometimes other manifestations such as splenomegaly and hepatitis.

- Taking amoxicillin provokes a maculopapular rash in >95% of cases so it is advised to avoid amoxicillin for pharyngitis especially in adolescents and young adults when EBV is especially likely. Penicillin and cephalosporins are far less likely to cause this reaction in EBV infection.

- The blood film usually shows atypical lymphocytes, and the diagnosis is made by demonstrating heterophile antibodies ('monospot' test), or more specifically by demonstrating anti-VCA (viral capsid antigen) IgM antibodies.

- Occasional manifestations of latent EBV infection include malignancies (lymphoproliferative diseases, Burkitt's lymphoma, nasopharyngeal carcinoma, primary CNS lymphoma, especially seen in immunosuppression), chronic EBV disease, EBV-associated hemophagocytic lymphohistiocytosis and X-linked lymphoproliferative syndrome. These diseases require the requisite histology plus demonstration of EBV, usually by PCR.

- There are no antivirals with sufficient activity to be therapeutically useful.

- There is no vaccine.

Cytomegalovirus (CMV)

- Cytomegalovirus is a human herpesvirus (HHV-5) which commonly causes an infectious mononucleosis-like illness in young adults. Fever, sore throat, lymphadenopathy and hepatitis are the common symptoms, although infection may be asymptomatic.

- Like all herpesviruses, primary CMV infection is followed by latency, which results in a particular risk of reactivation disease in the immunosuppressed host. Patients with cellular immune deficiency, such as in acquired immune deficiency syndrome (AIDS) or post organ transplant, are at risk of invasive CMV disease of lungs, retina and gastrointestinal tract. These are life-threatening situations.

- CMV is also a major cause of congenital infection (see Chapter 24).

- Acute CMV infection can be confirmed by the presence of specific IgM followed by IgG with low avidity, and/or by detection of viral DNA. In the reactivation illness in the setting of immunosuppression, serum viral DNA levels may be useful, but tissue biopsy with typical histological appearance of intranuclear inclusions, or positive viral culture, is diagnostic.

- Treatment is not required in the immunocompetent host as the disease is self-limiting. In the immunosuppressed patient, treatment is necessary with intravenous ganciclovir, valganciclovir, cidofovir and/or oral valganciclovir. Foscarnet may be used if ganciclovir is contraindicated (bone marrow suppression) or if resistance is suspected or proven.

Adenovirus

Adenoviruses are small ribonucleic acid (RNA) viruses that are implicated in common human infections such as upper respiratory infections. Diagnosis of adenoviruses is by PCR immunofluorescence on respiratory specimens, or demonstration of a serological response. PCR is not widely available.

Human parvovirus B19

- Parvovirus B19 most frequently causes a benign exanthem of childhood, erythema infectiosum (fifth disease, 'slapped face syndrome'), or peripheral arthralgia and rash in adults.

- Infection can also result in red-cell aplasia—in the fetus this causes profound anemia leading to hydrops fetalis, and in those with hematological dyscrasias or immunosuppression infection can be prolonged, leading to pure red cell aplasia.

- Diagnosis is by detecting an IgM response or by PCR.

Enteroviruses

- The most common manifestation is a systemic infection with fever, and sometimes end-organ disease such as myocarditis and aseptic meningitis.
  » Aseptic meningitis is manifested by headache, photophobia, neck stiffness and fevers. Bacterial meningitis is the important differential diagnosis. CSF examination reveals raised protein and normal glucose with a mononuclear pleocytosis, but occasionally on the first day or two of illness there can be neutrophil pleocytosis.

- Enteroviruses are an uncommon cause of gastroenteritis.

- The diagnosis is made by exclusion of bacterial pathogens and demonstration of enterovirus RNA in CSF by PCR. Serology is insensitive and nonspecific.

- Severe systemic infection with myocarditis and hepatitis can occur in infections acquired during birth. Pleconaril has been trialed in neonatal disease.

Selected fungi

Yeasts

Candida species

Candida spp. are commensals of the human GI and genitourinary tracts, and can cause clinical infections in those exposed to broad-spectrum antibiotics and those with either neutropenia or T-cell immune deficiency.

- *C. albicans* is the most common species, but other species of *Candida* are increasingly seen due to the increasing use of antifungals to which these other species are often resistant.

- Clinical infections include diaper rash, vaginitis, oral candidiasis, and infection of skinfolds ('intertrigo'), particularly in the obese.
  » Immunodeficiency states see more severe cutaneous manifestations, esophagitis and bloodstream infections—the latter particularly seen in patients with long-term IV catheters while receiving broad-spectrum antibiotic treatment.

CLINICAL PEARL

Approximately 20% of cases of candidemia are complicated by retinitis. Request an ophthalmology consultation on every patient with candidemia.

- Upper GI tract surgery can be complicated by deep infections with *Candida* spp.
- Candidemia is seen in patients with total parenteral nutrition and patients with extensive mucositis (usually due to chemotherapy).
  - » Candidemia can be complicated by seeding of the retina (leading to endophthalmitis).
- Hepatosplenic candidiasis manifests with multiple liver and spleen lesions in neutropenic patients.
- *C. albicans* is usually sensitive to a wide range of topical and systemic antifungals; however, with widespread use of azoles some resistance is seen, and *Candida* spp. not susceptible to fluconazole are increasingly seen. Here it is important to take specimens for fungal culture to confirm species and sensitivities. Candida endocarditis and other invasive syndromes are typically treated with an echinocandin agent.
- Table 20-9 lists candidal species encountered clinically, with corresponding susceptibility profiles which to some extent are predictable from the species, but susceptibility testing is required if treatment is necessary. It is important to take specimens for fungal culture to confirm the presence of candida, determine the species and perform antifungal susceptibility testing.
- *C. auris* is an emerging candida species, typically seen in immunosuppressed patients particularly those exposed to antifungal agents. This species is hard to identify in the laboratory, and is typically multidrug resistant, being usually resistant to azoles, sometimes (30% in the US) resistant to amphotericin and occasionally (5% in the US) resistant to echinocandins as well.

Cryptococcus *species*

Three species of *Cryptococcus* are clinically significant: *C. grubii* (serogroup A), *C. neoformans* (serogroup D), and *C. gattii* (serogroup B or C).

- *C. grubii* and *C. neoformans* are found in bird guano, and *C. gattii* is associated with river red and forest red gum trees (*Eucalyptus camaldulensis*).
- Acquisition of *Cryptococcus* is by inhalation of airborne forms, causing pulmonary infection, followed by hematogenous dissemination to other sites, usually the leptomeninges and/or brain parenchyma.
- Cryptococcomas (Figure 20-3) and obstructive hydrocephalus are more common with *C. gattii*.
- Diagnosis involves demonstrating cryptococcal antigen in blood or CSF, or culturing the organism.
- Amphotericin B (usually a lipid formulation) is the mainstay of treatment; results are better if flucytosine is co-administered. Flucytosine levels are measured, as clearance is variable and accumulation is typical if amphotericin causes renal failure. Patients require prolonged amphotericin B and flucytosine, followed by oral fluconazole.

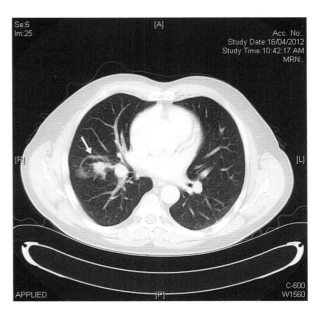

Figure 20-3 Cryptococcoma of the right lung

- Elevated CSF pressure is an important complication of cryptococcal meningitis, associated with severe sequelae including blindness. This is managed with serial lumbar punctures and if the pressure is not reduced, CSF shunting is often required.

CLINICAL PEARL

All patients with *Cryptococcus* species identified from any specimen should be investigated further for invasive disease, including MRI brain, CSF analysis and serology for cryptococcal antigen.

Molds

Aspergillus *species*

Aspergillus spp. are ubiquitous environmental fungi, the spores of which are continuously inhaled but in normal hosts are rapidly cleared. Higher levels of airborne spores are seen where there is decaying vegetation, such as compost heaps, and when moldy materials are disturbed, for example during building demolition works. T-cell immunosuppressed and neutropenic individuals are advised to avoid such scenarios.

- Colonization with *Aspergillus* spp. is frequently seen in patients with underlying processes such as bronchiectasis or lung cavities. Colonization *per se* does not require specific treatment.
- Allergic bronchopulmonary aspergillosis manifests with cough and wheeze, peripheral eosinophilia and an elevated IgE level. Specific *Aspergillus* spp. antibodies in high titer helps to confirm the diagnosis. The treatment is to modify the immune response with inhaled, and sometimes systemic, corticosteroids.
- Aspergillomas are fungal balls in cavities, usually seen on CT scan (Figure 20-4). Treatment of this is difficult: excision is best, but often such patients will not tolerate the extensive surgery that is typically required for cure.

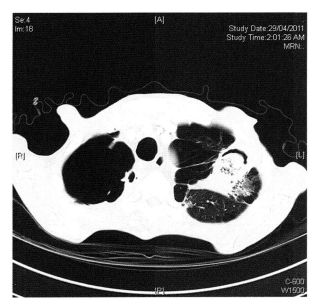

Figure 20-4 Computed tomography scan showing aspergilloma in a patient with underlying chronic obstructive pulmonary disease

Invasive disease is more likely if there is immunosuppression, particularly profound and prolonged or recurrent neutropenia.

- Diagnosis is difficult: accurate diagnosis requires demonstrating fungi invading lung tissue on biopsy, which is often not performed or is delayed until after commencement of empiric therapy.
- High-resolution CT scanning can demonstrate suspect lesions, especially progressive cavities with a crescent sign.
- Isolation of *Aspergillus* from respiratory tract specimens in the setting of neutropenia, especially with a suspicious CT scan, is suggestive.
- *Aspergillus* is rarely isolated from blood.
- Serial blood galactomannan levels or PCR can be useful in diagnosing invasive aspergillosis.

Voriconazole is more efficacious than amphotericin B in treatment; however, it is pivotal that the patients have a loading dose, to avoid delaying therapeutic steady-state levels. Alternative drugs include amphotericin B, echinocandins, and posaconazole.

Agents of mucormycosis

Mucormycosis is caused by *Rhizopus* spp., *Rhizomucor* spp., *Cunninghamella* spp., *Saksenaea* spp., *Absidia* spp., and *Mucor* spp.

- Invasive rhinocerebral mucormycosis occurs in diabetics, typically presenting with diabetic ketoacidosis, and rapidly progressive invasive disease including severe facial pain, periorbital edema, invasive infection emanating from sinuses destroying bone, and progressive cranial nerve palsies.
- Aggressive debridement and systemic antifungals are essential, but despite this death is frequent.
- More recently, pulmonary mucormycosis is an emerging infection in those who are profoundly neutropenic and in organ-transplant recipients.

- Diagnosis usually requires a tissue sample, and is often post mortem.
- The agents of mucormycosis are intrinsically (i.e. naturally) resistant to azoles and have been emerging since the use of widespread prophylaxis with broad-spectrum antifungals in severely immunosuppressed people. Successful therapy involves reversal of immunosuppression, and high-dose liposomal amphotericin B.

Dimorphic fungi

- Dimorphic fungi (*Histoplasma capsulatum*, *Blastomyces dermatitidis* and *Coccidioides imitis*) are associated with specific ecological regions around the world. Well-known regions include the southwest of the United States for *C. imitis*, the mid-west for *H. capsulatum* and many parts of North America for *B. dermatitidis*. The incidence of infection due to *H. capsulatum* is particularly associated with proximity to bird and bat colonies and caves infested with bat guano. Another species, *Penicillium marneffei*, is seen in Southeast Asia.
- When cultured in the laboratory these agents are hazardous to laboratory personnel, who need to be forewarned.

Histoplasma capsulatum

- Acute primary infection is usually manifested by fever and malaise, headache, and respiratory symptoms. There are usually few clinical signs; chest X-rays may show a patchy multilobar pneumonia, and lymph nodes may be enlarged.
- Acute histoplasmosis usually resolves, but can progress to chronic pulmonary infection, disseminate to any part of the body, or reactivate in immunosuppression, especially in patients with AIDS.
- Diagnosis is by isolation of fungus, demonstration of antigen, demonstration of typical findings on histology enhanced by special stains, the histoplasmin skin test, and serological response.
- Self-limited infections require no treatment. Azoles should be used in mild disease, and liposomal amphotericin B in severe infections.

Blastomyces dermatitidis

- Inhalation results in pulmonary infection, which may disseminate to skin, bones and the genitourinary system or other sites.
- Diagnosis is suggested by finding granulomas and compatible yeasts in microscopy of involved tissues, confirmed by culture and PCR. Serology is unhelpful.
- Azoles are used in mild to moderately severe cases, and amphotericin B for severe disease.

Coccidioides imitis

- Seroprevalence is high in the southwestern United States.
- Infection is usually pulmonary, but can disseminate.
- Neurological disease presents with headaches, confusion and seizures, and focal neurological signs.
- Diagnosis is based on isolation of this fungus from involved tissues and/or CSF, demonstrating a serological response, or a delayed hypersensitivity skin reaction.

- Treatment was previously with amphotericin B, but azoles can be used.

Selected parasites

Strongyloides stercoralis

Strongyloides stercoralis is commonly found in underdeveloped regions, particularly in tropical areas. Infection occurs via the skin from feces-contaminated soil.

- Infection is long-term; rarely, T-cell immunosuppression can result in rhabditiform larvae invading the gut and carrying *Enterobacteriaceae* into the blood, causing an overwhelming bloodstream infection.
- It is important to screen patients for *Strongyloides* in endemic areas who require immunosuppression. Screening typically relies on serology. Ivermectin is used for treatment, with follow-up serology being of some use in monitoring response.

CLINICAL PEARL

Three other soil-based helminths together contribute substantially to childhood malnutrition and anemia in lower and middle income countries: hookworm, *Ascaris lumbricoides* and the whipworm *Trichuris trichiuria*. Early *Ascaris* infection is also one of the causes of 'PIE' syndrome—pulmonary infiltrates with eosinophilia. All are readily treated in soil helminth elimination programs.

Malaria

Malaria is a systemic infection caused by one or more of five species of *Plasmodium*: *P. falciparum*, *P. vivax*, *P. malariae*, *P. ovale* and *P. knowlesi*, which are transmitted by mosquitoes in tropical areas.

- *P. falciparum* can cause rapidly progressive parasitemia in those who are nonimmune, such as young children or travelers to endemic areas.
- *P. knowlesi* is a recently described zoonotic species; recent studies show it is common in Southeast Asia and causes appreciable morbidity and some mortality.
- The other *Plasmodium* spp. also cause significant morbidity and some mortality, particularly in children.
- All species are acquiring resistance to drugs active in prophylaxis and treatment.

Diagnosis of malaria has traditionally been via thick and thin films of blood. The sensitivity is dependent on the experience and skill of the microscopist.

- Immunochromogenic tests are available for *P. falciparum* and *P. vivax*; this rapid test does not require a microscope.
- PCR is the best test with a much lower limit of detection, sensitivity and specificity than light microscopy or immunochromogenic tests, and allows ready diagnosis of mixed infections, usually simultaneous *P. falciparum* and *P. vivax*. Unfortunately, it is not readily available in most jurisdictions.
- All returned travelers with fever should have blood taken for malaria tests (blood films and antigen tests),

routine culture, and serology for common and potentially life-threatening infections such as dengue fever, leptospirosis and the various forms of typhus and spotted fevers. Admission to hospital is typically required and empiric antimicrobial treatment may be indicated. Malaria treatment for all species now typically involves the use of an artemether-lumefantrine combination product (common names being Coartem and Riamet). The former component is rapidly acting and the latter slow acting. Local treatment guidelines should be consulted.

- Pre-travel advice is important for those traveling to malarious areas.
  - » Mosquito bite prevention is important, as high levels of drug resistance are common. Use of insecticide-impregnated mosquito nets and mosquito repellent that contains 20–40% *N,N*-diethyl-3-methylbenzamide (DEET) is strongly recommended. Although travelers should be aware that *Anopheles* spp. mosquitoes bite between dusk and dawn, mosquitoes transmitting common arboviral infections such as dengue bite during the day, indicating that around-the-clock protection is required for most tropical locations. Sandflies and other vectors may also need to be taken into account.
  - » For chemoprophylaxis, up-to-date information is available via internet services from the WHO, CDC and other groups. Specific recommendations depend on the itinerary and planned activities, which will determine the likelihood of being bitten by malarious mosquitoes and the local drug resistance.

ANTI-INFECTIVE TREATMENT

CLINICAL PEARL

Principles of anti-infective treatment:
1. Establish whether or not infection is present.
2. Predict or identify the likely organisms.
3. Decide whether antibiotics are required.
4. Prescribe empirical and then definitive anti-infectives.
5. Consider host factors.
6. Decide whether other therapy is required.
7. Evaluate progress and further information to modify treatment.
8. Define treatment duration and endpoints.

Antibiotics are unique among pharmacological agents in that the effect on living organisms, including pathogenic micro-organisms, is not confined to the patient being treated. Humans and animals share their microflora quite widely. Antibiotic resistance is driven by widespread use of antibiotics in people and animals.

Is infection likely?

As always, history and examination are the most pivotal aspects of medical assessment.

- Constellations of symptoms might suggest the possibility of an infection, and what is involved or whether it might be a systemic infection.
- Vital signs indicate whether fever and/or shock are present.

- Physical examination might reveal signs suggesting a particular organ system.
- In general, for trivial infections it is probably not necessary to do diagnostic testing, but if testing may alter therapy, particularly where the possibility of drug-resistant bacteria exists or if confirmation of a viral infection means that antibiotics could be terminated, it is worth performing these tests. In addition, in patients who are moderately to severely unwell, tests are critical to first establish the diagnosis, and then to establish what organism is present and whether it might be resistant to empirical antibiotics.

What are the likely pathogen(s)?

Once the presence of infection is established, common causative organisms are quite predictable, as shown in Table 20-2.

Table 20-2 Some causes of common infections in normal hosts

INFECTION	COMMON PATHOGENS
Undifferentiated systemic sepsis	Organisms that can cause rapidly fatal infections need to be covered: *Streptococcus pneumoniae, Neisseria meningitidis, Staphylococcus aureus, Streptococcus pyogenes* Immunosuppression increases the list of likely pathogens Need to consider whether meningitis might be also present Children <4 months of age: group B streptococci, *Escherichia coli*, other Gram-negative bacilli
Upper respiratory tract infection (URTI)	Rhinovirus, coronavirus, metapneumovirus, respiratory syncytial virus Influenza virus
Pharyngitis	URTI viruses Epstein–Barr virus *Streptococcus pyogenes*
Community-acquired pneumonia	Adenovirus, metapneumovirus, respiratory syncytial virus Influenza virus *Streptococcus pneumoniae* *Haemophilus influenzae, Moraxella catarrhalis* *Staphylococcus aureus* 'Atypical' causes: *Mycoplasma pneumoniae, Chlamydia pneumoniae, Chlamydia psittaci, Legionella* spp., *Pneumocystis jiroveci*
Urinary tract infection (UTI)	*Escherichia coli* *Staphylococcus saprophyticus* *Proteus* spp., other Gram-negative bacilli
Skin and soft-tissue infections	*Streptococcus pyogenes*, other beta-hemolytic streptococci *Staphylococcus aureus, Fusobacterium* spp. (typically complicating pharyngitis)
Intra-abdominal infections	Usually mixed infections with fecal flora, i.e., *Enterobacteriaceae* (coliforms), anaerobes, various streptococci and enterococci
Bone and joint infections	Classically *Staphylococcus aureus* Sometimes *Streptococcus pyogenes*
Infective endocarditis	*Staphylococcus aureus*, especially in IV drug users and individuals with prosthetic valves, pacemakers and other long-term intravenous devices. Other staphylococci and enterococci—prosthetic valves and intravenous devices. *Viridans streptococci*—the classic cause of subacute bacterial endocarditis (SBE) in rheumatic heart disease, but may also infect prosthetic valves. *Candida* spp.—typically seen in debilitated hospitalised patients on broad-spectrum antibiotics and with long-term intravenous devices and total parenteral nutrition.
Meningitis and meningoencephalitis	Enterovirus Herpes simplex viruses Various exotic viruses, e.g. Japanese encephalitis, tick-borne encephalitis *Neisseria meningitidis* *Streptococcus pneumoniae* *Listeria monocytogenes* Gram-negative bacilli

The list of pathogens is broader in immunosuppressed hosts, as discussed in a later section.

Are anti-infective drugs required?

- Invasive bacterial infections, especially if severe, must prompt prescription of antibiotics. However, most infections are viral and/or trivial and do not require antibiotics; prescribing here adds to antibiotic resistance and exposes patients to the risk of side-effects.
- Antibiotics have not been shown to confer benefit in acute otitis media.
- In influenza, oseltamivir and zanamivir are mostly indicated in immunocompromised individuals, including those with chronic cardiorespiratory disease, particularly within the first couple of days of illness and if clinical features indicate severe disease.
- Minor boils can be treated with a 'drain and refrain' strategy. Larger and coalesced boils (carbuncles) can also be treated with a specific antibiotic such as trimethoprim/sulfa.

Choice of empirical and definitive antibiotics

CLINICAL PEARL

Considerations in choosing empirical antibiotics:
- Likely bacteria
- Likely site of infection
- Host factors such as age and immunosuppression
- Pharmacokinetics (e.g. oral bioavailability, elimination half-life)

Numerous guidelines exist for choosing empirical and definitive antibiotics, which take into consideration local antibiotic resistances and available antibiotics. Many hospitals and health services have their own policies and guidelines for antibiotic prescription and use. It is recommended to use the local guidelines as these have input from local infectious disease physicians, microbiologists, other relevant doctor groups, and consider local patterns of likely pathogens and resistance profiles, and recommend anti-infectives that are readily available locally.

What host factors need consideration?

Table 20-3 shows a number of host factors that need consideration in the selection of anti-infective drugs.

What therapy other than antibiotics is required?

Proven ancillary treatments are shown in Table 20-4. Immune modulators have been extensively trialed in sepsis, and have mostly been found to not improve outcome.

Ongoing assessment and further results

If the initial therapy appears not to be working, consider the possibilities listed in Table 20-5.

Table 20-3 Host factors affecting anti-infective agent selection

FACTOR	EFFECT
Previous adverse drug reaction	May recur on rechallenge with same or similar drug
Age	Altered pharmacokinetics
Gastric pH	Ultra-absorption of drugs affected by gastric acidity
Renal dysfunction	Profound effects on drugs eliminated by renal excretion
Hepatic dysfunction	Profound effects on drugs eliminated primarily by hepatic excretion
Binding to bone/teeth	Binding causes staining of non-erupted teeth, which is permanent
Genetic or metabolic abnormalities	Slow acetylators G6PD (glucose-6-phosphate dehydrogenase) deficiency
Induction of hepatic cytochromes	Increased metabolism of other drugs affected by these enzymes
Inhibition of hepatic cytochromes	Decreased metabolism of other drugs affected by this enzyme system
Pregnancy	Increased clearance and volume of distribution
Effects on fetus	Multiple different effects—guidelines exist for specific antibiotics in pregnancy and lactation (e.g from the Therapeutic Guidelines Group)
Increased clearance and V_d (volume of distribution)	Burns Adolescents and young adults Septicemia
Concentration in breast milk	Breastfeeding infants will probably receive a low dose of the drug
Site of infection hard to penetrate	Central nervous system/eye Abscesses Vegetations, bones, devitalized tissues Biofilm infections Intracellular pathogens

What is the duration and endpoint of treatment?

- Most of the common infections have a standard duration of treatment. For conditions such as endocarditis, these durations have been established by clinical trials. Giving shorter courses has a high failure rate, and longer courses do not appreciably increase the success rate.

Table 20-4 Proven ancillary measures used in treatment of specific infections

INFECTION	MEASURE
Abscess	Drainage (radiological or surgical)
Endocarditis	Valve replacement
Pneumococcal meningitis	Administration of corticosteroids prior to antibiotics
Tetanus	Anti-tetanus immunoglobulin

Table 20-5 Reasons for apparent failure of anti-infective treatment

REASON FOR FAILURE	SPECIFIC PROBLEM
Diagnosis wrong	Incorrect infection diagnosed
	Illness is not due to infection
Inadequate treatment	Pathogen is not susceptible to anti-infective agent
	Undrained pus
	Wrong dose, dosing interval or route of administration
	Infection at hard-to-reach site
	Non-adherence
Host factors	Patient is immunosuppressed
	Chronic disease such as diabetes, alcoholism, chronic organ disease
Inadequate blood levels	Malabsorption (e.g. shock, short gut syndrome)
	Increased hepatic clearance
	Interaction with other drugs
Infected foreign body	Intravenous lines, surgical and intravascular implants
Complication of infection	Undrained pus
	Spread of infection
	Superinfection at original site, including by multidrug-resistant organisms (MROs)
New problem	New infections such as urinary tract infection or pneumonia
	Thromboembolic disease
Treatment complication	Infected intravenous line
	Non-infective thrombophlebitis from intravenous line
	Drug fever
	Surgical site infection

- For serious infections that do not have endpoints defined by clinical trials, the progress can be followed by the history (the symptoms have resolved), clinical examination (signs of inflammation have subsided), and investigations such as acute phase reactants and imaging.
- If indices such as white cell count, neutrophils, platelet count, C-reactive protein, and pro-calcitonin are raised in the acute infection, normalization in the context of clinical resolution probably indicates resolution.
- Organ imaging such as CT and MRI scanning can detect formation of new abscesses and collections, and other destructive complications of the infection. However, MRI and radionucleotide scans detect inflammation long after micro-organisms have been killed, and if used as a primary endpoint can prolong therapy.

ANTI-INFECTIVE AGENTS

Antibiotics

Beta-lactams

- Beta-lactams bind to penicillin-binding proteins in the bacterial cell wall and inhibit cell–wall synthesis and repair.
- These drugs are usually bactericidal.
- A summary of the classification and activity of common beta-lactams against commonly encountered bacteria is shown in Table 20-6 (overleaf).
- Penicillins are divided into groups, as shown in Table 20-6. The main potential adverse reactions include hypersensitivity, diarrhea, GI tract intolerance, hemolytic anemia, and hepatitis (particularly with flucloxacillin).
- Cephalosporins are better tolerated and cause fewer allergic reactions than penicillins and generally have longer half-lives thus less frequent administration which is helpful clinically, but they select out bacteria that are intrinsically resistant to them such as enterococci, MRSA, multiresistant Gram-negative bacilli, and *Clostridium difficile*.
  - » They are arbitrarily divided into five generations, with the early generations having good Gram-positive activity but lesser Gram-negative activity, and with Gram-negative activity increasing down the generations.
  - » Most recently, some cephalosporins ('fifth generation') with anti-MRSA activity have been developed, e.g. ceftaroline.
- Aztreonam, a monobactam, has good Gram–negative activity including against *Pseudomonas aeruginosa*, but has poor activity against Gram-positive organisms and anaerobes. It has a niche role in being able to be given to patients with major penicillin allergies, including anaphylaxis.
- Carbapenems include imipenem, meropenem, ertapenem and doripenem. These are the most broad-spectrum antibiotics covering *Staphylococcus aureus*, *Enterococcus* spp., *Enterobacteriaceae* including most that have broad-spectrum beta-lactamases, *P. aeruginosa* (not ertapenem), and anaerobes. The major gaps in the coverage of carbapenems are: MRSA, VRE, Gram-negatives with

metallo-beta-lactamases, *C. difficile*, *Stenotrophomonas maltophilia*, and nonbacterial pathogens such as yeasts. Adverse reactions from carbapenems include hypersensitivity, diarrhea including *C. difficile* colitis, hemolytic anemia, hepatitis, and cholestasis.

Beta-lactam allergy

- 10–20% of patients are labeled as being allergic to penicillin, but only about one-tenth of these are truly allergic. The cost of the alternative drug therapy is commonly much higher than with beta-lactams. Alternative drugs such as vancomycin are inferior to beta-lactams for serious infections with organisms such as methicillin-sensitive *S. aureus*.
- Establishing the presence or absence of true penicillin allergy is desirable (see Chapter 16).

CLINICAL PEARL

Most patients labeled with penicillin allergy are not allergic to penicillin. Always check the nature of the allergy and consider referral to an immunologist for further evaluation if the history indicates an immediate-type or other severe reaction. Lesser, unconvincing reactions can often be managed with a small test-dose of antibiotic.

Table 20-6 Activity of beta-lactams against selected bacteria commonly encountered in clinical practice

ANTIBIOTIC	*Staphylococcus aureus*[a]	*Streptococcus* spp.	*Enterococcus* spp.[b]	Coliforms[c]	ESCAPPM/ SPACE	*Pseudomonas aeruginosa*[d]	Anaerobes[e]
Penicillins							
Penicillin	5%	+++	+++	–	–	–	V
Ampicillin, amoxycillin	5%	+++	+++	±	–	–	V
Flucloxacillin, nafcillin	+++	+	–	–	–	–	–
Ticarcillin, piperacillin	5%	+++	+++	V	–	++	V
Amoxycillin/clavulanate	+++	+++	+++	++	–	–	+++
Piperacillin/tazobactam	+++	+++	+	+++	–	++	+++
Cephalosporins							
Cefazolin, cephalexin	+++	+++	–	+	–	–	–
Cefotetan	+	++	–	++	–	–	–
Cefoxitin	+	+	–	++	–	–	+
Ceftriaxone, cefotaxime	++	++	–	+++	–	–	–
Ceftazidime	–	–	–	+++	–	+++	–
Cefepime, cefpirome	++	+++	–	+++	+++	+++	–
Monobactams							
Aztreonam	–	–	–	+++	+++	+++	–
Carbapenems							
Meropenem	+++	+++	+	+++	+++	+++	+++
Ertapenem	+++	+++	+	+++	+++	–	+++

[a] Methicillin-resistant *S. aureus* (MRSA) strains are resistant to all beta-lactams (except new anti-MRSA cephalosporins such as ceftaroline).

[b] Vancomycin-resistant enterococci (VRE) are virtually always resistant to penicillins and carbapenems.

[c] Coliforms are common *Enterobacteriaceae*, i.e. *Escherichia coli, Klebsiella pneumonia, K. oxytoca* and *Proteus mirabilis*.

[e] *Pseudomonas aeruginosa* is intrinsically resistant to most antibiotics; it can also acquire resistance to anti-pseudomonal antibiotics.

[f] Anaerobes are considered as a group, as most infections are polymicrobial and speciation is not performed by diagnostic laboratories except in special circumstances.

+++, >90% effective; ++, 50–90% effective; +, 10–50% effective; –, <10% of strains are susceptible; ESCAPPM, *Enterobacter* spp., *Serratia* spp., *Citrobacter* spp., *Acinetobacter* spp., *Proteus vulgaris, Providentia* spp. and *Morganella* spp.; SPACE, *Serratia* spp., *Proteus vulgaris, Acinetobacter* spp., *Citrobacter* spp. and *Enterobacter* spp.; V, variable, depending on strain.

Non-beta-lactams

A summary of the activity of common non-beta-lactams against commonly encountered bacteria is shown in Table 20-7.

Aminoglycosides

Aminoglycosides include streptomycin, gentamicin, netilmicin, tobramycin and amikacin.

- Aminoglycosides cover aerobic Gram-negative organisms (*Enterobacteriaceae* and *P. aeruginosa*), but not Gram-positive organisms or anaerobes.
- Gentamicin is the most commonly used aminoglycoside, and tobramycin and amikacin are reserved for infections with gentamicin-resistant bacteria. Amikacin also has a special role in atypical *Mycobacterium* and *Nocardia* infections.
- Synergy between aminoglycosides and cell-wall-active agents such as glycopeptides and penicillins is seen in most enterococci, hence the use in enterococcal endocarditis.
- Aminoglycosides are rapidly bactericidal and are important drugs in treating Gram-negative bacteremia, but they have considerable renal and 8th nerve toxicity.
- Risk factors for toxicity include age, excessive dosing, or prolonged regimens, but vestibular toxicity can occur after just a single dose.
- Deafness and loss of vestibular function is often permanent and very disabling. As a consequence of this, it is recommended to use aminoglycosides empirically for short courses only. Commonly, a single dose of gentamicin is administered (with or without additional Gram-negative cover) while awaiting blood and urine cultures to guide ongoing therapy. It is important to ensure that the dose is sufficient for a patient's weight.
- Prolonged treatment is not justified except in the synergistic role for enterococcal endocarditis, and for treatment of some unusual infections such as extremely resistant Gram-negative bacilli, atypical mycobacteria and nocardioforms.

CLINICAL PEARL

If aminoglycosides are given for more than 2 days, it is essential to perform therapeutic drug monitoring. With once-daily dosing, trough levels are hard to interpret and various other methods are advised, with the most accurate being methods that calculate area under the curve.

Glycopeptides

These include vancomycin and teicoplanin.

- They inhibit cell wall synthesis of Gram-positive organisms.
- Both drugs are eliminated by renal excretion.
- They cover most Gram-positive organisms, but are less efficacious than beta-lactams for sensitive organisms and should be reserved for MRSA and coagulase-negative streptococci.
- Adverse drug reactions include renal and 8th nerve toxicity regimens in which higher doses are used to increase efficiency. Neutropenia and drug rashes (including DRESS syndrome) are seen.
- Therapeutic drug monitoring of trough levels is indicated to assess therapeutic efficacy.

CLINICAL PEARL

Too-rapid infusion of glycopeptides can cause a non-Ig-E-mediated histamine release from mast cells—the 'red person syndrome'.

Lipopeptides

- Lipopeptides include daptomycin, which acts by binding to the cell wall of Gram-positive bacteria in a calcium-dependent way, resulting in potassium efflux from the cell, loss of membrane potential and cell death.
- The spectrum of activity is very similar to that of vancomycin.
- Toxicity includes myalgias and pulmonary eosinophilia.
- Daptomycin is inactivated by pulmonary surfactant and should not be used in pneumonia; however, it is efficacious in hematogenous lung abscesses caused by *S. aureus*.
- It is equally efficacious as vancomycin for the treatment of MRSA endocarditis.

Macrolides/lincosamides

Macrolides and lincosamides, while chemically different, are grouped together because of their biological similarities.

- They bind to the 50S ribosomal subunits and inhibit protein translation.
- They cover *Staphylococcus aureus*, most strains of *Streptococcus pyogenes*, and have variable activity against *Streptococcus pneumoniae*.
- They also cover some anaerobes, *Legionella* species, *Mycoplasma pneumoniae* and have variable activity against *Chlamydia* species, but do not cover *Haemophilus influenzae*, *Moraxella catarrhalis* and Gram-negative bacilli.
- Erythromycin can cause problems with GI intolerance and can also cause hepatitis, deafness with high-dose IV regimens, and is quite irritating to veins. It has been largely superseded by newer macrolides.
- Lincomycin and clindamycin cover most strains of *S. aureus* and *S. pyogenes*, and have quite good activity against anaerobes but do not cover Gram-negatives. The most common side-effect is a maculopapular rash. They can cause GI upset, and clindamycin was the first drug to be reported to cause pseudomembranous colitis due to *Clostridium difficile*. Clindamycin also has the somewhat unique role as an inhibitor of superantigen synthesis when combined with penicillins in the treatment of severe infections caused by *Strep. pyogenes*.

Table 20-7 Activity of non-beta-lactams against bacteria commonly encountered in clinical practice

ANTIBIOTIC	*Staphylo-coccus aureus*[a]	MRSA[b]	*Strepto-coccus* spp.	*Entero-coccus* spp.[c]	Coli-forms[d]	ESCAPPM/ SPACE	*Pseudo-monas aerugi-nosa*[e]	Anae-robes[f]
Aminoglycosides	−[g]	−[i,g,h]	−	−	+++	+++	++	−
Vancomycin, teicoplanin	+++	+++[i]	+++	+++	−	−	−	Gram+
Daptomycin	+++	+++	+++	+++	−	−	−	Gram+
Erythromycin	++	V	V	−	−	−	−	V
Clindamycin	+++	V	+	−	−	−	−	++
Azithromycin	++	−	++	−	++[i]	−	−	−
Nalidixic acid	−	−	−	−	+++	+++	−	−
Ofloxacin	+++	V	++	−	++	++	−	−
Ciprofloxacin	+++	V	V	−	+++	+++	+++	−
Moxifloxacin	+++	+	+++	−	+++	+++	++	++
Linezolid	+++	+++	+++	+++	−	−	−	−
Co-trimoxazole	+++	V	+	V	V	V	−	+
Tetracycline	+++	V	V	V	V	V	−	++
Tigecycline[j]	+++	+++	+++	+++	+++	+++	−	++
Rifampicin	+++	+++	−	−	−	−	−	−
Fusidic acid	+++	+++	−	−	−	−	−	−
Chloramphenicol	+++	+++	++	−	++	++	−	++
Colistin	−	−	−	−	+++[k]	+++[k]	+++	−
Fosfomycin	−	−	−	−	+++	+++	−	−
Mupirocin[l]	+++	+++	−	−	−	−	−	−
Metronidazole	−	−	−	−	−	−	−	+++

[a] Methicillin-sensitive *Staphylococcus aureus*.

[b] Methicillin-resistant *Staphylococcus aureus* (MRSA) strains have variable susceptibilities to non-beta-lactams and these are strain-dependent, vary between geographical locations and on whether the acquisition is community- or healthcare-related. Typically, nosocomial strains are multidrug-resistant but retain susceptibility to glycopeptides, lipopeptides, linezolid, quinupristin/dalfopristin, tigecycline, rifampicin, fusidic acid, chloramphenicol and mupirocin; community strains are typically susceptible to most or all non-beta-lactams with the most common resistance being to macrolides/lincosamides.

[c] Vancomycin-resistant enterococci (VRE) are resistant to most drugs but usually retain susceptibility to linezolid, quinupristin/dalfopristin, daptomycin, and tigecycline.

[d] Coliforms are common *Enterobacteriaceae*, i.e. *Escherichia coli*, *Klebsiella pneumonia*, *K. oxytoca* and *Proteus mirabilis*.

[e] *Pseudomonas aeruginosa* is intrinsically resistant to most antibiotics; it can also acquire resistance to anti-pseudomonal antibiotics.

[f] Anaerobes are considered as a group, as most infections are polymicrobial and speciation is not performed by diagnostic laboratories except in special circumstances.

[g] Some strains of *S. aureus* test susceptible *in vitro*, but aminoglycosides are ineffective as monotherapy and there is no impact on mortality or length of stay in combination with cell-wall-active agents.

[h] Some rare strains of MRSA have reduced susceptibility to vancomycin.

[i] Azithromycin is active against *Salmonella enterica* Typhi, including multidrug-resistant strains and *Shigella* spp.

[j] Tigecycline has low blood levels and therefore is ineffective for bloodstream infections.

[k] *Proteus* spp. are highly resistant.

[l] Topical only.

+++, >90% effective; ++, 50–90% effective; +, 10–50% effective; −, <10% of strains are susceptible; ESCAPPM, *Enterobacter* spp., *Serratia* spp., *Citrobacter* spp., *Acinetobacter* spp., *Proteus vulgaris*, *Providentia* spp. and *Morganella* spp.; Gram+, Gram-positive anaerobes only; SPACE, *Serratia* spp., *Proteus vulgaris*, *Acinetobacter* spp., *Citrobacter* spp. and *Enterobacter* spp.; V, variable, depending on strain.

- Azithromycin has good coverage against atypical respiratory pathogens and *Chlamydia* species, and is usually well tolerated but can cause GI upset. Azithromycin has activity against some *Enterobacteriaceae*, and has a new role in the treatment of multiresistant *Salmonella enterica* subspecies Typhi.
- Roxithromycin is an orally available macrolide, with coverage against atypical pneumonia agents such as *M. pneumoniae* and *Chlamydia* spp., and is also active against *Haemophilus* and *Moraxella* spp. and has variable activity against *S. aureus*, *S. pyogenes* and *S. pneumoniae*. It is usually well tolerated.
- Clarithromycin is active against atypical respiratory pathogens, has variable activity against *S. pneumoniae*, is active against *M. pneumoniae* and *Chlamydia* spp., and is the most active macrolide against atypical mycobacteria. Clarithromycin is usually well tolerated, but can cause GI intolerance and hypersensitivity reactions.

Quinolones

Quinolones include nalidixic acid, early-generation fluoroquinolones including norfloxacin, ciprofloxacin and ofloxacin, and newer-generation fluoroquinolones including levofloxacin and moxifloxacin.

- These drugs have a dual ring structure and differ in their side-chain moieties, which affect the antibacterial spectrum and pharmacokinetic properties. They act by inhibiting type II isomerases, DNA gyrase and topoisomerase IV, causing degradation of DNA and cell death.
- Most quinolones have good oral bioavailability, such that IV use is not indicated except in malabsorption states.
- Norfloxacin has low blood levels and is only used for urinary tract infection and enteric fever.
- Ciprofloxacin and norfloxacin had excellent coverage against *Enterobacteriaceae* and *P. aeruginosa* when introduced, but resistance is now common in many parts of the world. Later-generation compounds have better Gram-positive coverage, and also are active against anaerobes, *M. pneumoniae*, *Chlamydia* spp. and *Mycobacteria* spp., including the tubercule bacillus.
- The most common adverse drug effect is GI tract intolerance.
- Rupture of the Achilles' tendon has been reported, due to interference with cross-linking of type IV collagen.
- Quinolones can also cause neurological manifestations including confusion and seizures, particularly in the elderly, and more unusually can cause hepatitis and acute renal failure.
- QTc prolongation can occur with later-generation quinolones.

Oxazolidinones

- Linezolid is the first oxazolidinone, which acts by a novel mechanism to inhibit protein synthesis by binding to the 50S ribosome at its interface with the 30S

sub-unit, preventing formation of the 70S initiation complex.
  - » It has consistent activity against Gram-positive bacteria.
  - » It has no activity against most Gram-negative organisms except *Neisseria* spp.
  - » There is *in vitro* activity against some atypical mycobacteria and nocardioforms.
- Despite being bacteriostatic, it is efficacious in serious *S. aureus* infections; including endocarditis, where it has been used in treatment of strains with reduced vancomycin susceptibility.
- It might be superior to vancomycin for MRSA pneumonia.
- It is also useful for VRE infections.
- Resistance is rare, but is increasingly seen.
- Anemia and thrombocytopenia are commonly seen in patients treated for >2 weeks, and occasionally irreversible peripheral and optic neuropathy is seen.

Folate antagonists

- Sulfonamides and trimethoprim inhibit sequential steps of folic acid synthesis. They are absorbed orally with high bioavailability, and penetrate into most tissues including bone, and the CNS.
- Due to resistance, coverage of commonly encountered staphylococci, streptococci and coliforms is uneven; it does not cover *Haemophilus* spp., *Moraxella* spp. or *P. aeruginosa*.
- Co-trimoxazole (trimethoprim/sulfamethoxazole) has a special role in the treatment of *Pneumocystis jirovecii*, *Listeria monocytogenes*, and *Nocardia* spp. infections.
- The sulfonamide moiety is responsible for most of the serious side-effects, including skin rashes, Stevens–Johnson syndrome, erythema multiforme, hepatitis, interstitial nephritis, and drug fever.
- 50% of patients with AIDS treated with high-dose co-trimoxazole develop a rash; roughly half can be desensitized.

Tetracyclines and tigecycline

- Tetracyclines bind to the 30S ribosomal sub-unit, inhibiting protein synthesis.
- These drugs are well absorbed orally and penetrate into all tissues except the CNS.
- Many different tetracyclines have been available, and mainly differ in their half-life.
- They are broad-spectrum antibiotics, but widespread resistance has emerged by several mechanisms including active efflux, ribosomal mutations, and changes in permeability. An interesting historical observation is that the introduction of tetracycline in 1948 is believed to have resulted in the global dissemination of the clone of group B streptococcus that today causes most invasive disease in neonates.

- Coverage of *S. aureus*, *Streptococcus* spp., *Enterobacteriaceae* and anaerobes is patchy, but these drugs are particularly useful for *Chlamydia* spp., *Mycoplasma* spp., *Rickettsia* spp. and prophylaxis of malaria.
- They also have non-antimicrobial uses in dermatology and for pleurodesis.

CLINICAL PEARL

Adverse drug reactions to tetracyclines include staining of non-erupted teeth, and thus these drugs are contra-indicated in pregnancy, lactation and in children less than 8 years of age. Doxycycline is thought to be safe, although it is generally best to use an alternative agent where possible.

- Tetracyclines can cause photosensitization and GI upset.
- Doxycycline must be taken in the upright position with plenty of fluids to avoid lodgement in the esophagus, causing a severe burn.
- Minocycline can also cause benign intracranial hypertension, skin pigmentation and vertigo.
- Tigecycline is only available intravenously and is extremely broad-spectrum, covering most Gram-positive and Gram-negative pathogens (except *P. aeruginosa*) and anaerobes, and also has activity against MRSA, VRE, multiresistant *Enterobacteriaceae*, and atypical mycobacteria. It can cause severe gastrointestinal intolerance.

Rifamycins

- Rifamycins include rifampicin and rifabutin. These agents inhibit DNA-dependent RNA polymerase. They are well absorbed orally, and can be given intravenously. They have a short half-life, but a long post-antibiotic effect and are given once daily.
- These drugs penetrate most tissues including bone, but do not penetrate into the CNS. Coverage is broad, including *S. aureus*, *Mycobacteria* spp., selected Gram-negative organisms (e.g. *N. meningitidis* and *H. influenzae*, where they have a public health but not a treatment role), and anaerobes. They have no activity against streptococci.
- Rifampicin penetrates well into the nasopharynx, and thus is useful in eradicating staphylococcal carriage states (in combination treatment), and as monotherapy in prophylaxis against *N. meningitidis* and *H. influenzae* type B.
- High-level resistance by single base-pair mutation occurs rapidly if monotherapy is given, so combination treatment is given, e.g. in the treatment of tuberculosis or MRSA infections.
- Rifamycins are potent inducers of hepatic cytochrome enzymes, and thus diminish the activity of drugs such as warfarin, hormonal contraceptives, and anticonvulsants. These agents stain the urine and tears. Other side-effects include hepatitis, drug fever, rashes, and interstitial nephritis.

Fusidic acid

Fusidic acid is a steroid antibiotic which interferes with cell wall synthesis and elongation factor G.

- It is well absorbed orally. It can be given intravenously, but can cause significant hepatitis given in this way.
- It penetrates into most tissues, including bone and the CNS.
- Fusidic acid covers *S. aureus*, including most MRSA strains, but it does not cover streptococci or Gram-negative organisms, and anaerobes.
- Adverse drug reactions include GI tract intolerance, hepatitis, and rashes.

CLINICAL PEARL

The combination of fusidic acid and HMG-CoA reductase inhibitors is associated with rhabdomyolysis, including fatal cases. If fusidic acid must be used, e.g. for treatment of multiresistant MRSA infections, it is recommended to stop the HMG-CoA reductase inhibitor for the period the patient takes fusidic acid.

Chloramphenicol

Chloramphenicol binds to the 50S ribosomal sub-units, inhibiting protein synthesis.

- This drug is bacteriostatic.
- It is very well absorbed and universally distributed in the body, including into the CNS.
- It has very broad spectrum of coverage of most aerobic and anaerobic organisms, and had roles in invasive infections with *S. enterica* Typhi, *H. influenzae* and *N. meningitidis* until superseded by other drugs.
- Chloramphenicol induces reversible myelosuppression commonly, but has a 1:10,000 risk of aplastic anemia, and accordingly is rarely used in Western countries. Topical preparations remain widely used and do not incur this risk.

Colistin

Colistin is a detergent which disrupts bacterial cell walls, and is particularly active against aerobic Gram-negative bacilli, except *Proteus* spp.

- Due to significant renal toxicity it was relegated to topical use until the emergence of extremely drug-resistant Gram-negative pathogens such as *Acinetobacter baumannii* and *P. aeruginosa*, where there were few other options.
- A major problem with this drug is that blood levels are usually just above the minimum inhibitory concentration (MIC) of infecting organisms.
- The drug is efficacious in bloodstream infections, but not in other infections such as ventilator-associated pneumonia, where lung tissue levels are less than the MIC.
- Colistin has also been shown to be efficacious and nontoxic when administered intrathecally in the treatment of multi-antibiotic resistant *A. baumannii* meningitis.

Fosfomycin

Fosfomycin inhibits an enzyme which catalyzes the first step in bacterial cell wall synthesis.

- It is a bactericidal agent with a broad spectrum of activity, including MRSA and multidrug-resistant *Enterobacteriaceae* and *P. aeruginosa*.
- The drug is readily absorbed following oral administration and achieves moderate blood levels with a half-life of 6–12 hours.
- It is excreted unchanged in urine and feces and penetrates into most sites except the CSF. As an oral agent it is mostly only used in the treatment of multidrug-resistant UTIs.
- When administered intravenously, it has been used in the treatment of urinary tract infection, and has also been used in small groups of patients with other infections such as osteomyelitis or severe staphylococcal infections, and has been trialed in surgical prophylaxis.

Nitroimidazoles

Metronidazole and tinidazole are commercially available nitroimidazoles.

- These are well absorbed after most routes of administration, and have excellent tissue penetration, including the CNS and bone. Activity is high against most anaerobes except *Peptostreptococcus* spp., and they also cover protozoans such as *Giardia intestinalis* and *Gardnerella vaginalis*.
- Adverse drug reactions include metallic taste, and a disulfiram–like interaction with ethanol, which is to be avoided during therapy with this agent.

CLINICAL PEARL

When considering empiric treatment for anaerobic infections, a useful rule is to use metronidazole 'below the diaphragm', i.e. for intra-abdominal sepsis, and to use clindamycin or a beta-lactam/beta-lactamase inhibitor combination 'above the diaphragm', i.e. for lung abscess or orofacial sepsis.

Antibiotic resistance

Resistance to antibacterial agents can be coded for by genes on the bacterial chromosome and/or plasmids. There are four basic mechanisms of resistance, as shown in Table 20-8.

Table 20-8 Mechanisms of antibiotic resistance, with typical examples

MECHANISM	SPECIFIC ENTITY	ANTIBIOTIC	TYPICAL SPECIES
Inactivating enzymes			
Beta-lactamases	Penicillinase	Penicillin	*Staphylococcus aureus*
	TEM/SHV beta-lactamase	Amoxicillin	*Escherichia coli*
	Extended-spectrum beta-lactamase (ESBL)	Ceftriaxone	*Klebsiella pneumoniae*
	Metallo-beta-lactamase (MBL)	Meropenem	*Enterobacteriaceae*
Aminoglycoside-modifying enzymes		Gentamicin	*Klebsiella pneumoniae*
Acetyl transferases	Chloramphenicol acetyl transferase (CAT)	Chloramphenicol	*Salmonella enterica*
Altered target sites			
Penicillin-binding proteins (PBPs)	Modified PBP2a	Methicillin	Methicillin-resistant *Staphylococcus aureus*
DNA gyrase		Ciprofloxacin	*Staphylococcus aureus*
Ribosomes	MLS$_B$	Erythromycin	*Staphylococcus aureus*
RNA polymerase	*rpo*B	Rifampicin	*Staphylococcus aureus*
Dihydrofolate reductase	Various	Sulfonamides	*Escherichia coli*
Decreased permeability			
Altered porins	Various	Meropenem	*Pseudomonas aeruginosa*
Active efflux			
	*tet*M	Tetracyclines	*Enterobacteriaceae*

DNA, deoxyribonucleic acid; MLS$_B$, macrolide, lincosamide and streptogramin B; RNA; ribonucleic acid; *rpo*B, gene encoding RNA polymerase; SHV, sulfhydryl variable specificity; *tet*M, tetracycline resistance gene.

Antiviral agents

CLINICAL PEARL

Antiviral agents are virustatic rather than virucidal, and thus efficacy relies on the host immune system. Thus in the immunosuppressed, especially with herpes viruses, ongoing antiviral suppression is often required.

Drug susceptibility testing is problematic with antiviral agents, because readily available *in vitro* systems to test this do not exist in clinical laboratories. However, with the maturation of molecular technology, testing for known resistance determinants in specific viruses can be done. Additionally, in infections such as HIV, hepatitis B and hepatitis C, viral load can be quantitated by PCR, which can be used to ascertain disease activity and gauge the efficacy of therapy.

Drugs used in the treatment of HIV/AIDS are discussed in Chapter 16; other antivirals are discussed below.

Interferons

Interferons are part of the antiviral immune response.

- Synthetic alpha-interferon has activity against hepatitis B, hepatitis C, HIV and human papillomaviruses.
- Interferons are not absorbed orally, and are administered generally by subcutaneous injection, or intralesionally for warts.

Treatment usually causes significant symptomatology, including influenza-like illness, depression, and reactivation of dormant autoimmune processes. Interferons are now little used in the treatment of chronic viral infections.

Nucleoside analogs

Aciclovir, famciclovir, valaciclovir

- Valaciclovir is a pro-drug of acyclovir (aciclovir).
- Famciclovir is the pro-drug of penciclovir.
- Aciclovir and penciclovir are phosphorylated by virally encoded thymidine kinase to monophosphate forms, which are phosphorylated to triphosphates by cellular kinases, which are then incorporated into DNA as a false base and terminate replication.
- These drugs are highly active against HSV-1 and HSV-2, and to a lesser degree against VZV. They do not inhibit CMV or EBV at levels achievable in humans.
- These drugs are well tolerated, with the main toxicity being renal impairment due to crystallization in the renal tubules, particularly with high-dose IV administration. This is less likely in adequately hydrated patients.
- Oral treatment is sufficient for minor HSV and VZV infections, but in severe disease, especially in immunosuppressed individuals, IV aciclovir is used.
- Resistance to these agents is seen in HSV in severe immunosuppression, such as untreated HIV infection.

- There is cross-resistance to all members in this category and also to ganciclovir, but not foscarnet, which is used in this situation.

Ganciclovir and valganciclovir

- Valganciclovir is the pro-drug of ganciclovir.
- Ganciclovir is not well absorbed orally, unlike valganciclovir.
- Ganciclovir is phosphorylated within infected cells by the CMV UL97 protein, and after further phosphorylation by cellular kinases inhibits CMV DNA polymerase, and thus viral replication.
- Ganciclovir is quite potent against HSV and VZV, but aciclovir and analogs are clinically effective and far less toxic, and thus ganciclovir is not used here.
- For CMV disease in the immunocompetent patient, ganciclovir is usually considered too toxic to use, but disease in the immunocompromised can be very severe and treatment normally consists of induction therapy with IV ganciclovir and then maintenance therapy. Recent guidelines now allow initial therapy with oral valganciclovir for certain conditions.
- Ganciclovir also has activity against EBV and the human herpesviruses HHV-6, HHV-8 and HHV-7, but this is not clinically useful.
- Ganciclovir causes bone marrow suppression. It is renally excreted, and dosage reduction is required in renal impairment.

Nucleotide analogs

Cidofovir

Cidofovir is a nucleotide analog active against HSV-1, HSV-2, CMV and VZV.

- It is nephrotoxic, and thus less frequently used than ganciclovir or foscarnet.
- It has a long half-life, allowing weekly dosing.
- It has a niche use in progressive vaccinia virus infections.

Direct DNA polymerase inhibitors

Foscarnet

Foscarnet is a pyrophosphate analog directly inhibiting herpesvirus DNA polymerase.

- It is particularly useful in aciclovir-resistant strains of herpes simplex and ganciclovir-resistant CMV.
- Foscarnet is eliminated by renal excretion, and dose reduction is required in renal impairment.
- The main adverse drug reaction is renal failure, and sometimes hypercalcemia and pancreatitis can occur.

Assembly/maturation/release agents

Oseltamivir and zanamivir

- These agents are active against influenza A and B, and work by inhibiting neuraminidase, which impairs virion assembly and release from infected cells.

- Despite widespread use in the H1N1/09 influenza pandemic, resistance was remarkably rare.
- Strains that are resistant to oseltamivir remain sensitive to zanamivir.
- Oseltamivir is available only as an oral formulation, which was problematic during the influenza pandemic where an IV neuraminidase inhibitor would have been useful. IV peramivir has become available in some countries.

Other antivirals

Ribavirin

- Ribavirin is a purine analog requiring intracellular phosphorylation for antiviral activity, the exact mechanism of which is unclear.
- *In vitro* activity against many DNA and RNA viruses is seen, but this is not replicated clinically for most of these.
- Respiratory syncytial virus (RSV) infections respond to nebulized ribavirin; however, ribavirin is quite toxic, teratogenic, and possibly carcinogenic to healthcare workers. Administration requires the use of a tent apparatus to isolate the patient from the healthcare workers for occupational health. It is therefore usually given orally or intravenously for this indication, a route that does not have demonstrated efficacy.
- Ribavirin was used in the early stages of the severe acute respiratory syndrome (SARS) epidemic in 2002/2003 but was found to lack efficacy.
- Although ribavirin exhibits activity against hepatitis C virus, it has been superseded by the newer directly-acting agents.
- Ribavirin has been used in severe measles and viral hemorrhagic fevers, and had been used in influenza prior to the availability of neuraminidase inhibitors.

Antifungals

Antifungal drugs were slow in development because of the similarities of complicated fungal cell metabolism to that of mammalian cells. Early agents were far too toxic to be clinically useful. Antifungal therapy was revolutionized by the development of azoles, which are considerably less toxic as well as efficacious, and most recent agents have very broad-spectrum activity. The classification and activity spectra of modern antifungals against selected fungal pathogens are shown in Table 20-9 (overleaf).

Azoles

- Azoles inhibit C14 alpha-demethylase, which interferes with the synthesis of an important cell wall constituent, ergosterol.
- A wide repertoire of systemic azoles is now available, including ketoconazole, fluconazole, itraconazole, voriconazole and posaconazole.
- Miconazole is only used as a topical agent.

Ketoconazole

Ketoconazole is an early azole with significant hepatotoxicity and GI intolerance. It also inhibits P450 cytochrome enzymes, resulting in drug interactions. It is mostly only used now as a topical agent, e.g. for treatment of seborrheic dermatitis.

Itraconazole

Itraconazole is active against yeasts and molds, including *Aspergillus* spp.

- Patients with AIDS and bone-marrow transplants have decreased absorption.
- Blood levels are quite variable, and in serious infections therapeutic drug monitoring is recommended.
- There is low penetration into the CNS, but good penetration into most other tissues.
- The drug inhibits P450 cytochrome enzymes.

Fluconazole

Fluconazole is a triazole drug with good activity against yeasts, particularly *Candida* spp. (except some intrinsically resistant species: *C. krusei*, *C. parapsilosis* and most *C. glabrata*) and *Cryptococcus* spp.

- Intravenous and oral formulations are available.
- Oral bioavailability is excellent, so this route is preferred except in malabsorption states.
- Penetration into all tissues is excellent, including vitreous humor, subarachnoid space and brain parenchyma.
- The drug is eliminated by the kidney.
- The drug is well tolerated usually, with much less hepatotoxicity than with other azoles.
- Like other azoles, it inhibits cytochrome P450 enzymes, resulting in drug interactions.

Voriconazole

Voriconazole has significant activity against molds, especially *A. fumigatus*, and emerging mold species such as *Scedosporium* spp.

- There is good oral absorption, and there is also an IV preparation.
- It is necessary to give a loading dose to get patients to therapeutic levels, which is particularly important in systemic infections.
- Voriconazole is used prophylactically in acute myeloid leukemia (AML) and transplantation patients experiencing severe immunosuppression.
- While suppressing infections with *Candida* spp. and *Aspergillus* spp., emerging infections with species resistant to voriconazole, such as agents of mucormycosis, are now being seen.
- Pharmacokinetics are highly variable between individuals, necessitating therapeutic drug monitoring.
- Toxicity includes visual disturbances and hallucinations due to effects on the retina, but only last a day or two; this is more likely in patients with high blood levels.

Table 20-9 Activity of antifungal agents against selected yeasts and molds seen in systemic fungal infections

| | YEASTS | | | | | DIMORPHIC FUNGI | MOLDS | | | |
| | Candida spp. | | | | Crypto-coccus spp. | Histo-plasma capsulatum | Asper-gillus fumigatus | Scedos-porium prolificans | Fusarium solani | Agents of mucor-mycosis |
	C. albicans	C. glabrata	C. krusei	C. parapsilosis						
Azoles										
Ketoconazole	+	–	–	–	–	–	–	–	–	–
Itraconazole	++	–	–	–	–	++	++	–	–	–
Fluconazole	+++	+	–	–	+++	–	–	–	–	–
Voriconazole	+++	++	++	++	+++	++	+++	+++a	++	–
Posaconazole	+++	+++	++	++	+++	++	+++	+++	++	++
Polyenes										
Amphotericin B	+++	+++	+++	+++	+++b	+++	++	–	+	+++
Echinocandins										
Caspofungin	+++	+++	+++	+++	–	not used	++	–	not used	–
Allylamines										
Terbinafine	–	–	–	–	–	not used	not used	+++a	–	–
Miscellaneous										
5-Flucytosinec	not used	not used	not used	not used	+++b	not used	not used	not used	not used	–

a The combination of voriconazole and terbinafine shares *in vitro* synergy; case reports demonstrate clinical efficacy of this combination.
b The combination of flucytosine with amphotericin B results in better outcomes in non-immunocompromised patients with cryptococcal meningitis.
c 5-Flucytosine monotherapy results in the rapid emergence of resistance in most fungi.

- Voriconazole can derange liver function tests, and is an inhibitor of cytochrome P450 enzymes, causing important interactions with many of the drugs used in transplantation.

Posaconazole

Posaconazole has a similar spectrum of activity and side-effects to voriconazole. It is only available as an oral preparation, and absorption is better if given with fatty foods.

Therapeutic drug monitoring for azoles

Pharmacokinetics of azoles are highly variable, particularly for itraconazole, voriconazole and posaconazole, and thus for serious infections in which these agents are used, therapeutic drug monitoring is recommended. It is typically used as a prophylactic agent during treatment for acute leukemias and in bone marrow transplantation.

Ampholenes

Amphotericin B intercalates between phospholipids, disrupting the lipid structure of the cell membrane of fungi, causing cell death.

- Amphotericin B deoxycholate is the original formulation. It is considerably toxic, causing predictable short-term and long-term renal impairment, and fever and rigors with infusion. It is now rarely used.
- More recent lipid preparations are less toxic but considerably more expensive.
- Amphotericin B is broadly active against most molds and yeasts, except for *Scedosporium* spp. and *Fusarium* spp.

Echinocandins

Echinocandins (caspofungin, anidulafungin and micafungin) inhibit glucan formation in the fungal cell wall, terminating cell replication.

- Although not absorbed orally, good levels are obtained following IV administration, and these drugs penetrate well into most tissues, the main exception being the urinary tract.
- They are eliminated by hepatic excretion, but do not interact with the cytochrome P450 system.
- Side-effects have been relatively few; they do not appear to interact with many medications, unlike the azoles, and thus are particularly useful in transplantation.
- Echinocandins have excellent activity against most *Candida* and *Aspergillus* spp., but are not active against fungi lacking glucan such as *Cryptococcus* spp.

SPECIFIC SYNDROMES

Acute fever

The steps in Table 20-10 are suggested in managing those with acute onset of fever.

Table 20-10 Management of acute fever

STEP	COMMENT
Identify patients requiring urgent intervention	Vital signs consistent with shock Confusion, seizures, dehydration Meningitis Sepsis in asplenic patients Infective endocarditis Febrile neutropenia
Identify people with localized or easily diagnosed infection	Many infections have a typical clinical syndrome, for example pneumonia, gastroenteritis
Identify patients potentially harboring serious infection	Rapid progression Rigors Muscle pain Decreased level of consciousness Vomiting, especially with abdominal pain or headache Unexplained rash Jaundice Elderly patients Injection-drug users Diabetes mellitus Travel history Possibility of zoonosis Contact with meningococcal disease
Investigations	'Septic work-up': —Full blood count —Chest X-ray —Urine analysis and urine microscopy and culture —Blood cultures —Imaging
Admission	Patients with possibility of serious infection or presence of risk factors, as outlined above Patient re-presenting with febrile illness Temporal course suggesting progression

Pyrexia of unknown origin (PUO)

Pyrexia or fever of unknown origin is defined as a patient with an unexplained fever despite an extensive set of investigations, generally over at least 1 week for a hospitalized patient, and 2 or 3 weeks for one investigated as an outpatient. Such investigation would include the usual septic work-up (shown in Table 20-10), plus organ imaging and investigation for autoimmune disease. Positron emission tomography (PET) is being increasingly used in the assessment of patients with PUOs.

Common causes of PUO are shown in Table 20-11, overleaf.

Table 20-11 Common and important causes of fever of unknown origin

INFECTIONS		
TYPE	**EXAMPLES**	**COMMENT ON DISEASE MANIFESTATIONS**
Bacterial/ mycobacterial	Tuberculosis (TB)	Typically has a focus that should be evident on physical examination or imaging. Miliary TB usually evident on chest X-ray but requires mycobacterial culture of blood for confirmation.
	Non-tuberculous mycobacteriosis	Mycobacterium avium complex is a classic cause of persistent fever in advanced HIV infection (and other rarer causes of immunodeficiency), accompanied by hepatitis, weight loss and diarrhea.
	Endocarditis	Classic viridans streptococcal endocarditis may be remarkably sub-acute (hence 'SBE'), with diagnosis compounded by the fact that blood culture is sometimes omitted from the work-up of FUO in ambulatory care settings. Culture-negative endocarditis is commonly related to prior/ongoing antibiotic treatment; less commonly caused by unusual pathogens such as Coxiella (Q fever), Bartonella, etc.
	Implanted cardiac device infection	Both the generator pocket and the lead may become infected, with non-specific focal signs and negative cultures of blood.
	Deep abscess	Typically discovered on abdominopelvic CT. Repeated imaging often required.
	Osteoarticular infections	In children, as a cause of FUO, mostly occurs as long bone osteomyelitis. In adults, occurs with vertebral osteomyelitis (although usually with focal pain), or following fracture fixation, joint replacement or reconstructive procedures, including sternotomy for cardiac surgery.
	Urinary tract infection	Chronic pyelonephritis (although now less common than in times past) may present with little in the way of typical lower urinary tract symptoms. Often caused by resistant pathogens and associated with multiple prior courses of antibiotic treatment. May be associated with underlying structural abnormalities such as vesicoureteric reflux.
	Pericarditis	Requires ECG and echocardiography.
	Enteric fever (typhoid, paratyphoid)	Requires culture of blood and, occasionally, bone marrow.
	Syphilis	Secondary syphilis in particular can be a cause of FUO, typically accompanied by fever, rash, 'mucous patches' and lymphadenopathy.
	Brucellosis	Exposure history important: travel and occupational exposure to parturient or slaughtered grazing animals.
	Psittacosis	Often associated with history of exposure to sick caged birds (typically parrots and budgerigars).
	Q fever	Typically associated with exposure to parturient or slaughtered animals.
	Whipple's disease	Fever may accompany the classic tetrad of arthralgia, weight loss, diarrhea and abdominal pain. Other manifestations may occur.
Viral	CMV	Fever typically accompanied by elevated transaminases and lymphocytosis.
	EBV	Commonly evident as subacute pharyngotonsillitis, but may present with just fever, lymphadenopathy and splenomegaly.
	HIV	Seroconversion illness may be accompanied by fever, sore throat, rash, lymphadenopathy. Advanced, untreated disease complicated by opportunistic infections (see elsewhere). Newly treated disease may be associated with immune restoration inflammatory syndromes (IRIS).
Fungal	Histoplasmosis	An endemic mycosis that can have pulmonary, extrapulmonary and disseminated manifestations. Limited to certain geographic regions.

The approach to a patient with PUO is essentially that of any infectious disease, involving a very thorough history and examination. Diagnostic work-up generally starts with noninvasive tests, then works through imaging, and then more invasive tests involving tissue biopsies. The rapidity with which one would escalate through this range of tests depends on how unwell the patient is, and whether there are symptoms, signs or blood tests that are consistent with serious organic illness.

CLINICAL PEARL

When the cause of a patient's fever is not immediately obvious, cross-checking to make sure all elements of the history, examination and investigations, as described in the 'Clinical Approach to Infectious Diseases' above, is pivotal.

The initial round of investigation should ensure that pivotal sections of the history and examination and septic work-up are not being missed.

- The **history** of each symptom needs to be established with respect to time course, duration and severity.
- Collaborative history is often useful, and a history of occupational and animal exposures, overseas travel, sexual history and drug use should be sought.
- Physical **examination** is to be thorough, and as well as the usual cardiovascular, respiratory and abdominal examination, examination of the integument, lymph glands, eyes including fundi, temporal arteries, and thyroid gland for evidence of hyperthyroidism is necessary.
- Rectal, pelvic and breast examinations should be considered, and evidence of thrombosis sought.

Investigations should include:
- Full blood count and blood film examination.
- 3–4 sets of blood cultures.
- Acute phase reactants, including ESR, C-reactive protein and possibly pro-calcitonin.
- Urine analysis, urine microscopy, and culture.
- Chest X-ray.
- Liver function tests.
- Electrolytes, creatinine, and urea.
- Immunological tests, including anti-nuclear antibodies (ANA), rheumatoid factor, ANCA (anti-neutrophil cytoplasmic autoantibody), anti-double-stranded DNA (ds-DNA) antibodies, and antiphospholipid antibodies.
- HIV testing should be performed on any patient with unexplained illness, after appropriate counseling and obtaining of consent. Not all patients with HIV have typical risk factors, and occasionally patients are not aware of or deny the presence of risk factors. Missing the diagnosis of HIV will have untoward consequences as the real diagnosis of HIV will be delayed, resulting in more investigations including invasive ones being performed, and definitive effective treatment will not occur until the correct diagnosis is made, and

HIV complications may develop if HIV treatment is delayed.

- Serological testing should include an HIV antibody test and testing for EBV and CMV, and, depending on likelihood, entities such as Q-fever, brucellosis, leptospirosis, syphilis, psittacosis, toxoplasmosis and hepatitis A, B and C.
- Tuberculosis should be sought specifically with a full range of tests.
- Organ **imaging** is pivotal in evaluating PUO. Many occult diagnoses of yesteryear such as liver abscesses are readily diagnosed by CT.
- Nucleotide imaging is sometimes useful. Gallium scanning can help elucidate which organ system may be responsible in more obscure cases. Occasionally, a bone scan can detect inflammatory conditions of the bones such as osteomyelitis, and entities such as SAPPHO syndrome (synovitis, acne, palmo-plantar pustulosis, hyperostosis, osteitis). The role of SPECT scanning in diagnosing PUO is being researched; it may have a role similar to gallium scanning.
- Echocardiography is essential to rule out endocarditis.

If the diagnosis is not forthcoming, further rounds of investigation and their invasiveness will depend on how ill the patient is, and whether there is evidence of serious organic disease. If this is so, more invasive tests such as tissue biopsies should be considered. Note that it is important to revisit the history and examination as a vital piece of information may be detected, or a helpful symptom or sign may develop, which might help in making the diagnosis.

- Tissues such as skin, lymph nodes, muscle and bone marrow are generally safely sampled. Repeat biopsy of enlarged lymph nodes should be considered if initial biopsies are non-diagnostic and a PUO remains unresolved.
- Other more invasive biopsies should be reserved for those in which the diagnosis is elusive and imaging or blood tests suggest a particular organ is involved such as the liver.

Occasionally, diagnostic laparotomy has been used in the past to diagnose PUO. This has been supplanted by laparoscopy, which is much safer for the patient, allows direct visualization of most intra-abdominal organs and allows for sampling under controlled conditions.

CLINICAL PEARL

The longer a PUO remains undiagnosed, the more likely it is to have a non-infective cause, e.g. lymphoma, auto-inflammatory or autoimmune condition. Do not forget long-term medications (e.g. phenytoin) as potential causes of PUOs.

Skin and soft tissue infections

A wide range of skin and soft tissue infections are seen in clinical practice, as shown in Table 20-12 (overleaf).

Table 20-12 Skin and soft tissue infections, and common pathogens

INFECTION	USUAL PATHOGENS	LESS-COMMON PATHOGENS
Impetigo	*Streptococcus pyogenes* *Staphylococcus aureus*	
Folliculitis	*Staphylococcus aureus*	*Pseudomonas aeruginosa* (spa pools) *Malassezia furfur*
Boils and carbuncles	*Staphylococcus aureus*	
Erysipelas (skin infection confined to the upper dermis; Figure 20-5)	*Streptococcus pyogenes*, group G streptococci	Group B streptococci
Cellulitis	*Streptococcus pyogenes* Group G streptococci Group C streptococci Group B streptococci (especially diabetics) *Staphylococcus aureus*	*Pseudomonas aeruginosa*; other resistant Gram-negative bacilli (immunosuppressed patients) *Pasteurella multocida* (cat or dog bites) *Aeromonas* spp. (fresh/brackish water; patients with cirrhosis) *Vibrio* spp. (salt/estuarine water; patients with cirrhosis) *Erysipelothrix rhusiopathiae* (injury from saltwater fish or crustaceans) *Mycobacterium marinum* (indolent infection after water exposure)

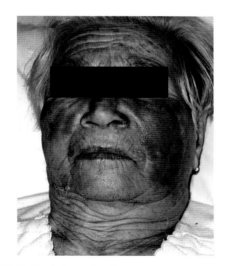

Figure 20-5 Facial erysipelas

Furuncles and carbuncles

- A *furuncle* is extension of folliculitis into the dermis.
- A *carbuncle* is the confluence of several furuncles, usually seen in areas of hairy skin.
- They are classically caused by *S. aureus*, and are the hallmark of community MRSA.

Treatment involves incision and drainage, and hygiene measures.

- It has been shown that for lesions less than 5 cm in diameter, incision and drainage alone is just as good as incision and drainage followed by antibiotics. Additionally, the widespread use of antibiotics increases resistance in MRSA.
- However, if the lesion is greater than 5 cm and/or systemic sepsis is present, systemic antibiotics should be used in addition to the main treatment of draining the lesion(s).
- It is important to take swabs, because many of these lesions are now due to MRSA strains, and the susceptibility to non-beta-lactams in MRSA strains is becoming less predictable.
- It is important to detect a history of recurrent boils in the patient or family members. If this is present, then a staphylococcal eradication regimen should be applied once all acutely pyogenic lesions are controlled.

CLINICAL PEARL

8-point plan to eradicate *Staphylococcus aureus* carriage:

1. Control all the patient's pyogenic lesions first.
2. Treat all family members simultaneously.
3. Take showers, not baths, and use an anti-staphylococcal soap or body cleanser.
4. Do not share towels, clothing, or other linen that comes into contact with the skin.
5. Wear clean clothes and pyjamas daily during the treatment period.
6. Avoid shaving affected areas.
7. Wash clothes and bed linen in hot water.
8. Apply nasal mupirocin ointment for 10 days.

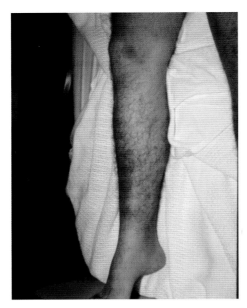

Figure 20-6 Cellulitis of the anterior aspect of the right leg

Failure of the above regimen usually means inadequate adherence, or a new staphylococcal carrier has been introduced to the group.

- If there has been adequate adherence and no identified re-introduction of *S. aureus*, then it is reasonable to consider repeating the regimen but also using systemic antibiotics, usually containing rifampicin in combination with another drug.
  - » Note that rifampicin has important drug interactions such as interfering with the oral contraceptive pill, which is usually an issue in these family groups.
  - » It is necessary to use a second agent in conjunction with rifampicin to prevent the emergence of resistance.

Cellulitis

Cellulitis is a pyogenic infection of the skin and soft tissue, and is usually caused by beta-hemolytic streptococci, sometimes in conjunction with *S. aureus*.

- Mostly it involves the lower limbs (Figure 20-6), and risk factors for this infection include obesity, tinea, ulcers, chronic venous disease, and diabetes mellitus.
- Gram-negative organisms can be introduced by certain exposures such as to water.
- Patients with hepatic cirrhosis are predisposed to infections with *Vibrio* and *Aeromonas* spp., which can be rapidly progressive.

In the case of mild cellulitis, blood cultures are generally negative, but in cases of sepsis then blood cultures can be very informative.

- Any purulent or ulcerated lesion should be swabbed. Sometimes the pathogen can be obtained by aspirating the leading edge.

- In *S. pyogenes* cellulitis the anti-streptolysin O titer (ASOT) and/or DNase B may be positive, but is not helpful if negative.

With respect to empirical therapy, anti-staphylococcal penicillins or 1st-generation cephalosporins cover both beta-hemolytic streptococci and *S. aureus*.

- If there are boils or abscesses, the possibility of MRSA should be covered. Non-beta-lactam antibiotics such as trimethoprim-sulfamethoxazole or clindamycin may be indicated.
- If there are risk factors for Gram-negative organisms, cover should be broadened.

It is vitally important to recognize abscess collections, infected foreign bodies and surgical hardware, and necrotizing fasciitis, all being conditions that may require urgent surgical management. Necrotizing fasciitis is suggested by rapid progression with severe pain, and a much discolored limb in a septicemic patient. This should prompt referral to a surgeon for urgent debridement, sending samples to the laboratory for microbiological examination. Hyperbaric oxygen should be considered. *S. pyogenes* and polymicrobial coliform/anaerobe infections need to be covered, generally with a carbapenem plus a lincosamide (such as clindamycin) to inhibit ribosomal translation of exotoxins should the etiology be *S. pyogenes*. Once the pathogen is identified, antibiotics can be modified.

Drug fever

It is important to recognize drug fevers to avoid to avoid unnecessarily long and repeated courses of antibiotics and series of investigations. It is important to have a full history of the drugs that have been taken in the past few weeks, including those that have been discontinued. Certain drugs, such as phenytoin, may cause fever only after long periods of treatment.

Table 20-13 lists some drugs known to cause drug fever, classified by pathological mechanism.

Factors suggesting the possibility of drug fever:

- Patient taking medication known to cause fever
- Initiation of possible offending agent within the last week or two before fever
- Absence of a clinical source of infection
- Patient looks relatively well
- Relative bradycardia
- Rash
- Eosinophilia
- Particular organ dysfunction which may be part of the drug reaction, including derangement of liver function tests and elevated creatinine
- Fever resolves within days of terminating the offending drug
- Re-challenge that causes fever is highly suggestive (but could result in a more serious reaction and is generally best avoided).

Table 20-13 Drugs known to cause drug fever

TYPE OF REACTION	IMPLICATED DRUGS
Hypersensitivity	Phenytoin, carbamazepine
	Penicillins, cephalosporins
	Sulfonamides
	Nitrofurantoin, minocycline
	Abacavir
	Allopurinol
	Alpha-methyldopa
Thermoregulator interference	Major tranquilizers, tricyclic antidepressants
	Methylenedioxymethamphetamine (Ecstasy), amphetamines, cocaine
Direct pyrogens	Amphotericin B
	Pharmacological drug action
	Tumor lysis syndrome following chemotherapy and/or radiotherapy
	Jarish–Herxheimer reaction following treatment of spirochete and mycobacterial infections
Idiosyncratic	Malignant hyperthermia: succinylcholine, halothane
	Neuroleptic malignant syndrome: major tranquilizers
	Serotonin toxicity: selective serotonin reuptake inhibitors, lithium, L-tryptophan

INFECTIONS IN SPECIAL HOSTS AND POPULATIONS

Infections in immunosuppressed patients

Immunocompromised patients are increasingly seen as more patients are subjected to more aggressive immunosuppressant therapies.

In infections in the immunosuppressed:

- Localizing information may be minimal or absent, and presentations can be atypical.
- Symptoms and signs may appear or increase on restitution of the immune deficit.
- Physical examination must be thorough, is needed regularly, and includes sites such as the perianal region and CNS including the fundi.
- The range of pathogens is considerably broader.
- There can be more than one cause of fever, such as more than one infection or an infection plus a non-infective cause.

- Empirical treatment needs to be broad-spectrum, but can be tailored to specific pathogens when microbiology results become available.
- A wide range of diagnostic tests, including invasive ones, needs to be applied.

CLINICAL PEARL

The clinical assessment of infections in immunosuppressed patients should be approached by considering three main areas of inquiry: the Syndrome (key symptoms, signs and results of investigations); the Host (age, gender, type and duration of immunosuppression, implanted devices, medication history); and the Exposures (contacts, hospital, recent procedures, animals, travel).

Neutropenia

Neutropenia induced by cytotoxic chemotherapy, especially for acute myeloid leukemia (AML) and in bone marrow transplantation, is commonly seen. As the neutrophil count drops below 1.0×10^9 cells/L, opportunistic infection becomes much more common, and below 0.1×10^9 cells/L rapidly overwhelming bacterial infections may occur. With severe and prolonged neutropenia, invasive fungal infections are seen.

- With the onset of fever in a neutropenic patient, it is important to do a full clinical examination including perianal areas and eyes, IV lines, plus chest, cardiovascular and abdominal examinations.
- Multiple sets of blood cultures, urine examination, and chest X-ray should be done, and broad-spectrum anti-pseudomonal beta-lactams instituted immediately. It is important that the regimen covers *Pseudomonas aeruginosa*, because this pathogen can be rapidly lethal and is resistant to many of the commonly used antibiotics.
- Common sites of infection are the lungs and IV devices, and so high-resolution CT scanning of the chest is very important.
- About 20% of patients will have positive blood cultures but negative blood cultures do not rule out invasive infections, especially from fungi and/or viruses.

The diagnosis of invasive fungal infections is problematic, as the 'gold standard' tissue for diagnosis is usually not available.

- Bronchoscopy may yield potential pathogens.
- Biomarkers such as galactomannan levels are unreliable in isolation, although serial galactomannan assays or PCR assays of blood have some utility.
- PCR for various respiratory pathogens can be done on various respiratory specimens, and is very useful to diagnose viral agents and *Pneumocystis jirovecii*.
- Consultation with the microbiology/infectious diseases department can facilitate choosing appropriate tests and reduce the turnaround time in getting results.

Box 20-1 shows pathogens that should be considered in febrile neutropenic patients with pulmonary infiltrates.

Box 20-1
Causes of pulmonary infiltrates and lesions in neutropenia

Bacteria
- *Streptococcus pneumoniae*
- *Pseudomonas aeruginosa*
- *Enterobacteriaceae*
- *Staphylococcus aureus*
- *Legionella pneumophila*

Viruses
- Influenza
- Human metapneumovirus
- Respiratory syncytial virus
- Rhinovirus
- Parainfluenza virus

Fungi
- *Aspergillus* spp.
- Agents of mucormycosis
- *Scedosporium* spp.
- *Pneumocystis jirovecii*

Reactivation
- *Strongyloides stercoralis*
- *Mycobacterium tuberculosis*
- Dimorphic fungi

Non-infectious causes
- Pulmonary edema
- Neoplasm
- Pulmonary hemorrhage
- Pneumonitis (drug-induced)
- Pneumonitis (radiation-induced)

Humoral immunodeficiency

Patients with multiple myeloma, chronic lymphocytic leukemia, nephrotic syndrome and protein-losing enteropathy have defective humoral immunity, and are at greater risk of infection with encapsulated bacteria (such as *S. pneumoniae* and *N. meningitidis*). Although the response is impaired, it is recommended to vaccinate such patients against these organisms, and consider infusions of gammaglobulin.

Cellular immunodeficiency

Patients with HIV/AIDS, or those on various immunosuppressant drugs administered as part of transplantation regimens or in the treatment of autoimmune and hematological disorders or primary cellular immune defects, have defective cellular immunity and are predisposed to infections with intracellular pathogens, both primary infections and reactivation with the agents shown in Table 20-14.

Splenectomized patients

Patients who are asplenic are unable to clear opsonized bacteria and are particularly prone to overwhelming infections with *S. pneumoniae*, but also with *N. meningitidis* and (historically) *H. influenzae*. It is recommended to vaccinate such patients against these pathogens, give prolonged prophylactic beta-lactams, and counsel them to present immediately for antibiotics should fever and rigors occur.

Sexually transmitted infections (STIs)

General points

- The term 'sexually transmitted infections' denotes infections in which the primary mode of transmission is sexual.
- Some infections not classified as STIs can be transmitted sexually (e.g. hepatitis B virus, CMV, *C. albicans*, *Shigella* spp.). These infections often involve a period of latency and a high proportion of asymptomatic cases, which facilitates transmission, or are associated with male-to-male anal sex. They also feature a lack of protective immunity at the mucosal level, allowing for repeated infections.
- Contact tracing is very important in the control of STIs. There can be important cultural considerations here, such as with culturally and linguistically diverse people, Indigenous people, or sexual minority groups. It is often useful to engage the assistance of social workers and STI nurses in counseling and contact tracing.
- Drug resistance is known to be a serious issue with treating gonorrhea and *Shigella* spp., and may well be a serious issue in treating other STIs.
- Many isolates of *N. gonorrhoeae* from certain geographical areas are resistant to what were first-line drugs, and have to be treated with parenteral drugs; and pan-resistant strains are emerging.

CLINICAL PEARLS

- Patients with sexually transmitted infections (STIs) may have multiple sexually transmitted infections, including asymptomatic ones. All STI patients should be tested for HIV, syphilis, gonorrhea, *Chlamydia trachomatis*, and hepatitis B as a minimum, plus other STIs that are locally prevalent.
- Prompt empirical treatment and contact tracing are essential in disease control.

History

History taking and examination, as in all areas of medicine, are pivotal in the evaluation of a patient for STIs.

- The key to taking a proper sexual history is taking a proper and thorough history in the first place, including an appropriate social history. This will then lead to more detailed and sensitive inquiry relevant to the patient's needs.
- In particular, elucidation of symptomatology pertaining to the genitals can be delicate, and achieving rapport with patients and gaining their confidence are

Table 20-14 Opportunistic pathogens seen in cellular immunodeficiency

TYPE OF ORGANISM	SPECIES	TYPICAL INFECTIONS
Viruses	Cytomegalovirus	Viremia End-organ disease
	Herpes simplex virus	More severe local diseases May disseminate
	Varicella zoster virus	Severe primary infection Severe reactivation often with secondary dissemination
	Epstein–Barr virus	Various malignancies
	JC virus	Progressive multifocal leukoencephalopathy (PML)
Bacteria	*Mycobacterium tuberculosis*	Reactivation Can be atypical
	Non-tuberculous mycobacteria	Pulmonary Disseminated
	Salmonella enterica	Disseminated
	Listeria monocytogenes	Meningitis Hepatitis Disseminated
	Nocardia spp.	Pulmonary Brain abscess Disseminated
Fungi	*Cryptococcus* spp.	Meningitis Disseminated
	Pneumocystis jirovecii	Pneumocystis pneumonia
	Dimorphic fungi	Reactivation (sometimes years after exposure)
Parasites	*Strongyloides stercoralis*	Autoinfection Can have secondary Gram-negative bacteremia
	Toxoplasma gondii	Cerebral abscesses

important in getting full details of sexual partners and sexual acts undertaken.

- Confidentiality is very important in this area, and in STI clinics clients are often identified by a number rather than by name and date of birth, to facilitate attendance and specific questioning about sexual history, sexual acts including vaginal, anal and oral sex, use of sex toys, accessory drugs and substances.
- A past history of STIs is important, as is a travel history that includes places visited and sexual activities during the trip. The geographical area where the patient was exposed influences diagnostic considerations; acquisition in less-developed countries increases the chance of HIV and syphilis, for example.
- Medications and allergies are important, especially if the patient might have a drug-resistant pathogen or the

symptomatology might be an adverse consequence of a drug.

Examination

The examination needs to involve a full examination of the anogenital region as well as the rest of the body. It is important to have a private area with a comfortable examination couch and good lighting, and a full range of equipment (i.e. swabs and speculae) on hand. STI clinics typically have culture media and a basic microbiology setup in-house to facilitate rapid provisional diagnoses and maximise sensitivity of culture of what are often fragile organisms.

- The presence of HIV can be suggested by wasting, oral candidiasis and/or seborrheic dermatitis.

- Rashes can occur in HIV seroconversion, acute CMV and EBV (especially if antibiotics have been taken), and also secondary syphilis.
- Lymphadenopathy and/or hepatosplenomegaly can occur in systemic viral infections including HIV, EBV and CMV.
- With respect to genital examination, the presence of vesicles on a red base suggests herpes simplex virus (HSV) infection.
- A painless red lesion could be a syphilitic chancre.
- Painful red lesions could suggest lymphogranuloma venereum.
- Urethral or cervical discharge suggests gonococcal or chlamydial infection.
- Warts can be found on the genitals or anal region. And be mindful that a proper anogenital examination is more than just a digital rectal examination—commonly known as a 'DRE' or 'PR exam'. The external examination is very important.

A full set of diagnostic specimens should be taken during the physical examination.

- Diagnostic specimens include urethral or cervical swabs for Gram stain, culture and PCR for *N. gonorrhoeae* and *C. trachomatis*, swab of ulcers for darkfield examination for *T. pallidum*, and high vaginal swab for wet film (*Trichomonas* spp.) and culture (*C. albicans*).
- PCR on urine for *N. gonorrhoeae* and *C. trachomatis* is extremely sensitive, and can mean avoiding internal examinations in some patients. Note that not culturing *N. gonorrhoeae* means there will be no antibiotic susceptibility testing, so in cases where resistance is suspected epidemiologically or because of treatment failure, culture specimens should also be taken.

Investigations

Table 20-15 shows diagnostic tests for specific STIs.

Management—general

- The general principles of STI management include counseling, advice about safe sex and prevention of STIs, contact tracing, and provision of empirical treatment.
- Empirical treatments are aimed at likely pathogens and usually select agents that have a higher adherence.
- Partner notification is important, as is notification to the relevant public health authorities, and follow-up for test-of-cure specimens and definitive results.

Table 20-15 Diagnostic tests for sexually transmitted infections

PATHOGEN	SPECIMEN	DIAGNOSTIC TESTS	COMMENTS
Herpes simplex virus HSV-2 or HSV-1	Viral swab	PCR	PCR is the best test and is now widely available
		IF	Quick, high sensitivity and specificity
		Culture	Slower, superseded
	Blood	IgG, IgM, WB	Usual in seroprevalence surveys but not helpful in routine diagnosis of HSV
Neisseria gonorrhoeae	Vaginal or urethral swab	PCR	Fast and sensitive; no antibiotic data
	First pass urine	PCR	Fast and sensitive; no antibiotic data
	Vaginal or urethral swab	Culture	Bacterium is fragile and can die before reaches laboratory; could inoculate plates at bedside Culture allows for susceptibility testing Special swabs facilitate survival of organism during transport to laboratory
Chlamydia trachomatis	Vaginal or urethral swab; first-pass urine	PCR	Sensitive, specific and widely available
Treponema pallidum	Swab	Dark-field examination	Some utility in diagnosing genital chancre Not useful in pharynx or anus as spirochetes are part of normal flora
	Blood	EIA (ELISA)	Usual screening test; if positive, traditional tests (RPR, TPPA, etc) performed to confirm Like all syphilis serological tests, can be falsely negative in early primary disease so retest if primary disease possible

PATHOGEN	SPECIMEN	DIAGNOSTIC TESTS	COMMENTS
		RPR (VDRL)	'Reaginic' test, titer some reflection of disease activity, falls with successful treatment RPR supersedes VDRL which requires microscopy
		TPPA/TPHA	Specific test, quite sensitive, stays positive for life
		FTA-ABS	Used as confirmation of new diagnosis
		WB	Used as confirmation of new diagnosis
Human immunodeficiency virus (HIV)	Blood	EIA	Current '4th-generation' HIV tests include HIV-1, HIV-2 and p24 antigen
		WB	Used as confirmation of EIA; can be positive, negative or indeterminate Although WB is still done as a routine confirmatory test, a confident diagnosis can now usually be made with current standard HIV tests
		VL/Nucleic acid tests	Useful in determining blood level and also response to antiretroviral treatment. For some indications such as blood transfusion and transplantation, and in some jurisdictions such as the US (but not Australia currently), nucleic acid tests are licensed for the diagnosis of HIV infection (in conjunction with serology). A person recently infected will be RNA positive just prior to seroconversion and developing the various bands on the western blot.
Gardnerella vaginalis	Vaginal swab	Wet film	Coccobacilli replace lactobacilli and adhere to squamous epithelial cells ('clue cells')
Trichomonas vaginalis	Vaginal swab	Wet film	Typical morphology and motility on wet film
Haemophilus ducreyi	Swab of lesion	Gram stain	Typical small Gram-negative coccobacilli
		Culture	Culture of organism. PCR is not widely available but sensitive and specific
Klebsiella (formerly Calymmatobacterium) granulomatis	Swab/biopsy/impression smear of lesion	PCR is the best test; Wright's or Giemsa stain	Donovan bodies (unculturable)
Chlamydia trachomatis (LGV strains)	Blood	Serology	
Human papillomavirus	Papanicolaou smear	Cytology stain	Atypical or malignant cells
	Tissue or smear	PCR	Recently replaced Pap smears as the screening test of choice for cervical cancer

EIA, enzyme immunoassay; ELISA, enzyme-linked immunosorbent assay (old term for EIA); FTA-ABS, fluorescent *Treponema* antibody absorption test; IF, immunofluorescence test; IgG, immunoglobulin G; IgM, immunoglobulin M;; LGV, lymphogranuloma venereum; p24 Ag, p24 antigen; PCR, polymerase chain reaction; RPR, rapid plasma reagin test; TPHA, *Treponema pallidum* hemagglutination test; TPPA, *Treponema pallidum* particle agglutination test; VDRL, Venereal Diseases Reference Laboratories test; VL, viral load; WB, western blot.

Specific entities

Urethritis

- Patients with urethritis are treated empirically for gono-coccal and chlamydial infection.
- Antibiotic resistance is highly variable between countries, and within countries, being common in underdeveloped countries and still unusual in isolated communities.
  - » Sex worker movement between countries can import STIs, including drug-resistant strains of *Neisseria gonorrhoeae*.
- Many strains of *N. gonorrhoeae* seen today are resistant to all oral agents, including quinolones, necessitating the use of 3rd-generation cephalosporins.
- *Chlamydia trachomatis* lacks a cell wall and so is not affected by beta-lactams, but is susceptible to tetra-cyclines and macrolides.
- If *N. gonorrhoeae* or *C. trachomatis* is not demonstrated, the patient is considered to have non-specific urethritis. Agents such as *Mycoplasma genitalium*, *Ureaplasma urea-lyticum*, *Trichomonas vaginalis*, *Neisseria meningitidis* and *Haemophilus* spp., and viruses such as HSV and human papillomavirus (HPV), can be implicated.
- *N. gonorrhoeae* infects any columnar epithelium, and so infections of the rectum, pharynx and conjunctiva can occur. Anti-gonococcal drugs such as penicillin or specti-nomycin do not clear pharyngeal carriage, and so quinolo-nes or 3rd-generation cephalosporins need to be used here.

Proctitis

- Patients with proctitis present with tenesmus, anal dis-charge, and blood and mucus in the stools.
- Etiologies include *N. gonorrhoeae*, HSV, *C. trachomatis*, *Shigella* spp. and *Campylobacter* spp.
- Diagnosis is confirmed at proctoscopy, at which time swabs can be taken for Gram-stain for gonococci within neutrophils, culture and/or PCR, and viral swabs taken for HSV PCR.
- Stools should be submitted for *Shigella* spp. and *Campy-lobacter* spp. culture.

Cervicitis

- Cervicitis presents with discharge, and during specu-lum examination pus can be seen coming out of a friable uterine os.
- Etiology is usually *N. gonorrhoeae* or *C. trachomatis*.
- Investigation and treatment is as per urethritis.

Pelvic inflammatory disease

- The etiology of pelvic inflammatory disease is often sex-ually transmitted organisms such as *N. gonorrhoeae* and *C. trachomatis* in young women, and ascending infec-tions with rectovaginal flora in older women.
- Actinomycosis can complicate those with intrauterine contraceptive devices.
- Lower abdominal pain and fever, and tenderness on rock-ing the cervix during pelvic examination, are characteristic.

- Specimens for *N. gonorrhoeae* and *C. trachomatis* should be taken (urine and/or cervical swabs), and antibiotics covering STI organisms and ascending normal flora initiated (such as cefoxitin + doxycycline, ceftriaxone + metronidazole + doxycycline).

Vaginal infections

Three common vaginal infections are candidiasis, bacterial vaginosis, and *Trichomonas* spp.

- **Candidiasis** is usually due to *C. albicans* but can be due to other *Candida* species, particularly in immunocom-promised people. The diagnosis is made when typical inflamed areas are seen with curd–like deposits or there is a positive fungal culture. Candidal organisms can also be seen on gram stain and wet films. Treatment is with topi-cal antifungal creams, but more recently fluconazole orally 150 mg as a single dose has proved to be highly effective.
- **Bacterial vaginosis** is an alteration of normal vaginal flora, where the normal lactobacilli are replaced by organ-isms such as *Gardnerella vaginalis*, *Mycoplasma hominis*, *Mobi-luncus* species and anaerobes. Diagnosis is by observing a clear or frothy discharge with a fish-like odor, and a wet film that shows replacement of the normal bacilli with coc-cobacilli organisms, often found adherent to the surface of squamous epithelial cells ('clue cells'). Bacterial vaginosis is associated with premature labor, and ascending infections in pregnant women. Treatment is with oral metronidazole 500 mg twice daily for 7 days, although a significant num-ber of cases will resolve without treatment.
- ***Trichomonas vaginalis*** is a protozoan that is transmitted sexually, and the diagnosis is readily made by observa-tion of motile protozoans on a wet film. The patient and partners are treated with metronidazole, tinidazole or clindamycin.

Genital ulceration

STIs causing genital ulceration include HSV, syphilis (see later section), chancroid, donovanosis, and lymphogranu-loma venereum.

Herpes simplex virus

- HSV typically is revealed as small vesicles on a red base, which may burst to form ulcers which can coalesce.
- Primary infections range from asymptomatic to severe, with bilateral lesions, and also systemic features such as fever and enlarged inguinal lymph nodes. On occasion there is urinary retention, and sometimes neurological complications such as aseptic meningitis.
- Recurrences are usually less severe and vary consider-ably in frequency.
- Diagnosis is made by observation of classic lesions with virological confirmation. PCR is highly sensitive and specific and is the test of choice, superseding immuno-fluorescence and culture.
- Serology is not usually useful in the diagnosis of herpes genitalis.
- Treatment is with a thymidylate kinase inhibitor (fam-ciclovir, valaciclovir or acyclovir/aciclovir).

- Suppressive treatment can be considered for frequent recurrences.
- Disease tends to be more severe, prolonged, and sometimes progressive in the immunosuppressed, and in this group drug resistance can also occur.

Chancroid

- Chancroid is caused by *Haemophilus ducreyi* and is seen in northern Australia, Asia and Africa.
- It presents with multiple tender ulcers and inguinal lymphadenopathy.
- The diagnosis is made by swabbing the lesions and observing typical organisms on Gram stain, and sometimes positive culture. There is no serological test.
- Therapy is with a 3rd-generation cephalosporin, quinolone or azithromycin.

Donovanosis

- Donovanosis is caused by *Klebsiella* (formerly *Calymmatobacterium granulomatis*), an unculturable organism, which causes beefy red exuberant lesions on the glans penis or in the perianal area.
- Diagnosis is made by seeing classic lesions and performing PCR on surface swabs of the lesion. Historically observing Donovan bodies on Wright's or Giemsa stain of swabs or tissue.
- Donovanosis requires a prolonged course of antibiotics to be adequately treated. Erythromycin or tetracycline should be taken for 3 weeks.
- Current treatment involves a weekly dose of azithromycin for at least 3 weeks, with alternative treatments being doxycycline, ciprofloxacin, erythromycin or co-trimoxazole.

Lymphogranuloma venereum (LGV)

Lymphogranuloma venereum is caused by LGV strains of *Chlamydia trachomatis*.

- This disease manifests with transient genital ulceration followed by increasing inguinal lymphadenopathy.
- Diagnosis is made by demonstrating a raised antibody titer to this organism and sometimes culture or immunofluorescence of fluid from a bubo.
- Treatment is with tetracyclines or macrolides.

Human papillomavirus (HPV)

- 70 types of HPV are described.
  - » Types 6 and 11 cause asymptomatic infections or genital warts that are not associated with malignancy.
  - » Types 16, 18, 31, 33, and 35 cause asymptomatic anogenital infections, which can lead to the development of squamous cell carcinomas of the cervix but also of the anus.
- Treatment of genital warts can be challenging; it involves ablation with cryotherapy, diathermy, application of podophyllin residues, and sometimes intralesional interferon injection.
- A vaccine was developed with Australian research, and initially was rolled out for adolescent females. Currently a 9-valent vaccine is used in the Australian Immunisation Schedule, and the target group has been widened to include all people aged 9-18 years, those with immunosuppression other than asplenia, and men who have sex with men.
- Widespread uptake of HPV vaccines has resulted in a dramatic decrease in the incidence of cervical cancer.
- This disease can be detected by screening with PCR of cervical smears, with Pap smears and biopsy reserved for further investigation of positive tests.
- HPV can be detected in tissue biopsies by various techniques, with the most sensitive being nucleic acid detection.
- For subclinical cervical infection, PCR is superseding Papanicolaou smears due to the ease of specimen collection and high sensitivity. If a lesion is biopsied, the light microscopy appearance is suggestive of HPV and histochemical stains and PCR can confirm the presence of HPV.

Molluscum contagiosum

- Molluscum contagiosum is caused by a poxvirus that causes centrally umbilicated raised lesions on the skin. In a normal host these regress spontaneously, but can progress in the immunosuppressed.
- Treatment if required is with cryotherapy, diathermy, curettage, or de-roofing lesions and applying glacial acetic acid or trichloracetic acid.

Syphilis

Syphilis is caused by *Treponema pallidum* and has been famous in the past as a great mimic of various diseases.

- In more recent times its incidence and prevalence has been increasing, particularly in men who have sex with men, and it is also highly prevalent in the developing world and in some indigenous communities.
- **Primary infection** may be manifested by a chancre, which is a painless red sore found on the genitals or sometimes perianally. This lesion resolves.
- A few weeks later, patients may manifest **secondary syphilis**, which is usually characterized by vasculitis, typically including a maculopapular rash that involves the palms and soles (Figure 20-7), and often a febrile illness with lymphadenopathy and hepatosplenomegaly.
- This will eventually resolve, and the disease becomes quiescent or **latent**. Latent disease of less than 2 years' duration is considered early latent disease, and beyond this it is late latent disease.
- Years after initial infection, **vasculitis** can be manifested by neurological manifestations such as cognitive impairment, tabes dorsalis, and Argyll Robertson pupils. More commonly, it is detected on a screening test of patients with unexplained symptoms.
- Co-infection with HIV can result in atypical manifestations of syphilis and false-negative diagnostic tests, and increases the chance of relapse after treatment.
- *T. pallidum* crosses the placenta, and congenital syphilis may develop. Manifestations are protean, and include stillbirth, rash, fever, hepatosplenomegaly, jaundice, coryza, and various deformities. Untreated, manifestations such

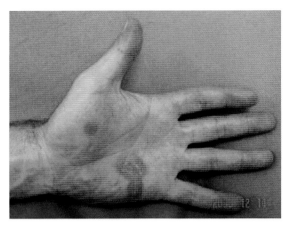

Figure 20-7 Maculopapular rash on the palms from secondary syphilis

From Ortega KL, Rezende NPM and Magalhães MHCG. Diagnosing secondary syphilis in a patient with HIV. Br J Oral Maxillofacial Surg 2009;47(2):169–70. © The British Association of Oral and Maxillofacial Surgeons.

as Hutchinson's teeth, interstitial keratitis, deafness, saddle nose, saber shins, and other manifestations can develop in early childhood. Children born to mothers with syphilis need expert follow-up and serial testing and, if the diagnosis is made or likely, treatment with penicillin instituted.

CLINICAL PEARL

Do not miss the typical features of secondary syphilis: fever, lymphadenopathy, rash and 'mucous patches' on the tongue and buccal mucosa. Iritis may also be observed.

Diagnosis

Occasionally, if a chancre is seen then diagnosis can be made by dark-field examination of fluid from this lesion. For most cases, the diagnosis is made serologically.

- Usually enzyme immunoassay (EIA) is used as a screening test. This is quite sensitive and specific, but like all syphilis tests can be falsely negative in early syphilis.
  - » If the index of suspicion is high, tests should be repeated several weeks later.
  - » If the EIA is positive, this is confirmed with traditional syphilis tests which include reaginic and treponemal tests.
- Reaginic tests use cardiolipin antigen, which cross-reacts against antibodies produced in syphilis but also in other diseases, especially autoimmune disease.
  - » Reaginic tests include the traditional Venereal Diseases Reference Laboratory (VDRL) test, which is very labor-intensive, utilizing light microscopy, and thus has been replaced by the rapid plasma reagin (RPR) test.
  - » Reaginic tests achieve high titers in active disease, especially secondary or tertiary, and the success of treatment can be measured by the extent of fall in titer.

- Treponemal tests utilize spirochete antigen. These include *Treponema pallidum* hemagglutination (TPHA) and *Treponema pallidum* particle agglutination (TPPA) tests. These tests are more specific for syphilis infection, and remain positive for life following infection.
- To gain greater specificity with the diagnosis, sera yielding positive reaginic and/or treponemal tests are usually confirmed with a further fluorescent *Trepenoma* antibody absorption (FTA-ABS) test, or sometimes with other tests such as a western blot.

It is important to note that in early primary syphilis, and sometimes in late disease in patients with AIDS, that false-negative results can occur with all of these tests.

Treatment

- Penicillin is the only drug of proven efficacy to treat syphilis.
- Different intensities in durations of treatment are recommended for the different stages of syphilis.
- 3rd-generation cephalosporins have been recommended in some regimens, particularly for HIV-positive individuals as this facilitates outpatient parenteral treatment, but evidence of efficacy in trials is lacking.
- Alternatives for penicillin-allergic patients such as doxycycline are unproven. It is generally recommended that patients said to be allergic to penicillin should be evaluated, and if found to truly be allergic to consider desensitization, particularly if the patient has late latent or tertiary syphilis and/or is immunosuppressed, especially due to HIV infection.
- All patients treated for syphilis require follow-up RPR at 3, 6, 12 and 24 months. The lack of a fourfold decrease in RPR titer at 6 months usually requires repeat treatment. Patients can be reinfected with *Treponema pallidum*.

SYSTEMIC VIRAL INFECTIONS

HIV

See Chapter 16 for HIV/AIDS. All patients with an STI should have HIV testing.

Hepatitis viruses

- Hepatitis A infection can be seen in men who have sex with men, sometimes causing outbreaks, and is particularly seen in people who have fecal–oral contact.
- Hepatitis B can be transmitted sexually, and should be screened for when evaluating patients with STIs.
- Vaccines against hepatitis A and hepatitis B are available, and should be given to those at risk.
- Hepatitis C is rarely transmitted sexually.

See Chapter 12 for additional information on the diagnosis and treatment of hepatitis virus infections.

Herpesviruses

- EBV and CMV exposures are more common in those with multiple sexual contacts. These infections can be manifested as primary infection. Diagnosis is usually readily made serologically.

- All herpesviruses have latent states, and can reactivate in immunodeficiency states such as in AIDS.

Diagnosis and treatment are covered earlier in the chapter.

Zoonoses

General

Zoonoses are caused by a complex group of pathogens, numbering in the hundreds.

- The definition is usually considered to be an infection that derives from vertebrate animals.
- Most emerging infectious diseases begin as zoonoses. Infectious diseases such as AIDS, tuberculosis and measles began as zoonoses, and common infections such as influenza are still predominantly zoonotic.
- Transmission can be via many routes, such as eating uncooked or cooked tissues of an animal, contact with the excreta of an animal, inhaling aerosolized material from an animal, the bite of an animal, or by transmission from animal to human by the bite of an invertebrate such as an insect.

History

The history of exposure is important in evaluation of all infectious diseases.

- The possibility of zoonotic infection is usually elucidated from the history.
- An extensive history of all travel, both recent and in the past and including immigration, is important.
- Occupational exposures, and hobbies and interests including pets other than dogs and cats kept at home and interest in hunting, bushwalking and other such activities, needs to be explored.

The following suggest the possibility of a zoonosis:

- Travel history
- Occupation as veterinarian, farmer or abattoir (slaughterhouse) worker
- Unusual food ingestion
- Hobbies such as hunting, trapping, bushwalking, adventure holidays
- Characteristic skin lesions
- Eating, being bitten by, or being exposed to particular animals
- Sometimes the possibility of zoonotic infection is not considered until clinical features, imaging or diagnostic test results are suggestive, and specific questioning then reveals possible or definite animal exposure.
- Additionally, there is extensive trade, both legal and illegal, in animals and animal products, which in conjunction with increased air travel results in greater range and frequency of exotic zoonoses being encountered.
- Animal bites can transmit flora from an animal's mouth (*Pasteurella multocida, Capnocytophaga* spp., anaerobes,

Clostridium tetani) or inoculate a patient's endogenous flora (*S. aureus*).

- Patients at higher risk of sepsis from animal bites include those with asplenia, diabetes, cancer, cirrhosis and lymphedema.
- Tissue destruction and late presentation increase the risk of infection.

Management

- Given the great variety of zoonotic syndromes encountered, management will vary greatly from one problem to the next.
- Irrigation and/or debridement and/or surgical exploration of bites and other wounds.
- Tetanus prophylaxis for bites and other wounds.
- Antibiotics are aimed at flora of animal mouths and human, e.g. the use of penicillin/beta-lactamase inhibitor combinations, or a 3rd-generation cephalosporin + metronidazole.
- Rabies post-exposure prophylaxis should be given if an animal from a country with rabies is involved.

Specific examples of zoonoses

Selected zoonotic infections are considered in Table 20-16, overleaf.

Lyme disease (*Borrelia burgdorferi*)

Lyme disease is a tick-borne illness endemic in the United States (north central and northeast) and Europe.

- In stage I (early, delayed), a red lesion (erythema migrans; Figure 20-8), often with a bull's-eye appearance, develops. Serology is of no value in this stage and treatment is usually doxycycline.
- If untreated, early disseminated disease (stage II) may manifest with fever, myalgia, lymphadenopathy,

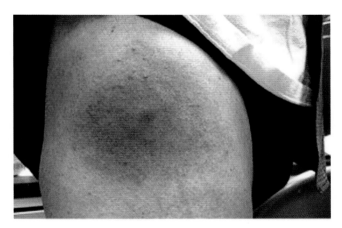

Figure 20-8 Erythema migrans in Lyme disease

From Bhate C and Schwartz RA. Lyme disease. Part I: advances and perspectives. J Am Acad Dermatol 2011;64(4):619–36. © American Academy of Dermatology, Inc.

Table 20-16 Selected zoonoses from specific animals

ANIMAL	TYPICAL PATIENT	PRESENTATION	ORGANISMS	INVESTIGATION	TREATMENT
Cat	Cat owner	Infected cat bite or scratch	*Pasteurella multocida* *Capnocytophaga* spp. Anaerobes *Staphylococcus aureus* *Clostridium tetani*	Wound swab	Tetanus prophylaxis Penicillin, 3rd-generation cephalosporins, quinolone
Cat	Cat owner	Cat scratch fever	*Bartonella henselae*	Serology; blood culture	Self-limited usually If prolonged, end-organ disease: azithromycin If immunosuppressed: get advice
Dog	Dog owner	Infected dog bite	As per cat bite	Wound swab	As per cat bite
Dogs, raccoons, cats, monkeys	Bite in a country that has rabid animals	Rabies	Rabies	Nil	Post-exposure vaccination
Cats, dogs, pigs, horses	Human in close contact	Staphylococcal infection	MRSA MRSA can be 'humanosis' then transferred to humans. Horses and pigs have own MRSA strains	Wound swabs, occasionally blood cultures	Anti-MRSA antibiotics
Monkey	Bite	Simian herpes	Simian herpesvirus	Nil	Aciclovir
Birds, esp. psittacine	Bird breeders, vet workers, tree workers, mowing lawn	Psittacosis	*Chlamydia psittaci*	Serology	Doxycycline; macrolides
Reptiles	Reptile owners	Salmonellosis	*Salmonella* spp.	Blood, stool cultures	Quinolones, 3GC, azithromycin
Monkeys	Airborne exposure	Tuberculosis (TB)	*Mycobacterium tuberculosis*	Sputa: Mantoux test; IGRA	Anti-TB treatment
Livestock	Abattoir (slaughter-house) worker	Systemic febrile illness: Q-fever, brucellosis, leptospirosis	*Coxiella burnetii* *Brucella* spp. *Leptospira interrogans*	Serology; culture for *Brucella* spp.	Doxycycline
Various	Highly contagious and exposure may not be recognized	Systemic illness, occasionally endocarditis	*Coxiella burnetii*	Serology; PCR	Resolved: no treatment Acute: doxycycline Endocarditis: rifampicin + doxycycline, surgery

Animal reservoir	Exposure/risk	Disease	Organism	Diagnosis	Treatment
Sheep, cattle, kangaroos	Rare lamb, beef or kangaroo meat eater	Toxoplasmosis Congenital toxoplasmosis Reactivation in immuno-compromised	Toxoplasma gondii	Serology Immunocompromised: CT brain, tissue biopsy	Primary disease: none Pregnancy: specialist evaluation and treatment Immunocompromised: sulfadiazine + pyrimethamine
Pigs	Pig hunter	Brucellosis	Brucella suis	Serology; blood cultures	Doxycycline + gentamicin
Ungulates (cattle, goats, sheep)	Drinkers of unpasteurized milk/milk products	Brucellosis	Brucella abortus, Brucella melitensis, Brucella ovis	Blood cultures; serology	Doxycycline + gentamicin
Fish	Fish handlers	Erysipeloid	Erysipelothrix rhusiopathiae	Characteristic lesions, biopsy for culture	Penicillin
Fish	Aquarium-keepers		Mycobacterium marinum	Biopsy for culture and histopathology	Antituberculous chemotherapy
Bats	Bat keeper	Contact or bite of bat: rabies-like illness	Australian bat lyssavirus	Exposure to bats	Post-exposure prophylaxis with rabies vaccine
Sheep	Farmer, shearer	Vesicle on hand	Orf virus	Nil; EM on biopsy	Nil; antibiotics if secondary infection
Sheep	Past farm contact	Hydatid disease	Echinococcus granulosus	CT: cystic lesions in liver, lung, other tissues Serology	Extirpation + albendazole ± praziquantel
Various	Farmers, bushwalkers	Fever, conjunctivitis, hepatitis, renal impairment, aseptic meningitis	Leptospira interrogans	Serology	Mild and settled: no treatment Not mild: doxycycline, penicillin or 3rd-generation cephalosporin

CT, computed tomography; EM, electron microscopy; IGRA, interferon-gamma release assay; MRSA, methicillin-resistant *Staphylococcus aureus*; PCR, polymerase chain reaction.

myocarditis (first-degree heart block) and aseptic meningitis (cranial neuropathy, retinopathy).

- Months to years later, migratory monoarthritis or rarely encephalopathy may occur (stage III).

Serology (enzyme immunosassay [EIA], then confirmatory western blot) is only useful in stages II or III. Testing should be reserved for those who live in an endemic area or have traveled to one, with clinically suggestive symptoms or signs.

Other tick-borne illnesses

Other tick-borne illnesses in the US include babesiosis (causing fever and hemolysis), southern tick-associated rash illness (a stage I Lyme-like disease) and ehrlichiosis (fever, myalgia, headache, lymphopenia, abnormal transaminases).

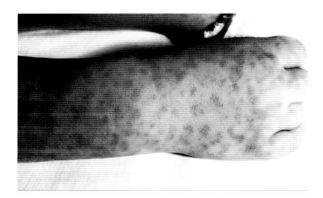

Figure 20-9 Rocky Mountain spotted fever

Photo courtesy of the CDC Public Health Image Library. © CDC.

CLINICAL PEARL

- There are a number of readily accessible on-line resources that facilitate a reasonably accurate assessment of zoonotic risk. The CDC website is typically a good place to start.

INFECTION PREVENTION AND CONTROL

Infection prevention and control is gaining center stage in modern hospitals due to the continually increasing problem of multidrug-resistant organisms (MROs). The patients themselves, the hospital environment, apparatus used on patients, and healthcare workers can be reservoirs of these organisms, and share organisms.

The major MROs of importance are given in Table 20-17.

Successful infection prevention and control programs involve all seven pillars of infection control:

1 Administrative support
2 Education
3 Judicious use of antibiotics
4 MRO surveillance
5 Infection control precautions
6 Environmental measures
7 Decolonization.

Administrative support

- All successful infection control programs have substantial administrative support. These programs are very expensive and require specific budgetary allocation.

Table 20-17 Multi-resistant organisms seen in modern hospitals

ACRONYM	ORGANISM	ANTIBIOTIC RESISTANCE	TYPICAL INFECTIONS
MRSA	Methicillin-resistant *Staphylococcus aureus*	All beta-lactams; usually multidrug-resistant Community MRSA usually non-multidrug-resistant	Bloodstream infection Surgical site infection Intravenous catheter infection
VRE	Vancomycin-resistant enterococci	Vancomycin; intrinsically resistant to most antibiotics	Bloodstream infection
ESBL	Extended-spectrum beta-lactamases (seen in *Enterobacteriaceae*)	Most penicillins and cephalosporins Usually resistant to other drugs also	Urinary tract infection Bloodstream infection Hospital-acquired pneumonia
MBL	Metallo-beta-lactamase (of pseudomonads, *Acinetobacter* spp., *Enterobacteriaceae*)	All beta-lactams including carbapenems Usually harbor resistance to most other drugs	Urinary tract infection Bloodstream infection Hospital-acquired pneumonia
Cdiff	*Clostridium difficile*	This species is intrinsically resistant to most antibiotics	Pseudomembranous colitis

- There also need to be management directives, and an organized program with buy-in from all members of staff.

Education

Continuous education is required of all levels of hospital worker, from senior management down through senior medical, nursing and allied health clinicians, to frontline workers, and probably also the patients and the public.

Judicious use of antibiotics

- Antibiotic stewardship programs are now integral to hospital prescribing practice in Western countries, as selection of MROs is enhanced by high uses of broad-spectrum antibiotics.
- Antibiotic stewardship programs must be supported by management and by senior clinicians.
- Computer programs are now available to facilitate antibiotic stewardship programs.

MRO surveillance

- With each MRO the numbers of asymptomatic carriers outnumbers those with overt infection, but both groups constitute the patient reservoir.
- Screening aims to detect the asymptomatic carriers in order to isolate them, and prevent transmission.

Infection control precautions

- These involve isolating patients with communicable pathogens (not just the MROs), wearing gowns and gloves, and the presence of effective hand hygiene.
- Hand hygiene requires a comprehensive program of education and auditing, and has been shown to decrease MRO transmission and hard endpoints such as MRSA bacteremias.

CLINICAL PEARL

The 'Five Moments of Hand Hygiene', as espoused by the World Health Organization, is pivotal in preventing transmission of pathogens between patients. These five moments are:

1 Before patient contact
2 Before a procedure
3 After a procedure or body fluid exposure risk
4 After patient contact
5 After contact with patient surroundings

Environmental measures

- The physical environment is an important reservoir of MROs, especially VRE, *C. difficile* and multiresistant Gram-negative bacilli.
- Eliminating this requires a rigorous program of environmental cleaning, involving adequate resources, training of cleaners, auditing of performance, and using the right disinfectants.
- Aerosolized hydrogen peroxide/silver nanoparticles have been found to eliminate MROs from hospital environments.

Decolonization

- Decolonization of many patients with MRSA is feasible if they do not have mitigating factors such as chronic ulcers or contaminated indwelling catheters.
- It involves skin decontamination with medicated soaps and/or body washes, and nasal mupirocin ointment for 7 days.
- If this fails, seek other carriers in the family group and treat them.
- Should this fail, re-treating with the addition of systemic antibiotics including rifampicin (noting the toxicity and drug interactions), plus another agent to prevent resistance, can be considered.
- It is not known how to eradicate VRE or multiresistant Gram-negative bacilli from the GI tract reservoir.
- Successful treatment of *C. difficile* involves eradicating the carrier state.

SELF-ASSESSMENT QUESTIONS

1 Which of the following drugs may cause fever?
   A Penicillin
   B Carbamazepine
   C Allopurinol
   D Gentamicin

2 Which cephalosporin has activity against methicillin-resistant *Staphylococcus aureus*?
   A Ceftazidime
   B Cefpirome
   C Ceftaroline
   D Ceftriaxone
   E Cephazolin (cefazolin)

3 A 23-year-old previous well woman presents with left lobar pneumonia. She says she can't have penicillin as she got wheezy and developed swollen lips when she was given this antibiotic for a sore throat last year. Which antibiotic can you prescribe for her which will cover likely bacterial pathogens and have minimal risk of causing a type I hypersensitivity reaction?
   A Amoxycillin
   B Gentamicin
   C Moxifloxacin
   D Amikacin
   E Ceftriaxone

4 *Staphylococcus aureus* causes a range of clinical manifestations ranging from asymptomatic carriage to minor skin and soft tissue infections to bacteraemia, endocarditis and death. What staphylococcal exotoxin is regarded as having a major role in patients developing large boils and sometimes lung abscesses, especially if the strain is methicillin-resistant (MRSA)?
   A Alpha haemolysin
   B Endotoxin
   C Panton-Valentine Leukocidin (PVL)
   D Staphylococcal scalded skin syndrome (SSSS) toxin
   E Staphylococcal toxic shock syndrome (STSS) toxin

5 In an era of increasing resistance to antibiotics, which pathogen has never been reported as resistant to penicillin?
   A *Staphylococcus aureus*
   B *E. coli*
   C *Streptococcus pyogenes*
   D *Neisseria gonorrhoea*
   E *Staphylococcus epidermidis*

6 What is the most sensitive test to diagnose chickenpox?
   A Serology for IgM against varicella-zoster virus
   B Serology for IgA against varicella-zoster virus
   C PCR on blood for varicella-zoster virus
   D PCR on a viral swab of lesion material for varicella-zoster virus
   E Taking a swab of lesion material for viral culture

7 With respect to the treatment of endocarditis due to *Enterococcus faecalis*, gentamicin is used in conjunction with penicillin because:
   A Gentamicin is bactericidal against enterococci
   B Enterococci are not killed by penicillins alone
   C Lower doses of both antibiotics can be used
   D Gentamicin increases penicillin levels by blocking renal elimination of penicillin

8 Infections by which agent below can be prevented by vaccination?
   A Influenza C
   B *E. coli*
   C Rotavirus
   D *H. influenzae* (non-typable)
   E *P. falciparum*

9 Which of the following are risk factors increasing the risk of cellulitis?

A Diabetes mellitus
B Chronic venous disease
C Tinea
D Ischemic heart disease
E Chronic obstructive pulmonary disease

10 Which organism is the most common cause of overwhelming sepsis in an asplenic patient?

A Community MRSA
B *Neisseria meningitidis*
C *Haemophilus influenzae* type B
D *Streptococcus pneumoniae*
E *Cytocapnophagia canimorsus* (DF-2)

ANSWERS

1 A, B, C.

Drug fevers may be caused by many drugs, and in the evaluation of a febrile patient, especially one where the cause is unclear, a full drug history is essential. Table 20-13 lists typical drugs that may cause drug fever.

2 C.

MRSA strains are resistant to all beta-lactams, except for new fifth-generation cephalosporins that bind specifically to penicillin-binding protein 2b, which is what makes MRSA resistant to beta-lactams.

3 C.

If she had a type I reaction to penicillin there is high risk of this happening with other penicillins, and some risk of this happening with cephalosporins, so these are contraindicated; so A and E are wrong. The most likely bacterial cause of lobar pneumonia is *S. pneumonia*; gentamicin and amikacin don't cover this pathogen, so are not recommended here. Moxifloxacin covers *S. pneumoniae*, as well as other bacterial pathogens, and is not a beta-lactam so there is no chance of a cross-reaction to this drug in this patient.

4 C.

Panton-Valentine Leukocidin (PVL) is produced by many *S. aureus* strains, especially community MRSA strains, and is associated with the tendency of these strains to form abscesses in the skin and subcutaneous tissues and the lung.

5 C.

S. pyogenes is the only common bacterial pathogen that has never been reported to be resistant to penicillin. However, it can be resistant to other classes of antibiotics such as macrolides. All the other species names have major problems with antibiotic resistance, to all beta lactams and other classes of antibiotics.

6 D.

The diagnosis of chickenpox is usually accurately made clinically, by observing the classic rash and its evolution over time. The rash and its evolution can be atypical in immunocompromised hosts, and here diagnostic tests are more important. The most sensitive and specific test is PCR on cellular material from the base of a de-roofed vesicle. The viremia is transient, and so PCR on blood may be negative. Serology is not particularly helpful except for determining immunity in contacts (with the IgG test). IgM is not particularly sensitive and specific for chickenpox on presentation, and IgA tests are not offered. Viral culture is slow and is superseded by PCR which provides a quick and accurate result.

7 B.

Antibiotics active against enterococci are bacteriostatic but not bactericidal alone, and in endocarditis antibiotics that are bactericidal fail to eradicate the causative organisms. The combination of penicillin and gentamicin is bactericidal. Gentamicin enters the cell when the cell wall is disrupted by penicillin, and thus able to access the ribosomes and kill the cell. Trials in enterococcal endocarditis have shown superior cure rates only if gentamicin is used with the penicillin. Given the morbidity and mortality of endocarditis, this is one of the few indications for a prolonged aminoglycoside course as these agents have significant nephrotoxicity and ototoxicity.

8 C.

Whilst the list of vaccine-preventable diseases is impressive and slowly growing, in the above list this includes only rotavirus. There are significant human pathogens for which a vaccine has proven elusive, such as bacteria that are normal human commensals such as *E. coli* and *Haemophilus influenzae* (non-type B). The *H. influenzae* type B vaccine only covers type B strains; deployment of this vaccine virtually eliminated childhood disease due to this bacterium, but has no impact on other stains of *H. influenzae*, such as the non-typable ones that are associated with acute and chronic bronchitis. The influenza vaccine is aimed at strains of influenza A and B but not C, which are predicted to circulate prior to each winter. A vaccine against malaria, especially *P. falciparum*, is proving difficult due to the ability of the parasite to continually change its surface antigens.

9 A, B, C.

Diabetes predisposes to cellulitis by interfering with the neutrophil response, causing micro- and macro-vascular diseases, because affected persons are often obese, amongst other reasons. Chronic venous disease affects the normal venous and lymphatic return from the legs, thus interfering with the local immune response; and also, if there is ulceration complicating this, then the skin barrier to microorganism entry is breached. Tinea causes breaching of the skin barrier, and needs to be specifically sought by carefully examining between the toes for typical lesions. Ischemic heart disease and chronic obstructive pulmonary disease are not predispositions to cellulitis in their own right unless complicated by peripheral edema.

10 D

Whilst B to E are all recognized complications of asplenia, *S. pneumoniae* is the most common cause of overwhelming sepsis in these individuals and is the primary agent against which the interventions of vaccination and prophylactic antibiotics are directed. Nonetheless, it is important to vaccinate against *meningococcus* and *H. influenzae* type B. *Cytocapnophagia canimorsus* sepsis can complicate dog bites to an asplenic person, and can be prophylacted by giving beta lactams in this scenario. Asplenic people are also susceptible to overwhelming malaria infection. There are guidelines including Australian ones to cover all these scenarios, and in some jurisdictions, a registry of splenectomized individuals has been established to improve the uptake of vaccinations and prophylactic antibiotics for these people.

CHAPTER 21

IMMUNIZATION

Robert W Pickles

CHAPTER OUTLINE

Globally, vaccination prevents at least 3 million deaths annually from diphtheria, tetanus, pertussis, and measles alone. Vaccination is responsible for the only successful global eradication of an infectious disease (namely smallpox), and the near eradication of polio. The introduction of *Haemophilus influenzae* type B immunization (Hib) in the early 1990s resulted in a greater than 90% reduction in cases of invasive *H. influenzae* type B disease.

No vaccine is 100% effective, nor 100% safe—in target populations, however, the benefits greatly exceed the risks. Benefits extend to both the individual and the community as a whole—with a sufficiently large proportion of the community vaccinated, unimmunized individuals are protected by a process of 'herd immunity'.

GENERAL PRINCIPLES

- *Active immunization* involves induction of immunity by the administration of live attenuated or inactivated organisms or their components, stimulating antibody or cell-mediated immunity against the disease.

- *Passive immunization* involves provision of temporary immunity via administration of exogenously produced antibody (including transplacental transfer from mother to fetus).

IMMUNIZING AGENTS

Immunizing agents may be vaccines, toxoids or immunoglobulins.

- *Vaccine*—a preparation of attenuated live or killed micro-organisms, consisting of either full organisms or components (e.g. surface antigen of hepatitis B) administered to induce immunity.
- *Toxoid*—a modified bacterial toxin rendered nontoxic but capable of inducing formation of antitoxin.

- *Immunoglobulin*—a sterile solution of antibody derived from human blood, indicated for passive immunization against hepatitis A and measles.
  » Intravenous immune globulin (IVIG) is used as replacement therapy in IgG-deficient states, as well as certain immunological conditions (e.g. immune thrombocytopenic purpura [ITP], Guillain–Barré syndrome).
  » Specific immunoglobulin comprises special preparations selected from donor pools with high levels of antibody content against a specific disease—hepatitis B immune globulin (HBIG), varicella immune globulin (VZIG), rabies immune globulin (RIG) and tetanus immune globulin (TIG).

Table 21-1 outlines the uses of vaccines in a range of diseases.

Table 21-1 Diseases prevented by vaccines available for use in Australia, the US and Europe, according to microbial and antigenic type

	'INACTIVATED' VACCINES				
	LIVE VACCINES	WHOLE MICROBE	SUB-UNIT	OTHER	TYPICAL PRIMARY POPULATIONS
Bacterial diseases					
Anthrax			Cell filtrate		Occupational
Cholera	Live (oral)	Whole			Endemic areas, travelers
Diphtheria				Toxoid	Throughout life
Haemophilus influenzae type B				Protein-conjugated polysaccharide	Infants, children
Meningococcus some or all of serogroups A, B, C, Y, W135			Polysaccharide, polyvalent	Protein-conjugated polysaccharide, polyvalent	Varies by country; children, adolescents, travelers
Pertussis			Multiple acellular components		Throughout life
Pneumococcus			Polysaccharide, polyvalent	Protein-conjugated polysaccharide, polyvalent	Infants, children, elderly; those with chronic disease
Tetanus				Toxoid	Throughout life
Typhoid	Live (oral)		Vi capsular polysaccharide		Endemic areas, travelers
Tuberculosis (Bacillus Calmette-Guérin [BCG])	Live				Varies by country; children, select other groups

	LIVE VACCINES	'INACTIVATED' VACCINES			TYPICAL PRIMARY POPULATIONS
		WHOLE MICROBE	SUB-UNIT	OTHER	
Viral diseases					
Hepatitis A		Whole			Varies by country; infants, children, adolescents, occupational, travelers, men who have sex with men, sex workers
Hepatitis B			Surface antigen		Varies by country; infants, children, adolescents, occupational, travelers, men who have sex with men, sex workers
Influenza A and B	Live (intranasal)		Split virus		Elderly, plus other groups such as children, adolescents, occupational
Japanese encephalitis		Whole			Endemic areas, travelers
Measles	Whole				Infants, children
Mumps	Whole				Infants, children
Papillomavirus (numerous types)			Virus-like particles		Adolescents, adults
Poliovirus	Whole	Whole			Infants, children
Rabies		Whole			Occupational, postexposure
Rotavirus (mono- or pentavalent)	Whole				Infants, children
Rubella	Whole				Infants, children
Tick-borne encephalitis		Whole			
Vaccinia (smallpox prevention)	Whole				Occupational
Varicella	Whole				Infants, children
Yellow fever	Whole				Endemic areas, travelers
Zoster	Whole		Surface glycoprotein E		Adults >50 and 65

*Multiple entries in a row indicate availability of more than one type of vaccine for that disease
Adapted from Cohen J, Powderly WG, and Opal SM. Infectious diseases, 4th ed. Elsevier 2017

CLINICAL PEARLS

- Immunization may be *active* (with induction of protective immune response), or *passive* (short-term passive antibody administration).
- Active vaccination may be achieved with toxoids (modified toxins), inactive products (killed organisms or sub-units), or live attenuated organisms.

FACTORS AFFECTING IMMUNOGENICITY

Chemical and physical properties of antigens (vaccines)

- Live attenuated viruses (e.g. measles, mumps, rubella) multiply in the body until checked by the immune response, and induce long-lasting immunity.
- Killed vaccines generally induce shorter-lived immunity, usually requiring subsequent booster doses to maintain immunity (diphtheria, tetanus, rabies, typhoid). Exceptions include hepatitis B and inactivated polio vaccination, where immunity lasts 10 years or more.
- Most vaccines are protein antigens that induce T-cell-dependent immunity with booster effects on repeat immunization. These vaccines produce good immune responses in all age groups.
- Purified bacterial polysaccharide capsule vaccines induce B-cell-dependent immunity, which is not long-lasting, requires frequent repeat vaccination and induces a poor immune response in children under 2 years of age (meningococcal, pneumococcal, and typhoid polysaccharide vaccines).
- Conjugation of a carrier protein to a polysaccharide vaccine induces a T-cell immune response, producing long-lasting immunity (Hib, pneumococcal conjugate vaccine).

Physiological attributes of individuals

Age, nutrition, immune status, pregnancy, stress, and infections all affect the immune response (see below).

Route of administration

- Intramuscular and subcutaneous administration results in mostly an IgG response.
- Oral or intranasal vaccination induces mostly a local IgA response with some systemic IgG response.
- Intradermal dosing allows reduction in dose, with potential cost savings.

Presence of adjuvants

- Adjuvants are particularly useful with inactivated vaccines such as diphtheria, tetanus toxoid, and acellular pertussis vaccine as well as hepatitis B vaccine.

- The mechanism of enhancement is unknown, but involves the innate immune system through pathogen-associated molecular patterns (PAMPs).

Contraindications

- Anaphylaxis to a prior dose of the same vaccine
- Intercurrent febrile illness (temperature >38.5°C) should prompt deferral of immunization
- Live vaccines:
  » severe immune deficiency
  » immunosuppressant drugs
  » immune globulin receipt within 3–11 months

False contraindications

- Family history of an adverse event
- Convulsions
- Previous illness similar to the target illness
- Prematurity
- Stable neurological conditions
- Intercurrent antibiotic treatment (except oral typhoid vaccine)

Egg allergy

- Egg allergy is not a contraindication for measles-mumps-rubella (MMR) vaccine.
- Caution should be exercised with influenza vaccine—a split-dose protocol should be considered.
- Yellow fever vaccine is contraindicated if a patient has anaphylaxis due to eggs.

CLINICAL PEARL

Polysaccharide capsule vaccines induce B-cell-mediated immunity, which is of short duration (2–3 years) and is ineffective in children under 2 years of age.

BOOSTER DOSES

General recommendations regarding the need for booster doses of specific vaccines are given in Table 21-2.

IMMUNIZATION IN SPECIFIC POPULATIONS

See Figure 21-1 later in this chapter for a summary of immunization recommendations.

Pregnancy

- Influenza vaccine (inactivated) is the only vaccine specifically recommended during pregnancy, due to the risk of severe infection.
- Additionally, the need for tetanus, diphtheria and pertussis vaccination (Tdap) is recommended in pregnancy, particularly pertussis between weeks 27–34 of gestation to help prevent infant pertussis.

Table 21-2 Booster doses for specific vaccines

VACCINE	COMMENTS REGARDING BOOSTERS
Diphtheria	DTPa at 4 years dTpa at 12–17 years dTpa at 10 and 20 years after primary immunization, then at age 50
Haemophilus influenzae type B	Booster at 12 months Single dose in splenectomy if not previously vaccinated
Hepatitis A	Single booster 12 months after primary dose
Hepatitis B	Not generally recommended
Human papillomavirus	Unknown
Japanese encephalitis	Unknown
Meningococcus	Single booster polysaccharide vaccine 3–5 years after initial dose Boosters not required for conjugate vaccine
Pertussis	Single booster at age 50 generally recommended, repeated at age 65; consider if undertaking high-risk travel and no booster within 5 years
Pneumococcus	23vPPV: single booster after 5 years; indigenous and other high-risk populations revaccinate 5 years after 2nd dose or at 65 years (whichever is later) 13vPCV: single booster at 2 years in high-risk and indigenous children
Poliomyelitis	Age 4 years; adults only if at especially high risk (travel)
Q fever	Revaccination contraindicated
Rabies	Every 2 years or if titer <0.5 IU/mL
Tetanus	DTPa age 4 years dTpa age 12–17 years, then age 50 (Australia); dTpa every 10 years (US)
Typhoid	Oral vaccine: booster at 5 years Vi capsule vaccine booster every 2–3 years if ongoing exposure

DTPa, diphtheria–tetanus–pertussis (acellular); dTpa, diphtheria–tetanus–pertussis (acellular; adult formulation); PCV, pneumococcal conjugate vaccine; PPV, pneumococcal polysaccharide vaccine.

- All other vaccines, particularly live attenuated vaccines, are generally contraindicated in the pregnant woman—fever is considered potentially teratogenic, whether vaccine- or illness-induced.
- Live attenuated vaccines are considered potentially teratogenic, although no definite risk has been demonstrated.

Preconception

- The preconception health check should review the need for measles, mumps, rubella, varicella, diphtheria, tetanus and pertussis vaccinations.
- Women should avoid becoming pregnant within 28 days of receipt of live vaccines.

Breastfeeding

Rubella vaccine virus is detectable in breast milk following vaccination, and has resulted in mild infection in the infant. No evidence of harm has been detected in breastfed infants where the mother has been vaccinated.

Immunocompromised hosts

Issues in the immunocompromised host include the risk of a reduced immune response to immunization, and the potential for disseminated infection with live vaccine organisms.

Factors to consider are:

- the degree of immunosuppression
- the risk posed by the target infection.

A corticosteroid dose >60 mg/day for >1 week requires delaying administration of live attenuated vaccines for 3 months after cessation of therapy.

Vaccines absolutely contraindicated are:

- Bacillus Calmette–Guérin (BCG)
- smallpox
- oral cholera
- oral typhoid.

Yellow fever vaccine requires caution in certain situations—the risk of disease versus the risk of vaccination (risk of developing viscerotropic disease) needs to be considered.

Figure 1. Recommended immunization schedule for adults aged 19 years or older by age group, United States, 2018

This figure should be reviewed with the accompanying footnotes. This figure and the footnotes describe indications for which vaccines, if not previously administered, should be administered unless noted otherwise.

Vaccine	19–21 years	22–26 years	27–49 years	50–64 years	≥65 years
Influenza[1]	1 dose annually				
Tdap[2] or Td[2]	1 dose Tdap, then Td booster every 10 yrs				
MMR[3]	1 or 2 doses depending on indication (if born in 1957 or later)				
VAR[4]	2 doses				
RZV[5] (preferred) ... or ... ZVL[5]					2 doses RZV (preferred) ... or ... 1 dose ZVL
HPV–Female[6]	2 or 3 doses depending on age at series initiation				
HPV–Male[6]	2 or 3 doses depending on age at series initiation				
PCV13[7]				1 dose	
PPSV23[7]		1 or 2 doses depending on indication			1 dose
HepA[8]	2 or 3 doses depending on vaccine				
HepB[9]	3 doses				
MenACWY[10]	1 or 2 doses depending on indication, then booster every 5 yrs if risk remains				
MenB[10]	2 or 3 doses depending on vaccine				
Hib[11]	1 or 3 doses depending on indication				

Recommended for adults who meet the age requirement, lack documentation of vaccination, or lack evidence of past infection | Recommended for adults with other indications | No recommendation

Figure 2. Recommended immunization schedule for adults aged 19 years or older by medical condition and other indications, United States, 2018

This figure should be reviewed with the accompanying footnotes. This figure and the footnotes describe indications for which vaccines, if not previously administered, should be administered unless noted otherwise.

Vaccine	Pregnancy[1-6]	Immuno-compromised (excluding HIV infection)[3-7,11]	HIV infection CD4+ count (cells/μL)[3-7,9-10] <200	HIV infection CD4+ count (cells/μL)[3-7,9-10] ≥200	Asplenia, complement deficiencies[7,10,11]	End-stage renal disease, on hemodialysis[7,9]	Heart or lung disease, alcoholism[7]	Chronic liver disease[7,9]	Diabetes[7,9]	Health care personnel[3,4,9]	Men who have sex with men[6,8,9]
Influenza[1]	1 dose annually										
Tdap[2] or Td[2]	1 dose Tdap each pregnancy	1 dose Tdap, then Td booster every 10 yrs									
MMR[3]	contraindicated			1 or 2 doses depending on indication							
VAR[4]	contraindicated			2 doses							
RZV[5] (preferred) ... or ... ZVL[5]	contraindicated		2 doses RZV at age ≥50 yrs (preferred) ... or ... 1 dose ZVL at age ≥60 yrs								
HPV–Female[6]		3 doses through age 26 yrs			2 or 3 doses through age 26 yrs						
HPV–Male[6]		3 doses through age 26 yrs			2 or 3 doses through age 21 yrs						2 or 3 doses through age 26 yrs
PCV13[7]		1 dose									
PPSV23[7]		1, 2, or 3 doses depending on indication									
HepA[8]		2 or 3 doses depending on vaccine									
HepB[9]		3 doses									
MenACWY[10]		1 or 2 doses depending on indication, then booster every 5 yrs if risk remains									
MenB[10]		2 or 3 doses depending on vaccine									
Hib[11]		3 doses HSCT recipients only	1 dose								

Recommended for adults who meet the age requirement, lack documentation of vaccination, or lack evidence of past infection | Recommended for adults with other indications | Contraindicated | No recommendation

Figure 21-1 Recommended immunization schedule for adults, United States, 2018

From Centers for Disease Control and Prevention, www.cdc.gov/vaccines/schedules/downloads/adult/adult-combined-schedule.pdf

Footnotes. Recommended immunization schedule for adults aged 19 years or older, United States, 2018

1. Influenza vaccination
www.cdc.gov/vaccines/hcp/acip-recs/vacc-specific/flu.html

General information
- Administer 1 dose of age-appropriate inactivated influenza vaccine (IIV) or recombinant influenza vaccine (RIV) annually
- Live attenuated influenza vaccine (LAIV) is not recommended for the 2017–2018 influenza season
- A list of currently available influenza vaccines is available at www.cdc.gov/flu/protect/vaccine/vaccines.htm

Special populations
- Administer age-appropriate IIV or RIV to:
  - **Pregnant women**
  - Adults with **hives-only egg allergy**
  - Adults with **egg allergy other than hives** (e.g., angioedema or respiratory distress): Administer IIV or RIV in a medical setting under supervision of a health care provider who can recognize and manage severe allergic conditions

2. Tetanus, diphtheria, and pertussis vaccination
www.cdc.gov/vaccines/hcp/acip-recs/vacc-specific/tdap-td.html

General information
- Administer to adults who previously did not receive a dose of tetanus toxoid, reduced diphtheria toxoid, and acellular pertussis vaccine (Tdap) as an adult or child (routinely recommended at age 11–12 years) 1 dose of Tdap, followed by a dose of tetanus and diphtheria toxoids (Td) booster every 10 years
- Information on the use of Tdap or Td as tetanus prophylaxis in wound management is available at www.cdc.gov/mmwr/preview/mmwrhtml/rr5517a1.htm

Special populations
- **Pregnant women**: Administer 1 dose of Tdap during each pregnancy, preferably in the early part of gestational weeks 27–36

3. Measles, mumps, and rubella vaccination
www.cdc.gov/vaccines/hcp/acip-recs/vacc-specific/mmr.html

General information
- Administer 1 dose of measles, mumps, and rubella vaccine (MMR) to adults with no evidence of immunity to measles, mumps, or rubella
- Evidence of immunity is:
  - Born before 1957 (except for health care personnel, see below)
  - Documentation of receipt of MMR
  - Laboratory evidence of immunity or disease
- Documentation of a health care provider-diagnosed disease without laboratory confirmation is not considered evidence of immunity

Special populations
- **Pregnant women and nonpregnant women of childbearing age** with no evidence of immunity to rubella: Administer 1 dose of MMR (if pregnant, administer MMR after pregnancy and before discharge from health care facility)

- **HIV infection and CD4 cell count ≥200 cells/µL for at least 6 months** and no evidence of immunity to measles, mumps, or rubella: Administer 2 doses of MMR at least 28 days apart
- **Students in postsecondary educational institutions, international travelers**, and **household contacts of immunocompromised persons**: Administer 2 doses of MMR at least 28 days apart (or 1 dose of MMR if previously administered 1 dose of MMR)
- **Health care personnel born in 1957 or later** with no evidence of immunity: Administer 2 doses of MMR at least 28 days apart for measles or mumps, or 1 dose of MMR for rubella (if born before 1957, consider MMR vaccination)
- Adults who **previously received ≤2 doses of mumps-containing vaccine and are identified by public health authority to be at increased risk for mumps in an outbreak**: Administer 1 dose of MMR
- MMR is contraindicated for pregnant women and adults with severe immunodeficiency

4. Varicella vaccination
www.cdc.gov/vaccines/hcp/acip-recs/vacc-specific/varicella.html

General information
- Administer to adults without evidence of immunity to varicella 2 doses of varicella vaccine (VAR) 4–8 weeks apart if previously received no varicella-containing vaccine (if previously received 1 dose of varicella-containing vaccine, administer 1 dose of VAR at least 4 weeks after the first dose)
- Evidence of immunity to varicella is:
  - U.S.-born before 1980 (except for pregnant women and health care personnel, see below)
  - Documentation of receipt of 2 doses of varicella or varicella-containing vaccine at least 4 weeks apart
  - Diagnosis or verification of history of varicella or herpes zoster by a health care provider
  - Laboratory evidence of immunity or disease

Special populations
- Administer 2 doses of VAR 4–8 weeks apart if previously received no varicella-containing vaccine (if previously received 1 dose of varicella-containing vaccine, administer 1 dose of VAR at least 4 weeks after the first dose) to:
  - **Pregnant women without evidence of immunity**: Administer the first of the 2 doses or the second dose after pregnancy and before discharge from health care facility
  - **Health care personnel without evidence of immunity**
- Adults with **HIV infection and CD4 cell count ≥200 cells/µL**: May administer, based on individual clinical decision, 2 doses of VAR 3 months apart
- VAR is contraindicated for pregnant women and adults with severe immunodeficiency

5. Zoster vaccination
www.cdc.gov/vaccines/hcp/acip-recs/vacc-specific/shingles.html

General information
- Administer 2 doses of recombinant zoster vaccine (RZV) 2–6 months apart to adults aged 50 years or older regardless of past episode of herpes zoster or receipt of zoster vaccine live (ZVL)

- Administer 2 doses of RZV 2–6 months apart to adults who previously received ZVL at least 2 months after ZVL
- For adults aged 60 years or older, administer either RZV or ZVL (RZV is preferred)

Special populations
- ZVL is contraindicated for pregnant women and adults with severe immunodeficiency

6. Human papillomavirus vaccination
www.cdc.gov/vaccines/hcp/acip-recs/vacc-specific/hpv.html

General information
- Administer human papillomavirus (HPV) vaccine to **females through age 26 years** and **males through age 21 years** (males aged 22 through 26 years may be vaccinated based on individual clinical decision)
- The number of doses of HPV vaccine to be administered depends on age at initial HPV vaccination
  - **No previous dose of HPV vaccine**: Administer 3-dose series at 0, 1–2, and 6 months (minimum intervals: 4 weeks between doses 1 and 2, 12 weeks between doses 2 and 3, and 5 months between doses 1 and 3; repeat doses if given too soon)
  - **Aged 9–14 years at HPV vaccine series initiation and received 1 dose or 2 doses less than 5 months apart**: Administer 1 dose
  - **Aged 9–14 years at HPV vaccine series initiation and received 2 doses at least 5 months apart**: No additional dose is needed

Special populations
- Adults with **immunocompromising conditions (including HIV infection)** through age 26 years: Administer 3-dose series at 0, 1–2, and 6 months
- **Men who have sex with men** through age 26 years: Administer 2- or 3-dose series depending on age at initial vaccination (see above); if no history of HPV vaccine, administer 3-dose series at 0, 1–2, and 6 months
- **Pregnant women** through age 26 years: HPV vaccination is not recommended during pregnancy, but there is no evidence that the vaccine is harmful and no intervention needed for women who inadvertently receive HPV vaccine while pregnant; delay remaining doses until after pregnancy; pregnancy testing is not needed before vaccination

7. Pneumococcal vaccination
www.cdc.gov/vaccines/hcp/acip-recs/vacc-specific/pneumo.html

General information
- Administer to immunocompetent adults aged 65 years or older 1 dose of 13-valent pneumococcal conjugate vaccine (PCV13), if not previously administered, followed by 1 dose of 23-valent pneumococcal polysaccharide vaccine (PPSV23) at least 1 year after PCV13; if PPSV23 was previously administered but not PCV13, administer PCV13 at least 1 year after PPSV23
- When both PCV13 and PPSV23 are indicated, administer PCV13 first (PCV13 and PPSV23 should not be administered during the same visit); additional information on vaccine timing is available at www.cdc.gov/vaccines/vpd/pneumo/downloads/pneumo-vaccine-timing.pdf

Figure 21-1 Recommended immunization schedule for adults, United States, 2018 *continued*

Special populations
- Administer to adults aged 19 through 64 years with the following chronic conditions 1 dose of PPSV23 (at age 65 years or older, administer 1 dose of PCV13, if not previously received, and another dose of PPSV23 at least 1 year after PCV13 and at least 5 years after PPSV23):
  - **Chronic heart disease** (excluding hypertension)
  - **Chronic lung disease**
  - **Chronic liver disease**
  - **Alcoholism**
  - **Diabetes mellitus**
  - **Cigarette smoking**
- Administer to adults aged 19 years or older with the following indications 1 dose of PCV13 followed by 1 dose of PPSV23 at least 8 weeks after PCV13, and a second dose of PPSV23 at least 5 years after the first dose of PPSV23 (if the most recent dose of PPSV23 was administered before age 65 years, at age 65 years or older, administer another dose of PPSV23 at least 5 years after the last dose of PPSV23):
  - **Immunodeficiency disorders** (including B- and T-lymphocyte deficiency, complement deficiencies, and phagocytic disorders)
  - **HIV infection**
  - **Anatomical or functional asplenia** (including sickle cell disease and other hemoglobinopathies)
  - **Chronic renal failure and nephrotic syndrome**
- Administer to adults aged 19 years or older with the following indications 1 dose of PCV13 followed by 1 dose of PPSV23 at least 8 weeks after PCV13 (if the dose of PPSV23 was administered before age 65 years, at age 65 years or older, administer another dose of PPSV23 at least 5 years after the last dose of PPSV23):
  - **Cerebrospinal fluid leak**
  - **Cochlear implant**

8. Hepatitis A vaccination
www.cdc.gov/vaccines/hcp/acip-recs/vacc-specific/hepa.html
General information
- Administer to adults who have a specific risk (see below), or lack a risk factor but want protection, 2-dose series of single antigen hepatitis A vaccine (HepA; Havrix at 0 and 6–12 months or Vaqta at 0 and 6–18 months; minimum interval: 6 months) or a 3-dose series of combined hepatitis A and hepatitis B vaccine (HepA-HepB) at 0, 1, and 6 months; minimum intervals: 4 weeks between first and second doses, 5 months between second and third doses

Special populations
- Administer HepA or HepA-HepB to adults with the following indications:
  - **Travel** to or work in countries with high or intermediate hepatitis A endemicity
  - **Men who have sex with men**
  - **Injection or noninjection drug use**
  - **Work with hepatitis A virus in a research laboratory or with nonhuman primates infected with hepatitis A virus**
  - **Clotting factor disorders**
  - **Chronic liver disease**
  - Close, personal **contact with an international adoptee** (e.g., household or regular babysitting) during the first 60 days after arrival in the United States from a country with high or intermediate endemicity (administer the first dose as soon as the adoption is planned)
  - Healthy adults **through age 40 years who have recently been exposed to hepatitis A virus**; adults older than age 40 years may receive HepA if hepatitis A immunoglobulin cannot be obtained

9. Hepatitis B vaccination
www.cdc.gov/vaccines/hcp/acip-recs/vacc-specific/hepb.html
General information
- Administer to adults who have a specific risk (see below), or lack a risk factor but want protection, 3-dose series of single antigen hepatitis B vaccine (HepB) or combined hepatitis A and hepatitis B vaccine (HepA-HepB) at 0, 1, and 6 months (minimum intervals: 4 weeks between doses 1 and 2 for HepB and HepA-HepB; between doses 2 and 3, 8 weeks for HepB and 5 months for HepA-HepB)

Special populations
- Administer HepB or HepA-HepB to adults with the following indications:
  - **Chronic liver disease** (e.g., hepatitis C infection, cirrhosis, fatty liver disease, alcoholic liver disease, autoimmune hepatitis, alanine aminotransferase [ALT] or aspartate aminotransferase [AST] level greater than twice the upper limit of normal)
  - **HIV infection**
  - **Percutaneous or mucosal risk of exposure to blood** (e.g., **household contacts** of hepatitis B surface antigen [HBsAg]-positive persons; adults younger than age 60 years with **diabetes mellitus** or aged 60 years or older with diabetes mellitus based on individual clinical decision; adults in predialysis care or receiving **hemodialysis or peritoneal dialysis**; recent or current **injection drug users**; **health care and public safety workers** at risk for exposure to blood or blood-contaminated body fluids)
  - **Sexual exposure risk** (e.g., sex partners of HBsAg-positive persons; sexually active persons not in a mutually monogamous relationship; persons seeking evaluation or treatment for a sexually transmitted infection; and **men who have sex with men** [MSM])
  - Receive care in **settings where a high proportion of adults have risks for hepatitis B infection** (e.g., facilities providing sexually transmitted disease treatment, drug-abuse treatment and prevention services, hemodialysis and end-stage renal disease programs, institutions for developmentally disabled persons, health care settings targeting services to injection drug users or MSM, HIV testing and treatment facilities, and correctional facilities)
  - **Travel** to countries with high or intermediate hepatitis B endemicity

10. Meningococcal vaccination
www.cdc.gov/vaccines/hcp/acip-recs/vacc-specific/mening.html

Special populations: Serogroups A, C, W, and Y meningococcal vaccine (MenACWY)

- Administer 2 doses of MenACWY at least 8 weeks apart and revaccinate with 1 dose of MenACWY every 5 years, if the risk remains, to adults with the following indications:
  - **Anatomical or functional asplenia** (including sickle cell disease and other hemoglobinopathies)
  - **HIV infection**
  - **Persistent complement component deficiency**
  - **Eculizumab use**
- Administer 1 dose of MenACWY and revaccinate with 1 dose of MenACWY every 5 years, if the risk remains, to adults with the following indications:
  - **Travel to or live in countries where meningococcal disease is hyperendemic or epidemic**, including countries in the African meningitis belt or during the Hajj
  - At risk from a **meningococcal disease outbreak attributed to serogroup A, C, W, or Y**
  - **Microbiologists** routinely exposed to *Neisseria meningitidis*
  - **Military recruits**
  - **First-year college students who live in residential housing** (if they did not receive MenACWY at age 16 years or older)

General Information: Serogroup B meningococcal vaccine (MenB)
  - May administer, based on individual clinical decision, to young adults and adolescents aged 16–23 years (preferred age is 16–18 years) who are not at increased risk 2-dose series of MenB-4C (Bexsero) at least 1 month apart or 2-dose series of MenB-FHbp (Trumenba) at least 6 months apart
  - MenB-4C and MenB-FHbp are not interchangeable

Special populations: MenB
- Administer 2-dose series of MenB-4C at least 1 month apart or 3-dose series of MenB-FHbp at 0, 1–2, and 6 months to adults with the following indications:
  - **Anatomical or functional asplenia** (including sickle cell disease)
  - **Persistent complement component deficiency**
  - **Eculizumab use**
  - At risk from a **meningococcal disease outbreak attributed to serogroup B**
  - **Microbiologists** routinely exposed to *Neisseria meningitidis*

11. *Haemophilus influenzae* type b vaccination
www.cdc.gov/vaccines/hcp/acip-recs/vacc-specific/hib.html
Special populations
- Administer *Haemophilus influenzae* type b vaccine (Hib) to adults with the following indications:
  - **Anatomical or functional asplenia** (including sickle cell disease) or undergoing elective splenectomy: Administer 1 dose if not previously vaccinated (preferably at least 14 days before elective splenectomy)
  - **Hematopoietic stem cell transplant** (HSCT): Administer 3-dose series with doses 4 weeks apart starting 6 to 12 months after successful transplant regardless of Hib vaccination history

Figure 21-1 Recommended immunization schedule for adults, United States, 2018 *continued*

Oncology patients

- If well and in remission and infection-free for >6 months, the following vaccines may be given:
  - » DTPa (acellular diphtheria–tetanus–pertussis; adult form is dTpa)
  - » hepatitis B
  - » MMR
  - » inactivated poliomyelitis vaccine (iPV)
  - » Hib (if patient <5 years of age)
  - » varicella after completion of therapy.
- If there are hematological malignancies associated with invasive pneumococcal disease, such as myeloma, Hodgkin lymphoma, non-Hodgkin lymphoma or chronic lymphocytic leukemia (CLL), vaccination should occur at diagnosis, before chemo/radiotherapy, or on completion of therapy.
- Influenza vaccination is indicated in all cancer patients over 36 months of age.

Solid-organ transplant patients

- Where possible, potential recipients should be immunized pre-transplant.
- Live vaccines are contraindicated post-transplantation.
- Inactivated vaccines can be given 6–12 months post-transplantation, although immune responses may be blunted.

Hemopoetic stem-cell transplant (HSCT) recipients

- Protective immunity to vaccine-preventable infections is partly or completely lost after allogeneic or autologous HSCT.
- Most vaccines are delayed for at least 12 months post-transplantation, due to poor immune responses during this time. Immunity testing is recommended before and after hepatitis B, measles, rubella and varicella to determine the need for future doses.

HIV/AIDS

- BCG is absolutely contraindicated in patients with human immunodeficiency virus (HIV) or acquired immune deficiency syndrome (AIDS).
- See Figure 21-1 (on previous pages) for other recommendations.
- Provided that CD4+ cells are >250/mm^3, many live attenuated vaccines can be administered safely.

CLINICAL PEARL

Live attenuated vaccines are generally contraindicated in immunosuppressed individuals.

Asplenia

- Patients with anatomical or functional asplenia (seen in some patients with systemic lupus erythematosus or celiac disease) should receive pneumococcal, meningococcal and Hib vaccination.
- Receipt of a conjugate vaccine should be followed by polysaccharide vaccine 6 months later.

Occupational exposure

Certain occupations are associated with an increased risk of some vaccine-preventable diseases.

- Infected workers (especially healthcare and child-care workers) are at risk of transmitting infections such as influenza, rubella, measles, mumps, pertussis, and others to susceptible contacts, with potentially serious outcomes.
- The current recommended vaccines for people at risk of occupationally acquired vaccine-preventable diseases are shown in Table 21-3.

Travel vaccines

- There is a need to consider routine immunization status as well as specific travel-related vaccine requirements in those embarking upon travel.
- Travelers visiting friends and relatives (VFRs) are generally at high risk of acquiring travel-related infections.
- Vaccines may be *required* (in order to cross international borders), or *recommended* (according to the risk of infection in the area of travel).
- Country-specific recommendations are available at http://www.cdc.gov/travel and http://www.who.int/ith/en.

POST-EXPOSURE PROPHYLAXIS (PEP)

Intramuscular immune globulin

Hepatitis A

- Hepatitis A vaccination is preferred over immune globulin for PEP and for protection of travelers.
- Patients aged <12 months or >40 years, the immunocompromised, and those with chronic liver disease, should be given immune globulin.
- Immune globulin is effective if given within 14 days of exposure.

Measles

Immune globulin is effective if given within 6 days of exposure to at-risk individuals.

Specific intramuscular immune globulin preparations (hyperimmune globulins)

Hepatitis B immune globulin (HBIG)

- Hepatitis B immune globulin is recommended following exposure to known hepatitis B (HBV)-infected sexual

Table 21-3 Vaccines for occupational exposure

OCCUPATION	DISEASE/VACCINE
Healthcare workers	Hepatitis B Influenza, pertussis (dTpa), MMR if not immune, varicella (if seronegative)
Working with children	Pertussis (dTpa) MMR, varicella (if not immune) Hepatitis A (child-care and preschool)
Carers	Hepatitis A and B (intellectual disability) Influenza (aged care)
Emergency service personnel (including in correctional facilities)	Hepatitis B Influenza
Laboratory personnel (routinely working with infectious tissues)	Q fever (veterinary specimens) Rabies Anthrax, vaccinia poxviruses, poliomyelitis, typhoid, yellow fever, meningococcal disease, Japanese encephalitis
Veterinarians (and students, nurses)	Q fever Rabies (lyssavirus)
Poultry workers	Influenza
Bat handlers, wildlife officers	Rabies (lyssavirus)
Abattoir (slaughterhouse) workers, livestock transporters, sheep shearers/farmers, goat farmers, saleyard workers	Q fever
Embalmers	Hepatitis B, BCG
Sex-industry workers	Hepatitis A and B
Tattooists, body piercers	Hepatitis B
Plumbers	Hepatitis A

BCG, Bacillus Calmette–Guérin; dTpa, diphtheria–tetanus–pertussis (acellular, adult formulation); MMR, measles-mumps-rubella.

partners or to HBV surface antigen (HBsAg)-positive blood by the percutaneous (72 hours) or mucous membrane (14 days) route.

- Children born to HBsAg-positive mothers should be given HBIG at birth as well as a dose of hepatitis B vaccine.

Rabies immune globulin (RIG)

- Rabies immune globulin is prepared from previously immunized humans.
- It should be given along with rabies vaccine in previously unvaccinated exposed individuals.
- RIG is unnecessary in those who received rabies vaccine more than 8 days earlier.

Tetanus immune globulin (TIG)

- Tetanus immune globulin is indicated for those with tetanus-prone wounds with no history of prior tetanus vaccination.
- Combined tetanus and diphtheria vaccination should be administered simultaneously at a different site, and a primary course of vaccination should be completed.

Varicella zoster immune globulin (VZIG)

- The decision to administer VZIG depends on:
  - » the likelihood that the exposed person is not immune

» the probability of exposure resulting in infection
» and the likelihood that complications of varicella will develop.

- VZIG should be given to neonates whose mothers develop varicella 5 days before to 48 hours after birth.
- VZIG should be administered within 96 hours of exposure.
- VZIG may not prevent infection but usually attenuates it, with resultant subclinical or mild infection.
- Subsequent varicella vaccination should be given 5 months after VZIG, unless contraindicated or clinical varicella develops.

Specific immune globulins for intravenous use

Cytomegalovirus (CMV IVIG)

This is given for prophylaxis of CMV disease in CMV-seronegative organ-transplant recipients.

Botulism IVIG

Botulism IVIG is indicated for infant botulism.

ROUTINE IMMUNIZATION OF ADULTS

A recommended schedule for adult immunizations is given in Figure 21-1 (earlier in chapter).

SELF-ASSESSMENT QUESTIONS

1 The following are all live attenuated vaccines *except*:
   A Yellow fever vaccine
   B Japanese encephalitis vaccine
   C MMR (measles-mumps-rubella)
   D Varicella vaccine
   E Oral typhoid vaccine

2 The following statements regarding pneumococcal polysaccharide vaccine (23vPPV) are correct *except*:
   A It is indicated in asplenic individuals.
   B HIV-infected individuals should be offered 23vPPV.
   C It stimulates T-cell-mediated immunity.
   D It is poorly immunogenic in children aged less than 2 years.

3 A 50-year-old man is being assessed for renal transplantation. His hepatitis B serology shows:
   i   HBsAg negative
   ii   HBsAb negative
   iii HBcAb positive.

   These results are consistent with all the following statements *except*:
   A The patient has immunity to hepatitis B from prior vaccination.
   B The patient has had prior hepatitis B infection.
   C This could be a false positive result.
   D The patient has chronic hepatitis B infection.
   E The patient has occult hepatitis B infection.

4 A 28-year-old woman with stable human immunodeficiency virus (HIV) infection is planning to travel to South America for 3 months. Her CD4+ cells are 450/mm^3 (32%) and she is stable on her current antiretroviral regimen. Which one of the following vaccines poses no risk of disseminated infection to her?
   A Oral typhoid vaccine
   B BCG (Bacillus Calmette–Guérin)
   C Varicella zoster vaccine
   D Yellow fever vaccine
   E Typhoid Vi vaccine

5 A 25-year-old pregnant woman known to be a carrier of hepatitis B virus wishes to discuss strategies to prevent transmission of HBV to her child. Which of the following statements is incorrect in the setting of a pregnant woman infected with hepatitis B?
   A Approximately 5% of children will acquire infection transplacentally.
   B Administration of hepatitis B vaccine at birth will prevent 90% of cases of vertical transmission.
   C A strategy of hepatitis B vaccine plus immune globulin will prevent at least 95% of cases of vertical transmission.
   D Antiviral therapy with entecavir given in the final trimester has been shown to prevent neonatal infection.
   E Elective Cesarean section has not been shown to prevent transmission from occurring at delivery.

6 The following statements about diphtheria vaccination are true *except*:
   A The vaccine is a live attenuated preparation, and is contraindicated in immunocompromised patients.
   B Protective levels of antitoxin are induced in more than 90% of recipients who complete the vaccination schedule.
   C The vaccine is a purified preparation of inactivated diphtheria toxin and is known as a toxoid.
   D Vaccination does not prevent acquisition or carriage of the causative organism.
   E The adult formulation has a lower concentration of the agent, as local reactions are thought to relate to age and dose.

7 Which of the following vaccines is contraindicated in those with a documented egg allergy?
   A Typhoid Vi
   B Cholera
   C Yellow fever
   D Varicella zoster
   E MMR(measles-mumps-rubella)

8 Which of the following is absolutely contraindicated in people with HIV/AIDS, regardless of CD4+ count?
   A BCG (Bacillus Calmette–Guérin)
   B Cholera
   C Smallpox
   D Typhoid
   E Varicella zoster

9 Which of the following is contraindicated in a renal transplant patient?
   A Oral typhoid vaccine
   B DTP (diphtheria–tetanus–pertussis) vaccine
   C Hepatitis A vaccine
   D Japanese encephalitis vaccine
   E Rabies vaccine

10 All of the following are specifically recommended for healthcare workers *except*:
   A DTP (diphtheria–tetanus–pertussis) vaccine
   B Hepatitis A vaccine
   C Hepatitis B vaccine
   D Influenza vaccine
   E MMR (measles-mumps-rubella) vaccine

11 A 27-year-old woman with no history of either varicella infection or vaccination attends following contact with a nephew with chickenpox. The contact occurred 36 hours ago and her screening varicella IgG is negative. The most appropriate action would be to:
   A Commence oral valaciclovir 1 g TDS for 7 days
   B Administer varicella vaccine
   C Administer zoster immune globulin and varicella vaccine at separate sites that day
   D Administer zoster immune globulin followed by varicella vaccine 5 months later
   E Administer zoster immune globulin

12 Which of the following statements are incorrect regarding the varicella vaccine?
   A It is a live attenuated virus vaccine
   B A lack of detectable varicella IgG following vaccination implies non-response
   C It is contraindicated in pregnancy
   D Patients with a history of shingles do not require varicella vaccination
   E It is possible to develop shingles after receipt of varicella vaccine.

13 Which one of the following vaccines is safe to administer to an HIV-positive woman who is intending to travel to rural Thailand to spend some time with her family? She is on antiretroviral therapy with a CD4+ cell count of 180/mm^3 (11%).
   A Oral typhoid vaccine
   B Japanese B encephalitis vaccine
   C BCG (Bacillus Calmette-Guérin)
   D Varicella zoster vaccine
   E Oral cholera vaccine

14 A 48-year-old man is being assessed for treatment for hepatitis C infection. His baseline hepatitis B testing shows:

HBsAg negative
HBcAb positive
HBsAb positive

These results are consistent with which one of the following statements?
   A The patient is immune from prior hepatitis B vaccination
   B The patient has chronic hepatitis B infection
   C The patient is immune from prior hepatitis B infection
   D The patient has acute hepatitis B infection
   E The patient has occult hepatitis B infection

15 Patients who have undergone splenectomy should consider all of the following except:
   A Pneumococcal polysaccharide vaccine followed by pneumococcal conjugate vaccine 6 months later
   B Meningococcal conjugate vaccine
   C *Haemophilus influenzae* type B conjugate vaccine
   D Prophylaxis with penicillin V for at least 2 years
   E Appropriate care in malaria-prone areas

16 A 21-year-old is about to start work in a rural Queensland veterinary practice. He has already been vaccinated against Q fever. Which one of the following vaccines would you recommend in addition?
   A Leptospirosis vaccine
   B Hendra virus vaccine
   C Q fever booster
   D Rabies vaccine
   E Anthrax vaccine

17 Which of the following statements is true regarding hepatitis A vaccination?
   A   Vaccination is recommended for plumbers and preschool workers
   B   Vaccination is contraindicated in those with reduced cell-mediated immunity
   C   Administration of immune globulin is preferred to vaccination in cases of post-exposure prophylaxis
   D   Administration of hepatitis A vaccine is preferred to immune globulin in cases of post-exposure prophylaxis in patients with chronic liver disease
   E   Post-vaccination serology should be performed after the 2nd dose to ensure efficacy

18 Which of the following statements regarding yellow fever vaccine is incorrect?
   A   It is a live attenuated virus vaccine
   B   A single dose is considered to be protective for life
   C   It is a requirement of travel to parts of Asia
   D   It may be safely administered to patients with HIV infection provided CD4+ cells are > 250/mm^3
   E   Care needs to be exercised in patients with anaphylaxis to eggs

19 Which one of the following is not a true contraindication to the receipt of a live virus vaccine?
   A   Receipt of immunosuppressant medications such as tacrolimus
   B   Receipt of oral prednisone at a dose of 7.5 mg/day
   C   Pregnancy
   D   Anaphylaxis to a prior dose of the vaccine
   E   An intercurrent febrile illness with fever of 38.5°C

20 A 26-year-old woman visits her GP to ask about vaccination during pregnancy. Which one of the following statements is incorrect regarding vaccination in pregnancy?
   A   Women should avoid becoming pregnant within 28 days of receipt of a live vaccine
   B   Pregnant women should be advised to have influenza vaccination
   C   If a pregnant woman is found to have a low titer of rubella IgG she should receive MMR vaccine as soon as practicable
   D   Booster vaccination with Tdap is advised during pregnancy if a woman has not had a booster within 10 years
   E   A pregnant woman traveling to an area with known yellow fever transmission may receive yellow fever virus vaccine

ANSWERS

1   B.

   Japanese encephalitis vaccine is an inactivated vaccine. Yellow fever, MMR and oral typhoid vaccines are all live attenuated vaccines. Varicella vaccine and varicella zoster vaccine (VZV) are both live attenuated vaccines—VZV is approximately 14 times as potent as varicella vaccine, and must only be given to people with prior immunity to varicella.

2   C.

   Polysaccharide capsule vaccines stimulate B-cell-mediated immunity. Pneumococcal polysaccharide vaccine is indicated in asplenic individuals (over 50 years of age) or with certain chronic diseases, as well as HIV-infected individuals, all of whom are at greater risk of invasive pneumococcal disease. Polysaccharide capsule vaccines stimulate B-cell immunity, and as such are poorly immunogenic in children under 2 years of age and require booster doses to maintain immunity.

3   A.

   Hepatitis B immunity due solely to vaccination is characterized by the presence of anti-surface-antigen antibodies (HBsAb) alone. Thus, a previously immunized patient who has HBcAb in addition to HBsAb is immune on the basis of natural infection rather than immunization. Isolated anti-core-antigen antibodies (HBcAb) may be due either to prior hepatitis B infection with loss of HBsAb over time, low-level chronic infection, or occult infection. Determination of HBV DNA levels are needed to exclude chronic or occult infection. Administration of a single dose of hepatitis B vaccine will lead to detection of HBsAb in the setting of prior infection, although in practice this is rarely seen. In some cases the presence of HBcAb alone represents a false-positive finding.

4   E.

   Typhoid Vi vaccine is a capsular polysaccharide vaccine and is quite safe to be given to an immunocompromised host. All the other vaccines are live attenuated vaccines which pose variable risks of disseminated infection in this setting. BCG in particular is absolutely contraindicated in all adults with HIV infection regardless of their CD4+ cell counts.

5   B.

   Administration of hepatitis B vaccine alone to a neonate whose mother is a carrier of HBV (especially if she is HBeAg-positive) will prevent about 70% of vertical transmissions. Addition of hepatitis B immune globulin to vaccination will result in 95% protection, with the remaining 5% of cases being transplacentally infected. Cesarean section has not been shown to add to the strategy of administration of vaccine plus immune globulin, while entecavir given during the third trimester in women with a viral load greater than log 6 copies/mL has been shown to have additive benefits to vaccination and immune globulin.

6 A.

Diphtheria vaccine is a toxoid preparation available only in combination with tetanus and other antigens. It results in protective levels of antitoxin in >90% of vaccines. Vaccination does not prevent acquisition or carriage of the causative agent, *Corynebacterium diphtheriae*, but reliably prevents clinical disease. Administration of pediatric formulations to adults results in a higher incidence of local reactions due to the higher dose of toxoid found in pediatric preparations.

7 C.

Yellow fever vaccine is derived from embryonated chicken eggs, and patients with egg-associated anaphylaxis should not receive yellow fever vaccine nor influenza vaccine. The other vaccines listed are not egg-derived and can be safely given to those with egg allergy.

8 A.

BCG vaccination in people with HIV infection may result in fatal disseminated BCG infection regardless of CD4+ cell counts, and as such is absolutely contraindicated. Smallpox, oral typhoid and varicella zoster vaccines may, after consultation and careful consideration of the balance of risk versus benefit, be given to patients with normal CD4+ cell counts. Varicella zoster vaccine may also be given to patients with documented immunity, although it is not generally recommended.

9 A.

Oral typhoid vaccine is a live attenuated vaccine, and is therefore contraindicated in immunosuppressed individuals such as solid-organ transplant recipients. All the other agents are inactivated agents or, in the cases of diphtheria and tetanus, toxoids and can safely be given to immunosuppressed individuals.

10 B.

All healthcare workers should receive MMR, annual influenza, DTP (adult formulation) and hepatitis B vaccines. Healthcare workers in the pediatric setting, or those working with the developmentally delayed, should also consider hepatitis A vaccine.

11 D.

There is little data to support prophylactic oral antivirals other than in children or pregnant women. Live vaccines and immune globulin cannot be administered together as the response to the vaccine is blunted; a period of at least 5 months is recommended between administration of immune globulin and live virus vaccines.

12 B.

Varicella IgG testing is not required after receipt of 2 doses of varicella vaccine, and the absence of detectable varicella IgG does not infer lack of protection. The other responses are all correct.

13 B.

Japanese B encephalitis vaccine is an inactivated vaccine, whereas all the others are live attenuated vaccines. Most live attenuated vaccines may be given to people with HIV provided their CD4+ cell counts are $> 250/mm^3$ although BCG vaccination is absolutely contraindicated regardless of CD4+ cell numbers.

14 C.

Immunity from natural hepatitis B infection induces antibodies to hepatitis B surface antigen (HBsAb) and anti-core antibodies (HBcAb), whereas immunity from vaccination alone would be marked by the sole presence of HBsAb. Patients with acute or chronic hepatitis B infection remain surface antigen positive (HBsAg) along with HBcAb, but negative HBsAb. Some patients have occult hepatitis B infection with low levels of viremia detected by HBV DNA PCR—they usually have anti-core antibodies (HBcAb) in the absence of other serological markers.

15 A.

Pneumococcal vaccination should occur first with pneumococcal conjugate vaccine (PCV) followed by the pneumococcal polysaccharide vaccine (23vPPV) 6 months later. Beta-lactam prophylaxis and standby antibiotics should be offered, as well as meningococcal and HiB vaccinations. Asplenic patients are particularly vulnerable to severe infection with malaria and should carefully consider malaria preventive strategies when traveling overseas.

16 D.

Rabies virus vaccination is recommended for veterinarians (including students and nurses) to protect against bat lyssavirus which is present in flying foxes in Australia. There are no licensed human vaccines against leptospirosis or Hendra virus, although they do exist for animal use. Q fever boosters are contraindicated. Anthrax vaccination may be considered in laboratory personnel at risk of exposure to anthrax.

17 A.

Hepatitis A vaccination is recommended for plumbers as well as those working with young children. It is also advised for men who have sex with men, commercial sex workers, and travellers to certain countries. As it is not a live virus vaccine it may be safely administered to immunosuppressed patients. Active vaccination is now the preferred option for post-exposure prophylaxis, rather than immune globulin, except in patients aged < 12 months or > 40 years, or in those with chronic liver disease or immune suppressed individuals where the risk of suboptimal response means that immune globulin is preferred. As response rates to the vaccine are so high, patients who have received 2 doses of vaccine do not require post-vaccination serology testing.

18 C.

All other statements are correct. Yellow fever is found in parts of sub-Saharan Africa and South America, although it has not been detected in Asia.

19 B.

Receipt of low doses of prednisone are not generally considered to be a contraindication to vaccination even with live virus vaccines. Patients receiving immunosuppressants such as tacrolimus, leflunamide, and azathioprine for example should not receive live virus vaccines. Pregnancy, anaphylaxis to a previous dose of the same vaccine, and an intercurrent febrile illness are all considered to be genuine contraindications to live virus vaccination.

20 C.

All statements are generally correct except for receipt of MMR vaccine in a non-immune pregnant woman which is generally not recommended (although no definite harm has been shown). If travel to a yellow fever endemic area is unavoidable then the benefits generally outweigh the risks of vaccination. Influenza vaccination is recommended in pregnancy due to the higher risks of severe infection and death, particularly in the third trimester.

CHAPTER 22

DERMATOLOGY FOR THE PHYSICIAN

Brad Frankum and Saxon D Smith

The skin and mucous membranes frequently reveal clues to underlying medical illnesses, and both a history of rash or skin lesions and an examination of the skin should be a routine part of the assessment of the medical patient.

The skin is easily accessible to biopsy. A low threshold should exist for a biopsy of abnormal skin in a patient with a systemic illness in whom there is diagnostic uncertainty.

A number of skin-related symptoms or signs may either be evidence of a primary dermatological disorder, or secondary to other systemic disease.

AUTOINFLAMMATORY DISEASES OF THE SKIN

Acne

It is important to distinguish acne vulgaris from rosacea and periorificial dermatitis (Box 22-1, overleaf).

Treatment comprises:

- Periorificial dermatitis: Cease all topical corticosteroids and topical calcineurin inhibitors. Oral antibiotics (doxycycline, minocycline or erythromycin).

- **Rosacea:** topical antibiotics (erythromycin, metronidazole) or long-term oral antibiotics (doxycycline,

Box 22-1

Differentiation of acne vulgaris, periorificial dermatitis and rosacea

Acne vulgaris	Periorificial dermatitis	Rosacea (Figure 22-1)
• Commences at puberty • Comedones, pustules, cysts • Affects face and trunk • Can be a sign of androgen excess in females; side-effect of steroid use, including corticosteroids	• More common 14 years old to 45 years old (can occur at any age) • Female preponderance • Background erythema with studded erythematous papules and pseudopustules (no comedones) • Affects one or more of the mouth, nose and eyelids • Spares the vermillion border • No systemic associations • May have a family history • Unknown initial trigger but made worse by topical corticosteroids and topical calcineurin inhibitors	• Generally occurs in middle age • Caucasian skin predominantly • Female preponderance • Papules, telangiectasia, pustules (no comedones) • Centrofacial, often with rhinophyma, and blepharitis • No systemic disease associations • Facial flushing, especially with alcohol use

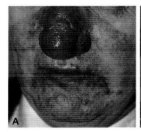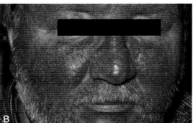

Figure 22-1 Severe rosacea with (**A**) scattered papules on the face and involvement of the nose, and (**B**) severe inflammation with redness and significant edema

From Ferri FF. Ferri's Clinical advisor 2014. Philadelphia: Elsevier, 2014.

minocycline); avoidance of caffeine, alcohol, UV radiation, spicy foods.

- **Acne vulgaris:**
  - » mild—topical benzoyl peroxide or retinoid
  - » moderate—add oral antibiotic (doxycycline, minocycline) or (in females) oral contraceptive pill (OCP)
  - » severe (cystic)—oral isotretinoin.

Atopic dermatitis

Clinical features

- Commonly affecting up to 20% of children and 4% of adults.
- Chronic patchy erythematous pruritic skin condition which typically has periods of flare.
- Part of the atopic tendency with asthma, allergic rhinitis, and predisposition to food and environmental allergies.
- Staphylococcal infections, keratoconus, sleep disturbance, depression and anxiety are more common in atopic dermatitis patients than the general population.

Treatment

- General skin measures (soap free wash, short luke warm showers and regular moisturiser).
- Reduction of known triggers
- Topical corticosteroids and topical calcineurin inhibitors
- Phototherapy (Narrow Band UVB)
- Oral systemic agents: oral corticosteroids (short term only), methotrexate, azathioprine, cyclosporine (ciclosporin). New Jak/Stat/Tyk2 small molecule agents will become increasingly available including baricitinib and upadacitinib.
- Biologic agents will become increasingly used such as interleukin (IL)-4/13 (dupilumab).

Hidradenitis suppurativa

Clinical features

- Hidradenitis suppurativa is an autoinflammatory disorder that commonly affects the intertriginous zones (axillary, inframammary, infraabdominal apron, groin and buttock).
- It is characterized by recurrent, painful, deep-seated erythematous pustules and nodulocystic lesions, rapid onset abscesses, odorous discharging sinuses and sinus tracts, scarring, and double-ended comedones (blackheads).
- It has a female predominance.
- It is more commonly seen in polycyctic ovarian syndrome, smokers, and overweight patients, or with a family history.
- There is an association with inflammatory bowel disease (Crohn disease) especially with anogenital involvement.
- Diabetes mellitus type 2, metabolic syndrome, cardiovascular disease, inflammatory arthropathies (such as PAPA syndrome), depression, and anxiety are more common in patients with hidradenitis suppurativa than the general population.

Treatment

- smoking cessation
- weight loss
- wound care and dressings for lesions
- topical clindamycin and resorcinol
- intralesional corticosteroids
- systemic antibiotics (doxycycline, minocycline, rifampicin + clindamycin)
- oral agents (spironolactone, metformin, retinoids)
- biologic agents are used for moderate to severe patients—TNF-α (tumor necrosis factor-alpha) inhibitors (adalimumab)
- surgery can also play a role in some patients.

The skin is an immunologically active tissue, with persistent exposure to an environment that contains both toxic and potentially allergenic substances. The skin is also the site of a number of primary and systemic autoimmune diseases.

Psoriasis

Clinical features

- Psoriasis is common, affecting up to 3% of the population.
- The rash has a predilection for the elbows, buttocks, knees, posterior aspect or the ears or external auditory canal, and scalp.
- The usual rash is plaque-like with a silvery scale and an erythematous base (Figure 22-2).
- Nail abnormalities are very common, especially onycholysis and pitting. Subungual hyperkeratosis and a pathognomonic yellow-brown discoloration known as 'oil spots' can also be seen.
- Erythrodermic psoriasis, generalized pustular psoriasis, and psoriasis associated with arthropathy can be classified as severe forms of the disease.
- Guttate psoriasis is an acute form of disease with small psoriatic lesions, often following streptococcal sore throat. Pustular psoriasis is an atypical form of disease with crops of sterile pustules occurring on one or both palms and/or soles of feet. It is associated with erythema, scale/crust and hyperkeratosis which can develop painful cracks or fissures. There is a rarer variant which can be more widespread on the rest of the body.
- Oral corticosteroids, interferons, beta-blockers, lithium, and antimalarial drugs can exacerbate psoriasis.
- Around 30% of psoriasis patients will develop psoriatic arthritis. This is a destructive sero-negative arthritis in which the severity can be divergent to the severity of the cutaneous psoriasis.
- Cardiovascular disease, obesity, and the metabolic syndrome are more common in psoriatic patients than the general population.

Treatment

- Topical corticosteroids.
- Topical tar preparations.

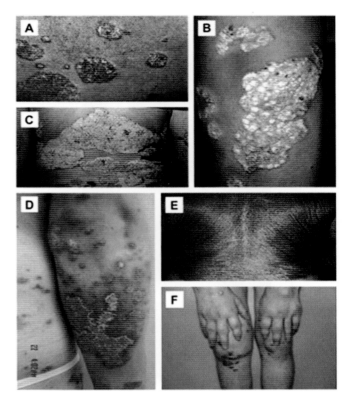

Figure 22-2 Psoriasis subtypes: (**A**) small plaque psoriasis, (**B**) localized thick plaque psoriasis, (**C**) large plaque psoriasis, (**D**) inflammatory localized psoriasis, (**E**) erythrodermic psoriasis, and (**F**) psoriasis and psoriatic arthritis

From Menter A et al. Guidelines of care for the management of psoriasis and psoriatic arthritis: Section 1. Overview of psoriasis and guidelines of care for the treatment of psoriasis with biologics. J Am Acad Dermatol 2008;58(5):826–50.

- Topical synthetic vitamin D analog (calcipotriol) products which are combined with a topical corticosteroid.
- Phototherapy (Narrow Band UVB)
- Topical calcineurin inhibitors for facial or flexural disease.
- Acitretin is a 2nd-generation retinoid that is used in the treatment of psoriasis. Adverse effects include teratogenicity, hepatitis, hypertriglyceridemia, cheilitis, xerosis, alopecia and bony hyperostosis.
- Methotrexate or cyclosporine (ciclosporin) may be used for treatment of severe skin disease and psoriatic arthropathy.
- Biological agents are increasingly being used with success in severe disease—TNF (tumor necrosis factor) inhibitors (infliximab, etanercept, adalimumab), interleukin (IL)-12/23 blockers (ustekinumab) include interleukin (IL)-17 blockers (secukinumab, ixekizumab) or interleukin (IL)-23 blockers (guselkumab, tildrakizumab, risankizumab).

Erythema nodosum (EN)

- Erythema nodosum is in fact a form of panniculitis.
- It presents with tender, red, palpable lesions predominantly on the pretibial area (Figure 22-3).

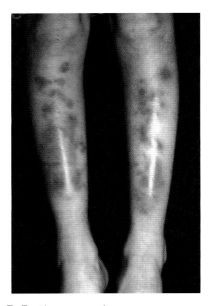

Figure 22-3 Erythema nodosum

From James WD, Berger T and Elston D. Andrews' Diseases of the skin: clinical dermatology, 11th ed. Elsevier, 2011.

- Typically occurs between 20 and 45 years old.
- Female predominance in adults but equal in pediatric population.
- May fluctuate in activity every 6–8 weeks.

Causes

- Sarcoidosis
- Streptococcal infections (beta-hemolytic)
- Inflammatory bowel disease
- Drugs, e.g. sulfonamides, penicillin, sulfonylureas, estrogen
- Tuberculosis
- Other infections (less common), e.g. lepromatous leprosy, histoplasmosis, blastomycosis, coccidioidomycosis, toxoplasmosis, *Yersinia*, *Chlamydia*, lymphogranuloma venereum
- Systemic autoimmune disease—systemic lupus erythematosus (SLE), antiphospholipid syndrome, scleroderma, autoimmune thyroid diseases
- Behçet's syndrome
- Pregnancy
- Idiopathic

Treatment

- The lesions often resolve spontaneously over weeks to months.
- Treatment is largely directed at the underlying cause. In idiopathic cases treatment includes: compression dressings, non-steroidal anti-inflammatories (NSAIDs), super saturated potassium iodine, or oral tetracyclines.

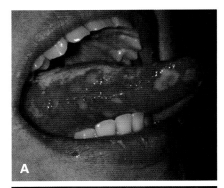

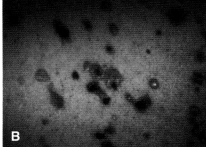

Figure 22-4 Pemphigus vulgaris: (**A**) painful tongue lesions; (**B**) typical skin bullae and ulcerations

From Edgin WA, Pratt TC and Grimwood RE. Pemphigus vulgaris and paraneoplastic pemphigus. Oral Maxilofacial Surg Clin North Am 2008;20(4):577–84.

- Rest and wet dressing bandaging with a hospital admission is sometimes used in severe acute cases.

Bullous lesions

Pemphigus vulgaris

Clinical features

- Pemphigus vulgaris usually presents in the 5th to 7th decade.
- Mucosal involvement is frequently present—oral, pharyngeal, conjunctival, and genital ulcers or blisters.
- Flaccid blisters (Figure 22-4) are seen on the scalp, face, axillae and upper trunk (especially at sites of trauma or pressure), rarely on the limbs, and are painful.
- Nikolsky's sign is positive (affected superficial skin can be moved over the deeper layer).
- Whilst most cases are idiopathic, drug-induced pemphigus and paraneoplastic pemphigus should be considered.

Pathology

- Skin biopsy reveals acantholysis (rounded keratinocytes resulting from detachment of intercellular adhesion), and intraepidermal vesicles/bullae.
- Immunofluorescence shows immunoglobulin G (IgG; intercellular substance antibody) and C3 deposits in the interepithelial spaces.
- Serum titer of IgG anti-desmoglein-3 antibody is useful to monitor disease activity.

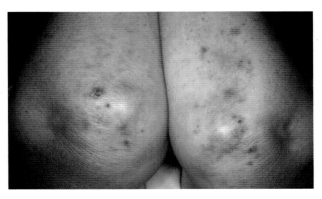

Figure 22-6 Dermatitis herpetiformis

From Kárpáti S. Dermatitis herpetiformis. Clin Dermatol 2012;30(1):56–9.

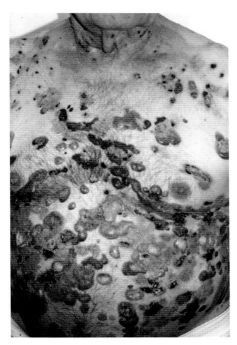

Figure 22-5 Bullous pemphigoid

From Brinster NK et al. Dermatopathology: a volume in the High-yield Pathology series. Philadelphia: Elsevier, 2011.

Treatment

Pemphigus vulgaris requires aggressive immunosuppression with high-dose corticosteroids, and frequently cyclophosphamide, mycophenolate or rituximab.

Bullous pemphigoid

Clinical features

- Bullous pemphigoid presents predominantly in the elderly.
- It features large, tense, not easily broken, sometimes hemorrhagic bullae, on an erythematous base (Figure 22-5).
- It may be localised to one area or widespread on the body and limbs.
- Oral ulcers are uncommon.
- Bullous pemphigoid is infrequently associated with malignancy.

Pathology

- Skin biopsy—subepidermal vesicles/bullae rich in eosinophils with IgG or IgM, and complement, in a linear pattern along the basement membrane zone.
- Immunofluorescence reveals IgG anti-basement-membrane zone antibodies in 70% of patients.
- Circulating anti-basement-membrane zone antibodies do not correlate with disease activity.

Treatment

High-dose, high-potency topical corticosteroids may be effective for localized or milder disease.

Failure to control disease with topical corticosteroids, and severe disease with extensive ulceration and blisters, will necessitate the addition of oral corticosteroids, and/or immunosuppressive agents such as azathioprine or methotrexate.

Dermatitis herpetiformis

Clinical features

- Dermatitis herpetiformis presents with intensely pruritic vesicles, or excoriations, on knees, elbows and buttocks (Figure 22-6). Mucosal involvement is not seen.
- It usually presents in the 3rd or 4th decade.
- Celiac disease (often asymptomatic) is almost always present.
- HLA DQw2 and DR3 are associated in >90% of cases.

Pathology

- Skin biopsy shows subepidermal vesicles, beneath which are found neutrophils in dermal papillae.
- Immunofluorescence reveals IgA in a granular pattern, and complement in the dermal papillae and along the basement membrane zone of involved and uninvolved skin rich in eosinophils.
- Serum IgA tissue transglutaminase antibodies are present in the majority of cases, and may be helpful to monitor disease activity.

Treatment

A gluten-free diet is the cornerstone of therapy. However, it can take up to 2 years for DH to settle with a gluten-free diet alone. Oral dapsone +/- topical corticosteroids are frequently used in the meantime.

CLINICAL PEARL

Any skin change noted by a patient, or detected by the physician, should prompt consideration of whether it represents a cutaneous manifestation of a systemic illness.

Livedo reticularis

Livedo reticularis is a spidery or lattice-like appearance that can be red or blue in coloration (Figure 22-7), and affects the skin of the limbs. It represents sluggish venular blood flow. A number of diseases may be associated with livedo reticularis (Box 22-2) although benign and physiologic forms exist.

SKIN PROBLEMS ASSOCIATED WITH UNDERLYING SYSTEMIC DISEASE

Acanthosis nigricans

Clinical features

Acanthosis nigricans is characterized by hyperpigmentation and velvety thickening of the intertriginous areas (Figure 22-8).

Causes

- Malignancy—adenocarcinoma, lymphoma
- Endocrine disease, e.g. acromegaly, Cushing's syndrome, hypothyroidism, diabetes mellitus and insulin resistance states, lipodystrophies (especially leprechaunism), Stein–Leventhal syndrome, polycystic ovarian syndrome
- Obesity
- Hereditary
- Benign/idiopathic
- Drug-induced (rare)

Box 22-2

Diseases associated with livedo reticularis

Autoimmune disease
- Systemic lupus erythematosus
- Antiphospholipid syndrome
- Dermatomyositis
- Scleroderma
- Sjögren's syndrome
- Rheumatoid arthritis
- Vasculitides

Neoplastic disease
- Pheochromocytoma
- Carcinoid
- Myeloma
- Polycythemia vera
- Leukemia
- Essential thrombocytosis

Infection
- Parvovirus B-19
- Hepatitis C
- Tuberculosis
- Syphilis

Drug reactions
- Amantadine
- Warfarin
- Quinidine

Vascular disease
- Cryoglobulinemia
- Cholesterol emboli
- Endocarditis
- Thrombotic thrombocytopenic purpura
- Disseminated intravascular coagulation

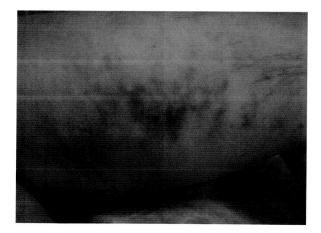

Figure 22-7 Livedo reticularis on the inner thigh

From Jorquera-Barquero E et al. Oxalosis and livedo reticularis. Actas Dermo-Sifiliográficas (Engl ed) 2013;104(9):815–18.

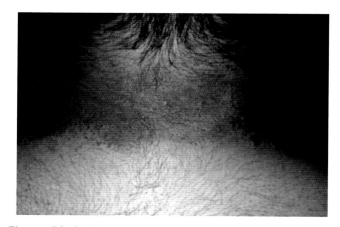

Figure 22-8 Acanthosis nigricans

From Lebwohl MG et al (eds). Treatment of skin disease: comprehensive therapeutic strategies, 4th ed. Elsevier, 2014.

Neutrophilic dermatoses

Pyoderma gangrenosum

This is a serious, painful, ulcerating disease of the skin and soft tissue, often affecting the lower legs. There are several common clinical presentations: deep ulcers, superficial ulcers, peristomal ulcers, and neutrophilic dermatosis of the dorsum of the hands.

Causes

- Inflammatory bowel disease
- Rheumatoid arthritis
- Paraproteinemia, e.g. IgA myeloma
- Myeloproliferative disorders
- Idiopathic

Clinical features

- Pyoderma gangrenosum usually starts quite suddenly and often at a site of minor injury. It causes pustules and sterile abscesses, which rupture and leave denuded, ulcerated lesions that may necrose.
- The edges of the ulcers are characteristically purple, and undermined (Figure 22-9).
- Lesions are painful with the pain often disproportionate to the area of the skin affected.
- Patients often experience pathergy, where new lesions appear at the sites of new or previous trauma.
- Without intervention, the disease often progresses and can be life-threatening.
- There is no diagnostic test for pyoderma gangrenosum.
- Diagnosis is made on appearance of the skin lesions, and exclusion of other causes of blistering, pustular or necrotic lesions, by other tests or skin biopsy.

Treatment

- Aggressive systemic immunosuppression is required.
- Corticosteroids are often effective, but moderate to high doses are required initially.

- Anti-TNF therapy or cyclosporine (ciclosporin) can be effective in some cases.
- Identified underlying disease should be treated.

Sweet's syndrome (acute febrile neutrophilic dermatosis)

This rare syndrome causes painful, erythematous papules or vesicles and nodules or plaques, typically in association with fever.

Causes

- It is more common in women, and in those who are pregnant.
- It may be idiopathic; however, in a significant proportion of patients there is an associated malignancy (especially hematological malignancies), infection, or an autoimmune or inflammatory disorder.
- Drugs including furosemide, trimethoprim-sulfamethoxazole, hydralazine, retinoic acid and minocycline have been implicated in this disorder.

Clinical features

- The cutaneous eruption has a predilection for the dorsa of the hands, and the head, neck and upper limbs, but can affect any part of the skin.
- Lesions are generally tender, erythematous, and papular or plaque-like (Figure 22-10). Vesiculation and pustulation can occur.
- Along with fever, multiple systemic features have been described, including malaise, lethargy, arthralgia, myalgia and ocular involvement.

Diagnosis

Leukocytosis and elevated acute phase reactants are generally evident, but diagnosis depends on histopathology.

Treatment

Although spontaneous resolution can occur in some patients over time, the severity of the symptoms requires the use of

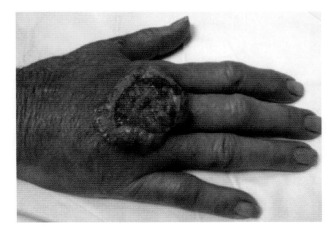

Figure 22-9 Pyoderma gangrenosum

From Wall LB and Stern PJ. Pyoderma gangrenosum. J Hand Surg 2012;37(5):1083–5.

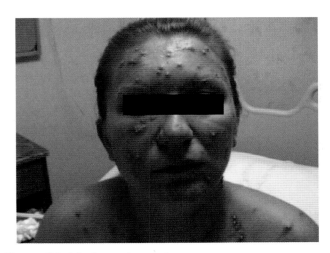

Figure 22-10 Sweet's syndrome

From Fazili T, Duncan D and Wani L. Sweet's syndrome. Am J Med 2010;123(8):694–6.

oral corticosteroids in moderate to high doses in most cases. This is generally effective for both cutaneous and systemic manifestations in Sweet's syndrome.

Pruritus

Any generalized persistent pruritus with scratch marks, that is unrelieved by emollients and wakens the patient from sleep, needs evaluation to exclude systemic disease. Systemic causes include:

- cholestasis, e.g. primary biliary cholangitis
- chronic renal failure
- pregnancy
- lymphoma, myeloma
- polycythemia rubra vera, mycosis fungoides
- carcinoma, e.g. breast, stomach, lung
- endocrine disease, e.g. diabetes mellitus, hypothyroidism, thyrotoxicosis, carcinoid syndrome
- iron deficiency
- medication.

Pigmentation

There are multiple causes of skin pigmentation:

- liver disease, e.g. hemochromatosis, Wilson's disease, primary biliary cholangitis, porphyria
- malignancy (related to cachexia, or ectopic adrenocorticotropic hormone [ACTH] production)
- endocrine disease, e.g. Addison's disease (Figure 22-11), Cushing's syndrome, acromegaly, pheochromocytoma, hyperthyroidism
- chronic kidney disease
- systemic autoimmune disease, e.g. SLE, scleroderma, dermatomyositis
- drugs, e.g. neuroleptics, hydroxychloroquine, busulfan, gold, lead, amiodarone, minocycline, heavy metals
- radiation
- malabsorption
- chronic infection, e.g. infective endocarditis

- increased levels of female hormones—pregnancy, oral contraceptive pill.
- familial.

Photosensitivity

Causes of photosensitivity include:

- drugs, e.g. neuroleptics, antibiotics (sulfonamides, tetracycline), sulfonylureas, NSAIDs, diuretics
- porphyria cutanea tarda (Figure 22-12)
- SLE
- solar urticaria
- polymorphous light eruption
- pellagra.

Rash on the palms and soles

Differential diagnosis of such rash:

- syphilis
- acute infections, e.g. infectious mononucleosis (nonspecific macular erythema), gonococcemia (purpuric tender pustules; Figure 22-13), toxic shock syndrome, hand, foot and mouth disease (linear or oval vesicles)
- erythema multiforme
- Reactive arthritis (formerly known as Reiter's syndrome) (erythematous pustular eruptions—keratoderma blennorrhagica)
- atopic dermatitis
- scabies
- pustular psoriasis
- drug reaction
- mercury or arsenic poisoning.

Red person syndrome (erythroderma or exfoliative dermatitis)

This refers to a confluent, generalized erythamatous rash that can be the result of any etiology. An example is shown in Figure 22-14 (overleaf).

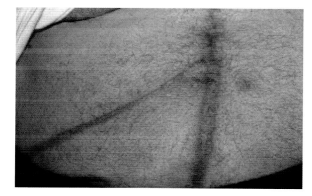

Figure 22-11 Pigmentation of scars in Addison's disease

From Ferri FF. Ferri's Clinical advisor 2014. Philadelphia: Elsevier, 2014.

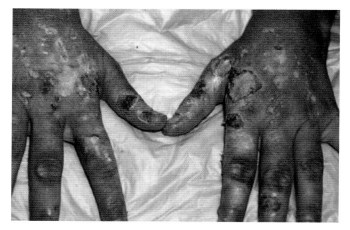

Figure 22-12 Porphyria cutanea tarda

From Brinster NK et al. Dermatopathology: a volume in the High-yield Pathology series. Philadelphia: Elsevier, 2011.

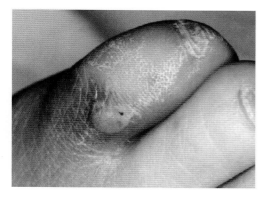

Figure 22-13 Pustular lesion on foot from gonococcal infection

Courtesy of the Graham International Dermatopathology Learning Center.

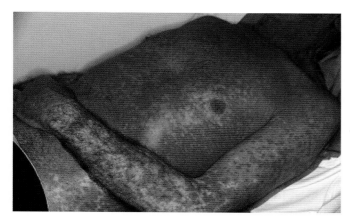

Figure 22-14 Erythroderma of red person syndrome

From Gawkrodger DJ and Ardern-Jones MR. Dermatology: an illustrated colour text, 5th ed. Elsevier, 2012.

Causes are:
- malignancy
- mycosis fungoides (infiltration of the skin by T cells)
- lymphoma, leukemia
- carcinoma (rare)
- drugs, e.g. phenytoin, allopurinol
- generalization of a pre-existing dermatitis, e.g. psoriasis, atopic dermatitis.

Regardless of cause, patients may present with edema (hypo-albuminemia from skin loss), loss of muscle mass, temperature dysregulation, and extrarenal water loss.

Excessive sweating (hyperhydrosis)

Causes of excessive sweating include:
- thyrotoxicosis
- pheochromocytoma
- acromegaly
- hypoglycemia

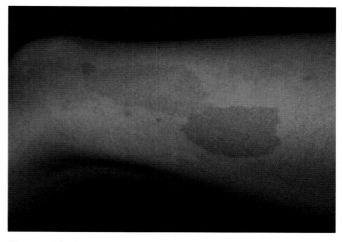

Figure 22-15 Café-au-lait spots

From Boyd KP, Korf BR and Theos A. Neurofibromatosis type 1. J Am Acad Dermatol 2009;61(1):1–14.

- autonomic dysfunction, e.g. Riley–Day syndrome and Parkinson's disease
- physiological causes, e.g. idiopathic, emotional stress, fever, menopause.

Facial flushing

Causes of facial flushing include:
- menopause
- rosacea
- mastocytosis
- carcinoid syndrome
- thyroid disease including medullary carcinoma of the thyroid
- drugs, e.g. alcohol.

GENETIC OR CONGENITAL SKIN DISEASES

Skin lesions may be manifestations of genetic or congenital diseases.

The phakomatoses

Neurofibromatosis

Type I (von Recklinghausen's disease: chromosome 17)
This is characterized by:
- neurofibromas of peripheral nerves
- more than six ≥1.5 cm café-au-lait spots (Figure 22-15)
- hamartomas of the iris (Lisch nodules)
- axillary freckling (Crowe's sign)
- pseudo-arthrosis of the tibia.

Patients are predisposed to nervous system neoplasms, including plexiform neurofibromas, optic gliomas, pheochromocytomas, ependymomas, meningiomas, astrocytomas, and change to sarcoma.

Type II (chromosome 22q)

- Type II neurofibromatosis is characterized by bilateral acoustic schwannomas.
- Patients are predisposed to meningiomas, gliomas, and schwannomas of peripheral and cranial nerves.
- The most common presentation is unilateral deafness. If detected early, surgery can preserve the auditory nerve.

Tuberous sclerosis

Clinical features are:

- the disease is autosomal dominant, or sporadic
- it presents with a triad of convulsions, cognitive developmental delay (with calcification in the temporal lobes), and adenoma sebaceum (fibromas on the cheeks and forehead)
- other features may include the shagreen patch (thick yellow skin on the lower back), cardiac rhabdomyoma, renal angioleiomyoma, and pulmonary fibrosis.

Von Hippel—Lindau disease

Clinical features are:

- autosomal dominant
- hemangioblastomas of the retina, cerebellum and spinal cord
- cysts in the kidney, epididymis or pancreas
- hemangiomas elsewhere (e.g. liver, pancreas, kidney)
- pheochromocytoma
- renal and pancreatic cancer.

Sturge—Weber syndrome

Clinical features are:

- a congenital, non-hereditary disorder
- capillary hemangiomas (port wine stains) in a cranial nerve V distribution, upper or middle branch, with an intracranial venous hemangioma of the leptomeninges
- association with seizures, glaucoma, and cognitive developmental delay.

Ataxia—telangiectasia

Clinical features are a triad of cerebellar ataxia, oculo-cutaneous telangiectasia on the bulbar conjunctiva and skin, and immunodeficiency (decreased IgA and IgE, and thymic atrophy).

SKIN DISEASE ASSOCIATED WITH MALIGNANCY

Primary or secondary malignancy

Skin lesions may at times represent primary or secondary malignancy, other than those that are typically a result of ultraviolet radiation exposure.

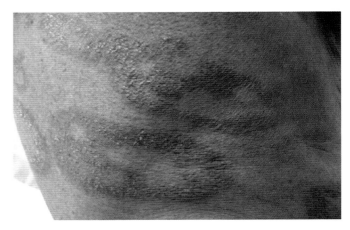

Figure 22-16 Mycosis fungoides

From Brinster NK et al. Dermatopathology: a volume in the High-yield Pathology series. Philadelphia: Elsevier, 2011.

Cutaneous T-cell non-Hodgkin lymphoma

Mycosis fungoides

Clinical features

- Initially, discrete patches and plaques on the skin. These are typically scaly and erythematous or hyperpigmented (Figure 22-16).
- Frequently occurs in the bathing trunk distribution of the central body. These may progress to coalescent lesions, nodules or even tumors which can ulcerate.
- Lymph nodes and viscera may become involved in time.

Diagnosis

Biopsy reveals monoclonal CD4+ T-lymphocytes in the epidermis and dermis (epidermotropism).

Treatment

This depends on the stage of disease. It may require:

- topical therapy with corticosteroids and retinoids
- radiotherapy
- narrow-band UVB therapy with or without oral retinoids
- systemic chemotherapy.

Sézary syndrome

Clinical features

- Generalized erythroderma
- Keratoderma of the palms and soles
- Pruritus
- Lymphadenopathy
- Sézary cell count of >1000/mm^3 in the peripheral blood

Diagnosis

Biopsy reveals monoclonal CD4+ T-lymphocytes in the epidermis and dermis (epidermotropism).

Treatment

- Topical therapy with corticosteroids and retinoids
- Oral retinoids
- Phototherapy (oral psoralen plus UVA or narrow band UVB)
- Radiotherapy
- Extracorporeal photopheresis
- Systemic chemotherapy

Underlying malignancy

Malignancies which metastasize to the skin include:

- carcinomas of the:
  » breast
  » gastrointestinal tract
  » lung
  » kidney
  » ovary
- melanomas
- leukemias (especially acute myeloid leukemia).

Clues to underlying malignancy are outlined in Table 22-1, below.

Table 22-1 Cutaneous clues to underlying malignancy

SKIN CHANGE	POSSIBLE UNDERLYING MALIGNANCY
Extramammary Paget's disease	Genitourinary or gastrointestinal
Acanthosis nigricans	Gastrointestinal, especially stomach
Pyoderma gangrenosum	Leukemia
Necrolytic migratory erythema	Glucagonoma
Torre's syndrome (multiple sebaceous tumors of the skin)	Carcinoma of the colon, breast
Cowden's syndrome (trichilemmomas, verrucous papules, oral fibromas)	Carcinoma of the breast, thyroid
Gardener's syndrome (soft-tissue tumors, sebaceous cysts)	Carcinoma of the colon
Acquired ichthyosis	Hodgkin lymphoma
Hirsutism	Adrenal or ovarian tumor
Hypertrichosis	Carcinoid; carcinoma of the breast, gastrointestinal, lymphoma
Erythema gyratum repens (concentric erythematous bands)	Carcinoma of the lung, breast
Sweet's syndrome (acute febrile neutrophilic dermatosis)	Leukemia
Dermatomyositis	Especially gastrointestinal
Multiple mucosal neuromas	Medullary carcinoma of the thyroid
Cutaneous amyloidosis	Myeloma
Tylosis (palmar–plantar keratoderma)	Carcinoma of the esophagus
Pemphigus	Thymoma
Paraneoplastic pemphigus (associated with erythema multiforme)	Lymphoma, leukemia
Epidermolysis bullosa acquisita	Myeloma

SELF-ASSESSMENT QUESTIONS

1   A 47-year-old woman complains of flushing for the past 18 months. Her menstrual periods have been irregular for 12 months, and she has been amenorrheic for the past 3 months. Her past medical history is unremarkable. The patient also complains that her bowel habit has changed over that period, with watery diarrhea occurring up to several times per day. On physical examination you observe signs of facial rosacea. What would be the most appropriate next step in this case?

A   Order 24-hour urinary collection for 5-HIAA (5-hydroxyindoleacetic acid) quantitation.
B   Commence hormone replacement therapy.
C   Commence topical antibiotics for treatment of rosacea.
D   Perform serum tryptase to exclude systemic mastocytosis.

2   A 45-year-old male presents with painful lesions on the lower limbs. On examination you observe tender, indurated lesions, predominantly over the pretibial area. On further questioning, the patient also has a dry cough. What further investigations would be appropriate at this stage?

A   Biopsy of lesion, anti-neutrophil cytoplasmic antibodies
B   Anti-neutrophil cytoplasmic antibodies, computed tomography (CT) mesenteric angiogram
C   CT mesenteric angiogram, chest radiograph
D   Chest radiograph, serum angiotensin-converting enzyme (ACE) level
E   Serum ACE level, biopsy of lesion

3   A 25-year-old female patient presents with extremely pruritic vesicles on the limbs, predominantly around the elbows, shoulders and knees. There is no mucosal involvement. This has been present for 2 months. The likely appropriate treatment in this case would be:

A   A gluten-free diet
B   High-dose oral corticosteroids
C   Liberal application of potent topical steroid creams
D   Oral valacyclovir (valaciclovir)

ANSWERS

1   **A.**

This patient has carcinoid syndrome—this is an example of a skin manifestation being the first sign of a systemic disease. It is important to take a thorough history with any new symptom, even if menopause is by far the most common cause of flushing in a female of this age. The symptom of new-onset watery diarrhea is always concerning, and must not be ignored. Systemic mastocytosis can certainly cause diarrhea, but the skin rash is urticarial and pruritic.

2   **D.**

Erythema nodosum is generally very characteristic in appearance, so biopsy can be avoided in most cases and a clinical diagnosis made. With the presence of a dry cough, one needs to be suspicious of sarcoidosis, and if bilateral hilar lymphadenopathy is present, with or without interstitial lung changes, this becomes more likely. A positive serum ACE level is moderately specific for sarcoidosis in this situation, but lacks sensitivity. An important differential diagnosis is tuberculosis, in which case a chest radiograph is also very important. The history would be important to screen for inflammatory bowel disease. Anti-neutrophil cytoplasmic autoantibody (ANCA)-associated vasculitis is not associated with erythema nodosum, but cutaneous polyarteritis nodosa can look similar in appearance.

3   **A.**

Dermatitis herpetiformis is the most likely diagnosis here, given the significant pruritus, the lack of mucosal involvement and the lack of bullae. Chickenpox would not last for 2 months and would be more generalized. Pemphigus vulgaris always involves the mucous membranes, and bullous pemphigoid results in large bullae and is usually seen in older age groups. A gluten-free diet is the first-line therapy for dermatitis herpetiformis.

CHAPTER 23

MEDICAL OPHTHALMOLOGY

Michael Hennessy, Brad Frankum, Peter McCluskey and Elisa Cornish

INTRODUCTION

Eye examination is an essential part of a comprehensive general medical consultation. Ocular symptoms and/or signs can:

- help determine an accurate diagnosis

- indicate disease severity when the diagnosis is established (e.g. a patient with diabetes mellitus)

- reveal ocular changes related to treatment.

Performing an accurate eye exam is based on understanding:

- the structure and function of the eye and visual system, recognizing that light is transmitted through living, effectively transparent tissues and optically clear extra-cellular material (aqueous and vitreous) to then activate the photoreceptors in the retina which then transmits light signals back to the visual cortex.

- that the manifestations of disease are determined by the unique features of the anatomy and physiology of the eye, and how these result in patients' symptoms and the examination signs.

Key concepts include:

- Transparency.
  » To be transparent, a healthy cornea and lens are free of intrinsic blood vessels, and the tissue structure renders it transparent.
  » The inner cellular layers of a healthy retina are transparent. Retinal vessels supply the inner retina in all but the central 0.5-mm–diameter foveal area which is supplied by the choroid. The retinal arterioles and venules, and the arterioles and venules are visible with the ophthalmoscope. The retinal color seen on fundoscopy is due to the retinal pigment epithelium (RPE) and choroid. The color of the fundus can change when the normal transparency of the retina changes to being opaque from ischemia resulting from a central retinal arterial occlusion. Clinically this appears as a 'cherry red spot' as the fovea has its regular choroidal red hue, however the surrounding retina is opaque.
- Manifestations of disease in the eye are directly visible at a cellular level with imaging techniques that involve illumination and magnification, as is achieved even with a basic tool such as the direct ophthalmoscope.

OCULAR HISTORY

- Common ocular symptoms are:
  » altered vision
  » pain, including photophobia
  » lacrimation
  » discharge
  » changed appearance including redness
  » diplopia (either monocular or binocular)
  » ptosis
  » anisocoria
  » leukocoria.
- The timing or tempo of symptoms, and how they developed or changed with time, should be explored carefully. 'Blurry' vision can mean different things, including double vision or blur, or it can mean decreased vision or double vision.
- Establishing the patient's refraction on history can guide you in your clinical differential. Patients who are myopic (short-sighted) are at higher risk of developing a retinal detachment, myopic retinal degeneration or, if a contact-lens wearer, keratitis. Whereas a patient who is hypermetropic (long-sighted) is at higher risk of developing angle-closure glaucoma.
- A comprehensive systemic history is essential, and should include:
  » allergies
  » drug reactions
  » medications, including use of eye drops
  » trauma to or near the eye, both recent or many years previous
  » general medical history, including diabetes, thyroid eye disease or rheumatological disease and both specific ocular and general surgical history.

OCULAR EXAMINATION

'Bedside' eye examination techniques include the following.

General inspection findings

This can include, where relevant:

- scars around the orbit or of the lids
- measurement of ptosis
- exophthalmos or enophthalmos
- areas of altered sensation
- exotropia or esotropia
- anisocoria
- facial trauma or scars.

The clarity of the cornea and the depth of the chamber can be assessed by gross inspection, directional illumination, and with minimal magnification. A blue filter for the light and the instillation of fluorescein stain can be used to detect corneal ulcers as part of a magnified external eye exam. A red reflex elicited by a direct ophthalmoloscope is useful to establish clear media to the retina.

CLINICAL PEARL

Test corneal sensitivity and the blink reflex prior to instillation of eye drops, specifically those with topical anesthesia.

Visual acuity

- Standard visual acuity (VA) assessment is performed at a distance of 6 m, with a 6 m Snellen chart—where the letter sizes on the test chart are standardized for the testing distances are available. A smart phone VA app is useful for bedside examination.
- If distance glasses are used, visual acuity is tested with glasses on.
- One eye is tested at a time with the other thoroughly covered, e.g. with the palm of the patient's hand or an occluder.
- Visual acuity is recorded for each eye as a fraction, with the test distance being the numerator and the smallest size letter achieved being the denominator (e.g. RVA [right eye visual acuity] with glasses: 6/6).
- If the vision is subnormal, a pinhole (PH) is used to check for improvement. Improvement with PH indicates that there is a refractive error.
- Near vision is tested with a reading card with fonts of different sizes.

Intraocular pressure

- Formal intraocular pressure readings are recorded with a tonometer.
- Gross estimation of intraocular pressure (hard, normal or very soft) is gained by palpation of the globe through the eyelid. Palpation should be avoided if there is a possibility of globe injury.

Field of vision

The visual field of each eye is tested by confrontation with the count fingers technique, each eye in turn.

- The examiner faces the patient at eye level at about a 1 meter distance. With the right eye covered, the examiner asks the patient to look at his/her nose and describe any scotoma in the field of view. This may detect large field defects such as a hemianopia or an altitudinal defect.

- Then the examiner systematically tests the four quadrants of left field in turn, equidistant between examiner and patient. The examiner will have his/her left eye covered when testing and comparing to the patient's left visual field. This is then repeated for the patient's right visual field.

- Visual field defects are interpreted by following the path first of the light onto the retina, and then of the nerve fibers from the eye to the visual cortex. Light from the right side of fixation in each eye reaches the left side of the retina in each eye (relative to the fovea); that is, the nasal retina in the right eye and the temporal retina in the left, and vice versa.

There are eight key features of visual field defects:

- Retinal and optic nerve lesions on one eye produce field defects for that eye. An inferior retinal or optic nerve pathology will produce a superior field loss and vice versa.

- A bi-temporal hemianopia is caused by a lesion of the optic chiasm that affects the nasal fibers crossing from the optic nerve to the contralateral optic tract.

- Lesions posterior to the chiasm (retro-chiasmal) cause homonymous field defects:
  » anterior retro-chiasmal lesions cause incongruous homonymous field defects
  » posterior retro-chiasmal lesions cause congruous homonymous field defects
  » temporal lobe lesions involving the optic radiation cause upper quadrantinopias—often slightly incongruous
  » complete homonymous hemianopias cannot be specifically localized along the contralateral retro-chiasmal visual pathway
  » unilateral homonymous hemianopia does not reduce visual acuity. In cortical blindness, the visual acuity should be equal in both eyes. If not, there is an additional cause for the difference in acuity.

Pupils

Pupil size and the response to light stimuli are determined by the combination of:

- nerve distribution in the afferent and efferent paths
- the central connections that establish the reflex arc
- the activity from higher brain centers
- the effects of some drugs.

The normal neurological reflex arc (optic nerve, midbrain, oculomotor nerve) function determines that:

1 the pupils will be the same size under any particular level of room illumination

2 the direct and consensual pupil responses are equal from the same torchlight stimulation on each side.

The elements of the reflex arc are: retina → optic nerve → optic chiasm (partial decussation) → superior brachium of the midbrain → Edinger–Westphal subnucleus (bilateral, equal innervation of both subnuclei by each side) → oculomotor nerve pre-ganglionic nerve fiber → post-ganglionic nerve → iris sphincter muscle.

Pupil size

- Pupil size is first observed and compared between the two sides, and with the patient's gaze directed to a specific point in the distance.

- The pupils should be of equal size and concentric, and constrict briskly in a smooth motion in response to a light stimulus from a torch directed through the pupil.

- Pupils of equal size will usually be first tested with the torchlight test. Alternatively, when unequal-sized pupils are present, the size difference of the pupils is first compared between bright and dim levels of room illumination.

- Pupil size can be affected by various drugs.

Direct pupillary response

The timing and characteristic of each pupil's response to direct torchlight stimulation is recorded in dim room light settings. The direct response for the other eye is tested the same way.

Swinging flashlight test

The pupil responses to light for the pair of eyes are best compared by using the swinging torch (swinging flashlight) test:

- The torch light is directed at one eye for about 3 seconds, then switched instantly to the other eye, and the second illuminated pupil is observed over the next 3 seconds to determine whether this pupil dilates.

- When the light first arrives after the switch, the pupil size is the result of the consensual response from the other eye, and the response that becomes evident after 3 seconds of illumination shows any relative change for the direct light response.

- Dilatation of the pupil after the switch of the torchlight signifies a relative afferent pupillary defect (RAPD) on the side that dilates (see the clinical pearl overleaf).

- If the size of one pupil does not change from either room illumination or direct light response, then rather than watching the pupil where the light shines, the examiner observes the responses of the pupil that has a reaction, including with instantaneous switches of the torchlight. This is useful in cases where the patient has had unilateral pharmacological dilatation or previous ocular disease process or surgery preventing pupil response.

Pupil accommodation response

The pupil response to the effort of accommodation should be tested with slightly dimmed room lighting:

- The patient looks into the distance with both eyes, then switches to read small print within an arm's length, and then switches fixation back to the distant object. Pupils should constrict on accommodation.

CLINICAL PEARL

A relative afferent pupillary defect (RAPD) is interpreted in relation to the visual acuity and the field of vision. An RAPD is a very sensitive sign of optic nerve pathology and can be present with relatively normal direct light responses. Thus if the pupils are the same size in room illumination and the direct response on each eye looks normal, the swinging torch test is essential and needs to be performed (See above description). A clinical example would be seen in a patient who has recovered from a unilateral episode of optic neuritis. The affected eye might regain essentially normal acuity, have a very subtle visual field defect, have a subtle sense of color desaturation and a subjective sense of reduced brightness, and demonstrate an RAPD.

- Sustained pupil constriction from near effort in the absence of normal pupil light responses is called a 'light near dissociation'.
- When the sign is present it usually occurs with normal vision. It signifies pathology of the dorsal midbrain affecting the afferent nerve fibers passing through the superior brachium, or aberrant regeneration of post-ganglionic parasympathetic nerve fibers from pathology of the ciliary ganglion.

Unequal pupils

If the pupil sizes are unequal, the difference in size is compared between normal and dim room lighting. Remember to ask about a history of ocular trauma, surgery or inflammation (uveitis) as these can all affect the pupils ability to react normally.

- A pupil that fails to dilate in the dark has a defect of sympathetic innervation, or a miotic agent has been used (e.g. pilocarpine) in the affected eye.
- A pupil that is not as constricted as its fellow, especially in brighter light, has a defect of parasympathetic innervation, or the eye shows the effect of a mydriatic agent (e.g. atropine).

Unequal pupil size is interpreted relative to the level of consciousness:

- In the conscious patient, associated signs should be noted such as ipsilateral ptosis in sympathetic paresis, or ipsilateral ptosis, diplopia and the unilateral down-and-out ocular deviation noted with oculomotor nerve palsy.
- When a dilated pupil is present with a down-and-out ocular deviation in an unconscious patient, and without the effect of a mydriatic agent in one eye, this sign indicates compression or injury of the 3rd cranial nerve and the upper brainstem, caused either by an extending intracranial mass lesion or by diffuse brain injury (Don't forget to check that a mydriatic agent hasn't topically been installed).

Color saturation

Red color saturation differences between two eyes is tested using a pin with a large red-colored head. Each eye is tested separately, and the patient is asked to compare the intensity of the red color between the two eyes.

Formal color testing can be done using a number of tests. Ishihara test plates are used for testing red–green color discrepancies. Farnsworth-Munsell 100 hue test is a more detailed test for overall color vision acuity.

CLINICAL PEARL

Red desaturation is interpreted in conjunction with visual acuity and visual field test results, and usually signifies optic neuropathy.

Ocular motility

Each eye is moved within the bony orbit by the action of the four recti and two oblique muscles of each eye.

- The oculomotor nerve (cranial nerve [CN] III) supplies the medial, superior and inferior recti, and the inferior oblique muscles.
- The trochlear nerve (CN IV) supplies the superior oblique muscle.
- The abducens nerve (CN VI) supplies the lateral rectus muscle.
- The lateral and medial rectus muscles in each eye control ocular abduction and adduction, respectively.
  » The ocular 'ductions' are the monocular movements, including abduction and adduction, elevation, depression and cyclotorsion.
  » The ocular 'versions' are the movements of both eyes together, and the movement is *conjugate* when the movement of both is coordinated to maintain visual fixation. Extraocular muscle action is controlled through voluntary and automatic ocular motility neural-control mechanisms that are manifest through the horizontal and vertical gaze centers, and then the respective brainstem cranial nerve motor nuclei.
  » The horizontal yoked pairs are controlled by the horizontal gaze center at the pontomedullary junction near the 6th cranial nerve nucleus, with interneurons travelling in the medial longitudinal fasciculus to the medial rectus nucleus in the midbrain.

CLINICAL PEARL

The 'primary gaze position' refers to the straight-ahead direction of gaze for both eyes, toward the horizon. Loss of alignment of the two eyes will result in diplopia, which will be visible objectively as different positions of the corneal reflection of a torchlight on each eye—called the 'corneal light reflex'.

Pursuit eye movements are used so that vision tracks a moving object. This voluntary movement is also coordinated by the cerebellum, acting on the horizontal and vertical gaze centers.

Involuntary eye movements can be initiated by:

- an optokinetic stimulus, whereby rapid movement of an object across the field of vision elicits physiological nystagmus
- a vestibular stimulus, whereby movement of endolymph in the semicircular canals of the inner ear provokes vestibular nystagmus.

Testing eye movement

Eye position, extraocular muscle action, and extraocular movement control are tested as part of a cranial nerve and cerebellar examination.

- Ocular motility is tested by first observing the alignment of the eyes in the primary gaze position. The corneal light reflex is a useful aid to assess ocular alignment.
- Eyelid position and movement, and the extent of the sclera visible between the eyelids, should be observed in conjunction with eye movement.
- Pursuit movement is used to test movement into the cardinal positions of gaze ('H' pattern), where the patient may describe increased object separation when there is diplopia. The ductions of each eye (unilateral testing) and the versions of the pair are observed.

When strabismus is present, the cover test is used in the primary and cardinal positions of gaze to test extraocular muscle action.

- The fixating eye (central corneal light reflex) is covered to test for movement of the eye that remains uncovered.
- Any movement of the eye that remains visible where it attempts to regain object fixation when the cover is applied confirms the under-action of the muscle responsible for the direction of movement of the visible eye.
- No movement indicates poor visual acuity of the uncovered eye (unable to fixate), or complete paralysis of the muscle responsible for the refixation movement.

The uncover test reveals the position that had been taken by the covered (non-paretic) eye when the eye with a paretic muscle action was being used for fixation. The uncover test makes evident the dramatic ocular deviation of the eye which has normal muscle actions, because of the extra drive needed for the paretic muscle of the fixating eye; that is, the yoked pair innervation means the same drive required for the weak muscle is also delivered to the normal 'mate' of the pair.

Vertical movement of both eyes is observed for:

- relative changes in eyelid position during pursuit, as can occur with lid lag in thyroid-related eye disease
- vertical gaze defect.

CLINICAL PEARL

Generalized ophthalmic muscle paresis occurs from reduced muscle action in multiple planes of action and can result from myopathies, such as chronic progressive external ophthalmoplegia, neuromuscular junction disease such as myasthenia gravis, and muscular dystrophies such as myotonic dystrophy.

Ophthalmoscopy

To facilitate ophthalmoscopy, mydriatic drops paralyze the pupil constriction to light and improve the examiner's field of view, however, a limited view of the patient's optic nerve head and macular can be obtained without a dilated pupil.

- The mydriatic drop tropicamide, an antimuscarinic agent which also produces cycloplegia, has about a 10-minute onset with 4- to 8-hour duration.
- Rarely, tropicamide can precipitate an acute attack of very high intraocular pressure from anterior chamber angle closure, with the associated risk of severe optic nerve damage (acute angle-glaucoma).

The examiner should first check for the red reflex (Figure 23-1). The examiner's focus is then directed to the disc, retinal vessels and macula, which are systematically inspected.

A diminished red reflex can be due to any loss of optical clarity from the cornea to the retina. Examples of which are: corneal scar, cataract or vitreous haemorrhage. Causes of cataracts are listed in Box 23-1.

Auscultation

Patients who complain of an audible buzzing, with proptosis, a red eye and diplopia (secondary to limitation of eye movements) may have an audible bruit on ausculataion. These are signs and symptoms of a carotid cavernous fistula.

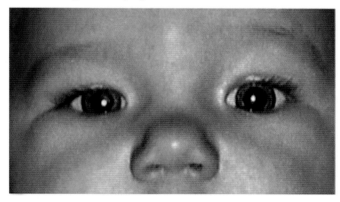

Figure 23-1 Loss of red reflex on ophthalmoscopy in the right eye of a child with cataract

From Hoyt CS and Taylor D. Pediatric ophthalmology and strabismus, 4th ed. Elsevier, 2013.

Box 23-1

Causes of cataract

- Idiopathic, especially with aging
- Congenital—familial, or due to maternal infection e.g. rubella, cytomegalovirus
- Metabolic—diabetes mellitus, hypothyroidism
- Drugs—corticosteroid therapy (systemic, topical, high-dose inhaled), quetiapine, miotics
- Trauma
- Genetic disorders, e.g. Down syndrome, Turner syndrome, myotonic dystrophy
- Secondary to other ocular disease, e.g. uveitis

OCULAR CONDITIONS

Retinal vascular disease

Systemic hypertension, dyslipidemia, diabetes mellitus, and tobacco smoking contribute to the risk of retinal vascular occlusive disease, namely central and branch retinal arterial and venous occlusion, and non-arteritic anterior ischemic optic neuropathy.

Arteriolosclerosis

A sign of chronic systemic hypertension, this is evident in the main retinal arterioles:

- copper and silver wire changes of the normal light reflex from the vessel (Figure 23-2A)
- attenuation of arteriolar caliber, either generalized or focal
- arteriovenous (AV) crossing changes—AV nipping (hourglass shape), venous banking, increased vascular tortuosity
- retinal hemorrhages.

Acute hypertensive retinopathy

Severe acute hypertension without preceding chronic hypertension affects terminal retinal arterioles, where acute-on-chronic hypertension will give a mixed picture of changes of the terminal and main retinal arterioles:

- focal intra-retinal peri-arteriolar transudates—small, white, focal oval dots deep in the retina, associated with major arterioles
- cottonwool spots (CWS)—nerve fiber layer infarct resulting from retinal arteriole obstruction, usually taking up to 6 weeks to fade (Figure 23-2B)
- capillary damage leading to microaneurysms, shunt vessels and collaterals.

Acute hypertensive optic neuropathy

Bilateral optic disc swelling and disc hemorrhages.

Acute hypertensive choroidopathy

- Focal retinal pigment epithelium (RPE) white dot changes
- Serous neurosensory retinal detachment, often in the macular region, and cystoid macular edema

Chronic hypertensive choroidal changes

- Diffuse RPE changes—granularity that looks 'moth-eaten'
- RPE clumping and atrophy (Elschnig spots)
- Larger atrophic patches
- Linear hyperpigmented flecks along choroidal vessels (Siegrist streaks)

Retinal arterial occlusion

Retinal arterial occlusion is a spectrum of clinical presentations, from amaurosis fugax to central retinal arterial occlusion, and visible retinal arterial emboli may or may not be evident.

- Amaurosis fugax is the painless, transient monocular loss of vision akin to a cerebral transient ischemic attack. Residual emboli may be visible with the ophthalmoscope. Irreversible retinal ischemia occurs after at least 100 minutes of occlusion.
- A central retinal arterial occlusion (CRAO) is painless and occurs with permanent monocular loss of vision. The retinal pallor from ischemia develops within about an hour of the onset of symptoms, and fades within a few days. The characteristic feature is the cherry red spot (Figure 23-3). A central spot of the macular remains the normal choroidal color because there is no inner retina

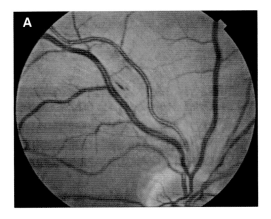 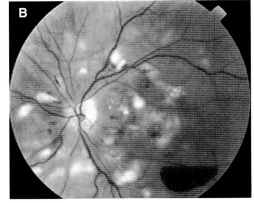

Figure 23-2 Retinal changes due to hypertension. (**A**) Acute—arterioles show silver wiring, vascular tortuosity, generalized reduced arterial caliber, and flame hemorrhage is evident. (**B**) Chronic—cottonwool spots, pre-retinal hemorrhage, flame and blotch hemorrhages, hard exudates, irregular venous caliber, venous banking, and arteriovenous crossing changes with arteriolar deviation

From: (A) Yanoff M and Duker JS (eds). Ophthalmology, 4th ed. Saunders, 2014. (B) Rogers AH and Duker JS. Rapid diagnosis in ophthalmology series: retina. Elsevier, 2008.

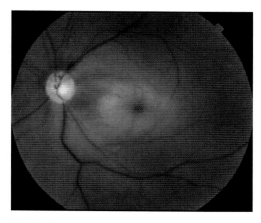

Figure 23-3 Central retinal arterial occlusion. Diffuse retinal pallor, except at the fovea, where the normal retinal (choroidal) colour looks cherry red by comparison with the 'sick' pale surrounding retina

From Duker JS, Waheed NK and Goldman D. Handbook of retinal OCT. Elsevier, 2014.

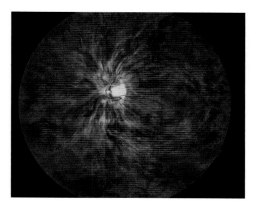

Figure 23-4 Diffuse retinal hemorrhages secondary to central retinal vein occlusion, predominantly involving the retinal nerve fiber layer, resulting in the arch-shaped pattern of hemorrhage. Retinal veins are tortuous. Optic disc swelling is present, with detail obscured. Macular edema is present

From Ryan SJ et al. (eds). Retina, 5th ed. Elsevier, 2013.

becuase there is no blockage from inner retina at the fovea. The surrounding retina becomes opaque secondary to the inner retinal ischemia. **This is an ophthalmic emergency.**

- » Embolism may occur from known or occult conditions such as atrial fibrillation, ipsilateral carotid stenosis, cardiac valve vegetations, or patent foramen ovale.
- » Urgent investigation and treatment will be required to attempt to restore circulation, recover vision, and avoid other embolic events. There is a poor prognosis, but some chance of visual recovery from early intervention.
- » In addition to emboli, CRAO can be due to thrombotic occlusion of atherosclerotic lesions, inflammatory arteritis (e.g. giant cell arteritis), vascular spasm, and occlusion secondary to low perfusion pressure.
- Branch retinal arterial occlusion (BRAO) arises from embolic occlusion of more-distal retinal vessels, often in the temporal retinal circulation. It may produce a defect in the field of vision that can be permanent.

Retinal venous occlusion

Retinal venous occlusion is a common retinal vascular disorder, with a variable pattern of monocular vision loss. Severe central retinal vein occlusion (CRVO) has devastating consequences, such as rubeotic glaucoma and painful monocular total blindness. The severity is usually related to the extent of retinal capillary non-perfusion; and the severity can change, becoming ischemic over time, making exact classification difficult.

- The characteristic findings in CRVO are (Figure 23-4):
  - » retinal hemorrhages in all four quadrants
  - » dilated, tortuous retinal veins
  - » cottonwool spots
  - » macular edema
  - » optic disc swelling.

- Ischemic CRVO is associated with a greater risk of proliferative retinopathy, vitreous hemorrhage and rubeotic glaucoma, and the diagnosis is based on:
  - » severe vision loss at presentation
  - » the presence of an RAPD
  - » extensive non-perfusion on a fluorescein angiogram.
- The non-ischemic form is usually milder, with less severe loss of vision, no RAPD, fewer hemorrhages and CWS, and good perfusion on a fluorescein angiogram. If it does not then progress to the ischemic form, non-ischemic CRVO can resolve and the patient achieves a relatively good visual outcome.
- CRVO is associated with a range of factors that impinge on the central retinal vein at the optic disc head, especially where the vein passes through the lamina cribrosa:
  - » external compression of the vein from structural changes of the lamina cribrosa, as can occur associated with glaucomatous cupping, from swelling of the optic nerve, or from pressure originating in the orbit from orbital swelling
  - » inflammation of the vessel wall in vasculitis
  - » changes in the blood, such as deficiency of thrombolytic factors and increase in clotting factors
  - » blood flow disturbances, either hyperdynamic or sluggish circulation from hyperviscosity.

The patient history should address the following areas:
- hypertension
- diabetes mellitus
- cardiovascular disorders
- bleeding or clotting disorders
- vasculitis
- autoimmune disorders
- use of oral contraceptives
- closed-head trauma
- alcohol consumption

- amount of physical activity
- primary open-angle glaucoma or angle-closure glaucoma.
- Vision loss in CRVO is usually secondary to macular edema. This is treated with intravitreal anti-vascular endothelial growth factor (VEGF) agents.

Diabetic retinopathy (DR)

Diabetes mellitus, whether type 1 or type 2, is associated with the risk of developing DR. The duration and severity of the diabetes can predict the severity of the DR.

- DR is a micro-vascular disease that can lead to retinal ischemia, macular edema and proliferative retinopathy. All of which can cause vision loss.
- The longer a patient has had diabetes, the poorer the glucose and cardiovascular risk factors are controlled, the higher relative risk of developing vision loss from DR.
- The early stages of DR (non-proliferative diabetic retinopathy (NPDR)) often has no symptoms, hence the importance of diabetic retinal screening.
- Macular edema, occurs due to leaking vessels, can occur at any stage of NPDR. Macular edema leads to visual deteriation and is treated with anti-VEGF intravitreally.
- Proliferative diabetic retinopathy (PDR) occurs when retinal ischemia drives the development of abnormal new blood vessels. These new vessels are fragile and can bleed causing sudden vision loss.
- There is proven benefit from optimal systemic control of diabetes to delay or prevent the onset and reduce the severity of retinopathy.
- Screening eye examination allows early detection of retinopathy, and institution of effective preventative treatment.
- Vision loss or disturbance associated with diabetes includes a range of pathological changes in addition to

DR and its sequelae. Examples of non-DR complications include cataract, isolated cranial nerve palsies, and the consequences of ocular and periocular infection.

Grading of DR (see below) establishes its severity and the presence of diabetic macular edema.

- The grade of retinopathy is used to set intervals for screening eye examinations, and the criteria for referral to an ophthalmologist.
- Management by an ophthalmologist is required when there is imminent risk of loss of vision, where either a shorter-interval screening schedule or ocular treatment is indicated.
- Prompt referral to an ophthalmologist is usually required where there are symptoms of altered vision, or reduced visual acuity is found during the screening examination.
- Pregnancy can accelerate the deterioration of DR grading, hence a pregnant patient with DR requires closer ophthalmic monitoring.

Features and grading of DR

Accurate classification of DR guides clinical management.

- No retinopathy—normal visual acuity and no retinopathy in a patient with diabetes mellitus. This usually requires 2-yearly visual acuity checks and a follow-up dilated fundus examination. In such a setting, there is a low risk of rapid progression of retinopathy by the next eye examination.
- Minimal NPDR—normal visual acuity and a few retinal microaneurysms. It requires a 12-month follow-up eye examination performed by a practitioner able to accurately detect retinopathy and maculopathy.
- Moderate & severe NPDR, PDR and maculopathy require referral to an ophthalmologist (Figure 23-5).

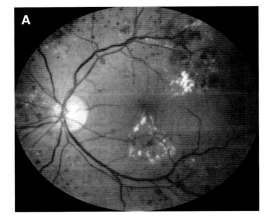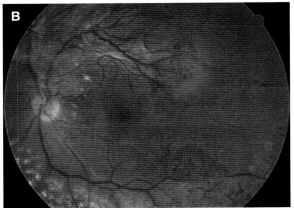

Figure 23-5 (**A**) Severe non-proliferative diabetic retinopathy, macular hard exudates, microaneurysms, dot and blotch hemorrhages, and venous beading. (**B**) Proliferative diabetic retinopathy that has had laser treatment: laser scars, new vessels at disc and elsewhere, retinal hemorrhages, and fibrosis overlying vessels superior to disc

From: (A) Ryan SJ et al. (eds). Retina, 5th ed. Saunders, 2013. (B) Rakel RE and Rakel DP. Textbook of family medicine, 8th ed. Elsevier, 2011.

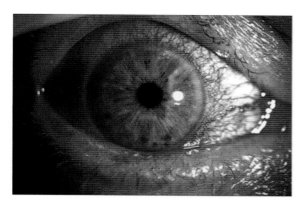

Figure 23-6 Anterior uveitis. Diffuse perilimbal vascular congestion; cornea is clear

From Phelps K and Hassad C. General practice: the integrative approach. Sydney: Elsevier Australia, 2011.

- Common features on fundoscopy seen in DR are:
  - » microaneurysms
  - » intra-retinal hemorrhages
  - » venous beading
  - » hard exudates
  - » intra-retinal microvascular abnormalities
  - » neovascularization at the disc or elsewhere
  - » vitreous or pre-retinal hemorrhages
  - » microaneurysms and intra-retinal hemorrhages in all four retinal quadrants
  - » venous beading in more than two retinal quadrants
  - » any prominent intra-retinal microvascular abnormalities (IRMAs)
  - » the presence of neovascularization either at the optic disc or elsewhere in the retina
  - » vitreous or pre-retinal hemorrhages.

UVEITIS

Uveitis is inflammation of the uveal tract—iris, ciliary body of choroid. It can be classified into its location such as anterior, intermediate, posterior or pan-uveitis. Its duration and time course is divided into acute or chronic. If bilateral it is important to exclude a systemic inflammatory condition. Uveitis is an important differential diagnosis in any case of 'red eye' (Figure 23-6).

CLINICAL PEARL

The symptoms of uveitis include acute pain, redness, photophobia, lacrimation, reduced vision, and/or floaters.

- Slit-lamp examination is generally required to make the diagnosis; The protein and cellular exudate of acute inflammation, or the intraocular signs of the consequences of chronic inflammation, are seen directly.
- A dilated retinal fundus examination is required in all cases of uveitis, and can establish whether there are intraocular features of previous uveitis—such as a posterior synechia, or a well-established chorio-retinal scar, with possibly acute reactivation of the scar, or retinal vasculitis.

CLINICAL PEARL

Common systemic conditions associated with uveitis include seronegative arthropathy, sarcoidosis, systemic lupus erythematosus, HLA-B27 associated disease, juvenile rheumatoid arthritis, herpesvirus group infections, toxoplasmosis, syphilis, tuberculosis, ANCA-associated vasculitis, and Behçet's disease.

- An infective cause of uveitis needs to be ruled out, prior to treatment with corticosteroids.
- Intensive topical steroids, and non-steroidal anti-inflammatory eye drops, through to local steroid injections and glaucoma treatment, require supervision by an ophthalmologist in conjunction with the physician treating the underlying systemic condition.
- Uveitis that cannot be controlled by local treatment may need systemic treatment starting with oral corticosteroids. Some conditions need further immunosuppression in coordination with a rheumatologist or immunologist.

Scleritis

Scleritis usually presents as a unilateral painful red eye. This is a rare potentially blinding chronic inflammatory condition characterized by:

- severe dull pain which typically gets worse at night and wakes the patient from sleep early in the morning.
- the involved eye is red, exquisitely tender and vision is typically normal
- there can be spillover involvement of other ocular structures such as the cornea
- it most commonly affects the anterior sclera but up to 20% involve predominantly the posterior sclera and may present with severe pain and minimal physical signs
- involvement of the sclera can be diffuse, nodular or necrotizing.

Scleritis is associated with rheumatoid arthritis, ANCA-associated vasculitis, inflammatory bowel disease, spondyloarthropathies, relapsing polychondritis and other autoimmune diseases.

THYROID-RELATED ORBITOPATHY

Orbital involvement can occur as part of Graves' disease.

- The orbital involvement can precede, coincide with, or follow thyrotoxicosis.

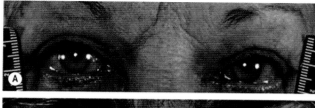

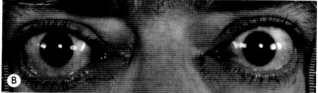

Figure 23-7 (**A**) Thyroid eye disease secondary to Graves' disease; convergent strabismus, conjunctival congestion, right palpebral aperture greater height than left. (**B**) Bilateral proptosis, left eyelid retraction, inferior scleral show, right > left

From Levin LA and Albert DM. Ocular disease: mechanisms and management. Elsevier, 2010.

- The ocular symptoms include tearing, through to epiphora, gritty dry eye symptoms, more severe ocular pain manifesting as both surface and deep ache, photophobia, proptosis, diplopia, and reduced vision.
- The autoimmune cellular infiltrate and associated edema of the orbital tissues is the underlying cause of the signs and symptoms of the increased orbital volume that develops as a consequence (Figure 23-7A) and causes:
  » diplopia because of decreased ocular motility
  » proptosis sometimes complicated by corneal exposure
- The eyes can be red, resulting either from the orbital inflammation or from dryness
  » apical crowding leading to optic nerve compression
  » eyelid retraction and scleral 'show' giving a staring, startled look (Figure 23-7B)
- Lid lag can be evident on downward-pursuit eye movement.
  » raised orbital pressure which can lead to increased intraocular pressure and glaucomatous optic neuropathy.

DRY EYE

'Dry eye' symptoms usually describe ocular surface irritation and grittiness, and commonly are accompanied by a sense of mild visual disturbance.

The composition of tears can be thought of in terms of the components that originate from different ocular adnexal structures:

- the superficial lipid layer derived from the eyelid meibomian glands
- an aqueous layer derived from the main and accessory lacrimal glands
- a hydrophilic mucin layer derived from the surface epithelium and conjunctival goblet cells.

Normal tears contain water, electrolytes, proteins such as immunoglobulin G (IgG) and secretory IgA, lysozyme, lactoferrin and lipocalin, as well as lipids, mucins and a range of other small molecules.

- The dry eye syndrome results from a variety of ocular surface conditions which alter the overall tear film composition and function.
- Conditions ranging from blepharitis and rosacea, to keratoconjunctivitis sicca will lead to the dry eye syndrome, with multiple factors often simultaneously at play.
- The hallmarks of the dry eye syndrome include increased osmolarity of the tear film and associated ocular surface inflammation, which exacerbates the instability of the tear film, and this diminishes the lubricating, protective effect of the tears for the mucosal ocular surface, and impairs the function of the epithelial cells.

Sjögren's syndrome is the triad of ocular and oral sicca, with autoimmune connective tissue disease.

- Dry eye will be prominent in both the primary and the secondary form of the disease.
- Schirmer's test will prove the reduction in tear production.
- Biopsy of lacrimal or salivary glands will reveal lymphocytic infiltration, but is usually not required in the setting of typical clinical symptoms and autoimmune serological abnormalities.

Treatment of dry eye syndrome is usually multifaceted, and addresses the range of underlying causative factors.

- Aqueous tear deficiency is remedied by the use of eyedrop lubricant supplements, and occlusion of lacrimal drainage with plugs placed into the nasolacrimal puncta.
- Topical cyclosporine A (ciclosporin A) is a topical immunosuppressive drug that effectively decreases ocular inflammation that characterizes dry eye disease. This gives symptomatic relief and may improve tear film quality and quantity.
- Severe dry eye can lead to filamentous strands of mucus and epithelium attached to the ocular surface that need to be removed with forceps and treated with acetylcysteine eye drops.
- Surgical treatment may be required if severe corneal ulceration occurs.

Severe dry eye syndrome can lead to a disabling level of ocular surface discomfort, through to a risk of blindness from corneal ulceration and infective keratitis, making early recognition and prompt treatment of dry eye syndrome essential.

NEOPLASIA AND THE EYE

Neoplasia can affect the eye as primary ocular disease:
- eyelid carcinomas
- rare ocular surface neoplasia
- primary melanoma in any of the melanin-pigment-containing tissues (conjunctiva and uveal tract)
- retinoblastoma
- optic nerve glioma

- optic nerve sheath meningioma
- orbital tissue tumors such as pleomorphic lacrimal gland adenomas, and orbital tissue sarcomas.

Secondary tumor metastases can develop within the eye, typically the uveal tract, or in the orbit.

Tumors developing within the eye cause visual disturbance, and tumors external to the eye cause visual disturbance, proptosis, diplopia, and pain. The diagnosis is usually made through a systematic ocular and general clinical examination addressing the presenting symptom.

NEURO-OPHTHALMOLOGY

Optic neuritis (ON)

Optic neuritis is a demyelinating inflammation of the optic nerve. Occasionally it occurs in association with orbital or paranasal sinus infections, or following a systemic viral infection.

- The onset of ON is usually unilateral, decreased vision with retro-orbital or ocular pain—especially associated with eye movement. The first attack of ON may occur in previously healthy young adults. Other visual symptoms such as altered color vision (dyschromatopsia) may precede reduced visual acuity.
- The diagnostic work-up of ON will also address conditions with similar ocular signs, such as anterior ischemic optic neuropathy, compressive optic neuropathy, or nutritional or hereditary optic neuropathy.
- ON can be a primary demyelination, or occur in association with multiple sclerosis (MS) or neuromyelitis optica (NMO).
  - » Optic neuritis that occurs in young adults (20–45 years) can be the first clinical manifestation of MS. It can also occur in older patients.
  - » Detecting antibodies to aquaporin 4 can differentiate NMO from MS.
  - » ON that occurs with other, sometimes previous, neurological symptoms suggests a diagnosis of either MS or NMO.
- A male with bilateral optic neuropathy, and relatively little recovery of vision and a family history, suggests Leber's hereditary optic neuropathy, and a family history with affected maternal uncles may be present.

> ### CLINICAL PEARL
>
> In assessing optic neuritis, the vision assessment includes testing visual acuity, visual fields, pupil responses to light including the swinging torch test for a relative afferent pupillary defect, and color vision testing.

- Ophthalmoscopy may reveal diffuse optic disc swelling. The absence of swelling does not rule out ON, as two-thirds of cases can have retrobulbar optic nerve involvement.
- Various patterns of visual field defects can be evident, altitudinal, arcuate defects, central scotoma or a diffuse field loss.

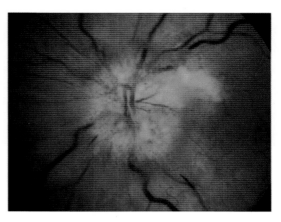

Figure 23-8 Anterior ischemic optic neuropathy; note the pale, diffuse optic nerve edema and retinal ischemia evidenced by pallor

From Kidd DP, Newman NJ and Blousse V (eds). Neuro-ophthalmology. Blue Books of Neurology, issue 32. Butterworth-Heinemann, 2008.

- Severe bilateral ON with chiasmal patterns of field defects (e.g. bi-temporal field loss) suggests NMO.
- Magnetic resonance imaging (MRI) of the brain and orbits with contrast may be required, in atypical presentations, to exclude compressive optic neuropathy, and confirm optic nerve enhancement and detect any other central nervous system (CNS) lesions.
- Spinal cord and brainstem MRI will be indicated where there are spinal cord signs, or NMO is a possibility.
- Intravenous steroid treatment will usually be considered for ON. The potential benefit is quicker recovery from the acute episode, with little benefit in 5-year visual outcomes.

Non-arteritic anterior ischemic optic neuropathy (NAION)

Anterior ischemic optic neuropathy (AION) is the most common acute optic neuropathy in older patients. Giant cell arteritis (GCA) must be excluded prior to giving this diagnosis. It is characterized by:

- sudden monocular visual loss associated with relatively pale disc swelling
- associated flame hemorrhage at the disc or in the nerve fiber layer (Figure 23-8)
- cottonwool spots in some cases.

Vision loss is usually permanent, with some recovery possible within weeks to months. A degree of optic atrophy results.

Common risk factors for NAION include: age, BP/hypercholesterolemia/diabetes, thrombophilia, obstructive sleep apnoea, some medications: sildenafil, amiodarone, and disc at risk (assess the other optic disc to see if is small and has no physiologic cup).

Arteritic anterior ischemic optic neuropathy (AAION)

Giant cell arteritis (GCA) is an important AION to be mindful of in patients over 50 years with acute vision loss. It

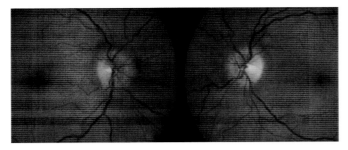

Figure 23-9 Papilledema: bilateral optic disc swelling (right > left); loss of disc margins, increased visibility of small capillaries crossing disc, peri-papillary hemorrhages (right)

is a medium to large vessel granulomatous disease that can lead to bilateral blindness or mortality if left untreated.

- Patients with symptoms of polymyalgia rheumatica (PMR) can develop GCA (15%), and half of those with GCA will have preceding PMR.
- GCA has a range of ocular effects, including external ophthalmoplegia and central or branch retinal artery occlusion.
- A localized headache of recent onset, with a high erythrocyte sedimentation rate (ESR) and C-reactive protein (CRP), in conjunction with AION can be highly suggestive of the diagnosis and the need for urgent treatment.

CLINICAL PEARL

Sudden monocular visual loss, associated with pale disc swelling, in a patient aged 50 years or older will require consideration for urgent systemic corticosteroid treatment, and possibly anticoagulation, because of the risk of imminent involvement of the second eye from giant cell arteritis, and thus the risk of sudden acute total blindness.

- The diagnosis is formally confirmed by a temporal artery biopsy that exhibits a chronic granulomatous inflammatory cell infiltrate in the elastic lamina of the arterial wall. Fluorescein angiography can demonstrate delayed and patchy perfusion of the choroid from the short posterior ciliary arteries.
- The symptoms and signs are related to the reduced perfusion caused by the vasculitis of the external carotid, and the ophthalmic arteries and their branches.

Papilledema

Bilateral optic disc swelling associated with raised intracranial pressure (ICP) is termed papilledema (Figure 23-9).

- Raised ICP is commonly accompanied by symptoms of headache, nausea and vomiting, and pulsatile tinnitus.
- The possibility of underlying severe systemic hypertension, with raised ICP, should be borne in mind.

The visual symptoms that may be present with papilledema include:

- transient visual changes (obscurations) such as 'gray out' of vision associated with posture change to a more elevated position, or transient visual flickering
- blurred vision associated with constricted visual fields and altered color vision
- diplopia due to a 6th nerve palsy due to the raised ICP.

Urgent CT or MRI neuro-imaging is required to identify intracranial causes for raised ICP, and magnetic resonance venography may need to be performed to detect venous sinus thrombosis.

Extraocular muscle paralysis

Paralysis of the extraocular muscles arises from pathology affecting the oculomotor, trochlear or abducens nerves. The primary symptom is diplopia:

- Oculomotor palsy has combined horizontal and vertical diplopia, with ipsilateral ptosis and dilated pupil, reflecting the combined extraocular motor and parasympathetic motor functions of the oculomotor nerve. The most common pathologies involve all fascicles of the nerve, and thus isolated under-action of individual extraocular muscles is uncommon.
- Trochlear nerve palsy gives vertical, torsional or oblique diplopia, especially on down-gaze and looking to the side away from the side of the affected superior oblique muscle ('down and in').
- Abducens nerve palsy gives horizontal diplopia that is worse looking to the side of the weak lateral rectus muscle, with esotropia in primary gaze, and a compensatory head turn to the side of the weak muscle.

The diagnosis of cranial nerve palsy causing extraocular muscle paralysis with symptoms of diplopia is primarily 'anatomical', and is achieved from identifying the symptoms and signs that arise from involvement of the nerve and associated structures along the path of each nerve from the brain stem nucleus to the muscle(s).

PHAKOMATOSES

The phakomatoses are a group of disorders where hamartomas are present in the nervous system (central or peripheral), and the eye, skin and viscera. Ocular features are given in Table 23-1.

OCULAR EFFECTS OF SYSTEMIC MEDICATION

Visual disturbance may result from the side-effects of medication, necessitating a careful drug history in any patient with such a symptom. Table 23-2 (overleaf) lists some ocular complications of systemic pharmacotherapy.

Table 23-1 Ocular features in the phakomatoses

	NEUROFIBRO-MATOSIS	TUBEROUS SCLEROSIS	VON HIPPEL—LINDAU SYNDROME	ATAXIA—TELANGIECTASIA	STURGE—WEBER SYNDROME
Inheritance	Autosomal dominant	Autosomal dominant	Autosomal dominant	Autosomal recessive	Sporadic
Ocular complications	Lisch nodules (hamartoma of iris melanocytes) Eyelid neurofibromas Prominent corneal nerves Optic nerve and chiasmal gliomas Retinal and optic disc hamartomas Compressive optic neuropathy Bony deformities Cataracts	Retinal and optic nerve hamartomas	Retinal angiomata Retinal detachment	Conjunctival telangiectasia Oculomotor apraxia	Hamartomatous angiomata of eye Glaucoma

Table 23-2 Medications that can exacerbate or cause ocular conditions

	MEDICATION
Cataract	Steroids Statins Amiodarone Phenothiazine Pilocarpine
Acute angle closure crisis	Topiramate Selective serotonin reuptake inhibitors
Optic disc edema	Tetracyclines Naproxen & ibuprofen Oral contraception/estradiol Isotretinoin
Optic neuropathy	Ethambutol, isoniazid
Non-ischemic optic neuropathy	Amiodarone, sildenafil
Keratopathy	Amiodarone
Maculopathy	Chloroquine Hydroxychloroquine Thioridazine Tamoxifen Fingolimod Niacin Interferons Prostaglandin analogs Epinephrine

SELF-ASSESSMENT QUESTIONS

1 A 45-year-old man presents with a painful, red left eye. Physical examination reveals reduced visual acuity, and an irregular pupil. He complains of a dry cough for the past 6 weeks. Which of the following investigations would be a priority in this case to ascertain the diagnosis? More than one answer may be correct.

 A Thyroid function tests, thyroid autoantibodies
 B Blood sugar level, fluorescein retinal angiography
 C Chest X-ray, serum angiotensin-converting enzyme (ACE) level
 D Antineutrophil cytoplasmic autoantibodies (ANCA), erythrocyte sedimentation rate (ESR)
 E C-reactive protein (CRP), rheumatoid factor (RF)

2 A 60-year-old woman presents with painful monocular blindness. Physical examination reveals a relative afferent pupil defect, and extensive retinal hemorrhages. Which of the following underlying illnesses may have led to this problem? More than one answer may be correct.

 A Antiphospholipid syndrome
 B Type II diabetes mellitus
 C Warfarin therapy for recent pulmonary embolus
 D Low-molecular-weight heparin thromboprophylaxis for recent orthopedic surgery
 E Nephrotic syndrome

3 You see a 22-year-old male who has had type I diabetes mellitus since the age of 5. Which of the following clinical findings would prompt you to refer him to an ophthalmologist for urgent review? More than one answer may be correct.

 A Mild reduction in the red reflex in the right eye
 B Detection of neovascularization near the macula but no change in vision
 C Intermittent visual blurring after recent introduction of insulin-pump therapy
 D Painful red eye with mucopurulent ocular discharge
 E Three new microaneurysms in the right eye

4 A 71-year-old woman presents with transient monocular visual loss. Which of the following may be a risk factor for this condition? More than one answer may be correct.

 A Multiple sclerosis
 B The presence of aquaporin-4 antibodies
 C Atrial fibrillation
 D Commencement of vasodilator therapy for hypertension
 E Giant-cell arteritis

5 Which of the following may explain a sudden deterioration of vision in a patient as a consequence of hypertension? More than one answer may be correct.

 A Retinal hemorrhage
 B Serous retinal detachment
 C Acute (closed-angle) glaucoma
 D Papilledema
 E Arteriovenous nipping of retinal vessels

ANSWERS

1 C.

A painful red eye with an irregular pupil and reduced vision is suggestive of uveitis. Sarcoidosis is a known cause of uveitis, and the presence of a dry cough must raise the possibility of this diagnosis. The presence of bilateral hilar lymphadenopathy or interstitial changes on a chest X-ray would strengthen the clinical suspicion. Serum ACE is only moderately sensitive and specific for sarcoidosis. An elevated result would, however, increase the likelihood of this diagnosis.

ANCA-positive vasculitis, especially granulomatosis with polyangiitis, can certainly cause a variety of ocular conditions, as well as lung disease, so answer D is not unreasonable. However, the ESR is too nonspecific in this situation to help narrow the diagnosis. Thyroid eye disease may cause proptosis and ophthalmoplegia, but should not produce uveitis. Rheumatoid arthritis can also be associated with autoimmune ocular complications and with pulmonary inflammation, but the RF and CRP are lacking in specificity. Diabetes mellitus should not be the cause of uveitis.

2 A, B and E.

The clinical scenario is describing central retinal vein occlusion. Any cause of hypercoagulability is a risk factor in this instance. Therefore, antiphospholipid syndrome due to the presence of anti-cardiolipin antibodies, and nephrotic syndrome due to loss of antithrombotic proteins in the urine, can lead to this problem. Diabetes mellitus is also a risk factor, probably through multiple mechanisms such as hypercoagulability associated with severe hypoglycemia with dehydration, or nephropathy with nephrotic syndrome. Anticoagulant therapy is not a cause of retinal vein occlusion.

3 **B and D.**

Features of severe diabetic retinopathy that require referral to an ophthalmologist include:

i   microaneurysms and intra-retinal hemorrhages in all four retinal quadrants
ii venous beading in more than two retinal quadrants
iii any prominent intra-retinal microvascular abnormalities (IRMAs)
iv the presence of neovascularization either at the optic disc or elsewhere in the retina
v   vitreous or pre-retinal hemorrhages.

In the above scenario, it would be important to arrange urgent ophthalmological assessment for option B, as the patient with proliferative retinopathy is at risk of hemorrhage and sudden loss of vision, which often can be prevented by laser photocoagulation therapy. Similarly, a longstanding diabetic with an infection in the eye, such as in option D, can lose the eye very quickly through development of endophthalmitis if prompt treatment is not instituted with appropriate anti-microbial therapy.

Early cataract (option A), transient changes in visual acuity secondary to lens distortion from rapid blood sugar level changes (option C), and background diabetic retinopathy (option E) are not emergencies.

4 **C and D.**

This scenario describes amaurosis fugax. Amaurosis fugax is usually the consequence of embolic occlusion of the central retinal artery, with subsequent dissolution and dislodgement of the clot. Atrial fibrillation with the formation of left atrial thrombus, as in option C, is therefore an important risk factor. It can, however, result from hypoperfusion due to a transient drop in blood pressure in the setting of pre-existing cerebral vascular disease, such as in option D.

Multiple sclerosis and neuromyelitis optica (NMO) can cause optic neuritis, which can result in reduced visual acuity, but not transient loss of vision. NMO is associated with aquaporin-4-antibodies. Giant-cell arteritis can cause arteritic retinal arterial occlusion or anterior ischemic optic neuropathy. The blindness is usually not transient.

5 **A, B, D.**

Hypertension, both acute and chronic, has multiple effects on the eye, and can affect the vasculature, optic nerves and retina, including the choroid. Some of these can acutely threaten the vision, such as retinal hemorrhage (option A), serous retinal detachment (option B), and papilledema (option D). Papilledema can result from acute severe hypertension. Acute (closed-angle) glaucoma does not result from hypertension. Arteriovenous nipping of vessels is a sign of hypertensive vascular change, but *per se* will not affect the vision.

CHAPTER 24

WOMEN'S HEALTH FOR THE PHYSICIAN

Steve Robson and Andrew Korda

CHAPTER OUTLINE

INFERTILITY

CLINICAL PEARL

Infertility is the failure of a couple to conceive:
- after 12 months of regular intercourse without use of contraception in women less than 35 years of age
- after 6 months of regular intercourse without use of contraception in women 35 years and older.

Primary infertility implies no previous pregnancy; *secondary infertility* is defined by an inability to conceive following a history of any antecedent pregnancy, including miscarriage, abortion, and ectopic pregnancies.

- Overall, the great majority (80–90%) of apparently normal couples will conceive within the first year of trying.
- The prevalence of infertility is approximately 7% in the general population.
- In developed countries, the various sources of infertility are classified as shown in Table 24-1 (overleaf).

Table 24-1 Types of infertility

TYPE	PREVALENCE
Female factor infertility	40–55%
Male factor infertility	25–40%
Both male and female factor infertility	10%
Unexplained infertility	25%

Table 24-2 Causes of infertility

CAUSE	APPROXIMATE INCIDENCE
Male factor hypogonadism, post-testicular defects, seminiferous tubule dysfunction	26%
Ovulatory dysfunction	21%
Tubal damage	14%
Endometriosis	6%
Coital problems	6%
Cervical factor	3%
Unexplained	28%

Age and infertility

An increasing number of women older than 35 years will seek treatment for infertility, as a woman's fertility is known to decline with age, and the number of women wishing to conceive between 35 and 45 years old is increasing.

- The possibility for oocytes to be fertilized and develop naturally is compromised with increasing age.
- There is a clear inverse relationship between fertility and female age, and spontaneous pregnancies are rarely reported after the age of 45.
- Significant changes in ovarian and uterine physiology also occur with advancing age, specifically loss of oocyte integrity, high rates of aneuploidy, and decreased uterine receptiveness.
- As women age, there is also an increase in the prevalence of gynecological and systemic disease, such as endometriosis, pelvic infection, fibroids, diabetes, obesity, hypertension and smoking-related diseases.
- In women older than 35 who seek infertility treatment, prompt and complete investigation of fertility should be offered so that any correctable conditions can be treated as soon as possible.

Some causes of infertility, such as azoospermia, longstanding amenorrhea, or bilateral tubal obstruction, are easy to determine. However, the situation is often less clear: the sperm count may be reduced but not absent; there may be oligomenorrhea with some ovulatory cycles; the woman may have partial tubal obstruction; or a menstrual history may suggest intermittent ovulation.

Table 24-2 outlines the likelihood of different causes of infertility

- Investigation of infertility should commence in couples who have not been able to conceive after 12 months of unprotected and frequent intercourse, but earlier assessment (after 6 months) can be started in women over 35 years of age or where there is a clinically-apparent cause, such as known tubal disease.
- The timing of the initial investigation into infertility also depends on the couple's risk factors.

Infertility is stressful for most couples. It is important to appreciate that couples may have multiple factors contributing to their infertility; therefore, a complete initial diagnostic evaluation, including a detailed history and physical examination, should be performed. This will detect the most common causes of infertility. Evaluation of both partners should be performed concurrently.

The following are valuable in most couples with infertility:

- menstrual history
- semen analysis
- imaging, such as hystero-contrast sonography to assess tubal patency and the uterine cavity
- day 3 serum FSH (follicle-stimulating hormone) and AMH (anti-Mullerian hormone) levels
- serum prolactin estimation
- evaluation of thyroid function
- pelvic ultrasound examination to determine the presence of uterine fibroids and ovarian cysts
- diagnostic laparoscopy and hysteroscopy to identify endometriosis, or other pelvic pathology such as tubal disease ± hydrotubation for tubal patency
- assessment of ovarian reserve in women over 35 years of age, which may involve ultrasound for early follicular antral follicle count, or AMH measurements.

The utility of measurement of anti-sperm antibodies is not established.

Once the cause of infertility is identified, therapy is aimed at correcting reversible causes and overcoming irreversible factors.

The couple should also be counseled on lifestyle modifications to improve fertility, such as cessation of smoking, reducing excessive alcohol consumption, achieving a normal body mass index (BMI), and the appropriate timing and frequency of intercourse (every 1–2 days around the expected time of ovulation).

Anovulatory infertility

Ovulatory dysfunction and anovulation affect 15–25% of all infertile couples seeking therapy.

- Treatment of ovulation disorders, if isolated, remains one of the most successful of all infertility treatments.
- Post-treatment conception at 2 years is between 78% and 96%.

- Initial treatment is most commonly with either the SPRM (selective progesterone receptor modulator) letrozole or clomiphene citrate (clomifene), a selective estrogen receptor modulator (SERM) which stimulates ovulation induction.
- Patients with some degree of insulin resistance might require some adjuvant therapy to clomiphene. Correction of hyperinsulinemia may increase the rate of spontaneous ovulation, and also increase the response to clomiphene. This is best achieved by the use of metformin, an insulin-sensitizing agent.
- In the event that patients do not conceive on clomiphene citrate and metformin, other medications have been useful; such as adrenal steroid therapy, and gonadotropins, with or without gonadotropin-releasing hormone (GnRH) agonists or GnRH antagonists.

Hyperprolactinemia

Hyperprolactinemia is present in 23% of patients with amenorrhea, and 8% of patients with oligomenorrhea. Elevated prolactin is believed to be a cause of anovulation by impairing gonadotropin pulsatility, and the arrangement of the estrogen-positive feedback effect of LH secretion.

CLINICAL PEARL

Prolactin can be increased by physiological events, such as stress, or a normal breast or pelvic examination.

- Patients who have persistently elevated prolactin levels should also be screened for hypothyroidism and for a pituitary gland mass.

The treatment of hyperprolactinemia depends on the cause. Prolactin suppression can be achieved with bromocriptine, an ergot-alkaloid dopamine-receptor agonist.

Infertility due to anatomical abnormalities of the reproductive tract

- In the event of tubal pathology, surgical treatment of tubal disease or assisted conception to overcome the tubal obstruction are the treatments of choice.
- If fibroids involve a significant portion of the endometrium or obstruct the tubal ostium, their removal is warranted. Submucous fibroids need careful evaluation and may need resection.
- Asherman's syndrome, a condition characterized by adhesive scarring of the endometrium, needs to be treated with hysteroscopic resection of adhesions.
- Endometrial polyps, which may be diagnosed by imaging studies, should be removed.
- Endometriosis, if minimal to mild, should be treated surgically. The management of endometriosis is complex and evolving, and should be individualized.

Male factor infertility

Only a small proportion of infertile men have conditions for which therapy of confirmed benefit is available.

- Treatment of most infertile men mostly involves techniques that use available sperm, rather than fruitless efforts to improve sperm concentration or motility.
- There is no evidence that repair of a varicocele improves pregnancy rates.
- Intra-uterine insemination may sometimes be used in cases of asthenospermia.
- In cases of non-obstructive azoospermia where viable sperm cannot be obtained surgically, donor sperm remains the only option for couples.

CLINICAL PEARL

At least 25–40% of infertility is attributable to abnormalities in male reproductive function. It is, therefore, important to evaluate the male partner as an integral part of the infertility work-up.

Unexplained infertility

Unexplained infertility is diagnosed when other causes have been excluded. It is a term applied to an infertile couple for whom standard investigations yield normal results.

- Without treatment, up to 60% of couples with unexplained infertility will conceive within 3 years.
- After 3 years of infertility, the pregnancy rate without treatment decreases by 2% every month of infertility.
- The most sensible option for ongoing unexplained infertility is assisted conception such as IVF (in-vitro fertilization).
- It is important to understand that women who use infertility therapies such as IVF appear to have a small but statistically significant increase in risk of pregnancy complications, such as pre-term birth and abnormal placentation.
- Compared with the general population, an increased risk of poor pregnancy outcomes has been observed among untreated subfertile women who conceive naturally.

CONTRACEPTION

About half of all pregnancies in the United States are unplanned and almost a half of these occur in women using contraception. About half of women aged 15–44 years have experienced an unwanted pregnancy.

Fertility control is an important contributor to reproductive health. It has been well documented that fertility regulation has significantly decreased maternal mortality.

An understanding of the available contraceptive methods allows clinicians to advise women about the methods that are most consistent with their routine and viewpoint, and therefore most likely to be successful.

The most popular contraceptive methods are given in Table 24-3 (overleaf).

Table 24-3 Methods of contraception

CONTRACEPTIVE METHOD	APPROXIMATE RATE OF USE
Oral contraception	31%
Female sterilization	27%
Condoms	18%
Injectables/implants/patch	9%
Male sterilization	9%
Other	8%

No method of contraception is perfect. The effectiveness of contraception is often quantified by the Pearl index, which is defined as the number of unintended pregnancies per 100 women per year of use (i.e. the number of pregnancies in 1200 observed months of use).

- The most effective contraceptive methods are intrauterine contraception, contraceptive implants, and sterilization.
- The next most effective methods are injectables, oral contraceptives, transdermal contraceptive systems, and the vaginal ring.
- The least effective contraception systems are diaphragms, cervical caps, condoms, spermicides, and withdrawal.
- Natural family planning, also known as the rhythm method, has a high failure rate of around 20–30% per year.

Steroidal contraception

Oral contraceptives

The development and widespread use of the oral contraceptive pill was a major breakthrough in reproductive health in the 20th century.

Benefits of oral contraception

Known benefits of oral contraception include:

- the very low likelihood of extrauterine pregnancies
- a reduction in pelvic inflammatory disease, ovarian cysts, and iron–deficiency anemia
- a decrease in the rate of ovarian and endometrial cancers.

Side-effects of oral contraception

Side-effects are a major source of patient non-adherence and discontinuation. Estrogen commonly produces breast tenderness and nausea; these symptoms usually decline after 3 months of use. Caution should be exercised when prescribing oral contraceptives to patients with certain underlying conditions.

Cerebrovascular disease

Oral contraceptives are contraindicated in the presence of cerebrovascular disease, as they increase the risk of stroke in women with other underlying risk factors.

Migraine and headache

Patients with a history of migraine and headache should use oral contraceptives circumspectly.

Most expert guidelines recommend against prescribing oral contraceptives to women who suffer focal migraines. This is partially because of an increased risk of ischemic stroke, but also because contraceptive use commonly increases headache severity and duration.

Epilepsy

Oral contraceptives have no impact on the pattern or frequency of fits; however, some anticonvulsants decrease serum concentrations of estrogen and thus increase the likelihood of intermenstrual bleeding and pregnancy. Women with epilepsy should use a high-dose oral contraceptive formulation.

Cardiovascular disease

Women who are older than 35 years, and who smoke, should not use oral contraceptives, as in this group there is an increased incidence of cardiovascular complications such as myocardial infarction.

Deep vein thrombosis

Care should be taken with the use of oral contraceptives in women who have deficiencies in protein C, protein S, or anti-thrombin 3. The newer oral contraceptives containing third-generation progestins and cyproterone carry an increased risk of thromboembolic disease.

Women with a body mass index of >29 kg/m^2 have an independent increased risk of venous thromboembolic disease, and in such women oral contraception should only be used if they are 35 years of age or younger.

Hypertension

Oral contraceptives have a potential to aggravate hypertension, hence blood pressure should be controlled prior to their commencement. If blood pressure is controlled and no vascular disease is present, the use of oral contraceptives is not contraindicated.

A history of pregnancy-induced hypertension is not a contraindication to the use of oral contraceptives, provided the blood pressure returns to normal after delivery.

Dyslipidemia

All oral contraceptives increase triglyceride levels to some extent. If a woman's triglycerides are ≥350 mg/dL (≥3.95 mmol/L), or in patients with familial hypertriglyceridemia, oral contraceptives should be avoided because they may precipitate pancreatitis or increase the risk of cardiovascular disease.

Angina

Oral contraceptives do not stimulate the atherosclerotic process, and may actually inhibit plaque formation. On the other hand, they are contraindicated in the presence of coronary artery disease. There is an increased incidence of cardiovascular disease secondary to atherosclerosis in past oral contraceptive users. Smoking, when combined with oral contraceptive use, markedly increases the risk of atherosclerosis.

Women with known angina and suspected atherosclerosis, but with no history of prior myocardial infarcts or additional risk factors, may safely use low-dose oral contraceptives.

Mitral valve prolapse

In general, oral contraceptives can be used in women with mitral valve prolapse who are symptom-free.

Diabetes mellitus

- Women with diabetes mellitus who do not have retinopathy, nephropathy or hypertension can use low-dose oral contraceptives.
- Women with a history of gestational diabetes during their last pregnancy can safely take low-dose oral contraceptives.

Sickle-cell disease

The risk of pregnancy in this condition is much greater than the risk posed by the use of oral contraceptives.

Cancer risk with oral contraception

Breast cancer

There is no association between oral contraceptive use and an increased relative risk of breast cancer. The risk of breast cancer in women who take oral contraceptives up until the age of 55 is no different to that of the rest of the population.

Oral contraceptive use in women with a history of breast cancer in a first-degree relative does not increase the risk of breast cancer.

Cervical cancer

There is no association between the use of oral contraceptives and the development of cervical cancer, except maybe for the potential higher exposure to human papillomavirus (HPV).

Endometrial cancer

It is well established that combined oral contraceptive use is protective against endometrial cancer.

Ovarian cancer

It is well established that oral contraceptive use for more than two years reduces the risk of ovarian cancer and this is an important strategy for women at increased heritable risk.

Estrogen dose

When choosing an oral contraceptive, the higher the dose of estrogen then the better the cycle control.

- In general, oral contraceptives with 25 microg of estrogen have an 11% incidence of intermenstrual bleeding, while 30–35 microg of estrogen reduces intermenstrual bleeding to 4%.

- The use of oral contraceptives containing 50 microg of estrogen should be reserved for women requiring additional estrogen to prevent intermenstrual bleeding, or women who have recurring functional ovarian cysts in order to significantly suppress ovarian function.

Breastfeeding

Breastfeeding women should avoid the use of combined oral contraceptive medications, as small amounts of steroids are excreted in the milk, and estrogen may suppress milk production.

Progestin-only contraception

Progestin-only contraception is useful for women who are breastfeeding, as progestins alone do not suppress lactation. They are also useful for women with other contraindications to the use of oral estrogens.

Interaction with other drugs

Certain antibiotics, particularly penicillins and tetracyclines, may diminish the effectiveness of oral contraceptives.

Discontinuation of an oral contraceptive

Fertility is restored quickly after cessation of oral contraceptives.

Long-acting reversible contraceptives (LARCs)

Injectable contraception is highly effective, reversible, and reduces the need for adherence. One injection is given every 12 weeks. Additionally, progestin injections reduce the risk of endometrial cancer and the volume of menstrual bleeding.

- There is no proven relationship between depot medroxyprogesterone acetate and weight gain.
- Women with sickle-cell anemia, congenital heart disease, or those older than 35 are excellent candidates for contraception with depot medroxyprogesterone acetate.
- Women with a history of long-term use of depot medroxyprogesterone acetate have a reduced bone density.
- Depot medroxyprogesterone acetate is not teratogenic, and is safe during lactation.

Intrauterine contraception

Intrauterine contraception is safe and effective.

- Currently, intrauterine contraceptives release either copper or a synthetic progestin.
- The progestin-releasing intrauterine contraceptives have additional advantages such as decrease in menstrual blood loss, relief of dysmenorrhea, and cure of endometriosis.
- Unlike previous models, modern intrauterine devices are not associated with a higher rate of expulsion or an increased risk of pelvic inflammatory disease.
- Intrauterine devices decrease the probability of pregnancy; however, if it occurs, the incidence of ectopic pregnancy increases. It is therefore important to determine the site of pregnancy, if it occurs.

Contraceptive vaginal ring

- Contraceptive vaginal rings are based on the principle that the vaginal epithelium can absorb steroids released from the silicone elastomer at a constant rate.

- The ring releases minimal amounts of estrogen into the circulation, yet maintains efficacy and cycle control comparable to that of oral contraceptives.

- The vaginal ring has an outside diameter of 54 mm, and is inserted by the woman and worn continuously for 3 weeks, after which time it is removed for 1 week to allow for withdrawal bleeding. After this week, a new device is inserted.

- A disadvantage of the ring is that some 18–30% of men report feeling the ring during intercourse and some women report an increase in leukorrhea. If this is a problem, the ring can be removed for intercourse but must be replaced within 3 hours. If the ring remains outside the vagina for longer than 3 hours, its effectiveness is compromised.

- Pregnancy rates are reported to be 1–2 per 100 women years of use.

Transdermal contraception

- Transdermal drug delivery provides continuous, sustained release of hormonal contraception over several days, thereby avoiding fluctuations in hormone levels and the need for daily patient action.

- The benefits, risks and contraindications of transdermal contraception are similar to those of combined oral contraceptives, except that the transdermal device is associated with more estrogen-related adverse events, including venous thromboembolism.

- Obese women should be counseled about reduced efficacy but obesity is not a contraindication.

Barrier methods

Barrier methods of contraception such as a diaphragm, cervical cap, male condom and female condom have a much higher pregnancy rate than hormonal methods. They are not recommended for women with serious medical conditions in whom pregnancy is life-threatening. Such women should be advised about the availability of emergency contraception.

Emergency contraception

Emergency contraception is also known as post-coital contraception. Women who have had unprotected intercourse, including those who have had a failure of another method, are potential candidates for this intervention. It has the potential to reduce abortion rates.

- This method of contraception is indicated after unprotected intercourse and for couples who experience, and recognize, a failure of a barrier method.

- Two methods of post-coital contraception are commonly used. The first is the SPRM ulipristal acetate; the other is high-dose progestin.

- Emergency contraception utilizing progestin-only pills is available without a prescription in many countries. The mechanism of emergency contraception is uncertain, and may vary depending upon the day of the menstrual cycle and the drug administered. It is likely to inhibit or delay ovulation, interfere with fertilization or tubal transport, prevent implantation by altering endometrial receptivity, and may cause regression of the corpus luteum.

CLINICAL PEARL

A routine follow-up visit with a pregnancy test is essential after emergency contraception to ensure that, if bleeding has not occurred, an intrauterine or ectopic pregnancy is not present.

MENOPAUSAL SYMPTOMS

Menopausal hormone therapy (MHT) continues to play a role in the management of menopausal symptoms such as hot flushes, vaginal atrophy and mood changes.

- While it is no longer recommended that hormone therapy in women over the age of 60 be used for primary prevention of cardiovascular and other chronic diseases, the use of hormone therapy to treat menopausal symptoms is safe and appropriate. This should, however, be re-evaluated after 5 years of use because of the increased risks of complications after this period.

- There is evidence for a benefit of unopposed estrogen use in women who have undergone hysterectomy, in that the incidence of breast cancer in this group is reduced.

Hormone therapy results in a definite reduction of recurrent urinary tract infection, and improves quality of life and balance, but with an increased risk of stroke, venous thromboembolism, and cholecystitis. Therefore, post-menopausal hormone therapy is currently only recommended for the short-term management of moderate to severe vasomotor symptoms.

- If there is no history of breast cancer, coronary heart disease, or a previous thromboembolic event, estrogen therapy is appropriate. Active liver disease and migraine headaches are also contraindications.

- If a patient has not had a hysterectomy then a progestin should be added, as endometrial hyperplasia and endometrial cancer can develop after as little as 6 months of unopposed estrogen therapy.

The best preparation to use is a combined preparation of conjugated estrogen and a synthetic progestin. The drugs can be delivered either orally or transdermally, as they are equally effective for the treatment of vasomotor symptoms.

The treatment should involve the lowest possible dose of estrogen and progestin that controls the symptoms.

Apart from vasomotor symptoms, menoposal hormonal treatment may be used to treat symptoms relating to vaginal atrophy.

- Vaginal atrophy results in vaginal dryness, itching, and dyspareunia.
- It can be treated with systemic hormone replacement therapy, but intravaginal estrogen in a cream, tablet or ring form is the most effective therapy and can be administered indefinitely, as systemic absorption is negligible.

PREMENSTRUAL SYNDROME

Premenstrual syndrome is characterized by symptoms that occur monthly in the second half of the menstrual cycle. Although most women experience mild emotional and physical symptoms just prior to the onset of menstrual periods, the term 'premenstrual syndrome' is restricted to when these symptoms occur for at least 5 days before the onset of menstrual period, and are associated with economic or social dysfunction. These symptoms may include:

- symptoms such as depression, anger, irritability, anxiety, breast pain, bloating, and headaches
- an impairment in quality of life, a decrease in productivity, and increased absenteeism.

There are no physical signs associated with premenstrual syndrome. Diagnosis is made when there is at least one symptom, either psychological or behavioral, that impairs functioning in some way.

If untreated, premenstrual symptoms can last throughout reproductive life and only disappear with the menopause.

- Treatment with selective serotonin reuptake inhibitors such as fluoxetine has been demonstrated to be better than placebo. These agents are usually administered during the luteal phase, and discontinued after the onset of the menstrual period.
- There is no evidence that other antidepressants and lithium have any benefit in the treatment of premenstrual syndrome.
- Benzodiazepines such as alprazolam are effective, but side-effects limit their use.
- GnRH agonists and danazol (an androgen) suppress ovulation and therefore control symptoms, but side-effects preclude their use on a prolonged basis.
- Hormonal oral contraceptives can also be effective.

ABNORMAL UTERINE BLEEDING

CLINICAL PEARL

Abnormal uterine bleeding is responsible for as many as one-third of all outpatient gynecological visits. The majority of cases occur just after the menarche or in the perimenopausal period.

Most cases of abnormal uterine bleeding are related to pregnancy, structural uterine pathology, anovulation or, rarely, disorders of hemostasis or neoplasia.

- Symptoms of ovulation should be noted, as well as the age of onset of abnormal bleeding. As an example, persistent menorrhagia since the menarche suggests a bleeding disorder, while abnormal uterine bleeding due to anovulation is more common around the menarche and the perimenopause.
- Any precipitating factor such as trauma should be sought, as well as a family history of bleeding or systemic disorders. The possibility of pregnancy should be considered.
- Changes in bodyweight should be elicited, as eating disorders, excessive exercise, illness or stress may interfere with ovulation.

The amount of bleeding is difficult to evaluate, as a patient's self-reports are often inaccurate indicators of the quantity of blood loss:

- around 25% of women with normal periods consider their blood loss excessive
- around 40% of women with excessive bleeding consider their periods as light or moderate
- about 33% of women who consider that their periods are heavy have blood loss which is truly excessive.

Diagnosis

Physical examination should involve a general examination to detect systemic illness, and then a gynecological examination which should determine any obvious bleeding sites on the vulva, vagina, cervix, urethra or anus.

- Suspicious findings such as a mass, ulceration, laceration or foreign body should be noted, and the size, contour and tenderness of the uterus as well as the possibility of an adnexal mass should be determined.
- All women of reproductive age should have a pregnancy test to exclude either an intrauterine or an ectopic pregnancy.
- Cervical cytology should be obtained to exclude cervical cancer, and any visible cervical lesion should be biopsied.
- After pregnancy is excluded, an endometrial sample should be obtained to exclude endometrial cancer or hyperplasia.
- Both transabdominal and transvaginal ultrasound examinations should be performed to demonstrate any subserosal or intramyometrial uterine pathology such as fibroids, adenomyosis or neoplastic change. An ultrasound examination can also detect an ovarian neoplasm.
- Hysteroscopy provides excellent visualization of the endometrial cavity. It also allows targeted biopsy or excision of pathologies such as polyps.
- Other investigations such as thyroid function tests, coagulation profile, full blood count, serum prolactin, and androgen levels may be indicated. The initial approach to the management involves treatment of underlying conditions such as fibroids, polyps or arteriovenous malformations, often with surgery.

Management

- Estrogen–progestin contraceptives are usually the first line of medical therapy in most women. In addition to reducing blood flow, they regulate cycles, provide contraception, prevent the development of hyperplasia in anovulatory patients and treat dysmenorrhea.

- The second line of therapy is the insertion of a levonorgestrel intrauterine device, which releases a high local concentration of progestin which thins out the endometrium. This treatment is more effective than hormonal oral contraception, and is as effective as systemic progestogens. It is superior to non-hormonal medical therapy.

- Non-steroidal anti-inflammatory drugs (NSAIDs) reduce the volume of menstrual blood loss by 20–50%, via reduction of the rate of prostaglandin synthesis in the endometrium, leading to vasoconstriction and reduced bleeding.

- Antifibrinolytic agents such as tranexamic acid reduce menstrual flow by 30-50% of baseline. The risk of thrombosis with these drugs is controversial, so they should be used when other therapies have failed in women who do not have an increased thrombotic risk.

If medical treatment fails, invasive treatments such as uterine artery embolization (UAE), endometrial ablation, and hysterectomy should be considered.

DYSMENORRHEA

Dysmenorrhea is a common problem experienced by women of reproductive age. When severe, it interferes with the performance of daily activities, often leading to absenteeism from school, work or other responsibilities.

- *Primary dysmenorrhea*, defined as abdominal pain during menses without any identifiable pathology, is mainly a clinical diagnosis.
  - » It is likely to be due to the release of prostaglandins from the endometrium during menstrual periods.
  - » Symptoms usually begin during adolescence, after ovulatory cycles become established.
- *Secondary dysmenorrhea* is due to pathological processes such as endometriosis, adenomyosis, ovarian cysts, intrauterine or pelvic adhesions, chronic pelvic inflammatory disease, cervical stenosis, or pelvic congestion syndrome.
  - » Inflammatory bowel disease, irritable bowel syndrome, and various psychogenic disorders can also generate secondary dysmenorrhea.

The goal of treatment of dysmenorrhea is to provide adequate relief of pain.

- In primary dysmenorrhea, the treatment is empirical. NSAIDs are the most effective agents.
- In secondary dysmenorrhea, the associated pathological entities will need to be specifically treated.
- Hormonal contraception to suppress ovulation is also effective.

> **CLINICAL PEARL**
>
> The prevalence of dysmenorrhea is very high; between 50% and 90% of women describe some degree of dysmenorrhea. The majority of these women are young, and have primary dysmenorrhea. The prevalence of primary dysmenorrhea decreases with age.

VULVAR CONDITIONS

> **CLINICAL PEARL**
>
> Benign conditions of the vulva and vagina are common. About one-fifth of women have significant vulval symptoms lasting for >3 months at some time in their lives.

Symptoms of vulvar conditions are common, often chronic, and can cause significant sexual dysfunction.

- Itch is a common symptom. If itching is worse before or during menstrual periods, then recurrent vulval candidiasis is likely.

- Various dermatoses can also be intermittent, with flare-ups associated with precipitant factors.

The history is sometimes difficult to elicit because of anxiety and frustration about ineffective treatment. A thorough examination with good illumination is vital. The diagnosis is often clued by information from the history, physical examination and the results of investigations.

- A vaginal or vulval swab for culture and sensitivity should be taken in all patients.

- If fissures or ulcers are present, testing for herpes simplex virus (HSV) should be performed.

- Biopsy is required for any abnormal findings that persist without a clear diagnosis, and is mandatory to rule out malignancy.

Management

- It is important to advise the woman that vulval conditions respond slowly to treatment, usually over weeks to months, and that the aim of treatment is to control symptoms rather than to cure the condition.

- Sometimes a multidisciplinary approach is required, such as a physiotherapist with experience in biofeedback, and sexual counselors, especially in the case of vulvodynia.

- Good vulval skin care should be part of the treatment of all conditions. This involves the avoidance of irritants, including soap, and moisturizing the skin with creams such as sorbolene or aqueous cream. If there is incontinence or a vaginal discharge, a barrier cream should be used. Scratching can be reduced by applying cold compresses.

Conditions with abnormalities on examination

Dermatitis

Dermatitis is common, and is present in about half of women who present with chronic vulval symptoms. It is even more common in individuals with vulval atrophy, in whom the skin is less able to tolerate environmental insults.

- Clinical signs may be subtle and are associated with erythema, scale, fissures, lichenification, and excoriation.
- Itch is a common presenting symptom, although burning can occur if the mucosa is involved.
- Contact allergens such as deodorant soaps, bubble-bath products, or perfumed feminine hygiene products can be irritating, and can intensify symptoms, and are therefore best to be avoided.
- If urinary incontinence is present it should be addressed, as urine is a major vulval irritant.

Initial treatment involves identification and elimination of the irritating agent, the use of cotton underwear washed in a bland detergent, the taking of sitz baths using plain tepid water twice a day, and applying a thin, plain petrolatum film or zinc oxide 10–20% ointment after bowel movements.

- Tricyclic antidepressants such as doxepin may be considered for treatment of pruritus.
- Topical corticosteroids may be used for 2–3 weeks to reduce inflammation and to promote healing.
- Methylprednisolone aceponate is useful until symptoms have resolved, after which, a weaker corticosteroid such as 1% hydrocortisone can be continued for a further 3 months. The cycle can be repeated if disease activity flares.

Recurrent vulvo-vaginal candidiasis

- Vulvo-vaginal candidiasis is considered to be recurrent if at least four discreet documented episodes occur in 12 months. The pathophysiology of recurrent infections is unclear.
- Recurrent vulvo-vaginal candidiasis presents primarily with itch; but burning, especially after intercourse, is also common. It is common for symptoms to worsen before menstrual periods.
- Examination usually reveals erythema of the vulva, with some swelling and occasional longitudinal fissures (Figure 24-1); a discharge is a common association.
- Some 50% of women have negative microscopy on swabbing.

Most cases are caused by *Candida albicans*, but *C. glabrata*, *C. tropicalis* and *C. parapsilosis* can also occur and may be difficult to treat.

- 90% of uncomplicated cases respond to topical antifungals.
- Resistant cases may respond to oral fluconazole or ketoconazole.
- If there is significant dermatitis, the addition of 1% hydrocortisone cream may be useful.

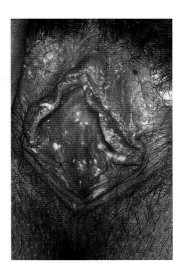

Figure 24-1 The most common presentation for acute vaginal candidiasis is a red inflamed vulva and vagina, and a white, thick discharge

From Habif TP. Clinical dermatology, 5th ed. St Louis: Elsevier, 2009.

- Women who have *C. glabrata* are usually not sensitive to standard antifungal treatment, and respond to intravaginal boric acid.
- There is no clinical evidence that dietary modification for the elimination of *Candida* spp. from the gastrointestinal tract, or the treatment of asymptomatic male sexual partners, is useful.
- Low-dose oral contraceptives can be used to prevent recurrence.

CLINICAL PEARLS

- Vaginitis due to bacterial vaginitis from *Gardnerella vaginalis* has a fishy odor when mixed with potassium hydroxide, and clue cells are present (epithelial cells with bacteria adhering).
- *Trichomonas vaginalis* causes a frothy, fishy-smelling discharge that is yellow-green, and a strawberry-colored cervix.

Lichen sclerosis

Lichen sclerosis is a common vulval disorder. The mean age of onset is 50 years, although it rarely occurs in children and pre-pubertal girls. The etiology is unknown.

- Lichen sclerosis presents most commonly with an itch; burning and dyspareunia can also occur.
- There is an association with autoimmune disease in 20% of patients.
- Lichen sclerosis is characterized by thinning and whitening of the perianal and perivaginal skin, with an accompanying loss of mucocutaneous markings and skin elasticity. There is atrophy of the involved tissues and a loss of vulval architecture (Figure 24-2).

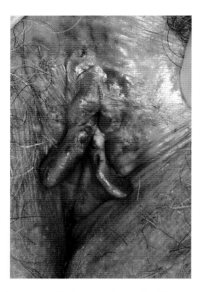

Figure 24-2 Vulvar lichen sclerosis. The crease areas are atrophic and wrinkled, the labia is hyperpigmented, and the introitus is contracted and ulcerated

From Habif TP. Clinical dermatology, 5th ed. St Louis: Elsevier, 2009.

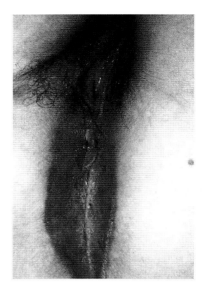

Figure 24-3 Psoriasis of perineum and vulva. Flexural psoriasis often lacks the typical parakeratotic scale of psoriasis on other body sites. Painful erosion of the natal cleft is common

From Robboy SJ, Anderson MC and Russell P (eds). Pathology of the female reproductive tract. Edinburgh: Elsevier, 2002.

» There may be associated purpura, hyperpigmentation, erosion, fissures and edema.
- Routine vulvar biopsy for diagnosis is debated. Biopsy only after failure of empirical treatment is acceptable.

Treatment should aim to control symptoms, minimize scarring, and detect malignant change early.

- Potent topical corticosteroids are effective in more than 90% of women, providing a rapid symptomatic relief.
- Betamethasone dipropionate ointment 0.05% should be used initially twice daily for a month, then daily for 2 months, and gradually tapered to use as needed.

Annual follow-up is recommended, as the lifetime risk of squamous cell carcinoma within the affected area is about 4%. Annual biopsy of the vulva is prudent.

Psoriasis

Psoriasis of the vulva occurs in about 5% of women who present with chronic vulval symptoms. It can be easily mistaken for atopic dermatitis. One-third of patients with psoriasis have a family history of the disease.

- Clinically, psoriasis on the vulva lacks the typical silver scale, and usually appears as red or reddish yellow pustules on the intertriginous areas (Figure 24-3).
- Genital psoriasis often appears in the mons and the labia.

Treatment usually requires mid- to high-potency topical steroids, injectable corticosteroids, as well as weak-potency preparations such as 3% liquor picis carbonis (coal tar) in aqueous cream twice daily. This helps to provide a break from prolonged corticosteroid use.

Vulvar intraepithelial neoplasia

Vulvar dysplasia, or vulvar intraepithelial neoplasia (VIN), is reported as VIN I, II or III. VIN III is synonymous with carcinoma-in-situ.

- The incidence of VIN has increased significantly in women who are young, and those who smoke. This increased incidence reflects the higher prevalence of the human papillomavirus in women.
- The most common symptom of VIN is localized itching and burning, although some 60% of cases are asymptomatic.
- VIN is usually multifocal and looks like raised or keratinized skin, or a macule usually on mucosal areas.
- VIN III can progress to vulvar cancer.
- A biopsy is necessary for any raised hyperpigmented lesion.

The treatment for VIN is wide local excision, or laser treatment where invasive malignancy has been ruled out.

Erosive vulvovaginitis

Chronic painful erosions and ulcers with superficial bleeding can be seen in the vulvar vestibule. Causes include:
- Crohn's disease
- Behçet's syndrome
- neurofibromatosis
- cicatricial pemphigoid
- pemphigus vulgaris
- vulvar pyoderma gangrenosum
- desquamative inflammatory vaginitis.

As vulvar and vaginal adhesions can occur in these conditions if they are not properly managed, specialist referral is recommended.

Atrophic vaginitis

Estrogen deficiency causes the vaginal epithelium to become thin, pale and dry. Symptoms include dyspareunia, minor vaginal bleeding, and pain from splitting caused by friction. Topical vaginal estrogen creams are useful.

Vulvar vestibular syndrome (vulvodynia)

Apart from dyspareunia, these patients usually have focal erythema and localized vulvar dysesthesia. Many women have associated urinary symptoms such as frequency and bladder irritability.

- This condition may be associated with the presence of interstitial cystitis.
- Diagnosis is usually made by the 'touch test'. A cotton-tip swab is used to firmly touch the labia majora, the sulci and the lateral labia minora. This is followed by firmly touching the ostia of the Skene's glands, and the major and minor vestibular glands. Women with vulvodynia classically have a heightened sensitivity associated with the touch of the gland openings.

Management is difficult and very often prolonged, and involves both behavioral and medical interventions that are common in many pain syndromes.

Dysesthetic vulvodynia

Dysesthetic vulvodynia, also known as generalized vulvodynia, occurs mainly in older patients.

- The etiology is unclear. Neuropathic pain, pudendal neuralgia, chronic reflex pain syndrome, pelvic floor abnormalities, and referred visceral pain have been suggested as causes.
- The predominant symptom is chronic, localized burning or pain in the vulva, with no abnormalities on examination but hypersensitivity and altered perception to light touch.
- Patients with this condition often have psychosexual dysfunction.
- Treatment with low-dose tricyclic antidepressants can be helpful.

SEXUALLY TRANSMITTED INFECTIONS (STIs)

CLINICAL PEARLS

- The sexually transmitted infections that present with vulvar ulceration are lymphogranuloma venereum, chancroid, herpes simplex, primary syphilis, and granuloma inguinale.
- The sexually transmitted infections that present with cervicitis are chlamydia, gonorrhea, and pelvic inflammatory disease.

- Sexually transmitted infections are more common in:
  - » the young
  - » the unmarried
  - » women who have recently had a new sexual partner
  - » those with multiple sexual partners
  - » women with a previous sexually transmitted infection
  - » recreational drug users
  - » women who have contact with sex workers
  - » women who meet partners on the internet.
- All patients who seek screening for STIs should receive testing and counseling for human immunodeficiency virus (HIV) and hepatitis B and C infection.
- The optimal interval for screening is uncertain, but rescreening at three months after a diagnosed infection is recommended.
- Other sexually transmitted diseases and infections include condylomata acuminata (genital warts), molluscum contagiosum, and pediculosis pubis.
- Complications of sexually transmitted infections include upper genital tract infections, infertility, cervical and vulvar cancer, and enhanced transmission of HIV.

Chlamydia

Chlamydia trachomatis is a small Gram-negative intracellular bacterium, and is the most common bacterial agent of sexually transmitted infections.

- A large percentage of women are carriers of *C. trachomatis* and are asymptomatic, thereby providing an ongoing reservoir. Rates of chlamydial infection are highest in adolescent women.
- The incubation period of symptomatic disease ranges from 7 to 14 days.
- Symptoms of chlamydial infection include cervicitis, discharge and urethritis.
  - » Cervicitis causes a vaginal discharge, and intermenstrual and post-coital bleeding.
  - » Cervical discharge is frequently mucopurulent.
  - » Urethritis commonly accompanies cervicitis, with concomitant symptoms such as urinary frequency and dysuria.
- Infants born to mothers who have an infected birth canal may develop conjunctivitis and pneumonia.

Chlamydia cannot be cultured on artificial media; traditionally, tissue culture has been required to establish a diagnosis. Although tissue culture is the 'gold standard' in identifying chlamydial infection, rapid diagnostic testing using nucleic acid amplification technology is now readily available, and reasonably accurate.

- The natural history of chlamydial infection is not clearly established. Rates of spontaneous resolution, persistence and progression are difficult to establish.
- Occasionally patients with chlamydial infection develop peri-hepatitis and inflammation of the liver capsule and adjacent peritoneal surfaces, known as Fitz-Hugh–Curtis syndrome.
- Approximately 30% of women with chlamydial infection develop upper genital tract involvement such as

pelvic inflammatory disease and, if left untreated, this results in infertility.

Treatment

Chlamydia trachomatis is highly susceptible to tetracyclines and macrolides. The first-line agents are doxycycline and azithromycin.

- The recommended regimen is 100 mg of doxycycline orally twice daily for 7 days, or azithromycin 1 g orally in a single dose.
- Alternative regimens include erythromycin, ofloxacin, or levofloxacin.

Except in pregnant women, it is not recommended that patients have a test-of-cure 3 weeks after completing treatment if the recommended or alternative regimens were used.

Gonorrhea

Gonorrhea is the second most commonly reported communicable disease in the United States, accounting for more than 300,000 cases annually. It is estimated that an equal number of cases are unreported.

- Although men are often symptomatic, and usually present early for therapy, symptoms in women may not be apparent until complications such as pelvic inflammatory disease develop.
- In women, the most common complaints are a vaginal discharge, dysuria and/or abnormal vaginal bleeding. Infection of Skene's glands, Bartholin's glands, the anus and the pharynx are common.
- Disseminated gonococcal infection occurs in 1–2% of women.
- Untreated gonorrhea is a common cause of infertility, chronic pelvic pain and an increased incidence of ectopic pregnancy.

Diagnosis of gonorrhea is made by either culture or nucleic acid amplification tests. Rapid diagnostic tests are highly sensitive, detecting up to 98% of infections. However, nucleic acid amplification tests of swabs taken from the rectum and pharynx yield poor results.

- Culture for *Neisseria gonorrhoeae* is processed on Thayer-Martin agar, which prevents the overgrowth of other endogenous flora.
- Swabs should be obtained from the urethra, cervix, rectum and pharynx for culture. Culture with sensitivity testing is particularly important for detection of resistant organisms.

Treatment needs to have an efficacy rate of greater than 95%, as treatment failure has significant public health implications.

- Approximately 20 drugs within the cephalosporin, quinolone, macrolide and tetracycline classes of antibiotics demonstrate high rates of gonococcal eradication with single-dose therapy. Single-dose therapy decreases the reliance on patient adherence.
- The preferred therapeutic agents are cefixime 400 mg orally in a single dose, ceftriaxone 250 mg intramuscularly in a single dose, ciprofloxacin 500 mg orally in a single dose, ofloxacin 400 mg orally in a single dose, or levofloxacin 250 mg orally in a single dose.
- Treatment should also include antibiotics for chlamydial infection, as coexistence of *C. trachomatis* is common.

PELVIC INFLAMMATORY DISEASE (PID)

Pelvic inflammatory disease is defined as sexually transmitted pelvic infection, between the menarche and the menopause. It does not include vulvar or vaginal infections. It is often used synonymously with salpingitis, but in fact is the infection of the uterus, uterine tubes, adjacent parametrium and overlying pelvic peritoneum.

- The list of causative organisms is long, but includes *C. trachomatis*, Gram-negative bacilli, *Haemophilus influenzae*, group B and D streptococci, *Mycoplasma hominis*, and various anaerobic organisms including anaerobic Gram-positive cocci and bacteroides species. Polymicrobial infection is common.
- It is possible that viruses including coxsackievirus B5, echovirus 6, and HSV may cause PID, but their role is not clearly established. Mycobacteria have also been implicated.
- Pelvic infection is found more frequently in some sectors of the community than others. It is most common between 15 and 19 years of age.
- Approximately 25% of women with PID will experience long-term complications such as infertility, chronic pelvic pain, dyspareunia, and an increased incidence of ectopic pregnancy.
- PID is never seen in prepubertal females, and very rarely seen after the menopause.

Clinical features

The most important presenting feature is abdominal pain. The pain is continuous and bilateral, involving both lower abdominal quadrants.

- While pain is usually present in patients with PID, not all patients with lower abdominal pain will have an infection.
- Pain is increased with movement and coitus.
- The pain is also present during menstruation and micturition.
- Some 35% of patients also have irregular bleeding, but this feature is not helpful when considering a differential diagnosis.
- Many patients have increased vaginal discharge.
- Those with severe infection have nausea, vomiting, malaise, and fever.

Examination may reveal pyrexia, tachycardia, abdominal tenderness and, during pelvic examination, pain on moving the cervix. An adnexal mass may be palpable.

- An increasing number of women with PID will not have classic features. It is estimated that cases of silent

PID now outnumber clinically apparent cases by a ratio of 3:1.

- Abdominal ultrasound is useful to differentiate an ectopic pregnancy or complications of early pregnancy from PID.
- Laparoscopy is the 'gold standard' for diagnosis.

CLINICAL PEARL

A pregnancy test is essential to exclude ectopic pregnancy in women with abdominal pain in the reproductive age range, even if pelvic inflammatory disease is the suspected cause.

To establish the diagnosis of PID, all three of the following clinical features must be met:

1 abdominal tenderness (and/or rebound)
2 tenderness with movement of the cervix and uterus
3 adnexal tenderness

and one or more of the following:

1 Gram stain of the endocervix positive for Gram-negative intracellular diplococci
2 temperature greater than 38°C
3 leukocytosis greater than 10,000/mm³
4 purulent material (white cells present) from the peritoneal cavity by laparoscopy or laparotomy
5 pelvic abscess of inflammatory complex on bimanual examination *or* observed by pelvic ultrasound.

Treatment

The aim of treatment is to prevent infertility, ectopic pregnancy, and other long-term sequelae. If the patient is extremely ill, hospitalization will be necessary.

- Treatment regimens include levofloxacin 500 mg orally once daily for 14 days, with metronidazole 500 mg twice a day for 14 days to enhance anaerobic coverage.
- If the patient is an inpatient, then intravenous cefotetan 2 g 12-hourly, and doxycycline 100 mg orally or intravenously every 12 hours, with intravenous metronidazole 500 mg every 8 hours should be administered.

SEXUAL PROBLEMS

Sexual problems are common. Approximately 40% of women have sexual concerns, and some 12% have distressing sexual problems.

- Although it is thought that the frequency of sexual activity declines with age, population-based studies indicate that sexual activity continues in women aged between 66 and 71 years, and in a third of women over the age of 78. With the advent of treatment of male sexual dysfunction, the likelihood that women will continue sexual activity well into their 80s will be a feature of modern life.

An understanding of normal sexual response is necessary for the evaluation and treatment of sexual problems, along with an open and non-judgmental approach. The sexual response is complex, involving social, psychological, neurological, vascular and hormonal processes, and includes complex interactions of sexual stimulation with the central nervous system, the peripheral neurovascular system, and hormonal influences that are not completely understood.

The female sexual response is divided into four phases:

1 *Desire*—the desire to have sexual activity, including sexual thoughts, images and wishes.
2 *Arousal*—which includes physiological changes such as genital vascular congestion, and systemic changes such as tachycardia, elevation in blood pressure, and increased respiratory rate.
3 *Orgasm*—which is a peaking of sexual pleasure and a release of sexual tension with rhythmic contractions of the perineal muscles and reproductive organs.
4 *Resolution*—which involves both emotional and physical satisfaction.

Within this framework, for many women there is a difference in sequence.

Most women report inability to achieve orgasm with vaginal intercourse, and require direct stimulation of the clitoris. About 20% have coital climaxes, and 80% climax before or after vaginal intercourse when stimulated. Only 30% of women almost always, or always, achieve orgasm with sexual activity, in contrast to 75% of men.

Female sexual dysfunction can be classified into four areas:

1 *Sexual arousal disorder*—the persistent inability to reach sexual excitement.
2 *Orgasmic disorder difficulty*—inability to reach orgasm after sexual stimulation and arousal.
3 *Sexual desire disorder*—the lack of desire for sexual activity and/or the absence of sexual thought and fantasy, as well as a fear of and avoidance of sexual thought and situations.
4 *Sexual pain disorder*, including dyspareunia, vaginismus, or genital pain that occurs with any type of sexual stimulation.

Female sexual dysfunction is multifactorial, often with several different etiologies contributing to the problem.

- Patients should be evaluated for associated physical or psychological issues.
- The medical history is important, as certain illnesses or medications affect sexual function. For instance, spinal cord injuries, thyroid disease, diabetic neuropathy, surgical or medical castration with accompanying decreased estrogen and testosterone levels, and depression may interfere with sexual function.
- Antidepressants, antipsychotics and sedatives alter the blood flow to the genitals, decreasing arousal and/or lubrication.
- Recreational drugs and alcohol are often associated with sexual dysfunction.
- Excessive smoking may lead to vascular insufficiency and decreased genital blood flow.

- A previous vaginal delivery or vaginal surgery may result in interference with nerve supply, and dyspareunia.
- Vaginal blood flow and vaginal secretions are estrogen-dependent. Low estrogen levels are associated with significant decreases in clitoral, vaginal, and urethral blood flow, and thinning of the mucosa in the genital region. Any medical condition or medication that interferes with estrogen levels can contribute to sexual dysfunction.
- Women with urinary incontinence, fecal incontinence, or uterovaginal prolapse often have difficulty with sexual function.

When assessing women with sexual dysfunction, routine laboratory testing is not recommended unless an endocrinopathy is suspected.

Treatment

The treatment of sexual dysfunction is complex and time-intensive, and requires special expertise.

- A team approach with the use of psychotherapists, sex therapists and physiotherapists is sometimes needed to address specific aspects of treatment.
- If associated medical conditions are found, these should be treated before or during sexual dysfunction therapy. For instance, a woman with depression may require an antidepressant.
- Relationship problems often exacerbate or underlie sexual dysfunction in women. Couples counseling may be effective when there is relationship conflict or poor communication.

Hormone therapy

- Estrogen improves vaginal and clitoral blood flow, increasing lubrication. Dyspareunia caused by atrophy is treated best by vaginal estrogens. The ability of systemic estrogens to enhance sexual function has not been established.
- Testosterone has been linked to increased libido, although the data on testosterone use for the treatment of female sexual function is poor, partly because of the side-effect profile.
- Dehydroepiandrosterone (DHEA) has been shown to improve sexual interest and satisfaction in some women.

It is important to counsel patients that androgen therapy can result in androgenic, metabolic and adverse endocrine effects, and therefore should be used with caution in women who are at risk of cardiovascular disease, hepatic disease, endometrial hyperplasia or cancer, or breast cancer. Additionally, women should be warned of the possibility of significant hirsutism, acne, voice deepening and clitoromegaly.

Pelvic-floor disorders

Pelvic-floor disorders such as urinary and fecal incontinence and pelvic organ prolapse are common, and have a negative impact on the sexual function of women. Multiple studies have shown that surgical treatment of the underlying disorder, such as repair of prolapse and treatment of urinary or fecal incontinence, improves sexual function.

Hysterectomy

- There is no evidence that hysterectomy alters sexual function. Multiple studies have demonstrated a positive effect from total and subtotal abdominal and vaginal hysterectomy on sexual function.
- Preservation of the cervix during hysterectomy has no benefit on sexual function.

Pregnancy and childbirth

- Sexual dysfunction is very common after childbirth; up to 86% of women report sexual problems in the first 3 months after vaginal delivery.
- Most women resume normal sexual function 6 months after childbirth.
- Continued breastfeeding, and severe genital tract trauma sustained during childbirth, may lead to prolonged sexual problems.

SELF-ASSESSMENT QUESTIONS

1 A 55-year-old woman is having hot flushes and is requesting hormone replacement therapy. She has a history of a previous deep vein thrombosis in her right calf. Which of the following statements is *true* for managing this patient?

   A This patient could use unopposed estrogen therapy for 5 years.
   B The best preparation to use is a combined preparation of conjugated estrogen and synthetic progestin.
   C Hormone therapy is recommended for the prevention of cardiovascular disease.
   D With a history of previous thromboembolic disease, hormone replacement is inappropriate.

2 A 70-year-old woman, a smoker with a previous history of cervical cancer, presents with vulval itching, burning and irritation. On examination of her vulva there is a raised hyperpigmented lesion visible on the labium majus. Which of the following statements is *true* for this woman?

   A A vulval biopsy should be performed to determine the exact pathology.
   B She should be treated with topical antifungal agents.
   C She should be treated with topical corticosteroids.
   D She should be encouraged to use oatmeal baths.

3 A 60-year-old obese woman who has hypertension and type 2 diabetes mellitus develops vaginal bleeding for the first time since the menopause 9 years previously. Which of the following statements is *true* for the management of this woman?

   A The most likely explanation for this woman's symptoms is the presence of an arteriovenous malformation in the uterine wall.
   B She probably has fibroids.
   C She has engaged in energetic sexual intercourse.
   D She needs to be evaluated with a pelvic examination and transvaginal ultrasound, and needs referral for endometrial sampling.

4 Which *four* of the following options are the investigations that are valuable in most couples with infertility?

   A Semen analysis
   B Measurement of testicular volume
   C Day 3 serum FSH (follicle-stimulating hormone)
   D Papanicolaou smear
   E Serum prolactin estimation
   F Magnetic resonance imaging of the brain
   G Thyroid function tests

5 Which *four* of the following can influence the measurement of serum prolactin level in the evaluation of infertility?

   A Sexual intercourse an hour before the measurement
   B Hyperthyroidism
   C Adenoma of the pituitary gland
   D Psychological stress
   E Breast examination
   F Pelvic examination

6 Which *two* from the following list are the most common causes of infertility?

   A Male factors
   B Tubal pathology
   C Fibroids
   D Endometrial polyps
   E Unexplained

7 Which *four* of the following options may be side-effects of hormonal oral contraceptive agents?

   A Cardiovascular disease
   B Migraine headaches
   C Epilepsy
   D Deep vein thrombosis
   E Worsening hypertension
   F Angina
   G Mitral valve disease
   H Diabetes mellitus
   I Stroke

8 Which of the following explains the mechanism of action of emergency contraception?

   A Inhibits or delays ovulation
   B Interferes with fertilization
   C Interferes with tubal transport
   D Prevents implantation
   E Causes regression of the corpus luteum
   F All of the above.

ANSWERS

1 D.

If there is a history of a previous thromboembolic event, the use of estrogen therapy is inappropriate. Unopposed estrogen therapy in a woman who still has a uterus is dangerous as it can predispose to endometrial cancer. There is no evidence that hormone replacement prevents any disease process except osteoporosis.

2 A.

Any woman with a history of previous papillomavirus infection, as evidenced by the diagnosis of cervical cancer, is at risk of developing vulvar intraepithelial neoplasia, and when this is associated with a raised hyperpigmented lesion the risk of malignancy is significant.

3 D.

In a postmenopausal woman, especially with diabetes, obesity and hypertension, the risk of endometrial cancer is high and needs to be excluded.

4 A, C, E, G.

5 C, D, E, F.

6 B, E.

7 B, D, E, I.

8 F.

While the mechanism is not fully known, all or any are possibly correct.

CHAPTER 25

OBSTETRIC MEDICINE

Annemarie Hennessy and Angela Makris

CHAPTER OUTLINE

GENERAL PRINCIPLES OF MEDICAL OBSTETRIC CARE

Pregnancy is commonly associated with several major medical problems. The most common of these are diabetes and high blood pressure, but respiratory disease, viral infections, thyroid disease and gastrointestinal disturbance are also not uncommon.

There are fundamental principles for considering any acute medical illness in pregnancy; these are outlined in Table 25-1.

The safety of medication treatment is defined by a classification system based on evidence of risk in pregnancy. This is applied to all medications and should be discussed in detail with any patient requiring medical management of their disease in pregnancy. There is some variation in classification systems throughout the world, but the following categories are widely used.

- A—safe in pregnancy, and have been used by a large number of pregnant women without harmful effect.
- B—animal reproduction studies have failed to demonstrate a risk to the fetus, and there are no adequate and well-controlled studies in pregnant women; *or* animal studies have shown an adverse effect, but adequate and well-controlled studies in pregnant women have failed to demonstrate a risk to the fetus in any trimester.
- C—animal reproduction studies have shown an adverse effect on the fetus and there are no adequate and well-controlled studies in humans, but potential benefits may warrant use of the drug in pregnant women despite potential risks. The adverse event is a reversible effect on the human fetus.
- D—drugs which have caused human fetal malformations or irreversible damage.

- X—studies in animals or humans have demonstrated fetal abnormalities and/or there is positive evidence of a human fetal risk based on adverse reaction data from investigational or marketing experience, and the risks involved in use of the drug in pregnant women clearly outweigh the potential benefits. These should not be used in pregnancy or where there is a possibility of pregnancy.

In Australia the B category is subdivided, and this has been adopted by some other countries also.

- B1—used by a limited number of women who are pregnant or of child-bearing age without an increase in malformation or other harmful effect, and no effect in animal studies.
- B2—as for B1 but where animal studies are lacking or inadequate.
- B3—as for B1, with an increase in fetal damage seen in animals, the significance of which is considered uncertain in humans.

The complexity of the disease–pregnancy interaction indicates that specialist care needs to be provided, and where possible this should include a fetomaternal specialist and an obstetric physician, or a specialist physician with particular knowledge of physiological and pathophysiological processes and treatments in pregnancy. For the most common conditions (diabetes mellitus, hypertension and thyroid disease), most major centers conduct 'high-risk' clinics which combine midwifery, obstetric, fetomaternal specialist and physician care, with the appropriate tertiary support as required.

DIABETES IN PREGNANCY

Diabetes is one of the most common medical complications of pregnancy, and is increasing in incidence due to higher rates of obesity and type 2 diabetes, and also a rise in

Table 25-1 Principles relating to acute medical illness in pregnancy

QUESTION	RELEVANCE
What is the potential adverse impact of being pregnant on the course of the disease?	Pregnancy → Disease Example: Increased possibility of maternal disability or death due to H1N1 influenza occurring in a pregnant woman
What is the potential adverse effect of the disease on the pregnancy?	Disease → Pregnancy Example: Increased risk of premature labor in a patient with genital infection or renal disease causing preeclampsia
What is the likely effect of either disease or pregnancy on the fetus/neonate?	Disease/Pregnancy → Fetus/Neonate Example: Increased risk of macrosomia in the fetus when a pregnant woman has diabetes mellitus
What are the likely implications of the necessary investigations on the pregnancy?	Investigations → Pregnancy Example: The danger from radiation exposure to the fetus, particularly in the 1st trimester, needs to be carefully considered if a pregnant woman needs radiological tests in the setting of a serious illness
What are the likely implications of the necessary treatment on the pregnancy?	Treatment → Pregnancy Example: An acute attack of asthma may require oral corticosteroid therapy, but early in pregnancy this would impart a very slight increased risk of congenital abnormality in the fetus (such as cleft lip)

maternal age at pregnancy. Current rates of gestational diabetes are approximately 12–14% depending on race, family history and high-risk comorbidities, but the changing demographics of women, higher screening rates and tighter criteria for diagnosis are likely to lead to greater numbers of women being diagnosed in pregnancy. Diabetes in pregnancy is classified as:

- gestational diabetes
- pre-existing diabetes, either:
  » type 1 diabetes in pregnancy or
  » type 2 diabetes in pregnancy.

The White classification, used to assess maternal and fetal risk, classifies diabetes as follows.

- Gestational diabetes:
  » Class A1—gestational diabetes controlled with diet
  » Class A2—gestational diabetes controlled with insulin.
- Pre-existing diabetes:
  » Class B—onset at age 20 or older or with duration of <10 years
  » Class C—onset at age 10–19 or duration of 10–19 years
  » Class D—onset before age 10 or duration >20 years
  » Class E—overt diabetes mellitus with calcified pelvic vessels
  » Class F—diabetic nephropathy
  » Class R—proliferative retinopathy
  » Class RF—retinopathy and nephropathy
  » Class H—ischemic heart disease
  » Class T—prior kidney transplant.

Gestational diabetes

The diagnosis of gestational diabetes mellitus (GDM) is made on the basis of elevated blood glucose concentrations in pregnancy only. This condition is largely discovered on screening blood tests in the target population, although universal screening is recommended. Risk factors for gestational diabetes are given in Box 25-1.

Mechanisms

- The metabolic derangement that leads to higher maternal blood glucose concentrations is insulin resistance conferred by the placenta, through production of cortisol and progesterone, as well as human placental lactogen, prolactin and estrogen.
- It is also thought that increases in fat deposits mediate some of the hormonal responses.
- There is a clear genetic component to these responses, with genetic risk tracking with insulin receptor, insulin-like growth factor and glucokinase gene variations.
- There is a prevailing view that there is pancreatic beta-cell impairment.

Clinical presentation, investigation and diagnosis

The majority of presentations are asymptomatic, and therefore diagnosis is determined by screening serum and urine

---

Box 25-1

Risk factors for gestational diabetes

Women at greatest risk of gestational diabetes mellitus include those:

- over 40 years of age
- with a family history of type 2 diabetes mellitus (1st-degree relative with diabetes or a sister with GDM)
- who are overweight (defined as pre-pregnancy body mass index of >35 kg/m²) (moderate risk factor if BMI 25–35 kg/m²)
- of racial background including Asian, Middle Eastern, Polynesian, Melanesian or Māori, African-American, Indian Subcontinent and Indigenous Australian
- with a previous history of gestational diabetes (moderate risk factor)
- with a previous adverse obstetric outcome such as macrosomia (birthweight more than 4500 g or >90th centile), shoulder dystocia or polyhydramnios
- previously elevated blood glucose level
- women with polycystic ovarian syndrome
- or women on certain medications e.g. corticosteroids

---

biochemical tests. First-trimester testing for overt disease can include fasting plasma glucose or random plasma glucose, and then glycosylated hemoglobin (HbA_{1C}) if glucose is elevated.

Screening typically occurs at 24–28 weeks of gestation for all pregnancies in some countries, and is recommended at 14 weeks of gestation for those at highest risk. The defining blood sugar concentrations for diagnosis are:

- A diagnosis of GDM is made if one or more of the following glucose levels are elevated:
  » Fasting glucose ≥ 5.1 mmol/L
  » 1-hr glucose ≥ 10.0 mmol/L
  » 2-hr glucose ≥ 8.5 mmol/L
- Women at high risk of GDM should have a glucose tolerance test at the first opportunity after conception.
- Women who should have an early GTT are those with one high risk factor or two moderate risk factors.

If symptoms and signs occur, they can be maternal, fetal or neonatal.

- Maternal (although these can be nonspecific symptoms of pregnancy):
  » thirst
  » polyuria
  » constant hunger.
- Fetal:
  » macrosomia
  » polyhydramnios, or oligohydramnios (uncommon).
- Neonatal:
  » hypoglycemia
  » hyperbilirubinemia
  » polycythemia.

However, it is most common that the diagnosis is made on biochemical screening.

Treatment and targets

Evidence-based targets for GDM require close attention to detail (diagnosis and treatment), and a multidisciplinary model of care.

- Early detection of gestational diabetes is optimal, from either universal or targeted screening at either 14 or 28 weeks of gestation.
- Patient education is very important, and a multidisciplinary team approach including midwives, dietitians, diabetic educators, obstetricians, and endocrinologists or obstetric physicians, if available, is beneficial.
- Dietary therapy is essential, with oral hypoglycemic agents or insulin added where required to achieve the minimum goals for glycemic control: fasting blood glucose <5.1 mmol/L, 1-hour postprandial <7.4 mmol/L, or 2-hour postprandial <6.7 mmol/L.
- Careful antepartum fetal surveillance is essential. Continuation of the pregnancy in uncomplicated GDM not on insulin and with controlled glycemia to 10 days beyond term is acceptable, provided that indications from fetal monitoring are reassuring. This may include regular fetomaternal assessment of fetal growth parameters and other markers of fetal wellbeing (amniotic fluid index, non-stress test, biophysical profile, and umbilical artery flow characteristics).
- Close neonatal monitoring is important, particularly for the detection of hypoglycemia.

CLINICAL PEARL

Maternal follow-up, with an oral glucose tolerance test, should be performed 6–8 weeks postpartum and then at least every 2 years, because of the increased risk of developing permanent diabetes.

Type 1 diabetes in pregnancy

Classes E–T of the White classification (overt diabetes mellitus with calcified pelvic vessels; diabetic nephropathy; proliferative retinopathy; retinopathy and nephropathy; ischemic heart disease; and prior kidney transplant) are associated with greater maternal and fetal adverse outcomes, and require great care in the pre-pregnancy planning phase as well as careful monitoring during the pregnancy.

Of particular note, women with diabetic proliferative retinopathy should consider having their retinal vessels treated with photocoagulation on specialist advice early in pregnancy to reduce the risk of retinal hemorrhage, which is increased in pregnancy. This is especially important in those being considered for prophylaxis with aspirin (for preeclampsia).

Treatment and targets

- A pre-pregnancy consultation should be undertaken, with appropriate specialist referral.
- Patients with diabetic nephropathy (White classes F and RF) are likely to be treated with renal protective antihypertensives such as angiotensin-converting enzyme inhibitors (ACEIs) and angiotensin II receptor antagonists (ATRAs), which are contraindicated in the 2nd and 3rd trimesters of pregnancy; they are usually ceased once pregnancy is detected. These drugs are associated with increased fetotoxicity (drug category D). They should be substituted with drugs that are safe in pregnancy.
- Other organ pathologies resulting from diabetes, such as ischemic heart disease, cardiac autonomic neuropathy or gastric autonomic neuropathy, can cause significant symptoms in pregnancy. These need to be carefully managed with optimal treatment and care for the course of the pregnancy.
- Early identification and treatment of diabetic ketoacidosis and acute hypoglycemia are major considerations in those on insulin. With early diagnosis and appropriate care, fluid management and insulin, the incidence of fetal death has now decreased to below 10%. Women should be taught signs and symptoms that require medical attention.
- Women should be prescribed high dose pre-pregnancy folate supplementation (5mg daily) that is continued till 12 weeks gestation.
- The risk of preeclampsia in these women is of the order of 30%, but relates to the degree of blood pressure control and renal function prior to the onset of the pregnancy.

Type 2 diabetes in pregnancy

- The most common form of established diabetes seen in pregnancy (>90% of cases) is type 2 diabetes mellitus. These women are generally overweight or obese, and have a familial and genetic tendency to diabetes.
- Insulin resistance is the hallmark of this disorder, which is worsened by the metabolic changes of pregnancy.
- Pregnancy may be the first time women have been tested for diabetes, so it may not be clear whether a woman has underlying type 2 diabetes or GDM.
- The presence of microalbuminuria (albumin/creatinine ratio of >15 mg/mmol Cr) can also increase the chance of additional renal dysfunction, and preeclampsia in the pregnancy.

Treatment and targets

In addition to the targets set above for gestational diabetes, weight control and ongoing dietary advice are important in the management of those with type 2 diabetes in pregnancy.

CLINICAL PEARL

Dramatic weight loss is not a target for the management of type 2 diabetes in pregnancy, but a focus on healthy diet, maintenance of weight, and a concerted effort not to gain significant weight during pregnancy are important in the overall management.

Pre-conceptual care includes:

- weight loss
- education in diet, and self-monitoring of blood glucose
- diagnosis and management of target organs affected by diabetes

- a target of HbA_{1C} of <7% to decrease risk of fetal malformations
- pre-conceptual high-dose (5 mg) folate supplementation that continues until 12 weeks.

Pregnancy care requires:

- fetal surveillance
- tight glycemic control, including with oral hypoglycemic agents or subcutaneous insulin.

HYPERTENSION IN PREGNANCY

Mechanisms of disease

- Hypertensive disorders of pregnancy (HDP) are classified as those that are present only in pregnancy (usually appearing after 20 weeks of gestation), and those present prior to, or after, pregnancy.
- The risk factors (Table 25-2) for gestational hypertension, preeclampsia and superimposed preeclampsia (in a patient with chronic hypertension) reflect the prevailing theories that preeclampsia is related to placental mass, placental dysfunction and some level of immunological activation in the presence of a toxic antiangiogenic response from the placenta.
- The epidemiological association noted in women who have been using barrier contraception, have short cohabitation times, new partners, and who use artificial reproductive techniques (and therefore non-exposed tissues) has sparked investigation into immunological mechanisms as a cause of preeclampsia. It is yet to be determined how this knowledge will affect the capacity to prevent preeclampsia.
- Our understanding of preeclampsia has been greatly enhanced by the recent discovery of abnormalities in the antiangiogenic molecules (soluble FMS-like tyrosine kinase-1), and their regulators (placental growth factors, vascular endothelial growth factor) which arise from the placenta as important causal molecules. The link between these molecules, alterations in innate immunity and regulation of innate immunity by cytokines has also advanced our understanding of preeclampsia, and the likelihood that focused treatment may be offered in the future.

Clinical presentation, investigation and diagnosis

While much attention has been paid in the past to the classification of the hypertensive disorders in pregnancy, the more recent classification into four categories has significantly simplified our understanding and capacity to determine the risk and prognosis in any given pregnancy:

1. Gestational hypertension.
2. Preeclampsia related to pregnancy.
3. Chronic hypertension and superimposed preeclampsia where blood pressure is elevated before or prior to 20 weeks of pregnancy or persists 3 months after delivery.
4. Chronic hypertension, either primary (essential) or secondary, and including 'white coat' hypertension. This group has an increased risk of superimposed preeclampsia which can be severe, occurring early in the pregnancy and leading to significant maternal and perinatal mortality and morbidity.

Gestational hypertension

Gestational hypertension is any increase in blood pressure (BP) after 20 weeks of gestation which is resolved by 3 months post-delivery. Any prior history, even of a transient increase in BP in the setting of oral contraceptive use, excludes women from this classification. Gestational hypertension requires two BP readings of ≥140 mmHg systolic or ≥90 mmHg diastolic taken more than 4 hours apart; an elevation in either is required.

Preeclampsia/eclampsia

Preeclampsia/eclampsia is any increase in blood pressure after 20 weeks gestation associated with at least one of the following:

- proteinuria >300 mg per 24 hours or a protein:creatinine ratio of 30 mg protein/mmoL Cr
- serum creatinine >0.09 mmol/L; oliguria
- elevated liver enzymes, a >30% reduction in platelet count or <100 × 10^9/L; hemolysis or disseminated intravascular coagulation (DIC)

Table 25-2 Risk factors for preeclampsia

RISK FACTOR	RISK
Renal transplant recipient, with an elevated creatinine, high blood pressure, and on high-risk immunosuppression such as cyclosporine (ciclosporin)	Approaching 100%
APS (antiphospholipid syndrome) severe, untreated	85% Also at risk of miscarriage
Renal disease	30%
Chronic hypertension	30%
Donor ovum	30%
Triplet pregnancy	22.7%
Twin pregnancy	14%
Primiparity	10%
New partner, donor sperm	10%
Interpregnancy interval >10 years	10%
Second pregnancy to a partner without preeclampsia	2%

- pulmonary edema
- persistent and/or severe headache; convulsions (eclampsia); persistent visual disturbance; stroke
- epigastric pain
- hyper-reflexia/clonus
- fetal growth restriction
- placental abruption.

Issues in diagnosis

Considerable discussion arises about the sensitivity and specificity of the urine testing regimen. However, a urinary protein excretion of ++ or more (+++ and ++++) on a dipstick test is reliable to diagnose significant proteinuria. Once identified, proteinuria, regardless of its progress, establishes the diagnosis of preeclampsia/eclampsia.

- The usual pattern is for the proteinuria to increase with time, although a sudden severe increase in proteinuria (often within hours) is very well described in preeclampsia.
- The difficulty rests with the diagnosis of no proteinuria on a dipstick test, and low-range proteinuria (trace and +), which has a false-negative rate of up to 9%. Here the sensitivity and specificity range from 27% to 89%. Normal urinary protein excretion is <300 mg/day in the 3rd trimester.
- The screening nature of this test can be improved by requesting a laboratory (or point of care) urine protein/creatinine ratio, which takes into account the concentration of the urine at the time of testing. A ratio of >30 mg/mmol Cr is considered significant.
- Ultimately, the 24-hour collection for urine quantification is the 'gold standard', but it needs to be recognized that up to 50% of the actual tests end in inaccurate collection, especially if done at home.
- Proteinuria confers additional risk of poor obstetric outcome but, in and of itself, does not confer severity.

Blood pressure discussions are similarly vexed.

- When the BP is >170/110 mmHg there is universal agreement about the diagnosis and need for treatment.
- When BP is under 140/90 mmHg, women do not reach the diagnostic threshold.
- The identification of at-risk women, particularly those in a younger age group, by a rise in systolic BP of 25 mmHg or a rise in diastolic BP of 15 mmHg should prompt the need for greater monitoring. BP readings between 140/90 and 170/110 mmHg (either systolic or diastolic) meet the criteria for gestational hypertension or preeclampsia.

The investigation for secondary hypertension in those with chronic hypertension, or occasionally in those with *de novo* hypertension, should be reserved for those with signs or symptoms suggestive of secondary disease:

- very high BP early in the 2nd trimester—pheochromocytoma
- radio-femoral delay—suggestive of coarctation of the aorta

- a renal bruit or discrepant renal size—suggestive of renal artery stenosis
- hypokalemia—suggestive of mineralocorticoid excess
- hypercalcemia—suggestive of hyperparathyroidism as a potential cause
- under- and over-active thyroid function—suggests thyroid disease as a target for treatment.

Overlap syndromes with diabetes and diabetic nephropathy are also important contributors to the risk of preeclampsia.

Treatment and targets

- The use of magnesium sulfate is safe for babies and mothers and has a proven benefit in preventing maternal seizures. Magnesium sulphate also decreases both the rate of cerebral palsy in the extremely premature neonate (<30 weeks of gestation) and the rate of maternal mortality. It is used in many women with severe-range hypertension or at lower BP readings when there is neurological irritability or seizure. Magnesium sulphate is also indicated for the fetus where no such maternal issues exist but delivery is to occur at extreme prematurity e.g. <30 weeks gestation.
- For those with a BP under 140/90 mmHg, even if this represents an increase in BP, treatment is not routinely recommended.
- Considerable debate exists about the need for treatment in the group with BP between 140/90 and 169/109 mmHg. Those who favor antihypertensive treatment recognize the worsening prognosis of hypertension with respect to risk of intracerebral hemorrhage and placental abruption. Those who oppose antihypertensive treatment identify risks to fetal weight gain and neonatal safety.
- Treatment of hypertension in pregnancy is important to allow safe progression of the pregnancy, timely and controlled delivery where possible, and a decrease in maternal and fetal morbidity and mortality.
- There is also increasing evidence that preeclampsia affects future maternal cardiovascular risk.

CLINICAL PEARL

Treatment of severe hypertension in pregnancy (especially if the blood pressure is above 170/110 mmHg) requires rapid blood pressure control and immediate fetal monitoring. Antihypertensive therapy including intravenous treatment is indicated in this group of women.

Antihypertensive drug choices in pregnancy are outlined in Table 25-3.

Prevention strategies for preeclampsia

There is increasing evidence that acetylsalicylic acid can be used prophylactically to decrease the risk of preeclampsia in the highest risk groups: those with renal disease, diabetes and chronic hypertension. The usual dose is 100 mg (low dose) per day, started in the 1st trimester and ceasing at 34 weeks of gestation.

Table 25-3 Antihypertensive drug choices in pregnancy

DRUG	MECHANISM OF ACTION	CATEGORY IN PREGNANCY
Alpha-methyldopa	Centrally acting, alpha-2 agonist	A
Clonidine	Centrally and peripherally acting, alpha-2 agonist	B3
Labetalol	Non-selective beta-blocker	C (fetal bradycardia)
Nifedipine	Calcium-channel blocker	C (fetal distress)
Diazoxide	Peripheral vasodilator	C (neonatal hyperglycemia)
Hydralazine	Peripheral vasodilator	C (fetal distress)
Prazosin	Peripheral vasodilator	B2

RESPIRATORY DISEASE IN PREGNANCY

Pneumonia

> ### CLINICAL PEARL
>
> Pneumonia is not more common in pregnancy, but the consequences of some forms of pneumonia, notably varicella pneumonia, include extremely high mortality in pregnancy.

- Risk factors for pneumonia in pregnancy include asthma and anemia.
- The bacterial pneumonias are typically those that are commonly seen outside of pregnancy; streptococci, *Haemophilus influenzae* and *Mycoplasma pneumoniae*. These are easily treated with both beta-lactam and macrolide antibiotics, which are considered safe in pregnancy.
- Viral infections, including varicella, and influenzas including avian influenza, severe acute respiratory syndrome (SARS) and more recently swine influenza, can be complicated by maternal pneumonia and have an increased mortality in pregnancy. The increased mortality in the swine influenza epidemic of 2009 was contributed to by obesity and increased susceptibility in some ethnic groups.
  - » Treatments include the rapid use of antiviral medication, and support for respiratory failure such as ECMO (extracorporeal membrane oxygenation).
- Apart from maternal respiratory failure, the other complications of pneumonia in pregnancy are premature labor and the increased risk of low-birthweight infants.

Early recognition of pneumonia is therefore critically important in pregnancy. The increasing availability of vaccination, particularly for influenzas, may decrease the associated morbidity and mortality in pregnancy. Women should be advised to receive the flu vaccine in pregnancy, especially due to their immunosuppressed state.

Asthma

Asthma is a common disorder, and therefore flares may occur in pregnancy. The consequences of uncontrolled asthma can have significant and surprising consequences on the fetus (increased risk of hypoxic injury) and the mother (increased risk of preeclampsia).

- The respiratory rate is essentially unchanged in pregnancy, but the increase in tidal volume, minute ventilation and minute oxygen uptake, and therefore the decrease in functional residual capacity and residual volume, can appear as a hyperventilatory state in the latter part of the pregnancy.
- The effect of pregnancy on partial pressure of carbon dioxide (pCO_2; a decrease), serum bicarbonate (a decrease), and pH (an increase) reflect a chronic respiratory alkalosis which needs to be taken into account when interpreting blood gases and biochemistry results in pregnant women.

> ### CLINICAL PEARL
>
> In the setting of asthma, a normal partial pressure of carbon dioxide (pCO_2) in a pregnant patient may signal impending respiratory failure.

Clinical presentation, investigation and diagnosis

The diagnosis of asthma in pregnancy uses the same criteria as in the non-pregnant state: breathlessness, cough, and wheeze. The demonstration of airway reactivity reversible with beta-mimetics is the pathognomonic feature of the disease.

Given that dyspnea is common in pregnancy, it is a challenge to sort out the physiological breathlessness in pregnancy from potentially dangerous diagnoses including:

- airway obstruction
- amniotic fluid embolism
- acute congestive heart failure (CHF), secondary to peripartum cardiomyopathy
- pulmonary thromboembolism.

Box 25-2

Adverse outcomes from severe and poorly controlled asthma in pregnancy

- Preeclampsia and gestational hypertension
- Uterine hemorrhage
- Pre-term labor
- Premature birth
- Congenital anomalies (especially related to drugs taken in the 1st trimester)
- Intrauterine growth restriction
- Low birthweight percentile
- Neonatal hypoglycemia, seizures, tachypnea, and neonatal intensive care unit admission

Asthma may worsen, improve or remain unchanged during pregnancy. The time of greatest risk for asthma flares is in the 3rd trimester when mechanical factors, such as diaphragmatic splinting and decreased functional reserve, limit respiratory reserve.

- The complications for the mother at this stage can include respiratory failure, barotrauma, and adverse effects of treatment including corticosteroids, causing, for example, pathological rib fractures secondary to osteoporosis.
- Left untreated, or under-treated, severe maternal morbidity and mortality can result (Box 25-2).

The use of standard asthma medication is recommended in pregnancy when required. The net effect of untreated asthma outweighs any perceived problems based on the use of regular anti-asthma medications. Women need to be encouraged to have their asthma adequately treated, including with the assistance of regular respiratory review and airflow testing.

VENOUS THROMBOEMBOLISM (VTE) IN PREGNANCY

Venous thromboembolism, including deep vein thrombosis (DVT) and pulmonary embolism (PE), is an uncommon but potentially life-threatening disorder in pregnancy. Pregnancy is associated with a 10-fold increase in the incidence of VTE due to an increase in several coagulation factors, increase in venous stasis and possible endothelial injury.

CLINICAL PEARL

Accurate diagnosis of venous thromboembolism is essential, and clinical symptoms alone should not be used in place of objective radiological diagnostic tests.

- Objectively diagnosed VTE, whether DVT or PE, requires immediate anticoagulation, with therapeutic-dose low-molecular-weight heparin preferred over unfractionated heparin given its increased bioavailability, its more predictable dose effect, and its better side-effect profile. Unfractionated heparin is associated with a risk of heparin-induced thrombocytopenia (HIT) and osteoporosis if used over several weeks.
- Warfarin is best not used to treat VTE during pregnancy due to its teratogenicity profile in the 1st trimester and its increased risk of bleeding (given prolonged half-life) in the 3rd trimester where delivery may occur.
- Risk factors for VTE in pregnancy may be pregnancy-specific, such as preeclampsia, cesarean section and post-partum hemorrhage; or general maternal risk factors, such as a personal or family history of thrombosis, increased body mass index (BMI), immobility or smoking.
- Thrombophilic patients are at risk, and pelvic surgery is an additional risk factor in the pregnancy setting.
- Women at increased risk of developing pregnancy-associated VTE will require antepartum and usually 6 weeks postpartum thromboprophylaxis, but there are very few data from clinical trials to give clear guidelines.
- Management of the bleeding risk in the peri-delivery period is particularly challenging. Anticoagulation should be discontinued for the shortest time possible in women at increased risk of developing thrombosis. Women who must be fully anticoagulated may need to be converted to intravenous unfractionated heparin around the time of delivery. Vaginal delivery should be the goal unless cesarean section is indicated for obstetric reasons and a safe plan for anticoagulation can be formulated.

THYROID DISORDERS IN PREGNANCY

All thyroid disease can present in pregnancy, but from the fetal wellbeing point of view the most important consideration is the functional thyroid hormone level.

Generally, thyroid function tests in pregnancy need to be considered in the context of the following normal physiological changes.

- Altered thyroid-hormone-binding globulin (TBG) production and sialylation from 2 weeks to 20 weeks of gestation.
- Increased triiodothyronine (T_3) and thyroxine (T_4) produced to match TBG increases.
- Iodine deficiency:
  - » increased renal clearance due to hyperfiltration of pregnancy
  - » reactive increase in thyroid uptake (may increase the size of the gland)
  - » direct competition by which the thyroid overrides fetal uptake of iodine
  - » inadequate oral maternal iodine intake.
- Increased beta human chorionic gonadotropin (beta-hCG):
  - » shares an alpha subunit with thyroid-stimulating hormone (TSH)

» stimulates the TSH receptor and decreases transiently the TSH concentration (may lead to false diagnosis of hyperthyroidism)

- Pregnancy specific reference ranges for TSH vary throughout pregnancy and differ to the usual reference range (e.g. 1st trimester TSH 0.1–2.5 mIU/L, 2nd trimester TSH 0.2–3.0 mIU/L and 3rd trimester TSH 0.3–3.0 mIU/L).

Hypothyroidism

Hypothyroidism occurs in 9/1000 of the young female population prior to pregnancy, and another 3/1000 are diagnosed during pregnancy.

- Symptoms can be very difficult to define in pregnancy, as the hormonal effects of pregnancy *per se* can lead to tiredness, lethargy, weight change, and cold intolerance.
- The usual pattern for recognition is biochemical, and includes elevated TSH and low free T_4.
- The most common cause is Hashimoto's thyroiditis.
- Pituitary causes of hypothyroidism are rare.
- Treatment is directed at adequately replacing thyroid hormone. Women already taking thyroxine replacement should have an increase in dose by two additional doses per week (or 30%) on confirmation of pregnancy.
- There are special concerns for the treatment of hypothyroidism relating to the possibilities of thyrotoxicosis or hypothyroidism in the neonate, with the attendant concerns for neurodevelopmental delay if not treated.
- Neonatal encephalopathy can be a complication of either hypothyroidism or its treatments.

Hyperthyroidism

Hyperthyroidism occurs in 2/1000 pregnancies.

- This is most likely (95%) to be due to autoimmune thyroiditis/Graves' disease, due to production of immunoglobulin G (IgG) thyrotropin-receptor-stimulating autoantibodies, also known as thyroid-stimulating immunoglobulins (TSIs).
- It can rarely be due to multinodular goiter, a functioning solitary nodule, subacute thyroiditis, or a thyroid carcinoma.

CLINICAL PEARL

The most common explanation for apparent hyperthyroidism in pregnancy, as evidenced by low levels of thyroid-stimulating hormone, is simply the artifactual biochemical result induced by beta human chorionic gonadotropin (beta-hCG).

- It is essential to assess women for tremor, tachycardia, nodular thyroid disease, and proptosis, and then test for functional thyroid concentrations and thyroid antibodies.
- Thyroid disease often decreases in the 2nd and 3rd trimesters due to changes in maternal immunity, but worsens again in the puerperium.

As with thyroid disease in non-pregnant individuals, the mainstay of treatment is with drugs which block the organification of iodine and the coupling of iodotyrosyl molecules.

- Propylthiouracil and carbimazole are the most commonly used drugs.
  » Both of these agents cross the placenta, although propylthiouracil seems to do so less readily.
  » Propylthiouracil also decreases the conversion of T_4 to T_3, in both the mother and the fetus. As deiodinases II and III are preserved, as long as iodine is sufficient then fetal brain development is not usually affected.
- Monitoring for side-effects is just as important in pregnancy as in the non-pregnant state. Methimazole has been reported to be associated with esophageal or choanal atresia as well as aplasia cutis when given in early pregnancy.
- As would be the principle in treating any chronic disease in pregnancy, a minimum dose should be used to control symptoms and signs, with close monitoring and dose reductions wherever possible.
- Control of thyroid function assists with managing hypertension, and thereby reduces the risk of superimposed preeclampsia.

COMMON GASTROENTEROLOGICAL AND LIVER DISORDERS IN PREGNANCY

Gastroesophageal reflux disease (GERD)

Dyspepsia in pregnancy is an almost universal symptom. Some risk factors are independent of pregnancy (e.g. obesity), but include the increase in production of relaxin, estrogen and progesterone in combination, and other relaxing hormones, which predispose the gastroesophageal junction to dysfunction resulting in symptoms of heartburn, 'hunger pains' and chronic chest pain.

- Treatment of GERD is problematic, as many treatments, other than delivery of the pregnancy, are not effective.
- Antacid medications are commonly prescribed.
- Increasingly, safety around the use of proton-pump inhibitors is being accumulated. Some studies have shown a non-significant increase in congenital abnormalities related to omeprazole. The advice at present is to reserve these medications for those with peptic ulceration and, perhaps, proven blood loss, and to give as late as possible in the pregnancy.

Constipation and irritable bowel syndrome (IBS)

The contribution of cyclical hormones to bowel motility is well known, and in pregnancy the effects of sex steroids and known physiological phenomena such as fluid shifts and increased bowel transit time contribute to clinical constipation.

- Constipation also possibly contributes to the increased rates of anal fissure, hemorrhoids and anal bleeding which occur in pregnancy. In the 1st trimester, constipation may exacerbate nausea and hyperemesis.
- IBS is common in women of reproductive age, but there is no clear evidence of increased rates in pregnancy. Symptoms can be worse, better or the same in pregnancy. No other complications or sequelae from IBS have been described in pregnancy.

Inflammatory bowel disease (IBD)

Inflammatory bowel disease, especially Crohn's disease, has an important impact in pregnancy. Symptoms of Crohn's disease that can be exacerbated by pregnancy include:

- chronic diarrhea
- rectal bleeding
- weight loss
- fever
- abdominal pain and tenderness (often on the right side of the lower abdomen)
- feeling of a mass or fullness in the lower, right abdomen.

Taking into account the lack of predictability of the condition in pregnancy, general wisdom would be to embark on a pregnancy when the disease is quiescent, when treatment is stable and/or while taking minimal, non-teratogenic medication. Joint counseling and care between obstetricians specializing in high-risk obstetrics, gastroenterologists or obstetric physicians, and colorectal surgeons is often necessary in preparing for and managing a pregnancy. Consideration needs to be given to:

- the state of disease activity at the time of the pregnancy
- the likelihood that the pregnancy will exacerbate the condition and what action will be taken if this occurs
- the possible effects of the disease on the pregnancy
- the possible effects of the disease and treatments on the baby, including likely prematurity
- the possibility of superimposed complications such as preeclampsia or gestational diabetes if the woman is on corticosteroids.

Cholestasis of pregnancy

CLINICAL PEARL

Acute or intrahepatic cholestasis of pregnancy is the most common cause of jaundice in pregnancy.

This is a condition related to the estrogen glucuronides that inhibit the bile salt export pump, and thus lead to a cholestatic pattern of liver function test abnormalities. There is an increased sensitivity of the bile tract membranes and hepatocytes to estrogen and progesterone. There are links to a diet low in selenium, and it is seen in the winter in temperate

---

Box 25-3

Differential diagnosis of jaundice in pregnancy

- Drug hepatotoxicity (can be seen with alpha-methyldopa)
- Viral hepatitis
- Autoimmune hepatitis (screen for antimitochondrial antibodies)
- Hyperemesis gravidarum (severe)
- Cholelithiasis
- Cholangiocarcinoma (extremely rare)
- Overlap syndromes:
  - » preeclampsia (HELLP syndrome) (liver rupture, and infarction in rare cases)
  - » acute fatty liver of pregnancy

---

climates, in those with HLA-B8/BW16 haplotypes, and with changes in the *ABCB4* phosphatidylcholine bile transporter gene. This can have effects on bile transport across the placenta, and is thought to contribute to the potential fetotoxicity of the disease.

- The condition is more common in those with thyroid disorders in pregnancy, and with multiple gestation.
- It occurs in 2% of all pregnancies, and in those who have had it once it recurs in 45–70% of subsequent pregnancies.
- Any jaundice in pregnancy should provoke a search for other diagnostic possibilities (Box 25-3).
- The diagnosis is confirmed by an increase in bilirubin concentration, and an increase in the transaminases to approximately twice normal concentrations.
- There is an increase in serum bile acids.
- There is often a prolongation of the prothrombin time, which is responsive to vitamin K.
- In interpreting liver function test results in pregnancy, it is important to remember that they are usually low, as there is a mild dilutional effect in the 1st and 2nd trimesters.

The fetal complications are the most worrying feature, and it is unclear whether sudden fetal demise (stillbirth) is related. For this reason there is a tendency to monitor carefully and induce delivery at the safest possible time for the baby, usually no later than 38 weeks, although there is no clear consensus. This can occur at an earlier gestation if the jaundice is severe and the mother intensely symptomatic.

- The other complications include preterm labor, fetal distress, fetal clotting, and meconium aspiration.
- It is recommended that fetal monitoring is increased to twice weekly from 30 weeks of gestation on the advice of a fetomaternal specialist.

The only proven treatment for the associated pruritus is ursodeoxycholic acid (UDCA). UDCA reduces sulfated metabolites of progesterone in serum and stimulates biliary transport, thereby increasing bile acid clearance.

- Other treatments have included guar gum, S-adenosyl-methionine, activated charcoal and cholestyramine, but have been less effective in relieving the itch.
- There is no effect of these treatments on improving fetal outcome.

Acute fatty liver of pregnancy (AFLP)

This is a much rarer but potentially life-threatening liver failure, specific to pregnancy.

- Risk factors include obesity, abnormal thyroid function, primiparity, multi-gestational pregnancy, and male fetus.
- There are crossover syndromes, where acute liver failure in the setting of hypertension and proteinuria creates confusion with preeclampsia as an alternative diagnosis.
- The condition is due to a defect of intramitochondrial fatty acid oxidation, more specifically long-chain 3-hydroxyacyl-CoA dehydrogenase deficiency (LCHAD).
- The discovery of these fatty acid oxidation pathway abnormalities in the offspring of the related pregnancy has indicated a potential genetic basis for the disease.

CLINICAL PEARL

Presentation of acute fatty liver of pregnancy (AFLP) is usually with right upper quadrant pain, fever, vomiting, headache, hypoglycemia and jaundice. Itch occurs in 30%. Ascites develops in 43%, and necrotizing enterocolitis can occur, as well as pancreatitis.

- The diagnosis is assumed when there is an elevated white cell count in the setting of jaundice, with elevated alkaline phosphatase (ALP) in excess of a rise in uric acid or aspartate transaminase.
- The transaminases are typically 3–10 times the upper limit of normal, and the serum bilirubin levels are also elevated.
- The identification of hypoglycemia, and its rapid treatment, is an essential part of the treatment.
- The maternal mortality is 18% and the fetal mortality 23%, and therefore this condition requires the highest level of tertiary care and multidisciplinary input. It is usually managed in an intensive care unit.
- Death usually occurs following complications of acute fulminant liver failure including bleeding, renal failure and hepatic encephalopathy.

Budd–Chiari syndrome in pregnancy

Budd–Chiari syndrome (1/1,000,000 pregnancies) is due to occlusion of the hepatic arteries, and presents in pregnancy as abdominal pain, ascites and hepatomegaly.

- The presentation can be *acute*, *fulminant*, *chronic*, or *asymptomatic*.
- Approximately 10–20% of women also have hepatic vein thrombosis.
- This rarely occurs in the setting of thrombophilia, and only limited screening for antiphospholipid antibodies and hematological malignancy is recommended.

CLINICAL PEARL

Any palpable liver is abnormal in pregnancy, as the liver is normally displaced upwards and to the right, and is not palpable.

Thrombophilia investigation in pregnancy should include testing for:

- protein S deficiency
- protein C deficiency
- antithrombin III deficiency
- activated protein C resistance (from the factor V Leiden mutation)
- antiphospholipid syndrome (coagulation profile, anti-cardiolipin antibody and lupus anticoagulant)
- prothrombin gene mutation
- paroxysmal nocturnal hemoglobinuria (in rarer cases where clinically indicated).

Some of these investigations may be affected by pregnancy itself and should be interpreted with regards to pregnancy specific reference ranges. Treatment requires transfer to a liver treatment hospital/unit which offers liver transplantation as an option. The mainstay of initial treatment is anticoagulation, but managing the pregnancy in the context of progressive liver failure requires a multidisciplinary team, including a high-level neonatal nursery in the event of premature delivery.

VIRAL INFECTION IN PREGNANCY

Although viral infections are no more likely to occur in pregnancy, they are conditions that require special consideration.

- The effect of the disease on the pregnancy relates to prematurity, usually due to pre-term delivery (spontaneous).
- The effects of the infection on the fetus can include increased rates of stillbirth and congenital abnormality. This is particularly relevant with cytomegalovirus (CMV) maternal infection, which is second only to parvovirus and herpes simplex virus (HSV) as the major viral cause of stillbirth.

Viral hepatitis

- In the case of viral hepatitis, the effect of pregnancy on the disease is the tendency for more severe disease.
- The fetal effects can include intrauterine growth restriction (IUGR), except for hepatitis A.
- Hepatitis A appears to have no increased rate of spontaneous abortion or stillbirth.
- No increase in congenital abnormalities has been described with viral hepatitis, except CMV where the complex syndrome includes IUGR, jaundice, hepatosplenomegaly, petechial rash, thrombocytopenic rash, chorioretinitis and encephalitis. CMV screening is an

important part of 1st trimester pregnancy screening for this reason.

CLINICAL PEARL

The typical viral screening strategies for early pregnancy include:

T Toxoplasmosis
O Other infections (including syphilis)
R Rubella
C Cytomegalovirus
H Herpes simplex virus and human immunodeficiency virus.

- Vertical transmission to the fetus is of major concern, with other agents as well as CMV. Hepatitis B transmission is of particular public health interest due to a high burden of disease, and its contribution to lifelong risk for chronic hepatitis and hepatocellular carcinoma (HCC). There are several therapeutic and preventative options for both mother and baby that should be explored to reduce the vertical transmission, e.g. hepatitis B immunoglobulin, vaccination or antiviral therapies.

Investigation of maternal serology is harmless to the fetus, and is the mainstay of diagnosis of the different possible viral agents.

- Confirmation of neonatal infection is usually undertaken after birth.
- Diagnostic liver biopsy is no more likely to develop complications than in the non-pregnant state, but should only be considered in severe cases where there is significant diagnostic uncertainty.

Most antiviral treatments are relatively contraindicated in pregnancy.

IMMUNOLOGICAL AND HEMATOLOGICAL DISEASE IN PREGNANCY

Systemic lupus erythematosus (SLE)

Systemic lupus erythematosus is a common disease in the reproductive-age female population.

- The immediate aspects of most relevance to pregnancy are renal disease, antiphospholipid syndrome, and respiratory complications of the disease.
- Functional status of the various organ components in SLE is essential to determine obstetric risk. The level of renal dysfunction is especially important.
- Creatinine clearance below 30 mL/min/1.73 m^2 and uncontrolled hypertension increase the likelihood of a poor pregnancy outcome. This level of chronic kidney disease is more likely with those who have had class 3 and 4 lupus nephritis, and who may have responded initially to treatment but progressed to renal scarring with time.

- The diagnosis of either of these forms of aggressive inflammatory lupus nephritis during pregnancy creates the ultimate dilemma for the parents and caring team: that of the need to terminate the pregnancy in order to treat the progressive renal disease.
  - » Generally, it would not be considered safe to administer alkylating agents, in pregnancy.
  - » In a similar way, chronic pulmonary fibrosis and poor respiratory reserve would be a relative contraindication to pregnancy, given the need to increase respiratory function in pregnancy.
- Symptomatic relief of lupus arthritis becomes problematic in pregnancy due to the intrinsic unsafe fetal profile of high-dose continuous corticosteroids (prednisone generally does not cross the placenta but has been implicated as a contributor to cleft palate in very high doses), antimetabolites, and even the non-steroidal anti-inflammatory drugs (NSAIDs) (premature closure of the ductus arteriosus, renal adverse drug reactions). Lower dose corticosteroids, e.g. 10 mg or less, may provide a therapeutic option without significant adverse fetal events as smaller doses do not cross the placenta.

Antiphospholipid syndrome (APS)

Miscarriage can be a feature of SLE, APS and other thrombophilias, uncontrolled hypertension, chronic kidney disease, infectious diseases, diabetes, drug and alcohol use, as well as some obstetric and genetic causes which lead to pregnancy loss.

CLINICAL PEARL

Late miscarriage (>10 weeks of gestation), 2nd-trimester loss and recurrent miscarriage as well as early severe preeclampsia are all indicators of possible antiphospholipid syndrome and should be investigated accordingly.

- The mechanism of pregnancy loss or complication (miscarriage or preeclampsia) is through antiphospholipid antibody binding to trophoblast in the placenta, causing microthrombi, which decreases placental perfusion and leads to placental insufficiency. These placentas are smaller, and consist of areas of small infarcts and calcification.
- The placental failure leads to loss in the 2nd trimester (weeks 12–28 weeks of gestation), IUGR, preeclampsia, and placental abruption.

APS is a clinical diagnosis supported by laboratory tests. The diagnostic criteria include one or more of the following clinical criteria:

- arterial, venous or small-vessel thrombosis without vessel inflammation and not in a superficial vessel
- ≥3 unexplained consecutive miscarriages (<10 weeks of gestation), excluding anatomical, genetic, infective or hormonal causes
- ≥1 unexplained death(s) of a morphologically normal fetus at or after 10 weeks of gestation

- ≥1 premature birth(s) of a morphologically normal neonate at or before 34 weeks of gestation, associated with severe preeclampsia or severe placental insufficiency, including IUGR.

Treatment

- Pregnant patients with confirmed APS should be fully anticoagulated.
- The risk of recurrent miscarriage in the patient with APS can be reduced by prophylactic-dose unfractionated heparin, or prophylactic-dose low-molecular-weight heparin plus low-dose aspirin.

Idiopathic thrombocytopenic purpura (ITP)

The normal physiological response to pregnancy is up to a 30% reduction in platelet count from baseline. An acute decline of platelet count within the setting of hypertension or proteinuria is supportive of a diagnosis of preeclampsia. In the absence of preeclampsia and with >30% drop in platelet count, ITP should be considered.

- The incidence of ITP is 1 in 10,000 pregnancies.
- Mild decreases in platelet count are not thought to be threatening to mother or baby, and can be just watched carefully.
- The neonatal effect of maternal antiplatelet antibodies is largely minimal, and has in some places led to an increased use of delivery by cesarean section with perception of greater fetal safety. This is not proven.
- ITP is only diagnosed with the exclusion of SLE, lupus anticoagulant and anti-cardiolipin antibody, and in a setting not suggestive of viral thrombocytopenia.
- The risk of bleeding with ITP is very low, and the risk of neonatal thrombocytopenia is minimal.
- In the absence of bleeding, the goal should be monitoring and anticipation of potential bleeding risk.
- The general rule of the platelet count needing to be >80 $\times 10^9$/L does not totally hold up in women with chronic ITP, and it is likely that ≥50 $\times 10^9$/L is sufficient for delivery and >70 $\times 10^9$/L for regional anesthesia.
- Therapeutic options for women include oral corticosteroids or intravenous immunoglobulin to increase the platelet count in preparation for delivery. This would only be indicated if the platelet count was significantly less than 50 $\times 10^9$/L.

Iron-deficiency anemia (IDA)

Anemia is common in pregnancy and is contributed to by the following physiological responses to pregnancy:

- iron deficiency in the 1st trimester leads to an increase in iron absorption in the 2nd and 3rd trimesters
- an increased iron requirement in the 2nd and 3rd trimesters (50% increase) due to an increase in fetal uptake of iron.

The consequences of IDA in any pregnancy are:

- preterm delivery

- infant small for gestational age (SGA)
- inferior neonatal health
- reduced ability to withstand the adverse effects of excessive blood loss should they occur during delivery
- bleeding during childbirth
- a higher risk of requiring transfusion in the postpartum period.

Anemia in multiple sequential pregnancies becomes a compounding problem, with progressive depletion of total body iron stores. The non-pregnant recommended daily intake of iron is 18 mg for menstruating women of reproductive age. In pregnancy the dietary requirement for iron increases to 27 mg/day, which is difficult to achieve by diet alone.

- It is routine to measure hemoglobin concentration in the 1st trimester, at 28 weeks and 36 weeks of gestation (depending on the country), in order to monitor the increasing iron requirements in the latter half of pregnancy and intervene if anemia is progressive.
- Appropriate levels of iron supplement (up to 100 mg/day) are recommended and can be titrated against the level of anemia.
- Intravenous iron can be used where oral iron is poorly tolerated. IV iron is currently contraindicated in the 1st trimester of pregnancy.

CARDIAC DISEASE IN PREGNANCY

Overall, although heart disease is relatively uncommon, it remains a great concern in pregnancy due to the risk of maternal death. It is still the biggest contributor of any chronic medical condition to maternal mortality. The specific entities which are of concern are as follows.

- Acquired conditions such as:
  - » cardiomyopathy
  - » postpartum cardiomyopathy
  - » aneurysm/dissection
  - » myocardial infarction
  - » valvular heart disease/rheumatic heart disease.
- Congenital disease:
  - » Congenital heart disease is a concern now that children are reaching reproductive age after corrective surgery.
  - » Non-structural heart disease in the form of arrhythmia is a common feature of pregnancy. Palpitations, most usually due to a sinus tachycardia, are common in pregnancy. In the absence of any structural abnormality these do not typically lead to increased risk of maternal mortality.
  - » The risk of a congenital cardiac lesion in the fetus is also increased.

Valvular heart disease

Valvular heart disease can be congenital, or acquired through rheumatic fever.

- The most common **congenital** abnormalities seen in the pregnant population are patent ductus arteriosus, atrial septal defect, pulmonary stenosis and ventricular septal defect.
- The rates of these conditions are similar to those seen in the general female population.
- In the advent of corrected major heart disease, such as tetralogy of Fallot, pregnancy outcomes can be very complicated, depending on the severity of the underlying heart condition. Treatment strategies should include pre-conceptual investigation to establish the level of left and right ventricular function, and history of arrhythmia.
- Occasions of heart failure from congenital abnormalities are rare in pregnancy.
  » Heart failure at the time of delivery is of special concern, and fluid shifts in the immediate postpartum period need to be carefully monitored.
- **Rheumatic heart disease** is common in some parts of the world by reason of socioeconomic disadvantage, as well as other infective factors. Rates have rapidly dropped in the past 40 years in many developed countries.
- The most common valvular lesion of concern is mitral stenosis, and this is the most frequent cause of heart failure in the setting of chronic rheumatic heart disease in pregnancy.
- In the presence of mitral stenosis, pulmonary edema occurs due to exaggerated physiological responses to pregnancy (outlined below).

CLINICAL PEARL

Contributors to acute pulmonary edema in pregnancy:
- increased heart rate preventing ventricular refilling
- increase in cardiac output
- increase in pulmonary blood volume
- increase in circulating blood volume.

As with congenital heart disease, pre-conceptual care, and assessment of left and right atrial and ventricular function and the degree of valve stenosis need to be determined prior to pregnancy.

- The appearance of pulmonary edema is potentially life-threatening and can be intractable, so it needs to be identified and treated early.
- Mitral valve stenosis may require surgical intervention in the pregnancy, and this may be achieved by closed valvuloplasty.

The other issue with valvular heart disease and the care of pregnant women who have had artificial valves is prophylaxis for thromboembolism, and endocarditis in selected cases, especially at delivery, and identification and treatment of arrhythmias.

- The general principle in heart disease is that it is a pregnancy effect on the disease, with the increasing fluid volumes, increased cardiac output, and heart rate that are part of the normal response to pregnancy causing a risk that the heart with valvular heart disease can fail.

- This is especially true of stenotic valvular lesions, with the regurgitant lesions faring better in pregnancy.

Arrhythmias and palpitations

Arrhythmias are more common in pregnancy, and palpitations occur in 50% of pregnant women although this rate is close to that in the normal population under 40 years of age.

- There is an increased awareness of even the benign arrhythmias such as sinus tachycardia in pregnancy, which increases the frequency of complaint.
- Sustained arrhythmias are less common and occur in 2–3/1000.
- As indicated above, it is the arrhythmia in the presence of a structural cardiac abnormality that increases the risk of maternal morbidity.
- Treatment decisions depend on the diagnosis, but also the duration, frequency and tolerability of the arrhythmias to the mother.
- The management of arrhythmias with pharmacotherapy is generally safe, with no clear contraindications.
  » Some of the highly selective beta-blockers (atenolol) have been associated with a marked reduction in birthweight, and should be replaced by non-selective beta-blockade unless there is no alternative.

Cardiomyopathy, including postpartum cardiomyopathy

- Biventricular cardiac failure is an uncommon complication of pregnancy.
- The most common time for heart failure seen in pregnancy is in the immediate postpartum period, and relates to a dilated, progressive and aggressive form of cardiomyopathy.

Other vascular conditions

Other vascular conditions likely to have cardiac consequences in pregnancy relate to those which cause chronic severe hypertension, such as coarctation of the aorta (Figure 25-1) and reno-vascular disease.

In coarctation of the aorta:

- identification of concentric left ventricular hypertrophy and appropriate pre-pregnancy treatment of hypertension is essential in management of a pregnancy
- there needs to be a clear pattern of BP-taking that is manageable in the pregnancy, with discrepant readings in the arms or legs identified early
- where the coarctation is corrected prior to the pregnancy, sometimes leaving a limited defect, a better outcome can be expected.

Reno-vascular disease causes an early and aggressive form of preeclampsia.

- This can be managed by correction of the stenosis—by arterioplasty of fibromuscular dysplasia in young women—and can dramatically improve the prognosis for pregnancy and reduce the risk of preeclampsia.

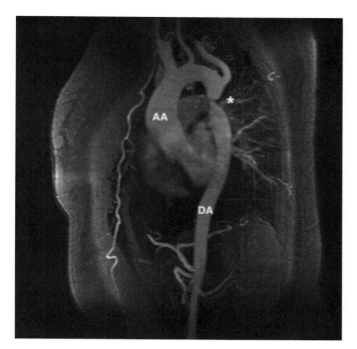

Figure 25-1 Coarctation of the aorta in a pregnant woman, seen on magnetic resonance imaging. AA, ascending aorta; DA, descending aorta

From Creasy RK, Resnik R et al. (eds). Creasy and Resnik's Maternal–fetal medicine, 7th ed. Philadelphia: Elsevier, 2014.

- The only clinical clues for reno-vascular disease are discrepant renal size (detected on renal ultrasound), and a renal bruit. However, a renal bruit is very difficult to ascertain in a pregnant abdomen, and sounds of uterine souffle can confuse the sign.

OBESITY IN PREGNANCY

A special mention needs to be made about the increasing worldwide trend for obesity in women of reproductive age.

Obesity is a major contributor to conditions which have altered prognoses for pregnancy:

- anovulatory infertility
- increased rate of miscarriage
- metabolic syndrome and diabetes mellitus
- gestational diabetes
- chronic hypertension
- risk for preeclampsia/gestational hypertension
- reduced respiratory function, primary hypoventilation
- obstructive sleep apnea and other forms of sleep-disordered breathing
- risk of venous thrombosis and pulmonary embolism
- increased infective risk
- increased risk of hemorrhage
- increased risk of caesarean-section-related complications including wound dehiscence
- increased rate of obstetric complications
- increased intraoperative risk if caesarean section is required
- increased birth risks—macrosomia, shoulder dystocia and birth trauma, increased rates of congenital abnormalities, fetal death.

NEUROLOGICAL CONDITIONS IN PREGNANCY

The most common neurological comorbidity managed in pregnancy is epilepsy.

- Although epilepsy does not seem to have an effect on the course of the pregnancy, it has been associated with an increased risk of cesarean delivery.
- Pregnancy *per se* can lower the seizure threshold and increase the frequency of seizures in some patients.
- By far the most significant issue is that of appropriate drug use in pregnancy. There are a significant number of new anticonvulsants with little long-term data about their safety in pregnancy.

SELF-ASSESSMENT QUESTIONS

1   Mrs K is a 29-year-old with a history of hypertension since the age of 20 years, who is taking the oral contraceptive pill. She is admitted to the obstetric ward at 30 weeks of gestation with a decrease in fetal movements, and is noted to have a blood pressure (BP) of 240/140 mmHg. She is otherwise asymptomatic. Mrs K is noted to have 300 mg/day of proteinuria. Her usual medications are alpha-methyldopa 250 mg three times daily, and labetalol 100 mg three times daily. Which of the following would *not* indicate the need to consider delivery of the pregnancy immediately?

   A   Inability to control the BP with additional intravenous antihypertensive, and magnesium sulfate.
   B   An increase in urinary protein excretion to 1500 mg/day.
   C   Sudden onset of headache and neurological irritability (clonus and hyper-reflexia) requiring magnesium sulfate.
   D   Elevation in serum creatinine and transaminases above the normal range.
   E   A baby that has not grown since the last fetal assessment scan 2 weeks prior to this admission.

2   A 26-year-old known asthmatic is now pregnant. She has noted an increase in exertional dyspnea in the 3rd trimester of her pregnancy (she is at 29 weeks of gestation). Her usual medication consists of inhaled budesonide twice daily, and inhaled salbutamol as required. She has considered changing to combined fluticasone/salmeterol, as per her doctor's recommendation. Which additional features of her lung function and capacity, in pregnancy, will influence your interpretation of her peak flow, forced expiratory time and FEV_1/FVC ratio?

   A   Peak flow remains unchanged, forced expiratory time is unchanged, and the FEV_1/FVC ratio is the same as non-pregnant readings.
   B   The decrease in respiratory muscle strength and decrease in functional residual volume make the peak flow and forced expiratory time unhelpful, but increase the reliability of the FEV_1/FVC ratio.
   C   Increase in respiratory rate and decreased residual volume make the partial pressure of carbon dioxide (pCO_2) a much more reliable marker.
   D   The increase in tidal volume and minute ventilation make the FEV_1/FVC ratio unreliable.

3   Jennifer is at 24 weeks of gestation in her second pregnancy. In her first she was noted to have increased blood pressure (BP) from week 12 and had been treated with labetalol; she is not asthmatic. Her BP remained managed in that pregnancy, and the delivery was uncomplicated by preeclampsia. In this, her second pregnancy, she has elected to try alpha-methyldopa for BP control, as she has heard that it is the only category A (i.e. safe) medication in pregnancy. She has a body mass index of 39 kg/m^2 and is known to have had a gallstone identified during an episode of right upper quadrant (RUQ) abdominal pain 3 months after the birth of her first child. An attempt to have this surgically corrected was halted when it was found that she was pregnant again. She now has new-onset RUQ pain and tenderness, and the results of liver function tests are shown in the following table. Her blood pressure is 130/80 mmHg and her urine shows 190 mg of protein. Her platelet count is 150×10^9/L.

Bilirubin	26 micromol/L	Reference range (RR) 3–15 micromol/L
Albumin	31 g/L	RR 36–47 g/L
Alkaline phosphatase (ALP)	201 IU/L	RR 30–150 U/L
Gamma glutamyl transpeptidase (GGT)	42 IU/L	RR 30–115 U/L
Aspartate aminotransferase (AST)	222 IU/L	RR 1–30 IU/L
Alanine aminotransferase (ALT)	260 IU/L	RR 1–40 IU/L

Which is the most likely diagnosis, and what course of action would be indicated?

   A   This is an episode of cholecystitis and she needs an abdominal ultrasound.
   B   This is likely to be an episode of alpha-methyldopa liver toxicity and the drug should be stopped immediately.
   C   Sclerosing cholangitis is likely, and urgent biliary tract stenting is indicated.
   D   She has preeclampsia and requires urgent delivery irrespective of the prematurity of the pregnancy.

ANSWERS

1   B.

   The markers of severity in terms of deciding the need to deliver urgently at any gestation in preeclampsia are:

   i   Inability to control the BP to <170/110 mmHg and preferably to at or below 140/90 mmHg.
   ii   Increase in maternal symptoms, especially seizure.
   iii Increase in liver enzymes, indicating cytotoxic edema of the liver (often associated with liver pain and enlargement, which can lead to liver rupture).
   iv   Rapidly decreasing platelet count (note whether the platelet count is <30% of baseline).
   v   Any significant increase in serum creatinine (remember that serum creatinine is below the normal range in pregnancy

(30–60 micromol/L)). A rise to within the (non-pregnant) reference range can be highly significant and represent a serious decrease in glomerular filtration rate (Figure 25-2).

vi   A baby that is failing to grow.

vii A baby that shows acute distress (ultrasound criteria and cardiotocographic criteria—consultation with obstetrician and neonatologist is required).

Although proteinuria is a marker of disease, i.e. a defining feature for the diagnosis of preeclampsia, it is not a criterion for delivery *per se*. Delivery may be required for the rapidly rising creatinine even though the absolute value is still within the 'normal' range.

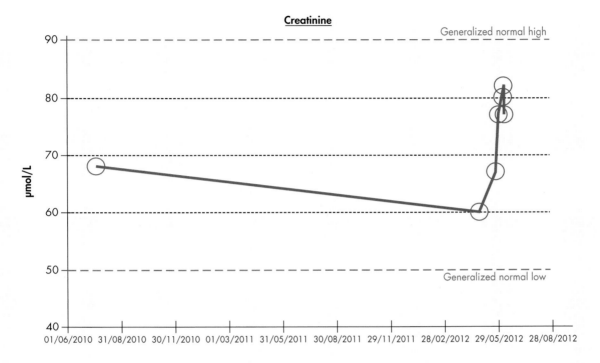

Figure 25-2 Note the dramatic rise in serum creatinine in this graph from a patient with preeclampsia. The maximum level remains within the 'normal' laboratory reference range, but the change indicates a rapid fall in glomerular filtration rate

2   A.

Respiratory rate is essentially unchanged in pregnancy, but the increase in tidal volume, minute ventilation and minute oxygen uptake, and therefore the decrease in functional residual capacity and residual volume, can appear as a hyperventilatory state in the latter part of the pregnancy. The effect of pregnancy on pCO_2 (a decrease), serum bicarbonate (a decrease) and pH (an increase) reflect a chronic respiratory alkalosis which needs to be taken into account when interpreting blood gases and biochemistry results in pregnant women.

Asthma needs to be identified and treated in pregnancy, and the usual monitors of peak flow, FEV_1/FVC ratio and forced expiratory time remain reliable indicators of disease state in pregnancy. Uncontrolled asthma has been associated with poor neonatal outcomes and with preeclampsia. Episodes of severe asthma in pregnancy are more likely in those with initial poor control, and infants small for gestational age are more common in this severe group.

3   B.

Many women who are fertile are at risk of cholecystitis, and this should be monitored in pregnancy. However, the pattern of liver function test abnormality, just as in non-pregnant cases, should reflect an obstructive jaundice. Her pattern of hepatocellular damage is consistent with a drug toxicity reaction as is seen in 1/200 cases with alpha-methyldopa. For this reason the drug should be stopped immediately, and another antihypertensive drug chosen, such as labetalol. It is unlikely that a new-onset cholangial disease is present in this case, as she has no risk factors (e.g. inflammatory bowel disease). Although she is at risk for preeclampsia, her current investigations are not diagnostic, and she should be watched for proteinuria (>300 mg/day) symptoms and fetal growth signs of placental dysfunction. Remember that the placenta produces alkaline phosphatase, which is always elevated in pregnancy.

CHAPTER 26

GERIATRIC MEDICINE

Will Browne, Balakrishnan Kichu R Nair, Elizabeth Whiting, Jeffrey Rowland, Paven Preet Kaur and Ramdeep Bajwa

CHAPTER OUTLINE

INTRODUCTION

The enormous scientific and social advances of the past and current centuries have resulted in a progressive rise in the number people living to an advanced age. At one time exceptional, survival beyond the age of 70 years is now commonplace. As many diseases rise in prevalence and incidence with age, this change in the population has had a profound impact upon the nature of medical practice—adult medicine, whether in a hospital or outpatient setting, cares for a predominantly elderly population of patients.

Safe and effective care of this growing cohort of older patients requires an understanding of the way human physiology changes with advancing age, and of the patterns of disease and their clinical expression in this population, as well as social, economic and ethical considerations relevant to them.

EPIDEMIOLOGY OF AGING

There is a global shift toward an older population due to declining fertility rates and increasing life expectancy. This is known as the 'demographic shift'. Figure 26-1 illustrates this process. While more advanced in developed countries, the same factors drive demographic transition in developing countries, where this represents a significant and growing economic burden.

THEORIES OF AGING

Processes underlying aging

Aging is a complex process, and it has proved challenging to determine which of the features associated with advanced age reflect accumulation of the effects of disease and which reflect a distinct process caused by tissue senescence and degeneration. In many cases, both degeneration related to aging and damage due to disease interact in the same organ

and tissues. Current theories of aging share the mechanism of progressive metabolic damage to cells driven by reactive oxygen species and also the damage associated with accumulation of amyloid, glycation end products, oxidized proteins and lipids (lipofuscin).

Homeostenosis

Homeostenosis refers to the aging-related loss of reserve capacity in maintaining homeostasis. This gradual decline in homeostatic reserve explains the typical presentation of the 'geriatric syndromes' described below, as well as the increased susceptibility of many older individuals to a wide variety of pathological processes.

Evolution and aging

It is likely that some of the diseases and degenerative changes seen in aging result from the failure of natural selection to act upon genes and traits that manifest after reproductive life.

As evolutionary processes act largely prior to the conclusion of childbearing, there is little selective pressure acting on processes that cause disease in the 50s, 60s, 70s and beyond. There is 'the grandmother theory' that would suggest there may be some benefit from a healthy second generation assisting in the upbringing of the grandchildren. An example might be seen in the case of Alzheimer disease—a disease with at least some component determined by genetic factors. The incidence of this disease rises sharply following the end of the typical reproductive span. Genes associated with the late life onset of Alzheimer disease are presumably therefore less influenced by selective pressure.

Telomere shortening and mitochondrial dysfunction

- It has been known since the 1960s that human cells in culture are able to undergo mitosis a finite number of times before losing the ability to divide further. In somatic cells, each cycle of mitosis is associated with progressive shortening of the telomeres.
- There is a definite functional link between mitochondria and telomeres. The latter are protective segments at the ends of chromosomes that shorten with repeated cellular divisions.
- Telomeres have long been thought to play some role in the senescence of rapidly dividing tissues. The suggestion of a link between them and mitochondria implicates both in some aspects of aging.
- Telomere failure may result in impaired mitochondrial function.

Endocrine factors associated with aging

- Hereditary factors contribute to aging processes, and there is evidence that IGF1 levels may have an inverse effect on the rate of aging. Despite this, falling circulating levels of IGF1 are associated with both aging and cognitive decline.

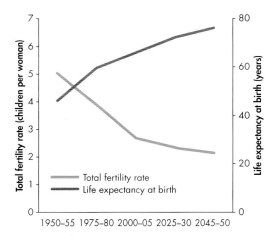

Figure 26-1 Total fertility rate and life expectancy at birth: world, 1950–2050

From Population Division, DESA, United Nations. World Population Ageing 1950–2050. Geneva: United Nations, 2007.

- IGF1 pathways are important regulators of lifespan in animal models. It is likely that IGF1 plays a similar role in humans, and hence in human aging.
- Growth hormone is another endocrine factor influencing aging and longevity in animal models.
- Insulin, pathways involved in thyroid hormone secretion, testosterone, estrogen and many other hormones have been hypothesized to influence aging. Determining causal relationships has been challenging.

Inflammation and aging

- Inflammatory conditions are often associated with diseases common in older people, and contribute to sarcopenia and to other phenotypic changes characteristic of the syndrome of aging.
- Inflammation is correlated with diseases of aging, and markers of inflammation carry some value in stratifying risk for a number of conditions, including heart disease and the development of tumors and malignancy.

Free radicals and aging

- The production of oxyradicals (also called free radicals or reactive oxygen species) in many tissues, as well as their accumulation, increases with aging.
- Oxyradicals are potentially damaging to cellular structures. They are produced during mitochondrial metabolism, and are scavenged by a number of cellular systems.
- Superoxide dismutase, glutathione and catalase all play a role in the detoxification of oxygen, and variations in the efficiency of these repair systems may underlie some of the variable changes of aging seen between individuals.

Programmed aging

- It has been hypothesized that some aspects of aging may be programmed genetically, with a switching off of repair mechanisms after peak reproductive function has slowed or ceased.
- Enhanced longevity associated with changes in the expression of certain genes (such as histone demethylase JMJD-3.1 in *C. elegans*) possibly influenced by epigenetic factors, may provide evidence for programmed aging.

PHYSIOLOGY OF AGING

While there is compelling evidence that the process of homeostenosis (diminished reserve, and compensatory failure) occurs in the absence of specific disease, understanding changes in normal aging physiology is made more challenging by the problem of distinguishing the effect of disease from the consequences of aging.

The changes discussed in the following sections might be expected to occur in a healthy older individual.

Cardiovascular changes

In older individuals there are changes to many aspects of cardiac and vascular structure and function.

- In addition to the changes caused by disease, there is an increase in heart weight, left ventricular wall thickness, and hypertrophy in healthy aging.
- Of particular importance are the aging-related changes contributing to the very high prevalence of hypertension among the elderly. These include:
  » changes in endothelial function
  » low plasma renin
  » increasing arterial wall stiffness
  » changes in body fat percentage and distribution
  » changes in metabolism and insulin resistance.

Cardiac changes

These include:

- left ventricular diastolic dysfunction related to changes in the extracellular matrix
- changes in the mechanical properties of myocytes
- increases in mass, weight, and wall thickness of the heart
- altered connective tissue, with increased proportions of collagen and fibrinogen
- degenerative changes in the cardiac valves, including calcification and fatty changes
- fibrotic changes of the conducting system
- thickening and increasing tortuosity of many of the major blood vessels.

While these changes generally have only a modest impact on day-to-day cardiac function, they result in a lowered threshold for the development of disease. For this reason, cardiovascular disease is among the most important causes of serious illness in older people.

Renal changes

- There is a progressive decline in renal reserve with advancing age, which can become clinically important when an acute illness occurs.
- The same changes may have an impact on drug clearance.
- The effect of age on glomerular filtration is embodied in the Cockroft–Gault calculation for estimated creatinine clearance (eClCr):

$$eCrCl = \frac{(140 - age) \times mass\ (in\ kg) \times (0.85\ if\ female)}{72 \times serum\ creatinine\ (in\ mg/dL)}$$

- The decline in renal function with aging is greatly accelerated by the presence of hypertension, diabetes, vascular disease and a variety of nephrotoxic environmental exposures, including excessive use of analgesics.
- Atherosclerotic disease and heart failure are closely associated with decline in renal function in older people, and it is probable that at least part of the decline in renal function with aging is due to renal atherosclerosis.

Musculoskeletal changes

- Sarcopenia or progressive loss of muscle mass is typical in aging, and is one of the components of the important concept of frailty.

- Part of this loss of skeletal muscle tissue is driven by falling levels of androgen, a change which occurs in both genders with aging.
- IGF1 levels also fall with aging, and interestingly in this context are associated with greater sarcopenia.
- Bed rest is particularly concerning, resulting in an average loss of 5% of muscle mass per week. The skeletal muscle of aged individuals is particularly likely to undergo apoptosis or atrophy.
- Inflammation is probably contributory to the loss of muscle mass in many people, and possibly to the aging process itself.
- A decline in bone density with aging due to alterations in bone turnover contributes to the development of the disease osteoporosis in many people.
- Loss of articular cartilage and resulting progressive impairment in joint function is closely associated with aging.

Neurological changes

Numerous neurological changes associated with aging have been proposed.

- At a cellular level there is loss of nerve cells, changes in dendritic function, and alterations in glial cell reactivity.
- Some of these changes may relate to accumulation of protein metabolites. Amyloid-beta accumulates in hippocampal and medial temporal structures in normal aging but does so to a far greater extent in Alzheimer disease.
- Cognitive changes do occur with aging and can be measured with neuropsychological tests. When severe, such changes are usually associated with a neurodegenerative disorder. Milder changes in speed of processing, executive functioning, and memory changes are common and are usually unassociated with serious dysfunction.
- The combination of change in the number of neurons and synaptic connections, as well as the effects of vascular and neurodegenerative disease, results in an increased susceptibility to the state of pathological cognitive dysfunction known as delirium.

Skin changes

Sometimes overlooked by physicians but seldom by patients, the skin undergoes important changes with aging.

- Even in the absence of drugs like corticosteroids that accelerate skin thinning, the epidermis becomes progressively thinner with aging.
- The inner surface of the skin is normally characterized by an undulating appearance to microscopy, with projections of epidermal tissue called rete ridges extending downward into the dermal layer. This distinctive undulation is progressively lost as aging advances.
- The epidermis has fewer melanocytes and Langerhans cells.
- The dermis undergoes atrophy. There are fewer fibroblasts, mast cells and blood vessels.

Metabolic and endocrine changes

The metabolic changes with aging are diverse, and include changes in tissue turnover, glucose utilization and endocrine function. Despite this, normal function in the absence of stressors is generally maintained in normal aging. Under stress, however, reserve capacity is reduced and important clinical consequences arise accordingly.

- Plasma glucose levels are well maintained in normal aging, while a glucose load causes a substantially higher plasma glucose level than in younger people.
- The production of some hormones may be increased to compensate for this waning in endocrine function. For example, levels of follicle-stimulating hormone (FSH) and luteinizing hormone (LH) increase in healthy older males in order to maintain serum testosterone.
- Cessation of ovulation with menopause is an important age-related milestone in women which is associated with significant fluctuations and changes in the production of a number of hormones including FSH, LH and oestrodiol.

Gastrointestinal changes

Gastrointestinal changes related to aging are complex, and their association with symptoms such as constipation is not clear.

- Fewer neurons are found in the myenteric plexus.
- There is a reduced response of the bowel to direct stimulation.
- Progressively higher collagen deposition is seen in the left colon, associated with lower rectal compliance.
- There is reduced colonic segmental motor coordination.
- There is greater binding of plasma endorphins to intestinal receptors.
- Fibro-fatty change, and thickening of the internal anal sphincter, is found.

PATHOLOGY: DISEASE IN OLDER PEOPLE

Concepts related to aging

The biological mechanisms of aging are complex. Simplistically the following concepts may be of use:

- Degeneration

  The body as a biological system is in a constant state of use resulting in wear and tear. The system response is to repair the damage. Over time, the ability to repair is outstripped by the rate of damage which may lead to dysfunction.

- Threshold

  As the system deteriorates, compensatory mechanisms come into play. When the level of dysfunction gets beyond a certain tipping point, then a level of failure is reached, manifesting with dysfunction.

- Summation

The body is a complex system comprised of multiple subsystems. Within this complex system, a single failure may not become obvious due to compensatory mechanisms. However, if enough systems are affected then the ability to compensate will be compromised and this will manifest as dysfunction.

Common problems typical to older people

CLINICAL PEARL

The giants of geriatric syndromes can be remembered as the 6 'I's and as the 6 'S's.

The 6 'I's
- Infection
- Instability
- Immobility
- Incontinence
- Impaired cognition
- Iatric

The 6 'S's
- Stability
- Sarcopenia
- Sad (depression)
- Sepsis
- Sore (pain)
- Social isolation

Frailty

Frailty is a syndrome used to describe vulnerable patients with declining physiological reserve and function. The decline is likely multi-factorial and related to the concepts of aging described above. Increasing frailty is associated with an increasing risk of morbidity and mortality. Frailty is independently linked to falls, poor mobility, hospitalisation and death. Given this, identifying frailty is a key skill, for which various tools have been developed. The Fried model is a phenotypic tool, which defines someone as frail if they meet three or more of the following five criteria:

- Unintentional weight loss of ≥4.5kg in the preceding year
- Self-reported exhaustion
- Weak grip strength
- Slow walking speed
- Low physical activity

Another commonly used tool is the Clinical Frailty Scale (Figure 26-2). There is a growing body of evidence around the management of patients with frailty to reduce risk. Evidence supports the benefit of various forms of exercise, nutritional supplementation and cognitive training to slow the progression of frailty and improve functional status.

Clinical Frailty Scale*

 1 Very Fit – People who are robust, active, energetic and motivated. These people commonly exercise regularly. They are among the fittest for their age.

 2 Well – People who have **no active disease symptoms** but are less fit than category 1. Often, they exercise or are very **active occasionally**, e.g. seasonally.

 3 Managing Well – People whose **medical problems are well controlled,** but are **not regularly active** beyond routine walking.

 4 Vulnerable – While **not dependent** on others for daily help, often **symptoms limit activities.** A common complaint is being "slowed up", and/or being tired during the day.

 5 Mildly Frail – These people often have **more evident slowing,** and need help in **high order IADLs** (finances, transportation, heavy housework, medications). Typically, mild frailty progressively impairs shopping and walking outside alone, meal preparation and housework.

 6 Moderately Frail – People need help with **all outside activities** and with **keeping house.** Inside, they often have problems with stairs and need **help with bathing** and might need minimal assistance (cuing, standby) with dressing.

 7 Severely Frail – Completely dependent for personal care, from whatever cause (physical or cognitive). Even so, they seem stable and not at high risk of dying (within ~ 6 months).

 8 Very Severely Frail – Completely dependent, approaching the end of life. Typically, they could not recover even from a minor illness.

9. Terminally Ill - Approaching the end of life. This category applies to people with **a life expectancy <6 months,** who are **not otherwise evidently frail.**

Scoring frailty in people with dementia

The degree of frailty corresponds to the degree of dementia. Common **symptoms in mild dementia** include forgetting the details of a recent event, though still remembering the event itself, repeating the same question/story and social withdrawal.

In **moderate dementia,** recent memory is very impaired, even though they seemingly can remember their past life events well. They can do personal care with prompting.

In **severe dementia,** they cannot do personal care without help.

* 1. Canadian Study on Health & Aging, Revised 2008.
2. K. Rockwood et al. A global clinical measure of fitness and frailty in elderly people. CMAJ 2005;173:489-495.

© 2007-2009. Version 1.2. All rights reserved. Geriatric Medicine Research, Dalhousie University, Halifax, Canada. Permission granted to copy for research and educational purposes only.

Figure 26-2 A Clinical Frailty Scale

Image courtesy of Geriatric Medicine Research, Dalhousie University, Halifax, Canada. © 2007-2009.

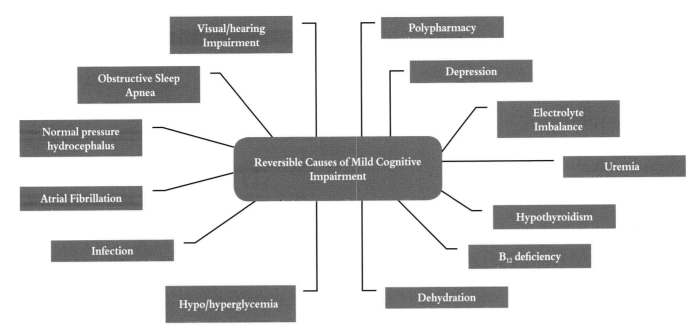

Figure 26-3 Reversible Causes of Mild Cognitive Impairment

Dementia and mild cognitive impairment

Dementia is characterized by a decline in cognition from the patient's baseline in one or more cognitive domains, significant enough to affect the patient's ability to function independently with day-to-day activities. In mild cognitive impairment, there has been a change from baseline above what is considered normal age-related cognitive decline but with preservation of independence and function. Although normal cognition, mild cognitive impairment and dementia are part of a spectrum of disease, mild cognitive impairment does not always progress on to dementia with a 5–10% rate of progression to dementia per year. Diagnosis and differentiation requires detailed history taking, clinical examination, objective cognitive testing, pathology and imaging. A detailed clinical assessment ensures identification of any reversible factors, which may affect the patient's cognition, for example depression, polypharmacy, and untreated obstructive sleep apnea. Reversible factors need to be addressed and the patient re-assessed prior to a diagnosis of dementia (Figure 26-3).

The most widely used cognitive screening tools include the Mini Mental State Examination (MMSE), the Montreal Cognitive Assessment (MOCA), the Mini-Cog, and the Rowland Universal Dementia Assessment Scale (RUDAS) for patients from non-English speaking backgrounds. Pathology testing is used to rule out potentially reversible causes including hypo- or hyperglycemia, vitamin B_{12} deficiency, hypercalcemia or hypothyroidism.

A non-contrast CT head or MRI is used to rule out a malignancy, chronic subdural or normal pressure hydrocephalus. Early diagnosis of dementia is important to allow patients and their families time to plan ahead while the patient has capacity to make decisions regarding their future health including advance care planning, enduring power of attorney and future living plans. Further detail on the topic of dementia can be found in Chapter 18.

Declining mobility, falls and fractures

Mobility

Changes in mobility are minimal in uncomplicated aging and should raise consideration of a disease, such as a neurodegenerative or musculoskeletal process. A detailed history looking at the course of the mobility change as well as associated symptoms or signs, including pain, limb weakness, bladder/bowel dysfunction or change in medication, can help determine the underlying cause. It is also important to consider the patient's environment including stairs and distance to bathroom. Determining complications due to the change in mobility, including the new use of walking aids, any falls or injuries, can help the clinician understand the impact on the patient and if they are safe in their current environment.

When examining the patient, the Timed Up and Go Test can be easily implemented either on the ward or in clinic to assess a patient's mobility (see Box 26-1). This simple test assesses proximal strength needed to stand from sitting, gait, gait speed, balance, fatigue and ability to follow instructions. The time taken to complete this task correlates with increasing dependence, falls, injury and increased care needs.

Falls

Worldwide, approximately 28–35% of people aged 65 and over fall per year with the frequency increasing with age, frailty and for those who reside in aged care facilities. Falls are a major source of fear for patients and stress for families with 20–30% leading to injuries and contributing to 10–15% of all emergency department visits. The duration of the ensuing hospital stay varies depending on the injury but tends to be longer than that related to other injuries. Post fall, patients can suffer from loss of independence, depression and isolation secondary to fear of falling, delirium and

Box 26-1
Timed up and go test

1 Equipment—armchair, tape measure, tape, stop watch.

2 Begin the test with the patient sitting correctly in a chair with arms; the patient's back should be resting on the back of the chair.

3 Place a piece of tape or other marker on the floor 3 m away from the chair.

4 Give the instructions 'On the word GO you will stand up, walk to the line on the floor, turn around and walk back to the chair and sit down. Walk at your regular pace.'

5 Start timing on the word 'GO' and stop timing when the patient is seated again correctly in the chair, with their back resting on the back of the chair.

6 Normal healthy elderly people usually complete the task in 10 seconds or less. Very frail or weak elderly people with poor mobility may take 2 minutes or more.

A score of ≥14 seconds has been shown to indicate a high risk of falls.

disability secondary to injuries. With over 400 risk factors associated with falling, some are modifiable and others are not. A prior history of falls in the past year is the most important risk factor and predictive of future falls. A holistic and multidisciplinary approach is necessary to minimize future risk of falls and should include strength and balance training, a home hazard review, vision testing and a medication review.

Fractures

Fragility fractures in the elderly are associated with a higher rate of comorbidity and complications and therefore an increased rate of mortality. Co-management between orthopaedic surgeons and geriatricians result in improved outcomes for patients with fragility fractures, with evidence for shorter inpatient lengths of stay, a reduction in rate of readmissions, shorter time to surgery and lower complications rate—all resulting in lower morbidity and mortality.

Urinary incontinence

The rates of incontinence increase with age with urinary incontinence affecting 15–30% of older adults living in the community. However, it is important to recognize incontinence is not a normal part of aging and is generally associated with underlying pathology or a causative factor. Urinary incontinence may be associated with adverse effects on a patient's mental health with feelings of embarrassment and fear of leakage resulting in social isolation, depression and a reduction in quality of life. The physical complications include pressure areas, frequent urinary tract infections and falls. Urinary incontinence can be divided into acute and chronic. Causes of acute and potentially reversible urinary incontinence include:

- Urinary tract infections as a result of urothelial inflammation leading to changes in bladder sensation
- Constipation with faecal impaction applying pressure on the bladder reducing its capacity
- Medication, including but not limited to diuretics, opioids, alpha blockers
- Atrophic vaginitis
- Delirium resulting in incontinence due to cognitive changes
- Psychological concerns including anxiety or depression can contribute to incontinence.

Chronic urinary incontinence can be divided into the following categories:

- Urge: the most common type of incontinence amongst the elderly, due to detrusor overactivity with symptoms of urgency and incontinence dominating. Treatment is with a combination of bladder retraining, lifestyle changes, the use of continence aids such as pads, and medications such as oxybutynin (an antimuscarinic) and mirabegron (a beta-3-adrenergic receptor agonist)
- Stress: incontinence secondary to increased intra-abdominal pressure, for example sneezing, laughing, coughing. Treatment is with pelvic floor exercises, lifestyle changes, the use of continence aids such as pads or in some cases surgery
- Mixed: a combination of stress and urge incontinence
- Overflow: due to an over-distended bladder with incomplete bladder emptying
- Functional: due to inability to access toileting amenities in time despite a functionally normal urinary tract, usually due to mobility limitations or cognitive impairment.

Fecal incontinence

Older adults with urinary incontinence are more likely to suffer from faecal incontinence as the neural pathways are closely related. Fecal impaction and severe constipation can present with diarrhea and fecal incontinence due to liquid moving around the impacted stool. Management begins with addressing the underlying precipitants, and then diet and lifestyle modification as well as use of pads and barrier creams. Bulking agents and anti-diarrheal agents are helpful in selected patients.

Depression

Depression in the elderly may be difficult to recognise. It may be difficult to identify neuro-vegetative features or feelings of sadness or isolation as reflecting a mood disorder rather than issues related to physical ill health or issues of loss associated with aging. In addition, depression in the elderly may present as cognitive impairment (pseudo-dementia) which may improve or resolve with treatment. Treatment challenges may include medication side-effects, medication non-compliance and impact on comorbidities. It should be noted the rate of suicide in men over the age of 85 is higher than in any other age group. The second peak in depression may be partly related to vascular risk factors. Psychotherapy, pharmacotherapy or a combination of treatment are effective much the same as in younger people. However, in older patients, monotherapy is recommended to minimize complications with a start low and go slow approach advised with regular monitoring for side-effects.

ATYPICAL PRESENTATION OF ACUTE ILLNESS

Elderly patients can often present with an altered clinical presentation; for example, sepsis may present without fever or an acute abdomen may present without pain. Well-known atypical presentations are known as the 'geriatric syndromes' and include:

- Delirium
- Declining mobility and falls
- New incontinence

Delirium

Delirium is a syndrome categorised by rapid onset of impaired, fluctuating attention with impaired cognition with or without altered consciousness. Delirium can be the sole sign on presentation of acute illness and should prompt an urgent and broad assessment. The Confusion Assessment Method (CAM) and the 4AT are the two most widely used screening tools. The 4AT screening tool is used clinically for rapid detection of delirium and consists of the following areas for testing:

1 Alertness
2 AMT4 (abbreviated mental test 4 – a tool for assessing cognitive impairment in older people)
3 Attention
4 Acute change or fluctuating change

History taking (usually a collateral) should be aimed at determining the following:

- Is it delirium or dementia?
- What is a trigger for delirium? Common causes include:
- Infection
  » Constipation. Although the role of constipation as a trigger for delirium is not strongly supported by available evidence, some clinicians remain confident it can nevertheless trigger or contribute to delirium.
  » Medications, in particular, new medications—as well as withdrawal
  » Pain
  » Hypoxia
  » Alcohol withdrawal
  » Surgery
  » Neurological insults
  » Recent change in environment

Examination:

- Is this hyperactive or hypoactive delirium?
- Neurological examination—could this be an aphasia?
- Look head to toe for a source of infection, including skin and sacral area

Investigations:

- Bloods looking for anemia, electrolyte imbalance, acute kidney injury and liver injury
- Urine microscopy, culture and sensitivity
- Chest X-ray for pneumonia
- Consider a CT head to look for intracranial causes, including hydrocephalus and hemorrhage
- Remember—older people may have an infection without fever.

Delirium is managed with a multicomponent non-pharmacological approach to reverse underlying triggering factors and reduce risk to the patient.

Declining mobility and falls

Walking is a complicated, higher order function with minor stress or illness affecting a frail person's mobility resulting in falls.

History should determine:

- Onset: is it new or recurrent?
- Is there a concurrent illness?
- Has there been a change in medications?
- Is polypharmacy a concern?
- History of symptoms prior to falling, including is it postural?
- Is it syncope with an associated loss of consciousness?
- Injuries from falling
- Is it environment related, including due to a lack of walking aids, vision related or ill-fitting shoes?

Examination:

- Look for injuries
- Assess for arrhythmia and brady/tachycardia
- Assess for postural hypotension
- Assess gait with and without aid
- Neurological examination, including peripheral sensation, cerebellar signs
- Assess vision
- Inspect feet

New incontinence

History should determine:

- Is it due to a urinary infection?
- Is it secondary to fecal impaction?
- Is it secondary to new medication?
- Is it due to cognitive concerns?
- Is it due to mental health concerns?

Examination:

- Abdominal examination +/- rectal exam for fecal impaction, prostatitis and prostate size.

GERIATRICS, THE 5M'S AND THE ROLE OF THE GERIATRICIAN

The goal of geriatric medicine is to manage the complex medical and social challenges faced by older people, in order to improve quality of life.

The GERIATRIC 5Ms were proposed by geriatricians in Canada and the United States in 2017. The 5Ms represent a restructuring of the concept of the 'Geriatric Giants' and are intended to communicate the areas where doctors specialized in the care of the elderly can contribute. The same broad approach should be applied by any physician caring for older adults.

The 5 Ms are:

1. Mind
   » Evaluation of mentation
   » Diagnosis and management of dementia
   » Diagnosis and management of delirium
   » Diagnosis and management of late life depression
2. Mobility
   » Addressing impairments of gait and balance
   » Minimizing falls, and the injuries which follow falls
3. Medications
   » Identification of polypharmacy and undertaking deprescribing
   » Ensuring appropriate prescribing of useful therapies
   » Identification and management of medication adverse effects
4. Multicomplexity
   » The care of older people often involves management of complex comorbidities and challenging social interactions
5. Matters most
   » Identifying goals and care priorities that matter to the individual patient

Geriatricians often combine evaluation with implementing strategies to address these 5 elements of care as part of the **comprehensive geriatric assessment**. This assessment is described in the next section. Optimally teams of practitioners, including physicians, occupational and physical therapists, pharmacists and nurses (as well as others) work together to structure individualized multifaceted interventions. Such an approach has been shown to reduce mortality, improve quality of life, and reduce risk of institutionalization.

CLINICAL PEARL

The discipline of geriatric medicine and its objectives can be summarized with The 5 'M's©:

Mind, Mobility, Medications, Multi-complexity, Matters Most

APPROACH TO COMPREHENSIVE GERIATRIC ASSESSMENT

Comprehensive Geriatric Assessment (CGA) is 'a multi-dimensional, usually interdisciplinary, diagnostic process used to quantify an elderly individual's medical, psychosocial and functional capabilities'.

The process involves:

- Generating a problem list as part of the diagnostic evaluation
- Formation of a holistic management plan for short-term and long-term goals.

As part of the process, several key principles are followed:

- The patient is at the center of care
- Application is to select patients, namely those who are likely to benefit, rather than indiscriminate application to all older patients
- A multidimensional and multidisciplinary approach is advised given problems faced by older patients are multi-factorial, with the following individual aspects needing careful consideration:
  » Medical
  » Psychological
  » Cognition
  » Function
  » Social

In younger patients, it is often appropriate to look for a single disease process, whereas in the elderly the interaction between comorbidities, physiology and medications makes evaluation more complicated with an increased likelihood of several overlapping problems at once. Diagnostic evaluation is further complicated as common pathologies can present in an atypical manner. A multidisciplinary evaluation of the above factors allows the team to take a broader approach when making diagnoses and to develop individualized goals of care. Implementation of Comprehensive Geriatric Assessments has been shown to improve survival and likelihood to return home after an inpatient stay. Geriatric Evaluation and Management (GEM) units provide care to older patients who are likely to benefit from CGA with evidence to show less functional decline at the time of discharge and a lower rate of institutionalization at one year post discharge.

CLINICAL PEARL

This important group of functional skills may be conveniently remembered with the somewhat ironic acronym DEATH:

D Dressing

E Eating

A Ambulating

T Toileting

H Hygiene

CLINICAL PEARL

The IADLs are best remembered with the acronym SHAFT:

S Shopping

H Housework

A Accounting

F Food

T Transport

SPECIAL CONSIDERATIONS

Undernutrition

Undernutrition occurs when energy intake is reduced and not adequate to meet energy requirements thus resulting in weight loss. This can lead to sarcopenia, which is the loss of muscle mass and function and affects approximately one in five adults aged over 80 years. Given sarcopenia is an independent risk factor for poor health outcomes and future disability, it is important to prevent undernutrition. The Malnutrition Screening Tool is used in clinical settings to identify those potentially at risk, using the following questions:

- Have you/the patient lost weight recently (over the last six months) without trying? If so, how much weight loss in kg?
- Have you/the patient been eating poorly because of a decreased appetite?

A score of two or more should prompt further assessment. The Subjective Global Assessment tool is commonly used for this purpose.

Undernutrition can be physiological and related to changes of ageing or pathological. Physiological changes in hormones, neurotransmitters, satiety and sense of taste and smell—all factors can change involved in food intake control, with age.

As with many other problems in the elderly, disease or other problems should be ruled out before attributing this to aging. The mneumonic 'MealsOnWheels' can be used to remember common contributors of malnutrition:

- Medications
- Emotion related
- Alcoholism
- Late life mental health issues
- Swallowing disorders
- Oral factors, for example dentition related, ulcers
- No money (poverty)
- Wandering or dementia related behavior
- Hyperthyroidism, hypothyroidism, hyperparathyroidism, hypoadrenalism
- Enteric pathology (malabsorption)
- Eating concerns (unable to feed self)
- Low salt, low cholesterol diet
- Social problems

A multidisciplinary approach is recommended for managing patients, with non-pharmacological and pharmacological options. Non-pharmacological management includes education for the patient and families, a medication review and a dental review. Pharmacological management includes nutritional supplementation to help meet protein needs and replenishing deficiencies, such as vitamin D. The complications of under-nutrition and sarcopenia include:

- Increased frequency of hospitalization and prolonged hospitalization
- Osteoporosis
- Poor wound healing
- Reduced quality of life
- Increased mortality

Advance care planning

'Advance care planning is a process of planning for future health and personal care whereby the person's values, beliefs and preferences are made known so that they can guide decision-making at a future time when that person cannot make or communicate his or her decisions.'

Planning ahead ensures the wishes of patients are respected and followed should they lose capacity. The benefit of planning ahead is in the improvement in the quality of end of life cares for the patient and a reduction in anxiety and worry experienced by family members. However, the number of older patients who have taken the steps to complete advance care planning remains low at approximately 5–8%.

Uptake can be improved by ensuring patients and families are educated on advance care planning in the context of their conditions, the likely disease course, treatment options and prognosis. Written information alone has been found to be inadequate and instead written information with individualized explanations by a trained facilitator has better success rates.

Capacity

Capacity refers to a person's ability to make decisions regarding their healthcare, personal affairs and finances. A person is assumed to have capacity until proven otherwise. There are four aspects to assessing if a person has capacity. These include the ability to:

- Understand the information given
- Retain the information
- Weigh up the information to make a decision
- Communicate the information.

A person is deemed competent if they can demonstrate all four of the above. Capacity is not a simple assessment and, importantly, is decision specific. For example, a patient may be deemed competent to make decisions regarding minor surgery but not for major surgery or deemed competent to make financial decisions but not all healthcare related decisions. Further, the existence of a neurodegenerative condition such as dementia does not automatically equate to not having capacity. If a person is deemed to no longer have decision capacity, to protect the individual, a substitute decision-maker is invoked. Substitute decision-makers in priority order are:

- The patient's valid Advance Health Directive
- Tribunal-appointed Guardian

- Attorney appointed under most recent enduring document
- The patient's statutory health attorney
- Public Guardian

End of life care

End of life care aims to treat the symptoms a patient may experience toward the end of life, such as pain or dyspnea, in order to maximize their quality of life to ensure comfort for the patient and their family. With an aging population, death may be a result of health issues not traditionally associated with poor prognosis such as dementia or frailty. Poor recognition of such conditions as terminal illnesses may lead to poor advance care planning and end of life care. Open and clear communication regarding the likely course of disease and prognosis is key to advance care planning and allowing the individual to establish goals of care and ceiling of care. A multidisciplinary approach is advised to ensure a holistic approach.

Immunizations

Age is associated with changes in the immune system and diminishing function of lymphocytes and hence an increasing risk of infection. Immunization in older age is linked with a reduction in hospitalization and a reduction in mortality. However uptake of immunizations in those aged over 70 is only 50%. The following vaccinations are recommended:

- Influenza
- Pneumococcal
- Herpes zoster
- Tetanus

Elder abuse

Elder abuse is an under-recognised behaviour from others such as family members or carers, resulting in harm to an older person. It is important healthcare professionals are able to identify patients suffering from abuse and are aware of the interventions available to help the patient within their healthcare system. The abuse can take place in the form of physical, psychological or financial abuse and can occur in any environment. Fear can prevent patients from reporting the abuse. There are multiple theories behind the cause of abuse but it is likely multi-factorial and may relate to the abuser's own personality, carer stress, increased dependency of the older person or family dynamics.

Management requires a multidisciplinary approach and is individualized to the needs of the patient. Options include:

- Hospital admission
- Urgent respite care
- Increase in community support services
- Counseling
- Legal intervention

TREATMENT CONSIDERATIONS

Polypharmacy

Most studies relating to medication trials exclude older patients and those with multiple comorbidities therefore making it difficult to interpret results in the context of older patients where comorbidity, frailty and age-related changes to pharmacokinetics and pharmacodynamics are present. The changes in pharmacokinetics and pharmacodynamics associated with age can result in increased exposure and toxicity at routinely used doses.

Polypharmacy (the concurrent use of greater than five medications) and hyper-polypharmacy (the concurrent use of greater than ten medications) are associated with an increased risk of adverse events including an increased rate of falls, delirium and mortality. As expected, an increase in the number of medications is associated with an increasing number of comorbidities but also with pain, dyspnea and dependence. The adverse events associated with polypharmacy increases with the total number of medications independent of the medication groups themselves. Sedating medication, antipsychotics, antidepressants, anticonvulsants and anti-hypertensives are associated with the risk of falling.

Delirium secondary to medications is common and easily modifiable. A medication review is needed for all patients with delirium, looking at new medications, changes in doses, abrupt cessation and use of over the counter or herbal medications.

The combination of polypharmacy with falls and/or delirium should prompt a review of medications and de-prescribing. De-prescribing should take life expectancy, time for the medication to achieve benefit and the goals of care into account.

Medications should be started one at a time, at the lowest possible dose and up-titrated slowly to response. The individual and their family should be counselled on the indication for new medication, monitoring needs and potential side-effects.

Bed rest

Both short-term and long-term bed rest has been shown to be detrimental to older patients with frail older patients being particularly at risk. Bed rest, related to hospital admission, can contribute to functional decline and deconditioning with loss of muscle mass, muscle strength and functional activity with a reduction in walking speed, stair ascent power and chair standing. Patients should be encouraged to mobilise during inpatient admissions throughout the day, if it is safe to do so, and to sit out during meal time.

Futility of treatment

'In end of life care, medically futile treatment can be considered to be treatment that gives no, or an extremely small, chance of meaningful prolongation of survival and, at best, can only briefly delay the inevitable death of the patient.' Understanding the limitations of healthcare is key to ensuring comfort and dignity at the end of life to minimize distress to the patient and family. Futility can be divided into quantitative and qualitative. Quantitative futility relates to the extended life expectancy with treatment being unacceptably low and qualitative futility relates to the quality of life outcome for the patient being unacceptably low. Decisions regarding futility of care are shared between patients, families and the treating team with the path of comfort cares explored as an alternative when appropriate.

SELF-ASSESSMENT QUESTIONS

1 A 75-year-old male presents with worsening self-care. He is brought in by his daughter. Symptoms began 18 months ago when his daughter noticed that her father was not remembering details of conversations. He has neglected to attend medical appointments recently, and his blood pressure control has deteriorated. He denies low mood. His blood pressure is 170/80 mmHg. Over the past 6 months, the patient's daughter has taken over payment of his bills. Which of the following statements is correct in this case?

  A Magnetic resonance imaging (MRI) of the brain should allow diagnostic confirmation.
  B The patient should be commenced on a low-dose selective serotonin reuptake inhibitor (SSRI) antidepressant.
  C Aggressive blood pressure control will reverse the cognitive deficits.
  D The patient should be commenced on risperidone 0.5 mg at night.
  E Discussion of strategies to manage current and future deterioration in memory is indicated.

2 An 80-year-old woman undergoes elective hip replacement for the management of disabling osteoarthritis. She has a background of diet-controlled type 2 diabetes mellitus, hypertension, and mild cognitive impairment/minor neurocognitive disorder. Two days after her surgery she becomes agitated, attempting to hit nursing staff attending to her care, and refusing food and medications. She claims the nursing staff are trying to poison her. Symptoms of confusion are noticeably worse at night, and have improved by morning. She sleeps and is drowsy and confused for much of the following day, but becomes agitated and aggressive again late in the afternoon. Her family say that she was forgetful at times before her surgery, but she was able to function essentially as normal. What is the most likely diagnosis?

  A Lewy body disease
  B Psychotic depression
  C Alzheimer disease
  D Manic phase of bipolar disorder
  E Acute delirium

3 A 79-year-old man is reviewed in the clinic because of recurrent falls. He has depression and was recently started on a selective serotonin reuptake inhibitor (SSRI) antidepressant with significant improvement in his symptoms and quality of life. He still experiences sleep disturbance. His serum 1,25-dihydroxycholecalciferol level is 65 pg/mL (156 pmol/L). His only medications are the antidepressant and a vitamin D supplement (1000 IU/day). Physical examination reveals the absence of orthostatic hypotension, a blood pressure of 130/70 mmHg, a normal cardiovascular examination, mild proximal weakness, and difficulty rising from a seated position without the use of the arms. He has impaired standing balance. He walks with a narrow-based, cautious gait, and tends to reach for furniture to steady himself. Which of the following interventions is most likely to reduce the risk of a subsequent fall in this patient?

  A A program that integrates balance and strength training into everyday home activities (functional exercise).
  B Increase in the dose of serum vitamin D supplementation to 2000 IU/day.
  C Commencement of low-dose benzodiazepine at night to improve sleep quality and duration.
  D Stopping the SSRI and commencing a tricyclic antidepressant.
  E A trial of levodopa/carbidopa combination.

4 A 70-year-old woman presents to her family physician with the complaint of new-onset urinary incontinence. She describes the sudden strong urge to urinate and finds that if she is unable to quickly reach a toilet she will involuntarily void a large volume of urine. She is embarrassed by this problem, and has stopped attending her local church and caring for her grandchildren as a consequence. She has the background problems of hypertension, ischemic heart disease, and type 2 diabetes mellitus. Her blood sugars have been well controlled on her current medication and with the implementation of a modified diet and exercise program. Her current medications include indapamide, aspirin, metoprolol, metformin, perindopril and atorvastatin. She is an ex-smoker of some 20 pack-years, and consumes a glass of wine most evenings. She was recently widowed, and has three supportive adult children. On examination she is a well-looking woman. Her body mass index is 31 kg/m^2. Her blood pressure is 120/80 mmHg and heart rate is 65 beats/min. The remainder of her physical examination is normal. Urinalysis is normal. What is the next step in the management of this patient's incontinence?

  A Commence oxybutynin.
  B Ask the patient to complete a voiding and fluid intake diary.
  C Refer patient for pelvic-floor exercises.
  D Refer patient for urodynamic studies.
  E Counsel patient to lose weight by diet modification and exercise.

5 Which of the following is not an alpha-synucleinopathy?

  A Idiopathic Parkinson's disease
  B Progressive supranuclear palsy
  C Multi-system atrophy—parkinsonian subtype
  D Multi-system atrophy—cerebellar subtype
  E Dementia with Lewy bodies

6 Which of the following statements regarding pharmacological management of hyperactive delirium is true?

A Risperidone is a typical anti-psychotic commonly used in the management of hyperactive delirium.
B Quetiapine causes a lower degree of sedation compared to risperidone.
C Quetiapine is contraindicated in patients with parkinsonism.
D Haloperidol causes a lower degree of sedation compared to quetiapine.
E Haloperidol and risperidone are less likely to cause extrapyramidal side-effects than quetiapine or olanzapine.

7 Three months ago, a 74-year-old man was admitted to hospital after having a fall. He spent several weeks in the rehabilitation ward and during this time, he was found to have bradykinesia and a shuffling gait. Levodopa/benserazide 100 mg/25 mg three times per day was commenced. At the time of discharge, he was mobilizing with the use of a single point walking stick.

He presents to your outpatient clinic for review, accompanied by his wife.

His mobility has deteriorated since discharge. He is now using a wheelchair to mobilize outdoors. He reports multiple near falls, particularly when trying to turn. He admits to daily freezing episodes. His wife is having to assist with transfers more frequently. He was reviewed by the general practitioner one month ago and the dose of levodopa/benserazide was increased to 100 mg/25 mg four times per day yet there has been little improvement.

There is past medical history of cerebrovascular disease. Six months ago he had a right middle cerebral artery ischaemic stroke that was treated with thrombolysis. He also has type 2 diabetes mellitus, hypertension, hypercholesterolemia and continues to smoke 20 cigarettes per day, with a 50-pack year history.

On examination, there is no resting tremor in the upper limbs. There is hyperreflexia at the knees bilaterally and plantar reflex is extensor bilaterally. On gait assessment, there is delayed initiation, followed by a shuffling gait and turning en bloc. There is dysarthric speech and a brisk jaw jerk reflex. There is no upward gaze palsy and no decrementation on rapid alternating movements in the upper limbs.

A magnetic resonance imaging (MRI) scan of the brain performed after the ischemic stroke showed extensive white matter lesions.

Which of the following is the most appropriate management of this patient?

A Increase the levodopa/benserazide dose with a view to up-titrate to the maximum tolerated dose
B Switch to a levodopa/carbidopa formulation
C Switch to a levodopa/carbidopa/entacapone formulation
D Add in a pramipexole
E Cease levodopa/benserazide, optimize mobility and reassess falls risk/prevention

8 A 75-year-old female presents to the Emergency Department. Her neighbor was concerned after she had not been seen for several days and called the police to perform a welfare check. On arrival, the police found the patient lying on the ground, confused, with evidence of urinary and fecal incontinence. She is transferred to the hospital by the paramedics.

A collateral history is provided by her daughter. There has been short-term memory impairment over the last 12 months but her mother continues to live at home independently and is able to manage all of her activities of daily living.

She has a past medical history of atrial fibrillation, chronic kidney disease, depression, urinary incontinence and gout.

Drug history includes digoxin, warfarin, amitriptyline, paroxetine, oxybutynin and allopurinol.

Which of the following statements regarding this patient is false?

A A fall with long lie is associated with increased morbidity and mortality.
B Cessation of allopurinol is likely to help in the resolution of the patient's delirium.
C Paroxetine is a risk factor for falls in older patients.
D Digoxin has anti-cholinergic properties.
E The prescription of amitriptyline, paroxetine and oxybutynin increases the probability of longer-term cognitive decline.

9 A 75-year-old man presents to the Emergency Department with diarrhea. He has a past medical history of idiopathic Parkinson's disease, mixed Alzheimer and Parkinson's dementia, hypertension, hypercholesterolemia, osteoarthritis and gastroesophageal reflux disease. He is confused and unable to provide a history.

A collateral history from his daughter reveals gradual weight loss over the last six months with no change in appetite. There is no history of vomiting, hematochezia, malena or mucus. The diarrhea is described as watery, has been present for the last four weeks, with associated urgency and fecal incontinence. The patient has been opening his bowels 4–6 times per day. There is no history of subjective fevers or chills.

The daughter is unsure of any recent medication changes. Drug history is therefore compiled from the Webster pack brought in with the patient and includes levodopa/carbidopa, donepezil, olmesartan, amlodipine, rosuvastatin, ibuprofen and lansoprazole.

On examination, the blood pressure is 130/80 mmHg and the temperature is 36 degrees Celsius. The patient is orientated to person but not to place. There is hypersalivation and cogwheel rigidity in upper limbs, which is worse in the left arm. There is a pill rolling tremor of the left hand. The abdomen is soft and non-tender. There are no palpable masses, lymphadenopathy or organomegaly and normal bowel sounds are present. A per rectum examination reveals soft brown stool in the rectum, with no masses, malena or fresh blood.

Which of the following is least likely to be contributing to the patient's diarrhea?

A   Levodopa/carbidopa
B   Donepezil
C   Olmesartan
D   Ibuprofen
E   Lansoprazole

10   A 78-year-old female presents to the emergency department. A collateral history is provided by the patient's husband. Five days ago, the patient reported a generalized headache. Initially this improved with paracetamol but more recently the headache is constant. There is no history of photophobia, neck stiffness or rash. There was development of subjective fevers and confusion two days ago. In the last 24 hours the patient has been asking about the location of her deceased mother and sister, with intervening episodes of drowsiness, which triggered presentation to the hospital.

Past medical history includes hypertension and rheumatoid arthritis.

Drug history includes amlodipine, methotrexate and prednisolone 5 mg.

On examination, vital signs reveal a blood pressure of 120/70 mmHg, heart rate 80/min, respiratory rate 14/min, oxygen saturation 98% on air and a temperature of 38 degrees Celsius. The patient is drowsy and but easily roused. She is not orientated to time or place and has confused speech. Neurological examination is unremarkable. Kernig's and Brudzinski's sign is negative. Cardiovascular and respiratory examination is unremarkable. There is no rash.

A chest X-ray is unremarkable.

Urine microscopy and cytology shows < 10 leucocytes, < 10 erythrocytes, < 10 epithelial cells and no bacteria seen.

A computed tomography (CT) scan of the brain is unremarkable.

A lumbar puncture is performed and the following results from cerebrospinal fluid (CSF) analysis are available:

White cell count 100×10^6/L—50% polymorphonuclear cells and 50% mononuclear cells

Glucose 3.4 mmol/L (serum glucose 7 mmol/L)

Protein 480 mg/L (normal range: 150–500 mg/L)

Gram stain negative

Bacterial culture proceeding

Viral PCR proceeding

Which of the following options is the most appropriate management?

A   Intravenous ceftriaxone
B   Intravenous ceftriaxone and intravenous vancomycin
C   Intravenous ceftriaxone and intravenous benzylpenicillin
D   Intravenous ceftriaxone, intravenous vancomycin and intravenous benzylpenicillin
E   Supportive management with intravenous fluids and anti-pyrexial medication

11   Which of the following would have the highest priority in providing consent for a patient who is deemed to lack capacity with regards to withholding or withdrawing life-sustaining measures?

A   A state tribunal appointed Guardian
B   An enduring power of attorney appointed under the most recent enduring document
C   The patient's statutory health attorney
D   The Public Guardian
E   The patient's paid carer

12   Which of the following regarding urinary incontinence is false?

A   Surgical management for urinary continence can worsen symptoms if there is an urge component.
B   Urge incontinence is the most common type of urinary continence in elderly men and women.
C   Pelvic floor exercises are first-line management for stress incontinence.
D   Mirabegron is a beta 3 adrenoceptor antagonist that can be used in the management of urge incontinence.
E   Patients with significant cognitive and/or physical impairment should not be considered for botulinum toxin A therapy for detrusor overactivity.

13   Which of the following regarding the normal physiology of aging is false?

A   There is a loss of atrial pacemaker cells.
B   There is decreased hepatic blood flow.
C   There is an increased response to pro-inflammatory cytokines such as interleukin-1 (IL-1), interleukin-6 (IL-6) and tumor necrosis factor alpha (TNF-alpha).
D   There is an increase in gradient between alveolar partial pressure of oxygen and the arterial partial pressure of oxygen (the A-a gradient).
E   There is increased deposition of neurofibrillary tangles and amyloid in the brain.

14 Which of the following regarding dementia with Lewy bodies (DLB) is true?
A Mini mental state examination is more likely to show visuo-spatial impairment in DLB compared to Alzheimer disease (AD).
B Visual hallucinations typically present as a late manifestation in DLB.
C Memory deficits typically present as an early manifestation in DLB.
D Fluctuating cognition typically presents as a late manifestation in DLB.
E DLB coexists with AD in 25% of cases.

ANSWERS

1 E.

The utilization of memory strategies in the setting of milder degrees of dementia can be helpful. In this case, the use of medication dosing devices, calendars, residential nursing support and automated reminder messages can improve patient safety. One possible reason for the patient's worsening blood pressure is the loss of adherence due to worsening memory impairment.

This patient most likely has Alzheimer dementia. While MRI can be helpful to rule out alternative diagnoses, it is not possible to make a specific diagnosis on imaging alone. Antidepressant medications can be helpful in the management of major depression in the elderly, with SSRIs currently considered the agents of choice. Depression can also mimic the features of a dementing illness in some patients. However, this patient does not have clinical features supporting a diagnosis of depression. Management of hypertension is an important goal of care, but is unlikely to reverse the patient's cognitive disturbance. Risperidone can be useful for managing psychotic symptoms complicating a dementing illness. However, this patient does not have a history suggesting psychosis.

2 E.

This patient's presentation is most consistent with an episode of acute agitated delirium. This common neurological disturbance is frequent in hospitalized patients. Both the CAM (Confusion Assessment Method) and the 4AT are validated tools that can help to screen for delirium. Diagnostic features captured in the CAM include:

i   acute onset and fluctuating course
ii   inattention
iii altered level of consciousness
iv   disorganized thinking.

Psychotic depression can be associated with altered behavior and delusions. However, the acute nature of this change in the setting of recent surgery suggests this is not the most likely cause of this patient's symptoms. Alzheimer disease is frequently associated with psychotic symptoms, but this is seldom the presenting form of this form of dementia. Furthermore, the acuity of the patient's behavior change argues against the more indolent progression of a pure dementia. An underlying cognitive disorder, perhaps mild Alzheimer disease or mild cognitive impairment, is a major risk factor for the development of delirium. Lewy Body Disease characteristically produces greater fluctuation in mental state than is seen in Alzheimer disease and can be associated with psychotic symptoms as well as visual hallucinations. In this case, however, the onset of symptoms only following illness or surgery makes delirium far more probable. Mania is associated with agitation and altered behavior, but its manifestation for the first time in an elderly person would be unlikely, and again the onset immediately after surgery strongly suggests delirium.

3 A.

Strength and balance training integrated with daily activities, also called functional training, has been demonstrated to lower the risk of falls in community-dwelling older people by as much as 30%.

While treating vitamin D deficiency has been shown to reduce the risk of falls, this patient's level is already acceptable and is unlikely to improve with the provision of further supplementation. Benzodiazepines can increase the risk of falls and should be avoided if possible. Tricyclics are generally less well tolerated than SSRIs. This patient's depressive illness is responding to his current agent and there is no indication for a change at this time. This man has a cautious and unsteady gait and does not have features of Parkinson's disease. The use of levodopa/carbidopa is therefore not indicated.

4 B.

The next step in the evaluation of this patient's new-onset symptoms is asking the patient to complete a voiding and fluid intake diary. Correlation of the timing of episodes of incontinence with the amount and type of fluids consumed, and association or otherwise with activities and medications can often yield potential strategies to reduce or prevent the problem.

This patient's symptoms suggest the onset of urge incontinence, associated with detrusor instability and increased bladder sensation. Oxybutynin and other anticholinergic agents can be useful in managing these symptoms as can beta3 adrenergic agonist mirabegron, but their use should not precede evaluation of the problem. Pelvic floor exercises can improve symptoms in patients with mixed or stress incontinence. They are less likely to be helpful in this patient with predominant urge symptoms, and their use should not precede evaluation of the complaint. Urodynamic studies are helpful in the evaluation of selected patients with urinary incontinence, but are time-consuming and expensive. They would be indicated in patients with prior or planned surgery to the urogenital system, or in patients where the diagnosis remained unclear after an appropriate evaluation. Weight loss with diet and exercise is a desirable goal in this patient with a body mass index of 31, and can improve urinary incontinence symptoms. However, this patient has already engaged in such a program.

5   B.

Progressive supranuclear palsy is a tauopathy. The remaining options are all alpha-synucleinopathies.

6   D.

Risperidone is an atypical anti-psychotic that is commonly used in the management of hyperactive delirium. Haloperidol is a typical anti-psychotic that is also commonly used and has the best evidence base in terms of larger clinical trials. Both risperidone and haloperidol cause low degrees of sedation but carry a higher risk of extrapyramidal side-effects, especially in patients with parkinsonism. Quetiapine and olanzapine are atypical anti-psychotics which are less likely to cause extrapyramidal side-effects but are more sedating than haloperidol and risperidone.

7   E.

This patient has vascular parkinsonism which rarely responds to dopaminergic therapy.

Parkinsonism can be caused by several aetiologies and the most common form is idiopathic Parkinson's disease.

Vascular parkinsonism is sometimes referred to as 'lower body parkinsonism', due to the condition most commonly presenting with lower limb findings and relative preservation of the upper limbs.

Clinical signs include bradykinesia, a shuffling gait, turning en bloc and freezing. It is common for mobility to deteriorate rapidly. There is often no tremor in the upper limbs as seen in tremor predominant idiopathic Parkinson's disease. Pyramidal signs are also more pronounced in the lower limbs compared to the upper limbs.

Other clinical features are seen in vascular parkinsonism are pseudobulbar palsy and poor response to dopaminergic therapy, both of which are described in this case.

Ischemic and less commonly hemorrhagic strokes can lead to vascular parkinsonism, particularly if lesions are in the subcortical white matter, basal ganglia, thalamus and/or the upper brainstem.

Patients with vascular parkinsonism rarely respond to dopaminergic therapy. Escalation of dose or changing to different formulation will unlikely yield any benefit yet expose the patient to side-effects, such as nausea, vomiting and hallucinations.

The focus of management in this case should be optimizing mobility and reassessing falls risk/prevention, which is best achieved with a multidisciplinary approach with physiotherapy and occupational therapy advice. An assessment of cognition, continence, mood and carer stress should also be performed.

8   B.

This patient has mild cognitive impairment and is prescribed multiple medications with anti-cholinergic properties. While oxybutynin and paroxetine have the most potent anti-cholinergic effects, digoxin, warfarin and amitriptyline also have anti-cholinergic properties. Anti-cholinergic medications are known to be risk factors for the development of delirium and long-term worsening of cognition.

Selective serotonin reuptake inhibitors (SSRIs) such as paroxetine are strongly associated with increased falls risk in older patients.

A fall with a long lie is associated with increased morbidity and mortality in older patients. Falls with or without prolonged immobilization is the most frequent cause of rhabdomyolysis in the elderly. The greater the number of medications at the time of admission, the shorter the overall survival in elderly patients with rhabdomyolysis. This highlights the impact of polypharmacy on both causing and complicating falls.

Of all the medications listed, allopurinol is the only drug with no anti-cholinergic properties and therefore its cessation would be unlikely to be affecting the patient's delirium.

9   A.

Donepezil is a cholinesterase inhibitor used in the treatment of mild Alzheimer dementia. Its pro-cholinergic properties can lead to hypersalivation and diarrhea. The diarrhea tends to be seen shortly after commencing the medication whereas onset of hypersalivation can occur much later.

Olmesartan is associated with sprue-like enteropathy that is characterized by watery diarrhea and weight loss. The mechanism of the enteropathy is unclear and management is to cease olmesartan indefinitely.

Proton pump inhibitors (particularly lansoprazole) and non-steroidal anti-inflammatory drugs (NSAIDs) are associated with microscopic colitis, which can present with watery diarrhea, urgency, incontinence and nocturnal defecation. Diagnosis is based on histology following colonoscopy and is subclassified into collagenous, lymphocytic or incomplete microscopic colitis. Management is to cease offending medications, smoking cessation if relevant, anti-diarrheals and a course of oral steroids (usually budesonide).

Diarrhea is not a known side-effect of levodopa/carbidopa. Autonomic dysfunction secondary to idiopathic Parkinson's disease tends to lead to constipation rather than diarrhea.

10 C.

This patient should receive empirical treatment for bacterial meningitis and importantly should receive benzylpenicillin which is active against *Listeria monocytogenes*.

Bacterial meningitis from *Listeria monocytogenes* has a spectrum of presentations from a subacute illness as in this case, to a fulminant course with coma. The most common presenting symptoms are fever, confusion and headache.

Risk factors for developing the condition include immunocompromise, age >50 years and malignancy. Approximately one-third of cases have no identifiable risk factors.

Acute meningitis from Listeria infection can present very differently when compared to other pathogens such as *Streptococcus pneumoniae* and *Neisseria meningitidis*.

Approximately 40% of patients do not have signs of meningism on examination at admission. The CSF profile is less likely to have a high white cell count or a high protein concentration. Gram stain is negative in two-thirds of cases. Listeria is the one cause of bacterial (nontuberculous) meningitis in which a substantial number of lymphocytes (>25%) can be seen in the CSF differential count in the absence of antibiotic therapy.

Intravenous ceftriaxone alone would not be sufficient as Listeria is intrinsically resistant to cephalosporins.

Indications for vancomycin include Gram-positive diplococci seen on Gram stain, if the pneumococcal antigen assay of CSF is positive, if the patient has suspected otitis media/sinusitis, or has been recently treated with a beta lactam—none of which are applicable in this case.

The patient requires anti-microbial therapy; therefore supportive management is not appropriate.

Continuing ceftriaxone, in addition to benzylpenicillin, is important given that Gram stain sensitivity for bacterial meningitis in general ranges from 50–90%. Once the results of bacterial culture are available, the antibiotic choice can be rationalised. While waiting for these results, empirical therapy with ceftriaxone and benzylpenicillin is the most appropriate management step from the options available.

11 A.

Dealing with patient capacity issues, particularly in the context of withholding or withdrawing life-sustaining measures, can become very complex. Different clinical scenarios also generate different time pressures to make such decisions. For example, an elderly patient who is deemed to lack capacity that presents with ischemic bowel requires a very urgent assessment and decision regarding surgical intervention. Whereas the process of withdrawing nasogastric feeding in an elderly patient who has made poor neurological recovery after a large ischemic stroke can take place over a longer time period, having multiple meetings with substitute decision-makers.

With regards to the options above, an advanced health directive (AHD) would have 'trumped' all the other options listed. Options A–D are in fact listed in the correct order of priority. Paid carers cannot be considered as a statutory health attorney.

12 D.

Surgical management for urinary incontinence can worsen symptoms if there is an urge component and is the reason why urodynamic studies are performed in patients being considered for surgical intervention.

Urge incontinence is the most common type of urinary incontinence in elderly men and women.

Pelvic floor exercises are first-line therapy for patients with stress incontinence. They can also be utilized in patients with urge incontinence but are less effective than in stress incontinence.

Mirabegron is a beta-3 adrenoceptor agonist which can be used in the management of urge incontinence. Beta-3 receptor activation causes detrusor muscle relaxation and can therefore be effective in those with detrusor overactivity.

Approximately 10% of patients that receive botulinum toxin A therapy for detrusor overactivity develop urinary retention that requires self-catheterization. Therefore, patients who are unable to perform self-catheterization should not be considered for botulinum toxin A therapy.

13 C.

Aging is associated with multiple changes in many organ systems.

There is a loss of atrial pacemaker cells and this contributes to the increased risk of developing atrial fibrillation with increasing age.

There is decreased hepatic blood flow, which leads to decreased first pass metabolism and therefore contributes to altered pharmacokinetics of medications in the elderly.

There is a decreased response to pro-inflammatory cytokines and this is a reason why fevers are less commonly seen in the elderly despite the presence of infection.

Changes in the respiratory system, such as increased anatomical dead space, reduced compliance and elastic recoil of the lungs and flattening of the diaphragm, lead to a reduced arterial partial pressure of oxygen and thus an increased A-a gradient. An estimated normal A-a gradient with age correction can be calculated as (age + 10)/4. For example, an estimated normal A-a gradient in a 75-year-old patient would be approximately 21 mmHg. This would be considered to be an elevated A-a gradient in a 45-year-old patient. In younger patients, a normal A-a gradient is 5–10 mmHg.

Neurofibrillary tangles (phosphorylated Tau protein) and amyloid deposits in the brain are normal in aging. However, the levels of deposition are significantly higher in disease states, such as Alzheimer disease.

14 A.

Patients with DLB tend to have pronounced visuo-spatial deficits when compared to patients with AD. Fluctuating cognition and visual hallucinations are core clinical features of DLB and both tend to occur early in the disease process.

Patients with AD tend to have pronounced deficits in short-term memory early in the disease process, whereas memory impairment tends to occur late in DLB.

These differences reflect the different neuropathology of DLB and AD. In DLB, there is early involvement of frontal subcortical structures and later involvement of the temporal and parietal areas. Whereas in most cases of Alzheimer disease, neurofibrillary tangles initially involve medial temporal lobe structures such as the hippocampus and then extend to other temporal, parietal and frontal lobe structures.

Differentiating DLB and AD in routine clinical practice is challenging, as they coexist in 80% of cases. The differences in their presentations are derived from patients with 'pure' DLB, which only represent 20% of cases.

Page numbers followed by 'b' indicate boxes, 'f' indicate figures, and 't' indicate tables.

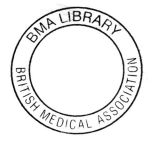
BMA LIBRARY
BRITISH MEDICAL ASSOCIATION